FOR INSTRUCTORS

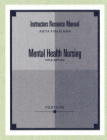

Instructor's Resource Manual
ISBN: 0-13-098028-5

This manual contains a wealth of material to help faculty plan and manage the Mental Health nursing course. It includes chapter overviews, detailed lecture suggestions and outlines, learning objectives, a complete test bank, answers to the textbook critical thinking exercises, teaching tips, and more for each chapter. The IRM also guides faculty how to assign and use the text-specific Companion Website, **www.prenhall.com/fontaine**, and the CD-ROM that accompany the textbook.

Instructor's Resource CD-ROM
ISBN: 0-13-098027-7

This cross-platform CD-ROM provides illustrations in PowerPoint from the new Fifth Edition of this textbook for use in classroom lectures. It also contains the Test-Gen electronic test bank, answers to the textbook critical thinking exercises, and animations and videos from the Student CD-ROM. This supplement is available to faculty free upon adoption of the textbook.

Companion Website Syllabus Manager
www.prenhall.com/fontaine

Faculty adopting this textbook have *free* access to the online **Syllabus Manager** feature of the Companion Website, **www.prenhall.com/fontaine**. Syllabus Manager offers a whole host of features that facilitate the students' use of the Companion Website, and allows faculty to post syllabi and course information online for their students. For more information or a demonstration of Syllabus Manager, please contact a Prentice Hall Sales Representative.

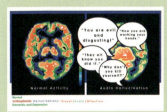

Online Course Management Systems

Also new to this package are online course companions available for schools using course management systems. The online course management solutions feature interactive modules, electronic test bank, PowerPoint images, and animations and videos. For more information about adopting an online course management system to accompany **Mental Health Nursing, 5th Edition** please contact your Prentice Hall Health Sales Representative or go online to www.prenhall.com/demo.

BRIEF CONTENTS

FIFTH EDITION

Mental Health
Nursing

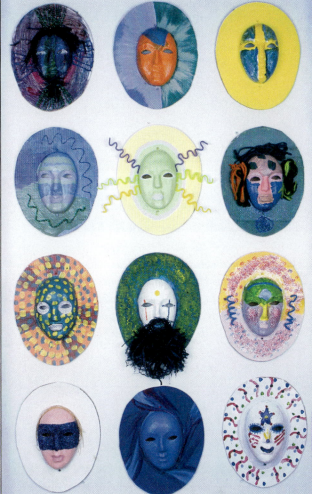

Karen Lee Fontaine, RN, MSN, AASECT
Professor, Purdue University Calumet
Hammond, Indiana

Prentice
Hall

Upper Saddle River, NJ 07458

Library of Congress Cataloging-in-Publication Data

Fontaine, Karen Lee.
    Mental health nursing / Karen Fontaine.—5th ed.
      p.; cm.
    Includes bibliographical references and index.
    ISBN 0-13-097992-9
    1. Psychiatric nursing. I. Title.
    [DNLM: 1. Mental Disorders—nursing. 2. Psychiatric nursing—
    methods. WY 160 F678m 2003]
    RC440 .E82 2003
    610.73'68—dc21

                                                    2002022005

Publisher: *Julie Levin Alexander*
Assistant to Publisher: *Regina Bruno*
Executive Editor: *Maura Connor*
Managing Development Editor: *Marilyn Meserve*
Development Editor: *Elisabeth Garofalo*
Assistant Editor: *Yesenia Kopperman*
Editorial Assistant: *Sladjana Repic*
Director of Production and Manufacturing: *Bruce Johnson*
Managing Production Editor: *Patrick Walsh*
Production Liasion: *Danielle Newhouse*
Production Editor: *Linda Begley, Rainbow Graphics*
Manufacturing Manager: *Ilene Sanford*
Design Director: *Cheryl Asherman*
Design Coordinator: *Maria Guglielmo*
Interior Designer: *Amanda Kavanagh*
Cover Designer: *Cheryl Asherman*
Electronic Art Creation: *ElectraGraphics*
Photographer: *Al Dodge, AD Productions*
Manager of Media Production: *Amy Peltier*
New Media Project Manager: *Stephen Hartner*
New Media Production: *Jack Yensen, Synergy*
Marketing Manager: *Nicole Benson*
Marketing Coordinator: *Janet Ryerson*
Production Information Manager: *Rachele Strober*
Composition: *Rainbow Graphics*
Cover printer: *Phoenix Color Corp.*
Printer/Binder: *RR Donnelley & Sons*

Pearson Education LTD.
Pearson Education Australia PTY, Limited
Pearson Education Singapore, Pte. Ltd
Pearson Education North Asia Ltd
Pearson Education, Canada, Ltd.
Pearson Educación de Mexico, S.A. de C.V.
Pearson Education–Japan
Pearson Education Malaysia, Pte. Ltd

Notice: Care has been taken to confirm the accuracy of the information presented in this book. The authors, editors, and the publisher, however, cannot accept any responsibility for errors or omissions or for consequences from application of the information in this book and make no warranty, express or implied, with respect to its contents.

The authors and the publisher have exerted every effort to ensure that drug selections and dosages set forth in this text are in accord with current recommendations and practice at time of publication. However, in view of ongoing research, changes in government regulations, and the constant flow of information relating to drug therapy and drug reactions, the reader is urged to check the package inserts of all drugs for any change in indications of dosage and for added warnings and precautions. This is particularly important when the recommended agent is a new and/or infrequently employed drug.

The authors and publisher disclaim all responsibility for any liability, loss, injury, or damage incurred as a consequence, directly or indirectly, of the use and application of any of the contents of this volume.

DEDICATION

This book is dedicated to Al Renslow, who continues to teach me the power of optimism, hope, and cheerfulness in the face of catastrophic illness, and Elisabeth Garofalo, who always goes the extra mile with a smile on her face and laughter in her voice.

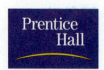

10 9 8 7 6 5 4 3 2

ISBN 0-13-097992-9

FIFTH EDITION

Mental Health Nursing

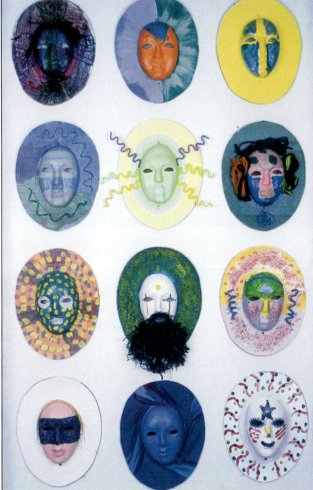

Karen Lee Fontaine, RN, MSN, AASECT

Professor, Purdue University Calumet

Hammond, Indiana

Prentice Hall

Upper Saddle River, NJ 07458

Library of Congress Cataloging-in-Publication Data

Fontaine, Karen Lee.
  Mental health nursing / Karen Fontaine.—5th ed.
    p.; cm.
Includes bibliographical references and index.
ISBN 0-13-097992-9
  1. Psychiatric nursing. I. Title.
  [DNLM: 1. Mental Disorders—nursing. 2. Psychiatric nursing—
methods. WY 160 F678m 2003]
RC440 .E82 2003
610.73'68—dc21

                                                    2002022005

Publisher: *Julie Levin Alexander*
Assistant to Publisher: *Regina Bruno*
Executive Editor: *Maura Connor*
Managing Development Editor: *Marilyn Meserve*
Development Editor: *Elisabeth Garofalo*
Assistant Editor: *Yesenia Kopperman*
Editorial Assistant: *Sladjana Repic*
Director of Production and Manufacturing: *Bruce Johnson*
Managing Production Editor: *Patrick Walsh*
Production Liasion: *Danielle Newhouse*
Production Editor: *Linda Begley, Rainbow Graphics*
Manufacturing Manager: *Ilene Sanford*
Design Director: *Cheryl Asherman*
Design Coordinator: *Maria Guglielmo*
Interior Designer: *Amanda Kavanagh*
Cover Designer: *Cheryl Asherman*
Electronic Art Creation: *ElectraGraphics*
Photographer: *Al Dodge, AD Productions*
Manager of Media Production: *Amy Peltier*
New Media Project Manager: *Stephen Hartner*
New Media Production: *Jack Yensen, Synergy*
Marketing Manager: *Nicole Benson*
Marketing Coordinator: *Janet Ryerson*
Production Information Manager: *Rachele Strober*
Composition: *Rainbow Graphics*
Cover printer: *Phoenix Color Corp.*
Printer/Binder: *RR Donnelley & Sons*

Pearson Education LTD.
Pearson Education Australia PTY, Limited
Pearson Education Singapore, Pte. Ltd
Pearson Education North Asia Ltd
Pearson Education, Canada, Ltd.
Pearson Educación de Mexico, S.A. de C.V.
Pearson Education–Japan
Pearson Education Malaysia, Pte. Ltd

Notice: Care has been taken to confirm the accuracy of the information presented in this book. The authors, editors, and the publisher, however, cannot accept any responsibility for errors or omissions or for consequences from application of the information in this book and make no warranty, express or implied, with respect to its contents.

The authors and the publisher have exerted every effort to ensure that drug selections and dosages set forth in this text are in accord with current recommendations and practice at time of publication. However, in view of ongoing research, changes in government regulations, and the constant flow of information relating to drug therapy and drug reactions, the reader is urged to check the package inserts of all drugs for any change in indications of dosage and for added warnings and precautions. This is particularly important when the recommended agent is a new and/or infrequently employed drug.

The authors and publisher disclaim all responsibility for any liability, loss, injury, or damage incurred as a consequence, directly or indirectly, of the use and application of any of the contents of this volume.

DEDICATION

This book is dedicated to Al Renslow, who continues to teach me the power of optimism, hope, and cheerfulness in the face of catastrophic illness, and Elisabeth Garofalo, who always goes the extra mile with a smile on her face and laughter in her voice.

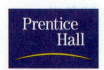

10 9 8 7 6 5 4 3 2

ISBN 0-13-097992-9

CONTENTS

Goals of *Mental Health Nursing*

Mental, behavioral, and social health problems are increasing throughout the world. According to recent world studies, four of the ten leading causes of disability worldwide are mental illnesses. In the United States, mental illnesses are the nation's second leading cause of disability, and mental illness has been classified as a public health crisis.

My goal is that nursing students and nurses in all professional practice specialties incorporate psychiatric nursing skills as they work with a variety of clients to improve the quality of life and achieve the highest possible level of functioning. Strong interpersonal and communication skills are critical to every area of practice. In addition, nurses encounter people with mental illnesses in inpatient, outpatient, and community sites including medical–surgical settings, intensive care units, emergency departments, obstetrics, and pediatrics. Thus, wherever you practice nursing, your mental health nursing skills will help you think critically and creatively.

The fifth edition of *Mental Health Nursing* is designed to appeal to both traditional and nontraditional nursing students. The text is written in a user-friendly style for undergraduate students with the understanding that students and clients encompass a wide range of ages and ethnic groups, both genders, and a variety of sexual identities. This diversity is reflected throughout the text.

This text is based on the belief that the practice of mental health nursing means taking time to be with clients and their families in deeply caring ways. To that end, nursing students are encouraged to engage in self-analysis in order to increase their self-understanding and self-acceptance. This is important because nurses who are able to clarify their own beliefs and values are less likely to be judgmental or to impose their own values and beliefs on clients.

Language is a powerful tool that reflects our beliefs and values. When we refer to someone with a disability by a label, we profess a belief that the disability is the most important feature about that person. This attitude is reflected when we label people as alcoholics, schizophrenics, or quadriplegics. In contrast, I use "people-first" language. I acknowledge the person first by saying, "a person with schizophrenia" or "a person who has a substance abuse problem." In the same spirit, I use the words "client" and "consumer" interchangeably. I believe these terms reflect people with options and choices who have the right to determine their own direction in life.

Philosophical and Theoretical Frameworks

Many theories and models are relevant to the practice of mental health nursing. It is the integration of these theories that creates the unique domain of mental health nursing as we respond to the social, cultural, environmental, and biological components of mental illness. It is important that we maintain the art of nursing, which is being there, with another person or persons, in a context of caring. It involves compassion and sensitivity to each person within the context of her or his entire life.

The model basic to this text is one of competency. This is based on the belief that individuals and families are resourceful and have the capacity to grow and change. The competency model does not ignore pathology and dysfunction but emphasizes strengths and adaptation. The role of nursing is to empower people to respond and adapt to life circumstances. In this spirit, nurses develop collaborative partnerships with clients and families. The overall goal is to provide the support, education, coping skills training, and advocacy necessary for successful living, learning, and working in the community. Consumer-sensitive nursing care helps people assume personal responsibility for where they are in their lives and for where they are going.

Traditional Strengths of *Mental Health Nursing*

In the fifth edition, *Mental Health Nursing* retains many of the strengths that have made it a popular "user-friendly" text for nursing students.

There is a heavy emphasis throughout the text on the development of effective communication skills. Chapter 2, **Relating, Communicating, and Teaching,** includes a new example of a student–client interaction and an analysis thereof in the form of a process recording. Each chapter in Part IV, Mental Disorders, features Clinical Interactions, illustrating a therapeutic interaction between a nurse and client.

The nursing process is the organizing framework for Chapters 11 through 23. This organizational consistency is extremely effective in helping students begin to assess, analyze, plan, implement, and evaluate in a systematic manner. The **Focused Nursing Assessment** feature aids students in learning the type and range of assessment questions to ask particular clients. **NANDA diagnoses** are correlated with **Nursing Outcomes Classification (NOC)** and with **Nursing Interventions Classification (NIC)** in tables. These taxonomies model a systematic use of the nursing process. At the same time, students are not limited to these taxonomies as the information flows well within other internal models of the nursing process.

Clinical Interactions present a brief patient history and then provide clinical interactions between client and nurse to promote effective therapeutic communication skills.

Vignettes give insights into brief client scenarios and their applications relevant to chapter topics.

Key Concepts are listed at the end of each chapter. Students who read these concepts before reading the chapter will find this helpful in focusing their attention. Key concepts are also a useful tool to quickly review the chapter content.

Culture-Specific Content continues to be a feature of Chapters 11 through 23. In addition to Chapter 5, **The Role of Cultural Diversity in Mental Health Nursing,** culture-specific characteristics are highlighted throughout these chapters to show students the importance of cultural considerations when caring for a variety of clients.

New Features in the Fifth Edition

While retaining many of the strengths of the previous edition, this new fifth edition of *Mental Health Nursing* includes much new and significantly updated material, new pedagogical features, and new emphases.

Learning Objectives and **Key Terms** introduce each chapter. Page numbers are included with each key term to identify the place where the term first appears in the chapter, in bold blue type. In addition, other important terms are bolded within the chapter content. The glossary on the student CD-ROM, is expanded to twice the previous size.

Critical Thinking Exercises are integrated in every chapter in the text. Answers to these exercises are found on the accompanying Student CD-ROM and the Instructor's Resource CD-ROM and Instructor's Resource Manual.

Complementary/Alternative Therapies describe the use of and "how to" apply complementary therapy as an adjunct to traditional psychiatric care.

Books for Clients & Families provide a listing of useful books for clients and their families.

Community Resources include names and addresses of agencies and organizations that may provide additional information to students about a variety of topics.

Lengthy clinical pathways have been eliminated with the expansion of the nursing process section. A sample of a **clinical pathway** is provided in Chapter 11, **Anxiety Disorders.** Evaluation is linked to outcome criteria, enabling the student to see the ongoing process of professional nursing practice. **Interactive Care Plan activities** on the Companion Web site allow students to develop their own care plans based on a specific client scenario. Students can e-mail these custom care plans to their instructors as homework assignments.

A new feature, **MediaLink,** introduces each chapter of the text and lists additional specific content, animations, NCLEX Review, tools, and other interactive exercises that appear on the accompanying Student CD-ROM and the Companion Web site. MediaLink icons appear throughout the chapter to indicate topics in the textbook that are further explained on the accompanying media supplements. Finally, at the end of each chapter, the section entitled **EXPLORE MediaLink** encourages students to use the CD-ROM and the Companion Web site to apply what they have learned from the text in case studies, practice NCLEX questions, and use additional resources. The purpose of the MediaLink feature is to further enhance the student experience, build on knowledge gained from the textbook, prepare students for the NCLEX, and foster critical thinking.

Chapter 17, a new chapter on **Spectrum Disorders,** focuses on attention deficit hyperactivity disorder, oppositional defiant disorder, conduct disorder, Tourette's disorder, bipolar disorder, Asperger's syndrome, and autistic disorder. These disorders are grouped together not only because they begin in childhood but also because they are linked by overlapping signs and symptoms and genetic similarities.

Chapter 19 is a new chapter on **Neuropsychiatric Problems.** While these are not mental disorders per se, the disorders covered in this chapter have significant psychiatric symptoms as part of the clinical picture. This chapter is designed to help students see the application of psychiatric nursing principles to medical conditions.

A new chapter on **Community Violence,** Chapter 23, focuses on the perpetrators and victims of violence in American culture, including the effects of terrorism. The emphasis is on children and adolescents as they are the largest demographic group involved in and affected by violent behavior.

Chapter 1, **Introduction to Mental Health Nursing,** includes new material on the human genome, diathesis-stress model, nature versus nurture, genetic anticipation, and behavioral genetics.

The fifth edition of the text increases emphasis on family and community mental health by expanding it to two chapters. Chapter 3, **The Family in Mental Health Nursing,** focuses on the competency model of mental health nursing. New or expanded material includes boundaries, family burden, family pain, family recovery, expressed emotion, and cultural assessment of families. Chapter 4, **The Community in Mental Health Nursing,** reflects today's changing health care environment. New or expanded material includes the Americans with Disabilities Act, Individual with Disabilities Education Act, least restrictive environment, homeless populations, crisis response services, recovery-oriented nursing interventions, and community-based nursing practice.

Chapter 7 on **Neurobiology and Behavior** has been extensively revised, including new artwork illustrating structures of the brain, pathways of fear, and ligands and neurotransmission. New or expanded content includes neuroplasticity, free radicals and antioxidants, executive functions, reward deficiency syndrome, feedback and feedforward, working memory versus long-term memory, emotions, language and self-talk, motivation, and psychoneuroimmunology.

Chapter 10, **Treatment Modalities,** has been extensively revised and includes the negative impact of seclusion and restraints. Suggestions are provided to prevent the use of these aversive "interventions." New or expanded content includes civil rights protection, crisis intervention, 12-step programs, online support groups, social skills training, self-esteem interventions, physical exercise, group therapy, and play and art therapy. An overview of the major alternative therapies is provided, with a focus on how these are used in mental health settings.

Most chapters have been revised to include new information from the neurobiological sciences, DSM-IV-TR boxes, community resources, and suggested books for clients and families. **Age-Specific Characteristics** are integrated into each chapter, appearing as a distinct head in the chapter content and replacing the chapters on children and adolescents and older adults from the fourth edition. This is a separate chapter feature apart from the childhood disorders presented in Chapter 17, **Spectrum Disorders.**

About the Artwork and Poetry

All of the artwork and corresponding descriptions at the opening of each unit and chapter are creative expressions of psychiatric patients involved in the Expressive Therapy program at Four Winds–Saratoga, Saratoga Springs, New York. In the Expressive Therapy groups, patients are encouraged to utilize a range of art media to depict and explore their internal landscapes, clarify and communicate their struggles, and identify obstacles, as well as discover their strengths and create the ways to more effectively direct the journey toward a more gratifying life. Giving shape, form, and color to feelings promotes an increased sense of mastery over even the most painful affect. The communication through art then promotes the sharing of experiences in a safe and nonthreatening manner. The transformation of overwhelming feelings into the constructive communication embodied in the art object nurtures the patients' spontaneity and problem-solving skills in life, thereby promoting increased understanding of self and connection to others.

Submission of work for this book was voluntary and offered to patients at the end of each Expressive Therapy group over a period of six weeks. Once submitted, the appropriate legal releases of the work were secured from the individuals or their guardians, if under age 18. Many patients submitted work and were enthusiastic and appreciative of the invitation to contribute to the further education of professionals. By sharing their use of the modality of Expressive Therapy, they are sharing a very intimate dynamic expression of their search for direction, connection, strength, and hope in their individual healing process. Expressive Therapy makes manifest our belief that each individual is unique, as is his or her vision of life experience. To share that vision sparks our recognition of our common human experience. With that recognition comes the possibility of a society of greater benevolence, human dignity, and respect *(Catharine Sanderson, Expressive Arts Therapist, Four Winds–Saratoga).*

All New Comprehensive Teaching and Learning Package

To enhance the teaching and learning process, the following supplements have been developed in close correlation with the new edition of *Mental Health Nursing.* The full complement of supplemental teaching materials is available to all qualified instructors from your Prentice Hall Health Sales Representative.

Student CD-ROM. A new addition to this package, the Student CD-ROM includes NCLEX-style multiple-choice questions that emphasize the application of nursing care. Students can test their knowledge and gain immediate feedback through rationales for right and wrong answers. The CD-ROM also provides several animations to help students understand and visualize more difficult concepts in mental health nursing care. Answers to the critical thinking exercises from the textbook NOC and NIC classifications, and the glossary are provided on the CD-ROM, with complete discussions of these topics. Finally, the CD-ROM allows access to the Companion Web site described below. This CD-ROM is packaged free with every copy of the textbook.

Clinical Companion. This clinical companion serves as a portable, quick reference to psychiatric–mental health nursing. Topics include DSM-IV-TR classifications, common diagnostic studies, over 20 clinical applications for mental health disorders, medications, and much more. This handbook will allow students to bring the information they learn from class into any clinical setting.

Instructor's Resource Manual. This manual contains a wealth of material to help faculty plan and manage the mental health nursing course. It includes chapter overviews, detailed lecture suggestions and outlines, learning objectives, a complete test bank, answers to the textbook critical thinking exercises, teaching tips, and more for each chapter. The IRM also guides faculty on how to assign and use the text-specific Companion Web site, *www.prenhall.com/ fontaine,* and the CD-ROM that accompany the textbook.

Instructor's Resource CD-ROM. New to this package, the Instructor's Resource CD-ROM provides many resources in an electronic format. First, the CD-ROM includes the complete test bank in Test-Gen format. Second, it includes a comprehensive collection of images from the textbook in PowerPoint format, so faculty can easily import these photographs and illustrations into their own classroom lecture presentations. Finally, the CD-ROM provides instructors with access to the same animations that appear on the Student CD-ROM, so faculty can incorporate these visual accents into their lectures.

Companion Web Site and Syllabus Manager®. New to this package is a free Companion Web site at *www.prenhall.com/fontaine.* This Web site serves as a text-specific, interactive online workbook to ***Mental Health Nursing, Fifth Edition.*** The Companion Web site includes modules for Learning Objectives, Audio Glossary, Chapter Summary for lecture notes, NCLEX Review Questions, Case Studies, Care Plan activities, Message Board discussion questions, Web Links, and Nursing Tools, such as Standards of Practice, NANDA Nursing Diagnoses, and more. Instructors adopting this textbook for their courses have free access to an online Syllabus Manager with a whole host of features that facilitate the students' use of this Companion Web site and allow faculty to post their syllabi online for their students. For more information or a demonstration of Syllabus Manager, please contact your Prentice Hall Health Sales Representative or go online to *www.prenhall.com/demo.*

Online Course Management Systems. Also new to this package are online course companions available for schools using Blackboard, WebCT, or Course Compass course management systems. For more information about adopting an online course management system to accompany *Mental Health Nursing, Fifth Edition,* please contact your Prentice Hall Health Sales Representative or go online to *www.prenhall.com/demo.*

Karen Lee Fontaine

ACKNOWLEDGMENTS

I would like to express thanks to the many of those who have inspired, commented on, and in other ways assisted in the writing and publication of this book. On the publishing and production side at Prentice Hall, I was most fortunate to have an exceptional team of editors and support staff. Developmental Editor Elisabeth Garofalo was a godsend. Barely a day went by without her questions, insight, and support. She made a Herculean effort in attending to the myriad of necessary details and made my life as an author much easier. Maura Connor not only helped with the birth of this text as Executive Nursing Editor, she concurrently birthed her new son, Conor—quite a dual accomplishment. Thanks go to Sladjana Repic, Editorial Assistant, who was always willing to answer questions and find information. Patrick Walsh and Danielle Newhouse are thanked for their commitment to the project and attention to detail. Linda Begley and Rhonda Peters of Rainbow Graphics kept the book on schedule as the staff worked diligently to prepare the pages.

I would like to extend a very special thanks to Catharine Sanderson and Rolfe Lawson, Expressive Arts therapists, at Four Winds–Saratoga. Their commitment, enthusiasm, generosity, sense of humor, and creative expertise combined with the dedication and hard work of their Expressive Art therapy patients, are the result of the beautiful artwork and soulful poetry found in the part and chapter openers of this fifth edition. Al Dodge, our photographer, worked his usual magic to capture this artwork and poetry in its greatest light and composition.

I am greatly appreciative of Anita Finkelman, who developed the new critical thinking exercises, and Carol Green-Nigro for the previous critical thinking exercises. I am indebted to the past contributors for sharing their special knowledge of the discipline: Suzanne Beyea, Patriciann Brady, Brenda Lewis Cleary, Carol Green-Nigro, Kathryn H. Kavanagh, Paula G. LeVeck, Pamela Marcus, Valerie Mattheisen, Susan F. Miller, Mary D. Moller, Ellen Marie Moore, Leslie Rittenmeyer, Mary J. Roehrig, Shirley Sennhauser, Joseph E. Smith, and Karen G. Vincent-Pounds. A special thanks is due to the reviewers for this fifth edition.

It has been two years fraught with my partner Al's bouts with acute leukemia and devotion to writing this text. The staff at the University of Chicago Hospitals willingly helped me make space for my "office" in the hospital room!

I appreciate the encouragement and support from many friends and family including Beata Halter, Elaine Stahl and Jim Spicer, Patti Cleary, Brenda Ashley and Gary Johnson, Wayne Nagel, Mary Ann and George McGuan, Matt and Geanie Dilts, Bill and Jean Robinson, Jack Rowe and Paul Vaclavik, and Ann Uttech. I could not have done it without you. Appreciation also goes to my immediate family: Al Renslow, Jean-Marc, Danielle and Christopher Fontaine, Simone Fontaine, Shawn Hampton and Jaycee, Marcel and Jen Fontaine, Jessie, Mandi, and Andrew Renslow, John Lee, and Sandy and Carl Werth.

Karen Lee Fontaine
Purdue University Calumet

Karen Lee Fontaine received her bachelor's degree from Valparaiso University, Valparaiso, Indiana, a nursing degree from Luthern Hospital in St. Louis, Missouri, and her master's degree in psychiatric nursing from Rush University, Chicago, Illinois. Karen is currently a Professor of Nursing at Purdue University Calumet, where she has been teaching for 20 years. She is also a certified sex therapist and maintains a private practice counseling individuals and couples.

Karen's publishing awards include the AJN Book of the Year Award 2000 for her text entitled *Healing Practices: Alternative Therapies for Nursing,* Prentice Hall, and the Annual Nursing Book Review, Sigma Theta Tau 2000 for *Mental Health Nursing 4e,* Addison Wesley. Karen's distinguishing academic honors include the Luther Christman Excellence in Published Writing Award, Gamma Phi Chapter, Sigma Theta Tau, Rush University, Chicago, Illinois, in 1997 and Distinguished Lecturer 1994–1995 from Sigma Theta Tau, International.

Karen is a frequent presenter at national and regional seminars covering psychiatric–mental health nursing practice, alternative therapies, sexuality, and sex therapy. She is a member of several professional associations, which include the International Society of Psychiatric–Mental Health Nurses, the National Alliance for the Mentally Ill (NAMI), and the American Association of Sex Educators, Counselors, and Therapists.

Karen has also served on the Editorial Advisory Board for the *Journal of Couple and Relationship Therapy* since 2000.

Karen lives on a sand dune in Miller Beach with her soul mate, Al, and their Greater Swiss Mountain dog, Whitney. She has three children, Jean-Marc, Simone, and Marcel, and three grandchildren, Danielle, Christopher, and Jaycee. Karen enjoys spending time with her family, art, reading, walking on the beach, and throwing "Goddess" parties with her friends.

Media Consultant

Anita Finkelman, MSN, RN, is founder and president of Resources for Excellence, a health care consulting firm. She is currently adjunct Associate Professor/Clinical Nursing at the University of Cincinnati College of Nursing, and has also served as Director of Continuing Education and Associate Professor/Clinical Nursing at the college as well. Her 30 years of experience in psychiatric nursing includes clinical, educational, and administrative roles in a variety of health care settings. Ms. Finkelman has authored many books and lectured frequently on administration, managed care, continuing education, and psychiatric nursing, and has also been actively involved in many professional organizations such as the American Psychiatric Nursing Association and Sigma Theta Tau.

REVIEWERS

Marjorie Baier, RN, PhD, CS
Associate Professor
Southern Illinois University-Edwardsville
Edwardsville, Illinois

Bonny J. Barr, BSN, MN, CS
Department of Nursing
Boise State University
Boise, Idaho

Barbara Mathews Blanton, MSN, RN
College of Nursing
Texas Woman's College
Dallas, Texas

Jane C. Brenden, PhD, RN
Instructor
Mississippi Gulf Coast Community College
Gautier, Mississippi

Barbara Shelton Broome, PhD, RN, CNS
College of Nursing
University of South Alabama
Mobile, Alabama

Bernice W. Carmon, RN, MPH, MS
Associate Professor
University of Alaska Anchorage
Anchorage, Alaska

Jeanneane L. Cline, MS, RN, CS
Lead Teacher Psychiatric-Mental Health Nursing/
    Clinical Instructor
University of Texas
Arlington, Texas

Ronald E. Drake, MS, APRN, BC
Assistant Professor
Idaho State University
Pocatello, Idaho

Catherine Emley-Akanno, RN, MN, CS
Assistant Professor
Santa Ana College
Santa Ana, California

Anita W. Finkelman, MSN, RN
Associate Professor/Clinical Nursing
University of Cincinnati
Cincinnati, Ohio

Mary Jo Gagan, PhD, RNCS, FNP
Clinical Associate Professor
University of Arizona
Tucson, Arizona

Tamara George, RN, PhD
Associate Professor
Hope College
Schoolcraft, Michigan

Judy A. Glaister, PhD, RN, CS, LMFT, BCETS
Assistant Professor
University of Texas Medical Branch
Galveston, Texas

Rebecca Crews Gruener, MS
Associate Professor
Louisiana State University at Alexandria
Alexandria, Louisiana

Patsy Klose, MS, RN, CS
Clinical Associate Professor
Statewide Psychiatric Nursing Education Program
Jamestown, North Dakota

Merryle Parns, MS, MSN, ARNP, CS
Assistant Professor
Barry University School of Nursing
Miami Shores, Florida

Kathleen Rose-Grippa, PhD, RN
School of Nursing
Ohio University
Athens, Ohio

Marsha Snyder, PhD, RN, CS
Assistant Professor
University of Illinois College of Nursing
Skokie, Illinois

Patricia R. Teasley, MSN, RN, CS
Nurse Educator
Central Texas College
Killeen, Texas

Patricia R. Wahl, PhD, RN, FAAN
Professor & Director
San Diego State University
San Diego, California

Barbara Jones Warren, PhD, RN, CNS, CS
Associate Professor
The Ohio State University
Columbus, Ohio

Joan Wilk, PhD, RN
Associate Professor
University of Wisconsin-Milwaukee
Kenosha, Wisconsin

A GUIDE TO
MENTAL HEALTH NURSING
FIFTH EDITION

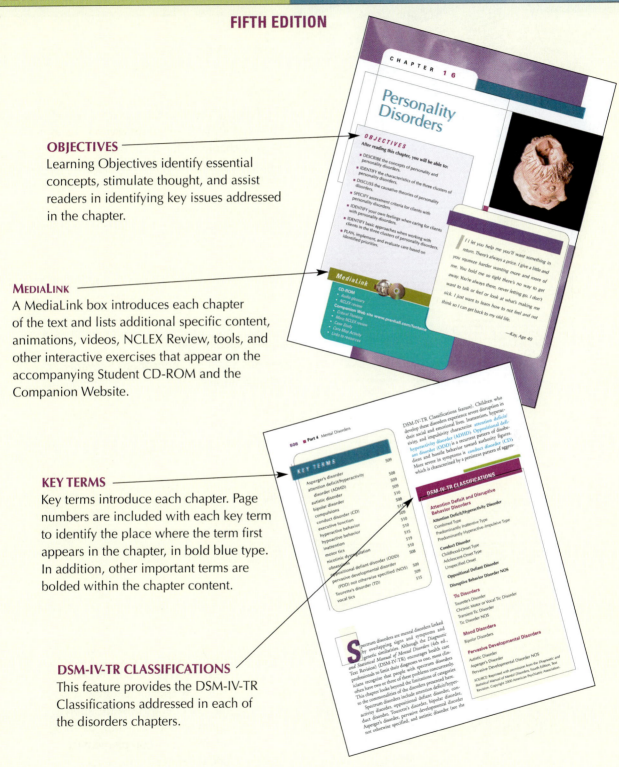

OBJECTIVES

Learning Objectives identify essential concepts, stimulate thought, and assist readers in identifying key issues addressed in the chapter.

MEDIALINK

A MediaLink box introduces each chapter of the text and lists additional specific content, animations, videos, NCLEX Review, tools, and other interactive exercises that appear on the accompanying Student CD-ROM and the Companion Website.

KEY TERMS

Key terms introduce each chapter. Page numbers are included with each key term to identify the place where the term first appears in the chapter, in bold blue type. In addition, other important terms are bolded within the chapter content.

DSM-IV-TR CLASSIFICATIONS

This feature provides the DSM-IV-TR Classifications addressed in each of the disorders chapters.

Your clinical group is meeting for a conference in your clinical site, which is a medical unit. Your instructor announces that he thinks a good topic to discuss is neuropsychiatric disorders. All of the students are continued and comment that they are not taking psychiatric nursing. The instructor asks all of the students to list the types of problems that their clients have at this time. The diagnoses listed are HIV/AIDS, stroke, and Parkinson's disease, and one client is hospitalized with diabetes. The instructor also has epilepsy. The instructor continues the discussion by asking you to list some of the symptoms you have identified in your assessment of these clients.

You finally arrive at the conclusion that your clients may have psychiatric problems associated with specific neurological disorders. You discuss how the disruption of the central nervous system affects client behavior, cognition, and social interaction. You begin to realize the psychiatric content has relevance wherever you are practicing.

1. How would you compare and contrast the cognitive and affect characteristics related to HIV/AIDS, stroke, epilepsy, and Parkinson's disease?

2. Based on the data about the illnesses/disorders noted in question 1 and this case, what key outcomes would you identify that would relate to all of them?

3. You are working with the family of the patient who has Parkinson's disease. How might you explain the patient's emotional response?

4. How might you intervene to assist the families of these clients?

5. One or your students states that she would expect to see depression as the virus affects the...

Cognitive Ability

Clients remain safe from harm. They verbalize an understanding of what is being communicated to them. Clients remain oriented.

Anxiety Control

Individuals demonstrating improved anxiety control plan and implement effective coping strategies. They rehearse and use techniques such as slow, deep breathing, muscle relaxation, guided imagery, distraction techniques, and a quiet environment to manage their feelings of anxiety.

Family Normalization

Family members verbalize their perspective of the disease process and prognosis. They are able to express fears and describe home management problems. Clients seek out peer and group support. They utilize respite care when necessary.

To build a care plan for a client with a neuropsychiatric problem, go to the Companion Web site for this text.

CRITICAL THINKING

Critical thinking exercises are integrated in every chapter of the text. Answers to these exercises are found on the Instructor's Resource CD-ROM and in the Instructor's Resource Manual.

---

and forcing them to take medication contribute to staff–client conflicts. When these actions are used with people who are used to controlling their environment through aggression and violence, one can predict an escalation of violent behavior.

Curtis, age 17, lives in a residential setting for severely emotionally handicapped adolescents. He was physically and emotionally abused as a child, and his family environment is very chaotic. He has a cyclical pattern of aggressive and passive behaviors. Curtis had talked to his mother by phone earlier in the day. At the time he was supposed to be in group therapy, he was in the kitchen with the staff. The staff told him to leave the kitchen and go to the group room. Curtis refused. As they repeated their directions, he began to posture aggressively, stare without blinking, and refused to move. More staff members were called to the kitchen to defuse the situation. One staff member took the lead and began talking to Curtis in a calm, nonthreatening manner, while the other staff members remained in the background. The staff member helped him identify his feelings of abandonment that resurfaced following the phone conversation with his mother. After a period of time, the intervention was successful and Curtis was able to join the group for the remainder of the therapy session.

It is believed that the increase in violence is related to increased substance abuse by people with mental disorders. Tardiff (1997) describes the relationship of violence to substance use:

- Direct effect of the substance on the brain—especially crack cocaine, which is associated with irritability, impulsiveness, and paranoid delusional thinking
- Exposure to a dangerous environment, such as drug dealing and crack houses
- Activities, such as robbery and prostitution, through which money is obtained for drugs

ASSESSMENT

Aggressive behavior can range from slaps, pushes, or shoves in play or in irritation to serious attempts to hurt another person. The threat of imminent violence is very frightening to staff, other clients, and, indeed, to the aggressive person him- or herself. The best predictor of future violence in a client is a *history of violent behavior.* In assessing for the potential, keep in mind the following situations in which violence is more likely to occur:

- First one or two days after admission: Person may not be completely evaluated and treatment may not have begun
- Auditory hallucinations: Telling person to strike out
- Visual hallucinations: Protecting self from what is being seen
- Tactile hallucinations: Disengage self from what is being felt
- Delusion: May perceive violence as the only option; may believe they are fighting for their life
- Affective dysfunction: Motivated by fear, frustration, or rage
- Poor impulse control: In response to limit setting by caregivers
- Drugs or alcohol: Intoxication can contribute to aggressive behavior
- Secondary gains: Motivated by power and control
- Environmental cues: Violence may be reinforced through encouragement by peer group
- Poor impulse control: Overreact to intrusions or insults from other clients
- Alzheimer's disease: Aggression usually unplanned and reactive; often during ADLs
- General medical problems triggering aggression: Hypoglycemia, acute febrile illness, temporal lobe epilepsy, head trauma

It is important that you continually assess for ongoing signs of escalation of aggressive behavior. If you assess accurately and respond early and appropriately, you may be able to halt the progression of aggressive behavior (see Table 9.3 ■).

Warning signs of aggression include (Shea, 1998):

- Speaking more quickly with subtly angry tone of voice

VIGNETTES

Vignettes give insights into brief client scenarios and their applications relevant to chapter topics.

---

family.

Often, family members have secondary gains that interfere with the growth and development of the family system. They must understand how the illness may, in fact, perpetuate existing family dynamics. Family members need help labeling feelings and sharing them with one another. You can teach the use of "I" language to express thoughts and feelings, such as "I think . . ." or "I feel. . . ." "I" statements help people assume responsibility for their own feelings rather than blaming others with "you" statements, such as "You make me feel. . . ." or "You never do anything right."

Physiological: Basic: Nutrition Support

Nutritional Counseling

Nutritional interventions include teaching clients about balanced diets, how to shop wisely, and how to cook simple meals. Because caffeine, chocolate, and alcohol may increase anxiety, strongly encourage them to stay away from these substances.

L-tryptophan (TRY) is an amino acid that is essential for the production of both 5-HT and niacin. If clients increase their intake of niacin, TRY will be forced to produce more 5-HT. Available in time-release capsules, it should not be taken by those suffering from peptic ulcer, liver impairment, diabetes, or gout. Vitamin B_6 is necessary for the conversion of TRY to 5-HT. It is important for clients to recognize that vitamin B_6 is depleted from the body by the use of antidepressants, birth control pills, and antihypertensive agents. Clients may need to supplement their vita...

...discover how this type...in a pattern of...

...with meals) in...

...um (600 to...and tension,...d doses) and...l supplements) has a calming...

...Zinc (not to exceed a...divided doses)...

...the central nervous system.

Physiological: Basic: Activity and Exercise Management

Exercise Promotion

Exercise has an overall relaxing effect on the body and may be used to manage anxiety. Discuss with clients the benefits of exercise and design a program that fits their lifestyle. Assist clients to prepare and maintain a...

Complementary/Alternative Therapies

How to Help Clients Decrease Anxiety

The next time you feel anxious, try this procedure to decrease your anxiety:

1. Hold your frontal eminences on your forehead with the first two fingers of your hands—the right and the left at the same time—or place the palm of your hand flat on your forehead.

2. While applying light pressure, in your mind go over exactly what you are thinking and how you are feeling. Continue holding these points and going over what is bothering you for a few minutes or until you feel the anxiety becoming less strong.

3. Let go with your hands and look around you. Mentally review the issue again. If anxiety is still there or has changed to other stressful feelings of frustration or anger, for example, go back and begin the process again. After a further few minutes, release the pressure and check your feelings about the situation again.

Hopefully your mind feels clearer and the anxiety no longer has the same stressful impact.

SOURCE: Fontaine, K. L. (2000). *Healing practices: Alternative therapies for nursing.* Upper Saddle River, NJ: Prentice Hall.

COMPLEMENTARY/ ALTERNATIVE THERAPIES

This new special feature describes the use of and "how to" apply complementary therapy as an alternative or complementary choice of treatment.

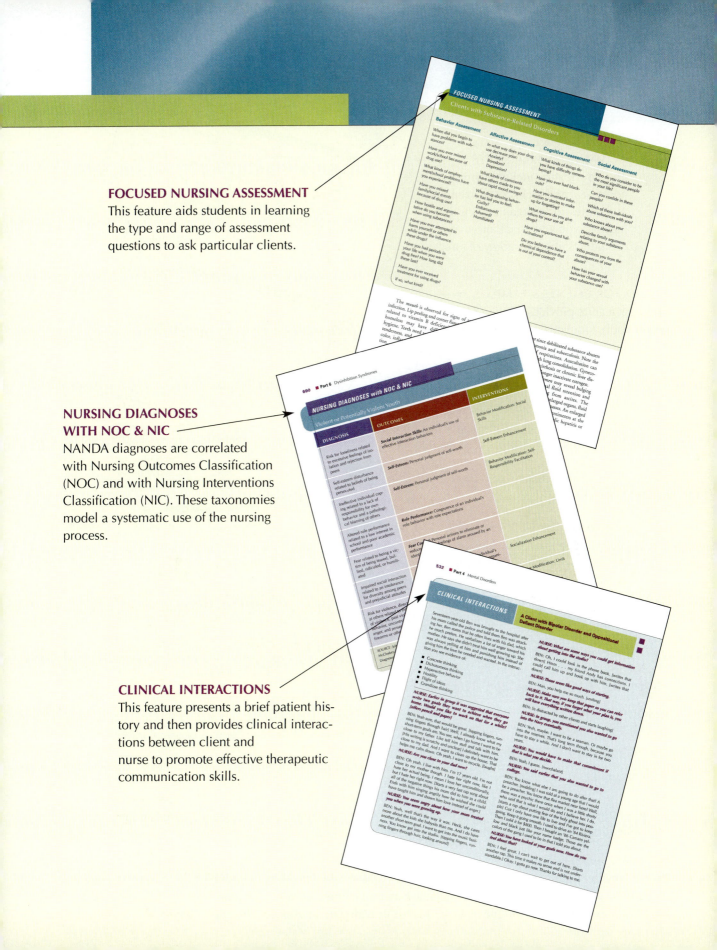

FOCUSED NURSING ASSESSMENT

This feature aids students in learning the type and range of assessment questions to ask particular clients.

NURSING DIAGNOSES WITH NOC & NIC

NANDA diagnoses are correlated with Nursing Outcomes Classification (NOC) and with Nursing Interventions Classification (NIC). These taxonomies model a systematic use of the nursing process.

CLINICAL INTERACTIONS

This feature presents a brief patient history and then provides clinical interactions between client and nurse to promote effective therapeutic communication skills.

COMMUNITY RESOURCES

This new feature includes names, addresses, and Websites of agencies and professional organizations that may provide additional information to students about a variety of topics.

BOOKS FOR CLIENTS & FAMILIES

This new feature provides a listing of useful books for clients and their families.

KEY CONCEPTS

Key Concepts are listed at the end of each chapter. Students who read these concepts before reading the chapter will find this helpful in focusing their attention. Key concepts are also a useful tool to quickly review the chapter content.

EXPLORE MediaLink

Found at the end of each chapter, EXPLORE MediaLink encourages students to use the CD-ROM and the Companion Website to apply what they have learned from the text in case studies, practice NCLEX questions, and other additional resources.

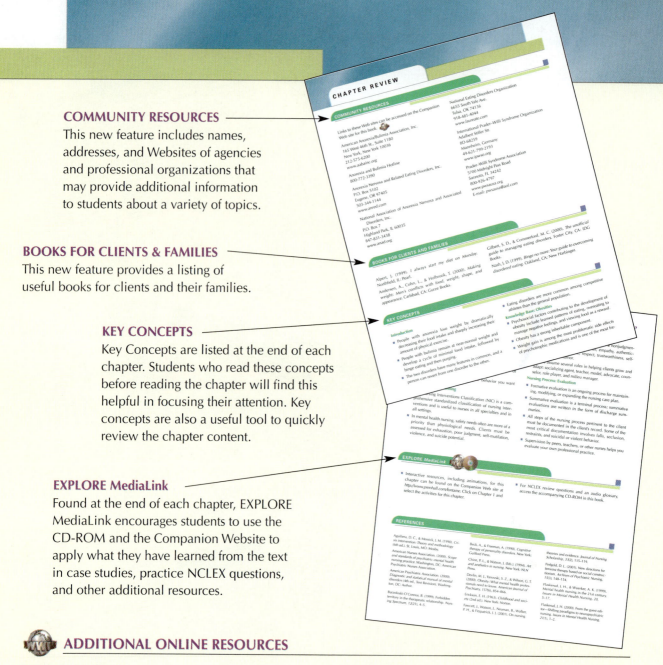

ADDITIONAL ONLINE RESOURCES

RESOURCE LINKS

Special icons refer the reader to the Companion Website where links to other sources of useful information are provided.

CASE STUDIES

A special icon found at the end of each Critical Thinking box, refers the reader to the Companion Website where a case study is provided for that chapter. The case study allows students to apply concepts and principles addressed in the chapter to realistic practice situations.

CARE MAP ACTIVITIES

Interactive Care Map Activities on the Companion Website allow students to develop their own care plans based upon a specific client scenario. Students can e-mail these custom care plans to their instructors as homework assignments. A sample of a care plan is provided in the Anxiety Disorders chapter.

PART ONE

FOUNDATIONS of Mental Health Nursing

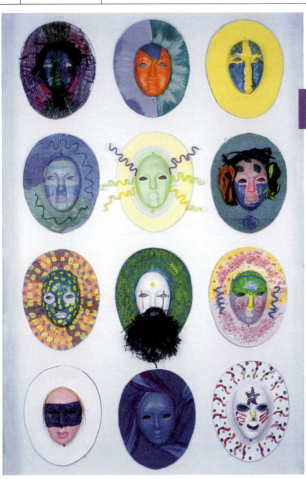

*T*he faces of many, together creating the courage to give vision and voice to their sense of self.

—An artistic collaboration from several patients at Four Winds-Saratoga

INTRODUCTION to
Mental Health Nursing

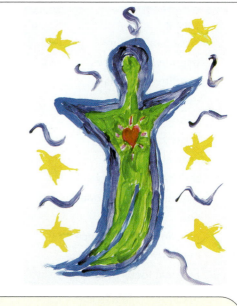

OBJECTIVES

After reading this chapter, you will be able to:

- DESCRIBE the continuum of mental illness–mental health.
- DESCRIBE the value of theories and models to mental health nursing practice.
- EXPLAIN the basic theoretical assumptions of the intrapersonal, social–interpersonal, behavioral, cognitive, and neurobiologic models.
- RELATE the theories presented to the practice of mental health nursing.
- DISCUSS personal concerns about the clinical setting.
- SPECIFY ways to care for yourself.
- ASSESS clients using psychosocial assessment and neuropsychiatric assessment.
- DIFFERENTIATE between nursing diagnoses and DSM-IV-TR diagnoses.
- IDENTIFY the most common priorities of care in mental health nursing.
- IDENTIFY a variety of nursing roles.
- EVALUATE care on the basis of identified outcomes.
- DESCRIBE challenges of the twenty-first century.

MediaLink

CD-ROM
- *Audio Glossary*
- *NCLEX Review*

Companion Web site www.prenhall.com/fontaine
- *Critical Thinking*
- *More NCLEX Review*
- *Case Study*
- *Care Map Activity*
- *Links to Resources*

I am breaking out of the black ring of trauma that surrounds me. My inner core is secure.

—Sharon, Age 43

KEY TERMS

One of the first questions students ask at the beginning of their psychiatric nursing course is, "What is mental illness, or, for that matter, what is mental health?" It is not an easy question to answer. Cultural, family, and individual beliefs strongly influence what is defined as mental illness or mental health. For example, in one culture, seeing things others do not see (hallucinations) is a valued part of religious experience and something to be desired. In another culture, hallucinating is considered evidence of insanity and is something to be avoided. Cultures, families, and individuals often define mental illness as behaviors, feelings, or ways of thinking that are unusual to them or not easily understood by them.

This lack of understanding often leads to moral judgments about people who are labeled "mentally ill." American attitudes toward and stereotypes about mental illness include the belief that it is incurable or that people are capable of bringing on, or turning off, their illness at will—and that it is caused by bad parenting or sinful behavior. These social attitudes determine how people with mental illness are treated. For example, if we believe someone is evil, we will punish her or him. Other examples of attitudes and resulting treatment are:

Attitude	Treatment
Evil	Punish
Possessed	Exorcise
Inhuman	Abandon, disenfranchise
Bizarre	Avoid, degrade
Weak	Institutionalize
Sick	Medicate, hospitalize
Dangerous	Confine, control
Incompetent	Assume responsibility

Unfortunate stereotypes like these often keep people from seeking treatment or contribute to them feeling ashamed of needing treatment.

Mental disorders are biologically based brain disorders that variably affect aspects of cognition, emotion, and behavior. The tragedy, however, is that these disorders continue to be cloaked in stigma and discrimination, the effects of which are often more damaging than the day-to-day struggles of living with an impairment.

As you begin the study of mental health nursing, you may believe many of society's myths and stereotypes about psychiatric consumers. As you progress through your course, you will begin to realize that there is neither a universally accepted definition of "normal" or "abnormal" nor clear parameters of mental health versus mental illness.

MENTAL HEALTH AND MENTAL ILLNESS

Mental health and mental illness can be viewed as end points on a *continuum*, with movement back and forth throughout life. You will be studying the continuum from several levels:

- Physical level, in the structure and function of the brain
- Personal level, in caring for and about the self
- Interpersonal level, in interactions with others
- Societal level, in social conditions and the cultural context

These levels interact in such a way that it is often difficult to separate the impact of each level. If a person's neurotransmitters are not functioning correctly, that person may have great difficulty organizing his or her thoughts. Disorganized thinking may interfere with the ability to perform activities of daily living (ADLs). Because of poor hygiene and the inability to communicate clearly, others may shun this individual. As the person becomes more isolated, there may be a further loss of contact with reality. If adequate community resources are not available, the person may become homeless.

In some cases, disruption to mental health may begin at the cultural level. An example is the impact of sexism on the mental health of women. Cultural sexism allows men to treat women as less worthy members of society. This treatment contributes to low self-esteem. Negative thoughts about oneself alter the amount and function of the neurotransmitters.

Disruptions can occur at any level; however, each level is so intertwined with the others that it is often difficult to pinpoint the original source of the distress. Personal, interpersonal, and cultural factors interact in ways that produce movement toward mental health or mental illness (Figure 1.1 ■). If there are more factors on the mental illness side of the continuum, the balance will shift toward that end of the continuum. Likewise, the presence of more factors associated with mental health will shift the balance toward mental health.

Movement toward the **mental illness** end of the continuum may begin with a sense of disharmony with aspects of living that may be distressing to the individual, family, friends, or community. Some aspects may be primarily distressing to the individual, such as feeling miserable, spending a great deal of time worrying, and suffering from multiple fears and anxieties. Other aspects may be distressing to family and friends, such as withdrawal from relationships, an inability to communicate coherently, manipulation, and emotional outbursts. Other aspects are distressing to society, such as violence and substance abuse and dependence. Contributing cultural factors include racism, classism, sexism, inadequate access to health care, and disenfranchisement of many individuals and groups. All these aspects are interdependent and interactive. They influence the development of disorders, clinical signs and symptoms, the course and prognosis of the disorders, and responses to therapeutic interventions.

Mental health is not a concrete goal to be achieved; rather, it is a lifelong process and includes a sense of harmony and balance for the individual, family, friends, and community. It differs from the mere absence of a mental disorder in that it is a growing toward potential, an inner feeling of aliveness. Movement toward the mental health end of the continuum brings with it a sense of harmony and balance, with a general feeling of vitality. Individual aspects may be a feeling of self-worth, a positive identity, and a sense of accomplishment. Aspects relating to family and friends may include a balance between separateness and connection, the ability to be intimate, and the desire or willingness to help others in need. Societal aspects may include tolerance for others who are different from oneself and the development of a sense of community. These aspects are also interdependent and interactive in the process of mental health.

One aspect of mental health is **emotional intelligence**. This idea puts emotions at the center of skills for living. Emotional intelligence encompasses the following five abilities (Goleman, 1995):

1. Recognizing your emotions as they occur
2. Managing your emotions internally

3. Emotional self-control

4. Recognizing emotions in others

5. Handling relationships

We send and receive emotional signals in every interaction we have. Emotional contagion is our tendency to automatically mimic the emotions we see in the other person. This transmission of emotion is often subtle and outside of our awareness. Just seeing someone express an emotion can bring on that same feeling in us.

Another aspect of mental health is that of **resiliency** or the ability to emerge relatively unscathed from negative life events. Resiliency includes personality and temperament factors along with specific skills and abilities that help people adapt and cope effec-

tively. The resilient person adapts to changes, forms nurturing relationships, has good social skills, and is able to utilize the problem-solving process. Resilient people have a number of strengths:

- *Insight*: They are able to ask themselves tough questions and give honest answers.

- *Independence*: They recognize their own and others' boundaries.

- *Relationships*: They develop intimate relationships that balance a mature regard for one's own needs with the capacity to give to someone else.

- *Initiative*: They take charge of and solve problems.

- *Creativity*: They find order and purpose in the midst of troubling experiences and painful feelings.

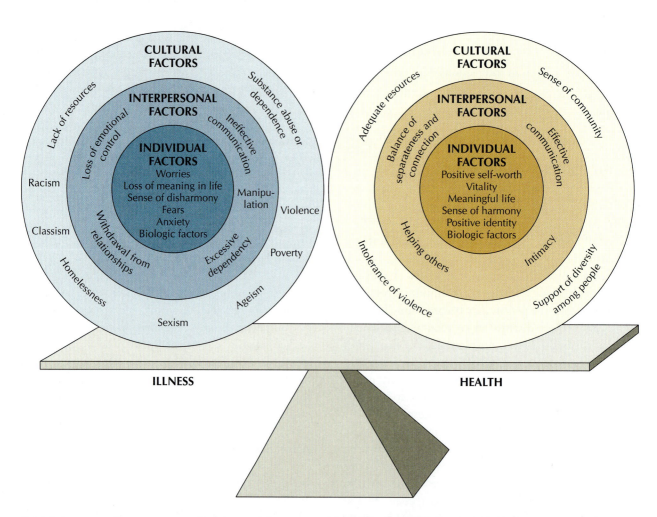

FIGURE 1.1 ■ Factors contributing to the mental health–mental illness continuum.

■ *Humor*: They find the comic in the tragic.

■ *Optimistic approach to life*: They expect the best outcome.

■ *Morality*: They have an informed conscience that works toward a good personal life for themselves and all humankind.

To be healthy means to be whole, and to be whole has a spiritual quality to it. **Spirituality** is that part of us that deals with relationships and values and addresses questions of purpose and meaning in life. Spirituality unites people and is inclusive in nature, not exclusive. It is not loyal to one group, continent, or religion. Although spirituality is not a religion, being involved in a particular religion is a way some people enhance their spirituality. Yet people can be very spiritual and not religious. Spirituality involves individuals, family, friends, and community. Individual aspects are the development of moral values and beliefs about the meaning and purpose of life and death. The development of our spirituality provides a grounding sense of identity and contributes to our self-esteem. Spiritual aspects relating to family and friends include the search for meaning through relationships and the feeling of being connected with others and with an external power often identified as God, a Supreme Being, or The Great Mystery. Community aspects of spirituality can be understood as a common humanity and a belief in the fundamental sacredness and unity of all life. It is that which motivates people toward truth and a sense of fairness and justice to all members of society. Our spiritual health is expressed through humor, compassion, faith, forgiveness, courage, and creativity. Spirituality enables us to develop healthy relationships based on acceptance, respect, and compassion.

Spiritual activities may include meditating or praying, religious activities, mystical experiences, self-help groups, caring for others, or enjoying nature. Health care professionals often consider spiritual problems to be those that question spiritual values, which may or may not be related to organized religion, the loss or questioning of faith, or problems associated with converting to a new faith (American Psychiatric Association [APA], 2000; North American Nursing Diagnosis Association [NANDA], 1999). In a broader sense, spiritual problems are related to fear, anger, greed, guilt, and worry. These barriers can be described as those daily problems that drain our energy and immobilize us. Left unresolved, they can prevent our development as healthy, spiritual beings (Lauver, 2000).

SIGNIFICANCE OF MENTAL DISORDERS

Mental, behavioral, and social health problems are increasing throughout the world. According to recent world studies, 4 of the 10 leading causes of disability worldwide are mental illnesses (see Table 1.1 ■). Hundreds of millions of women, men, and children suffer from mental illnesses; others experience distress from the consequences of violence, abuse, dislocation, poverty, and exploitation. The number of persons with major mental illnesses will continue to grow in the decades to come. One contributing factor is the increase in population, which brings a corresponding increase in the number of people with mental illness. Also, the rates of depression have increased worldwide in recent decades. Depression is now being seen at younger ages and in greater frequency in countries as different as Lebanon, Taiwan, the United States, and countries of Western Europe (Murray & Lopez, 1996; Special Research Section, 2000).

In the United States, mental illnesses are the nation's second leading cause of disability, and mental illness has been classified as a public health crisis. Although a range of effective, well-documented treatments exist for most mental disorders, nearly half of all Americans who have a severe mental illness fail to seek treatment. Financial barriers, stigma, and the complexity of the mental health delivery system fail those in our country who suffer from a psychiatric disability (*Mental Health*, 1999).

THEORIES OF MENTAL DISORDERS

Many theories and models are relevant to the practice of mental health nursing. One theory is not more "correct" than another, and practitioners choose the theory or model that is most appropriate for the client. The use of theories and models enables us to practice within a scientific framework, thereby providing scien-

TABLE 1.1

Leading Causes of Disability Worldwide (1990)

(As measured by years of life lived with a disability, YLD)	Total YLDs	Percent of Total
All Causes	*472.7*	
1. Unipolar major depression	50.8	10.7
2. Iron deficiency anemia	22.0	4.7
3. Falls	22.0	4.6
4. Alcohol use	15.8	3.3
5. Chronic obstructive pulmonary disease	14.7	3.1
6. Bipolar mood disorder	14.1	3.0
7. Congenital anomalies	13.5	2.9
8. Osteoarthritis	13.3	2.8
9. Schizophrenia	12.1	2.6
10. Obsessive–compulsive disorders	10.2	2.2

SOURCE: Reprinted with permission from Lopez, A. D., & Murray, D. J. L. (1998). The global burden of disease, 1990–2020. *Nature Medicine, 4,* 1241–1243.

tifically based care. Using them also ensures humanistic practice because the concepts are rooted in humanistic philosophies. The theoretical models presented in this chapter are used in mental health nursing as:

- Guides for understanding clinical problems
- Prescriptions for practice
- Aids in predicting outcomes of that practice
- Models for research and evidence-based practice

These theories and models focus on many different aspects of the person as a biopsychosocial being. Some focus on personality, others on behavior, and still others on learning. Some theories and models are based on principles of psychological development, and some on neurobiologic theories. They all provide a way of interpreting clinical data. The theories are organized under these headings, with representative theorists for each category: intrapersonal, social–interpersonal, behavioral, cognitive, and neurobiologic. It is the integration of these theories that creates the unique domain of mental health nursing as we respond to the social, cultural, environmental, and biological components of

mental illness. As Flaskerud and Wuerker (1999) have said: "Mental health nursing in the 21st century will have an expanding neuropsychiatric emphasis; it will, however, maintain its nursing focus, its caring, and its sensitivity to the human condition" (p. 15).

INTRAPERSONAL THEORY

Intrapersonal theory focuses on the behaviors, feelings, thoughts, and experiences of each individual person. Mental disorders are viewed as arising from within the individual. The intrapersonal theory of Sigmund Freud was the first to be developed. One of his great contributions was to identify components of the mind. The concepts of consciousness, id, ego, superego, and defense mechanisms are still widely used today, although there are many different versions than the original model. Erik Erikson expanded on Freud's theory of psychosexual development to include the entire life cycle.

The most essential aspect of contemporary intrapersonal theory is the idea of the importance of early experience. Intrapersonal theorists believe that personality is more strongly shaped by events occurring in the earliest years of life than by those occurring later in development. It is believed that symptoms of mental disorders have their roots in events in the first five years of life (Paris, 1999).

Sigmund Freud

Freud divided all aspects of consciousness into three categories: conscious, preconscious, and unconscious. The first category, **conscious**, includes thoughts, feelings, and experiences that are easily remembered, such as certain addresses, phone numbers, anniversaries and birthdays, and recent enjoyable events. The second category, **preconscious** (sometimes called subconscious) includes thoughts, feelings, and experiences that have been forgotten but that can easily be recalled to consciousness. Examples are old phone numbers or addresses, the feeling a woman had during the birth of her first child, the name of a first girlfriend, and the animosity one felt toward a former boss. The third category, **unconscious**, encompasses thoughts, feelings, experiences, and dreams that cannot be brought to conscious thought or remembered (Freud, 1935).

Freud theorized that there are three components to the personality: the id, the ego, and the superego. Each component has individualized functions, but the three are so closely interrelated that it is difficult to separate their individual effects on a person's behavior.

The biological and psychological drives with which a person is born constitute the id. The **id** holds in reserve all psychic energy, which in turn furnishes the power for the operations of the ego and superego. It has no knowledge of outside reality and functions totally within its own subjective reality. The id is self-centered, and its major concern is the instant gratification of needs. The **ego** is the component of the personality that mediates the drives of the id with objective reality in a way that promotes well-being and survival. The ego does not concern itself with moral values or societal taboos. The **superego** is the component of the personality that is concerned with moral behavior. The structural relationship formed by the id, ego, and superego is the accumulation of societal rules and personal values as interpreted by individuals (Figure 1.2 ■). The emphasis of the superego is not reality but the

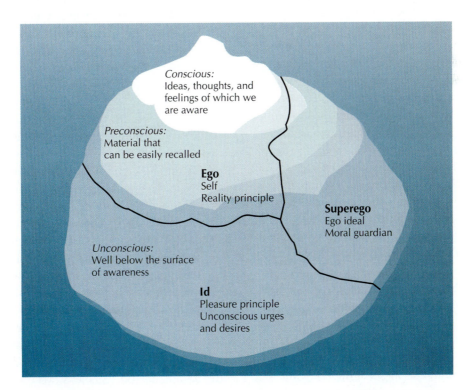

FIGURE 1.2 ■ The structural relationship formed by the id, ego, and superego.

SOURCE: Morris, C. G., & Maisto, A. A. (2001). *Understanding psychology* (5th ed). Upper Saddle River, NJ: Prentice Hall.

ideal, and its goals are perfection as opposed to the id's pleasure or the ego's reality (Freud, 1935).

The id operates according to what Freud called the *pleasure principle*: the tendency to seek pleasure and avoid pain. As this is not always possible, the demands of the id must be modified by the reality principle. The ego has learned to use the *reality principle* to delay the immediate achievement of pleasure. It also functions to keep tension at a manageable level until an appropriate object can be found to meet the person's needs.

Freud saw the interplay between the three components of the personality as having great significance in determining human behavior. He also saw conflict arising when the components tried to meet different goals. Freud believed that the way in which people resolved these conflicts determined the status of their mental health.

The concept of anxiety is a thread that runs consistently through Freud's intrapersonal theory. **Anxiety** is defined as a feeling of tension, distress, and discomfort produced by a perceived or threatened loss of inner control rather than from external danger. The feelings brought about by anxiety are so uncomfortable that they force a person to take some type of corrective action. Anxiety is a warning of impending danger and a clear message to the ego that unless some palliative steps are taken, it is in danger of being overcome. The ego copes with anxiety by consistently applying rational measures to reduce feelings of discomfort. This process is often successful in healthy people, but there are times in the lives of all of us when the ego is unable to cope and resorts to less rational ways of handling anxiety. These processes are called defense mechanisms.

Defense mechanisms operate at an unconscious level and alleviate anxiety by denying, misinterpreting, or distorting reality. Defense mechanisms prevent painful feelings and ideas from entering conscious awareness. Not all defense mechanisms distort reality to the same degree (see Table 1.2 ■).

Freud called the process by which personality develops from birth to adolescence *psychosexual development* (see Table 1.3 on page 13 ■). Each of five stages is differentiated by characteristic ways of achieving libidinal, or sexual, pleasure. The psychosexual stages correspond to the maturational stages of the body: the oral stage, anal stage, phallic stage, latency stage, and genital stage. Readiness to move through each depends on how well the needs of the previous stage were met.

Erik Erikson

Erik Erikson saw personality as developing throughout the entire life span rather than stopping at adolescence. He differed with Freud in that he believed people could move backward to achieve developmental tasks that they were unable, for whatever reason, to achieve earlier. Erikson's perspective, the developmental theory of personality, offered the hope of achieving a healthy development pattern sometime during a life span.

Although Erikson accepted Freud's intrapersonal perspective of the importance of basic needs and drives in children, he believed personality was shaped more by conflict between needs and culture than by conflict between the id, ego, and superego. He based this philosophy on the assumption that drives are much the same from one child to another, and cultures differ from one part of the world to another. He also believed that cultures, like humans, are capable of developing.

Erikson believed that the ego is much more important than the id or superego in determining personality. He saw the ego as the mediating factor between the individual and society and felt that this relationship is at least as important as the influence of the basic drives. He also believed in the importance of social relationships in the development of individuals. Erikson expanded the determinants of personality development from merely instinctual and biological to social and cultural.

Another area where Erikson expanded intrapersonal theory is in his view of the future. Whereas Freud saw the most significance in past events, Erikson felt there was more significance in the future. He believed people's abilities to anticipate future events made a difference in the way they acted in the present. Many feel Erikson's theory is more hopeful and positive than Freud's theory. By expanding on the intrapersonal perspective, Erikson acknowledged the chance to develop through the life span and to grow in a variety of ways.

According to Erikson, every person passes through eight developmental stages (see Table 1.4 on page 14 ■): (1) infancy (0–1 year), (2) infancy (1–2 years), (3) early childhood (3–5 years), (4) middle childhood (6–11 years), (5) adolescence (12–19 years), (6) young adulthood (20s, 30s), (7) middle adulthood (40s, 50s), and late adulthood (60 years and over) (see Figure 1.3 on page 15 ■). Each stage is characterized by conflicts and a set of tasks that a person must accomplish before moving on to the next developmental stage. Erikson believed

TABLE 1.2

Defense Mechanisms

Defense Mechanism	Example(s)	Use/Purpose
Compensation Covering up weaknesses by emphasizing a more desirable trait or by overachievement in a more comfortable area.	A high school student too small to play football becomes the star long-distance runner for the track team.	Allows a person to overcome weakness and achieve success.
Denial An attempt to screen or ignore unacceptable realities by refusing to acknowledge them.	A woman, though told her father has metastatic cancer, continues to plan a family reunion 18 months in advance.	Temporarily isolates a person from the full impact of a traumatic situation.
Displacement The transferring or discharging of emotional reactions from one object or person to another object or person.	A husband and wife are fighting, and the husband becomes so angry he hits a door instead of his wife. A student gets a C on a paper she worked hard on and goes home and yells at her family.	Allows for feelings to be expressed through or to less dangerous objects or people.
Identification An attempt to manage anxiety by imitating the behavior of someone feared or respected.	A student nurse imitates the nurturing behavior she observes one of her instructors using with clients.	Helps a person avoid self-devaluation.
Intellectualization A mechanism by which an emotional response that normally would accompany an uncomfortable or painful incident is evaded by the use of rational explanations that remove from the incident any personal significance and feelings.	The pain over a parent's sudden death is reduced by saying, "He wouldn't have wanted to live disabled."	Protects a person from pain and traumatic events.
Introjection A form of identification that allows for the acceptance of others' norms and values into oneself, even when contrary to one's previous assumptions.	A 7-year-old tells his little sister, "Don't talk to strangers." He has introjected this value from the instructions of parents and teachers.	Helps a person avoid social retaliation and punishment; particularly important for the child's development of superego.
Minimization Not acknowledging the significance of one's behavior.	A person says, "Don't believe everything my wife tells you. I wasn't so drunk I couldn't drive."	Allows a person to decrease responsibility for own behavior.
Projection A process in which blame is attached to others or the environment for unacceptable desires, thoughts, shortcomings, and mistakes.	A mother is told her child must repeat a grade in school, and she blames this on the teacher's poor instruction. A husband forgets to pay a bill and blames his wife for not giving it to him earlier.	Allows a person to deny the existence of shortcomings and mistakes; protects self-image.
Rationalization Justification of certain behaviors by faulty logic and ascription of motives that are socially acceptable but did not in fact inspire the behavior.	A mother spanks her toddler too hard and says it was all right because he couldn't feel it through the diapers anyway.	Helps a person cope with the inability to meet goals or certain standards.

(Continued on next page)

TABLE 1.2

Defense Mechanisms *(continued)*

Defense Mechanism	Example(s)	Use/Purpose
Reaction Formation A mechanism that causes people to act exactly opposite to the way they feel.	An executive resents his bosses for calling in a consulting firm to make recommendations for change in his department but verbalizes complete support of the idea and is exceedingly polite and cooperative.	Aids in reinforcing repression by allowing feelings to be acted out in a more acceptable way.
Regression Resorting to an earlier, more comfortable level of functioning that is characteristically less demanding and responsible.	An adult throws a temper tantrum when he does not get his own way. A critically ill client allows the nurse to bathe and feed him.	Allows a person to return to a point in development when nurturing and dependency were needed and accepted with comfort.
Repression An unconscious mechanism by which threatening thoughts, feelings, and desires are kept from becoming conscious; the repressed material is denied entry into consciousness.	A teenager, seeing his best friend killed in a car accident, becomes amnesic about the circumstances surrounding the accident.	Protects a person from a traumatic experience until he or she has the resources to cope.
Sublimation Displacement of energy associated with more primitive sexual or aggressive drives into socially acceptable activities.	A person with excessive, primitive sexual drives invests psychic energy into a well-defined religious value system.	Protects a person from behaving in irrational, impulsive ways.
Substitution The replacement of a highly valued, unacceptable, or unavailable object by a less valuable, acceptable, or available object.	A woman wants to marry a man exactly like her dead father and settles for someone who looks a little bit like him.	Helps a person achieve goals and minimizes frustration and disappointment.
Undoing An action or words designed to cancel some disapproved thoughts, impulses, or acts in which the person relieves guilt by making reparation.	A father spanks his child and the next evening brings home a present for him. A teacher writes an exam that is far too easy, then constructs a grading curve that makes it difficult to earn a high grade.	Allows a person to appease guilty feelings and atone for mistakes.

people had difficulty developing normally if they were unable to accomplish the tasks of the previous stage (Erikson, 1963).

Importance of the Intrapersonal Model

Freud's intrapersonal theory provides a systematic way of looking at how people develop in the early years of their lives and how they learn to cope with uncomfort-

able feelings of anxiety. Understanding this theory is beneficial for you because it provides a framework for assessing behavior. For example, using this theory makes it possible for you to distinguish clients' use of defense mechanisms. Anger directed at you is much easier to understand when you can identify the use of displacement or projection.

Using Erikson's developmental stages, you will discover that many of your clients are still trying to

TABLE 1.3

Stages of Psychosexual Development According to Freud

Stage of Development	Period	Defining Characteristics
Oral	Birth–18 months	Principal source of pleasure from month, lips, and tongue. Dependent on mother for care, so feelings of dependency are developed.
Anal	18 months–3 years	Focus on muscle control necessary to control urination and defecation. Expulsion of feces gives a sense of relief. Learns to postpone gratification by postponing the pleasure that comes from anal relief.
Phallic	3–6 years	Develops an awareness of the genital area. Sexual and aggressive feelings associated with functioning of the sexual organs are emphasized. Learns sexual identity during this stage. Masturbation and sexual fantasy are common.
Latency	6–12 years	Sexual development dormant. Focus of energy on cognitive development and intellectual pursuits.
Genital	12 years–early adulthood	Abundance of sexual drive. Primary goal is to develop satisfying relationships with members of the opposite sex.

achieve developmental tasks in any number of stages. With this recognition and understanding, you can help them achieve tasks so they can move on to a higher level of development.

SOCIAL–INTERPERSONAL THEORY

The theories of Freud started a revolution in the field of psychology. During the late nineteenth century, other disciplines began to emerge and develop their own scientific bodies of knowledge. Sociologists and anthropologists started to believe that human development was more complex than previously thought. It was not long before these beliefs started filtering into the knowledge that had come primarily from the advances in psychology. A number of theorists began to recognize the importance of the social context of personality development. The focus shifted away from forces within the individual to interpersonal relationships and events in the social context. Social–interpersonal theory was the result of this broader perspective.

Harry Stack Sullivan

The work of Harry Stack Sullivan had its beginnings under the umbrella of the intrapersonal perspective. But Sullivan created a developmental system markedly different from that of Freud. Sullivan believed personality was an abstraction that could not be observed apart from interpersonal relationships. Therefore, the unit of study for Sullivan was not the person alone but the person in the context of relationships. According to *interpersonal theory*, personality is manifested only in a person's interactions with another person or with a group. Sullivan acknowledged heredity and maturation as parts of development but placed far more emphasis on the organism as a social rather than a biological entity (Sullivan, 1953). Although Sullivan saw personality more abstractly than Freud did, he still viewed it as the axis of human dynamics in the interpersonal sphere. He identified three principal components of this sphere: dynamisms, personifications, and cognitive processes.

A *dynamism* is a long-standing pattern of behavior. You may think of a dynamism as a habit. In Sullivan's theory, dynamisms highlight personality traits. For instance, a child who is mean can be said to have a dynamism of hostility. The important idea is that any habitual reaction of one person to another or to a situation constitutes a dynamism. Sullivan viewed most

TABLE 1.4

Stages of Social Growth and Development According to Erikson

Stage of Development	Period	Developmental Task	Defining Characteristics
Sensory	Birth–18 months	Trust versus mistrust	Child learns to develop trusting relationships.
Muscular	1–3 years	Autonomy versus shame and doubt	Child starts the process of separation; starts learning to live autonomously.
Locomotor	3–6 years	Initiative versus guilt	Learns about environmental influences; becomes more aware of own identity.
Latency	6–12 years	Industry versus inferiority	Energy is directed at accomplishments, creative activities, and learning.
Adolescent	12–20 years	Identity versus role confusion	Transitional period; movement toward adulthood. Starts incorporating beliefs and value systems that have been acquired previously.
Young adulthood	18–25 years	Intimacy versus isolation	Learns the ability to have intimate relationships.
Adulthood	24–45 years	Generativity versus stagnation	Emphasis on maintaining intimate relationships. Movement toward developing a family.
Maturity	45 years–death	Integrity versus despair	Acceptance of life as it has been; acceptance of both good and bad aspects of past life. Maintaining a positive self-concept.

dynamisms as meeting the basic human needs of an individual by reducing anxiety.

Sullivan believed that an infant first feels anxiety as the anxiety is transferred from the mother. As the person grows older, anxiety is felt as a response to a threat to his or her own security. Sullivan called the dynamism that develops to reduce anxiety the dynamism of the self, or the *self-system*. The self-system is the protector of one's security.

A *personification* is an image people have of themselves and others. Every person has many such images, which are made up of attitudes, feelings, and perceptions formed from experiences. For example, a child develops a personification of a good teacher by having the experience of being taught by one. Any relationship that leads to "good" experiences results in a favorable personification of the person involved in that rela-

tionship. Unfavorable personifications develop in response to bad experiences. Sullivan believed that personifications are formed early in life to help people cope with interpersonal relationships. As a person gets older, however, very rigid personifications can interfere with interpersonal relationships.

The third component of the interpersonal sphere, **cognitive processes** are the development of the thinking process from unconnected to causal to symbolic. Sullivan believed that cognitive processes, like personifications, are functions of experiences. He believed experiences could be classified into three types. A *protaxic* experience is an unconnected experience that flows through consciousness. Examples are images, sensations, and feelings. Infants experience these most often, and protaxic experiences must occur before the other types. A *parataxic* experience is when a person sees a causal relationship

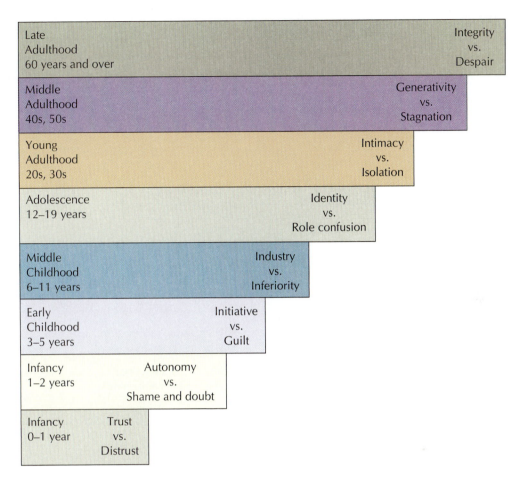

Late Adulthood 60 years and over	Integrity vs. Despair
Middle Adulthood 40s, 50s	Generativity vs. Stagnation
Young Adulthood 20s, 30s	Intimacy vs. Isolation
Adolescence 12–19 years	Identity vs. Role confusion
Middle Childhood 6–11 years	Industry vs. Inferiority
Early Childhood 3–5 years	Initiative vs. Guilt
Infancy 1–2 years	Autonomy vs. Shame and doubt
Infancy 0–1 year	Trust vs. Distrust

FIGURE 1.3 ■ Erikson's eight developmental stages.

SOURCE: Rice, F. P. (2001). *Human development* (4th ed). Upper Saddle River, NJ: Prentice Hall.

between events that occur at about the same time but are not logically related. Suppose, for example, a child tells his mother he hates her and later she becomes ill. Parataxic thinking leads him to conclude that every time he tells his mother he hates her, she will become ill. *Syntaxic* experience, the highest cognitive level, involves the validation of symbols, particularly verbal symbols. These symbols become validated when a group of people understands them and agrees on their meaning. This level of cognition gives a logical order to experiences and enables people to communicate. According to Sullivan, there are six stages of development from childhood through adolescence (see Table 1.5 ■).

Abraham Maslow

Abraham Maslow viewed personality as self-actualizing; that is, the ideal individual is one who is at peak capac-

ity for fulfilling his or her potential. However, before fulfillment can occur, more needs must be met. Maslow devised a hierarchy of needs (see Figure 1.4 on page 17 ■). *Basic needs* are physiological, such as the need for food, water, and sleep. *Metaneeds* are growth-related and include such things as love and belonging, esteem, and self-actualization. Under most circumstances, basic needs take precedence over metaneeds. A person who is hungry is less concerned with truth and justice than a person whose basic needs have been met. Maslow felt that fulfilling metaneeds enables people to rise above an animal level of existence. People who are unable to meet their growth needs, Maslow postulated, have the potential of becoming psychologically disturbed (Maslow, 1968).

Maslow looked primarily at the healthy, strong side of human nature. His is a *humanistic theory*, in which

TABLE 1.5

Stages of Interpersonal Development According to Sullivan

Stage of Development	Period	Defining Characteristics
Infancy	Birth–18 months	Oral zone is the main means by which baby interacts with environment. Breast-feeding provides the first interpersonal experiences. Having needs met helps develop trust.
Childhood	18 months–6 years	Transition to this stage is achieved by child's learning to talk. Starts to see integration of self-concept. Gender development during this time. Child is learning delayed gratification.
Juvenile	6–9 years	This is a time for becoming social. Child learns social subordination to authority figures. Social relationships give a sense of belonging.
Preadolescence	9–12 years	Need for close relationships with peers or same sex. Learns to collaborate. This stage marks the beginning of the first genuine human relationships.
Early adolescence	12–14 years	Development of a pattern of heterosexual relationships. Searching for own identity. Ambiguity about dependence–independence issues.
Late adolescence	14–21 years	Prolonged introduction to society. Self-esteem becomes more stabilized. Will learn to achieve love relationships while maintaining self-identity.

people are defined holistically as dynamic combinations of physical, emotional, cognitive, and spiritual processes. Maslow emphasized health rather than illness, success rather than failure. He even viewed basic drives, such as sex drive, as natural rather than as unhealthy urges that should be controlled. Maslow believed that people have an inborn nature that is essentially good or, at worst, neutral.

Hildegard Peplau

Hildegard Peplau is known as the "mother of psychiatric nursing." She was one of the first nurses to analyze nursing action using an interpersonal theoretical model and published this in her 1952 book, *Interpersonal Relations in Nursing*. She defined nursing as a "significant therapeutic interpersonal process that makes health possible for individuals and groups" (p. xx). The major concepts of her theory include growth, development, communication, and roles.

Communication, described in detail in Chapter 2, is a problem-solving process that takes place within the nurse–client relationship. Problem solving is a collabo-

rative process in which the nurse may assume many roles in helping clients meet their needs and continue their growth and development. As client conflicts and anxieties are resolved, their personalities are strengthened. Peplau noted that both nurses' and clients' culture, religion, ethnicity, education, past experiences, and preconceived ideas influence their interpersonal relationships.

Peplau believed that psychodynamic nursing liberated nurses from a tradition of being task oriented and gave them permission to focus on their excellent interpersonal skills. Hers is a humane and compassionate perspective, encouraging nurses to listen carefully and develop the empathy essential for the therapeutic relationship. Peplau's work continues to be the essence of psychiatric nursing.

Feminist Theory

Feminist theory has evolved out of a new focus on the events and themes that are important in women's lives. Women have been labeled pathological when in fact many of their thoughts, feelings, and behaviors are the

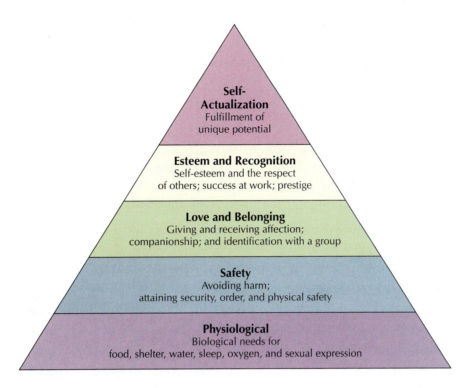

FIGURE 1.4 ■ Maslow's hierarchy of needs.

SOURCE: Adapted from Maslow, A. *Toward a psychology of being* (2nd ed.). Copyright 1968 by Van Nostrand Reinhold.

result of social, political, economic, psychological, and physical oppression. The consequences of this oppression are low self-esteem, powerlessness, and general unhappiness.

Feminist theory is a model of mental health for both women and men. The differences between nonfeminist and feminist approaches are in the definition of what it is to be a mentally healthy woman or man. For many years, there has been a double standard of mental health. Men and traditional male stereotypes were the model for a mentally healthy adult. Women and traditional female stereotypes were viewed as inadequate and mentally inferior. Feminist theory examines how gender roles limit the psychological development of all people and inhibit the development of mutually satisfying and noncoercive intimacy.

Feminism strives to:

- Help people develop egalitarian rather than dominant–submissive relationships
- Embrace the worth and dignity of all (children, women, men, and the elderly)
- Listen to the stories of people's lived experiences

- Implement social change through equality and justice for all groups of people
- Eliminate the disparities in health status experienced among groups in our communities
- Advocate change in social, political, economic, educational, and health services for a safer society (Gary, Sigsby, & Campbell, 1998)

Feminist therapy is gender-sensitive family or relationship therapy and is not restricted to female therapists. Since women value and focus on relationships, feminist therapists are caring, empathetic, and nonauthoritarian. This sense of being cared about and well regarded helps women to achieve greater feelings of self-worth. The concept of self-help encourages women to be assertive and take control of their own lives (Finfgeld, 2001; Lauver, 2000).

Crisis Theory

Crisis theory provides another perspective for understanding people's responses to life events. A **crisis** is a turning point in a person's life, a point at which usual resources and coping skills are no longer effective and the person enters a state of disequilibrium. All people experience psychological trauma at some point in their lives. Neither stress nor an emergency situation necessarily constitutes a crisis. It is only when an event is perceived subjectively as a threat to need fulfillment, safety, or a meaningful existence that the person enters a crisis state. A number of variables determine a person's potential for entering a crisis state (Aguilera & Messick, 1990). These variables, known as *balancing factors*, include:

- How the person perceives the event
- What experiences the person has had in coping with stress
- The person's usual coping abilities
- The support systems available to the person

To understand the development of a crisis state, you must be aware of the process of a crisis. Initially, people experience increased anxiety about the traumatic event and are unable to adapt to the situation. As their anxiety increases to high levels, they recognize the need to reach out for help. When both inner resources and external support systems are inadequate, they enter an active crisis state. During this time, they have a short attention span and are unproductive and impulsive. They look to others to solve their problems because they are consumed with feelings of "going crazy" or "losing their mind." Often, their interpersonal relationships deteriorate.

Because a state of disequilibrium is so uncomfortable, a crisis is *self-limiting* and usually lasts about 4 to 6 weeks. It is during this time that people are most receptive to professional intervention. Because people experiencing crisis are viewed as essentially healthy and capable of growth, changes may be made in a short period of time by focusing on the stressor and using the problem-solving process. The *minimum goal* of intervention is to help clients adapt and return to the precrisis level of functioning. The *maximum goal* is to help clients develop more constructive coping skills and move on to a higher level of functioning.

Importance of the Social–Interpersonal Model

Social–interpersonal theory provides another perspective from which you can view human behavior. This theory conceptualizes development within a social context and enables you to assess the influences of culture, social interaction, gender stereotypes, and support systems on the behavior of clients. The emphasis is on what is observable.

BEHAVIORAL THEORY

The focus of behavioral theory is on a person's actions, not on thoughts and feelings. Behavioral theorists believe that all behavior is learned and can therefore be modified by a system of rewards and punishments. They think that undesirable behavior occurs because it has been learned and reinforced, and that it is possible for people to learn to replace undesirable behaviors with desirable ones.

B. F. Skinner

Behavioral theory, particularly that of B. F. Skinner, had a major impact on the way scientists looked at personality development. Like the social–interpersonal theorists, Skinner rejected many of the conceptualizations of Freud and his followers. In addition, he questioned the validity of ideas such as instinctual drives and personality structure; he felt these could not be observed and therefore could not be studied scientifically.

The major emphasis of Skinner's theory is functional analysis of behavior, which suggests looking at behavior pragmatically. What is causing a person to act in a particular way? What factors in the environment reinforce that behavior? Behavioral theory is less concerned with understanding behavior in relation to past events than with the immediate need to predict a trend in behavior and control it. Skinner did not attribute much importance to unconscious motivations, instincts, and feelings; he did attribute importance to a person's immediate actions.

Skinner thought a person's behavior could be controlled by rewards and punishments, that all behavior has specific consequences. Consequences that lead to an increase in the behavior he called *reinforcements*, or *rewards*, and consequences that lead to a decrease in the behavior he called *punishments*.

One of the assumptions of the behavioral perspective is that behavior is orderly and can be controlled. Skinner believed people become who they are through a learning process and by interacting with the environment. Personality problems are the result of faulty learning and can be corrected by new learning experiences that reinforce different behavior.

One of the major concepts within Skinner's system is the *principle of reinforcement* (sometimes referred to as operant reinforcement theory). The ability to reinforce behavior is the ability to change the number of times a particular behavior occurs in the future. Skinner believed certain operations would decrease certain behaviors and increase other behaviors. According to the principle of reinforcement, a response is strengthened when reinforcement is given. Skinner referred to this as an *operant response*, that is, a response that works on the environment and changes it. An example of *operant conditioning* results when a nursing instructor teaches students it is all right to hand in papers late by always accepting late papers. However, handing in papers late can be minimized if the instructor prohibits this behavior. Another way for the instructor to diminish the behavior is by handing out punishments for it; this is called a *punishing response* (Skinner, 1953).

Skinner's theories have been criticized by some and embraced by others. To some, the idea of controlling people's behavior by a systematically applied reward–punishment system is abhorrent. One argument in defense of the theory is that using punishment is not necessary to reinforce desirable behaviors. In other words, a systematic application of rewards can reinforce desirable behaviors, and punishment does not necessarily have to be part of the process.

Importance of the Behavioral Model

Skinner's theories can be beneficial to you in two major areas. The first area is client education. One of the ways people learn is through positive reinforcement of correct responses. One of Skinner's philosophies is that people do not usually fail to learn, but that teachers fail to teach. If the client receives praise and nurturing feedback from you, success will be more likely. For this principle to work, goals must be clearly established so that success can be measured.

The second area in which behavioral principles might be applied is in the practice of mental health nursing. Behavioral therapies are frequently used with adolescents, with those who abuse alcohol or drugs, and with those who wish to control eating or smoking behavior. Behavioral theory can help both you and your clients understand more clearly what is being gained by acting a certain way.

COGNITIVE THEORY

Cognitive theory gives us a blueprint for the process of learning. The ability to think and learn makes us uniquely human. It enables us to be rational, make good judgments, interpret the world around us, and learn new skills. Without cognitive functions, we could not interpret our daily lives, adapt and make changes, and develop the insights to make those changes.

Jean Piaget

Jean Piaget believed that intelligence grows by exposing children to the world around them. He hypothesized that children's experiences and perceptions are challenged by constantly changing stimuli, whereby they recognize discrepancies between their own reality and the environment. Resolving these discrepancies helps children learn new relationships between objects and therefore develop a more mature understanding (Piaget, 1972).

Piaget identified four major stages of cognitive development: the sensorimotor stage, preoperational stage, concrete operational stage, and formal operational stage (Figure 1.5 ■). Piaget emphasized the range of personal differences in rates of development. The speed by which a child moves through each period depends on biological, intrapersonal, and interpersonal factors.

Aaron Beck

Cognitive theory according to Aaron Beck focuses not on what people do but rather on how they view themselves and their world. He believed that much emotional upset and dysfunctional behavior is related to misperceptions and misinterpretations of experiences. Cognitive theory does not speak to ultimate "causes" of mental disorders but describes how negative thinking (cognitions) can be the first link in the chain of symptoms of mental disorders.

Two important constructs of Beck's cognitive theory are schemas and the cognitive triad. **Cognitive schemas** are personal controlling beliefs that influence the way people process data about themselves and others. For example, you may believe that you are unlovable. When your partner left for work this morning, he slammed the door. The way you processed this event was: "If John slams the door, it means he is angry with me. If he is angry with me, he will reject me. If he rejects me, I will be all alone. If I am all alone, I will not survive." In this example, your core belief led you to misinterpret the significance of the slamming door,

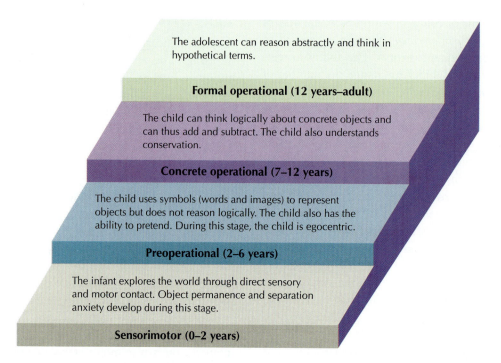

The adolescent can reason abstractly and think in hypothetical terms.

Formal operational (12 years–adult)

The child can think logically about concrete objects and can thus add and subtract. The child also understands conservation.

Concrete operational (7–12 years)

The child uses symbols (words and images) to represent objects but does not reason logically. The child also has the ability to pretend. During this stage, the child is egocentric.

Preoperational (2–6 years)

The infant explores the world through direct sensory and motor contact. Object permanence and separation anxiety develop during this stage.

Sensorimotor (0–2 years)

FIGURE 1.5 ■ Piaget's stages of cognitive development. Piaget portrayed development as a staircase in which the different steps, or stages, are distinguished by specific kinds of thinking.

SOURCE: Kassin, S. (2001). *Psychology* (3rd ed.). Upper Saddle River, NJ: Prentice Hall.

which, in fact, was caused by a sudden gust of wind. It is thought that cognitive schemas become activated during depression, anxiety, panic attacks, and personality disorders. These distorted views of the self and the world appear to be reality to a person who is ill.

Cognitive schemas contribute to the development of Beck's *cognitive triad*. Included in this process is (1) a view of the self as inadequate, (2) a negative misinterpretation of current experiences, and (3) a negative view of the future. When clients become caught up in this process, a number of cognitive distortions may occur (Beck & Freeman, 1990).

One type of distortion is *selective abstraction*, or focusing on certain information while ignoring contradictory information. Another distortion is *overgeneralization*, in which the person takes information or an impression from one event and attaches it to a wide variety of situations. Using such words as *always, never, everybody,* and *nobody* indicates that the client is overgeneralizing. People who use *magnification* attribute a high level of importance to insignificant events. Through the distortion of personalization, or ideas of

reference, clients believe that what occurs in the environment is related to them, even when no obvious relationship exists. There is also a tendency for *superstitious thinking*, in which the person believes that some unrelated action will magically influence a course of events. A further distortion is *dichotomous thinking*, an all-or-none type of reasoning that interferes with people's realistic perception of themselves. Dichotomous thinking involves opposite and mutually exclusive categories such as all good or all bad, celibacy or promiscuity, depressed or euphoric (see Table 1.6 ■).

Importance of the Cognitive Model

Cognitive theory provides a framework for assessment and intervention. It focuses on the educative nature of nursing practice. Because client/family education is extremely important, it is vital for you to be proficient in the assessment of the learning capabilities of consumers. Cognitive theory provides criteria on which to base these judgments. Cognitive distortions are symptoms of a number of mental disorders. Analyzing clients' cognitive schemas and triads will help you

TABLE 1.6

Examples of Cognitive Distortions

Distortion	Example
Selective abstraction	"Even though my husband says he loves me, I don't believe him. Look at how he never picks up his laundry."
Overgeneralization	"Women always turn mean after you marry them."
Magnification	"I know he saw the spot of coffee on my tie. Now I'll never get the job because he thinks I'm a slob."
Personalization	"I walked into the classroom and everyone stopped talking. I know they were talking about me."
Superstitious thinking	"If I never take off my wedding ring, my husband will never leave me."
Dichotomous thinking	"Either my life has to be absolutely perfect or I will commit suicide."

design individualized plans of care. For assessment questions based on the theories of Freud, Erikson, Sullivan, Maslow, Skinner, and Beck, see Box 1.1.

NEUROBIOLOGIC THEORY

Neurobiologic theory focuses on genetic factors, neuroanatomy, neurophysiology, and biological rhythms as they relate to the cause, course, and prognosis of mental disorders (see Chapter 7). Increasingly, we understand how mental disorders arise from neurodevelopmental or neurodegenerative processes, how life experiences intersect with these processes to help or hinder the development of disease processes, and how genes, molecules, and circuits interact dynamically in health and disease. Box 1.2 lists the various brain imaging techniques used to assess pathological structure or function.

In the past, nurses have talked about psychological problems as separate from biological processes in the brain. It was as if the mind and the brain were separate entities. This mind–body dualism argued that the processes and products of the mind had little to do with the processes and products of the body. The new framework believes that all functions of the mind reflect functions of the brain. We still do not, however, understand the details of the relationship between the brain and mental processes. Although we speak of the mind–body–spirit interaction, they are in fact inseparable. Kandel (1999) identifies *five principles* regarding the relationship of the mind to the brain:

1. All mental processes, including those conscious and unconscious, result from operations of the brain. Behavioral disorders are disturbances of brain function.

2. Genes are important determinants of how neurons function and thus exert significant control over behavior.

3. Social and developmental factors modify the expression of genes and thus the function of the neurons. All of nurture is ultimately expressed as nature.

4. Learning creates changes in neuronal connections. Abnormalities of behavior can be induced by social conditions.

5. Counseling and therapy can create long-term changes through learning, which produces change in gene expression.

Genetic Factors

Research teams throughout the world are attempting to track down the causes of mental disorders. They hope not only to identify the genes in such diseases,

BOX 1.1

Assessment Questions Using Specific Models

Freud's Intrapersonal Theory

What is the developmental stage of the client?

What tasks should the client be accomplishing?

Is there anything that is preventing the accomplishment of tasks?

What are the biological and psychological threats to the client?

What needs of the client are not being met?

What are the client's perceptions of his or her personal situation?

Is there an obvious use of defense mechanisms?

What purpose are those defense mechanisms serving for the client?

What signs of anxiety can be observed in the client?

Can the client's anxiety be validated?

Erikson's Developmental Theory

What is the developmental stage of the client?

What tasks should the client be accomplishing?

Was the client successful in accomplishing the tasks of previous developmental stages?

During what stages did the client fail to accomplish the developmental tasks?

What effect does this have on the client's psychosocial development?

How is this affecting the immediate problems confronting the client?

What are the environmental factors affecting the client and the client's present problems?

Sullivan's Interpersonal Theory of Development

At what stage of development is the client?

What development tasks should the client be accomplishing?

Did accomplishing previous developmental tasks meet the interpersonal needs of the client?

If interpersonal needs were not met, what effect did this have on the client?

What is the client's personification of self? How does the client describe self?

In what way does the client exhibit anxiety?

What are the client's coping mechanisms?

How does the client relate to other people?

What social networks are available to the client?

How can these social networks affect outcomes of the present situations?

Maslow's Humanistic Theory

Is the client meeting his or her basic needs?

How does the client describe these basic needs?

What obvious needs are being frustrated at this time?

Other than basic needs, what needs does the client consider important?

What is your description of the metaneeds being met by the client?

How does the client express self creatively?

What types of behaviors can be described that indicate the client is moving toward self-actualization?

How does the client describe his or her capabilities and resources?

Skinner's Behavioral Theory

What specific behaviors of the client need to be changed?

What new behaviors are desired to replace the old ones?

Does the client agree that certain behaviors need to be changed?

How is the behavior that needs to be changed reinforced?

Who or what is doing the reinforcing?

What types of things are important to the client?

What types of rewards would reinforce the new, desired behaviors?

Is the client willing to do mutual goal setting?

Does the client clearly understand the goals?

Beck's Cognitive Theory

What are the cognitive schemas or controlling beliefs that the client holds about self and others?

In what ways does the client have inadequate views of self?

What evidence is there that the client misinterprets current experiences?

How positively or negatively does the client view the future?

Is there evidence of cognitive distortions?

BOX 1.2

Brain Imaging Techniques

Positron Emission Tomography (PET)

Mapping via computer imaging that measures physiological processes in the brain such as blood flow, metabolic functions based on glucose utilization, density of neurotransmitters, location of neuroreceptors, and intricate brain circuitry.

Single Photon Emission Computerized Tomography (SPECT)

Measures the same physiological processes as PET but costs less and is more widely available; useful in monitoring the effects of medications on brain functions.

Neurometrics

Measures the electrophysiology of the brain, especially increased or decreased beta, alpha, theta, and delta waves.

Cerebral Blood Flow (CBF)

Measures the circulation of blood in a given brain region; blood flow to both gray matter and white matter can be determined.

Computer Electroencephalographic Tomography (CET)

Converts electrical signals into an electrical activity map of the brain; less accurate than PET but costs less and can be repeated without risk.

Magnetic Resonance Imaging (MRI)

Distinguishes gray and white matter in three dimensions; identifies structural abnormalities.

Magnetic Resonance Spectroscopy (MRS)

Expands MRI readings by adding radioactive tracers; identifies structural abnormalities in three dimensions as well as physiological abnormalities.

but also to design therapies that can better treat or even cure the victims. The **genome**, a word for the full complement of genetic information, is tightly packed into 23 pairs of chromosomes, each of which carries thousands of genes. All told, humans have about 30,000 genes. All genes are made up of just four different chemicals linked together in myriad combinations and lengths. Those chemicals, which scientists represent

with the letters A (adenine), C (cytosine), G (guanine), and T (thymine), make up a sort of genetic alphabet. Now that the Human Genome Project is almost complete, we know that 99.9 percent of this sequence is shared among every human being. What we do not know yet is all the differences in the remaining 0.1 percent that make us individuals, and more important, which of those differences make us susceptible to disease.

This is the mystery that gene hunters are trying to solve. To do that, scientists compare the DNA of both healthy and ill people. Using sophisticated technology to slowly sift through the 3.1 billion pairs of A's, C's, G's, and T's, they hope to identify the subtle differences that affect disease.

Genes determine *phenotype*—the structure, function, and other biological characteristics—of the cell in which they are expressed. In any given cell, 80 to 90 percent of the genes are repressed or inactive. The 10 to 20 percent of the genes that are expressed, or active, make specific proteins that specify the character of that cell and determine, for example, if the cell is a liver cell or a brain cell. Everything we do affects the activity of our genes in every cell. Genes are not destiny. Genes set boundaries for behavior, but within the boundaries is immense room for variation determined by experience, choice, and chance (Kandel, 1999).

Genes convey only *susceptibility* to mental disorders, not disease per se. It is also believed that multiple genes combine with one another and with environmental factors to cause mental illness. Given this, it is possible for people to have low, moderate, or high "doses" of the risk factors that predispose to mental illness. Using schizophrenia as an example, those with very high "doses" may experience the classic symptoms such as disorganized thinking, bizarre behavior, inappropriate affect, hallucinations, and delusions. Other individuals with only moderate "doses" of the risk factors may merely demonstrate seemingly benign characteristics such as odd speech, social dysfunction, or impaired attention. In general, the more severe the psychopathology, the stronger the genetic loading for the disorder (Paris, 1999).

Genetic anticipation may be apparent in some families. Genetic anticipation means that there is a progressively earlier onset of mental illness in successive generations and/or an increase in the severity of the disorder in successive generations.

The *nature versus nurture* dilemma poses the question: Are we mainly products of our genes or of our environment? Both of these models are reductionistic and based on very narrow theories. Those who say mental disorders are primarily caused by nature (neurobiology) fail to address the role of psychosocial precipitating factors. Those who say mental disorders are primarily caused by nurture (environment) oversimplify the role of stressors and do not address the interaction of environment with biology. Mental disorders are a result of the interaction between genes and environment.

The **diathesis-stress model** proposes that a biologically vulnerable person, when exposed to stressors or triggers, develops the disease. It is as if there needs to be a "second hit" to convert genetic vulnerability into brain disorders. This "second hit" could be a perinatal injury, a toxin, and/or life experiences. Many of these stressors appear to be of normal intensity but lead to catastrophic symptoms. It is noteworthy that genetic influence is not static but rather reacts to and interacts with environmental experiences. Most people go through life with predispositions to mental disorders that are never expressed. The relationship between stress and mental disorders is nonspecific. That is, the same illness can be brought on by a variety of stressors, and the same stressors can bring on a wide variety of illnesses (Paris, 1999; Pratt, Gill, Barrett, & Roberts, 1999; Price & Ingram, 2001).

Recent studies demonstrate that exposure to stressful life events is significantly influenced by genetic factors. In other words, people do not randomly experience stressful life events; rather, some people have a persistent tendency to put themselves into situations with a high probability of stressful outcomes. It is believed that this personality trait has a genetic basis (Kendler, Karkowski, & Prescott, 1999).

We must be careful not to equate "running in families" with hereditary causation. For example, if one of your parents is a nurse, there is a higher chance you will end up being a nurse. The simplistic and erroneous conclusion is that being a nurse is genetically determined. In studying the genetic factors in mental disorders, researchers must first establish that there is a higher-than-expected rate of incidence within families. The next step is identifying what parts are due to genetic factors and what parts are due to environmen-

tal factors. Studying monozygotic (identical) and dizygotic (fraternal) twins helps determine possible genetic influences. If the incidence of a mental disorder is greater among monozygotic twins than dizygotic twins, there is at least some degree of genetic influence. However, environmental variables are also a factor, even with monozygotic twins. The best twin studies available at this time are those in which monozygotic twins have been separated at birth and reared separately. When these twins demonstrate a higher-than-expected incidence of a mental disorder, a strong degree of genetic influence is likely. It is important to understand the genetic mapping, since hereditary factors appear to play a role in the development of many mental disorders.

Research in *behavioral genetics* has lagged behind other research in understanding health and illness. Behavioral genetics looks at the contribution of genetic variability to behaviors. For example, the desire to engage in physical activity, the choice of intervals between meals, and a dietary preference for fats may have a genetic component that relates to the tendency toward thinness or obesity. With continuing research, we will better understand how genetically determined preferences interact with environmental factors. The degree to which certain behaviors are genetically or environmentally based may vary both among individuals and among populations (Devlin, Yanovski, & Wilson, 2000).

Gender

Much of who we are, as female or male, is defined by brain differences, physiology, and hormones as well as society's efforts at socialization into gender roles and expectations. Every human's personality is genetically driven and individually developed. The male brain is 10 percent larger than the female brain. The female brain has a larger corpus callosum, which connects both hemispheres. Female brains produce more serotonin (5-HT), the neurotransmitter that inhibits aggressive behavior. Males have much higher levels of testosterone and lower levels of 5-HT, creating more potential for aggressive behavior. We have much to learn regarding gender and brain organization and cognitive functioning. There are gender differences in prevalence of most of the mental disorders. At this time, we do not know the specifics of why women and men are more vulnerable to different disorders (APA, 2000).

Females
 Anxiety disorders
 Schizoaffective disorder
 Depression
 Dysthymic disorder
 Eating disorders
 Borderline, histrionic, dependent personality disorders
 Alzheimer's disease

Males
 Learning disorders
 Autistic disorder
 Asperger's disorder
 Attention deficit/hyperactivity disorder
 Tourette's disorder
 Conduct disorder
 Substance use disorders
 Schizophrenia
 Antisocial, schizoid, schizotypal paranoid, narcissistic, obsessive–compulsive personality disorders
 Vascular dementia

Both Genders
 Bipolar disorder
 Oppositional defiant disorder (after puberty)
 Avoidant personality disorder

Neurotransmission

Theories of **neurotransmission** in mental disorders are concerned with the levels of norepinephrine (NE), serotonin (5-HT), dopamine (DA), acetylcholine (ACh), and gamma-aminobutyric acid (GABA) in the brain. As an electrical impulse travels to the nerve endings, neurotransmitters (chemical messengers) are released at the synaptic junction. These neurotransmitters react with the neuronal receptors, which allow the impulse to be conducted through the next nerve cell. Mental disorders are often related to either a deficiency or an excess of neurotransmitters, or to an imbalance among the various neurotransmitters. In other cases, there is a change in the sensitivity or the shape of the neuronal receptors, resulting in altered transmission of

impulses. Neurotransmission is described in greater detail in Chapter 7.

Biological Rhythms

Circadian rhythms are regular fluctuations of a variety of physiological factors over a period of 24 hours. Temperature, energy, sleep, arousal, motor activity, appetite, hormones, and mood all demonstrate circadian rhythms. The "biological clock" is located in the suprachiasmatic nucleus (SCN) in the hypothalamus and may be desynchronized by external or internal factors. An example of external desynchronization is jet lag: decreased energy level, reduced ability to concentrate, and mood variations resulting from rapid time zone changes. Internal desynchronization is demonstrated in some mental disorders when there are alterations in adrenal rhythm, temperature patterns, and sleep patterns. (Further information on circadian rhythms is covered in Chapter 7.)

Importance of the Neurobiologic Model

Our understanding of mental disorders has been revolutionized by contemporary knowledge of the biological components of behavior, affect, cognition, and interpersonal relationships. Recognizing genetic factors in mental disorders minimizes the tendency to blame the victim or family for the disorder. Understanding neurotransmission helps you comprehend how psychotropic drugs affect the brain to reduce or eliminate the symptoms of many mental disorders. It is impossible to practice mental health nursing without knowing and applying biological principles.

All nurses should be prepared to integrate genetic knowledge into professional practice. One study (Jenkins, Dimond, & Steinberg, 2001) found that nurses need to be able to:

■ Recognize indications for genetic referral

■ Complete a basic genetic health assessment

■ Apply ethical and societal issues in relationship to collecting, reporting, and recording genetic information

■ Assess the psychological effects of genetic information and technology on individuals and families

■ Update knowledge as new genetic methods become available

PERSONALITY

Personality is neither a model nor a theory of mental health nursing. It is, however, a concept that is common to a variety of theories. The concept of personality can also illustrate the interconnections between the different theories.

Personality is perhaps the most unique aspect of our individuality. **Personality** is the unique way we respond to the environment and includes our patterns of behavior, emotion, and cognition that remain consistent from one situation to another. *Temperament*, or personality traits, is the behavioral dispositions that are present at birth such as social responsiveness, fear, irritability, or level of physical activity. This is considered to be the inheritable component of personality.

But there is much more to personality than genetics. We are not robots who are shaped by our genes, nor are we infinitely adaptable to our environment. It is the interactions between temperament and social learning that creates our personality. In some ways, we are who we learn to be. Parents reinforce behaviors and children imitate parental behaviors. Siblings may receive differential treatment from parents or assume different niches in the family group. Children with different temperaments perceive the same environment differently. Children influence the quality of their environment by how others respond to their temperament. For example, temperamental excesses in children are amplified by the difficulties they create for the family, which may be one explanation for why irritable and/or impulsive children are more likely to experience abuse and neglect in the family (Paris, 1999).

Throughout this text you will find evidence of significant genetic influences in mental disorders. The same is true for *normal traits*. For example, the inheritability of intelligence is about 50 percent, with environmental influences accounting for the other half. If we look at sexual orientation we find that male monozygotic (identical) twins have a concordance rate of 52 percent for homosexual orientation while only 22 percent of male dizygotic (fraternal) twins are both homosexual. There are similar statistics for women: Monozygotic twins have a 48 percent concordance rate for homosexuality while there is only a 16 percent concordance rate among dizygotic twins (Grigsby & Stevens, 2000). Understanding the interaction between genes and environment in normal personality will help you understand the relationship in disorders

such as schizophrenia, bipolar disorder, and depression.

NURSING RESEARCH

A major aim of science is to evolve theory. This is considered essential to a scientific discipline because theories draw together groups of concepts and interrelate them so that meaning and understanding can be gleaned from them. These theories may then be used by practitioners to provide answers to questions and concerns. Because nursing is a practice discipline, theories are developed not only to name and explore concepts but also to offer a prescription for practice and an ability to predict outcomes of that practice. The **nursing process** is a way to organize that scientific data to prescribe practice criteria. It is the vehicle the nursing profession has chosen to divide the abundant information into a workable system. Research and theories, by their nature, provide a great deal of information that can be applied in many different situations. Nurses are becoming more adept at using and applying research to particular practice situations.

All research endeavors involve *values*. Societal, professional, and personal values can influence the outcomes of studies in the following ways:

- *Topic of study*: What is worth studying is a value judgment; attention is drawn to what is being studied and away from multiple other issues. *Example*: Studying stressors and the coping strategies of homeless individuals does not look at society's attitudes toward homeless people.

- *Unit of study*: Choice of studying the individual, family, or community narrows the way issues are conceptualized. *Example*: Studying the family of people who have bipolar disorder does not speak to intrapersonal issues.

- *Definitions*: Determine which interactions are counted. *Example*: Specific behaviors define what is labeled as child abuse, and related behaviors are not studied.

- *Choice of variables*: Selection of variables such as age, income, and ethnic identity used to organize the data. *Example*: Studying community violence in urban areas does not speak to community violence in rural areas.

The National Institute for Nursing Research has developed directions for psychiatric nursing research including the identification of biologic–behavioral factors in mental disorders and the testing of biobehavioral interventions. In the words of Jacquelyn H. Flaskerud (2000): "Psychiatric nursing can lead the way in establishing research designs and methods that are truly reflective of the synthesis of biology, behavior, and environment that characterizes nursing science" (p. 2).

THE THERAPEUTIC RELATIONSHIP

Therapeutic relationships are established to help the client. The way you establish the relationship depends on your reactions to the clinical setting and how you are able to care for clients. In mental health nursing, you examine the relationship to ensure that it is goal directed and therapeutic.

STUDENT CONCERNS

At the onset of your course in mental health nursing, you may be quite comfortable in the clinical setting, or you may experience uncertainties and concern relating to both yourself and your clients. Your personal concerns may stem from being in an unfamiliar environment, not knowing what to talk about, believing you have nothing to offer, and/or thinking you might say the wrong thing. Your concerns about clients may be rooted in your stereotypes of people with mental illness, your fear of rejection, your discomfort with anger, or your fear of being physically harmed by a client. Box 1.3 lists common student concerns and strategies for dealing with them.

CARING: THE ART AND ESSENCE OF NURSING

Caring is the essence of nursing and the foundation on which the nursing process is based. It is more than merely liking or comforting other people. It involves commitment and a binding together of individuals in interpersonal connections. Before nurses can care for clients, they must first learn to value and care for themselves. As Keen (1991) states: "If we are unable to care first for ourselves as individuals, and then for our nursing colleagues, the caring we give to our patients is not as good as it could be" (p. 173). One of your educational goals in mental health nursing might be discovering how to care for yourself more effectively. Caring for yourself means reducing unnecessary stress, managing conflict more effectively, communicating with family and friends more clearly, and taking time out for yourself. Caring for your colleagues means respecting cultural differences, asking for collaboration, and responding to constructive criticism.

The *art of nursing* is in being there, with another person or persons, in a context of caring. It is the capacity "to receive another human being's expression of feelings and to experience those feelings for oneself" (Chinn & Watson, 1994, p. xvi). Caring involves compassion and sensitivity to each person within the context of her or his entire life. Caring is the way we enter the world of our clients. In the past, nurses have been urged not to care too much or get too involved. However, caring, successful nurses do get involved with clients because they practice nursing as an art instead of nursing as just a day-to-day job. Clients have a right to competent nursing care, but they also desire a nurse who is committed to clients. In many schools of nursing over the past 50 years, the art of nursing has been devalued and separated from the science of nursing. Consequently, caring has often been a minimal part of the curriculum. With consumer expectations and demand, nursing is beginning to restore its caring–healing art as the basis of nursing practice (Jackson & Stevenson, 2000; Sadler, 2000; Sanford, 2000).

As caring nurses, we are also keepers of *hope*. It is a privilege to be intimately present with other human souls at some of their darkest and brightest moments. With this privilege comes a profound responsibility— to have a deep respect for that person who is our client. Hope is meaningfulness and dignity, even in the face of death. Hope is a way of relating to oneself and one's world. Hope is often attached to something or someone. Some people place hope in others such as their primary care provider. Some people place hope in their own abilities, called self-confidence. Some people place hope in a higher power. Hope can be highly specific regarding a particular outcome. Hope implies openness to experience and possibilities. Hope is acting in spite of circumstances.

Hope is also a way of being with our clients. Sometimes clients need to borrow our hope until they can regain their own. We see clients not merely as they are but as they can be. They need to hear about their

BOX 1.3

Student Concerns and Strategies for Dealing with Them

Sterotypical Ideas About People with Mental Health Problems

Identify cultural stereotypes and discuss your expectations in the first clinical preconference.

Identify specific concerns about clients and/or their families of origin or their current families.

Approach the client as a person rather than as a diagnosis.

Identify healthy aspects and resources of clients; they *are* able to cope effectively in many areas of life.

Fear of Not Knowing What to Talk About

When first meeting a client, introduce yourself by name and position.

Follow the client's lead in topics to be discussed in the initial interaction; pay attention to the client's nonverbal communication signals indicating comfort or discomfort.

Give up the unrealistic expectation that you have to be absolutely right before you offer any observations to clients.

Share your perceptions with clients and seek validation, by asking, for example, "Am I hearing you correctly, that you are very frustrated over this situation?" or "It sounds as if you are becoming more comfortable with being in the hospital."

Using your nursing care plan, decide on specific topics and goals for your one-to-one interaction; be flexible if the client has different priorities.

Concern About Having Nothing to Offer

Identify your own fears of inadequacy by listening to your self-statements: "How can I help this person when I don't know what's wrong with him?" "These clients are too sick/well, so how can I help them?"

If clients question your qualifications, simply state why you are here and what your role is on the unit.

Recognize that your knowledge and theory base will be increasing throughout the course.

Identify the energy and enthusiasm you bring as a positive quality to be used therapeutically.

Recognize that a positive interpersonal relationship is therapeutic because it increases self-esteem, develops interactional skills for clients, and promotes your own professional growth.

Involve clients in the nursing process and work together as a team toward specific goals; solutions come from working *with* clients, not from doing something *to* clients.

Concern About Hurting Clients by Saying the Wrong Thing

The quality of a caring relationship overcomes verbal mistakes; you will not destroy a client with a few ill-chosen words.

Recognize that clinical experience is an opportunity to learn and that verbal mistakes will be made; opportunities for more appropriate interventions are seldom lost—they're just postponed.

If you have made a mistake, apologize to the client and identify what would have been a more therapeutic response.

Use process recordings or audiotapes to evaluate, improve, and increase your communication skills.

Concern About Rejection by the Client

Identify your own characteristic response to rejection. Do you become angry? Feel hurt? Feel resigned to it? Withdraw from the person? In what other ways might you respond?

Identify what is the worst thing that will happen to you if a client refuses to work with you.

If a client is exhibiting behavior that indicates unwillingness to work with you, validate this behavior with her or him.

Remember that you will have opportunities to work with other clients.

Concern About Client Anger

Know and understand your own response to the feeling and expression of anger: "Nice people don't get angry," "It's okay to feel angry but it should be talked about calmly," "I'm uncomfortable if people shout when they are angry."

Accept the client's right to be angry; feelings are real and cannot be discounted or ignored.

Try to understand the meaning of the client's anger.

Ask the client in what way you have contributed to the anger; help the client "own" the anger—do not assume responsibility for her or his feelings.

BOX 1.3

Student Concerns and Strategies for Dealing with Them *(continued)*

Concern About Client Anger *(continued)*

Let clients talk about their anger.

Listen to the client, and react as calmly as possible.

After the interaction is completed, take time to process your feelings and your responses to the client with your peers and instructor.

Concern About Physical Harm from Clients

Ask your instructor about the reality of this concern.

Avoid being in a "trapped" position, e.g., isolated in a client's room.

Recognize the early signs of an impending violent outburst.

Seek help immediately from a staff member or instructor before a client gets out of control.

If a client begins to act out physically, stay out of the staff members' way as they implement their plan of action.

---

own competence and about their ability to grow and change, especially in times of stress and discouragement.

THE NURSE–CLIENT RELATIONSHIP

Throughout the text, the terms *client* and *consumer* will be used to refer to individuals experiencing mental disorders as well as their families and significant others. The nurse–client relationship is the key factor throughout the nursing process. It is the means by which nurses are able to assess clients accurately, formulate diagnoses, help them establish outcomes, plan and implement interventions, and evaluate the effectiveness of the nursing process. The nurse–client relationship is therapeutic, not social. Social relationships are reciprocal in that both people expect their individual needs to be met as fully as possible. The therapeutic relationship, on the other hand, exists for clients, and the focus is on their needs. To minimize the possibility of client dependency, do not try to meet all the needs of every client; support them in meeting their own needs whenever possible. In the professional role, you collaborate with your client as a team, forming a therapeutic alliance with the goal of the client's growth and adaptation. The *therapeutic relationship* is client centered, goal specific, theory based, and open to supervision by your peers, instructors, and supervising nurses.

In this era of sophisticated technology, managed care, and cost containment, the nurse–client relationship is often devalued. Health care is increasingly taking place outside of traditional institutions and moving into places where people live, work, and play. As the boundaries become more diffuse, health care is becoming less formal and demands greater attention to the relational dimensions of care. As you learn the art of mental health nursing, you will be in a unique position to bridge the gap between technology and therapeutic relationships (Krauss, 2000).

Nursing theorist Hildegard Peplau describes the nurse–client relationship as evolving through three phases: introductory, working, and termination. These phases are more easily identified in nurse–client relationships that last more than a few days. The phases often overlap and are thought of as interlocking. There are goals to be achieved in each phase of the relationship.

Introductory Phase

The introductory phase usually begins when you initiate the therapeutic relationship with your client. Start by introducing yourself by name and position and your role in helping the client identify problems and work toward resolving them. A mutually acceptable agreement or contract is established to guide the relationship. This contract, which is typically verbal, should include the purpose of the relationship; the duration of the relationship; and where, when, and for how long you will meet. It is critical that the issue of confidentiality is discussed. (See Chapter 6 for guidelines on confidentiality.)

Although client assessment continues throughout the therapeutic relationship, it is extremely important during the introductory phase. The introductory phase, which may last minutes to hours, ends with the development of preliminary diagnoses and outcome identification.

Working Phase

The second phase of the therapeutic relationship is the working phase. The nursing process is dynamic; assessment, diagnosis, outcome identification, planning, implementation, and evaluation are continuous throughout this phase. Parts of the care plan are revised, expanded, or eliminated according to the individual client's needs. The conscious process of working together toward mutually established goals is referred to as the **therapeutic alliance**. Ineffective behaviors and thoughts are identified as problems, and you and your clients work together to establish more effective ways of coping. It is during the working phase that the majority of client education and problem solving is accomplished.

Two phenomena that may occur during any phase of the relationship (but that are more likely to be noticed during the working phase) are transference and countertransference. **Transference** is a client's unconscious displacement of feelings for significant people in the past onto the nurse in the current relationship. These displaced feelings can be positive or negative and may be highly emotional. Transference that is not identified and managed may decrease the effectiveness of the working phase because the meaning of the nurse–client relationship becomes misinterpreted. When transference occurs, the nurse and client must explore it and separate past relationships from the present one.

Sue, 20 years old, is being seen in the clinic for depression. She was sexually abused by her father from age 7 to 12. Miguel is Sue's nurse–therapist. Sue states that she trusts Miguel, but her nonverbal communication indicates a great deal of fear and suspicion. Sue's feelings about her father have been unconsciously displaced onto Miguel.

Countertransference is the nurse's emotional reaction to the client based on significant relationships in the nurse's past. Countertransference may be conscious or unconscious, and the feelings may be positive or negative. Awareness of countertransference is critical because it could interfere with understanding the client and providing effective care. Discussing your feelings about your client with your instructor will help bring countertransference into conscious awareness.

Colleen's son was killed in an accident several years ago when he was 15 years old. Colleen is taking a course in psychiatric nursing and has been assigned to work with Brendan, who is 15 years old. Brendan is very manipulative, but Colleen has difficulty setting limits on his behavior. Through the process of supervision with her instructor, Colleen begins to realize that her inability to recognize Brendan's manipulation is because he reminds her of her dead son. She has displaced her feelings about her son onto Brendan and has attributed to him positive qualities he really doesn't have at this time.

Termination Phase

The third phase of the therapeutic relationship is the termination phase. Information about when and how this will occur is included in the introductory phase and discussed at times during the working phase. The primary goal of the termination phase is to reminisce about the relationship experiences in order to review the client's progress. With the client, review plans for the immediate future. Termination can be a traumatic experience for clients. Those who have had difficulty ending other relationships will likely have problems ending your shared therapeutic relationship. You must understand their sense of loss and help them express and cope with their feelings. In an effort to continue the relationship, clients may introduce new problems or try to extend the relationship beyond the clinical setting. Here is an example of part of the termination process between Colleen (the nurse) and Brendan (the client):

Brendan: *Colleen, I know this is your last day on the unit, and I'm going to be out of here* *next week. How about if you give me your phone number so I can call you sometime?*

Colleen: *Our relationship was a professional one and is restricted to the time we worked together here at the hospital.*

Brendan: *But Colleen, you really understand me. My own mother doesn't understand me. I just want to be able to call you if things get a little tough. Is that too much to ask?*

Colleen: *Yes, Brendan, it is. I cannot continue to be your nurse outside of the hospital. Let's talk about choices you do have if things get tough when you go home. I would also like to talk about feelings you're having right now as we are about to end our time together.*

COMPONENTS OF THE RELATIONSHIP

The *physical component* of the nurse–client relationship includes all the procedures and technical skills that you do with or for clients. This technological component of nursing education is easily defined and described for you. As a student, you are praised and evaluated for tasks that can be observed, which reinforces the task orientation prevalent in the medical model of health care.

The *psychosocial component* of the nurse–client relationship, which is as important as the physical component, involves your response to the client as one human being to another. You bring many qualities to these relationships: positive regard, a nonjudgmental attitude, acceptance, warmth, empathy, authenticity, and congruity of communication. (These attributes are discussed in further detail in Chapter 2.) You encourage clients to share their thoughts on how they perceive the world, their past experiences and expectations, and their hopes and dreams for the future.

Together with the psychosocial component, the *spiritual component* of the nurse–client relationship comprises the caring relationship. The spiritual component is the feeling of being connected between you and the client. It is that inner sense of being a part of something more than yourself. It is respect for the client's cultural values and religious views. Spirituality is what allows us to connect with clients who may be very different from ourselves. We may not be able to see clearly

the person who lives behind the mask of substance abuse or who is experiencing delusions or who has been forced into living on the streets, but responding to that person's spirit is what allows us to connect to them. Your role in providing spiritual care includes allowing clients to express important spiritual needs, such as the need for meaning in life, belief in God, or relief from fear, doubt, or loneliness. The important point is to recognize that spiritual needs are as diverse as our clients, their cultures, and their illnesses.

The *power component* of the nurse–client relationship is related to your and your clients' beliefs in locus of control. If you reflect an **external locus of control**, you expect clients to give up control to the staff, who then do "to" and "for" clients, stripping from them the right to choose their own healing journey and the quality of their life experiences. The focus of the nurse–client relationship has traditionally been one of curing, with health care professionals as the heroes. When clients have an external locus of control, they view their disease or disability as a "thing" that has been imposed on them and believe they are not responsible for either the cause or the cure.

If you believe in an **internal locus of control**, you welcome your clients' feelings, respect their wishes, and honor their needs for self-expression. Your role is to empower consumers through providing skills, information, and support as they choose options that are in their best interests. The relationship is built around clients' needs to shape and control their own lives as much as possible. Clients who have an internal locus of control feel powerful rather than victimized and are participants in their own healing process. They recognize behaviors, thoughts, and feelings that influence their own movement toward health or illness.

BOUNDARIES OF THE RELATIONSHIP

The boundaries of the nurse–client relationship are those edges that maintain a clear distinction between nurses and clients. The establishment of clear boundaries is designed to create an atmosphere of safety and predictability within which the nursing process can be implemented. Nurses are in a position of power within the relationship because of their specialized skills, the access to private information about the client, and because of the client's vulnerability.

Violation of boundaries includes behaviors such as burdening the client with personal problems, spending excessive amounts of time with a client beyond that which is expected, exchanging gifts, or flirting and acting secretive or defensive toward others in terms of the relationship. Much of the current concern about professional boundaries has grown out of a wish to prevent sexual misconduct by health care providers (Barzoloski-O'Connor, 1999).

NURSING PROCESS IN MENTAL HEALTH NURSING

CRITICAL THINKING

As nurses, we must be critical thinkers because of the nature of the discipline and the nature of our work. We are expected to solve client problems by performing critical analyses of the factors associated with the problems. This analytical process, or **critical thinking**, enables us to make better decisions. Thus, critical thinking, problem solving, and decision making are interrelated processes, with creativity enhancing the result.

Because nursing decisions may profoundly affect the lives of our clients and their families, we must think critically. But critical thinking is not limited to problem solving or decision making; we use critical thinking to make reliable observations, draw sound conclusions, create new ideas, evaluate lines of reasoning, and improve our self-knowledge.

To think critically, you must have cognitive skills and be willing to use them. Critical-thinking attitudes provide the motivation to use cognitive skills. These attitudes are interrelated and integrated, rather than used in isolation. For instance, it takes courage to acknowledge that you do not know something and to develop an inquiring attitude.

Characteristics of Critical Thinking

- *Thinking independently.* Critical thinking requires that we think for ourselves. As we mature and acquire knowledge, we must examine beliefs we acquired as children, holding those we can rationally support and rejecting those we cannot.
- *Humility.* Intellectual humility means having an awareness of the limits of our own knowledge. As critical thinkers, we are willing to admit what we don't know; we are willing to seek new information

and to rethink our conclusions in the light of new knowledge.

- *Courage.* With an attitude of courage, we are willing to consider and fairly examine ideas or views, especially those to which we may have a strongly negative reaction. This type of courage comes from recognizing that our own beliefs are sometimes false, misleading, and prejudicial.
- *Integrity.* Intellectual integrity requires that we question our own knowledge and beliefs as quickly and as thoroughly as we will challenge those of another.
- *Perseverance.* As critical thinkers, we strive to find effective solutions to client and nursing problems. We resist the temptation to find a quick and easy answer. Important questions tend to be complex and therefore often require a great deal of thought and research.
- *Empathy.* It is easy to misinterpret the words or actions of a person who is from a different cultural, religious, or socioeconomic background. It is also difficult to understand the beliefs or actions of a person experiencing a situation that you have never experienced. Empathy is the ability to see the world from another's perspective and to communicate this understanding for validation or correction.
- *Fair-mindedness.* As critical thinkers, we are fair-minded, assessing all viewpoints with the same objectivity. Fair-mindedness helps us consider opposing points of view and work to understand new ideas before rejecting or accepting them (see Table 1.7 ■).

Acting knowledge is outcome of assessment, critical thinking, moral reasoning, and creativity. It is translating what one knows into what one does. Knowing how to do something focuses only on a task. Acting knowledge goes beyond knowing how, to knowing what, when, where, by whom, and why (Whittemore, 1999).

After gaining an idea of what it means to think critically, solve problems, and make decisions, you need to become aware of your own thinking style and abilities. Acquiring critical-thinking skills and an attitude of inquiry then becomes a matter of practice. Critical thinking is not an "either–or" phenomenon; it exists on a continuum, along which people develop and employ the process of inquiry. Solving problems and making decisions are risky. Sometimes the outcome is not what was desired. With effort, however, everyone

> **TABLE 1.7**
>
> Characteristics of Critical Thinking

Characteristic	Description
Rational	Based on logic rather than prejudice or fear
Reflective	Collect data; think through in disciplined manner
Inquiring	Examine claims; determine truth and validity
Analytical	Analyze issues for understanding; decide which authorities are credible
Objective	Attempt to remove bias from own and others' thinking; aware of own values and feelings
Evaluative	Evaluate arguments; decide on course of action; solve problems; use accepted standards

can achieve some level of critical thinking in order to become effective problem solvers and decision makers (Kozier, Erb, Blais, Wilkinson, & Van Leuven, 2000).

THE NURSING PROCESS

The nursing process is the same in all clinical areas of professional practice. In the 2000 *Scope and Standards of Psychiatric–Mental Health Nursing Practice,* the American Nurses Association (ANA) delineates the standards to which nurses are held, both legally and ethically. These standards, based on the steps of the nursing process, are covered in Box 1.4. Such data can also be viewed on the American Nurses Association Web site, which can be accessed through a resource link on the Companion Web site for this book.

Standard I: Assessment

Assessment in mental health nursing is based on the collection of data from multiple sources, such as the client, family and friends, other health care providers, past and current medical records, and community agencies. The client's immediate condition or needs determine the order in which assessment data is collected. Clinical skills include observation, psychosocial history taking, neuropsychiatric assessment, and physical assessment. The assessment process provides the database for clinical decision making: diagnosis, outcomes, interventions, and evaluation.

Interview   The interview is often the initial step in the assessment process. The setting for the interview and the length of time are determined by the client's

mental and physical status. Prior to meeting the client you should ask yourself: What are the assumptions I have about this person, by virtue of her/his diagnosis, history, and lifestyle? We must first recognize our assumptions and predictions in order to put them aside and be fully present to the situation and the individual.

All nurses, no matter which field they choose as a specialty, must be able to gain the client's cooperation and collaboration. Thus, one of the first goals of the initial interview is to establish and maintain rapport with clients. Clients should not feel as if they are "being interviewed" but rather that they are "talking to someone" who is sensitive and compassionate. As you gather information, you must constantly attend to rapport with the client (Shea, 1998).

Observation   Careful, accurate observation is vital during the assessment process. You begin to observe the moment you meet clients and their families. Observation involves all the senses, but seeing and hearing are the most critical. In the chapters on disorders (Parts IV and V), you will learn how to assess clients for the behavioral, affective, cognitive, sociocultural, and physiological characteristics of each disorder. In general, here is how observations are used in each of those categories.

When observing clients *behaviorally*, answer the following questions:

- Where is the client, and what is she or he doing?
- Is the behavior appropriate to the setting (own home, public place)?

CRITICAL THINKING

The time has finally come for your first day of clinical on the psychiatric unit. Yesterday you went to the unit to find out your patient assignment. As you travel in your car to the hospital, you ask yourself what you know about your patient, Mrs. Johansson. The medical record indicated that her admitting DSM-IV-TR diagnosis is major depressive disorder. You did your reading on this diagnosis, but for some reason this gives you little comfort. You are anxious and concerned about the experience. You try to focus again on what you know about Mrs. Johansson before you meet her. You remember the nurses told you that Mrs. Johansson's husband recently told her he wanted a divorce, but Mrs. Johansson refuses to acknowledge this and continues to talk about her wonderful marriage and her two children. You have a feeling that her behavior should mean something to you.

You enter the unit, and a nurse introduces you to Mrs. Johansson, who is having breakfast. Now, what do you do? You wonder if she will want to talk to you, and you wonder why she would talk with you. You sit down next to her and begin a conversation. You remember that your instructor told you that you did not have to have a "heavy" conversation, and so you and Mrs. Johansson discuss her breakfast, which she seems to be avoiding eating, and what she did last night on the unit. She mentions that she has trouble sleeping. You know she has been in the hospital for two days. You observe that she has not combed her hair, and her blouse is dirty.

As you begin to feel just a little bit comfortable, a patient at the next table begins to yell at another patient. You immediately think, "This is more what I expected—screaming, out-of-control patients."

1. Based on this description and what you know about typical student concerns, what concerns are you experiencing and what are some strategies you can use to cope with them?

2. Your instructor meets with you and asks you about Mrs. Johansson. She asks you to identify a defense mechanism that the patient is using and to support your conclusion with data. You know this is an important aspect of the assessment. What do you tell her?

3. What is your initial impression of Mrs. Johansson?

4. What do you know about the nurse–client relationship that you need to think about now as you meet with Mrs. Johansson? Consider the phases of the relationship, components, and roles you might play?

5. How would you respond to the following statement: "Mental health is usually achieved by adulthood, and mental illness has little relationship to mental health."?

For an additional Case Study, please refer to the Companion Web site for this book.

- Is the client dangerous to self or others?
- Is any bizarre or unusual behavior occurring?

When observing for *affective* characteristics, answer the following questions:

- Is there any evidence of intense emotions, such as loud laughter, crying, yelling, or screaming?
- Is the affect appropriate to the situation?

When observing for *cognitive* characteristics, answer the following questions:

- Is the client going over and over the same topic (ruminating)?
- Can you follow what the client is saying?
- Are there themes recurring during the interaction?

When observing for *sociocultural* characteristics, answer the following questions:

- Does the client interact with others? Who? Staff? Peers? Family?
- Is the client assertive or passive with others?
- Is the client having any problems in living at home, in a residential setting, or on the inpatient unit?
- How does the client manage conflict with others?

When observing for *physiological* characteristics, answer the following questions:

- What is the client's motor behavior—for example, pacing, sitting in one position for a long period of time, foot swinging, teeth grinding?
- What does the client's nutritional status appear to be?
- Is the client sleeping at night? Taking naps during the day?
- Are there any physical complaints?

2000 ANA Standards of Care

Standard I. Assessment: The psychiatric–mental health nurse collects patient health data.

Rationale:
The assessment interview, which requires linguistically and culturally effective communication skills, interviewing, behavioral observation, record review, and comprehensive assessment of the patient and relevant systems, enables the psychiatric–mental health nurse to make sound clinical judgments and plan appropriate interventions with the patient.

Standard II. Diagnosis: The psychiatric–mental health nurse analyzes the assessment data in determining diagnoses.

Rationale:
The basis for providing psychiatric–mental health nursing care is the recognition and identification of patterns of response to actual or potential psychiatric illnesses, mental health problems, and potential comorbid physical illnesses.

Standard III. Outcome Identification: The psychiatric–mental health nurse identifies expected outcomes individualized to the patient.

Rationale:
Within the context of providing nursing care, the ultimate goal is to influence mental health outcomes and improve the patient's health status.

Standard IV. Planning: The psychiatric–mental health nurse develops a plan of care that is negotiated among the patient, nurse, family, and health care team and prescribes evidence-based interventions to attain expected outcomes.

Rationale:
A plan of care is used to guide therapeutic interventions systematically, document progress, and achieve the expected patient outcomes.

Standard V. Implementation: The psychiatric–mental health nurse implements the interventions identified in the plan of care.

Rationale:
In implementing the plan of care, psychiatric–mental health nurses use a wide range of interventions designed to prevent mental and physical illness, and promote, maintain, and restore mental and physical health. Psychiatric–mental health nurses select interventions according to their level of practice. At the basic level, nurses may select counseling milieu therapy, promotion of self-care activities, intake screening and evaluation, psychobiological interventions, health teaching, case management, health promotion and health maintenance, crisis intervention, community-based care, psychiatric home health care, telehealth, and a variety of other approaches to meet the mental health needs of patients. In addition to the intervention options available to the basic-level psychiatric–mental health nurse, at the advanced level an APRN-PMH may provide consultation, engage in psychotherapy, and prescribe pharmacological agents in accordance with state statutes or regulations.

Standard VI. Evaluation: The psychiatric–mental health nurse evaluates the patient's progress in attaining expected outcomes.

Rationale:
Nursing care is a dynamic process involving change in the patient's health status over time, giving rise to the need for data, different diagnoses, and modifications in the plan of care. Therefore, evaluation is a continuous process of appraising the effect of nursing and the treatment regimen on the patient's health status and expected outcomes.

SOURCE: Reprinted with permission from American Nurses Association, American Psychiatric Nurses Association, International Society of Psychiatric-Mental Health Nurses, *Scope and Standards of Psychiatric-Mental Health Nursing Practice,* © 2000 American Nurses Publishing, American Nurses Foundation/American Nurses Association, Washington, DC.

The above question sets are general guidelines. As you learn about the mental disorders, you will gather more specific information to guide your observations.

Psychosocial Assessment Agencies often have specific forms to be completed as part of the psychoso-cial assessment. In general, the following information is gathered from the client and significant others:

- Client and family's definition of present problem
- History of present problem, including health beliefs and practices

- Family history of psychiatric and medical illnesses
- Family interactions including support systems and ethnic and cultural factors
- Social history, including communication skills, social networks, work/school roles, economic stressors, and legal stressors
- Living conditions including the availability of food and shelter
- Spiritual considerations, including beliefs, values, and religious concerns
- Strengths and competencies

In each chapter in Parts IV and V, you will find a Focused Nursing Assessment table to help you learn the types of questions to ask and the particular characteristics for which to assess. Observing experienced nurses is a great way to learn basic interviewing skills, as well as seeing more advanced techniques implemented. Be sure to discuss with the nurse what you observed, and clarify anything you did not understand.

Neuropsychiatric Assessment   The neuropsychiatric assessment provides information about the client's appearance, behavior, speech, emotional state, and cognitive functioning. See Box 1.5 for the neuropsychiatric assessment. Box 1.6 describes signs of pathology when assessing clients' perceptions, form of thought, and content of thought.

Physical Assessment   Clinical skills include conducting a detailed physical assessment. In many community settings, psychiatric nurses are the only mental health care providers prepared to complete a physical assessment. Details of physical assessment are not included in this text since you learn those skills in other courses in the curriculum.

Standard II: Diagnosis

Analysis of the significance of the assessment data results in the formulation of nursing diagnoses.

Psychiatric Nursing Diagnosis   Standardized labels are applied to clients' problems and responses to mental disorders. These standardized labels come from the list of approved nursing diagnoses accepted by the *North American Nursing Diagnosis Association* (*NANDA*). Appendix B on the CD-ROM contains the current list of approved NANDA diagnoses. When we use standardized language to document the diagnoses of our clients, we can begin to build large databases

that will expand nursing knowledge. Such data can also be viewed on the NANDA Web site, which can be accessed through a resource link on the Companion Web site for this book.

BOX 1.5

Neuropsychiatric Assessment

General
- Age
- Relationship status
- Family composition
- Employment
- Living situation

Appearance
- General state of health
- Grooming and hygiene
- Posture

Activity
- Motor activity (appropriate; increased/decreased)
- Tremors, dystonias
- Hyperactivity (activity is purposeful)
- Agitation (activity is purposeless)

Speech and Language
- Fluency
- Comprehension
- Pace (fast, slow)
- Volume
- Tone (calm, hostile)

Emotional State
- Mood (sustained emotional state; what client describes; depression, anxiety, sadness, calmness, anger)
- Affect (immediate emotional expression; what others observe; appropriateness, intensity, lability, range of expression)

Perceptions
- Five senses: seeing, hearing, smelling, tasting, feeling

Cognitive Functioning
- Orientation (person, time, place)
- Concentration
- Memory (recent, remote)
- Intellectual functioning (general grasp of information, reasoning and judgment, insight)
- Form of thought
- Content of thought

BOX 1.6

Signs of Pathology

Perception

- Illusions (the misinterpretation of an environmental stimulus of sight, sound, touch, smell, or taste)
- Hallucination (occurrence of a sight, sound, touch, smell, or taste without any external stimulus)
- Depersonalization (feel sense of identity has been altered and therefore feel strange and unreal)
- Derealization (feel the environment has changed and is unreal)

Form of Thought

- Blocking (sudden stop in speech or train of thought)
- Circumstantiality (overly detailed, tedious; eventually reaches goal)
- Confabulation (unconsciously filling in memory gaps with imagined material)
- Derailment (speech is blocked and then begins again on unrelated topic)
- Flight of ideas (rapid, fragmented thoughts manifested in pressured speech)
- Loose association (disconnected thoughts)
- Neologism (making up new words; not understood by others)
- Tangential (thoughts veer from main idea and never get back to it)

Content of Thought

- Disorders range from transient preoccupations to intractable delusions
- Ruminations (recurring mood-congruent concerns usually related to anxiety or depression)
- Obsessions (unwanted, repetitive thoughts that lead to feelings of fear or guilt)
- Compulsions (thoughts or behaviors used to decrease the fear or guilt associated with obsessions)
- Delusions (grandiosity, persecution, control, sin and guilt; religious, erotomanic, somatic)
- Experiences of influence (ideas of reference, thought broadcasting, thought withdrawal, thought insertion)

In developing the nursing diagnoses further, it is necessary to describe the related or contributing factors. These include behavioral symptoms, affective changes, and disrupted cognitive patterns that accom-

pany the mental disorders. Spiritually, people with psychiatric disabilities often have difficulty with interpersonal relationships and may feel a lack of connectedness with others. Some people suffer from a lack of meaning in life, while others attempt to find meaning in their response to their mental disorder. Cultural pressures and expectations may be contributing factors in the development and prognosis of mental disorders. Signs and symptoms, referred to as *defining characteristics*, are subjective and objective data that support the nursing diagnosis. Defining characteristics are identified during the assessment process but are not usually written as part of the diagnostic statement. The following are examples of nursing diagnoses you may use during your clinical experience:

- *Hopelessness*: Related to chronic effects of poverty and racism; dire expectations of the future

- *Self-care deficit: bathing/hygiene*: Related to low energy and decreased desire to care for self; distractibility in completing ADLs.

- *Impaired verbal communication*: Related to retardation in flow of thought; flight of ideas; altered thought processes; obsessive thoughts; panic level of anxiety.

- *Altered family processes*: Related to rigidity in functions and roles; enmeshed family system; demands of caring for a family member with dementia; use of violence to maintain family relationships.

Nursing Diagnoses Versus DSM-IV-TR Diagnoses Mental disorders are classified in the *Diagnostic and Statistical Manual of Mental Disorders, 4th Edition* (*DSM-IV-TR*), published by the American Psychiatric Association. All members of the health care team use the DSM-IV-TR, which groups client information into five categories, called axes. (See Box 1.7 for a listing of the axes.) Axis I includes the majority of the mental disorders. Axis II lists long-lasting problems, including personality disorders and developmental disorders. Both Axis I and Axis II describe the intrapersonal area of functioning. Axis III describes the physical problems of disorders that must be considered when planning the client's treatment program. If there are no physical problems, the diagnosis on Axis III will be stated as "none." Axis IV describes the psychosocial stressors (acute and long lasting) occurring in the past

---

BOX 1.7

DSM-IV–TR Axes

Axis I:	Adult and child clinical disorders
	Conditions not attributable to a mental disorder that are a focus of clinical attention
Axis II:	Personality disorders
	Mental retardation
Axis III:	General medical conditions
Axis IV:	Psychosocial and environmental problems
Axis V:	Global assessment of functioning

SOURCE: Reprinted with permission from the *Diagnostic and Statistical Manual of Mental Disorders, Fourth Edition, Text Revision*. Copyright 2000 American Psychiatric Association.

---

year that have contributed to the current mental disorder. Nurses should be aware of how many stressors have occurred and how much change each stressor caused in the life of the client. Axis V rates the highest level of psychological, social, and occupational functioning the client has achieved in the past year, as well as the current level of functioning. It is especially important to be sensitive to cultural differences and expectations when rating clients on Axis V. Appendix A lists and describes the diagnostic categories of the DSM-IV-TR. Such data can also be viewed on the American Psychiatric Association Web site, which can be accessed through a resource link on the Companion Web site for this book.

The basis of nursing diagnoses and DSM-IV-TR diagnoses evolves from problem solving, which begins with data collection. Data collection includes reviewing signs and symptoms exhibited by clients. With nursing diagnoses, those signs and symptoms are translated into related and contributing factors. With the DSM-IV-TR, the signs and symptoms are translated into diagnostic criteria, including the essential and associated features of specific mental disorders, and a differential diagnosis ultimately results.

There are some similarities between psychiatric nursing diagnoses and the DSM-IV-TR diagnoses. They both serve to guide practice by synthesizing data leading to appropriate interventions. They are both communication tools basic to client care and research activities, and they are both international in scope. There are also significant differences between the two. DSM-IV-TR diagnoses are applicable only to individuals, while nursing diagnoses are applicable to individuals, families, groups, and communities. Nursing diagnoses are generally directed toward problems in daily living, while DSM-IV-TR diagnoses are oriented toward the "disease and cure" model.

Standard III: Outcome Identification

The widespread use of NANDA's nursing diagnoses has increased awareness of the need for standardized classifications of nursing outcomes. Outcomes are positive or negative changes in health status that can be credited to nursing care. They allow us to evaluate the appropriateness of our decision-making process in selecting nursing interventions. Outcomes are important for the quality of nursing care and clinical evaluation research. **Nursing Outcomes Classification (NOC)** is a list of standardized measures that reflect the current status of clients. Outcomes are descriptive, on a continuum from the least desirable to the most desirable states or behaviors. Goals, on the other hand, are prescriptive—the state or behavior you want the client to achieve. Outcomes tell you where the client is at any given moment, and goals tell you where you want the client to end up (Johnson, Maas, & Moorhead, 2000).

Definitions for each outcome are also supplied. NOC is a three-level taxonomy. The highest level contains seven *domains* (or supercategories):

- Functional Health
- Physiologic Health
- Psychosocial Health
- Health Knowledge & Behavior
- Perceived Health
- Family Health
- Community Health

Each domain includes *classes* (or subcategories) that are groups of general outcomes. The third level in the taxonomy is more specific *outcomes*. Third-level outcomes have specific indicators that nurses use to determine the client's status. The following is an example of the NOC taxonomy: (Johnson, Maas, & Moorhead, 2000):

Domain: Psychosocial Health
Class: Psychological Well-Being
Outcome: Hope
Definition: Presence of internal state of optimism
  that is personally satisfying and life supporting
Scale: 5-point scale from none to extensive
Indicators: (Sample from a list of 13 indicators)
- Expression of a positive future orientation
- Expression of will to live
- Expression of reasons to live
- Expression of meaning in life
- Expression of inner peace

You are encouraged to look over this classification system in Appendix D, which is on the CD-ROM, before reading any further.

Once your have established outcomes, you and the client mutually identify *goals* for change. Mutual goal setting is the process of collaborating with clients to identify and prioritize care goals and develop a plan for achieving those goals. Underlying this process is respect for clients' cultural values. You begin by assessing the clients' degree of insight into their problems. If clients are too acutely ill to be actively involved in the initial goal formulation, or if they are in denial of mental health problems, they must at least be informed of the goals and given an opportunity to express their opinions (McCloskey & Bulechek, 1996).

Clients are encouraged to identify strengths and abilities that they bring to this problem-solving process. You help them identify realistic, attainable goals and break down complex goals into small, manageable steps. After goals become manageable, work with clients on prioritization so they try to modify only one behavior at a time. Finally, help clients develop a plan to meet their goals, which includes identifying available resources, setting realistic time limits, and clarifying the roles of the nurse and client. Regular review dates are established with clients and families to review progress toward outcomes and goals (McCloskey & Bulechek, 1996).

Standard IV: Planning

Once the nursing diagnoses, outcome criteria, and goals have been identified, the plan of care is developed to assist the client toward a higher level of functioning and improved mental health. Planning consists of establishing nursing care priorities, identifying interventions, and selecting appropriate nursing activities.

Priorities of Care   In mental health nursing, safety needs are often more of a priority than physiological needs. There are many *safety* issues you need to be aware of at all times. Frequently ask yourself if the client is in danger of the following:

- Exhaustion related to excessive exercise; lack of sleep; panic level of anxiety
- Inability to exercise good judgment related to problems in thinking or perceiving
- Self-mutilation based on past or current behavior
- Violence directed toward others based on past or current behavior
- Suicide related to hopelessness; command hallucinations

Interventions   The widespread use of NANDA's nursing diagnoses has increased awareness of the need for standardized classifications of nursing interventions or treatments. Until very recently there has been no uniform way to define and document nursing care. The **Nursing Interventions Classification (NIC)** is the first comprehensive standardized classification of nursing interventions and is useful to nurses in all specialties and in all settings. Most of the interventions are for use with individuals, but many are for use with families, and a few are for use with entire communities (McCloskey & Bulechek, 1996). Appendix C on the CD-ROM is a partial list of the NIC taxonomy with the most common interventions used in mental health nursing. Definitions for each intervention are also supplied. NIC is a three-level taxonomy. The highest level contains six *domains* (or supercategories):

- Physiological: Basic
- Physiological: Complex
- Behavioral
- Safety
- Family
- Health System

Each domain includes *classes* (or subcategories) that are groups of related interventions. The third level in the taxonomy is the *interventions*. Supplementing the interventions is a list of nursing activities for each intervention. This is not a list of specific procedures as not all activities apply to every client. In addition, nurses may modify or add to the list of activities. The following is an example of the NIC taxonomy: (McCloskey & Bulechek, 1996):

Domain: Behavioral

Class: Coping Assistance

Intervention: Hope Instillation

Definition: Facilitation of the development of a positive outlook in a given situation

Activities: (Sample from a list of 18 activities)

- Assist patient/family to identify areas of hope in life.
- Expand the patient's repertoire of coping mechanisms.
- Help the patient expand spiritual self.
- Encourage therapeutic relationships with significant others.
- Provide patient/family opportunity to be involved with support groups.

The taxonomy is not linked to any specific nursing theory and can easily be used with NANDA and DSM-IV-TR diagnoses. You are encouraged to look over this classification system in Appendix C, which is on the CD-ROM, before reading any further.

This text uses the NIC format in organizing the planning and implementation of nursing care. You will find the domains, classes, and interventions in bold type. Each intervention is accompanied by text that describes the nursing activities you consider when planning and implementing your care (see Table 1.8 ■).

Standard V: Implementation

Caring is a way of relating to people that enables them to grow toward their full potential. Your nursing interventions should be implemented in a manner that recognizes the worth and dignity of people and considers the physical, emotional, social, cultural, and spiritual needs of your clients and their families.

Roles of a Psychiatric Nurse   No matter what mental disorder the client is experiencing, you will assume several roles in helping your clients grow and

---

TABLE 1.8

Comparisons of NANDA Diagnoses, NOC Outcomes, and NIC Interventions

DSM-IV-TR Diagnosis: Major Depressive Disorder

NANDA Diagnosis	NOC Outcomes/Indicators	NIC Interventions/Nursing Activities
Hopelessness: Related to negative expectations of self and future	**Hope:** Presence of internal state of optimism that is personally satisfying and life supporting ■ Expression of positive future ■ Expression of will to live ■ Expression of reasons of live ■ Expression of inner peace **Mood Equilibrium:** Appropriate adjustment of prevailing emotional tone in response to circumstances ■ Exhibits appropriate affect ■ Exhibits nonlabile mood ■ Exhibits impulse control ■ Exhibits concentration ■ Speech at moderate pace ■ Exhibits absence of grandiosity ■ Absence of suicidal ideation	**Hope Instillation** ■ Assist patient/family to identify areas of hope in life. ■ Help patient expand spiritual self ■ Employ guided life review and/or reminiscence, as appropriate ■ Avoid masking the truth ■ Encourage therapeutic relationships with significant others **Mood Management:** Determine whether patient presents safety risk to self or others ■ Provide opportunity for physical activity ■ Assist patient to identify precipitants to dysfunctional mood ■ Teach new coping and problem-solving skills ■ Provide cognitive restructuring as appropriate

SOURCES: Johnson, Maas, & Moorhead, 2000; McCloskey & Bulechek, 1996, North American Nursing Diagnosis Association, 1999.

adapt. The appropriate role at any given time is determined by the planned interventions. The various roles of a nurse are described below.

Socializing Agent The nurse functions as a socializing agent with clients. Working one-to-one with your client, you will focus on difficulties she or he may have in communicating thoughts and feelings to others. Socializing helps to model appropriate interpersonal behavior. Informal conversations such as these give clients the opportunity to discuss nonstressful topics and provide some relief from anxiety.

Teacher Another nursing role is that of teacher. A great deal of teaching occurs in connection with the treatment plan (see Chapter 2 for information on client and family education). Depending on client diagnoses, you may be involved in teaching ADLs. Some clients may need to learn basic cooking, laundry, or shopping skills in order to be able to live independently. Those who have no diversions or hobbies may need help selecting appropriate activities and learning the skills associated with them. Some clients will need to learn and practice assertiveness skills, anger management skills, and/or conflict resolution strategies. The problem-solving process is discussed in detail in Chapter 2.

You will also teach clients and families about the purpose of medication: expected therapeutic effects, the length of time after taking the medication before a change, and the usual side effects. Clients must be informed about any dietary or activity restrictions related to their medications, as well as what to do if they forget to take a dose. In addition, you must instruct clients about any related blood testing or situations in which the client should notify the physician immediately. In addition to oral instruction, written material (in the appropriate language) or pictures should be provided as a reference.

Model People learn by imitating models. Modeling enables clients to observe and experience alternative patterns of behavior. It helps clients clarify values and communicate openly and congruently. As a student nurse, you are a model for your clients, and you must not impose your own value system on impressionable individuals.

Advocate Nurses also act as advocates for clients. As an advocate, you will use a variety of communication techniques to reach clients in ways they can understand and to which they can respond. Nurse advocates serve as links between clients and other professionals or people in the community. As community members, nurses serve as advocates for all recipients of mental health care by striving to remove the stigma of mental illness.

Advocacy in nursing is based on a client's right to make decisions and a client's responsibility for the consequences of those decisions. You must respect the decisions even when you disagree with them. However, if the decisions involve danger to self or others, you must try to prevent the client from acting on the decision. As an advocate, you allow clients to express their feelings appropriately without censure or criticism. You teach responsible behavior of one person toward another, and you protect those clients temporarily unable to protect themselves.

Counselor Another nursing role is that of counselor. The counseling role is most typically assumed during regularly scheduled one-to-one sessions. The counseling interaction is directed toward specific goals and is based on the nursing care plan. As a counselor, you will create opportunities for clients to talk about thoughts, feelings, and behaviors that affect themselves and others. Effective verbal and nonverbal communication is both modeled and practiced during the interactions. The effectiveness of counseling is seen when clients exhibit improved coping skills, increased self-esteem, and greater insight into and understanding of themselves.

Role Player As role players, nurses help clients recreate and enact specific past or future situations as if they were occurring in the present. You will create an environment in which new behaviors can be practiced in a nonthreatening way. Role playing can strengthen a client's self-confidence in coping with problematic interactions, which in turn will increase the desire to implement what was learned in real-life situations. Through role playing, you will help clients express themselves directly, clarify feelings, act out fears, and become more assertive. Clients who think at a concrete level, however, may not be able to transfer the role-playing experience to real-life situations. Role playing is contraindicated with psychotic clients who are unable to comprehend "pretend" situations.

Milieu Manager Because of the round-the-clock contact with clients in some residential or hospital clinical settings, nurses have a unique opportunity to become milieu managers. The **therapeutic milieu** refers to the client's physical environment as well as all the interactions with staff members and other clients. The unit or facility is not just a place but is an active part of the treatment plan for each client, where there is a balance between the needs of each individual and the needs of the group. The environment influences client and staff behavior, and client and staff behavior changes the environment. You must be aware of this interactive process at all times. Think about what you are doing and saying, and evaluate the impact on the therapeutic milieu.

The therapeutic milieu has many group activities and is as *democratic* as possible. In some settings, clients will elect officers from the client population. Community meetings provide opportunities for clients to solve problems related to living with a large group of people, to experience leadership, to help develop policies and rules, and to make decisions for themselves.

As milieu manager, you will be providing clients with a *safe environment* in terms of self-mutilation, suicide, or violence to others. For some clients, you will have to set limits on behaviors that are not appropriate to the setting. Some clients require periods of privacy, while others need to be encouraged to socialize. You manage the milieu by your presence and your contact with clients. To help them learn new behaviors, you give support and direction, along with modeling appropriate behaviors.

The *goal* of a therapeutic milieu is to increase clients' sense of belonging, improve their interpersonal skills such as socialization or conflict management, and help them recognize the impact of their own behavior on others and grow toward autonomy as much as possible. (Characteristics of the therapeutic milieu are covered further in Chapter 10.)

Standard VI: Evaluation

The final step in the nursing process is evaluation. In this step, nurses evaluate and document client progress toward the outcome criteria, as well as evaluate their own clinical practice.

Evaluation of Client Progress   As you compare client behavior to previously established goals and outcome criteria, you should be able to answer the following questions:

1. Was the assessment adequate?

2. Were the nursing diagnoses accurate?

3. Was the client involved in setting goals? Were the goals appropriate? Were the goals attained?

4. Were the planned interventions effective?

5. Were the outcome criteria demonstrated?

6. What changes took place in the client's behavior?

7. Which nursing interventions were effective?

8. Which nursing interventions need revision?

9. Was the client satisfied with the nursing care?

10. What plans need to be modified?

11. Are new care plans necessary?

12. Has adequate documentation of the client's progress been completed?

There are two types of evaluation: formative and summative. *Formative evaluation* is an ongoing process based on the client's responses to care. From the formative evaluation, you maintain, modify, or expand the nursing care plan. *Summative evaluation* is a terminal process and is used to determine whether the client has achieved the mutually set goals. Summative evaluations are done in the form of discharge summaries.

Documentation   Documentation is a critical component of nursing practice. The general rule is: If it is not documented, it has not occurred. All steps of the nursing process pertinent to the client must be documented in the client's record. *Documenting assessment* includes the recording of psychosocial histories, focused nursing assessments, neuropsychiatric assessments, and client/family education needs. *Documenting diagnosis and planning* is typically accomplished in one or more of the following formats: critical pathways, individual nursing care plans, standard nursing care plans, and multidisciplinary care plans. Further documentation includes specific plans for client/family education. *Documenting implementation* includes writing progress notes in the form of narrative and flow sheets. Inpatient agencies require that nursing progress notes be entered at specific times, such as once every shift or once every 24 hours. Any significant events must also be documented, as well as the client's participation in and influence on the therapeutic milieu. Some of the most critical documentation issues in inpatient nursing involve falls, seclusion, restraints, and suicidal or violent behavior. Each clinical setting has specific routines and forms for close observation of these episodes. *Documenting evaluation* is done when progress toward the outcome criteria and goals is charted in the record. The client's level of knowledge achieved through the teaching plan must be included in the documentation. Discharge summaries are written when contact with the client has ended.

Self-Evaluation   It is important not only to evaluate client progress but also to evaluate yourself. Self-evaluation will increase your self-understanding and improve your clinical practice. You may use a variety of methods in this process such as process recordings, one-to-one interactions with your instructor, and group supervision during preconferences and postconferences.

Dealing with client desires, needs, and emotions can lead to feelings of discomfort or burnout for mental health nurses. Therefore, both beginning and experienced nurses need support and supervision to maintain their effectiveness. Supervision is the process of having a peer, teacher, head nurse, clinical specialist, or mentor evaluate your clinical practice to increase your knowledge and competence. It is an opportunity to share your feelings about yourself and your clients and to receive emotional support and guidance. From peers, you can determine the image you project and how others view you. Supervisors can assist in your process of self-evaluation by sharing their perceptions and offering suggestions for change.

MEETING THE CHALLENGES OF THE TWENTY-FIRST CENTURY

EVIDENCE-BASED PRACTICE

Evidence-based practice bridges the gap that often exists between clinical research and everyday practice. Nurses using **evidence-based practice** use critical thinking skills and relevant research to improve the quality of client care and promote clinical judgment. As students and beginning practitioners, you will need guidance from faculty and nursing researchers on how to obtain, interpret, and integrate the best available research.

When evidence-based practice is limited to randomized clinical trials as the only admissible evidence, nursing loses its diverse theories and diverse kinds of evidence. In this narrow sense, evidence-based practice reduces and distorts nursing into a simplistic practice (Fawcett, Watson, Neuman, Walker, & Fitzpatrick, 2001; Jennings & Loan, 2001).

Psychiatric nurses use both quantitative and qualitative research to support their decision-making process. In an effort to help nurses shift from traditional practice to evidence-based practice, Rosswurm and Larrabee (1999) developed the following model:

Step 1: Identify a Specific Problem with One Area of Nursing Practice

- Involve nursing staff, other health care providers, administrators, and interested clients.
- Examine data that indicates a need for a change in practice.

Step 2: Link the Problem with Outcomes and Interventions

- Use the language of standardized classifications: NANDA, NOC, and NIC.

Step 3: Synthesize Best Evidence

- Using critical thinking skills, review the research to determine if there is strong evidence to support a change in nursing practice.
- If there is no strong evidence to change practice, assess the benefit versus risk factors to change.

Step 4: Design a Change in Practice

- Develop a protocol or procedure, keeping the change as simple as possible to increase the chances that it will be accepted.
- Identify what resources are needed to make the change.
- Plan how change will occur.
- Define the outcomes of the change.

Step 5: Implement and Evaluate the Practice Change

- Analyze the data and interpret the results.
- Decide to adopt, adapt, or reject the change based on results of research and feedback.

Step 6: Integrate and Maintain Change in Practice

- Get people involved.
- Maintain open communication channels.
- Provide the necessary resources.
- Monitor process and outcomes.
- Reward quality performance with incentives.

INFORMATION TECHNOLOGY

There probably has not been a time when societal change has been as rapid as in the latter three or four decades of the twentieth century. In terms of nursing issues, there have been dramatic alterations in the way health care is organized and delivered: technology has changed the way we practice our profession, and there have been massive changes in the number of ethical issues related to health care.

There have also been changes in nursing education. Computer knowledge is almost a prerequisite for taking nursing classes. Many courses use fiber optics and satellites to beam lessons to remote connections. Nursing students can acquire information using technological advances such as online search engines on the Internet, computerized reference databases, CD-ROMs, and videodiscs. Many nursing journals are offering their issues online, and we are seeing the advent of electronic journals and books that are available only online.

This explosion of knowledge shows no sign of diminishing. Technology allows nurses to access information, select and use the data obtained, make sound decisions about the appropriateness of the data, and create solutions that meet clients' needs.

Across the country, and indeed the world, clients are learning about their own medical conditions and bringing that knowledge with them to their health care provider's office. As nurses, we are not only a resource for health information but we also help clients find sources of health information that are well-researched. Many clients find online support groups invaluable for their convenience, practical coping suggestions, and health care referrals. Online consumer health sites change frequently. The following are some respected sites that are likely to be around for some years:

Centers for Disease Control and Prevention, *www.cdc.gov*

U.S. Department of Health and Human Services, *www.healthfinder.gov*

Mayo Clinic Health Oasis, *www.mayohealth.org*

U.S. National Library of Medicine, *www.nlm.nih.gov*

Medscape, *www.medscape.com*

Mental Health Net, *www.mentalhelp.net*

Links to these Web sites can be accessed on the Companion Web site for this book.

NURSING TODAY

As nursing moves into the twenty-first century, it is advancing beyond the Western biomedical model to incorporate many healing tools used by our Asian, Latino, Native People, African, and European ancestors. Some see this movement as a "return to our roots." Other believe it is a response to runaway health care costs, growing dissatisfaction with high-tech medicine, and increasing concern over the adverse effects and misuse of medications. The growth of consumer empowerment also fuels this movement.

The rise of chronic disease rates in Western society has motivated consumers to increasingly consider self-care approaches. As recently as the 1950s, we lived in a world of curable disease, largely infectious, where medical interventions were both appropriate and effective and only 30 percent of all disease was chronic. Now, 80 percent of all disease is chronic. Western medicine, with its focus on acute disorders, trauma, and surgery, is considered to be the best high-tech medical care in the world. Unfortunately, it cannot respond adequately to the current epidemic of chronic illness. As nurses, we must become active in reforming the current health care system to be able to meet the challenges that lie ahead.

CHAPTER REVIEW

KEY CONCEPTS

Introduction

- Cultures, families, and individuals often define mental illness as behaviors, feelings, or ways of thinking that are unusual to them or not easily understood by them.

- Mental health and mental illness are end points on a continuum, with movement back and forth throughout life.

- Mental illness is a sense of disharmony with aspects of living that may be distressing to the individual, family, friends, and community.

- Mental health is a lifelong process and includes a sense of harmony and balance for the individual, family, friends, and community.

- Resiliency is a person's ability to emerge relatively unscathed from negative life events.

- Spirituality is a belief system that addresses questions of purpose and meaning in life, moral values, feelings of connectedness with others and an external power, and a belief in a common humanity.

Intrapersonal Theory

- Intrapersonal theory focuses on the behaviors, feelings, thoughts, and experiences of each individual.

- Freud divided all aspects of consciousness into three categories: conscious, preconscious, and unconscious. He theorized that there were three components to the personality: the id, ego, and superego.

- Freud defined anxiety as a feeling of tension, distress, and discomfort produced by a perceived or threatened loss of inner control. He identified processes called defense mechanisms, which alleviate anxiety by denying, misinterpreting, or distorting reality. For the most part, defense mechanisms operate at an unconscious level.

- Erikson saw personality as developing throughout the entire life span rather than stopping at adolescence. He believed personality was shaped by conflict between needs and culture. Erikson identified eight developmental stages: sensory, muscular, locomotor, latency, adolescence, young adulthood, adulthood, and maturity.

- Intrapersonal models provide a way of looking at how individuals develop, how they are still trying to achieve developmental tasks, and how they have learned to cope with anxiety.

Social–Interpersonal Theory

- The focus of social–interpersonal theory is on relationships and events in the social context.

- Sullivan believed that personality could not be observed apart from interpersonal relationships. He identified three principal components of the interpersonal sphere: dynamisms, personifications, and cognitive processes.

- Maslow identified basic physiological needs and growth-related metaneeds. His humanistic theory emphasizes health rather than illness.

- Peplau saw nursing as an interpersonal process, with the therapeutic nurse–client relationship at its core. The major components of her theory are growth, development, communication, and roles.

- Feminist theory is an androgynous model of mental health. Theorists examine how gender roles limit the psychological development of all people and inhibit the development of mutually satisfying and noncoercive intimacy.

- A crisis is a turning point in a person's life at which usual resources and coping skills are no longer effective and the person enters a state of disequilibrium. Variables, or balancing factors, determine a person's potential for entering a crisis state.

- Crises are self-limiting and usually last about 4 to 6 weeks. It is during this time that people are most receptive to professional intervention.

- Social–interpersonal models enable the nurse to assess the influences of culture, social interaction, gender stereotypes, and support systems on the behavior of clients.

Behavioral Theory

- The focus of behavioral theory is on a person's actions, not on thoughts and feelings.

- The major emphasis of Skinner's theory is the functional analysis of behavior. Reinforcements are consequences that lead to an increase in a behavior, and punishments are consequences that lead to a decrease in the behavior. The principle of reinforcement states that a response is strengthened when reinforcement is given.

- Behavioral models are helpful in planning client education and designing programs for a variety of mental health clients and families.

Cognitive Theory

- Cognitive theory explains how we interpret our daily lives, adapt and make changes, and develop the insights to make those changes.

- Piaget thought that children learn by the changing stimuli that challenge their experiences and perceptions. He identified four major stages of cognitive development: sensorimotor, preoperational, concrete operational, and formal operational.

- Beck's cognitive theory focuses on how people view themselves and their world. He identified cognitive schemas as personal controlling beliefs that influence the way people process data about themselves and others. Cognitive distortions result from the cognitive triad of an inadequate view of self, a negative misinterpretation of the present, and a negative view of the future.

- Cognitive models help you assess clients' learning capabilities. They also help you analyze cognitive distortions that are symptoms of a number of mental disorders.

Neurobiologic Theory

- Neurobiologic theory looks at how genetic factors, neuroanatomy, neurophysiology, and biological rhythms relate to the cause, course, and prognosis of mental disorders.

- All functions of the mind reflect functions of the brain.

- Multiple genes combine with one another and with environmental factors to cause mental illness.

- The diathesis-stress model proposes that a biologically vulnerable person, when exposed to stressors or triggers, develops the disease.

- Mental disorders are often related to dysfunctional neuronal receptors or a deficiency, excess, or imbalance of neurotransmitters.

- Personality is the unique way we respond to the environment and includes our patterns of behavior, emotion, and cognition that remain constant from one situation to another.

The Therapeutic Relationship

- The art of nursing is the ability to be compassionate and sensitive to each client within the context of that person's life.

- A therapeutic relationship focuses on client needs and is goal specific, theory based, and open to supervision.

- The introductory phase of the therapeutic relationship includes establishing a contract, discussing confidentiality, assessing thoroughly, and developing the preliminary nursing care plan.

- During the working phase, the care plan is implemented through the process of therapeutic alliance.

- Client transference is the unconscious process of displacing feelings for significant people in the past onto the nurse in the present relationship.

- Countertransference is the nurse's emotional reaction to clients based on feelings for significant people in the past.

- The primary goal of the termination phase of the therapeutic relationship is to review the client's progress and plans for the immediate future.

- The physical component of the relationship includes all procedures and technical skills that you do for clients.

- The psychosocial component involves qualities such as positive regard, nonjudgmental attitude, acceptance, warmth, empathy, and authenticity.

- The spiritual component is the feeling of connectedness with your clients and the respect for the diversity of spiritual needs among clients.

- The power component includes beliefs about external and internal locus of control.

- Boundaries of the nurse–client relationship are those edges that maintain a clear distinction between nurses and clients.

Nursing Process: Assessment

- Critical thinking helps us make reliable observations, draw sound conclusions, solve problems, create new ideas, evaluate lines of reasoning, and improve our self-knowledge.

- One of the first goals of the initial interview is to establish and maintain rapport with clients.

- Observation is extremely important in assessing clients with mental illness. Clients are observed in terms of their behavior, affect, cognition, interpersonal relationships, and physiology.

- The psychosocial assessment includes the client's and family's definition of the problem, history of the present problem, family and social history, spiritual considerations, physical assessment, and strengths and competencies.

- The neuropsychiatric assessment provides more specific information about the client's appearance, activity, speech, emotional state, cognitive functioning, and perception.

Nursing Process: Diagnosis

- The DSM-IV-TR is used by all members of the health care team. It categorizes client information into five axes: mental disorders, personality or developmental disorders, complicating physical problems, psychosocial stressors, and the client's past and current level of functioning.

■ Psychiatric nursing diagnoses are applicable to individuals, families, groups, and communities. They include the etiologies and standard nursing interventions.

Nursing Process: Outcome Identification

■ Outcomes are positive or negative changes in health status that can be credited to nursing care.

■ Nursing Outcomes Classification (NOC) is a list of standardized measures that reflect the current status of clients.

■ Goals are prescriptive—the state or behavior you want the client to achieve.

Nursing Process: Planning

■ The Nursing Interventions Classification (NIC) is a comprehensive standardized classification of nursing interventions and is useful to nurses in all specialties and in all settings.

■ In mental health nursing, safety needs often are more of a priority than physiological needs. Clients must be assessed for exhaustion, poor judgment, self-mutilation, violence, and suicide potential.

Nursing Process: Implementation

■ Characteristics of caring helpers include a nonjudgmental approach, acceptance, warmth, empathy, authenticity, congruency, patience, respect, trustworthiness, self-disclosure, and humor.

■ Nurses assume several roles in helping clients grow and adapt: socializing agent, teacher, model, advocate, counselor, role player, and milieu manager.

Nursing Process: Evaluation

■ Formative evaluation is an ongoing process for maintaining, modifying, or expanding the nursing care plan.

■ Summative evaluation is a terminal process; summative evaluations are written in the form of discharge summaries.

■ All steps of the nursing process pertinent to the client must be documented in the client's record. Some of the most critical documentation involves falls, seclusion, restraints, and suicidal or violent behavior.

■ Supervision by peers, teachers, or other nurses helps you evaluate your own professional practice.

EXPLORE *MediaLink*

■ Interactive resources, including animations, for this chapter can be found on the Companion Web site at *http://www.prenhall.com/fontaine.* Click on Chapter 1 and select the activities for this chapter.

■ For NCLEX review questions and an audio glossary, access the accompanying CD-ROM in this book.

REFERENCES

Aguiliera, D. C., & Messick, J. M. (1990). *Crisis intervention: Theory and methodology* (6th ed.). St. Louis, MO: Mosby.

American Nurses Association. (2000). *Scope and standards of psychiatric–mental health nursing practice.* Washington, DC: American Psychiatric Nurses Association.

American Psychiatric Association. (2000). *Diagnostic and statistical manual of mental disorders* (4th ed., Text Revision). Washington, DC: Author.

Barzoloski-O'Connor, B. (1999). Forbidden territory in the therapeutic relationship. *Nursing Spectrum, 12*(21), 4–5.

Beck, A., & Freeman, A. (1990). *Cognitive therapy of personality disorders.* New York: Guilford Press.

Chinn, P. L., & Watson, J. (Eds.). (1994). *Art and aesthetics in nursing.* New York: NLN Press.

Devlin, M. J., Yanovski, S. Z., & Wilson, G. T. (2000). Obesity: What mental health professionals need to know. *American Journal of Psychiatry, 157*(6), 854–866.

Erickson, E. H. (1963). *Childhood and society* (2nd ed.). New York: Norton.

Fawcett, J., Watson, J., Neuman, B., Walker, P. H., & Fitzpatrick, J. J. (2001). On nursing theories and evidence. *Journal of Nursing Scholarship, 33*(2), 115–119.

Finfgeld, D. L. (2001). New directions for feminist therapy based on social constructionism. *Archives of Psychiatric Nursing, 15*(3), 148–154.

Flaskerud, J. H., & Wuerker, A. K. (1999). Mental health nursing in the 21st century. *Issues in Mental Health Nursing, 20,* 5–17.

Flaskerud, J. H. (2000). From the guest editor—Shifting paradigms to neuropsychiatric nursing. *Issues in Mental Health Nursing, 21*(1), 1–2.

REFERENCES *(continued)*

Freud, S. (1935). *A general introduction to psychoanalysis.* New York: Simon & Schuster.

Gary, F., Sigsby, L. M., & Campbell, D. (1998). Feminism: A perspective for the 21st century. *Issues in Mental Health Nursing, 19,* 139–152.

Goleman, D. (1995). *Emotional intelligence.* New York: Bantam Books.

Grigsby, J., & Stevens, D. (2000). *Neurodynamics of personality.* New York: Guilford Press.

Jackson, S., & Stevenson, C. (2000). What do people need psychiatric and mental health nurses for? *Journal of Advanced Nursing, 31*(2), 378–388.

Jenkins, J. F., Dimond, E., & Steinberg, S. (2001). Preparing for the future through genetics nursing education. *Journal of Nursing Scholarship, 33*(2), 191–195.

Jennings, B. M., & Loan, L. A. (2001). Misconceptions among nurses about evidence-based practice. *Journal of Nursing Scholarship, 33*(2), 121–127.

Johnson, M., Maas, M., & Moorhead, S. (Eds.). (2000). *Nursing outcomes classification (NOC)* (2nd ed.). St. Louis, MO: Mosby.

Kandel, E. R. (1999). Biology and the future of psychoanalysis: A new intellectual framework for psychiatry revisited. *American Journal of Psychiatry, 156*(4), 505–524.

Keen, P. (1991). Caring for ourselves. In R. M. Neil & R. Watts (Eds.). *Caring and nursing: Explorations in feminist perspective* (pp. 173–188), Pub. No. 14-2369. New York: NLN Press.

Kendler, K. S., Karkowski, L. M., & Prescott, C. A. (1999). Causal relationship between stressful life events and the onset of major depression. *American Journal of Psychiatry, 156*(6), 837–841.

Kozier, B., Erb, G., Blais, K., Wilkinson, J., & Van Leuven, K. (2000). *Fundamentals of nursing* (6th ed.). Upper Saddle River, NJ: Prentice Hall.

Krauss, J. B. (2000). Protecting the legacy: The nurse–patient relationship and the therapeutic alliance. *Archives of Psychiatric Nursing, 14*(2), 49–50.

Lauver, D. R. (2000). Commonalities in women's spirituality and women's health. *Advanced Nursing Science, 22*(3), 76–88.

Maslow, A. (1968). *Toward a psychology of being* (2nd ed.). New York: Van Nostrand Reinhold.

McCloskey, J., & Bulechek, G. M. (Eds.). (1996). *Nursing interventions classification (NIC)* (2nd ed.). St. Louis, MO: Mosby.

Mental Health: A Report of the Surgeon General (1999). Rockville, MD: US Department of Health and Human Services, Substance Abuse and Mental Health Services Administration. Center for Mental Health Services, National Institutes of Health, National Institute of Mental Health.

Murray, C. J. L., & Lopez, A. D. (1996). *The global burden of disease.* Cambridge, MA: Harvard School of Public Health on behalf of the World Health Organization, Harvard University Press.

North American Nursing Diagnosis Association. (1999). *Nursing diagnoses, definitions and classification 1999–2000.* Philadelphia: Author.

Paris, J. (1999). *Nature and nurture in psychiatry.* Washington, DC: American Psychiatric Press.

Peplau, H. E. (1952). *Interpersonal relations in nursing.* New York: Putnam.

Piaget, J. (1972). *The psychology of the child.* New York: Basic Books.

Pratt, C. W., Gill, K. J., Barrett, N. M., & Roberts, M. M. (1999). *Psychiatric rehabilitation.* San Diego, CA: Academic Press.

Price, J. M., & Ingram, R. E. (2001). Future directions in the study of vulnerability to psychopathology. In R. E. Ingram & J. M. Price (Eds.), *Vulnerability to Psychopathology* (pp. 455–466). New York: Guilford Press.

Rosswurm, M. A., & Larrabee, J. H. (1999). A model for change to evidence-based practice. *Image, 31*(4), 317–322.

Sadler, J. (2000). Suffering: Nurses heeding the call. *Leadership,* Second Quarter, 8–9.

Sanford, R. C. (2000). Caring through relation and dialogue: A nursing perspective for patient education. *Advanced Nursing Science, 22*(3), 1–15.

Shea, S. C. (1998). *Psychiatric interviewing: The art of understanding* (2nd ed.). Philadelphia: Saunders.

Skinner, B. F. (1953). *Science and human behavior.* Riverside, NJ: Macmillan.

Special Research Section. (2000). The decade of the brain in its final year—and what a year it was! *NAMI Advocate, 21*(4), 1–4.

Sullivan, H. S. (1953). *The interpersonal theory of psychiatry.* New York: Norton.

Whittemore, R. (1999). To know is to act knowledge. *Image, 31*(4), 356–366.

CHAPTER 2

Relating, Communicating, and Educating

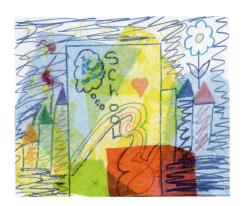

OBJECTIVES

After reading this chapter, you will be able to:

- DESCRIBE the use of self as a therapeutic tool.
- DISCUSS the characteristics of caring helpers.
- EXPLAIN the significance of nonverbal communication.
- DESCRIBE effective communication techniques.
- ASSESS client areas of learning.
- IDENTIFY informal and formal teaching methods.
- HELP clients implement the problem-solving process.

I will be a good teacher and help kids and be there for them.

—Crystal, Age 12

MediaLink

CD-ROM
- *Audio Glossary*
- *NCLEX Review*

Companion Web site www.prenhall.com/fontaine
- *Critical Thinking*
- *More NCLEX Review*
- *Case Study*
- *Care Map Activity*
- *Links to Resources*

*T*he art of nursing is caring and the foundation on which the nursing process is based. This is true for any setting in which the profession of nursing is practiced. The fundamental components of therapeutic support are: rapport and relating, communicating, educating, and problem solving. Your experiences in mental health nursing help you fine-tune and incorporate these caring skills into your professional practice.

RELATING

The ability to relate to clients effectively depends to some extent on your ability to translate caring into nursing action. Caring implies compassion and sensitivity to each person within the context of her or his entire life. Caring involves a deep respect for the individual who is our client. Caring is also the way we enter the world of our client.

Therapeutic nurse–client relationships have a sense of harmony and understanding, which is referred to as **rapport**. From the introductory phase through the termination phase, the relationship evolves as the client experiences your caring approach (Forchuk et al., 2000; Isenalumhe, 2000).

CHARACTERISTICS OF CARING HELPERS

The ability to integrate the characteristics of caring helpers into nursing practice will increase growth and satisfaction for both you and your clients. These interpersonal qualities and skills are critical to the therapeutic relationship through which nursing interventions are implemented. Used in isolation from the nursing process, they become characteristics of a social rather than a professional relationship.

Nonjudgmental Approach

One characteristic of caring nurses is a nonjudgmental approach to clients. It may be impossible for you to be completely nonjudgmental about clients. You make cognitive judgments when you assess clients and formulate reasonable plans of care. Emotional judgments are evidenced by such statements as "I really like her" or "He frightens me." Clients are also judged within the social context of appropriate or inappropriate behavior. Spiritual judgments include moral approval or condemnation of another person. Cultural judgments include being critical of behaviors, beliefs, and values that are different from yours.

A nonjudgmental approach to clients means that you are not harshly critical of them. Develop sufficient self-awareness to identify pejorative thoughts and feelings about particular clients. With this insight, you can avoid acting on negative judgments. Nonjudgmental nurses allow clients to talk about thoughts and feelings, and they respect clients as responsible people capable of making their own decisions.

Acceptance

Acceptance of clients is another characteristic of caring nurses. Acceptance is affirming people as they are and recognizing that clients have the right to emotional expression. Accepting nurses respect clients' thoughts and emotions and help them achieve self-understanding. As internal responses to one's perception of others and the environment, feelings are genuine and cannot be criticized, argued with, or denounced. To tell clients how they should or should not feel is to discount their past experiences, present state, and future potential. Being uncomfortable with one's own feelings often leads to discrediting the feelings of others.

Unless it is detrimental to the client or to others, accept client behavior. Certain behavior, such as masturbating in public, causes social embarrassment and discomfort to others and may later be a source of shame for the person. Protect clients by providing them with private space and time for this normal human activity. Set limits on activities that will lead to a client's complete exhaustion. Do not accept a client's violence toward self or others.

In determining whether or not a behavior is acceptable, first assess the probable consequences of the behavior. If you think it will be detrimental to the client or others, formulate a plan for intervention. Remember that if a client is incapable of changing behavior or chooses not to change it, physical force may be necessary. Ask the following questions during assessment: "Is this behavior detrimental, or is it just a source of irritation to me?" "Are the rules and regulations of the unit more important than the client's rights and dignity?" "Is this behavior dangerous enough to use physical force to stop it?" "Am I willing and able to use physical force to change the behavior?" The examples below illustrate this process.

Maria is a nurse in the emergency department. She is assigned to a client, Tom, whom the police have arrested for intoxication and disorderly conduct. He has been placed in a room designed to be safe for this type of client. When Maria enters the room, she finds Tom smoking a cigarette, which is against the rules of the department. When he ignores her requests to put out the cigarette, she attempts to take it away from him forcefully. Tom strikes out in anger, and Maria ends up with a facial cut that requires stitches.

Connie is a nurse on the psychiatric unit. She has been attempting to intervene with Roberta, a client who has become very angry with her roommate. When it is obvious that Roberta is losing control, Connie calls for help from other staff members, and they quickly formulate a plan for intervention. As Roberta picks up a chair and threatens her roommate, three staff members surround her and firmly take the chair away from her. She is then escorted to the quiet room, where two staff members remain with her until she has better control over her behavior.

It is apparent that Maria attempted to enforce the rules of the department without pausing to plan and prioritize. Since Tom was in a room by himself where there was no danger of fire, his smoking a cigarette did not constitute a fire hazard. Maria might have made the decision to remain with him while he finished his cigarette, to prevent any accidents with the smoking material, but using physical force to stop the behavior was inappropriate because the incident wasn't dangerous. If Maria was determined to stop Tom's behavior, she should have sought help and thought of a plan to accomplish this outcome.

In contrast, Connie identified that Roberta's behavior was unacceptable because there was the danger of her roommate's being injured. A plan was formulated and implemented so that no one on the unit was injured, and Roberta was given the opportunity to talk about the feelings underlying her unacceptable behavior.

Warmth

Another characteristic of caring nurses is warmth, the manner in which concern for and interest in clients is expressed. This does not mean that you should be effusive with clients or attempt to be their buddy. Warmth is primarily expressed nonverbally, by a positive demeanor, a friendly tone, and an engaging smile. Simply leaning forward and establishing eye contact are expressions of warmth, as is physical touch, as long as it is acceptable and not frightening to the client.

Empathy

Much has been written about empathy as a necessary characteristic of caring nurses. Empathy is the ability to see another's perception of the world and it is accepting how clients see themselves, what they are feeling, and what they are striving to become. Empathy is a two-step process of understanding and validating. The *first step* is careful consideration of the meaning of what clients are communicating and the feelings being expressed. The *second step* is communicating your acceptance verbally so that clients are able to validate or correct your perceptions. Most clients are not searching for a person who feels as they do. Rather, they are searching for someone who is trying to understand what they feel. Empathy can facilitate therapeutic collaboration and help clients experience and understand themselves more fully (Shea, 1998).

Authenticity

To be a caring nurse means you rely on your authenticity—being genuinely and naturally yourself in therapeutic relationships. When you make a commitment to clients, you take on a professional role. This is different from "playing" the professional role, which makes a pretense of helping clients. When you are more concerned about how you appear than what you are and do, you erect a façade of helping and are incapable of being authentic with clients, peers, and supervisors.

Congruency

Nurses are genuine when their verbal and nonverbal behavior indicates congruency. Clients can quickly sense when you are incongruent, or saying one thing verbally and another thing nonverbally. Congruency is a necessary ingredient to building trust.

It is Steve's first day on the psychiatric unit as a nursing student. He is in the day room, interacting with a group of clients and two other students. He appears tense, with upright body posture, clenched hands, and a swinging foot. His voice is pitched higher than normal. One of the clients jokingly asks him, "What's the matter? Are you afraid of us crazies?" Steve quickly replies, "No, I'm not afraid. I like being here." The clients respond to him with looks of disbelief and change their focus to the other two students. Steve seeks out his instructor for help with this problem. The two of them discuss how his verbal and nonverbal communication did not match and the effect this incongruity had on the clients.

Several weeks later, Steve finds himself becoming increasingly frustrated with a client who has consistently refused to participate in any unit activities. This time he is able to be congruent and express his frustration directly to the client rather than trying to cover up his feelings.

Patience

It is essential that you have patience with consumers, to give them the opportunity to grow and develop. Patience is not passive waiting, but active listening and responding. By allowing them to grow according to their own timetables, patience gives clients room to feel, think, and plan what changes need to be made. You must also be patient with yourself. Look for opportunities to develop self-awareness and gain new knowledge. Moreover, recognize that professional competence is not simply a goal; it is a long-term process of learning and developing as a nurse.

Respect

Respect for clients is another characteristic of caring nurses. Respect includes consideration for clients, commitment to protecting them and others from harm, and confidence in their ability to participate actively in solving their own problems. Do not let the nurse–client relationship become a dependent, parent–child relationship.

Trustworthiness

Trustworthiness is a characteristic of caring nurses toward which all the preceding characteristics build. By using good interpersonal skills, you help clients attach to you emotionally, which in turn helps build trust. This therapeutic attachment is facilitated through the nursing process. When you are trustworthy, you are dependable and responsible. You adhere to time commitments, keep promises, and are consistent in your attitude. Clients learn they can rely on you. Trust is also built when you demonstrate your willingness to continue working with clients who show little progress.

When you are trustworthy, you respect the confidentiality of the nurse–client relationship. Clients need to have their privacy protected because of the stigma associated with mental disorders. Reassure clients that information will not go beyond the health care team. Because you and your clients may live in the same community, some clients may fear that people will learn they are receiving mental health care. To minimize this fear, emphasize the issue of confidentiality. (Confidentiality is covered further in Chapter 6.)

Distrust may develop when consumers are denied access to the information in their records. Consumers have the right to read their records; this right protects them by ensuring that all viewpoints, including their own, are represented. Sharing nursing notes can be beneficial in that further discussion can develop from your initial observations and interpretations. Every clinical agency has regulations for sharing record information with clients, and you must adhere to these rules.

Self-Disclosure

Trust develops when nurses offer appropriate self-disclosure. In order to establish trust and openness, beginning students often believe they should be no more than passive, nonjudgmental listeners. But trust cannot be achieved if you withhold your own thoughts and feelings. Only when relationships are open and active can real progress be made. Appropriate self-disclosure is always goal directed and determined by the client's needs, not yours. Nurses frequently ask clients to talk about their feelings as a therapeutic intervention. For clients who have minimal interpersonal skills, however, it is equally important to teach them how to perceive other people's feelings and to validate this perception. Through your self-disclosure, clients can improve their interpersonal relationships. For clients, self-disclosure can lead to further self-exploration; they are often reassured that their feelings are real and shared by others.

Self-disclosure is not always appropriate. Clients who are acutely ill may not be able to see themselves as separate individuals from the staff. Self-disclosure in this situation may be a source of confusion because these clients may believe that you are talking about them. Self-disclosure about personal details is often inappropriate and should be avoided. If clients ask for information about your personal life, simply say you are uncomfortable sharing that information, and refocus the conversation on the client's issues.

Berta, a nursing student, is having a one-to-one session with Jim, her client of one week.

Jim: I notice you don't have a wedding band on. Does that mean you aren't married?

Berta: That's right.

Jim: Do you have a boyfriend, or are you dating anyone right now?

Berta: Jim, I'm not comfortable talking about my private life. We were just discussing your recent divorce. Could we go back to that topic, please?

Jim: I just want to know if you're available, that's all. I mean, maybe we could go out for dinner sometime after I get out of here.

Berta: Jim, you know that our relationship is a

professional one and is limited to my time here in the clinic with you. It is not possible to continue it after your discharge.

Jim: Well, I'm so lonesome since my wife left me, and you seem so nice and friendly.

Berta: Let's talk about your loneliness and see if we can find more appropriate ways to deal with this problem.

Humor

Humor is a useful tool in effective nurse–client relationships. Some nurses erroneously consider humor to be "unprofessional." Healthful humor must be distinguished from harmful humor. Harmful humor ridicules other people by laughing at them. Humor is also potentially harmful if it is used to avoid resolving genuine problems. Healthful humor, on the other hand, is a way to elicit laughter. It occurs when you laugh with other people. Healthful humor is appropriate to the situation and protects a person's dignity. A good sense of humor is a mature coping mechanism and can help people adapt to difficult situations.

Humor creates and invites laughter; as such, it is a communication process. Humor is a cognitive communication that creates an affective response, such as delight or pleasure, followed by a behavioral response, such as smiling or laughing. Humor reduces anxiety and fear. It diffuses painful emotions, which the person cannot experience when laughing, and decreases stress and tension. Humor may also be a safety valve for the energy generated by anger. If people are able to look at an irritating situation and laugh rather than explode in anger, the energy is discharged in an adaptive manner.

There are cultural differences in expressing humor. All people laugh, and people of all cultures have a sense of humor. The greatest difference between cultural groups is the content of humor. For example, the Irish make jokes about drinking, whereas the Israelis do not. American humor tends to have sexual and aggressive themes, which are not present in Japanese humor. People from so-called pioneer countries, such as the United States, Australia, and Israel, express humor with exaggeration and tall tales; in contrast, British humor is understated and intellectual. Jews and Britons tell many jokes revolving around self-mockery (Robinson, 1991).

A client's sense of humor may be a diagnostic cue for you. Changes in patterns of laughter may indicate other difficulties in adaptation. Clients who are depressed retain a cognitive sense of humor, but they receive no pleasure and are unable to laugh. Clients who are in a manic phase find everything funny, but because of their lack of judgment, their humor can turn into sarcastic wit and be potentially harmful to others. Those experiencing suspicious thoughts cannot laugh about their situation and are so frightened that they view humor as evidence of a personal attack. Clients who have difficulty with abstract thinking have problems understanding jokes. The influence of alcohol or other drugs may reduce a person's inhibitions so that nearly all stimuli in the environment appear funny. In assessing clients, it is appropriate to ask, "What is your favorite joke?" Responses to this question will give you an indication of the client's sense of humor.

COMMUNICATING

Communication is the foundation of interpersonal relationships and is a key factor in the nursing process. The purpose of communication is twofold: to give and receive information, and to make contact between people. As a student in mental health nursing, you use communication to assess clients and families as well as to implement your plan of care (giving and receiving information). Communication is also the means by which you initiate and establish relationships with clients (interpersonal contact). Clients use communication to share their feelings, express their thoughts, and tell you about their lives. Through interpersonal contact with you, clients and families learn more effective and adaptive ways of communicating with others.

THE NATURE OF COMMUNICATION

People often assume that communication is merely one person giving information to another person. However, communication is much more complex than the transfer of information. Communication takes place in the context of the people involved. To analyze communication, you must consider spoken words, paralanguage (sounds), the thinking process, emotions, nonverbal behavior, and the culture of the person who is sending the message. How the message is

heard depends on the listening skills, analysis of the message, emotions, and culture of the person who is receiving the message (see Figure 2.1 ■).

Effective communicators analyze their own and others' communication in terms of the behavioral, affective, and cognitive messages implied in the transfer of information. *Behavioral analysis* considers how accompanying nonverbal actions modify or enhance the verbal message. *Affective analysis* includes understanding the emotions involved in the communication, which are imparted both verbally and nonverbally. *Cognitive analysis* involves comprehension of the stated words as well as the thinking process of the person communicating. The cognitive component is communicated verbally or in writing.

Analysis of **paralanguage**, or sounds, provides additional information about the message that is being transmitted: the rate of speech, tone of voice, and loudness of the voice. Paralanguage also includes sounds that are not words, such as laughing, sobbing, snorting, and clicking of the tongue. You must also analyze how *culture* influences communication. Much of our communication is influenced by our cultural norms, for example, the use of personal space, acceptable body language, the amount of eye contact, and the types of paralanguage.

Nonverbal Communication

Because two thirds of communication is considered to be nonverbal, it is critical that you observe, understand, and respond to the nonverbal cues of your clients (see Table 2.1 on page 56 ■). You must also be a "self-observer," paying attention to what messages you are communicating nonverbally. **Body language** includes your position, posture, and movements. Sitting face to face with a person will encourage more interaction than sitting side by side. Removing barriers between the two of you, such as desks or tables, will facilitate communication. Standing over a client who is sitting is a dominating or intimidating position and will often interfere with effective communication. A rigid body posture may express anger or fear, while a relaxed body posture expresses openness and a feeling of safety. Leaning back may convey a message of distance and withdrawal; learning forward indicates warmth and receptivity. People who sit with their arms and legs tightly crossed appear to be protecting themselves from some real or perceived danger. A person whose body seems to be

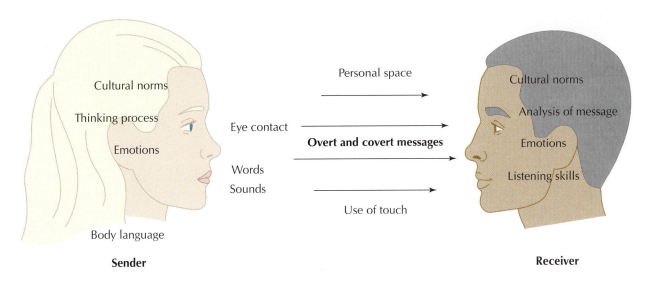

FIGURE 2.1 ■ The communication process.

pulling in on itself may be experiencing depression and low self-esteem. Body movements such as finger tapping, leg swinging, and nail biting may signal frustration, anxiety, anger, or embarrassment. Gestures such as pointing fingers, hands on hips, and shoulder shrugs are all aspects of communication.

Eye contact is extremely important in initiating, encouraging, and terminating communication. The listener usually maintains more eye contact than the speaker. Raised eyebrows may indicate interest, while frowning eyes may express disagreement. Suspicion is often communicated with narrowed eyes. Increased eye contact may be a cue that a person is anxious. Minimal eye contact may be evidence of shyness, low self-esteem, or boredom with the interaction.

Remember that different cultural and subcultural groups have varying patterns of nonverbal communication. Validate impressions and inferences with clients

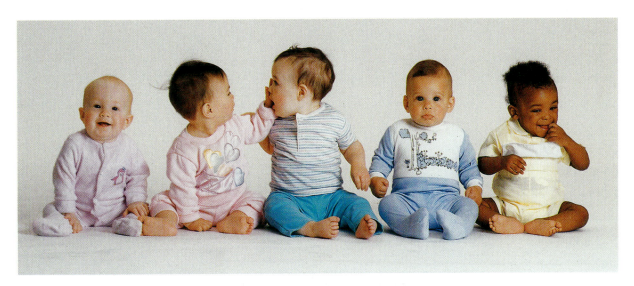

PHOTO 2.1 ■ Infants communicate with body language long before they speak.

SOURCE: Barbara Campbell/Getty Images, Inc.

TABLE 2.1

Forms of Nonverbal Communication

Behavior	Possible Meaning
Standing	
At beginning or end of the interaction	Initiation or termination of the interaction
Over other person while talking	Intimidation or domination
Sitting	
Face to face	Interest
Side by side	Neutrality
Turned away	Termination of the interaction
At the edge of the chair	Anxiety or eagerness
Body Posture	
Relaxed	Friendliness, warmth
Rigid or tense	Fear or anger
Leaning back	Withdrawal, distance
Leaning forward	Interest, friendliness
Arms and/or legs tightly crossed	Self-protection, withdrawal
Shrinking in	Depression, low self-esteem
Turned away	Distance, withdrawal
Gestures	
Leg or foot shaking, finger tapping	Anxiety, frustration, anger
Fidgety, restless movements	Anxiety, embarrassment
Finger shaking, hands on hips	Authority, intimidation
Hiding hands	Shyness, insecurity
Fist-clenching	Anger, frustration
Wringing hands	Hopelessness, helplessness
Eyes	
Frequent eye contact	Interest, honesty
Minimal eye contact	Low self-esteem, shyness, boredom
Rapidly shifting eye contact	Confusion
Frequent blinking	Anxiety
Touch	
Touching arm or hand	Interest, concern

during the observing and interviewing processes. This is even more important when you and your client are from different cultural backgrounds. For example, in some cultures, minimal eye contact does not indicate low self-esteem or boredom but is considered polite and respectful.

Personal space and *boundaries* are culturally determined and may range anywhere from 2 inches to 2 feet (5–61 cm). In mental health nursing, it is essential to respect clients' boundaries and their need for personal space. This respect includes how closely you sit with clients, how much space you give them when walking together, and asking their permission before entering their room.

Touch is related to personal space and boundaries and is determined by cultural norms and previous experiences. In mental health nursing, the use of touch must be well thought out, so as to avoid misunderstandings. You must think about if, how, or when you might use touch with each client. It is usually better to ask people if you may touch their hands, for example, than to make assumptions as to how comfortable they are with touch. Before touching others, ask yourself: What is the purpose of the touch? Is it appropriate? How might this person interpret the touch? With this kind of analysis, touch can be another form of nonverbal communication. (Table 2.2 ■ gives clues to what might be the reasons behind certain cultural behaviors.)

Listening

The art of nursing is the art of good listening. Good nurses listen for more than what is said by words alone. Every sentence has a meaning beyond the words.

TABLE 2.2

Nonverbal Communication of Major Ethnic Groups in the United States

Group	Nonverbal Patterns
African	Touch is common with family, extended family members; close personal space
Chinese	Not accustomed to being touched by strangers; avoid direct eye contact when listening; distant personal space
Eastern Indian	Handshakes between men only; direct eye contact considered disrespectful
Europeans	Eye contact acceptable; noncontact people; distant personal space; Southern countries have closer contact and touch
Filipino	Touch is stressed; some may fear eye contact; if eye contact is established, maintain it
Iraqi	Touch and embrace on arrival and departure
Israeli	Touch is demonstrative
Japanese	Handshakes acceptable; not accustomed to physical contact; distant personal space; direct eye contact shows lack of respect
Mexican	Touch often used, especially between those of same sex; close personal space
Native American	Periods of silence during communication shows respect; eye contact very limited; close personal space—no boundaries
Saudi	Male may touch only females in family; handholding by men acceptable

SOURCES: Shea, S. C. (1998). *Psychiatric interviewing: The art of understanding* (2nd ed.). Philadelphia: Saunders; and Spector, R. E. (2000). *Cultural diversity in health and illness* (5th ed.). Upper Saddle River, NJ: Prentice Hall.

Successful communication occurs when you hear what people mean, not just what they say.

If you are rehearsing what you are going to say next when the other person is talking, you are not listening. Many of us think we are good listeners, but more often than not, we talk too much. Often, we talk too much because we think we are supposed to "make things better" for our clients. We cannot solve people's problems for them. It is egocentric to think we can instantaneously analyze problems and fix them on the spot. It is important to realize the other person is not really looking for an answer. They are seeking empathy, sensitivity, and understanding.

In order to listen well, we must interrupt our preoccupation with ourselves and enter into the experience of the other person. Listening well is often silent but it is never passive. Listening means paying attention to what the person is saying, acknowledging feelings, holding back on what you have to say, avoiding interruption, and controlling the urge to give advice.

Better listening does not start with a set of techniques. It starts with making a sincere effort to pay attention to what is going on in the other person's experience. Listeners who pretend interest do not fool anyone for long—except, perhaps, themselves. Practice listening whenever your partner, family member, or friend speaks to you. Listen to them with the sole intention of understanding what that person is trying to express. Listen to yourself, get to know something about your own ways of communicating. Self-understanding will enable you to relate more effectively to other people.

Failure to be heard and understood is painful. No one loses the need to communicate what it feels like in our own private world of experience. The importance of listening, as a part of communication, cannot be overestimated. Being listened to means that we are taken seriously, and the gift of someone else's attention and understanding makes us feel validated and valued. In opposition, not being listened to makes us feel ignored, unappreciated, cut off, and alone.

Levels of Messages

To understand consumers' experiences, you must listen to both overt and covert levels of the message being transmitted. **Overt messages** are conveyed by spoken words and are heard in the context of the person's feelings. Tone of voice, rate of speech, body posture, gestures, eye contact, and facial expression convey **covert**

messages, which clarify or modify the overt message. For example, two hours ago, Jorge, age 22, was admitted for the first time to an acute care psychiatric facility. He asks the nurse, "What time are visiting hours?" The overt message is a simple request for information. If his words are spoken angrily and loudly or if his body posture is visibly tense, Jorge may be trying to assume some degree of control in an environment in which he feels uncomfortably dependent. If he speaks those same words in a frightened tone of voice, he may be terrified at being separated from his loved ones. Problems in communication can arise not from a lack of technical communication skills but from an insensitivity to covert messages.

Communication Difficulties

Listening In general, you will be more effective if you focus on listening and understanding clients' communication rather than trying to plan how you will respond. A common concern of nursing students is: What am I going to say next, and what is the client going to say then? Beginning students frequently focus on trying to say the "right thing" or use the "right technique" and may therefore appear either distant or oversupportive. More beneficial to clients is simply being yourself. As you become more comfortable with communication skills, saying the right thing will become secondary to listening and understanding.

Be aware of the pitfalls of being merely a polite listener, in which the listener goes through the motions of listening without truly hearing or understanding. Often seen in social interactions, this pattern can extend to nurse–client interactions. This may occur if you fear being regarded as inadequate or unintelligent. The polite listener is bored or impatient, and more interested in talking than in listening.

Nurses often assume that most of their communication has been listened to and understood by clients. However, feelings such as anxiety and anger may interfere with a client's ability to listen. Frequently ask yourself: Has the client listened to and understood what I have said? If you suspect that a client has not understood you, ask questions such as "Could you tell me what you heard me saying?" or "I'm not sure I said that very clearly. What did you hear?"

Questioning Nurses are taught to ask many questions during the history-taking and assessment processes. When this continues into the implementation phase, difficulties will usually develop. The nurse and client become simply questioner and questionee. The relationship becomes *unequal* because the questioner has the power to determine the course of the interaction. There is a tacit understanding that the questioner is the authority figure and the questionee must be submissive. A clue that too many questions are being asked is when clients give short answers or seldom take the initiative during interactions.

Silence   One of the most difficult aspects of communication is periods of silence. Students often feel uncomfortable with silence because of a belief that they should always have something therapeutic to say. With silent clients, the tendency among anxious students is to be excessively verbal. Silence has many meanings. Among them are:

- I am too tired to talk right now.
- I don't want to talk to you.
- I can't hear you; I'm listening to the voices.
- I don't know what you want from me.
- I'm lost and don't know what to say next.
- I don't know where this discussion is going.
- I would like to think about what was just said.
- I'm comfortable just being with you and not talking.

To respond appropriately, try to understand the reason for the client's silence. An observation such as "I've noticed that you have become very quiet. Could you tell me something about that quietness?" may encourage clients to share more.

Verbosity   Verbose clients may also pose problems. Just as students tend to be verbal with silent clients, they tend to be passive with talkative ones. You may be reluctant to interrupt for fear of being thought disrespectful or feeling inadequate in the face of such unrelenting talk. You may also feel a sense of relief that clients are finally talking to you. Some students mistakenly interpret clients' incessant verbalizing as evidence that the interactions are therapeutic. It is difficult to understand nonstop talk for more than 30 seconds. Interrupting will allow you to focus on the concerns being expressed and to convey a sense of involvement with the client's problems. Here are some examples of helpful interruptions:

- "You are bringing up a number of concerns. Could we discuss them one at a time?"
- "Let me interrupt you for a minute to make sure I understand what you are saying."
- "I don't want to stop you, but I need you to slow down so that I can understand better."

Deafness   Of the 20 million hearing-impaired people in the United States, about 10 percent are profoundly deaf. Significant hearing loss impairs language and communication. Those who use American Sign Language may have difficulty with English. Deaf individuals often learn mental health terminology from deaf friends, family, and/or reading. They may recognize concepts such as "depression" or "addiction" but are less likely to understand the concept of "psychosis." Since language fluency is essential for psychotherapy, interpreters may be necessary. The use of an interpreter then raises concerns about confidentiality. Group therapy may also become a problem when several people speak at the same time and the deaf person, being able to follow only one speaker at a time, misses much (Steinberg, Sullivan, & Loew, 1998).

The Americans with Disabilities Act prohibits discrimination against people who are deaf. Health care facilities must provide deaf clients with the means to communicate clearly with the staff. This may mean hiring an interpreter, writing notes, using flash cards, and a telecommunication device for the deaf. All staff should be alerted to the form of communication the client and family prefer (Sheehan, 2000).

Effective Communication

Effective communication is not an inborn skill but rather a learned process. Many instructors have their nursing students write up their one-to-one interactions (1:1) with clients—called process recordings—in order to analyze the communication process. This type of evaluation will help you understand yourself and your clients. The consistent use of analysis, along with input from peers and supervisors, will heighten your level of expertise (see Table 2.3 ■).

Questions   Questions can be either closed ended or open ended. *Closed-ended questions* can be answered with a yes, a no, or a simple fact. They are useful for finding out exact information or for helping a client focus on a topic more clearly. You will find that clients who are experiencing a high level of anxiety or

TABLE 2.3

Process Recording of Client Interview with a Student Nurse

Student's name: Jaimie

Client's name: Jeff

Client profile: Jeff is in the process of getting a divorce. He has a 14-year-old daughter but cannot see her due to a restraining order. Jeff has made threats to kill her and also threatens his wife. He believes that if all three of them die, "it will be a better ending to the story." He is currently unemployed and homeless since he left home to go to Arizona to "clear his head" from all the fighting and physical aggression happening at home. He stayed there for a short period of time and then drove from state to state before returning home. Jeff feels he has nothing to offer his family. After trying several times to have a meaningful relationship with his daughter, and failing, he feels she does not care for him. In return, he refuses to do anything for her. He has, at present and in the past, no close relationships with anyone. He states he prefers being by himself. Jeff states that he grew up in an emotionally abusive home. His mother attempted suicide two years ago. He has two brothers, one of whom is currently in a psychiatric hospital in another state. Jeff came to the hospital because he thought he had a heart attack due to all of his stress. He was anxious, depressed, and experiencing delusions. He also had suicidal and homicidal ideations.

Client's Communication	Analysis of Client's Response	Student's Communication	Analysis of Student's Response
		Jeff, can you tell me what brought you here?	*Focusing.*
Well (sits up and puts his right ankle on his left knee), I am just really stressed out. I am up to here in problems. (Puts his hand up to his head and shakes his head)	*Jeff does not believe that he has severe problems. He thinks he is just experiencing a very stressful time in his life due to the recent changes.*	What kind of problems are you experiencing?	*Exploring. Looking to start understanding what he is going through.*
(Runs his hands through his hair) Phew . . . you name it, I'm dealing with it.	*Accepts that he is currently facing many problems.*	Can you give me some examples? (Fold hands in lap)	*Clarifying. Wanted to learn about Jeff's problems so we could begin discussing how to work on them.*
Well to start, my wife and I are getting a divorce, I don't have a job or a home, and the FBI is after me.	*Seems calm when discussing these rather upsetting topics. Wonder if he is trying to distance himself from the pain through detachment.*	The FBI is looking for you? (Eyebrows raised)	*Restatement. This allows Jeff to elaborate on the topic.*
(Nods) Yeah, there were some guys at my work that were constantly around me, they were from the FBI. They didn't think I knew, but I did, that's why I quit. I told them I was quitting because I was going to be moving since I was getting a divorce. (Shrugs) Haven't seen those guys since.	*Delusions of persecution. If he was having any problems at work, they could be the fault of these harmful others. A drastic and self-defeating response to the delusions.* *Still enough in touch with reality to make up a story that would be understandable to the boss. Believes his quitting was an effective solution.*	What do you believe the FBI wants from you?	*Exploring. Curious to hear why he believes the FBI is after him. May have some significance or somehow relates to other stories that may arise later in the 1:1.*

TABLE 2.3

Process Recording of Client Interview with a Student Nurse *(continued)*

Client's Communication	Analysis of Client's Response	Student's Communication	Analysis of Student's Response
They have all of these charges against me, but I didn't do anything. They are after the wrong guy. I think the cops that were at my house that one night my wife and I were having an argument got the FBI after me. They didn't like me very much. (Good eye contact)	*Jeff has spent some time thinking about the delusion. Wonder if this ties into the fact that there is a restraining order against him. This may feed into his paranoid thinking.*	The cops were involved in one of the arguments?	*Restatement. Hoping he explains more about this event.*
(Rolling eyes) Yeah . . . she called them up when things started heating up. I was trying to talk to her about all the problems that are going on and all she ever wanted to do was yell. Then when I got frustrated and raised my voice, she called the cops and told them I was being aggressive toward her and our daughter.	*I know from the chart that Jeff believes his real wife died 3 months ago when he left, and now someone from the FBI is posing as her. More delusions concerning the FBI. This night was all set up so they could take him in. The plan was that he would get mad at his wife, become aggressive, and the cops could arrest him and then the FBI could do whatever they wanted to do with him (so he believes).*	You have a daughter?	*Changing the topic. Should have stayed focused on him.*
Yeah (nodding head). But I can't see her anymore since they got the restraining order against me.	*Sounds angry. He probably thinks this is more evidence of people acting against him.*	That must really upset you.	*Reflection.*
Yeah, but she doesn't mind it. She likes that I can't see her.	*Jeff is certain his daughter wants nothing to do with him. This could be accurate or more paranoid thinking.*	Has she said that to you?	*Clarifying. I wasn't sure if he was assuming or if she had told him this.*
You know, that girl is rotten. I know every teenager goes through this stage to some extent, but she is out of control. It's to the point where I just feel like giving up with her. I've tried everything—that girl just doesn't listen.	*Ignores what I asked him—changes the topic and blames daughter. He understands she may act the way she does just because of her age, yet he believes she is worse than a "typical" teen. He feels helpless. Calling her "that girl" depersonalizes her in a way.*	Does she not listen to you when you are disciplining her or when you just try talking to her?	*Clarification about when she doesn't listen.* *(Continued on next page)*

TABLE 2.3

Process Recording of Client Interview with a Student Nurse *(continued)*

Client's Communication	Analysis of Client's Response	Student's Communication	Analysis of Student's Response
Both. When we argue about her going out, she doesn't listen to me and even when I ask her a simple question, she ignores me.	*He believes that no matter what he does, she is not willing to communicate with him. Possibly contributes to low self-esteem—feels unneeded and unwanted.*	Let's talk about what happens when you two argue about her going out or not. Do you want her to stay in because you just don't want her going out with her friends sometimes or because you are concerned with her safety?	*Focusing. I wanted to focus on one topic at a time. I may have given him a "reason" for keeping her at home.*
(Pushing sleeves up) Well, of course I'm concerned for her safety, but if I tell her she can't go out because I worry about her—she laughs and calls me stupid. And on the nights when I would like her to stay home since she went out every night of the week already, just like every other parent, she tells me that she doesn't have to obey me and sneaks out.	*Sounds concerned for her safety.* *Feels inadequate as a parent. Has an external locus of control in terms of parenting.* *Tries to normalize his experience by comparing himself to all other parents.*	How do you react to her behavior?	*Exploring. Want to see if ways he handles situations are effective or need some work.*
We usually end up fighting— yelling that is—and I get so mad at her that I tell her to leave because I can't deal with it anymore. She said she's not going to listen to me because I'm not even supposed to be near her.	*Increased feelings of anger and frustration make him lose control. Daughter often wins the power struggle that occurs between the two of them.*	Teenagers often test how far they can push their parents. Do you think she may be doing this with you?	*Validating perception.*
I know she is—I just can't deal with it when she does.	*Recognizes his inability to deal appropriately with this problem.*	Have you ever thought of alternative ways to approach this situation?	*Encouraging formulation of plan of action—want to see if he has started problem solving.*
I always go into the situation thinking I will stay calm and be the strong one—but she just aggravates me so much, I lose it.	*Jeff expects the situation to improve even though he does nothing to change things and doesn't try different approaches. External locus of control—he's not responsible for his behavior.*	OK, how about learning new techniques of how to keep your cool and be the strong one when faced with these problems? Have you thought of ways to accomplish this?	*Encouraging formulation of a plan. Did not mean this to sound like I was advising him. I wanted him to identify goals to work toward.*

TABLE 2.3			

Process Recording of Client Interview with a Student Nurse *(continued)*

Client's Communication	Analysis of Client's Response	Student's Communication	Analysis of Student's Response
Hmmm . . . no, I don't think I ever went that far into it—never even thought about that.	*Honest. Seems interested in learning how to do this.*	Can you list some things that you could do to keep your anger under control?	*Suggesting collaboration. Talking about this together could help him get off to a good start in learning problem-solving skills.*
I could do that. Let's see . . .	*Willing to engage in the process.*		

The next five minutes Jeff lists, discusses, and predicts consequences regarding new techniques to keep control of his anger. All of his ideas were very appropriate. I basically accepted and gave him encouragement to follow along with his ideas throughout the one-to-one. Jeff's doctor then came in to talk with him.

SOURCE: Contributed by Jaimie Rzab, Purdue University Calumet.

disorganized thinking respond more easily to closed-ended questions. Examples are: "How long have you been married?" "Are you still living with your wife?" "Are you hearing voices right now?" *Open-ended questions* cannot be answered in a few short words. They are useful for increasing the client's participation in the interaction and for encouraging the client to continue the discussion. Examples are: "Would you tell me more about your relationship problems?" "How is that similar to your family when you were growing up?" Use both open-ended and closed-ended questions during interactions, but use open-ended questions whenever possible or appropriate. If several closed-ended questions are asked in succession, the interaction takes on an atmosphere of cross-examination, and the client may become reluctant to continue.

Questions beginning with *"What"* are generally used to evoke facts. Examples are: "What kind of work do you do?" "What do you argue about?" Questions beginning with *"How"* lead to a discussion of feelings and may elicit a client's personal view of a situation. Examples are: "How did you feel when he gave you that ultimatum?" "How do you think your work should be supervised?" Questions beginning with *"Could"* allow the client to have some control over the interaction and are the most open-ended of questions. Examples are:

"Could you give me an example of how he mistreats you?" "Could you tell me what is the most important problem to focus on today?" Questions beginning with *"Why"* lead to a discussion of reasons and often put clients on the defensive. "Why" questions do not typically help clients understand their situation more clearly but rather forces them to explain and justify their behavior. Examples are: "Why did you skip group today?" and "Why did you say that to your husband?"

Questioning is basic to critical thinking, problem solving, and creativity. Skillful questioning is basically an interactive process. Asking the right questions can help clients move beyond their usual patterns of thinking and responding. Questions can be used for *gathering information.* As stated earlier, you must be careful not to overuse this type of questioning. Nurses formulate their questions on the basis of their theoretical framework (Goldberg, 1998). See Chapter 1 for assessment questions using specific theoretical models. Consider the following interaction as the nurse gathers information:

Sonja: I am so tired of being depressed. I just don't want to be depressed anymore.

Nurse: Tell me, how will you know when you are no longer depressed?

Sonja: I'll be happy.

Nurse: But I'm not sure how you will know when you are happy. Give me a word picture of what you will be like when you are happy.

Sonja: Well, I would play with my daughter, I would smile and laugh more, I would enjoy my garden, and I would visit with my friends.

Nurse: What are you going to do to get started?

Sonja: Maybe I will try to play a little bit with my daughter this afternoon.

Questions can also be used as *interventions*. When you pose these types of questions, you invite the client to gain insight and explore new possibilities. They often center around choices people make throughout their lives. Examples of questions as interventions include: "Where do you hope to be in six months? One year? Five years?", "In what way could you make your relationship more satisfying?", "Could you help me understand more about your reasons for making that decision?", "In thinking back, what might you have done differently?", "What do you think might happen if you did . . . ?"

Skillful use of questions helps guide clients through the problem-solving process. Clients become empowered as they learn from situations they have encountered. Questions also help clients assume responsibility for their own actions.

Facilitating Techniques Effective communication techniques are those that communicate your listening, understanding, and caring. You must analyze the behavioral, affective, and cognitive components of communication in order to respond to overt and covert messages. Effective communication also encourages clients to examine feelings, explore problems in more depth, build on existing strengths, and develop new coping strategies (see Table 2.4 ■).

Broad openings are open-ended questions or statements. The purpose of a broad opening is to acknowledge clients and to let them know you are listening and concerned about their interests. But the overuse of broad openings will force the relationship to remain on a superficial level.

Giving recognition is noting something that is occurring at the present moment for clients. It is a fairly superficial level of communication but indicates attention to and care for individuals.

Minimal encouragements are verbal and nonverbal reinforcers that indicate active listening to and interest in what clients are saying. They prompt clients to continue with what is being said.

Offering self is a way of informing clients of care and concern. It is used to offer emotional and moral support.

Accepting lets clients know that you are comprehending their thoughts and feelings. It is one of the ways you express empathy.

Making observations moves the interaction to a deeper therapeutic level. It involves paying very close attention to the behavioral component of communication and connecting it to the affective and cognitive components. When communication is incongruous, you comment on the inconsistency and, with the client, explore the underlying meaning of the mixed messages. Clients who are experiencing disorganized thinking may be unable to take part in this process.

Validating perceptions gives clients an opportunity to validate or correct your understanding of what is being communicated. Using this technique will decrease confusion and affirm your genuine interest in understanding your clients.

Exploring helps clients feel free to talk and examine issues in more depth. As they organize their thoughts and focus on particular problems, their understanding of themselves and others increases.

Clarifying is useful when you are confused about clients' thoughts or feelings. It is appropriate to acknowledge your confusion and ask clients to rephrase what they just said.

Placing the event in time or sequence helps clients sort out what happened to them in what order. The goal is to help them understand the progression of events.

Focusing allows clients to stay with specifics and analyze problems without jumping from topic to topic. You may choose to focus on the main theme, to facilitate exploring the problem in more depth. Clients are often unaware of how they contributed to and participated in the development of their problems. By focusing on their feelings, thoughts, and behaviors, you pave the way for increased understanding and responsibility. Clients with disorganized thinking usually need help in staying focused.

Encouraging the formulation of a plan of action is the process of helping clients decide how they plan to proceed. In general, avoid telling clients what they should do. Instead, asking them what they will or might do will reinforce that they are in control of and responsible for themselves. If they are unable to formulate

TABLE 2.4

Effective Communication Techniques

Technique	Examples
Broad opening	"What would you like to work on today?" "What is one of the best things that happened to you this week?"
Giving recognition	"I notice you're wearing a new dress. You look very nice." "What a marvelous afghan that is going to be when you finish."
Minimal encouragement	"Go on." "Ummm." "Uh-huh."
Offering self	"I'll sit with you until it's time for your family session." "I have at least 30 minutes I can spend with you right now."
Accepting	"I can imagine how that might feel." "I'm with you on that [nodding]."
Making observations	"Mr. Robinson, you seem on edge. You are clenching your fist and grinding your teeth." "I'm puzzled. You're smiling, but you sound so resentful."
Validating perceptions	"This is what I heard you say. . . . Is that correct?" "It sounds like you are talking about sad feelings. Is that correct?"
Exploring	"How does your girlfriend feel about your being in the hospital?" "Tell me about what was happening at home just before you came in the hospital."
Clarifying	"Could you explain more about that to me?" "I'm having some difficulty. Could you help me understand?"
Placing the event in time or sequence	"Which came first . . . ?" "When did you first notice . . . ?"
Focusing	"Could we continue talking about you and your dad right now?" "Rather than talking about what your husband thinks, I would like to hear how you're feeling right now."
Encouraging the formulation of a plan of action	"What do you think you can do the next time you feel that way?" "How might you handle your anger in a nonthreatening way?"
Suggesting collaboration	"Perhaps together we can figure out. . . ." "Let's try using the problem-solving process that was presented in group yesterday."
Restatement	*Client*: Do you think going home will be difficult? *Nurse*: How difficult do you think going home will be?
Reflection	*Client*: I keep thinking about what all my friends are doing right now. *Nurse*: You're worried that they aren't missing you? *Client*: He laughed at me. My boss just sat there and laughed at me. I felt like such a fool. *Nurse*: You felt humiliated?
Summarizing	"So far we have talked about . . ." "Our time is up. Let's see, we have discussed your family problems, their effect on your schoolwork, and your need to find a way to decrease family conflict."

a plan of action, implement the problem-solving process. If clients are highly anxious or experiencing disorganized thinking, they may be unable to problem-solve or make appropriate judgments.

Suggesting collaboration is one technique of introducing the problem-solving process. It is an offer to help clients work through each step of the process and to brainstorm alternative solutions to their problems. Suggesting collaboration stresses the team effort of you and your client to develop more adaptive coping skills.

Restatement is the use of newer and fewer words to paraphrase the basic content of client messages. Restatement focuses on the cognitive component of communication and creates an opportunity to explore facts or reinforce something important clients have said.

Reflection involves understanding the affective component of communication and reflecting these feelings back to clients without repeating their exact words. Reflection helps clients focus on feelings and allows you to communicate empathy.

Summarizing is the systematic synthesis of important ideas discussed by clients during interactions. The goal is to help them explore significant content and emotional themes. Summarizing may also be used to move from one phase of the interaction to the next, to conclude the interaction, or to begin the interaction by reviewing the previous session. (See Table 2.5 ■ for use of clarifying techniques when clients use unclear or nonspecific language.)

TABLE 2.5

Unclear, Nonspecific Communication

Common Problem	Meaning	Verbal Example	Clarifying Technique
Deleting	Object of the verb is left out	"I'm afraid."	Inquire: "Afraid of what in particular?"
		"I'm really uncomfortable."	"What is making you uncomfortable?"
Unspecified verbs	Verbs in which the action needs to be more specific	"He really frustrates me."	Inquire: "How, exactly, does he frustrate you?"
		"They ignored me."	"In what way did they ignore you?"
Universal qualifiers	Words that generalize a few experiences to a multitude of experiences (all, every, never, always, nobody, only)	"I never do anything right."	Inquire: Has there ever been a time that you did do something right?"
		"You always hurt me."	"Has there ever been a situation in which I haven't hurt you?"
Necessity and possibility	Statements that identify rules or limits to a person's behavior and that often indicate no choice (have to, must, can't, no one can, not possible, unable)	"I have to take care of other people."	Inquire: "What would happen if you didn't take care of other people?"
		"No one can get me out of this mess."	"What would happen if you got out of this mess?"
		"I can't do it."	"What stops you from doing it?"
		"It's not possible."	"What do you need?" "What will have to happen so it is possible?"

TECHNIQUES THAT CONTRIBUTE TO INEFFECTIVE COMMUNICATION

Nurses who worry about what they are going to say next, who do not listen carefully, and who do not focus on trying to understand what clients are attempting to say are often ineffective communicators. Ineffective communication is also described as communication that avoids underlying feelings, remains on a superficial level, tells people what to do, or moralizes and expresses judgment (see Table 2.6 ■).

Stereotypical comments indicate that you care little about the individual experiences of clients and are relying on folklore and proverbs to communicate. Additional problems occur for clients whose thinking is concrete because many stereotypical comments rely on abstract understanding. Stereotypical comments are culture specific and therefore make little sense to people with different cultural backgrounds.

Parroting is simply repeating back to clients the words they themselves have used. When you merely

---

TABLE 2.6

Ineffective Communication Techniques

Technique	Examples
Stereotypical comments	"What's the matter, cat got your tongue?" "Still waters run deep."
Parroting	*Client*: I'm so sad. *Nurse*: You're so sad.
Changing the topic	*Client*: I was so afraid I was going to have another panic attack. *Nurse*: What does your husband think about your panic attacks?
Disagreeing	"I don't see any reason for you to feel that way." "No, I think that is a silly response to your mother."
Challenging	"Is that a valid reason to become angry?" "You weren't really serious, were you?"
Requesting an explanation	"Why did you react that way?" "Why can't you just leave home?"
False reassurance	"Don't worry anymore." "I doubt that your mother will be angry about your failing math."
Belittling expressed feelings	"That was four years ago. It shouldn't bother you now." "You shouldn't feel that all men are bad." "It's wrong to even think of your mother like that."
Probing	"I'm here to listen. I can't help you if you won't tell me everything." "Tell me what secrets you keep from your wife."
Advising	"You sound worried. I think you'd better talk to your doctor or your rabbi." "I think you should divorce your husband."
Imposing values	*Client*: [With head down and low tone of voice] I was going to go on the cruise, but my mother is coming to stay with me. *Nurse*: You must be looking forward to her arrival.
Double/multiple questions	"What makes you feel that you should stay? How would you get along if you left? Would you rent an apartment or move in with a friend?"

repeat what clients have said, the communication becomes circular, clients do not progress in understanding, and the interaction grinds to a halt.

Changing the topic occurs when you introduce topics that might be of interest to you but are not relevant to the client at that particular time. This technique can be a way of avoiding topics that make you uncomfortable. If you change the topic often, clients will begin to feel that what they are trying to say is not important. Clients may also change the topic if they are highly anxious about the topic being discussed or if their thinking is disorganized.

Disagreeing with clients' ideas and emotions denies them the right to think and feel as they do. Disagreeing provides clients with no opportunity to increase self-understanding.

Challenging clients forces them to defend themselves from what appears to be an attack by you. When you challenge clients, they are forced to offer reasons for their feelings, thoughts, or behaviors.

Requesting an explanation is similar to challenging and usually begins with "Why." The implication is that the client should not be behaving a certain way or experiencing a particular feeling.

False reassurance is another way of telling clients how to feel and ignoring their distress. They feel patronized when you act as if you know better and more than they do.

Belittling expressed feelings gives the message that you have not listened carefully, that you are ignoring the importance of their problems.

Probing occurs when you fail to respect clients' decisions regarding privacy of feelings and thoughts. Probing implicitly accuses them of keeping secrets and blames them for not progressing in treatment.

Advising occurs when you tell clients what to do, preventing them from exploring problems and using the problem-solving process to find solutions. Advising makes you, rather than the client, responsible for the outcome.

Imposing values is demanding that clients share your own biases and prejudices. It is preaching and moralizing rather than accurately understanding their values.

Double/multiple questions are ineffective because they tend to confuse clients. When asked a series of questions with no intervening opportunity to respond, clients may end up feeling bewildered or cross-examined.

COMMUNICATING WITH FAMILIES AND GROUPS

Nurses are involved with a variety of family systems, as well as informal and formal groups, in every clinical setting. Communication within families and communication within groups are presented together here because, for the most part, they are similar. To help people become more effective communicators, you must be able to analyze communication patterns.

The overall process to use in understanding family and group communication is as follows:

1. What do I see and hear? (Perception of nonverbal and verbal communication)
2. How do the members feel? How do I feel? (Affective analysis)
3. What does this mean? (Cognitive interpretation)
4. Is my assessment correct? (Validation by asking others, gathering more information)
5. How shall I respond? (Interventions based on your assessment)

The *significance of nonverbal communication* must always be considered. When working with families or groups, ask yourself the following questions, and then interpret the significance of the answers:

■ How closely together do people sit?
■ Are some members physically isolated from others?
■ Can each person see all the other members fairly easily?
■ Do members look at the person who is speaking?
■ Do members behave in a distracting manner while a person is speaking?
■ How is touch used within the group?
■ Are nonverbal behaviors directed toward a particular member or the entire group?
■ How do facial expressions change throughout the interaction?
■ What kind of gestures are used?
■ Are there changes in voice tone?

Another consideration is the *significance of verbal communication*. Ask yourself the following questions, and interpret the significance of the answers:

■ Is somebody refusing to talk?

- Who speaks to whom, about what, and when?
- Are there individuals who are speaking for others?
- Who interrupts others?
- Who is talkative?
- Who contributes little?
- Who asks questions?
- Who gives the answers?
- Who gives opinions?
- Who tries to clarify misunderstandings?
- Who initiates problem solving?
- If English is not the native language, how fluent are various family members?
- Are one or two members expected to interpret for others?

Affective expression among family and group members can be analyzed by answering these questions:

- To what extent is the communication of feelings encouraged?
- Are feelings expressed directly or indirectly?
- What happens when a member breaks the group's "rules" about expressing feelings?
- How much does the group encourage members to be sensitive to each other's feelings and to communicate this awareness?
- What are the feelings underlying the members' communication with one another?
- Who is helpful and friendly?

As a nurse, you help members improve their listening skills and their ability to be congruent in their communication by modeling and teaching effective communication. As they gain more adaptive skills, they will be better able to cope with individual, family, and group problems.

COMMUNICATING WITH CHILDREN AND ADOLESCENTS

You may be wondering: How do I communicate therapeutically with a child or adolescent? What do I say? How can I get this person to talk to me? Start by asking yourself what you are feeling. In what context have you interacted with people in this age group before? What emotions does this child or teen stir up in you? What do you feel your role is when working with children or adolescents? Are you there to guide, direct, teach, advise, or protect? Answering these questions is the first step toward communicating effectively with children and adolescents.

Rather than probing for details, listen for feelings. It is more important to help children learn how to interact effectively with you than to gather particulars. Children easily fall into superficially answering adults' questions and simply waiting for the next one. In this routine way, you set the pattern of a question-and-answer session. There are two problems with this pattern: The child will give you only short answers and not expand on the topic, and you will be frustrated when you run out of questions and haven't achieved any therapeutic purpose.

You will learn more by listening than by questioning. When you want information, use an open-ended format. For example, rather than asking, "Do you have friends?" say, "Tell me about the friends you like to do things with." Respect children's periods of silence. They may need this time to sort out thoughts and feelings and will be unable to do so if you bombard them with questions. Children soon discover whether or not you are a good listener. Some children do not respond to "talking" therapy because they have never experienced an adult really listening to them, they may not have been encouraged or allowed to express feelings, or they may not have the cognitive development to express their problems.

Children and adolescents recognize fake sentiments and insincere platitudes. They want to know that you are genuine, that you are trustworthy, and that your word is good. Explain what you expect of them and what they can expect from you. The clients you work with may have heard mixed messages throughout their lives and probably have learned to expect that adults make promises they do not keep. In working with young clients, you have an opportunity to model honest, adult behavior.

COMMUNICATING WITH OLDER ADULTS

When communicating with children and adolescents, you have the knowledge of personal experience regarding those ages and thus have some understanding of appropriate conversation. When communicating with older adults, you have not had that developmental experience to enrich your understanding, and in some ways it is new territory.

CRITICAL THINKING

Mary, a nursing student, has been assigned to care for Ifle, a 44-year-old client undergoing treatment on the psychiatric unit. Mary sits down close to Ifle, introduces herself, compliments Ifle on her appearance, and asks, "Are you doing okay today?" Ifle leans away from Mary, maintains a rigid posture, avoids eye contact, and nods her head yes. After several minutes of silence, Mary explains to Ifle that she has an hour that she can spend with her today. Following another long period of silence, Mary says, "I guess you're not in the mood to talk today, so I'll see you tomorrow." Mary leaves after spending 25 minutes with Ifle.

1. What actions by Mary demonstrated respect for Ifle?

2. What actions by Mary, if any, did not represent therapeutic communication skills and could decrease Ifle's confidence or trust in Mary?

3. Had you been Mary, how might you have interpreted Ifle's body language and silence during this first session?

4. How could Mary's interaction with Ifle been improved?

5. Why do you think Mary decided to leave after 25 minutes?

For an additional Case Study, please refer to the Companion Web site for this book.

Older adults are sometimes the targets of patronizing speech such as slow speech, simple sentences, concrete vocabulary, and demeaning emotional tone. Some health care professionals even use baby talk, especially with elderly persons who live in nursing homes. Patronizing speech implies that there is a question regarding the competence of the older person; this communicates a lack of respect that undermines self-esteem and dignity.

Patronizing speech is the result of age-related stereotypes. Some of these negative beliefs are that older adults are feeble, egocentric, incompetent, and/or abrasive. It is important that you examine your beliefs about older people and how they communicate. You must also examine how you talk to older individu-

als. Asking for feedback from others is helpful in the process of examining your communication skills.

Older people take longer to decode and encode messages and therefore take longer to react during conversation. At times, they may also have difficulties in word retrieval and name recall. The key to interacting in this situation is patience. People's senses play an important role in communication with others. Loss of hearing can make interactions more difficult. Do not cover your mouth or chew gum when you speak, since many older adults rely on lip reading to clarify what is being spoken. Since lip reading at best is 45 percent accurate, hearing impaired adults may guess at what was said. If people respond inappropriately, it may be that they did not hear any or part of the message. Slow your speech down because speech sounds are more difficult to hear when you speak at a fast rate. Consider the external environment when interacting with people who are hearing impaired since external noise is very distracting when struggling to listen to speech. Eyesight also has an important role in conversation. Nonverbal cues that expand on the spoken message may be missed by those whose vision is impaired (Nussbaum, Pecchioni, Robinson, & Thompson, 2000).

EDUCATING

Education of consumers and families is basic to nursing care. Knowledge empowers people to make informed decisions regarding their health status, plan for maintaining wellness, and illness care choices. Communication is the most important skill in the effective education of psychiatric consumers and their families. Good communication contributes to thorough assessment and accurate diagnosis of learning needs, and it is the major tool for implementing the teaching plan. You evaluate your teaching through verbal and (sometimes) written communication with your clients. Documentation is the written communication in records.

Education in the mental health care setting involves more than giving information to passive people. Education is an active process that is done with people, not to people. The steps of the nursing process are used in the educational process: assessing the learning needs, diagnosing the knowledge deficit with contributing factors, planning content, implementing the most effective methods of education, evaluating the effectiveness of the teaching, and documenting the entire process.

ASSESSMENT

The first step in the client/family teaching process is assessment. It is important that you understand their views of psychiatric disability. Clients and families often believe the cultural stereotypes—mental illness means being possessed by a demon, mental illness occurs only in people who are "bad," or families cause mental illness. These stereotypes need to be countered with factual data. Through assessment, determine what they have learned in previous contact with mental health professionals. If you have the erroneous view that psychiatrically disabled people cannot possibly understand their disorders and their medications, you will be surprised to learn how much they know.

Assessment also involves determining what consumers want and feel they need to know. Ask what they consider to be their most important problems at this time. Little progress will be made if you assume authority for prioritizing their problems. People are not likely to be open to learning about difficulties they consider unimportant; they will only learn material that is meaningful to them. You may need to help some individuals be specific if they have described their problems in vague terms.

Max has been readmitted to the psychiatric unit because he stopped taking his medication six months ago. Ryan, his nurse, has determined that Max needs to learn why it is important to keep taking his medication. Max says the reason he doesn't do it is that his wife is always nagging him to take it. He believes if she would just leave him alone, he would not have a problem taking it. It is more important to Max to learn skills that will help him get along with and communicate better with his wife than to learn the facts about how his medication works.

DIAGNOSIS

The nursing diagnosis often used in client/family education is "knowledge deficit." There are, however, any number of other diagnoses that can be used, such as "ineffective individual coping," "ineffective management of therapeutic regimen," or "altered role perfor-

mance." When forming a nursing diagnosis, you must specify exactly what people need to learn and what the related factors may be. Examples are:

- *Knowledge deficit*: Lithium therapy related to initiation of the drug
- *Knowledge deficit*: Basic cooking skills related to mother's doing all the cooking and her recent death
- *Ineffective individual coping*: Related to work stress that is contributing to high levels of anxiety and increased conflict at work
- *Ineffective management of therapeutic regimen*: Related to noncompliance with medications
- *Altered role performance*: Related to recent divorce and becoming a single parent

Diagnosis also includes specifying what, if any, barriers exist that might hinder the teaching and learning process. Clients who are experiencing a great deal of anxiety have a very short attention span, an extremely narrowed perceptual field, and very little capacity to learn. Attempting to teach clients when they are in a manic phase, delusional, or experiencing hallucinations may not be practical. Disorganized thinking, obsessional thoughts, and other cognitive impairments make it very difficult for clients to learn. Those who are depressed and feel hopeless and helpless about the present and future may have no motivation to learn. Clients or family members who are angry and hostile need to find a way to manage their emotions before effective learning can take place. People who deny the reality of mental disorders will not be open to increasing their knowledge or improving their coping skills.

PLANNING

Preparing clients for as much self-care as possible in order to live in the least restrictive setting is both the focus and the goal of client/family teaching. Planning must be designed to meet the specific needs of the client and family. The educational plan should be directed not only toward increasing knowledge but also toward improved problem solving and more adaptive coping skills. Helping clients learn from their situations and take responsibility for the results of their actions is empowering.

Outcome criteria are developed in order to evaluate the behavioral, affective, and cognitive changes resulting from effective teaching and learning.

To help people learn to cope with their current problems, emphasize the present: Change is possible only in the here and now. The past and future are also important, but only as perspectives on the present. Meanings attached to the past and expectations of the future influence present perceptions. But it is in the present that one evaluates the past, anticipates the future, and changes behavior. People who brood over past problems and pain without attending to the present are in danger of accepting the problems as permanent, with no hope for change. People who have dire future expectations and ignore the present potential for change will probably have their expectations fulfilled.

IMPLEMENTATION

Two of the most important skills you bring to client/family education are the ability to communicate clearly and the capacity to develop a relationship that is warm and caring. A humanistic approach has proven more successful than a technical approach in terms of client/family understanding and their willingness to participate in the process.

Family and friends often have questions about the disorder and want to know how they can best help. Including supportive others in education may improve the rehabilitative process because the living environment often affects the course of many mental disorders.

Education is both formal and informal. Examples of formal teaching are psychoeducational groups and audiovisual tools. The effectiveness of group education depends on a high level of skill on the part of the group leader. Consumers must be carefully assessed for appropriateness to the group. Those whose thinking is disorganized and those who are hyperactive, highly anxious, or hallucinating may not be appropriate for an educational group. One advantage of the group format is the ability to reach more people in a limited amount of time. Another advantage is that consumers interact with others who have similar problems and concerns. Sharing solutions to problems and coping behaviors can foster the learning process. The group should not have so many members that individuals have little opportunity to ask questions and provide answers. The best physical arrangement is a circle of chairs, to encourage a sense of connectedness.

Probably the most effective education format is the informal process. Every interaction you have with clients and their families is an opportunity to facilitate their learning. An example of informal teaching is when you discover a learning need and respond to it immediately. Examples are explaining the need for a new medication and helping a client control anger in response to an immediate situation.

General Areas of Learning

Client and Family Education may be the single most important factor in promoting healthy lifestyles. There are six general areas of learning to consider when implementing teaching plans. The first area relates to *knowledge of the mental disorder*. Clients and families who have struggled to live with psychiatric disabilities may be very knowledgeable in this area, in contrast to those who are experiencing disorders for the first time. Topics typically discussed are an explanation of the diagnosis, myths and folklore surrounding the disorder, goals of treatment, and the overall treatment plan. Clients and their families should also learn the signs and symptoms of relapse and know when to call the physician. A list of books for clients and families accompanies each of the disorders chapters.

The second general area of learning is *medications*. Most clients and families are able to understand basic neurotransmission, which helps them understand how the medication works and why they need it. If they are caring for themselves, they should know when to take each medication and have a system for accurate administration at home. Teach them about the possible side effects and how to manage them. If there are any special precautions for a particular medication, emphasize them. General medication teaching principles are covered in Chapter 8.

Some clients will need to learn activities relating to *managing activities of daily living (ADLs)*. They may never have had the opportunity to learn how to grocery shop, plan menus, prepare food, and do laundry. Some clients benefit from grooming groups, which reinforce basic hygiene, teach makeup and hair care, and help clients plan appropriate clothing, such as for job interviews and leisure activities. Some clients will need to learn how to use public transportation. Teach clients about available community resources for leisure activities, support groups, and religious expression.

Many clients and families need to learn the basics of *interpersonal communication*. They must be able to identify and express their own feelings and respect and listen to those of others. Family conferences and family therapy provide opportunities to help family members learn to communicate more effectively.

Clients often need to learn more effective skills for *coping with life*, including family, social, and vocational aspects. It is helpful if clients can identify how their illness has affected their lives and move on to a discussion of what the future might look like. Clients need to learn stress-avoidance and stress-management techniques, and how to manage any symptoms they may be experiencing. They often need to learn assertiveness skills and the problem-solving process. Some will need to develop a plan to avoid social isolation.

Another area of general learning is *community resources*. Types of programs are intermediate care facilities, partial-hospital programs, outpatient centers, respite care, transport resources, financial aid, pharmacies, and food programs. Self-help and support groups exist in most communities. Each chapter in Parts Four and Five includes a box with the names and addresses of community resources specific to each disorder or crisis situation.

Some useful general information Web sites for you, your client, and his or her families include:

- National Library of Medicine
  http://www.nln.nih.gov
- Mayo Health Clinic *http://www.mayohealth.org*
- Medscape *http://www.medscape.com*

These Web sites can be accessed through a resource link on the Companion Web site for this book.

The Problem-Solving Process

The *most important process* for clients and families to learn is how to solve problems. As they become increasingly skilled at problem solving, they will expand their coping skills and enhance the quality of their lives. In teaching the problem-solving process, focus on one problem at a time, and measure progress by observing small changes.

Because all problems are connected, changes in one problem will cause changes in others. Remind people that in the past they have done their best to deal with problems, and that now new solutions may be found. Your role is to listen, observe, encourage, and evaluate. More effective coping behavior will be the ultimate result of the problem-solving process. But before the process can begin, you must help them identify their problem. Identification includes the person's definition of the problem, the significance of the problem, and the influence of the past and future. Box 2.1 describes the steps in problem identification.

Throughout the problem-solving process, it is extremely helpful to have clients keep a written list of all the ideas generated. The list can be modified as time goes on.

After problem identification has been completed, the steps of the problem-solving process consist of the following:

1. Identifying the solutions that have been attempted
2. Listing alternative solutions
3. Predicting the probable consequences of each alternative
4. Choosing the best alternative to implement
5. Implementing the chosen alternative in a real-life or practice situation
6. Evaluating outcomes

Box 2.2 lists sample questions for each step.

BOX 2.1

Steps in Problem Identification

1. Client definition
   - How would you describe the problem?
   - For whom is this a problem? You? Family members? Employer? Community?
2. Significance of the problem
   - When did this problem begin?
   - What are the factors that cause this problem to continue?
3. Past and future influence
   - What past events have influenced the current problem?
   - What are your future expectations and hopes concerning this problem?
   - What is the most you hope for when this problem is resolved?
   - What is the least you will settle for to resolve this problem?
4. Concrete problem definition
   - Is there more than one problem here?
   - Which part of the overall problem is most important to deal with first?

The first step is identifying what *solutions* have been *tried* thus far. The specifics of the attempts, how the attempts were implemented, and what occurred as a result must all be clarified. Because the problem continues to exist, these solutions were not effective, so they should be either modified or discarded.

The second step is having the client list *alternative ways* of solving the problem. Frequently, the client will have only one or two ideas. You can propose brainstorming sessions to increase creativity in problem solving. All possible solutions, even those that are unrealistic or absurd, are written down. Thinking of absurd solutions often opens the mind to other creative, realistic solutions to the problem. Finally, after the client has listed all his or her ideas for solving the problem, you can add your own suggestions.

The third step is *predicting* the *probable consequences* of each alternative, which helps clients anticipate outcomes of behavior.

After thorough discussion, you and your client go on to the fourth step: choosing the *best alternative* to implement. Do not make this decision for clients; doing so would undermine the process by placing them in a childlike, dependent position. Using action-oriented terms, develop the selected solution further, as concretely and specifically as possible. At the same time, formulate measurable outcomes to use in evaluating the process.

The fifth step is *implementing* the proposed solution in either a practice or a real-life situation. Clients must be allowed to make mistakes during this step. If you rescue them, you are giving the message that they are incapable of taking charge of their lives.

Evaluation is the sixth step in the problem-solving process. Review the outcomes, and determine the degree of success or failure in achieving them. Successfully achieving an outcome means that the solution was effective and that it can continue to be implemented. Failing to achieve an outcome means you and your client need to analyze how and why the solution was ineffective. Then return to step 4, and either select a new solution or modify the old one.

As clients experience the steps of the problem-solving process, they increase their skills, which then can be applied to other problematic areas of life. With an improved ability to make and assume responsibility for decisions, they develop an internal locus of control, leading to competence and self-esteem.

BOX 2.2

Steps in the Problem-Solving Process

1. Identify attempted solutions
   - What have you done to try to solve the problem thus far?
   - How exactly did you do this?
   - What happened when you tried this?
2. List alternatives
   - What other ideas do you think you could try?
   - What might be some absurd solutions to this problem?
   - What else might be effective?
   - Have you thought about . . . ?
3. Predict consequences
   - What might happen if you tried the first idea?
   - Is there anything else that might happen?
   - What might happen if you tried the second idea (etc.)?
4. Choose the best alternative
   - Which alternative seems like the best decision at this time?
   - What specific behaviors are you going to try with this alternative?
   - Specifically, how will things be different if you are successful?
5. Implement the alternative
   - With whom are you going to attempt this solution?
   - When are you going to practice this new behavior?
   - Is there anything you need from me to help you try this out?
6. Evaluate
   - What was the result of your attempted solution?
   - Were your expectations met successfully?
   - Is there anything that needs to be modified?
   - If you were not successful, what other alternative idea from the list could you try?

When clients are acutely ill and unable to think logically, the problem-solving process is not an appropriate intervention. The interaction below illustrates the problem-solving process in action with a nurse and client.

Beth, a 25-year-old graduate student, has been seeing Miyuki, a nurse therapist, for several months. Beth has been in a long-term relationship with a married man who has been physically and emotionally abusive to her.

Beth: *It's really time now to end the relationship. I've known for a long time that it's not good for me to stay with Todd. I just don't know how to do it.*

Miyuki: *What have you tried to do so far in ending the relationship?*

Beth: *In the past two years, I've told Todd several times that I don't want to see him any more. Then he doesn't call me for a month and I start to miss him, so I give in when he finally calls me.*

Miyuki: *So, when you say no to Todd, he punishes you by not calling, with the end result that he manipulates you into going back to him.*

Beth: *Yes, I guess that's what happens. What's really unbelievable is that I don't even like him very much anymore. What I really miss is the sex after a while. So I just give in because of the sex.*

Miyuki: *If you really want to end this relationship, how might you go about doing it differently since just telling him hasn't seemed to work?*

Beth: *All my friends have been telling me to dump Todd. I guess I could tell some of them that I'm finally going to do it.*

Miyuki: *What might happen if you did that?*

Beth: *Well, when I would be tempted to go back to Todd, I could call them up for some moral support not to go back. I guess I would have to tell them ahead of time that's what I'd want them to do.*

Miyuki: *Are there some friends who would be better than others to depend on in this situation?*

Beth: *I think Carmela and Grace would be the best. They would try and help me, but they also wouldn't make me feel like a fool if I failed*

again. Leslie and Eva would just yell at me and be very critical.

Miyuki: *What else might help you break up with Todd?*

Beth: *I suppose I could try and do things with different friends. I always sit at home waiting for Todd to call me. I haven't gone out much with my friends in a long time.*

Miyuki: *How would that help you not go back to Todd?*

Beth: *At least I wouldn't be so lonesome. Maybe it's the loneliness as much as the sex that makes me go back to him.*

Miyuki: *What are some of the things that might get in the way of your staying away from Todd?*

Beth: *He has told me for years that no one else would want me because I'm fat and ugly and the only thing I'm good for is sex. I guess I really believe that after hearing it for so long. What if no one else will ever love me for the rest of my life?*

Miyuki: *It's understandable how you believe what he has told you. Men who are abusive undermine their victim's self-esteem to prevent the victim from leaving. It seems to me that is another aspect of the problem we should also try to solve. Let's finish discussing the loneliness and friends issues first, and then move on to your self-esteem issue.*

EVALUATION

Client and family education is effective if the outcome criteria are met. The only way to discover what people have learned is through evaluation. Evaluation must be measurable; that is, people must be able to hear or see evidence that they did or did not meet the outcome criteria. If criteria were not met, look for where the problem might be. The difficulty could be in any of the steps of the nursing process. Box 2.3 describes common problems that prevent meeting the outcome criteria. Use this box as a guide for locating problems in education. Revise your teaching according to evidence from the evaluation.

BOX 2.3

Problems in Client Education

Assessment

- Teaching material was not meaningful to the client.

Diagnosis

- Barriers to learning were not identified.

Planning

- Areas of learning were stated in vague terms.
- Outcome criteria were vague and unmeasurable.
- The focus remained on the past rather than on present problems.

Implementation

- Communication skills were ineffective.
- The nurse displayed a distant, uncaring attitude toward the client.
- The family and significant others were not included.
- The teaching methods and tools were not appropriate for the client.

Evaluation

- Areas of learning were no longer appropriate for the client's circumstances.

Evaluation can be done in a number of ways. You can have people verbalize attitudes, values, feelings, and facts. Written tests may be appropriate for cognitive information. Interpersonal skill achievement can be evaluated by role playing. Psychomotor skill achievement can be evaluated by having the learner demonstrate the skill for you. This final step of the nursing process is critical to effective education.

DOCUMENTATION

Documentation is an important step in the process of education. Communication between all members of the multidisciplinary team is essential to the effectiveness of the process. Much of that communication is through documentation. Documentation also provides legal protection for the staff. The rule is the same as with any other nursing activity: If it is not written down in the chart, it did not happen.

Documentation should include areas of learning, what has been taught, client/family response to the teaching, degree of success in meeting the outcome criteria, and what further areas of teaching are required. Any one of a number of forms may be used to document education, including narrative notes and teaching flow sheets. It is your responsibility to document all phases of client education in which you are involved.

CHAPTER REVIEW

Introduction

- Relating, communicating, educating, and problem solving are the foundation of interpersonal relationships and are key factors in the nursing process.

Relating

- Characteristics of caring helpers include a nonjudgmental approach, acceptance, warmth, empathy, authenticity, congruency, patience, respect, trustworthiness, self-disclosure, and humor.

Communicating

- To analyze communication you must consider spoken words, paralanguage, the thinking process, emotions, nonverbal behavior, and the culture of the person sending the message.

- Nonverbal communication includes body language, eye contact, personal space, and the use of touch.

- Listening means paying attention to what the person is saying, acknowledging feelings, holding back on what you have to say, avoiding interruption, and controlling the urge to give advice.

- Characteristics of effective helpers include a nonjudgmental approach, acceptance, warmth, empathy, authenticity, congruency, patience, trustworthiness, self-disclosure, and humor.

- Closed-ended questions determine specific information and may be helpful to clients experiencing high levels of anxiety or disorganized thinking. If these are overused, however, the interaction takes on an atmosphere of cross-examination.

- Open-ended questions help increase the client's participation in the interaction and encourage the client to continue the discussion.

- Techniques that facilitate effective communication include broad openings, giving recognition, minimal encouragements, offering self, accepting, making observations, validating perceptions, exploring, clarifying, placing the event in time or sequence, focusing, encouraging the formulation of a plan of action, suggesting collaboration, restatement, reflection, and summarizing.

- Techniques that contribute to ineffective communication include stereotypical comments, parroting, changing the topic, disagreeing, challenging, requesting an explanation, false reassurance, belittling expressed feelings, probing, advising, imposing values, and double/multiple questions.

- Understanding family and group communication includes the perception of communication, affective and cognitive interpretation, validation, and interventions.

- The interpretation of nonverbal communication, verbal communication, and affective expression will enable you to help families and groups become more effective communicators.

- You will learn more by listening than by questioning children and adolescents.

- Older people take longer to react during conversation. Hearing and vision difficulties can complicate the communication process.

Educating

- Communication is the most important skill in effective education.

- Assessing areas of learning includes the client's and family's view of mental illness, knowledge of medications, and what they want and need to know.

- You must diagnose any barriers to learning such as anxiety, manic behavior, delusions, hallucinations, disorganized thinking, obsessional thoughts, depression, anger, hostility, and denial of the mental disorder.

- The goal of teaching is to prepare clients and families for as much self-care as possible in order to live in the least restrictive setting.

- The six general areas of learning are knowledge of the mental disorder, medications, managing ADLs, interpersonal communication, coping with life, and community resources.

- The steps of the problem-solving process are identifying the problem, identifying attempted solutions, listing alternative solutions, predicting consequences, choosing the best alternative, implementing the alternative, and evaluating the outcome.

- Client/family education is effective if the outcome criteria are met.

- All steps of the education process must be documented in the client's record.

EXPLORE *MediaLink*

- Interactive resources, including animations, for this chapter can be found on the Companion Web site at *http://www.prenhall.com/fontaine.* Click on Chapter 2 and select the activities for this chapter.

- For NCLEX review questions and an audio glossary, access the accompanying CD-ROM in this book.

REFERENCES

Forchuk, C., Westwell, J., Martin, M., Bamber-Azzapardi, W., Kosterewa-Tolman, D. & Hux, M. (2000). The developing nurse–client relationship: Nurses' perspectives. *Journal of the American Psychiatric Nurses Association, 6*(1), 3–10.

Goldberg, M. C. (1998). *The art of the question.* New York: John Wiley & Sons.

Isenalumhe, A. E. (2000). Using therapeutic support. *Journal of Psychosocial Nursing, 38*(1), 23–26.

Nussbaum, J. F., Pecchioni, L. L., Robinson, J. D., & Thompson, T. L. (2000). *Communication and aging* (2nd ed.). Mahwah, NJ: Lawrence Erlbaum.

Robinson, V. M. (1991). *Humor and the health professions* (2nd ed.). Thorofare, NJ: Slack.

Shea, S. C. (1998). *Psychiatric interviewing: The art of understanding* (2nd ed.). Philadelphia: Saunders.

Sheehan, J. P. (2000). Caring for the deaf. *RN, 63*(3), 69–72.

Spector, R. E. (2000). *Cultural diversity in health and illness* (5th ed.). Upper Saddle River, NJ: Prentice Hall.

Steinberg, A. G., Sullivan, V. J., & Loew, R. C. (1998). Cultural and linguistic barriers to mental health service access: The deaf consumer's perspective. *American Journal of Psychiatry, 155*(7), 982–984.

CHAPTER 3

The Family

in MENTAL HEALTH NURSING

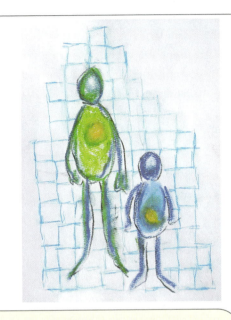

OBJECTIVES

After reading this chapter, you will be able to:

- EXPLAIN the competency model of family nursing.
- DESCRIBE the communication style, boundaries, cohesion, flexibility, and emotional availability of the family system.
- DESCRIBE the impact of loss on the family unit.
- DIFFERENTIATE between disenfranchised grief, uncomplicated grief, and complicated grief.
- ASSIST families through the process of family transformation.
- DESIGN family nursing interventions in the areas of psychoeducation, referral, and spiritual caregiving.

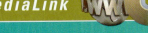

MediaLink

CD-ROM
- *Audio Glossary*
- *NCLEX Review*

Companion Web site www.prenhall.com/fontaine
- *Critical Thinking*
- *More NCLEX Review*
- *Case Study*
- *Care Map Activity*
- *Links to Resources*

*F*amily

born into family
left to be rebuilt
when closets open

a new family
to be searched out
and discovered

a family
born of respect and love

—Heather, Age 30

This chapter provides an overview of family competency, presents the impact of psychiatric disabilities on the family system, discusses mental disorders across the life span, and uses grieving as a model to illustrate mental health and developmental issues. The remainder of the chapter is devoted to family nursing practice.

For the majority of us, families are our earliest and most enduring social relationship. Families are the fabric of our day-to-day lives and shape the quality of our lives by influencing our outlooks on life, our motivations, our strategies for achievement, and our styles for coping with adversity. It is within our families that we develop our sense of self and our capacity for intimacy. Through family interactions we learn about relationships and roles and our expectations of others and ourselves. Each of us is simultaneously independent of and part of our families. We are both individuals and family members. We are part of our family and the family is part of us.

Families are considered to be two or more persons related by birth, marriage, formal or informal adoption, or by choice. This definition includes couples, traditional families, lesbian and gay families, communal families, families with cohabiting parents, extended families, multigenerational families, and even friends living together. Some families are protected by legal ties, whereas others are not. A family is an intimate group with a shared past, present, and future. No one family form necessarily provides an environment better for people to live or raise children in.

Labels indicate how we view families, and labels also have a tendency to become a self-fulfilling prophecy. In the past, health care professionals have used a deficit model in looking at families. Families were labeled functional or dysfunctional with the focus on fixing what needed repair. Psychiatric nursing has now moved to viewing families through a competency model. The **competency model** is based on the belief that all families are resourceful and have the capacity to grow and change. The model does not ignore pathology and dysfunction but emphasizes strengths, adaptation, and resources. The focus is one of building on competence rather than correcting deficits. Focusing on family strengths and resources, helps empower families to respond and adapt to life's circumstances (Mohr, Lafuze, & Mohr, 2000).

Family life becomes increasingly complex as the family responds to life events. Births, deaths, and illness, such as psychiatric disability, have a profound effect on family members and relationships. As nurses, it is important that we understand how the family relates to each other and struggles with a variety of life issues. Each family has a unique story and each family makes sense. No matter how dysfunctional they may appear on the surface, each family has a finely tuned style of living and interacting with one another. This does not mean that all families' way of living is healthy, effective, or even enjoyable. But the family does make sense when seen as a whole.

FAMILY SYSTEMS

In understanding the complexity of family systems, you consider how family members communicate, how they establish and maintain boundaries, how cohesive and flexible they are, and how emotionally available they are to one another. Understanding these interactions will provide you with a general idea of how well the family is able to adapt and function both in everyday life and in the face of adversity, such as the occurrence of a mental illness.

FAMILY COMMUNICATION

Family communication is measured by focusing on the family as a group with regard to their listening skills, speaking skills, self-disclosure, and tracking. The focus of *listening* skills is on empathy and attentive listening. *Speaking* skills include speaking for oneself and not speaking for others. *Self-disclosure* is the ability to share feelings about oneself and the relationship. *Tracking* is the capability to stay on topic.

Families who communicate well find themselves better able to adapt and cope. Families who find communication difficult, may experience lower levels of expressiveness, more vague requests to one another, an inability to comprehend each others' messages, frequent interruption of one another, speaking for others, and high levels of verbalized hostility.

Another aspect of family communication is the family's strategies to *resolve conflict*. The ability to resolve differences is based on the family's capacity to talk about areas of disagreement and their mutual willingness to negotiate and reach acceptable solutions. Problem-solving skills are critical to smooth family functioning. Without these skills, families seem to use strategies such as confrontation or avoidance, which are ineffective in reducing stress and do not resolve conflict satisfactorily.

Boundaries

Boundaries are the invisible lines that define the amount and kind of contact allowable among members of the family and between the family and outside systems. Boundaries determine the patterns of how, when, and to whom family members relate. Boundaries define the division between the spousal, parental, and sibling subsystems. *Clear boundaries* are firm yet flexible, and members are supported and nurtured but also allowed a certain degree of autonomy. *Rigid boundaries* isolate family members from one another

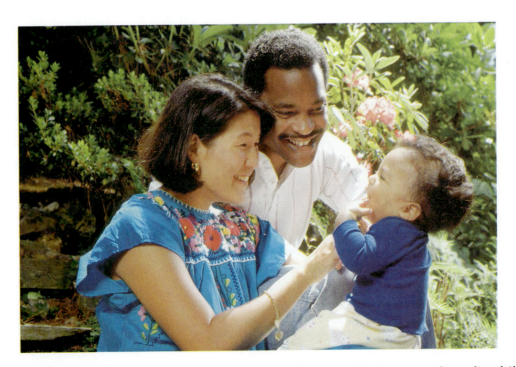

PHOTO 3.1 ■ Competent families have an emotional climate of intimacy and predictability.

and there is little room for negotiation and individual development. *Diffuse boundaries* are the opposite, where everybody is into everybody else's business. There is little distinction between members and too much negotiation, resulting in a loss of autonomy.

Competent families have clear hierarchical boundaries between generations in terms of power, authority, and responsibility. Competent adult leadership provides an emotional climate that considers everyone's needs and provides a sense of security. Members spend time apart as well as time together. Mutual respect is also a boundary issue. Competent families respect and value individuals' opinions and feelings. The family system tolerates individual differences and honors differing opinions.

Boundaries are a social construction and as such are culturally determined. What appears to be a boundary violation in one culture may be acceptable in another culture. For example, cultures vary in how family members respect privacy in regard to toileting, bathing, changing clothes, and sleeping arrangements. Multigenerational boundaries in terms of power and authority vary from culture to culture.

FAMILY COHESION

Family cohesion is defined as the emotional bonding that family members have toward one another. There are four levels of cohesion, ranging from disengaged (very low) to separated (low to moderate) to connected (moderate to high) to enmeshed (very high) (see Figure 3.1 ■). It is believed that the central ranges of cohesion (separated and connected) contribute to optimal family competency. The extremes (disengaged or enmeshed) are generally seen as less adaptive. Disengaged families seem almost like a group of strangers who happen to be living together. There is little loyalty or closeness. Members of enmeshed families cannot develop a separate identity, and each person must yield autonomy in order to belong to the family. Differentness is experienced as distance, and individuality is viewed as alienation and disloyalty (Olson, 1996). See Box 3.1 for characteristics of family cohesion.

FAMILY FLEXIBILITY

Family flexibility is the amount of change in a family's leadership, role relationships, and relationship rules.

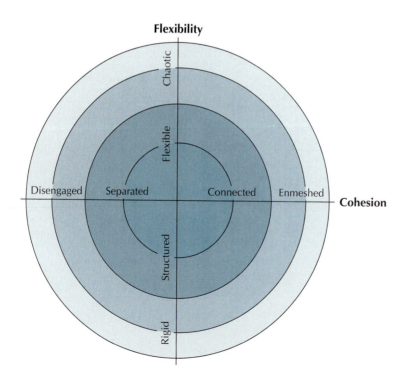

FIGURE 3.1 ■ Circumplex model.

BOX 3.1

Characteristics of Family Cohesion

Disengaged
- Little closeness
- Little loyalty
- High independence

Separated
- Low-moderate closeness
- Some loyalty
- Interdependent with more independence than dependence

Connected
- Moderate-high closeness
- High loyalty
- Interdependent with more dependence than independence

Enmeshed
- Very high closeness
- Very high loyalty
- High dependency

BOX 3.2

Characteristics of Family Flexibility

Chaotic
- Lack of leadership
- Dramatic role shifts
- Erratic discipline
- Too much change

Flexible
- Shared leadership
- Democratic discipline
- Role-sharing change
- Change when necessary

Structured
- Leadership sometimes shared
- Somewhat democratic discipline
- Roles stable
- Change when demanded

Rigid
- Authoritarian leadership
- Strict discipline
- Roles seldom change
- Too little change

Flexibility also refers to the family's ability to respond to stress. There are four levels of flexibility, ranging from rigid (very low) to structured (low to moderate) to flexible (moderate to high) to chaotic (very high) (see Figure 3.1). As with cohesion, it is believed that the central ranges (structured and flexible) are more conducive to family adaptation, with the extremes (rigid and chaotic) being the less competent (Olson, 1996). See Box 3.2 for characteristics of family flexibility.

Rules determine appropriate roles and relationship patterns within the family. Rules express the values of the family and form a boundary around each family, which then screens outside information for compatibility with the family's value system. If the message is not congruent with the family's values, you will hear such statements as: "That is not the way we do things in this family" or "I don't care what Marc is allowed to do; in this family, we . . ." To understand rules more clearly, reflect for a moment on the family in which you grew up. There were certain things that you just did, that you knew were expected. There were other things that were not permitted. For purposes of assess-

ing a few of the rules in your family of origin, complete the statements in Box 3.3.

EMOTIONAL AVAILABILITY

All members in competent families freely express a wide variety of feelings. The emotional climate is one of intimacy and predictability. In less competent families the emotional climate may be angry, cold, or distant.

Emotional availability is another way to describe the quality of parent–child interactions. Areas for assessment include parental sensitivity, structuring, nonintrusiveness, and nonhostility. *Parental sensitivity* is assessed by how parents pick up children's emotional signals and how appropriately they express their own emotions. *Parental structuring* refers to the ability of parents to support learning and exploration without overwhelming the child's autonomy. *Parental nonintrusiveness* refers to the ability to be available to the child without being interfering, overprotective, or overwhelming. *Nonhostility* refers to ways of interact-

BOX 3.3

Assessing Rules in Your Family of Origin

In my family, we were never allowed to . . .

In my family, we were always expected to . . .

In my family, girls were required to . . .

In my family, girls were allowed to . . .

In my family, girls were forbidden to . . .

In my family, boys were required to . . .

In my family, boys were allowed to . . .

In my family, boys were forbidden to . . .

In my family, household responsibilities were determined by . . .

In my family, we handled conflict by . . .

In my family, the most important thing in life for women is . . .

In my family, the most important thing in life for men is . . .

ing with the child that are generally patient and pleasant. When angry, parents express the anger in an appropriately controlled manner (Biringen, 2000).

FAMILY COMPETENCY

Competency is found in a wide diversity of family arrangements. More important than the form or type of family, are the family's relational resources and adaptive abilities. The most distinctive trait of competent families is the ability to productively manage stress. Simply put, adaptive families evolve and shift with changing situations, often referred to as *resiliency*. Walsh (1998) describes family resiliency as the "process of coming to terms with all that has happened, reaching new emotional and relational equilibrium with changed circumstances, and becoming more resourceful in facing whatever lies ahead" (p. 75). Life crises and developmental transitions can stimulate family growth and transformation. Resilient families make it through crises such as disability and death with a renewed sense of confidence and purpose in their lives.

PSYCHIATRIC DISABILITY AND THE FAMILY SYSTEM

Individuals with mental illness often have family members who share in the many losses that accompany the illness. Families are the major source of support and rehabilitation for their loved ones. Of clients discharged from acute care, 65 percent return to their families. At any given time, 40 to 50 percent of the 48 million Americans who are psychiatrically disabled live with their families on a regular basis. Even when consumers do not live at home, their families are often the only source of support. Care for the mentally ill has become as much family based as community based in the United States. This situation can result in overwhelming emotional and economic stress on the family system (Allen, Fine, & Demo, 2000; Johnson, 2000).

FAMILY BURDEN

Families have important needs of their own, in response to their loved one's mental illness. Psychiatric disability often puts the family under catastrophic levels of stress. As families respond to the grief and trauma, they need empathy and support from health care professionals (Mohr & Regan-Kubinski, 2001).

Family burden is the overall level of distress experienced as a result of the mental illness. The **objective family burden** is related to the actual, identifiable family problems associated with the person's mental illness. One burden the family must manage relates to *symptomatic behaviors*. Deficit behaviors of their loved ones such as lack of motivation, difficulty in completing tasks, isolation from others, inability to manage money, poor grooming and personal care, and poor eating and sleeping behavior can be of great concern to families. Intrusive or acting-out behaviors such as lack of consideration for others, excessive arguing, conflicts with neighbors and friends, damaging material possessions, inappropriate sexual behavior, suicide attempts, and substance abuse are very disturbing to family members. These behaviors may be more episodic than the deficit behaviors but may have more severe immediate consequences. This family burden may lead to loss of independence and increased responsibility as families try to cope with day-to-day living. This burden includes disruption in household functioning, restriction of social activities, and financial hardship due to medical bills and the cost of their loved one's economic burden.

Another objective burden related to family problems is *caregiving*. Families may find that community services are not always available and not always satisfactory. Inadequate funding results in lack of treatment programs and lack of services for families themselves. Families also find themselves negotiating with the legal and criminal justice system. With few long-term psychiatric facilities available, many people who were previously cared for in state hospitals now find themselves in jails and prisons. Often, the "crimes" with which they are charged are misdemeanors resulting from their symptoms of mental illness, such as disorderly conduct, trespassing, and drunkenness.

Families must also cope with the burden of *stigma*. Much to the shame of our country, people with mental illness continue to be ostracized from mainstream society. As their loved one faces multiple discriminations, families may feel isolated and shameful, lose self-esteem, and run the risk of self-stigmatization (Marsh, 1998).

The **subjective family burden** is defined as the psychological distress of the family members in relation to the objective burden. Families often experience intense feelings of **grief** and **loss**. They must mourn for the person they knew before the onset of the illness

and the loss of hopes, dreams, and expectations. They live with a sense of *chronic sorrow* as their loved one experiences periods of remission and relapse. There is also a sense of *empathetic pain* as they watch their family member become a victim of the illness. Living with and caring for a person with mental illness can have a tremendous impact of the family. Some families cope fairly well while others are easily exhausted and give up (Teschinsky, 2000) (see Table 3.1 ■).

FAMILY RECOVERY

Stage 1 of family recovery is one of *discovery and denial.* Family members are often the first to notice that their family member is exhibiting unusual behavior. The family's initial response may range from minimizing (it's not so serious) to denial (it's just a phase). Rather than maladaptive, this response is a temporary reaction to avoid painful reality. As the family attempts to explain the changes to others, they may attribute them to something more socially acceptable than mental illness. For example, they might tell others that the person is suffering from exhaustion or an endocrine problem or that stress at school or work is causing the difficulties. This avoidance of stigma and prejudice on the part of others can lead to family isolation and loss of relationships outside the immediate family system.

Stage 2 of family recovery is one of *recognition and acceptance.* As it becomes more evident that there is a

TABLE 3.1
The Language of Family Pain

Catastrophe: Watching as your loved one slips away. This is like a horror movie, in which the hero/heroine (loved one) is utterly transformed by some unseen, monstrous force.

Torture: The agony of watching a loved one experience relentless pain and suffering without being able to make it stop. The absolute panic when he or she refuses your assistance, rejects your help, resists your protection at the time when it is most needed.

Anguish: The pain of having loved ones turn on those who are trying to help them, attack them angrily, or blame them for their difficulties.

Horror/Fear: A dread that the ill person will do something terrible to self or others.

Nightmare: Rejection, labeling, and ostracism by the mental health system when we are trying to help.

SOURCE: Reprinted with permission from Burland, J. (1999). *NAMI provider education program.* Arlington, VA: National Alliance for the Mentally Ill.

significant problem, the family begins to search for reasons and solutions by gathering available information. Families begin to develop their own image of the disease process and expectations of mental health professionals. Many families also hope for what was in the past and for what might be in the future. It is very sad to lose a close family member to the world of mental illness. Many people do not believe that mental illness is a brain disease. If the disorder begins in childhood, it is easier to think that it is a result of bad parenting because that means good parenting should fix it. That is like telling parents of a child with leukemia that if they were better parents they could stop those white cells from growing. When a person experiences a mental disorder, the loss of ideal family dreams occurs. The expectation of a meaningful and productive individual and family life is shattered. All family members must be supported as they grieve the loss of their hopes and dreams (Badger, 1996).

Stage 3 of family recovery is one of *coping and competence.* This includes the day-to-day efforts to cope with all the changes in the family. When people become psychiatrically disabled, they often find they cannot carry out their family roles and responsibilities. Thus, other family members must assume those role functions and come to terms with an altered family lifestyle. Family members develop cognitive, emotional, and behavioral coping strategies to be able to live with their loved one who is experiencing a mental disorder. As they take stock of the challenges, constraints, and resources, they are better able to make the most of their options.

Coping strategies protect the affected family member and maintain the stability of family functioning. Some of these strategies include expressing affection, suggesting alternative choices, reducing conflict, seeking social support, and trying to make the best of their experiences by focusing on the positive parts of the relationship with the disabled family member.

Rose (1997) describes four family support sources: professional support, friend support, family support, and spiritual support. *Professional support* includes a nonblaming, respectful attitude toward families, information on how to respond to symptoms, and help in locating community resources such as housing or vocational training. *Friend support* comes from non–family members such as close friends and co-workers. It is most valued when the concern is genuine and stigma is

minimized. *Family support* often comes in the way of tangible assistance such as respite care for family members and physical presence in times of crisis. Many families find emotional strength from their religious faith. They find *spiritual support* as they search for meaning through relationships and the feeling of connectedness with others. Supportive relationships build and sustain courage, helping families make the best of their difficult lives.

As families learn to cope effectively, the intense focus on the ill family member lightens up as other members begin to focus on taking care of themselves and reconnecting with others outside the family as they move through the process of grief. The family adapts to their changed circumstances and continues to function successfully.

The final stage of family recovery is *personal and political advocacy.* This stage involves working with the mental health system to obtain treatment. Family members want to be seen as partners in treatment and do not want to be excluded from discussions and treatment recommendations. Ideally, professionals, clients, and families all work together in joint problem solving. At times, the issue of client confidentiality is raised. Family members generally respect confidentiality but do need information about treatments, medications, and ways to cope with certain behaviors.

Some families go on to educate the public about mental illness and lobby for improved public policy and legislation often through the National Alliance for the Mentally Ill (NAMI), an organization comprised of consumers, families, and professionals. NAMI actively lobbies for improved legislation and improved health care benefits at local, state, and federal levels (Pratt, Gill, Barrett, & Roberts, 1999; Sveinbjarnardottir & de Casterle, 1997).

MENTAL DISORDERS ACROSS THE LIFE SPAN

PREGNANCY AND CHILD CARE

Pregnancy, childbirth, and parenting are major issues for all women. For the psychiatrically disabled woman, who already has problems in adjustment and coping, pregnancy and parenting can be sufficient strain to exacerbate symptoms of the mental illness. Women with a history of mental illness must be monitored closely throughout their pregnancy. Although 10 to 15 percent of pregnant women meet criteria for depression, they often remain undiagnosed because the symptoms of depression are similar to the somatic changes of pregnancy. For many women, the postpartum period is associated with mental health problems, including postpartum blues in as many as 80 percent of new mothers, postpartum depression in 10 to 15 percent of new mothers, and postpartum psychosis in about one in 1,000 women (Deater-Deckard, Pickering, Dunn, & Golding, 1998; Viguera et al., 2000). (See Chapter 13 for more information on postpartum and depression.)

In the general U.S. population, 50 percent of pregnancies are unplanned; the rate is higher among women who are psychiatrically disabled. For women with bipolar disorder whose manic episodes increase their sexual activity and impair their judgment, the risk of unplanned pregnancy is high. It is not uncommon for women and their families to be unaware of a pregnancy until the pregnancy is far advanced, which places both the woman and fetus at risk. Other problems may include a diminished ability to comply with prenatal care, an inability to plan realistically for the baby, an increased risk of substance abuse during the pregnancy, and poor nutrition. The woman may also feel overwhelmed and ambivalent about motherhood and may fear losing custody of the baby.

If the woman is pregnant and taking psychotropic medications, the primary health care provider must weigh the risk of fetal anomalies against the exacerbation of the illness, which may present a danger to herself and others, including the fetus. All effective mood-stabilizing agents pose risks during pregnancy. Carbamazepine and valproic acid are associated with increased risk of neural tube defects and an increased risk of neonatal hemorrhage due to low levels of vitamin K. The main risks of lithium are polyhydramnios, premature labor, neonatal toxicity, and neonatal hypothyroidism. Antipsychotic and antianxiety medications are often utilized, as they cause fewer fetal anomalies and problems with the pregnancy. Electroconvulsive therapy (ECT) is an effective and relatively safe treatment for some clients since uterine muscle does not contract as part of the generalized tonic–clonic seizure (Bailine, Dean, Weiner, & Tramontozzi, 2000).

Psychiatric disability among mothers of newborns and young children has far-reaching implications for the mother and the family. If the mother is acutely ill at childbirth, she is usually separated from her newborn, which may be deeply distressing for her and impede the bonding process. This separation may be temporary, but in some cases the loss of custody becomes permanent. Psychiatric hospitalization for acute illness leads to disruption of the family system as children suffer repeated separations and a chaotic and unpredictable environment.

In the future, when disease-related genes are identified for mental disorders, it will be possible to develop prenatal tests for these diseases. Individuals at high risk for passing on the disorder will have the option to take such tests and to abort an affected fetus. Serious ethical considerations are involved with such options, and appropriate guidelines must be developed for the eventual genetic testing for mental disorders.

Nursing interventions for young families include helping the family develop a social support system and use community resources. Programs such as Head Start, day care centers, and recreational programs can stimulate the children and provide a time of respite for the mother. Teaching includes providing information about normal growth and development, stress-management techniques, time-management skills, and problem-solving skills. Collaborating with the extended family may minimize the impact of psychiatric disability on the primary family.

YOUTH

An estimated 8 million children (12 to 13 percent of all children under age 18) have a serious emotional disturbance with substantial functional impairment, nearly half of which lead to serious disability. Children with mental disorders are at increased risk for dropping out of school and of being marginalized members of society in adulthood. Few young children are identified with mental disorders and most do not receive appropriate and timely treatment (*Mental Health*, 1999; "Landmark Study," 1999).

When a child or adolescent experiences a mental disorder, the entire family system is strained. When primary responsibility for caregiving falls to one person, the parental system is stressed, which often leads to increased conflict and a greater likelihood for parental separation. The siblings are often excluded, leading to confusion or misunderstanding of the problem. Siblings' feelings may range from shame to protectiveness. At times, they may feel superior for not having "problems," while at other times they may feel neglected if the child with the disorder receives more parental attention.

Family turmoil can trigger the onset of a disorder in a biologically and genetically predisposed child. Families' emotional and affective styles may be a factor in the onset. The parent–child relationship is often severely strained due to stressors related to the child's mental disorder. Some parents respond in ways that foster dependence, which contributes to separation/individuation problems or boundary issues. Some parents may be rejecting and critical of the child with the disorder. Other parents alternate between overprotection/overcontrol and rejection. Other families learn to adapt in ways that foster the growth and development of all the children. It must be remembered that family patterns are *not* the primary cause of childhood mental disorders; mental disorders have multiple etiologies, including the interaction of biological, genetic, psychological, and social factors.

COUPLES

Most people who are psychiatrically disabled at a fairly young age remain single. Their social functioning is so limited that they are unable to sustain a relationship. In contrast, research suggests that people with depression may be able to be part of a couple. Studies indicate, however, that as many as half of individuals suffering from depression report serious couple difficulties and hope to resolve these relationship problems in therapy. In addition, couples who are experiencing relationship distress are at higher risk for developing depression.

One of the hallmarks of relationship distress is poor communication. Partners who are depressed behave in ways that discourage social interaction and increase relationship conflict. They are less skillful socially and more withdrawn; they seem to express more hostility and criticism of themselves and others; they may engage in long and hateful arguments; and they often express dissatisfaction with sexual activity. Living with a depressed person can also increase the nondepressed partner's susceptibility to depression. The goal of relationship therapy is to decrease conflict, increase the degree of intimacy and relationship satisfaction, and

enhance effective coping and social competence (Johnson, 2000).

ADULT CHILDREN

The current focus of mental health care is returning clients to their communities to live in the least restrictive environment that is realistic. As a result, at least half of the psychiatrically disabled adult population are living with their families on a regular basis. Professionals are beginning to look at and respond to the burden of family caregivers. Some of the problems that families of these adult children face are the need for daily caretaking, lack of freedom, emotional drain, stress of the unexpected, and financial strain. Parents often struggle to find a good balance between supporting their adult child with an illness as a dependent and fostering her or his own independence to the greatest extent possible. This balance involves both the person with the disability and the caregiving parent.

Client symptoms of illness such as inappropriate behavior, labile emotions, hallucinations, delusions, and outbursts of rage are often difficult for families to manage. Other symptoms that strain the family are dependency, poor social skills and outlets, and difficulties in finding employment. Financial considerations may force the parents to delay their expected retirement. They are often concerned about the welfare of their child after their death. Family caregivers need support and practical knowledge to enhance their ability to cope and their ability to support their loved one (Mohr & Regan-Kubinski, 2001; Pickens, 1998).

DEATH AND THE FAMILY SYSTEM

Death is a choiceless event that leads to chaos and disorder for survivors. Coming to terms with death is the most difficult task families must confront. We live, die, grieve, and survive within a family context. Prior experiences with death and loss in the family influence how we grieve. Families teach us how to behave and the way we should express our feelings when a significant death occurs.

Bereavement is the feelings, thoughts, and responses that loved ones experience following a death of a person with whom they have shared a significant relationship. **Mourning** or *grieving* is the active process

Sara, a 32-year-old legal secretary, has been meeting with her nurse, Bill, for the past several weeks. Sara is being treated for depression following a series of long- and short-term relationships that have inevitably ended because Sara is distrustful. Sara comes from a broken home in which her father was domineering and controlling. He disapproved of Sara's friends and interfered with her attempts to become independent.

In their initial relationship, Sara and Bill identified specific problem areas that were of concern to Sara and determined when and how often to meet. They agreed that their relationship would continue for at least 4 to 5 months. Currently, they are in the working phase of the nurse–client relationship and concentrating on mutually agreed-upon goals.

During a recent session, Sara became very angry with Bill, accusing him of being a dominant and controlling man. Bill remained calm, listened to Sara, and without judgment expressed concern and warmth toward her. He then assisted Sara to explore the differences between her father and himself.

1. What data support that Sara and Bill have moved beyond the introductory phase of their relationship?

2. Compare and contrast Sara and Bill's relationship with a social relationship. How is it similar?

3. If you were Bill, how would you interpret Sara's outburst and accusations?

4. Evaluate Bill's response based on your knowledge of the nurse–client relationship.

5. What difference would it make to Sara's care if Bill did not recognize Sara's response?

For an additional Case Study, please refer to the Companion Web site for this book.

also occurs with any significant loss experience and is a process of learning to live with our feelings as we struggle to reestablish our self-esteem or self-confidence in the face of these personal losses. The process of grieving is essential for our mental and physical health as it allows us to cope with the loss gradually and to accept it as part of reality. Our families, our religious beliefs, and our cultural customs influence mourning and grieving. It is a social process and is best shared and carried out with the help of others. None of us grieves predictably or uniformly. As caring nurses, we must always respect individuality in the way persons grieve and mourn (McGoldrick & Walsh, 1999).

Family gender roles also affect reactions at times of loss. In North America, women are often the ones who grieve outwardly in the form of tears and sorrow, while men are expected to "be strong" and show minimal emotion during grief. Men may choose strategies such as logical reasoning or diversional activities to manage their unacknowledged feelings. Our families' spiritual beliefs and religious practices influence how we react to loss and death and our resulting behavior. Most religious groups have customs and practices, which can help survivors with the process of grieving.

Family systems, like individuals, experience symptoms of grief, including changes in communication patterns, changes in family structure and changes in relationships outside the family. The death of a family member radically disrupts the family system. The first priority in managing the crisis of grief is to reestablish a stable equilibrium that is necessary to support ongoing family development. This requires the resources of the individual, extended family, friends, and community.

Family members need to be able to talk with one another about their emotions concerning the death and its circumstances. A family's ability to *communicate* about death is partially determined by its members' previous patterns of communication. If individuals are unable to talk about the death, any misconceptions about the cause or circumstances cannot be corrected. For example, in some families the cause of death is never told to children, who then grow up with questions or distorted ideas. There may be a change in the pattern of communication, such as who talks to whom. Some families cut off or reject certain members, while others may reconnect with distant family members.

of learning to adapt to the loved one's death. Mourning is a progression through a series of phases that include recognition and acceptance of the death, the experience of emotional and physical pain, and the rebuilding of a life without the loved one. Grieving

In response to death, family *structure* often changes temporarily. All family members play roles both within and outside the family. There may be role confusion, which contributes to turmoil in the family's hierarchy. Realignment of roles is a necessary function of grieving, and the process of recovery includes redistribution of role functions. Roles may be reassigned on the basis of achievement and interest or on the basis of gender and age. Individuals must adapt and adjust to the new roles and the absence of the deceased member. The more flexible family will typically be more successful. Like individuals, families are unique in their mourning process. What is effective for one family may not be effective for another.

Relationships with people outside the family often change as death disrupts established patterns of interaction. Some families are able to reach out to others, but some withdraw from their friends and other support networks. At times, families may overprotect some or all members, effectively isolating individuals (McGoldrick & Walsh, 1999).

Children experience the same emotions of grief as adults but are less likely to show acute grief in the initial phase and more likely to experience the process over a much longer period of time. At each developmental level, children rework the meaning of a family member's death from more mature cognitive and emotional functioning. Preverbal children understand death as a separation, not as a finite end to life. They are often convinced the deceased person could come back if she or he really wanted to. When children develop language skills at 2 to 3 years, they can begin the process of comprehending death and its causes, although they still believe death to be reversible. School-age children tend to be more avoidant in speaking of their grief than either preschoolers or teens, resulting in an appearance of unconcern. Because they equate death with abandonment, this age group is especially vulnerable to depression, self-blame, and low self-esteem for some months. *Adolescents* cognitively can understand death in adult terms. They may associate the tragedy with their age-appropriate search for independence. Some teens may become closer to the family and may even feel responsible for their family's survival. Others may begin acting out as their attempts to become their own person are complicated with grief.

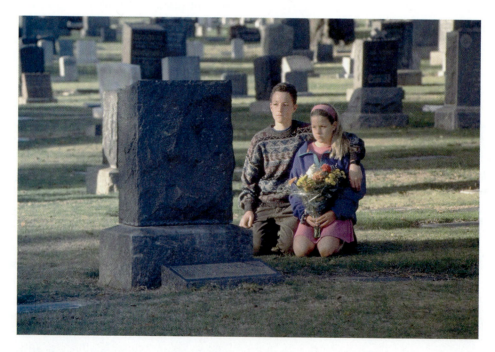

PHOTO 3.2 ■ Children experience the same emotions of grief as adults.

SOURCE: David Young–Wolff/PhotoEdit.

DISENFRANCHISED GRIEF

Every culture establishes grieving norms and denies such emotions to people who are deemed to have insignificant losses. These losses are not acknowledged or validated by others, and the survivors are deprived of their right to grieve. **Disenfranchised grief** means that the loss cannot be openly acknowledged, socially validated, or publicly mourned. Typically, there are three categories of disenfranchised grief: the relationship is not recognized, the loss is not recognized, or the griever is not recognized.

Often, *relationships are not recognized* when there are no kin ties. These would include close friendships, lovers, neighbors, or caregivers. Other unrecognized relationships are those that are not socially sanctioned, such as nontraditional relationships, extramarital affairs, or same-gender relationships. Relationships that existed primarily in the past are often not recognized as needing to be grieved, such as former friends, past lovers, or ex-spouses.

There are some *losses that cultures do not socially recognize.* These include elective abortions, perinatal deaths, giving up a child for adoption, and even the loss of a beloved pet.

The third category is *grievers who are not recognized.* In this instance, the person is not socially defined by the culture as capable of grief. The very old, who are thought to be too frail and fragile to cope with loss, and the very young, who are thought to be oblivious to loss, are often excluded from discussions and rituals. Sometimes it is assumed that people who are developmentally disabled are incapable of understanding death and have no need to mourn.

As nurses, we must remember that people exist in multiple relationships and form meaningful and significant attachments in different kinds of relationships. The dominant culture often ignores these in favor of the nuclear family, which is given a monopoly on mourning. Past relationships, such as those of ex-spouses, may still hold a degree of attachment, and thus there may be grief. When the promise of unborn children is terminated, parents experience grief. In our society, significant pet–human bonds develop, and there is grief when the pet dies. People are capable of a great capacity for attachments, so they are vulnerable to grief when these attachments are ended. The problem results when that fact is forgotten and the grief is minimized or ignored.

COMPLICATED GRIEF

The boundaries between normal and **complicated grief** are unclear. The judgment that a person's grief reaction is complicated is based not only on the individual but also on the range and tolerance of differences in grieving allowed by the culture. See Box 3.4 for factors that contribute to increased distress or to a good outcome during mourning.

Complicated grief may include symptoms such as intrusive images, severe feelings of emptiness, and neglect of activities at home and at work. Other symptoms include preoccupation with thoughts of the deceased person, yearning and searching for her or him, inability to accept the death, auditory and visual hallucinations of the person, bitterness and survivor guilt over the death, and symptoms of identification such as having pain in the same part of the body as the deceased person (McGoldrick & Walsh, 1999).

Individuals who experience complicated grief are at a higher risk for a variety of health problems. In American culture, grief is considered to be complicated

---

BOX 3.4

Factors Influencing Outcomes in Mourning

Increased Psychological Distress
- Predeath psychiatric disorder—coping with changes is especially difficult
- Manner of death—sudden, unexpected death more difficult to manage
- Family life cycle—loss of spouse for young parent with children
- Dysfunctional relationship with deceased person
- Constricted capacity to express feelings
- Financial problems

Increased Ability to Cope
- Sense of optimism
- Belief system that helps deal with death
- Self-sufficient
- Experience with loss
- Competent family interactions
- Supportive social network
- Adequate financial resources

TABLE 3.2

Differences Between Depression and Grief

Trait	Depression	Grief
Trigger	Specific trigger not necessary	Trigger usually loss or multiple losses
Active/passive	Passive behavior tends to keep them "stuck" in sadness	Actively feel their emotional pain and emptiness
Emotions	Generalized feeling of helplessness, hopelessness	Experience a range of emotions that are usually intense
Ability to laugh	Likely to be humorless and incapable of being happy or even temporarily cheered up; likely to resist support	Sometimes will be able to laugh and enjoy humor, more likely to accept support
Activities	Lack of interest in previously enjoyed activities	Can be persuaded to participate in activities, especially as they begin to heal
Self-esteem	Low self-esteem, low self-confidence; feels like a failure	Self-esteem usually remains intact; does not feel like a failure unless it relates directly to the loss
Feeling of the failure	May dwell on past failures, catastrophize	Any self-blame or guilt relates directly to loss; feelings resolve as they progress toward healing

when there is enormous social, psychological, and medical morbidity. Psychiatric complications include depressive episodes, anxiety-related symptoms and disorders, suicidal ideation, or psychotic denial of the death (see Table 3.2 ■). Medical problems include hypertension, cardiac problems, impaired immune function, and cancer. Some people develop chronic illness behavior and hypochondriasis, which leads to a preoccupation with health and an inability to reinvest energy or interest in social relationships.

FAMILY NURSING PRACTICE

Until recently, family members were sometimes utilized as a source of information about their ill members but were rarely involved in treatment, psychoeducation, or family therapy, and the idea of the family as a unit of care was controversial. With less restrictive

environments, shorter hospital stays, and fewer community programs, nurses must now develop a *collaborative partnership* with clients and their families. This collaborative relationship means that the family is viewed as the unit of care and as partners in treatment and rehabilitation. Thus, programs must be in place to provide support, education, coping skills training, social network development, and family therapy. As family nurses, it is critically important that we take the time to be with families in deeply caring ways. As we share our ideas and our strengths, our goal is to help families develop as more balanced and caring systems.

FAMILY ASSESSMENT

As nurses, we must focus our attention on the family both as the context for the individual as well as the unit of care. It is important to assess and involve families since they are in a position to be impacted by and to influence the course of individuals' problems. The questions we ask influence how we view the family. For example, if we ask only questions regarding problems, we are likely to "find" pathology in the family. On the other hand, if we also include questions about resourcefulness, we have an increased chance of discovering family competency. Questions shape our experience of and our interactions with clients and families. The following questions are examples of assessing the resourcefulness of the family system:

- What do you hope for in the future?
- How will your life be different when your concerns are no longer problems?
- What strengths, resources, and knowledge do you have to deal with the problems?

Assessment includes gathering information on how partners, parents, and children in the family experience or react to the client's symptoms. You need to learn how others are affected by problems and how they have attempted to cope with problems. If we want to know the family, we must listen to their story. The family's story will tell us who they are and what is meaningful to them. Telling their story also allows families to make sense out of any confusion.

Together, clients, families, and nurses collaborate to identify the family's strengths, resources, and social support, and try to identify problems that might cause stress for any of the family members. Factors in assessing clients and their families include family communication, boundaries, cohesion, flexibility, emotional availability, and overall family functionality.

ASSESSMENT OF VULNERABILITY TO RELAPSE

Understandably, families are very concerned with their loved one's vulnerability to relapse. Although families are not to be blamed for mental disorders, their interactions may influence the course of the disorder. Relapse is less common in families who see the client as ill (rather than lazy or manipulative) and provide support to one another. Relapse is more common in families who are highly critical, highly anxious, and preoccupied with their problems. Researchers have studied two family patterns, family *expressed emotion* (*EE*) and

family *affective style* (*AS*). Families rated as high EE tend to be hostile, critical, and emotionally overinvolved with the client. Families rated as high AS are intrusive and make guilt-inducing remarks during emotionally charged family discussions. Both high EE and SA families are predictors of relapse for people who are psychiatrically disabled. Families are more likely to be excessively critical or overinvolved when they lack information about the disorder and when they believe the symptoms are under the client's control. Family members who do not understand the nature of psychiatric disability may mistake the negative symptoms (see Chapter 14) as laziness (Teschinsky, 2000; Wuerker, 2000).

Medication noncompliance and substance abuse are other changeable factors related to relapse. Medication noncompliance is linked to lack of insight into the disorder, medication side effects, cost of medication, missed outpatient appointments, and negative client/family attitudes toward medication. Mental health status is further compromised by the use of alcohol or drugs. (See Chapter 15 for further information on substance abuse.) Clients who abuse substances also tend to be noncompliant with medication.

CULTURAL ASSESSMENT

Our culture shapes our concept of self. One way to look at the cultural self is along a continuum between egocentric and sociocentric orientations. The **egocentric self**, usually found in Western industrialized societies, exhibits characteristics such as individualism, separateness, autonomy, competition, and mastery of and control over one's environment. The **sociocentric self**, found in many non-Western societies, is interdependent and interconnected and values cooperation, cohesiveness, group identity, and harmony with one's environment. The person is defined by kinship and is seen in relationship terms.

African Americans, Asian Americans, Latinos, and Native People tend toward sociocentric orientations. There is a high value on interpersonal relationships, group membership, and cohesiveness. Relationships to others, family, and community are central to one's sense of well-being. An extensive kin network provides both economic and emotional support to its members. Mental illness is often viewed as a family affair as it affects all family members. These families express greater hope, optimism, and faith about long-term outcomes of their family member's mental illness. Siblings of disabled persons are more likely to be involved in caregiving and less likely to find their involvement burdensome than are Euro-American siblings.

A multicultural study of family caregiving found that 75 percent of Latino clients and 60 percent of African American clients lived with their families, compared with 30 percent of Euro-American clients. Cultural assessment of the family determines appropriate family-centered approaches to problem solving and treatment for mental disorders (Barrio, 2000; Johnson, 2000).

Generalizations about ethnic group families increase our level of awareness and alert us to the possibility of differences. It is very important, however, that you never assume that ethnic group generalizations accurately describe the family with whom you are working, as great variations exist. How a problem is viewed and how distress is handled vary with different family and cultural norms. You must also recognize and understand that differences are not pathology or dysfunction but simply another way of life. As a nurse, you take your families where they are, help them achieve their goals, and facilitate health in the way that is most useful for them. (See Chapter 5 for additional information on the role of cultural diversity.)

THE NURSE AS EDUCATOR

Psychoeducation has proven to be an important aspect of family nursing. (See Chapter 2 for more detailed information on psychoeducation.) We must be able to answer questions, help families identify feelings and reactions, and encourage them in their coping efforts.

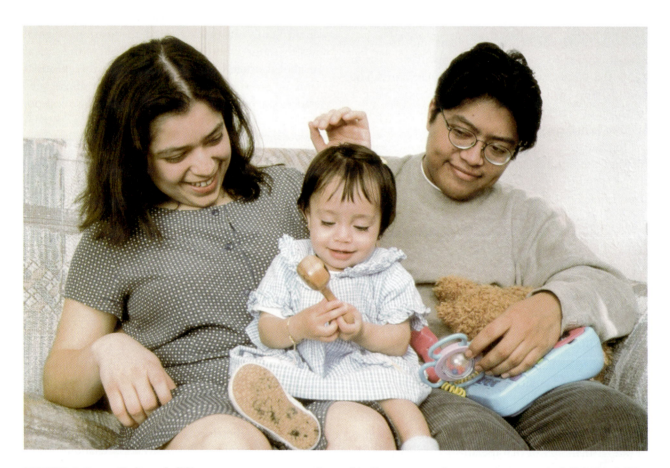

PHOTO 3.3 ■ Cultural differences exert a profound influence on how parents and children relate to one another.

SOURCES: Michael Newman/PhotoEdit.

Families need information about mental illness and service delivery programs. Illness education occurs in the context of the basic family unit and with multifamily groups. Information is provided on the disorder, symptoms, etiology, treatment, and relapse prevention and recognition.

Families also need skills to cope with the illness. Nurses help families identify problems and work out solutions that fit the family's current patterns of living. Family education programs include conflict-management skills and problem solving to help them resolve day-to-day living discord. Other skills include communication strategies and assertiveness training. Families can benefit from stress-management programs, which include relaxation exercises, visualization, affirmations, meditation, and physical exercise. (Information on alternative therapies is found in Chapter 10 as well as integrated throughout the text.)

As educators, we realize we cannot make decisions for others' lives. Clients and families know more about their lives and are the best judges for future direction. Through education we enhance the strengths and creativity of the family system and assist members in making changes and developing the lives they choose.

THE NURSE AS REFERRAL AGENT

Because families often feel stigmatized and alone, referrals to support groups are often helpful. Networking with other families who are struggling with similar issues normalizes the family's experiences.

Family nurses act as referral agents in making an effort to facilitate the transaction between family and community. As family advocates, we must be familiar with our local community resources such as crisis centers, community mental health centers, telephone hotlines, support groups, religious institutions, acute care facilities, and specific names of mental health professionals. The goal is to provide opportunities for people who are psychiatrically disabled to maximize their ability to live, work, socialize, and learn in communities of their choice. Working together, consumers, families, and health care providers can develop strategies to help clients achieve lives of value, meaning, and better health, and become contributing members of their communities.

The National Alliance for the Mentally Ill (NAMI) is a grassroots, self-help, support and advocacy organization of people with mental illness and their families and friends. NAMI's mission is to eradicate mental illness and to improve the quality of life for those who suffer from these brain diseases. Local self-help support groups enable members to share concerns, learn about mental disorders, and receive practical advice on treatment and community resources. NAMI provides up-to-date scientific information through publications, the Helpline, and an annual Mental Illness Awareness Week campaign. At federal, state, and local levels, NAMI demands improved services for people who are psychiatrically disabled, such as greater access to treatment, housing, and employment, and better health insurance. NAMI actively supports increased federal and private funding for research into causes and treatments of severe mental illnesses. See the Community Resources section at the end of this chapter for information on NAMI.

Mental health nurses are expected to systematically assess families; identify their structure, development, communication, and decision-making patterns; and recognize and refer multistressed families for family therapy. Family therapists should be specially educated in the practice of family therapy. Increasing numbers of psychiatric nurse practitioners and clinical specialists are being prepared in graduate programs that provide both theory and supervised clinical practice in this specialized area. Although undergraduate nursing programs focus on the importance of family nursing, they do not prepare nurses as family therapists.

THE NURSE AS SPIRITUAL CAREGIVER

Any serious illness, but perhaps especially a mental illness, is really a disease process. Both the illness and the associated stigma eat away at people's spirits, and they often feel beaten and broken. They begin to believe that their worth and value as a human being is diminished. As nurses, we must respond to the whole person, who is at once spirit, mind, and body. People who are psychiatrically disabled are entitled to dignified and meaningful lives.

Spiritual care includes developing caring and thoughtful relationships. We must foster family attitudes that arise out of people's spiritual dimension, such as love, forgiveness, hopefulness, and acceptance. Spiritual caregiving includes helping "patients" stop being patients and instead become active consumers and collaborators. Supporting individuals and families who seek ways to heal and achieve balance in their lives is an important aspect of spiritual nursing care.

CHAPTER REVIEW

COMMUNITY RESOURCES

Links to these Web sites can be accessed on the Companion Web site for this book.

American Association for Marriage and Family Therapy
1133 15th St. NW, Suite 300
Washington, DC 20005
202-452-0109
www.aamft.org

Federation of Families for Children's Mental Health
1021 Prince St.
Alexandria, VA 22314-2971
703-684-7710
www.ffcmh.org

National Alliance for the Mentally Ill (NAMI)
200 N. Glebe Rd., Suite 1015
Arlington, VA 22203-3754
800-950-6264
www.nami.org

National Resource Network on Child and Family Mental Health Services
777 N. Capital St., NE, Suite 800
Washington, DC 20002
202-408-9320
www.wbgh.com

BOOKS FOR CLIENTS AND FAMILIES

Brown, E. M. (1989). *My parents' keeper: Adult children of the emotionally disturbed.* Oakland, CA: New Harbinger.

Carter, R. E., & Galant, S. K. (1998). *Helping someone with mental illness: Compassionate guide for family and friends and caregivers.* New York: Time Books.

Secunda, V. (1997). *When madness comes home: Help and hope for the children, siblings, and partners of the mentally ill.* New York: Hyperion Books.

KEY CONCEPTS

Introduction

- Families include couples, traditional families, lesbian and gay families, communal families, families with cohabiting parents, extended families, and even friends living together.

- The competency model of family nursing is based on the belief that all families are resourceful and have the capacity to grow and change.

- Family communication is measured by focusing on the family as a group with regard to their listening skills, speaking skills, self-disclosure, tracking, and ability to resolve conflict.

- Boundaries define the amount and kind of contact allowable between family members and between the family and outside systems. Boundaries are described as clear, rigid, or diffuse.

- Family cohesion (emotional bonding) ranges from disen-

gaged to separated to connected to enmeshed, with the central ranges being the most functional.

- Family flexibility in leadership, roles, and rules ranges from rigid to structured to flexible to chaotic, with the central ranges most functional.

- Emotional availability is another way to describe the quality of parent–child interactions. Areas for assessment include parental sensitivity, structuring, nonintrusiveness, and nonhostility.

- Care for the mentally ill has become as much family based as community based in the U.S.

- Family burden is the overall level of distress experienced as a result of mental illness.

- Objective family burden includes managing symptomatic behaviors, caregiving responsibilities, and the experience of stigma.

KEY CONCEPTS *(continued)*

- Subjective family burden includes feelings of grief and loss, a sense of chronic sorrow, and empathetic pain for the loved one.

- The stages of family recovery are discovery and denial; recognition and acceptance; coping and competence; and personal and political advocacy.

Mental Disorders Across the Life Span

- Pregnancy may precipitate the onset of a mental illness or contribute to the exacerbation of a disorder.

- Problems to be addressed are medications and fetal defects, inadequate prenatal care, inability to care for a newborn, and disruption of the family system.

- When a child or adolescent experiences a mental disorder, the parental subsystem and the sibling subsystem may be severely strained.

- Depression can contribute to relationship problems and relationship problems can precipitate depression.

- The burden of family caregiving for adult children with mental disorders includes daily caretaking, emotional drain, and financial strain.

Death and the Family System

- Bereavement is the feelings, thoughts, and responses that happen to us when a person dies. Grief and mourning are active processes of learning to adapt to the death or loss.

- Families teach us how to behave and the way we should express our feelings when a significant death occurs.

- Family coping strategies include reestablishing a stable equilibrium, realigning family roles, and communicating clearly.

- Disenfranchised grief means that the loss cannot be openly acknowledged, socially validated, or publicly mourned.

- Complicated grief occurs when there is enormous social, psychological, and medical morbidity.

Family Nursing Practice

- Nurses must develop collaborative relationships with clients and families.

- Assessment questions share our experience of and our interactions with clients and families. We must actively assess the resourcefulness of the family system.

Assessment of Vulnerability to Relapse

- Both high EE and SA families are predictors of relapse for people who are psychiatrically disabled.

- Medication noncompliance and substance abuse are other changeable factors related to relapse.

Cultural Assessment

- The egocentric self, usually found in Western industrialized societies, exhibits characteristics such as individualism, separateness, autonomy, competition, and mastery and control over one's environment.

- The sociocentric self, found in many non-Western societies, is interdependent and interconnected and values cooperation, cohesiveness, group identity, and harmony with one's environment.

The Nurse as Educator, Referral Agent, and Spiritual Caregiver

- Psychoeducation includes illness education, conflict management skills, problem solving, and stress management.

- Clients and families know more about their lives and are the best judges for future direction.

- Mental health nurses are expected to systematically assess families and make appropriate referrals to community resources and, if appropriate, for family therapy.

- Spiritual caregiving includes developing caring and thoughtful relationships, fostering positive family attitudes, helping people become active consumers and collaborators, and supporting families who seek ways to heal and achieve balance in their lives.

EXPLORE *MediaLink*

- Interactive resources, including animations, for this chapter can be found on the Companion Web site at *http://www.prenhall.com/fontaine.* Click on Chapter 3 and select the activities for this chapter.

- For NCLEX review questions and an audio glossary, access the accompanying CD-ROM in this book.

REFERENCES

Allen, K. R., Fine, M. A., & Demo, D. H. (2000). An overview of family diversity. In D. H. Demo, K. R. Allen, & M. A. Fine (Eds.), *Handbook of family diversity* (pp. 1–14). New York: Oxford University Press.

Badger, T. A. (1996). Living with depression. *Journal of Psychosocial Nursing, 34*(1), 21–29.

Bailine, S. H., Dean, M. D., Weiner, R. D., & Tramontozzi, L. A. (2000). Comparison of bifrontal and bitemporal ECT for major depression. *American Journal of Psychiatry, 157*(1), 121–123.

Barrio, C. (2000). The cultural relevance of community support programs. *Psychiatric Services, 51*(7), 879–884.

Biringen, Z. (2000). Emotional availability: Conceptualization and research findings. *American Journal of Orthopsychiatry, 70*(1), 104–114.

Deater-Deckard, K., Pickering, K., Dunn, J. F., & Golding, J. (1998). Family structure and depressive symptoms in men preceding and following the birth of a child. *American Journal of Psychiatry, 155*(6), 818–823.

Johnson, E. D. (2000). Differences among families coping with serious mental illness: A qualitative analysis. *American Journal of Orthopsychiatry 70*(1), 126–134.

Landmark study reveals hellish lives for children with severe mental illnesses and their families. (1999). *NAMI Advocate, 21*(1), 25.

Marsh, D. T. (1998). *Serious mental illness and the family.* New York: John Wiley & Sons.

McGoldrick, M., & Walsh, F. (1999). Death and the family life cycle. In B. Carter & M. McGoldrick (Eds.), *The expanded family life cycle* (3rd ed.) (pp. 185–201). Boston: Allyn and Bacon.

Mental health: A report of the Surgeon General (1999). Rockville, MD: U.S. Department of Health and Human Services, Substance Abuse and Mental Health Services Administration. Center for Mental Health Services, National Institutes of Health, National Institute of Mental Health.

Mohr, W. K., Lafuze, J. E., & Mohr, B. D. (2000). Opening caregiver minds: National Alliance for the Mentally Ill's (NAMI) Provider Education Program. *Archives of Psychiatric Nursing, 14*(5), 235–243.

Mohr, W. K., & Regan-Kubinski, M. J. (2001). Living in the fallout: Parents' experiences when their child becomes mentally ill. *Archives of Psychiatric Nursing, 15*(2), 69–77.

Olson, D. H. (1996). Clinical assessment and treatment interventions using the family circumplex model. In F. W. Kaslow (Ed.), *Handbook of relational diagnosis and dysfunctional family patterns* (pp. 59–77). New York: John Wiley & Sons.

Pickens, J. (1998). Formal and informal care of people with psychiatric disorders. *Journal of Psychosocial Nursing, 36*(1), 37–43.

Pratt, C. W., Gill, K. J., Barrett, N. M., & Roberts, M. M. (1999). *Psychiatric rehabilitation.* San Diego: Academic Press.

Rose, L. E. (1997). Caring for caregivers: Perceptions of social support. *Journal of Psychosocial Nursing, 35*(2), 17–24.

Sveinbjarnardottir, E., & de Casterle, B. D. (1997). Mental illness in the family: An emotional experience. *Issues in Mental Health Nursing, 18*(1), 45–56.

Teschinsky, U. (2000). Living with schizophrenia: The family illness experience. *Issues in Mental Health Nursing, 21*(4), 387–396.

Viguera, A. C., Nonacs, R., Cohen, L. S., Tondo, L., Murray, A. B., & Baldesscrini, R. J. (2000). Risk of recurrence of bipolar disorder in pregnant and nonpregnant women after discontinuing lithium maintenance. *American Journal of Psychiatry, 157*(2), 179–185.

Walsh, F. (1998). Beliefs, spirituality, and transcendence. In M. McGoldrick (Ed.), *Revisiting family therapy* (pp. 62–77). New York: Guilford Press.

Wuerker, A. K. (2000). The family and schizophrenia. *Issues in Mental Health Nursing, 21*(1), 127–141.

The Community

in MENTAL HEALTH NURSING

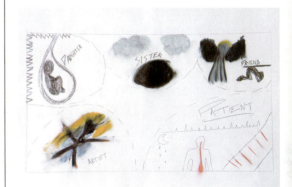

OBJECTIVES

After reading this chapter, you will be able to:

- ASSIST clients in making appropriate housing choices.

- DISTINGUISH among various community settings providing care.

- DESCRIBE the principles of psychosocial rehabilitation.

- IDENTIFY the characteristics of community mental health nursing practice and discuss the advantages for the consumer and the community.

*R*oles

Daughter: Created to become a creator

Sister: A rock to weather life's turmoil

Friend: The duty to protect and the comfort of protection

Artist: The gift of making an ugly world tolerable

Patient: To live a life of night scares, starvation, and mutilation

—Kate, Age 19

MediaLink

CD-ROM
- *Audio Glossary*
- *NCLEX Review*

Companion Web site www.prenhall.com/fontaine
- *Critical Thinking*
- *More NCLEX Review*
- *Case Study*
- *Care Map Activity*
- *Links to Resources*

Ideas about where and how treatment is rendered to clients in need of mental health care have changed drastically during the past five decades. Prior to the 1960s, most clients with mental disorders were institutionalized in long-term care facilities, some never leaving the institution in their lifetime. In 1955, the U.S. government established a commission to create a comprehensive plan for meeting the population's mental health care needs. In 1963, Congress passed an act that was the beginning of the *community mental health movement*. This act was based on the philosophy that individuals would receive better care if they remained in the local communities they knew and were not separated from their families and friends. The general plan was a complete array of community-based services available to all people seeking mental health care. Each community mental health center was expected to provide five basic services: inpatient care, outpatient care, emergency care, partial hospitalization, and consultation and education to the community. In addition to mental health centers, the plan included aftercare programs, halfway houses, and foster care.

The vision was a noble one, but by the 1990s it was clear that the system fell far short of the original goals. Programs such as individual or relationship therapy, employee assistance, crisis intervention, stress reduction, and grief therapy are usually available to people who can pay at least a minimal fee. Unfortunately, services for those who are psychiatrically disabled are often disorganized and poorly funded. People who are persistently mentally ill are often unable to cope with the complex public system of care. When one's thoughts are disorganized, it is difficult and frustrating to try to locate appropriate help. Because they have been ill for years and often unable to work, they frequently have extremely limited financial resources. As a result, those who are psychiatrically disabled may be homeless, live in shelters, or have rooms in cheap boarding hotels. At times, they may be brought to the acute care setting by case managers or the police. After being stabilized by medication, they are discharged back into the community, only to begin the vicious cycle over again. If individuals are a danger to themselves or others, they may be referred or court-ordered to a public long-term care facility. There is usually a waiting list for these facilities, and there is often inadequate funding for quality care. Following long-term treatment, clients are once again discharged back into the community.

With the passage of the *Americans with Disabilities Act (ADA)* in 1990, our society has made it a priority to promote full participation of people with psychiatric disabilities into the economic and social mainstream. To accomplish this goal, mental health services changed the focus from inpatient care to family and community care. In the past, professionals greatly underestimated the abilities of clients to make choices for themselves and determine the course of their lives. Through stressing the importance of consumer choice, the self-help and mental health consumer movements have demonstrated that psychiatrically disabled individuals can live successfully in local communities when given appropriate supports.

There are several principles that help guide how community mental health care is provided to consumers. The principle of **normalization** affirms that people with disabilities should be able to lead as normal a life as possible. This involves making modifications to both the physical environment, such as housing options, and the social environment, such as family respite care, community education, and employment opportunities. One goal of normalization is integration into the mainstream community. Integration is not simply physically housing disabled individuals within the community; it includes teaching necessary social skills to consumers as well as educating members of the community at large. With real integration comes *destigmatization* of those who are psychiatrically disabled. Another goal of normalization is one of *independence*. This means creating opportunities for clients to develop their own senses of autonomy and self-help. Professionals and family members don't "do for" clients but rather help them with doing (Pratt, Gill, Barrett, & Roberts, 1999).

Another principle of community mental health care is that of **contextualization**, or maintaining clients in their context. This means that clients are kept in as close contact as possible with their usual surroundings, both geographic and interpersonal. There may be temporary displacements, such as utilizing a transitional residential facility, but the long-range goal is living in their desired community. Another principle is *choice*. Consumer choice is critical to community mental health care. Having choices helps people cope with stressful situations and increases feelings of competence. The principle of **self-advocacy** arises out of the belief that those who are most affected by decisions should have the greatest impact on those decisions. This means advocating to be listened to when setting treatment goals and determining their own care.

In the recent past there has been a shift in relationships between mental health nurses and those who use their services. This shift is reflected in commonly used terms: Once it was *patients,* then it was *clients,* and now it is *consumers.* This change in language demonstrates an increasing awareness of persons with mental illnesses as autonomous individuals who have preferences and make choices (Pratt et al., 1999).

TREATMENT SETTINGS AND SERVICES

Prior to the 1950s, society believed that people with mental disorders could be treated only in hospitals. In the 1960s and 1970s, studies began to demonstrate that it was possible to treat even acutely ill people at home. Recent research provides evidence that community care is often as effective as hospital care and is significantly less costly.

Consumers of mental health services may receive their care in a variety of settings. These settings vary with regard to the types of services offered; the amount of support, structure, and restrictiveness; and the hours of operation. Community treatment for those who are psychiatrically disabled should focus on helping them learn basic coping skills necessary to live as autonomously and in the **least restrictive environment** as possible.

HOSPITALS

There are a small group of clients who require *long-term hospitalization* for their own safety as well as for the protection of family and community. These individuals profit most from treatment programs that emphasize highly structured behavioral interventions such as a token economy, point systems, and skills training that can improve their level of functioning.

Treatment in *acute care hospitals* has the advantage of providing a safe, structured, and supervised environment, lowering the stress on both consumers and family members. There are some situations in which inpatient care is the preferred setting: for consumers who are a danger to themselves or others, such as those who are acutely suicidal or homicidal; for those who are acutely psychotic and thus a serious danger to themselves because of confusion and disorganization; and for treatment of acute intoxicated states and withdrawal from alcohol or drugs. Stays have been reduced to three to eight days. Hospitalization allows the health care team to closely monitor the level of symptoms and reactions to treatments.

Day hospitalization can be used as an alternative to inpatient care or following a brief hospitalization. The advantage over inpatient care is less disruption of the person's life and treatment in a less restrictive environment. The person should not be at risk of harming self or others and should be able to cooperate minimally in treatment. People participating in day hospitalization programs typically attend the program for six to eight hours a day and are at home, work, or school the other hours. Services provided include medication administration and monitoring; group, individual, and expressive therapies; and opportunities for recreation and socialization.

OUTPATIENT SERVICES

Day treatment programs are used to provide ongoing supportive care and are usually not time limited. They provide structure and programs to help prevent relapse and to improve social and vocational functioning. They may also provide family therapy. There is a gradual introduction to the type of structured activities encountered in a full day of employment. Clients may be employed part-time while in the program. Day treatment programs have low staff-to-client ratios and minimal or no nursing staff.

Medication clinics are part of a more comprehensive program. They are helpful to clients who cannot manage their medications on their own. Nurses administer medications as well as monitor for side effects. Client education is a major focus of these clinics.

Psychosocial clubhouses are therapeutic communities where staff function as coaches whose role is to encourage decision making and socialization by the "members" of the club. Clubhouses exist primarily to improve the quality of life of their members. Members are accepted without regard to their symptoms, and they can stay as long as they like. Club activities focus on recreational, vocational, and residential functions. The approach is transitional, with individuals gradually assuming more responsibility and privileges.

HOUSING

Supportive housing is a program used for consumers who do not live on their own or with their families and who would benefit from some degree of assistance in self-care and self-management. These programs can increase social and vocational functioning, improve quality of life, and decrease homelessness and rehospitalization. Alternative housing often enables people with disabilities to increase their independence and develop the capacity to live as independently as possible.

Most consumers with psychiatric disabilities prefer their own residence and want autonomy over their housing choices. Most consumers prefer an apartment or a house that allows them to live independently. Consumers who live in transitional housing often see these arrangements as stepping-stones to greater independence. See Box 4.1 for types of residential facilities.

Studies have demonstrated that perceived choice over one's living arrangements is important to physical and psychological well-being. Increasing choice over housing can reduce the stress of repeated moves. When basic housing needs are satisfactorily met, consumers can begin to focus on other goals, such as employment, making friends, and participating in community activities.

BOX 4.1

Types of Residential Facilities

Transitional Halfway Houses
- Provide room and board until suitable housing is available

Long-term Group Residences
- On-site staff
- Appropriate for psychiatrically disabled person
- Length of stay is indefinite

Cooperative Apartments/Supported Housing
- No on-site staff
- Staff members make regular visits to assist residents

Intensive Care or Crisis Community Residences
- Used to help prevent hospitalization or shorten length of hospitalization
- On-site nursing staff and counseling staff

Foster or Family Care
- In private homes
- Close supervision of foster family to assure a therapeutic environment

Nursing Homes
- Appropriate for some psychiatric clients who are geriatric or medically disabled
- Psychiatric clients may have facilities or units separate from residents without a history of mental illness
- Activity programs and psychiatric supervision

The goal of consumer choice in supported housing has not yet been achieved. Many consumers believe that they have little or no choice and that their choices are highly or completely influenced by others. People who are psychiatrically disabled may be living on SSI (Supplemental Security Income) or SSDI (Social Security Disability Insurance), which are inadequate to rent even "affordable housing" in the United States. The vast majority receive less than $600 per month for total living expenses, which includes supplements provided by most programs to help pay rent. As nurses, we must become advocates at community, state, and federal levels to secure decent and affordable housing of choice in communities that consumers can call home.

Individuals who are psychiatrically disabled may need *social skills training* to enable them to live successfully in the community. Social skills training includes such things as personal hygiene and grooming skills, self-care, communication, time management, handling money, leisure activities, meal preparation, use of resources, and problem-solving skills. Consumers learn to interact appropriately with strangers, family members, and friends, both at work and at school. Social skills training fosters their ability to live and work in their communities just like anyone else. (See Chapter 10 for further information on social skills training.)

CRISIS RESPONSE SERVICES

In the traditional mental health system, the hospital is used to stabilize acute illness, but staff may have limited ability to help clients adapt to the real world on discharge. Psychiatrically disabled clients often cannot or will not follow up with services at a clinic, resulting in relapse into acute illness. Family or police bring them to the emergency department, where they are admitted to the acute care setting. This perpetuates the cycle of crisis–rehospitalization–discharge–crisis. Some people go into crisis because they are unable to understand their everyday problems and are unable to participate in a complex treatment plan. Some are unable to access their own care because the services are limited, expensive, and often inconvenient. Some go into crisis due to lack of housing, an absence of a social group, or relapse with drugs or alcohol. These problems result in feelings of shame, humiliation, and guilt. One person in crisis has an impact on the lives of others in the community—friends, family, neighbors, co-workers, and passersby. Those around the individual in crisis can be fearful, rejecting, or even hostile.

Residential crisis services are a new alternative to hospitalization and are provided in neighborhood homes that are staffed and organized to treat acutely ill clients. Consumers include adolescents with psychiatric problems, people in an acute psychiatric emergency resulting from a life crisis, or other individuals with acute psychiatric episodes. The residential crisis service offers a respite from their current living situation, which may be stressful or unsatisfactory, and provides intensive treatment in a program that utilizes medications, milieu therapy, and other forms of therapy.

Many acutely mentally ill people can be evaluated, treated, and stabilized by bringing therapists directly to clients in crisis. *Mobile emergency treatment* services bridge the gap between inpatient, outpatient, and family-based care. Some clients are too anxious, fearful, agitated, or depressed to come into traditional treatment settings. Visiting clients in their own environment helps the professional maximize clients' home and community resources. Emergency services need to be available when clients' coping skills are overwhelmed or when mental illness worsens and clients begin to experience dangerous symptoms.

Mobile crisis services are staffed by interdisciplinary teams of psychiatrists, nurses, social workers, psychologists, and counselors. The team is available 24 hours a day, 365 days a year. The mobile team may be called to private homes, group homes, shelters, hotels, street corners, malls, public buildings, recreational areas, police stations, or anywhere in the entire community. In the majority of requests for mobile assistance, professionals are at little, if any, risk. However, if the situation is potentially dangerous—an assaultive person, one who is suicidal, or a homicidal person with a weapon—the team members attempt to calm and support the client over the phone before or during their ride to the client's location. In this type of situation, the police are always asked to accompany the treatment team. The client must be informed that the police will be coming along and that the police will leave once everything is under good control. If clients are not manageable in the community setting, the team will bring them into the hospital (Turnbaugh, 1999). See Box 4.2 for intervention guidelines.

COMMUNITY SERVICES

CASE MANAGEMENT

The theory behind case management is effective collaboration with nursing, medicine, home care, ambulatory care, and administration. The goals are to increase appropriate use of resources, encourage collaborative team practice, facilitate continuity of care, and decrease length of need for services in order to promote quality and cost-effective outcomes. Case managers are currently employed in almost every imaginable health care setting, including acute care hospitals, rehabilitation facilities, community centers, outpatient clinics, and home care. Case managers are responsible for a number of activities. First, they *identify clients*, deter-

BOX 4.2

Intervention Guidelines for Mobile Crisis Services

Control Behavior

- Use the approach that is least restrictive but that maximizes safety for everyone.
- Make sure you are not alone, especially in a closed-in area.
- Remain calm and be observant as you approach the client.
- Remove items that could become harmful, such as ties, necklaces, large or dangly earrings, pens, and pencils. Stop about six feet away.
- Introduce yourself and address client by last name. Ask permission to use client's first name.
- If you do not feel endangered, ask whether client will shake hands with you.
- Explain procedures using simple, ordinary language, for example, "I need to check your blood pressure."

Assess Quickly

- Rule out a potentially life-threatening process that could be causing client's psychiatric signs and symptoms, such as hypoglycemia, head injury, or neurological illness.
- Look for Med-Alert bracelet, signs of injury.

Treat Specifically

- Psychotic and agitated behavior must be treated vigorously by ensuring a safe environment. Restraints are used only as a last resort.
- Appropriate medication will decrease violent symptoms and rapidly decrease the danger to self and others.

mining whose needs are congruent with the available services and resources. At times, they may increase access to services through outreach to difficult-to-reach people such as those who are homeless. At other times, they may limit services by ensuring that only those who are eligible will receive services. Once case managers identify clients, they must *assess individual needs and strengths*. Case managers work with other providers to determine the best way to meet those needs and support skills and strengths. This planning determines linkage, the next step in treatment. The case manager links clients to available services by helping them meet the qualifying criteria. If services are inaccessible, case managers may *broker for services*; that is, they create access to services. They also serve as advocates when they negotiate with agencies and policy makers in an effort to gain resources for consumers. Coordination ensures that providers deliver service in a consistent manner. Almost all case managers also provide *direct care* in the form of a therapeutic relationship, supportive psychotherapy, and crisis response (Nehls, 2000).

COMMUNITY-BASED NURSING PRACTICE

The goal of community mental health nursing is to promote health and provide opportunities for consumers to maximize their ability to live, work, socialize, and learn in the communities of their choice. Expanding consumer "voice" and choice continues to be the major focus for nurses working in the community. Successful support means that consumers of mental health services will be able to achieve lives of value and become contributing members of their communities.

Community-based nurses have distinct advantages in providing care, including a firsthand opportunity to observe clients and their families in a natural setting. These nurses are able to more accurately assess and intervene with clients when they understand the problems that are troublesome to people in their daily living encounters in the community. Understanding the social context of specific stressors, nurses can also identify possible pitfalls to effective interventions. In addition, community-based nurses focus on those problems identified by clients as most important in their daily lives.

SCREENING PROGRAMS

Community screening programs help provide early identification of mental health problems. Indications for using a screening test are that it is not readily apparent to people that they are suffering from the disorder, that the disorder is prevalent in the population and is treatable, and that early intervention will make a difference in the outcome. There must also be an accurate and cost-effective screening tool. A number of physical conditions meet these requirements, such as hypertension, breast cancer, lead screening, and stroke risk assessment. Screening for mental disorders is relatively new. National Depression Screening Day, begun in 1991, was the first national, community-based, voluntary screening program for mental illness. Research suggests that the program has been effective in bringing individuals with depression into treatment. Those clients who do not comply with screening recommendations to seek treatment often have misinformation about the disorder or lack financial means or insurance to seek additional evaluation and intervention. Other at-risk groups that would benefit from screening programs include single parents with young children, teen parents, victims of family and community violence, and older adults living alone. Community outreach must be increased to ensure that those who are at risk for or suffer from mental disorders receive appropriate and adequate assistance.

HOME SETTING

Providing mental health services to consumers and their families in their homes is a fairly new initiative in the mental health field. There are some distinct advantages of home care treatment. Direct observation of family interactions leads to more accurate evaluation of strengths and limitations. (See Chapter 2 for family assessment.) Home visits facilitate the participation of all family members including young children. Since the family is in their own home and the nurse is a guest, family members often feel more in control and empowered in the relationship. Consumers and families report more communication with staff, increased participation in treatment decisions, and being cared for with dignity and respect. Other advantages are that daily routines are less disrupted, relationships are less restricted, and levels of anxiety are minimized (Fagin, 2001).

Home treatment may be an alternative to inpatient treatment during the acute phase of a mental illness. Acute home care treatment involves the provision of intensive support through home visits by nurses, social workers, psychiatrists, and homemakers. Staff are available 24 hours per day and provide services such as medication management, interpersonal support for consumers and caregivers, behavioral management, maintenance of housing, assistance with activities of daily living (ADLs), reality orientation, and social/recreational activities. Once clients stabilize, they return to their case manager team for continuing support (Fagin, 2001).

Home health care nurses must always consider their own safety. If possible, they should call ahead and let the client know their arrival time. Family members or friends may be called on to escort the nurse from the car to the home if there are concerns about neighborhood safety. Portable phones should be turned on and programmed to speed-dial 911 in case of emergency. Once in the home, nurses must be alert to situations that might be risky, such as agitation, suspicious thinking, hostility, and threats. If calmness and nonthreatening support are ineffective in deescalating the threatening behaviors, calling for emergency assistance may be necessary (Worley, 1997).

SCHOOL SETTING

Nationwide, only one third of the children who need mental health services actually receive it. The main barriers to care are availability, accessibility, and affordability. In some cases, services may not be available; in others, families may be unaware of the available services. There may also be cultural barriers such as language differences or a poor ethnic match between consumers and providers of care. Access is a major problem for children since they are unable to seek mental health services for themselves and are dependent on adults, such as parents or teachers, to recognize this need and to initiate contact. Other accessibility problems are transportation, day care, and parental schedules. Many children and families cannot afford services and are unaware that care may be available at adjusted rates or even no cost (Armbruster, Gerstein, & Fallon, 1997; Fagin, 2001).

In a few locations, mental health services have teamed up with schools to provide services to behaviorally and emotionally disordered children. Services integrated into the school setting seem more natural for children and parents and improve access and limit barriers. Teachers often know the child and family well and are able to provide valuable information regarding strengths and weaknesses. The community mental health nurse is able to observe the child in the classroom, lunchroom, and playground, which provides a broader and more useful picture of both problems and assets. As communities broaden their outreach into the school system, an increased number of children with a wide range of psychiatric and behavioral problems will have their mental health needs met regardless of their ability to afford or access mental health care.

HOMELESS POPULATIONS

For the past 25 years, over one-half million Americans have been left **homeless**, living on city streets, and, if they are lucky, sleeping in emergency shelters each night. The homeless include people of every race, ethnic background, and educational level. It is difficult to estimate the number of homeless people with mental illness, but it is believed that one third have severe mental illness and up to one half of these have a concurrent substance use disorder. This is a deeply disadvantaged and difficult-to-reach-and-treat population (Rosenheck, 2000).

Chronic *substance abusers* may end up with no home if they are abandoned by families and friends. If the disease has interfered with the ability to maintain a job, the person may be forced to live on the streets. Homeless solitary women have higher rates of substance abuse than homeless mothers do.

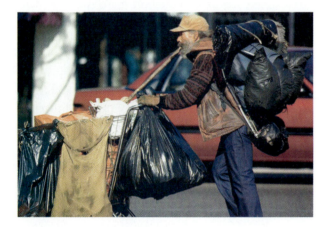

PHOTO 4.1 ■ Lacking adequate funding and staff, mental hospitals frequently failed to provide adequate treatment to their residents. Beginning in the 1950s and 1960s, the policy of deinstitutionalization led to the release of many individuals, who, without proper follow-up care, ended up living on the streets. Although not all homeless people are mentally ill, estimates suggest that between 30 and 50 percent of homeless persons suffer from some type of mental disorder.

SOURCE: Tom Prettyman/PhotoEdit.

Families now constitute 37 percent of the homeless population. Many homeless families are headed by women who take their children and flee from an abusive husband or partner. Homeless families may lose their sense of identity as a family, parents lose their sense of competence, and children lose the idea of home (Bassuk, Buckner, Perloff, & Bassuk, 1998).

Many *adolescents* find themselves living on their own as a consequence of running away from home or being thrown out by their families. Some have been physically or sexually abused in their homes. In other situations, parents of acting-out adolescents may force the teenager out of the home as a way to gain control in their own lives. Adolescents also become homeless because of family conflict, chaotic family systems, and unsuccessful foster care situations.

Nurses help the homeless population through outreach, social support groups, case management, and provision of transitional housing. Outreach to homeless people includes advertising in missions and shelters, using former "street people" as liaison staff, and using mobile crisis services. The purpose of outreach is to explain the available services and help homeless consumers negotiate the system.

Nurse-managed outreach clinics often provide care to homeless people. This is an appropriate setting as homelessness contributes to multiple health problems such as respiratory infections, tuberculosis, trauma, hypertension, and peripheral vascular disease. Vulnerability to infection places this population at higher risk for human immunodeficiency virus (HIV) and hepatitis B and C infections. Lack of access for good hygiene can lead to dental problems and skin problems such as lice, scabies, and impetigo. The inability to meet their self-care needs contributes to sustained feelings of despair and hopelessness (Gerberich, 2000).

Social support groups are set up in shelters, soup kitchens, drop-in centers, transitional housing units, and single-room occupancy (SRO) houses. Through these groups, nurses can empower consumers, increase their problem-solving skills, help them develop self-confidence, and support their identity with a group of people.

Through case management, nurses can help consumers negotiate appointments and services from a variety of agencies. Nurses may also monitor medication compliance, assist with ADLs, find appropriate shelter, and assist with the development of support systems.

RURAL SETTINGS

Increases in community-based services are needed in both rural and urban areas. However, rural communities face more severe challenges in meeting the mental health needs of their residents than do urban communities. Groups at greater risk for mental disorders, that is, those who are chronically ill, the poor, the dependent, and the elderly, are disproportionately represented in rural areas. Studies have consistently identified many rural services as fragmented, costly, and often ineffective. Poverty, inadequate transportation, and limited economic opportunities restrict treatment alternatives to the already insufficient numbers of mental health care providers.

Cost of services is a major barrier. Many of the newer psychotropic medications are very expensive. Of those individuals who have medical insurance, many lack coverage for psychotherapy even if they can find a therapist. Lack of quality inpatient care for acutely ill people is another problem in rural areas. These consumers are often hospitalized far from family and friends. Once discharged back into the community, there are limited psychosocial rehabilitation services available which frequently leads to repeat hospitalizations (National Institute of Mental Health [NIMH], 2000).

Although there are significant problems facing consumers who live in rural settings, there are also

---

CRITICAL THINKING

Marne has been working in a 10-bed psychiatric unit in a rural community hospital. The unit and the hospital's emergency services have experienced a gradual increase in demands for service over the last three years. The local community government and other community leaders, such as religious leaders and the school superintendent, have called for a review of psychiatric services and changes in the services provided. Marne has been asked to participate on the health care professional and community committee to develop a plan for change. Marne is excited about this opportunity as she feels that nursing concerns will be included in the final plan. She knows from her experience that rural services are often fragmented, costly, and often ineffective.

The committee collects data about the needs for mental health services in the community. Alcoholism is on the rise in two subpopulations: adolescents and young adults. There has been an increase in automobile accidents due to alcohol and admissions to emergency services for alcohol-related injuries and problems. In the past year, there was one adolescent suicide attempt and a suicide of a 16-year-old girl. This represents a substantial increase in suicidal behavior as there had not been any known attempts or suicides in the previous three years. Admissions to the inpatient unit have increased by 10 percent, and there have been times when patients have had to be sent to hospitals in other communities. Reviews of medical records indicate that some of these clients could have been treated in com-

munity settings if the settings had been available. Clients with long-term needs seem to get lost in the system. The committee was interested in obtaining more data about the prevalence of depression in the community.

1. At the first meeting of the committee, the chairperson mentioned the Americans with Disabilities Act (ADA). What is the relevance of this law to the purpose of the committee?

2. Marne brings up the importance of using the least restrictive environment for each client. One of the committee members, a teacher, asks Marne, "What do you mean by that? Are you talking about jail time? I thought everyone with mental illness needs to be hospitalized." How should Marne respond?

3. The chairperson felt that one of the first steps was to collect more data about community needs. What is one method that might be used to find out about community needs; for example, what is the number of people experiencing depression?

4. Based on the description of this rural community, what are some services that the committee might consider investigating to meet some of the community's needs?

For an additional Case Study, please refer to the Companion Web site for this book.

considerable community strengths in rural settings. Generally, rural communities have a strong loyalty to family, church, and community. This loyalty results in a higher degree of tolerance for perceived "abnormal behavior" among community members and a willingness to help those who are less fortunate. Depending on the rural community, there are indigenous care providers ranging from companion/aid to confidant/ therapist to healer/shaman. These natural helpers within the community may complement professional mental health providers and may also serve as a "bridge" between consumers and professionals.

COMMUNITY-BASED NURSING INTERVENTIONS

Community mental health services are often underused. It is estimated that about 28 percent of the U.S. population have significant mental health disorders, but half never seek treatment. In addition to the barriers previously mentioned, rigid bureaucratic guidelines and red tape are seen by consumers as derogatory or, at best, bothersome and unnecessary. Community-based services must be designed to minimize the problems of accessibility and promote entry into the care system. Staff must be educated about specific community issues. Treatment programs must actively involve consumers, such as developing outreach programs and home care programs, and offering comprehensive services, such as assistance with transportation and housing. Maintaining consumers in the community makes it possible for nurses to monitor the entire care process and remain involved until outcomes are achieved.

Community-based nursing interventions for diverse populations must be *culturally appropriate*. The egocentric orientation of Western cultures value independent action with the goal of psychosocial rehabilitation being one of autonomy and self-sufficiency. Those cultures with sociocentric orientations, however, typically reflect interdependence and family orientation. The rehabilitation goal of independence may not be culturally appropriate with these individuals. Thus, it is critically important that nursing interventions be relative to the culture of the consumers (Barrio, 2000).

Di, a 28-year-old Japanese American, came to the United States with his family when he was a teenager. He has continued to live at home while finishing college and starting his career. Having recently lost all his money and his job due to compulsive gambling, Di attempted suicide. He states that he cannot go back home because he has brought shame to his family, nor can he live apart from his family as he is unmarried.

BRIDGING STRATEGIES

Almost two thirds of the clients discharged from acute care facilities fail to keep outpatient referral appointments. Failure to engage in outpatient services increases the probability of relapse and rehospitalization. There are several strategies nurses can use to help people readjust to community living. These *bridging strategies* include sessions that make the family a part of the treatment team, linking family/friends to support services, communication regarding discharge plans between inpatient and outpatient staff, and enabling clients to begin outpatient programs before discharge. Successful community living means being adequately prepared for discharge and being linked to the appropriate community services (Boyer, McAlpine, Pottick, & Olfson, 2000).

COMMUNITY PROGRAMS

Assertive Community Treatment (*ACT*) allows consumers to live in their own communities while they receive the individual assistance they need with everyday life and managing their illness. ACT teams include a psychiatrist, nurses, social workers, peer specialists, a substance abuse specialist, and a vocational specialist. The team goes out to meet and work with the consumer, who does not have to make and keep office appointments. Team members help individuals find and keep housing and employment and manage everything from their medications to their money. Together, the ACT team and the consumer work to achieve the consumer's goals.

Psychogeriatric Assessment and Treatment in City Housing (*PATCH*) is an outreach program, in some areas of the country, for elderly public housing residents who need mental health care. Mental illness diagnosis and treatment is less likely to occur among the older population due to such factors as withdrawal, fearfulness, cognitive impairment, stigma, and decreased mobility. The PATCH team consists of two psychiatric nurses who are the service providers and two part-time psychiatrists who serve as consultants. PATCH has an extensive outreach program to identify individuals in need of care who are then provided with an in-home assessment by psychiatric nurses. Nurses serve as case managers and also provide direct care to the elderly residents. The program also has an educational arm geared toward lessening the stigma of mental illness and facilitating individuals' access to community services (Robbins et al., 2000).

SOCIAL NETWORK INTERVENTIONS

Social support has an effect on physical and mental status. Research indicates that people with more social resources, or networks, are better able to adapt to change and are in better health. Unfortunately, people who are psychiatrically disabled have fewer social networks and weaker support systems than people without mental illness do. This restricted network may not be able to provide the amount and type of support necessary for consumers to live in the community. Nursing can provide an important service: the enhancement of social support networks. This is accomplished by reinforcing existing ties, improving family ties, and building new ties.

Social network interventions are designed to improve the relationships within the consumer's social network. These interventions include peer consumer support, connection with indigenous healers, volunteer matching, family education and support, social skills training groups, and linkage with community resources. As networks increase in size and strength, consumers will be more able to remain in their communities of choice.

PSYCHOSOCIAL REHABILITATION

The field of psychosocial rehabilitation grew out of a need to create opportunities for people suffering from psychiatric disabilities. Psychosocial rehabilitation is the development of skills and supports necessary for successful living, learning, and working in the community. This approach creates collaborative partnerships with all interested people—consumers, families, friends, and mental health care providers. Recovery, a facet of reha-

bilitation, refers to incorporating the disability as part of reality, modifying dreams and aspirations, exploring new ideas, and eventually adapting to the disease. Each person's road to recovery is unique. It is assumed that the consumer will be "in charge" with regard to setting goals for where and how to live, work, learn, socialize, and recreate. Rehabilitation is a process, not a quick fix. This approach is quite different from the traditional approach to long-term consumers, where the assumption was that people with psychiatric disabilities needed to have decisions made for them.

People with mental illness differ little from the general population. They want work that is meaningful and self-enhancing and the opportunity to socialize with others. Psychosocial rehabilitation is anchored in the values of *hope* and optimism that people can grow, learn, and make changes in their lives. One essential element is *power*. People who have mental disorders need power and control in their relationships with professionals, in their own lives, and in the way resources are allocated. This allows them to take personal responsibility for where they are in their lives and where they are going (Test & Stein, 2000).

As a nurse, you not only provide care, but also work with clients to make decisions about treatment and about daily life. Recovery is about providing temporary support during hard times while working with clients to take responsibility for their own wellness. Box 4.3 lists guidelines for recovery-oriented nursing interventions.

Recovery is a personal choice. When you find resistance and apathy to recovery, you may feel frustrated as a nurse. It is important to recognize that severity of symptoms, motivation, and personality type can affect a person's ability to work toward recovery. Some people work at it intensely while others approach recovery more slowly. It is not up to you to determine when a person is ready to make progress—it is up to the person (Mead & Copeland, 2000). Box 4.4 lists the key aspects of recovery.

EDUCATION AND EMPLOYMENT

The 1990 *Individuals with Disabilities Education Act* (*IDEA*) mandates support for people with disabilities in educational settings. With the onset of a major mental illness in childhood or adolescence, educational programs are individualized to improve clients' level of academic functioning with the goal of enhancing quality

BOX 4.3

Guidelines for Recovery-Oriented Nursing Interventions

- Treat the person as an adult partner in care with the capacity and responsibility to learn, change, and make life decisions no matter how severe the symptoms.
- Make planning and treatment a truly collaborative process, with personal choice being most important.
- Accept that a person's life path is up to him or her.
- Never scold, threaten, punish, patronize, judge, or condescend to the person.
- Rather than focusing on a diagnosis or a label, concentrate on how the person feels, what the person is experiencing, and what the person wants.
- Limit the sharing of ideas. One idea a day or per visit is plenty. Avoid overwhelming the person.
- Pay close attention to individual needs and preferences.
- Implement evidence-based practice by learning about "best practices" based on scientific studies.

SOURCES: Adapted from Lehman, A. F. (2000). Putting recovery into practice. *Community Mental Health Journal, 36*(3), 329–331; and Mead, S., & Copeland, M. E. (2000). What recovery means to us: Consumers' perspectives. *Community Mental Health Journal, 36*(3), 315–328.

BOX 4.4

Key Aspects of Client Recovery

Hope
- Eliminate internalized dire predictions.
- Offer help as well as receive help.
- Take positive risks.

Self-Responsibility
- Work to heal oneself.
- Wellness is up to each individual.

Self-Advocacy
- Learn to see self as worthwhile and unique.
- Make treatment choices for self.
- Refuse treatments that are not in your best interests.
- Create your own advance directive.
- Create the life of your choice.

SOURCES: Adapted from Mead, S., & Copeland, M. E. (2000). What recovery means to us: Consumers' perspectives. *Community Mental Health Journal, 36*(3), 315–328; and Pratt, C. W., Gill, K. J., Barrett, N. M., & Roberts, M. M. (1999). *Psychiatric rehabilitation.* San Diego: Academic Press.

of life and developing career options. There are three types of supported postsecondary education programs. In the *self-contained classroom,* all the students have disabilities and the focus of the curriculum is on career planning and skill building. This is the least integrated model of the three. The *on-site support model* is the most common, with the goal of assisting students in utilizing resources that already exist within the college community. Services are provided through the Disabled Student Services or through Student Counseling Services. The *mobile support model* involves staff from the local mental health center as supports for individual students (Pratt et al., 1999).

The unemployment rate of people with psychiatric disabilities is 75 to 90 percent (Pratt et al., 1999).

However, many of these same individuals would benefit from work, as it can provide needed daily structure, an opportunity for socialization and meaningful activity, and self-sufficiency. Psychiatric disability and the accompanying unemployment, poverty, social stigma, hospitalizations, symptoms, and medication side effects contribute to lower quality of life. Being fired from a job or being persistently unemployed contribute to feelings of inadequacy and low self-esteem.

Not all consumers want to be employed, but many desire work and may need support in locating positions, filling out applications, role-playing interviews, and learning job expectations and behaviors. *Supported Employment (SE),* according to the Rehabilitation Act Amendments of 1998, means that ongoing support services are provided according to the needs of each individual. Some community mental health centers provide job coaches if necessary; these coaches work alongside consumers on the job until they can gradually be self-sufficient in the job. See Box 4.5 for vocational services.

BOX 4.5

Vocational Services

Transitional Employment

- Program of time-limited jobs in regular work settings
- Regular pay
- Agency staff provide training and support for that job
- When specified time of employment is over, job filled by another client

Job Club

- Structure and resources to assist members in own job search
- May not provide enough support for significantly disabled clients

Sheltered Workshops

- Workshop solicits manufacturing jobs from local business to provide work for people with disabilities
- May be a permanent placement or a step to competitive employment

Affirmative Industries

- Businesses are owned, managed, and operated by mental health agencies ranging from cleaning services to landscaping to bakeries and caterers.
- Clients are supervised by agency staff and paid by agency

Supported Employment

- Based on the philosophy that, given adequate supports, most people are capable of competitive employment
- Agency provides support services for people who are severely disabled

The financial disincentives to employment have yet to be addressed. Individuals receiving SSI or SSDI funds risk losing this financial assistance when they become employed, even in entry-level, low-wage positions. People who even take part-time work lose entitlement income including food stamps and rent subsidies, which amounts to an effective tax of 64 percent on their earnings. The greatest fear clients have is the loss of medical coverage. A way must be found to encourage employment while at the same time providing enough support to maintain community living and health care protection.

COMMUNITY RESOURCES

Links to these Web sites can be accessed on the Companion Web site for this book.

Association for Persons in Supported Employment
1627 Monument Ave.
Richmond, VA 23220
804-287-9187
www.apse.org

Center for Psychiatric Rehabilitation
Boston University
940 Commonwealth Ave. West
Boston, MA 02215
617-353-3549
www.bu.edu/sarpsych/reasaccom

Job Accommodation Network
West Virginia University
P.O. Box 6080
Morgantown, WV 26506-6080
800-526-7234
www.janweb.icdi.wvu.edu

National Association for Rural Mental Health
3700 W. Division St., Suite 105
St. Cloud, MN 56301
320-202-1820
www.narmh.org

National Coalition for the Homeless
1012 14th St. NW, Suite 600
Washington, DC 20005-3406
202-737-6444
www.nch.ari.net

National Rehabilitation Information Center
4200 Forbes Blvd., Suite 202
Lanham, MD 20706
800-346-2742
www.naric.com

National Resource Center on Homelessness
  and Mental Illness
Policy Research Associates, Inc.
262 Delaware Ave.
Delmar, NY 12054
800-444-7415
www.prainc.com/nrc

KEY CONCEPTS

Introduction

- The principle of normalization affirms that people with disabilities should be able to lead as normal a life as possible through integration into the mainstream community and support of independence.

- The principle of contextualization means that clients are kept in as close contact as possible with their usual surroundings.

Treatment Settings

- Treatment settings in the community include hospitals, day hospitals, day treatment programs, medication clinics, and psychosocial clubhouses.

- Types of residential facilities include halfway houses, long-term group residences, cooperative apartments, crisis community residences, foster care, and nursing homes.

- Most consumers prefer their own residence and want autonomy over their housing choices.

- Social skills training may be necessary to enable consumers to live successfully in the community.

Community Services

- The theory behind case management is effective collaboration with nursing, medicine, home care, ambulatory care, and administration.

- Case managers identify clients, assess individual needs and strengths, broker for services, and provide direct care.

- Residential crisis services offer a respite from the current living situation and provide intensive treatment in programs that utilize a variety of therapies.

- Mobile emergency treatment services are staffed by interdisciplinary teams and provide emergency mental health services anywhere in the community.

Community-Based Nursing Practice

■ Community screening programs help provide early identification of mental health problems.

■ Home treatment may be an alternative to inpatient treatment during the acute phase of a mental illness. This involves the provision of intensive support through home visits.

■ Mental health services within school systems improves access and affordability to children and parents in need of service.

■ Nurses help the homeless population through outreach, social support groups, case management, and provision of transitional housing.

■ Rural settings often have inadequate community-based services, but also provide more informal support to members of their communities.

Community-Based Nursing Interventions

■ Strategies to bridge inpatient with outpatient care include making the family a part of the treatment team, linking family to support services, staff communication, and enabling clients to begin outpatient programs before discharge.

■ Assertive Community Treatment (ACT) allows consumers to live in their own communities while they receive the individual assistance they need.

■ Psychogeriatric Assessment and Treatment in City Housing (PATCH) is an outreach program for elderly residents in need of mental health services.

■ Social network interventions are designed to improve relationships that helps clients better adapt to change.

■ Psychosocial rehabilitation emphasizes the development of skills and supports necessary for successful living, learning, and working in the community. It is anchored in the values of hope and power.

■ Recovery refers to incorporating the disability as part of reality, modifying dreams and aspirations, exploring new ideas, and eventually adapting to the disease.

■ Three types of educational programs for disabled persons are the self-contained classroom, the on-site support model, and the mobile support model.

■ Employment can provide needed structure and opportunity for socialization and meaningful activity.

EXPLORE *MediaLink*

■ Interactive resources, including animations, for this chapter can be found on the Companion Web site at *http://www.prenhall.com/fontaine.* Click on Chapter 4 and select the activities for this chapter.

■ For NCLEX review questions and an audio glossary, access the accompanying CD-ROM in this book.

REFERENCES

Armbruster, P., Gerstein, S. H., & Fallon, T. (1997). Bridging the gap between service need and service utilization: A school-based mental health program. *Community Mental Health Journal, 33*(3), 199–210.

Barrio, C. (2000). The cultural relevance of community support programs. *Psychiatric Services, 51*(7), 879–884.

Bassuk, E. L., Buckner, J. C., Perloff, J. N., & Bassuk, S. S. (1998). Prevalence of mental health and substance use disorders among homeless and low-income housed mothers. *American Journal of Psychiatry, 155*(11), 1561–1564.

Boyer, C. A., McAlpine, D. D., Pottick, K. J., & Olfson, M. (2000). Identifying risk factors and key strategies in linkage to outpatient psychiatric care. *American Journal of Psychiatry, 157*(10), 1592–1598.

Fagin, C. M. (2001). Revisiting treatment in the home. *Archives of Psychiatric Nursing, 15*(1), 3–9.

Gerberich, S. S. (2000). Care of homeless men in the community. *Holistic Nursing Practice, 14*(2), 21–28.

Lehman, A. F. (2000). Putting recovery into practice. *Community Mental Health Journal, 36*(3), 329–331.

Mead, S., & Copeland, M. E. (2000). What recovery means to us: Consumers' perspectives. *Community Mental Health Journal, 36*(3), 315–328.

National Institute of Mental Health. (2000). Rural mental health research at the National Institute of Mental Health. *http://www.nimh.gov/publicat/ruralresfact.cfm*

Nehls, N. (2000). Being a case manager for person with borderline personality disorder: Perspectives of community mental health center clinicians. *Archives of Psychiatric Nursing, 14*(1), 12–18.

REFERENCES *(continued)*

Pratt, C. W., Gill, K. J., Barrett, N. M., & Roberts, M. M. (1999). *Psychiatric rehabilitation.* San Diego: Academic Press.

Robbins, B., Rye, R., German, P. S., Tlasek-Wolfson, M., Penrod, J., Rabins, P. V., & Black, B. S. (2000). The psychogeriatric assessment and treatment in city housing (PATCH) program for elders with mental illness in public housing. *Archives of Psychiatric Nursing, 14*(4), 163–172.

Rosenheck, R. (2000). Cost-effectiveness of services for mentally ill homeless people. *American Journal of Psychiatry, 157*(10), 1563–1570.

Test, M. A., & Stein, L. I. (2000). Practical guidelines for the community treatment of markedly impaired patients. *Community Mental Health Journal, 36*(1), 47–60.

Turnbaugh, D. G. (1999). Crisis intervention teams. Curing police problems with people with mental illness. *NAMI Advocate, 21*(2), 11–12.

Worley, N. K. (1997). *Mental health nursing in the community.* St. Louis, MO: Mosby.

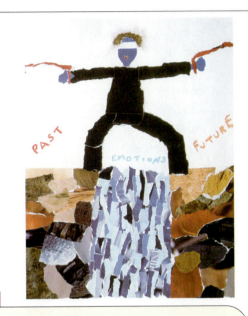

CHAPTER 5

The Role of Cultural Diversity

in MENTAL HEALTH NURSING

OBJECTIVES

After reading this chapter, you will be able to:

- EXAMINE ways in which values, attitudes, beliefs, and behaviors are related to health and illness.

- EXPLAIN the importance of understanding cultural diversity in mental health nursing.

- EXPLORE what happens when nurses and clients have different cultural values and social norms.

- DIFFERENTIATE between generalizations, stereotypes, prejudice, and discrimination.

- DESCRIBE racism-related stress factors.

- UTILIZE the heritage assessment tool.

*B*ridging Different Aspects of Identity

—*Kate, Age 19*

MediaLink

CD-ROM
- *Audio Glossary*
- *NCLEX Review*

Companion Web site www.prenhall.com/fontaine
- *Critical Thinking*
- *More NCLEX Review*
- *Case Study*
- *Care Map Activity*
- *Links to Resources*

KEY TERMS

A s a nation, the United States continues to change. As the new millennium begins, non–Euro-Americans comprise 29 percent of the U.S. population. By the year 2050, almost half of U.S. residents will trace their ancestry to Africa, Asia, the Pacific Islands, or the Hispanic or Arab worlds, rather than to Europe. That is a radical change for a country in which Euro-Americans have been the numerical majority and have held the bulk of the power, status, and wealth for several hundred years. In fact, even the term *minority status* is linked to power-lessness.

Some people find the trend toward increased ethnic and racial diversity threatening. Others view it as both an opportunity and a challenge to make the United States the type of democracy that it has idealized, but

that it has not, in fact, been. In any event, this transition, referred to as "the browning of America," is occurring. Nurses must be prepared to care for this diverse population, just as members of those diverse groups must be prepared to become nurses (Buerhaus & Auerbach, 1999; Zoucha & Husted, 2000).

The United States has more than 100 ethnic groups, whose members have thousands of beliefs and practices related to health and illness. There are over 500 Native People and native Alaskan tribes and nations alone, plus dozens of different Asian and Pacific Island cultures. Various subgroups of African Americans live in the United States, as do different "black" cultures from Africa, the Caribbean, and other parts of the world. There are also numerous Euro-American groups, each with its own ethnicity. The fastest-growing ethnic populations in the United States are Latino (also known as Hispanic), comprised of diverse nationalities, and Asian Pacific Americans, who include more than 50 distinct ethnic groups. Each of these major categories is so diverse that differences within groups may be as great as, or greater than, those among them. For instance, differences in the world-views and experiences of Oglala Sioux and Lumbee Indians, or of Puerto Ricans and Bolivians, or African Americans who are poor and those who are middle class, are often greater than differences between such visibly different groups as African Americans and Euro-Americans. In addition, many Americans cross group lines and have blended the identities of more than one racial and/or ethnic group. Therefore, it is simply not realistic to assume that nurses can know everything about groups that number in the millions and have great internal variation. However, we can educate ourselves to become culturally competent nurses.

Culture is a pattern of learned behavior based on values, beliefs, and perceptions of the world. Our culture teaches us how to view the world, how to experience it emotionally, and how to behave in relation to nature, higher powers, and other people. More important than a specific behavior are the underlying values, beliefs, and perceptions that encourage or discourage that particular behavior. Culture is taught and shared by members of a group or society. It is always in process and constantly changing. In contemporary social science, ethnic or national groups are loosely grouped together under the classification of modern or industrialized versus traditional or Western versus non-Western cultures.

A subculture is a smaller group within a large cultural group that shares values, beliefs, behaviors, and language. Although it is part of the larger group, a subculture is somewhat different. You may remember when you were a member of the teenage subculture. What you valued, what you believed in, and how you viewed the world may have been very different from your parents' subculture of adulthood. Your development and use of specific words, or informal language, may not have been understood by your parents. At the same time, both you and your family belonged to the larger cultural group with which you identified.

Ethnicity is ethnic affiliation, and a sense of belonging to a particular cultural group. Culture is so much a part of everyday life that it is taken for granted. We tend to assume that others share our own perspective, including those for whom we care. When we believe that our own culture is more important than, and preferable to, any other culture, we are expressing ethnocentrism. It is impossible to provide sensitive nursing care from an ethnocentric position.

Nursing must change to meet the needs of an increasingly diverse population. Diversity refers to variation among people. Customs and lifestyles that may seem strange to those outside a client's cultural group may be very important to that client. Valuing diversity in practicing nursing means helping clients reach their full potential, preserving their ways of doing things, and helping them change only those patterns that are harmful (Spector, 2000).

As people throughout the world become more mobile, both in traveling and resettling, nurses are increasingly faced with the prospect of caring for people from a culture different than their own. More than ever, there is a need for nursing care designed around unique cultural beliefs and the values and practices of clients. Therefore, understanding and respecting cultural diversity is basic to the individualization of nursing care through cultural competence.

A main reason for being flexible in handling diversity is that culture is only one way in which people differ. There are also differences in ethnicity, age, health status, experience, gender, sexual orientation, and other aspects of social and economic position. The same person might be Methodist, diabetic, Japanese American, a Democrat, a student, a sheet-metal worker, a bowler, and a parent. None of these characteristics describes the person's sex, family connections (being a son or daughter, sister or brother, cousin, etc.), educational level, socioeconomic status, or current health status. Yet just as each characteristic is part of whom this person is, each is worthy of recognition, and each has a potential impact on his or her mental health situation.

CULTURE AND MENTAL HEALTH

Ideas about mental health, mental illness, psychiatric problems, and treatments are based on cultural values and understanding. These ideas, called *explanatory models*, make sense out of illness as individual members of different groups understand it. Models delineate what is considered "normal" and "abnormal" in a particular population, explain how things happen, shape clinical presentations of mental disorders, and determine culturally patterned ways that mental disorders are recognized, labeled, explained, and treated by other members of that group. By talking with clients, you can learn, for example, whether mental illness in their culture is considered psychological, emotional, spiritual, physical, or a combination of these categories. Many cultural groups do not view the body and mind as separate, but as one (Mahoney & Engebretson, 2000; Spector, 2000).

What is considered normal or abnormal depends on the specific viewpoint. The same behavior may be seen as positive in one situation and pathological in another. Hallucinations, for instance, are typically viewed as abnormal by psychiatric standards but normal and even encouraged by certain Native People tribes as symbolic spiritual experiences called vision quests. Knowing about values and patterns of behavior helps us minimize the potential for imposing our expectations on people who come from different backgrounds and have different needs and goals.

Many beliefs about the cause of mental illness exist worldwide. Some people believe mental illness is a punishment for wrongdoing, the result of being "witched," or an illness that is "passed down" through the family. The belief that mental illness is a punishment for wrongdoing is quite common. Wrongdoings can range from minor infractions such as eating a taboo food to major violations such as killing a relative.

Another type of wrongdoing is offending ancestors, gods, and goddesses. The belief that another person can "witch" a person to have a mental illness is also common. People who have been offended put a sign, or hex, on the person who is at fault, who then goes "crazy." "Down-the-line" or inherited mental illness is another cultural belief. This is thought to be passed through only the mother, since she is the one who gives birth to the child. While most people believe that mental illness is not contagious, they also believe that the mentally ill should be avoided (Okasha, 2000).

PROBLEMS RELATED TO CULTURE

Alienation from Group

Psychosocial problems can include problems related to culture. People can become alienated from their cultural group for any number of reasons, including geographical moves or marriage into a different group. They may also be expelled from their religious or ethnic associations for many reasons such as sexual orientation, interracial marriage, or other violations of cultural norms. These types of problems result in loss of social status and self-esteem. Accurate assessment of culture-related factors is important in providing holistic care to clients and their families.

Socioeconomic Status

In the United States, the highest rates of mental disorders and psychological distress are found among groups with the lowest socioeconomic status (SES). One of the reasons is that all major psychosocial risk factors for mental illness are more prevalent in lower SES levels. These include acute and chronic stress, lack of community support services, lack of economic resources, and lack of control and mastery over one's life. Poverty has a powerful influence on mental disorders. For example, while poverty does not *cause* schizophrenia, poverty is strongly related to the experience of those who suffer from schizophrenia. The added stress of poverty may influence the rate of exacerbations and perhaps even the likelihood of recovery. With very limited community resources, many people living in poverty with schizophrenia find themselves homeless. Access to health care varies for them according to health insurance status. Research suggests that people in lower SES levels receive less mental health treatment, that is, fewer sessions, nonprofessional therapists, and less medication. All of these factors increase

the severity of the experience on mental illness (Flaskerud, 2000).

CULTURE-SPECIFIC SYNDROMES

Certain forms of mental illness are restricted to specific areas or cultures. These well-defined syndromes occur in response to certain situations in a particular culture. They are a heterogeneous group that can be further subdivided into three groups. **True syndromes** are illnesses with specific symptoms. **Illnesses of attribution** have a presumed cause but no specific signs and symptoms. An example in Western medicine might be an illness classified only as "infectious disease." **Idioms of distress** occur in people who are especially vulnerable to stressful life events. This vulnerability makes them susceptible to a wide variety of physical and mental illnesses. See Box 5.1 for information on culture-specific syndromes (Arboleda-Florez & Weisstub, 2000; Flaskerud, 2000).

VALUES

Values are a set of personal beliefs about what is meaningful and significant in life. Values provide general

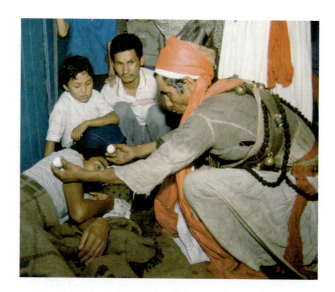

PHOTO 5.1 ■ This Nepalese shaman, known as Jhankari, treats a patient by holding eggs over his head to ward off evil spirits.

SOURCE: Earl & Nazima Kowall/CORBIS.

BOX 5.1

Culture-Specific Syndromes

True Syndromes—Dissociative Phenomena

Amok	Characterized by homicidal frenzy followed by amnesia; many different cultures.
Falling Out	Sudden collapse in which the eyes are open but the person cannot see or move; Southern United States and Caribbean.
Latah	Hypersensitivity to sudden fright with trance-like behavior; Malaysia.
Pibloktoq	Abrupt episodes of extreme excitement, followed by seizures, transient coma, and amnesia; Eskimo.
Grisi Siknis	Victim believes she is being attacked by devils and runs through the village; Nicaragua and Honduras.
Shin-Byung	Anxiety and somatic complaints followed by dissociation caused from possession by ancestral spirits; Korea.

True Syndromes—Anxiety States

Ataque de Nervios	Shaking, palpitations, flushing, and shouting or striking out; Latin America.
Dhat	Extreme anxiety associated with discharge of semen, which is thought to lead to depletion of physical and mental energy; Asia.
Koro	Man believes his penis is retracting into his body and that this will end in death; Asia.
Kayak Angst	Intense anxiety associated with fear of capsizing and drowning when going out to the open sea in a kayak; Eskimo.
Taijin Kyofusho	Intense anxiety about possibly offending, embarrassing, or displeasing others; Japan.

True Syndromes—Affective/Somatoform Disorders

Brain Fag	Pressure in the head, difficulty concentrating, anxiety, and visual complaints believed to result from too much thinking; West Africa.
Shenjing Shuairuo	Physical and mental exhaustion, difficulty concentrating, memory loss, sleeping and appetite problems, and irritability; China.
Anorexia Nervosa	Obsessive preoccupation with weight loss and delusional body image; Western cultures.

True Syndromes—Psychotic States

Boufee Delirante	Sudden outburst of aggressive behavior, confusion, agitation, paranoid ideation, and auditory and visual hallucinations; West Africa and Haiti.

Illnesses of Attribution—Induced by Anger

Bilis, Colera	Tension, somatic expressions, and fatigue; Latin America.
Hwa-Byung	Suppression of anger leads to indigestion, fatigue, fearfulness, and general dysphoria; Korea.

Illnesses of Attribution—Induced by Fright

Susto	Sudden fright believed to cause the soul to leave the body, leading to many physical and emotional symptoms; Latin America.

Illnesses of Attribution—Induced by Witchcraft

Ghost Sickness	An illness believed to be induced by witches, with symptoms such as delirium, nightmares, terror, anxiety, and confusion; Native American.
Voodoo	Illness ascribed to hexing, witchcraft, or the evil influence of another person; believed to cause a variety of symptoms and even death; Caribbean, Southern United States, Latin America.
Evil Eye	A fixed stare by an adult is believed capable of causing illness in a child or another adult; Mediterranean, Latin America.

Idioms of Distress

Nervios/ Nevra	A term describing people who are vulnerable to stress and who display a wide variety of physical and emotional illnesses; Latin America, Greece.
Locura	The most severe form of chronic mental illness; victim is incoherent, agitated, unpredictable, and possibly violent; Latin America.

SOURCES: American Psychiatric Association. (2000). *Diagnostic and statistical manual of mental disorders (4th ed., Text Revision)*. Washington, DC: Author; Guarnaccia, P. J., & Rogler, L. H. (1999). Research on culture-bound syndromes. *American Journal of Psychiatry, 156*(9), 1322–1327; and Levine, R. E., & Gaw, A. C. (1995). Culture-bound syndromes. *Psychiatric Clinics of North America, 18*(3), 523–536.

guidelines for behavior; they are standards of conduct that people or groups of people believe in. Values are the frame of reference through which we integrate, explain, and evaluate new ideas, situations, and relationships. Values may be *intrinsic*, internalized from a person's particular situation and experience, or *extrinsic*, derived from the culture's standards of right and wrong.

VALUE ORIENTATIONS

It has long been recognized that in every society, basic values emphasize shared ideals about the relationship between humans and nature, the relationship between humans and the universe, a sense of time, a sense of productivity and activity, and interpersonal relationships.

Humans and Nature

Values about the relationship between humans and nature fall along a continuum, as do values about each of the other subjects. The model relationship between humans and nature may be seen as predetermined, perhaps by God or fate or genetics, implying that some aspect of nature controls people. It may also be viewed as independent, with people controlling nature.

Humans and the Universe

Relationships with nature tend to reflect those between humans and the universe in being close and personal or distant and impersonal. Both orientations affect attitudes toward illness prevention and health care. For example, if we believe our fate is predetermined, we have little motivation for preventive strategies such as proper nutrition and immunization. In contrast, the more familiar value in the United States is mastery over the universe, the attitude that nature can be conquered and controlled if and when we learn enough about it. This attitude has led to the development of extensive technology focused on health care, along with the assumption that it is appropriate to intervene in what were traditionally viewed as natural phenomena—disease and death.

Sense of Time

Societies have values regarding time. People tend to be oriented toward the past, the present, or the future. They may emulate history and reclaim the *past*, such as through believing in ancestral spirits. If people focus too much on the past they may have little awareness of their present problems or joys and remain preoccupied with what has already happened. Others may live in the *present* moment. Living in the present allows us to be open to the possibilities of each moment as it unfolds. Living only in the present also has the potential for problems. Olympic contenders were asked if there were a magic pill that would guarantee a gold medal but would kill them within a year, would they take it? The 50 percent who said they would take the pill live only in the present moment, with little consideration for the future. On the same continuum is an orientation toward the *future* that encourages people to save money, to get an education and qualify for a career, and to set other long-range goals such as preventing diseases. Some people become preoccupied with a future that has not yet arrived and many spend hours upon hours worrying about future events.

The healthiest approach for most individuals is a *balance* of past, present, and future, with an awareness of exactly what we are doing in and with our lives and the effects our actions and thoughts have on what we do and don't do.

Productivity

Attitudes toward productivity are likewise varied. For some, it is enough to just exist; it is not necessary to accomplish great things in order to feel worthwhile. For others, a desire to develop the self is its own reward and requires no outside recognition. For still others, however, there is a belief that hard work will pay off materially as well as psychologically. As a result of their attitude toward productivity in life, people are relatively passive or active.

Interpersonal Relationships

Values about interpersonal relationships also exist on a continuum. One of the parameters is *dependency versus autonomy*. Certain cultures, for example, think that some people are born followers and others are born leaders. This belief implies that the follower need not assume responsibility for the self and can and should rely on others, such as health care professionals. Other cultures believe that all people have equal rights and should control their own destinies, become assertive, and take the lead, at least over their own lives. Between those two extremes are people who take their problems to close friends or family members, sharing the problem but keeping responsibility for it within a close personal group.

Values about interpersonal relationships are also reflected in the ideas people have about being individuals and members of groups. In some cultures, *interdependence*, affiliation, and loyalty to the family and community are more highly valued than individuality and personal achievement. The individual is inseparable from her or his status within the family and community, and many decisions of consequence are made in reference to the immediate social group. Shame thus becomes a driving force in these groups. Denial of the self for the sake of others is common in Indian, Asian, Arab, African, and Latin American cultures.

Scandinavian, European, and American cultures tend to value *individualism* highly, with members of families or communities a secondary priority. Autonomy and individuality are highly valued and people are perceived as being responsible for their own fate. Hard work is the basis for financial gain and personal advancement. Thus, guilt is a driving force in these groups. Interestingly, ethnic groups and women in the United States are more likely to define themselves in interdependent terms than are men or members of the Euro-American majority (Okasha, 2000).

Each of these sets of values exists along a continuum that illustrates wide human variation. No values are implicitly right or wrong; they simply shape ideas and responses. It is dangerously misleading if we assume that all clients share a given orientation.

PREDOMINANT AMERICAN VALUES

The most prominent values in the United States are reflected in our health care system, but those values tend to represent the dominant groups (Euro-American, middle class, Judeo-Christian, and male) and not the numerous and diverse subgroups within the country. The dominant set of values is oriented toward individuals, who are viewed as accountable for decision making, self-care, and many other self-oriented tasks. Hard work is regarded as the basis for personal achievement and financial gain. Privacy rights and personal freedom are based on the value of individualism. In many American subcultures, however, being individualistic is not a primary value.

Parrillo (1999) has created a useful list of values that predominate in the United States, as shown in Box 5.2. Consider ways in which each of these values is promoted not only in society in general, but in nursing practice in particular.

NURSING VALUES

Nursing reflects the society in which it exists. Nursing would not be accepted and utilized if it did not reflect the cultural values and social norms that predominate. While American values generally reflect those of the dominant culture, in reality, many cultural subgroups have quite different values and norms. Nursing as a discipline tends to have the same values as middle-class Americans of Euro-American background. Yet, as nurses, we must be flexible enough to meet the needs expressed by a very diverse population with widely varying values. In other words, standard nursing practice exhibits less diversity than our clients or we possess. We must be aware of the "standard" values and avoid assuming that they apply to everyone.

ATTITUDES AND PERCEPTIONS

Being knowledgeable about diversity includes understanding the attitudes and perceptions that perpetuate social equality and inequality. Attitudes and perceptions are formed from biases. Paul (1993) describes two different types of bias. The first type is **natural bias**, which refers simply to how our point of view causes us to notice some things and not others. The second type is **negative bias**: a refusal to recognize that there are other points of view. Natural and negative biases come into play when we organize or process information in such a way that we develop attitudes of open-mindedness and/or discrimination. As nurses, we must always be open-minded—learning what our natural and negative biases are, and changing those that prevent us from seeing and understanding the perspectives of other people.

GENERALIZATIONS, STEREOTYPES, AND PREJUDICE

We all work with huge amounts of information every day. To make it more manageable, we organize information into categories. One way we organize is through descriptive generalizations. **Generalizations**, which arise out of our natural biases, are changeable starting places for comparing typical behavioral patterns with what is actually observed. When we use generalizations to process information, we are more likely to remain open-minded: to develop open relationships with our clients, understand their point of view, and provide culturally competent nursing care.

BOX 5.2

Predominant American Values

Personal Achievement and Success

The emphasis is on competition, power, status, and wealth. What is good for the individual may be more important than what is good for the larger group, such as the community.

Activity and Work

People who do not work hard are considered lazy. It is assumed that hard work will be rewarded. Little consideration is given to people who have not had the same opportunities for success.

Moral Orientation

There is a tendency to moralize and to see the world in absolutes of right or wrong, good or bad. This pattern reinforces the inclination to stereotype.

Humanitarian Mores

Although quick to respond with charity and crisis aid, Americans often use these to limit deeper involvement with issues. Even professional "caring" relationships are typically kept impersonal.

Efficiency and Practicality

Solutions to problems are often based on short-term rather than long-term results.

Progress

Change is often seen as progress in which technology is highly valued and the focus is on the future rather than the present.

Material Comfort

The United States is a consumer-oriented society with a high standard of living.

Personal Freedom and Individualism

Individual rights are valued above the good of the group.

Equality

Personal freedom is a stronger value than equality, especially when there is competition for resources or opportunities.

External Conformity

Despite the value of personal freedom, there is pressure to conform to the Euro-American, middle-class, Judeo-Christian, and male values that predominate. Those differing are labeled deviant.

Science and Rationality

The medicalization of society has led to high expectations for "quick fixes," technology, and the efficiency of scientific medicine.

SOURCES: Adapted from Parrillo, V. N. (1999). *Strangers to these shores: Race and ethnic relations in the United States* (6th ed.). Riverside, NJ: Macmillan.

Another way to organize information is by using stereotypes, which arise out of our negative biases. **Stereotypes** are images frozen in time that cause us to see what we expect to see, even when the facts differ from our expectations. Stereotypes often capture characteristics that are real and common to a group. However, stereotypes may also be out of date and dangerously limited. They are particularly dangerous when they involve negative beliefs about a person or group, leading to "prejudgment" (or prejudice) that ignores actual evidence.

Prejudice is negative feeling about people who are different from us. Prejudicial attitudes are based on limited knowledge, limited contact, and emotional responses rather than on careful observation and thought. They are beliefs, opinions, or points of view that are formed before the facts are known or in spite of them.

Stereotypes can be favorable as well as unfavorable, although even favorable ones disregard facts and rely on preconceived notions. For example, Asian American students are often expected to excel in mathematics because of the stereotype that associates Asian Americans with technical accomplishments. Because every group has some individuals who do well in math and others who do not, Asian Americans who struggle with math must contend with a sense of failure. The same process occurs in many forms: A child is expected to

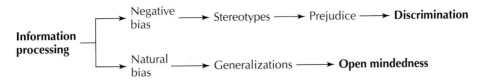

FIGURE 5.1 ■ Pathways to open-mindedness and discrimination.

do well because his or her older siblings did; people with glasses read a lot of books; all African Americans are good dancers or athletes. Although these are not negative stereotypes, they are potentially harmful because they impose expectations that are unrealistic.

There are two pathways of information processing—one leading to open-mindedness and the other leading to discrimination (Figure 5.1 ■).

DISCRIMINATION

Several types of prejudice are commonly observed in health care settings and can lead to discriminatory behavior. **Discrimination** is prejudice that is expressed behaviorally. Racism is one example of discrimination. Differentiating people according to racial characteristics has always been a pervasive social process in the United States. Despite nurses' extensive knowledge of biology, we tend to leave incorrect ideas about race unchallenged.

We are all members of the human race. Nonetheless, we use racial terms to divide and separate people. We often refer to skin color to group people into different races. Imagine somehow lining up the more than 5 billion people on this planet, starting on one end with the darkest-skinned and ending with the lightest-skinned. The very dark individuals would seem quite different from the very light, yet the vast majority would be in between in every shade of brown. Based on skin color, no one would be able to tell where one "race" ends and the next begins.

The time when African Americans, Asian Americans, Latinos, and Native People were prevented from entering the social and economic mainstream is officially over. However, despite formal integration, stereotypes and prejudices associated with white versus nonwhite status remain. For instance, negative stereotypes that associate African Americans with poverty, drugs, and violence ignore the fact that most African Americans are not poor and have nothing to do with either drugs or violence. Assuming that a client is on welfare because he or she is African American, or that substance abuse exists or physical aggression is a likelihood, may result in treatment different from that given to clients who are not African American.

Racism is defined as excessive and irrational beliefs regarding the superiority of a given group. Racism can traumatize, hurt, humiliate, enrage, and ultimately prevent optimal mental health of individuals and communities. Racism affects all people, both dominant and nondominant group members. People who are targets of discrimination experience unsolicited and unwarranted violence—whether physical or mental and covert or overt. Such experiences are significant stressors that interfere with mental, social, and physical adjustment. This is evidenced in part by the reality that one of the leading causes of death of African Americans is stress-related diseases (Dobbins & Skillings, 2000).

Likewise, those individuals of the dominant group who hold racist views have difficulty making a healthy adaptation to an increasingly multicultural society. They project blame to the victims in an effort to maintain a system of denial. Early on, they learn to feel justified in continuing the use of oppression of others. The continued use of projection and denial leads to maladaptive behaviors and poorer mental health. Harrell (2000) has identified ways in which racism increases people's stress and affects their well-being. Anxiety, depression, and hypertension are just a few of the many negative outcomes (see Table 5.1 ■).

A number of other forms of discrimination may be observed in health care settings. These patterns of interaction have acquired the label *"isms"* because of their common word ending. Each ism involves a tendency to judge others according to similarity to or dis-

TABLE 5.1

Racism-Related Stress Factors

Racism-Related Life Events
- Experiences are relatively time limited
- Occur in various settings/situations such as neighborhood, work, education, legal, health care
- Examples: being discriminated against in the emergency department, being harassed by the police, being rejected for a loan

Vicarious Racism Experiences
- Occur through observation and report
- Create a heightened sense of danger/vulnerability, anger, sadness
- May happen to family, friends, or strangers
- Example: the dragging death of James Byrd in Texas

Daily Racism Microstressors
- Subtle putdowns that are daily reminders that something racist can happen at any moment
- These slights and exclusions may be intentional or unintentional
- Experiences can feel demoralizing, disrespectful, or objectifying
- Examples: poor service in public accommodations, being followed by a store detective, being mistaken for someone who serves others (e.g., a maid, a janitor)

Chronic-Contextual Stress
- Political and institutional racism
- Unequal distribution of and access to resources
- Examples: lack of ethnoculturally diverse mental health service providers, out-of-date textbooks in schools, unchecked community violence

Collective Experiences
- Experiences of racism at the group level
- Examples: lack of political representation, stereotypic portrayals in the media

Transgenerational Transmission
- Historical context of the group and wider American society
- Examples: stories that are passed down through generations such as the slavery of African people, the internment of Japanese Americans during World War II, the removal of Native People from their tribal lands

SOURCE: Adapted from Harrell, S. P. (2000). A multidimensional conceptualization of racism-related stress: Implications for the well-being of people of color. *American Journal of Orthopsychiatry, 70*(1), 42–55.

similarity from a standard considered ideal or normal. Isms are shaped by personal or group judgment. For example, focusing on oneself is known as egocentrism. When an entire society promotes one way of behaving or thinking as the best way, it is called *sociocentrism*, as in Eurocentric or Afrocentric education. We frequently hear about ethnocentrism. Nearly every ethnic group sees itself as "best." However, in a society composed of multiple groups, we must counteract such biases, or isms, to prevent discrimination and social injustice. Table 5.1 can also be applied to victims of other forms of discrimination (see Table 5.2 ■).

TABLE 5.2

Forms of Discrimination

Form	Description	Example
Ableism	The assumption that the able-bodied and sound of mind are superior to those who are disabled or mentally ill.	A person who is psychiatrically disabled is not offered treatment choices.
Adultism	The assumption that adults are superior to youths.	Children are ignored and not given opportunities to learn decision making.
Ageism	The assumption that members of one age group are superior to those of other age groups.	Older people are assumed to be senile and incompetent.
Classism	The assumption that certain people are superior because of their socioeconomic status or position in a group or organization.	A poorly dressed high school dropout is not offered the same treatment facility as a well-dressed college graduate.
Egocentrism	The assumption that one is superior to others.	A person who has never experienced a mental illness thinks he or she is better than those who are diagnosed with a mental disorder.
Ethnocentrism	The assumption that one's own cultural or ethnic group is superior to that of others.	Everyone is expected to speak English and to know the rules for living in America.
Heterosexism	The assumption that everyone is or should be heterosexual.	When gays or lesbians experience a mental disorder, the cause is assumed to be their sexual orientation.
Racism	The assumption that members of one race are superior to those of another.	The color of one's skin determines educational and career opportunities.
Sexism	The assumption that members of one gender are superior to those of the other.	Women are viewed as less rational and more emotional, and therefore more likely to have a mental illness, than men.
Sizism	The assumption that people of one body size are superior to those of other shapes and sizes.	Obese people have fewer job opportunities and advancements.
Sociocentrism	The assumption that one society's way of knowing or doing is superior to that of others.	Biomedicine is expected to be effective, while folk medicine is discounted.

There is considerable evidence that even when the intent is to treat people fairly, they may be approached in ways that indicate subtle prejudice. In health care settings, one group tends to get treated well and another may get less attention, fewer choices, and generally less vigorous care. This unequal treatment is a reflection of the traits that society values. The YAVIS are Young, Attractive, Verbal, Intelligent, and Success-ful (or appear potentially successful). The QUOIDS, by contrast, are Quiet, Ugly, Old, Indigent (poor), Dissimilar (in lifestyle, language, or culture), and thought to be Stupid. Although someone carefully observing interactions in health care settings may readily discern preferential patterns involving YAVIS and QUOIDS, those who work there may be unaware of how their biases lead to behavior that is discriminatory.

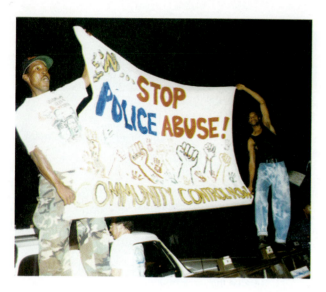

PHOTO 5.2 ■ Demonstrators protest the police acquittal in the Rodney King case in 1992.

SOURCE: Nick Ut/AP/Wide World Photos.

CARING FOR A DIVERSE POPULATION

To understand and care for diverse clients, you must learn to understand and appreciate multiple interpretations of events and behaviors. There are thousands of cultures and subcultures, and we cannot possibly know all there is to know about each one. Personal and group identities are very complex. Many people are exposed to or have been raised in more than one culture. Many others have altered their traditional cultural orientation to adapt to American society or specific life circumstances. We often hear about the importance of sensitivity to cultural differences. However, being only sensitive can leave you frustrated and powerless. You must also learn to become an advocate for diverse populations. Advocacy is supporting and defending people's rights to their beliefs, attitudes, and values. Effective advocacy depends on a balance of knowledge, sensitivity, and skills.

CULTURAL KNOWLEDGE

The first step in building knowledge is getting to know who we are. We cannot expect to understand others and help them achieve their full potential if we do not first develop an understanding of who we are as people and as nurses. This is not always simple, and it is an ongoing, never-ending process. Identifying our own attitudes, values, and prejudices helps us understand our feelings about people who are different. It helps us be nonjudgmental and may prevent us from exhibiting discriminating behavior when interacting with clients from a different cultural or subcultural group. Confronting our own ethnocentrism takes careful attention to our thoughts and behaviors. Self-understanding is enhanced when we ask for and listen carefully to feedback from clients, peers, faculty members, and supervisors. There is no easy way to acquire a depth of knowledge about cultural groups different from our own. Wherever we practice nursing, we must assume responsibility for learning about the culture of our clients. This can be done through reading, by talking to and listening to clients, and by attending workshops about diverse cultural groups. This begins the process of giving culturally competent nursing care. The list of community resources at the end of this chapter provides information sites for increasing your knowledge.

CULTURAL SENSITIVITY

Knowing ourselves is critical to becoming sensitive nurses. Once we become aware of our own attitudes, values, and prejudices, we must examine how they affect our nursing practice. Ask yourself: Do I pay more attention to clients who have a background similar to mine? Do I approach clients from a different background with initial suspicion or distrust? Does my body language change when I interact with someone from a different background? What are the stereotypes I have of people from various cultures? When I don't understand a client's behavior, do I ask for clarification or do I make assumptions about that behavior? Am I open to learning about alternative healing practices? Do I penalize clients whose values or behaviors are different from mine?

SKILLS IN IMPLEMENTING NURSING INTERVENTIONS

Knowledge empowers us to understand cultural differences. Sensitivity enables us to respect and honor differences. Sensitivity and knowledge must be combined with skills for appropriate and effective nursing intervention to occur.

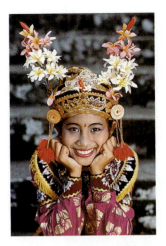 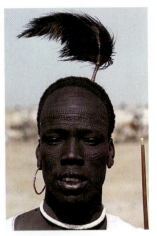 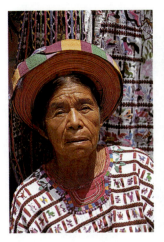 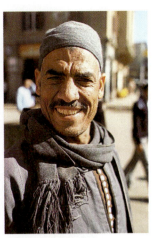

PHOTO 5.3 ■ To understand human behavior fully, we must appreciate the rich diversity of human beings throughout the world.

SOURCE: Pearson Education/PH College.

Communication is crucial to all nursing care, but it is especially important when caring for mental health clients from diverse backgrounds. To establish contact, present yourself in a confident way without seeming to be superior. Shake hands, if appropriate. Allow clients to choose their comfortable personal space. Respect their version of acceptable eye contact. Ask how they prefer to be addressed. Most people are pleased when others show sincere interest in them. Small things can often communicate acceptance. Making a setting comfortable by considering seating arrangements, background noises, and other environmental variables helps make clients feel welcome and recognized.

Talk with clients to determine their *level of fluency* in English, and arrange for an interpreter if needed. Speak directly to the client even if an interpreter is present. Choose a style of speech that promotes understanding and demonstrates respect for each client. Avoid the tendency to raise your voice, as if that will increase understanding or fluency. Avoid jargon, slang, complex sentences, and body language that may be offensive or misunderstood.

Before using any written materials, ask clients if they can read English. They may feel defensive about their reading ability. Softening the question can help. For example, asking "Are you comfortable reading this?" avoids the issue of ability and allows clients to say that they prefer to have printed materials read to them. The ability to read varies widely, and many people who speak English do not read it. Medications and the symptoms of mental disorders can also interfere with the ability and motivation to read.

To obtain information, use open-ended questions or questions phrased in several ways. Allow plenty of time for answers. Be aware that some people consider only open-ended questions to be acceptable, such as "How do you manage your job when you feel sick?" Others prefer closed-ended questions, such as "Do you sleep a lot when you feel sick?" Still others (members of certain Native American, Pacific Island, and African groups, for example) consider direct questions to be impolite. They may expect inquiries to be presented like a story, as in "One client told me that when he feels really bad, he wears a special shirt. I guess we all have things we do at certain times."

You may have to learn to use certain indirect styles of communication and wait to see if and how the client responds. Observe how the client communicates to others to learn what style is most appropriate. Ask family members or significant others if they can help with this information. It is important to avoid forcing clients to conform to communication patterns with which they are not comfortable.

Several different frameworks have been developed for assessment when planning health care services or programs within any multicultural group. The Heritage

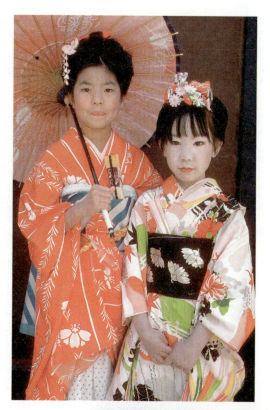

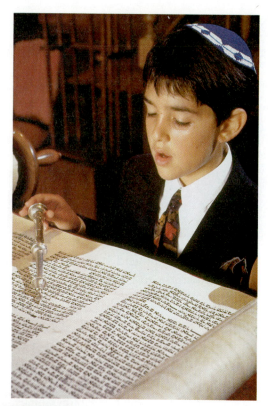

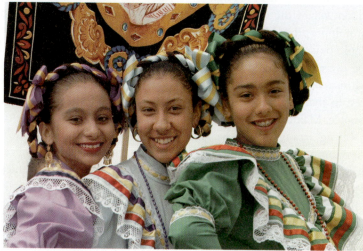

PHOTO 5.4 ■ Acknowledging the diverse environments in which people develop is essential to providing culturally competent care.

SOURCE: Pearson Education/PH College; Pearson Education/PH College; Skjold Photographs.

Assessment Tool (Box 5.3) is a practical and useful way for you to investigate a client's ethnic, cultural, and religious heritage (Spector, 2000).

Storytelling is a valuable approach to sharing views. Inviting clients to tell you stories about themselves and their problems is an excellent way to find out what is important to them and how they view their situations. "Can you tell me a story about when you were growing up?" "Would you tell me a story about coming to the hospital?" Communication is most productive when

CRITICAL THINKING

You and your classmates are doing your clinical in a community mental health clinic in an urban community. You have had several days of clinical working with your assigned clients. Your instructor has called for a conference with all of the students, and she has asked all of the students to consider cultural diversity issues within the clinic and with assigned clients.

At the beginning of the conference, your instructor asks for student observations related to cultural diversity. The group identifies that three students have been assigned clients who might experience cultural issues: African American, Hispanic, and Chinese. In addition, you note that the clinic tends to have clients from these three groups. One student notes that there is little interaction in the waiting room, but she wonders if this is due to the nature of the problems clients are experiencing rather than to the fact that clients are from different cultural groups. You comment that some clients and their families have had problems communicating with some staff when staff do not know Spanish or Chinese and the client knows little English.

The instructor comments that we have identified some good issues related to cultural diversity. We then begin to use our critical thinking skills to discuss the topic further. In the end, this will help us provide care that is more appropriate to the individual needs of our clients.

1. Why is it important for us to consider explanatory models when we work with different cultural groups?
2. If the clinic receptionist said to you, "Treatment for schizophrenia seems like a waste to me. Poverty causes schizophrenia. Look at all the poor people we have here with schizophrenia. We cannot do anything about poverty," how would you respond to these statements?
3. As the conference continues, your instructor asks the student group to compare and contrast generalization, stereotyping, and prejudice. As a group, we try to do this, and we find we are successful. How would you answer this request?
4. The two students who have been working with a Chinese client and a Hispanic client ask the following question. What should we consider when we develop our interventions so that we do not ignore cultural differences?

For an additional Case Study, please refer to the Companion Web site for this book.

you acknowledge that clients know more about their personal situation than you do. Having clients tell the story of their life and of their illness often provides information that will help you understand their experiences and views. Although this approach requires good listening skills and adequate amounts of time, it forms the core of effective care and treatment in many societies.

Client values, beliefs, and practices do not have to change simply because they are different from those of health care providers. You can help people recognize what to change and what not to change. To provide care that is both knowledgeable and sensitive, it is essential to identify the following (Leininger, 1991):

■ Those aspects of the client's life that mean a lot, are valuable just as they are, and should be understood and preserved without change.

■ Those aspects that can be partially preserved but need some adjustment, to be negotiated with the client.

■ Those aspects that require change and repatterning.

Analysis of the situation to clarify what is happening, and the probable consequences of each type of intervention, helps you make informed decisions. If your relationship is mutual and communication lines are open, it may quickly become clear that the client's value orientation can be maintained or will require only minor alteration. Lack of knowledge and insensitivity often leads to the conclusion that a client's approach is totally wrong and requires radical overhauling. In order to gain the client's cooperation, preserve the integrity of the client's view by being flexible, sensitive, knowledgeable, and skillful.

On the other hand, at times you must take a stand for substantive change, as in cases of illegal or injurious

BOX 5.3

Heritage Assessment Tool

This set of questions is to be used to describe a given client's—or your own—ethnic, cultural, and religious background. In performing a *heritage assessment*, it is helpful to determine how deeply a given person identifies with his or her traditional heritage. This tool is most useful in setting the stage for assessing and understanding a person's traditional health and illness beliefs and practices and in helping to determine the community resources that will be appropriate to target for support when necessary. The greater the number of positive responses, the greater the degree to which the person may identify with his or her traditional heritage. The one exception to positive answers is the question about whether or not a person's name was changed.

1. Where was your mother born? _____

2. Where was your father born? _____

3. Where were your grandparents born? _____

    a. Your mother's mother? _____

    b. Your mother's father? _____

    c. Your father's mother? _____

    d. Your father's father? _____

4. How many brothers _____ and sisters _____ do you have?

5. What setting did you grow up in? Urban _____ Rural _____

6. What country did your parents grow up in?

    Father _____

    Mother _____

7. How old were you when you came to the United States? _____

8. How old were your parents when they came to the United States?

    Mother _____

    Father _____

9. When you were growing up, who lived with you? _____

10. Have you maintained contact with

    a. Aunts, uncles, cousins?   (1) Yes _____   (2) No _____

    b. Brothers and sisters?   (1) Yes _____   (2) No _____

    c. Parents?   (1) Yes _____   (2) No _____

    d. Your own children?   (1) Yes _____   (2) No _____

11. Did most of your aunts, uncles, cousins live near your home?

    (1) Yes _____   (2) No _____

12. Approximately how often did you visit family members who lived outside of your home?

    (1) Daily _____   (2) Weekly _____   (3) Monthly _____

    (4) Once a year of less _____   (5) Never _____

13. Was your original family name changed?

    (1) Yes _____   (2) No _____

14. What is your religious preference?

    (1) Catholic _____   (2) Jewish _____

    (3) Protestant _____   Denomination _____

    (4) Other _____   (5) None _____

BOX 5.3

15. Is your spouse the same religion as you?

    (1) Yes _____   (2) No _____

16. Is your spouse the same ethnic background as you?

    (1) Yes _____   (2) No _____

17. What kind of school did you go to?

    (1) Public _____   (2) Private _____   (3) Parochial _____

18. As an adult, do you live in a neighborhood where the neighbors are the same religion and ethnic background as yourself?

    (1) Yes _____   (2) No _____

19. Do you belong to a religious institution?

    (1) Yes _____   (2) No _____

20. Would you describe yourself as an active member?

    (1) Yes _____   (2) No _____

21. How often do you attend your religious institution?

    (1) More than once a week _____   (2) Weekly _____   (3) Monthly _____

    (4) Special holidays only _____   (5) Never _____

22. Do you practice your religion in your home?

    (1) Yes _____   (2) No _____ (if yes, please specify)

    (3) Praying _____   (4) Bible reading _____   (5) Diet _____

    (6) Celebrating religious holidays _____

23. Do you prepare foods special to your ethnic background?

    (1) Yes _____   (2) No _____

24. Do you participate in ethnic activities?

    (1) Yes _____   (2) No _____ (if yes, please specify)

    (3) Singing _____   (4) Holiday celebrations _____

    (5) Dancing _____   (6) Festivals _____

    (7) Costumes _____   (8) Other _____

25. Are your friends from the same religious background as you?

    (1) Yes _____   (2) No _____

26. Are your friends from the same ethnic background as you?

    (1) Yes _____   (2) No _____

27. What is your native language? _____

28. Do you speak this language?

    (1) Prefer _____   (2) Occasionally _____   (3) Rarely _____

29. Do you read your native language?

    (1) Yes _____   (2) No _____

SOURCE: Spector, R. E. (2000). *Cultural diversity in health and illness* (5th ed.). Upper Saddle River, NJ: Prentice Hall.

behavior. It may be appropriate to consult the client's family or friends to help articulate a particular point of view. Many communities have rosters of organizations and individuals who will share information about the populations they represent. Getting help from these people is especially important when language or value differences create barriers between you and your clients.

Becoming competent and confident in managing diversity requires expertise and practice. Implementing knowledge, sensitivity, and skills in psychiatric nursing settings requires considerable time and energy. These efforts are rewarded, however, when difficult situations are handled as openly, mutually, and respectfully as possible, and by seeing clients respond favorably to such humanistic treatment.

DIVERSITY WITHIN THE PROFESSION

The challenge is not only to learn how to understand and uphold the cultures of clients. We must do the same with our co-workers so that cultural diversity is a positive force that enhances the nursing team. It is important that you take time to learn about those with whom you work through open dialogue, over time, and in a positive environment.

Because nondominant group members are underrepresented in all health professions, including nursing, it is important that we achieve greater representation in the nursing profession. Although minorities comprise 27 percent of the overall population, they account for only 9.7 percent of the total number of RNs. Native People are the least represented of all minority groups, including men, in the nursing profession. This lack of diversity in the nursing workforce is potentially harmful to the profession and the population it serves. Nursing programs must continue their efforts to recruit minorities into the field. This means that faculty must examine their programs for both barriers to success and support programs that enhance student–faculty communication and student academic success (Buerhaus & Auerbach, 1999; Dickerson, Neary, & Hyche-Johnson, 2000).

CHAPTER REVIEW

Links to these Web sites can be accessed on the Companion Web site for this book.

Association of Black Psychologists
P.O. Box 55999
Washington, DC 20040-5999
202-722-0808
www.abpsi.org

National Center for American Indian and Alaska Native Mental Health Research
University of Colorado Health Sciences Center
Campus Box AO11-13
4455 East 12th Ave.
Denver, CO 80220
303-315-9326
www.uchsc.edu/sm/ncaianmhr

National Coalition of Hispanic Health and Human Services Organization
1501 16th St. NW
Washington, DC 20036
202-797-4364
www.cossmho.org

Office of Minority Health Resource Center
P.O. Box 37337
Washington, DC 20013-7337
800-444-6472
www.omhrc.gov

Resources for Cross Cultural Health Care
www.DiversityRx.org

Transcultural Nursing Society
36600 Schoolcraft Road
Livonia, MI 48150-1173
888-432-5470
www.tcns.org

KEY CONCEPTS

Introduction

- Each of the major ethnic groups is so diverse that differences within groups may be as great as, or greater than, those between them.

- Culture is a pattern of learned behavior based on values, beliefs, and perceptions of the world. It is taught and shared by members of a group or society.

- A subculture is a smaller group within a large cultural group that shares values, beliefs, behaviors, and language.

- Ethnicity is ethnic affiliation, and a sense of belonging to a particular cultural group.

- Ethnocentrism is the belief that one's own culture is more important than, and preferable to, any other culture.

- Diversity refers to variation among people.

Culture and Mental Health

- Ideas about mental health, mental illness, psychiatric problems, and treatments are based on cultural values and understanding.

- What is considered normal or abnormal depends on the specific cultural viewpoint.

- Alienation from one's cultural group results in loss of social status and self-esteem.

- Major psychosocial risk factors for mental illness are more prevalent in lower SES levels including acute and chronic stress, lack of community support services, lack of economic resources, and lack of control and mastery over one's life.

Culture-Specific Syndromes

- True syndromes are illnesses with specific symptoms.

- Illnesses of attribution have a presumed cause but no specific signs and symptoms.

- Idioms of distress occur in people who are especially vulnerable to stressful life events.

Values

- Values are a set of personal beliefs about what is meaningful and significant in life. They provide general guidelines for behavior and are standards of conduct in which people or groups of people believe.

- Every society has basic values about the relationship between humans and nature, a sense of time, a sense of productivity, and interpersonal relationships.

KEY CONCEPTS *(continued)*

- Values about the relationship between humans and nature vary from predetermined to independent. These reflect beliefs about humans and the universe.

- Predominant American values tend to represent Euro-American, middle-class, Judeo-Christian, male values.

- Nursing as a discipline tends to have the same values as middle-class Americans of Euro-American background.

Attitudes and Perceptions

- Natural bias refers to how our point of view causes us to notice some things and not others.

- Negative bias is a refusal to recognize that there are other points of view.

- Generalizations are a way of organizing information. Arising out of natural biases, they are changeable starting places for comparing typical behavioral patterns with what is actually observed.

- Stereotypes are a way of organizing information. Arising out of negative biases, they are images frozen in time that cause us to see what we expect to see, even when the facts differ from our expectations. Stereotypes can be favorable or unfavorable, and either kind is potentially harmful.

- Prejudice is negative feeling about people who are different from us.

- Discrimination is prejudice that is expressed behaviorally. Examples are racism, egocentrism, and sociocentrism.

- Racism can traumatize, hurt, humiliate, enrage, and ultimately prevent optimal mental health of individuals and communities.

- People who hold racist views project blame on victims in an effort to maintain a system of denial.

- Even when the intent is to treat people fairly, they may be approached in ways that indicate subtle prejudice.

Caring for a Diverse Population

- Effective advocacy depends on a balance of knowledge, sensitivity, and skills.

- The first step in building knowledge is understanding ourselves and confronting our own ethnocentrism.

- You must acquire knowledge about clients' cultural groups that are different from your own.

- When we know ourselves, we are able to be nonjudgmental and sensitive to other's beliefs, feelings, and behaviors.

- Sensitivity includes examining how our own attitudes, values, and prejudices affect our nursing practice.

- Communication is an important skill in caring for clients from diverse backgrounds. It includes learning their level of fluency in spoken and written English, and determining the most important style of communication.

- Many aspects of the client's life should be understood and preserved without change. Some can be partially preserved but need adjustment, which is negotiated with the client. Other aspects require change and repatterning.

- Becoming competent and confident in managing diversity requires practice and patience. The reward is seeing clients respond favorably to such humanistic treatment.

Diversity Within the Profession

- It is important that we honor cultural diversity among our co-workers as well as our clients.

- Although minorities comprise 27 percent of the population, they account for only 9.7 percent of registered nurses. We must continue to recruit minorities into the nursing profession.

EXPLORE *MediaLink*

- Interactive resources, including animations, for this chapter can be found on the Companion Web site at *http://www.prenhall.com/fontaine.* Click on Chapter 5 and select the activities for this chapter.

- For NCLEX review questions and an audio glossary, access the accompanying CD-ROM in this book.

REFERENCES

American Psychiatric Association. (2000). *Diagnostic and statistical manual of mental disorders* (4th ed., Text Revision). Washington, DC: Author.

Arboleda-Florez, J., & Weisstub, D. N. (2000). Conflicts and crises in Latin America. In A. Okasha, J. Arboleda-Florez, & N. Sartorius (Eds.), *Ethics, culture, and psychiatry* (pp. 29–45). Washington, DC: American Psychiatric Press.

Buerhaus, P. I., & Auerbach, D. (1999). Slow growth in the United States of the number of minorities in the RN workforce. *Image, 31*(2), 179–183.

Dickerson, S. S., Neary, M. A., & Hyche-Johnson, M. (2000). Native American graduate nursing students' learning experiences. *Journal of Nursing Scholarship, 32*(2), 189–196.

Dobbins, J. E., & Skillings, J. H. (2000). Racism as a clinical syndrome. *American Journal of Orthopsychiatry, 70*(1), 14–27.

Flaskerud, J. H. (2000). Ethnicity, culture, and neuropsychiatry. *Issues in Mental Health Nursing, 21*(1), 5–29.

Guarnaccia, P. J., & Rogler, L. H. (1999). Research on culture-bound syndromes. *American Journal of Psychiatry, 156*(9), 1322–1327.

Harrell, S. P. (2000). A multidimensional conceptualization of racism-related stress: Implications for the well-being of people of color. *American Journal of Orthopsychiatry, 70*(1), 42–55.

Leininger, M. M. (Ed.). (1991). *Culture, care, diversity, and universality: A theory of nursing.* New York: National League for Nursing Press.

Levine, R. E., & Gaw, A. C. (1995). Culture-bound syndromes. *Psychiatric Clinics of North America, 18*(3), 523–536.

Mahoney, J. S., & Engebretson, J. (2000). The interface of anthropology and nursing guiding culturally competent care in psychiatric nursing. *Archives of Psychiatric Nursing, 14*(4), 183–190.

Okasha, A. (2000). The impact of Arab culture on psychiatric ethics. In A. Okasha, J. Arboleda-Florez, & N. Sartorius (Eds.), *Ethics, culture, and psychiatry* (pp. 15–28). Washington, DC: American Psychiatric Press.

Parrillo, V. N. (1999). *Strangers to these shores: Race and ethnic relations in the United States* (6th ed.). Riverside, NJ: Macmillan.

Paul, R. W. (1993). *Critical thinking: How to prepare students for a rapidly changing world.* Cotati, CA: Foundation for Critical Thinking.

Spector, R. E. (2000). *Cultural diversity in health & illness* (5th ed.). Upper Saddle River, NJ: Prentice Hall.

Zoucha, R., & Husted, G. L. (2000). The ethical dimensions of delivering culturally congruent nursing and health care. *Issues in Mental Health Nursing, 21*(3), 325–340.

Legal and Ethical Issues

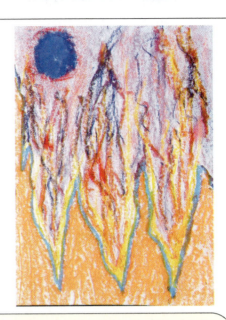

OBJECTIVES

After reading this chapter, you will be able to:

- DISTINGUISH between voluntary and involuntary admission.

- INTEGRATE the concepts of competency and informed consent into nursing practice and research.

- MAINTAIN confidentiality at all times.

- INSTITUTE precautions to prevent elopement.

- DISCUSS professional ethics in the mental health care setting.

*S*pectacular Frustration

—*Brian, Age 19*

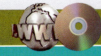

MediaLink

CD-ROM
- *Audio Glossary*
- *NCLEX Review*

Companion Web site www.prenhall.com/fontaine
- *Critical Thinking*
- *More NCLEX Review*
- *Case Study*
- *Care Map Activity*
- *Links to Resources*

Laws and ethical principles affect many decisions that nurses must make each day. It is important to be familiar with federal and state laws pertaining to nursing practice in general, and with those that have implications for the practice of psychiatric nursing in particular.

Mental disorders sometimes affect a person's ability to make decisions about his or her health and well-being. Whenever possible, client autonomy and liberty must be ensured by treatment in the least restrictive setting possible and by active client participation in treatment decisions. The challenge for nurses is maintaining the client's personal freedom in situations in which public welfare and/or the client's best interests are threatened.

TYPES OF ADMISSION

Voluntary admission occurs when a client, for the purpose of assessment and treatment of a mental disorder, consents to hospitalization and signs a document indicating as much. If clients choose to leave the hospital, they must give written notice of their intention to leave the facility. The number of hours or days between notice of intention and actual discharge is determined by individual states. This notification period provides the health care team with time to complete discharge arrangements or seek authorization for further hospitalization through the court system.

Parents of children can sign commitment papers requesting psychiatric treatment. In most states, when the individual is 18 or 21 years of age, she or he is considered to be an adult. An adolescent who has lived away from home for a certain period of time may be legally regarded as an emancipated minor. If the young adult or emancipated minor refuses hospitalization or treatment, the only recourse the parents have is to seek an involuntary admission.

Commitment, or **involuntary admission**—detaining a client in a psychiatric facility against his or her will—may be requested in most states on the basis of dangerousness to self or others. A few states have altered their laws by including the criterion of prevention of significant physical or mental deterioration. Some groups are lobbying for additions such as "grave disability" (people are unable to provide for their basic needs such as food and shelter), "need for treatment," and "lack of capacity" (people are unable to fully understand and make an informed decision regarding the need for treatment).

In most states, adults can be held temporarily on an emergency basis until there is a court hearing. At the judicial hearing, the health care team must present clear and convincing evidence of dangerousness or need for treatment. Commitment is for a specific time period, which varies by state. Commitment may be for inpatient or outpatient treatment, the decision being made by the committing judge. At the end of the specified time, the health care team must discharge the client or petition the court for continued hospitalization (Clark & Bowers, 2000).

Commitment is a controversial issue. In the United States, people have a fundamental right to make important decisions about their own treatment. At the same time, an individual may not be able to make treatment decisions when suffering from an acute episode of a mental disorder. There are legitimate concerns on both sides of the issue (Gardner et al., 1999; Lidz et al., 1998; Watson, Bowers, & Andersen, 2000).

Here are some of the reasons *for* commitment:

- Intervention will ease suffering and, in some cases, save lives.

- Commitment will alleviate embarrassment and rejection by the general public when grossly disturbed behaviors affect others.

- Commitment may reduce the length of a crisis, and that reduction seems to improve the prognosis for long-term recovery.

- In many instances, commitment is the only way to obtain treatment from the public mental health care system.

- In some cases, the family needs to protect itself against actual or threatened violence.

- The family may not be able to care for an acutely ill member and may see commitment as the only option.

Commitment is a very serious action because it restricts the freedom of someone who has not engaged in criminal activity. Here are some of the arguments *against* commitment:

- Commitment hearings are often perfunctory, and even though clients are entitled by law to an attorney, they often do not have one. Clients may not even be allowed to hear what is being said against them.

- The implicit promise of commitment is that the environment will be therapeutic, but many institutions dehumanize, degrade, and abuse clients.

- Coercion in mental health treatment does more harm than good, causing clients to distrust mental health caregivers.

- Commitment reinforces the stigma that mentally ill people are dangerous and unpredictable.

- It is a socioeconomic issue in that the majority of clients who are committed are poor and undereducated.

- If the family has requested commitment, the process damages trust among family members.

Commitment must never be viewed as a permanent or long-term solution. Alternatives must be explored. In some areas, mobile crisis teams or consumer-run services are offered as a substitute for hospital treatment. (See Chapter 4 for further information on alternative treatments and treatment settings.)

Because severe mental illness is often cyclical, stabilized clients may sign an **advance directive** indicating permission for treatment in the case of future incompetency. This plan is formulated between acute episodes and, while not legally binding in all states, advance directives assist family and caregivers who must make decisions for clients when they are unable to make them for themselves. Advance directives empower consumers who are psychiatrically disabled. Health care providers are given important information about the consumer's preferences for treatment. Family and friends experience less conflict and guilt during times of psychiatric crises.

The advance directive plan is initiated by the client and includes:

- Symptoms indicating that the person is not able to make decisions at this time

- The names and phone numbers of at least three people, including health care professionals and family members, who should make decisions on their behalf

- A listing of preferred, acceptable, and unacceptable medications, other treatments, and treatment facilities, including reasons

COMPETENCY

Competency is a legal determination that a client can make reasonable judgments and decisions about medical or nursing treatment and other significant areas of personal life. The principle is one of **autonomy** or self-determination. Autonomy is the freedom to choose and the ability to assume responsibility for one's own acts—in others words, freedom from pressures of any kind and the ability to govern one's own life. Clients are considered legally competent unless legally judged incompetent or temporarily incapacitated by a medical emergency. When a court rules an adult incompetent, it appoints a guardian or surrogate to make decisions on that person's behalf. Commitment is not a determination of incompetency. Clients who are committed for treatment are still capable of participating in health care decisions (Carpenter, 1999).

CONFIDENTIALITY

The primary reason for confidentiality is to encourage clients to be honest and open, to facilitate accurate diagnosis and effective treatment. As a nurse, you have a legal and ethical duty to protect client confidentiality. Confidentiality ensures that health care professionals, including nursing students, do not talk about clients with anyone who is not involved in their care. Going home and telling family members who is in the hospital and what happened on the unit is a serious breach of confidentiality. Discussing clients while in the hospital elevator or the cafeteria also breaches confidentiality. Nursing schools and hospitals have regulations regarding confidentiality. Breach of confidentiality is considered unprofessional conduct and is grounds for discipline by the state licensing board.

Under some circumstances, you have a legal and ethical duty *not* to protect client confidentiality. These circumstances include:

- The client is a danger to self or others
- The client is a minor, elderly, or disabled, and is believed to be a victim of abuse
- Disclosures to other professionals or supervisors directly involved in the treatment
- A therapist appointed by the court to evaluate the client
- A court order or other legal proceedings or laws requires disclosure of information

When you work with clients, you must discuss the subject of confidentiality. Explain to clients that what is discussed is shared only with the staff and the instructor. If you know the client from outside the hospital, reassure the client that his or her presence on the unit is absolutely confidential. In this situation, you should not provide care for this person nor read the chart.

There are federal regulations regarding chemical dependence (CD) programs. Everyone, including professionals and visitors, must sign a confidentiality statement before entering a CD unit. Staff members are not allowed to disclose any admission or discharge information. They may not even acknowledge whether the client is in the treatment facility.

Legally, a child does not have the right to confidentiality. In most cases, the parents, as legal guardians responsible for the child, have the right to know what is going on in treatment. Parents usually desire information and some level of involvement in their child's treatment plan. They often seek advice on how to cope with the day-to-day challenges they face, what they might expect in the future, and sources of community support.

Most states have laws regarding when human immunodeficiency virus (HIV) test results and/or the diagnosis of acquired immune deficiency syndrome (AIDS) may be disclosed. In many states, this information may not even be put in the medical record without the written consent of the client. In some states, clients must give written consent before HIV tests may be performed, while in other states, oral consent is sufficient. However, because oral consent is difficult to prove, most institutions require written consent.

INFORMED CONSENT

Informed consent is the client's right to receive enough information to make a decision about treatment and to communicate the decision to others. For consent to be given, the health care professional must inform the client of the objective, the benefit, and the risks of the proposed treatment. The client must also be told about any possible alternative interventions. The client must understand the information and be able to apply it to her or his own personal situation. The purpose of informed consent is to ensure that clients are not abused and that they are acknowledged as independent, responsible persons whose right and private space must be respected.

Clients may not be touched or treated without consent. If treatment is given without consent, the health care provider is held responsible for battery or offensive touching according to the law. In the event of an emergency situation with no time to obtain consent without endangering health or safety, a client may be treated without legal liability (Carpenter, 1999).

CLIENT RIGHTS

Clients do not lose their constitutional or legal rights when they are admitted to a facility for treatment of a mental disorder. Clients have the right to treatment with the *least restrictive alternative*, which means the

CRITICAL THINKING

Taneko is a 43-year-old woman who has been committed to a psychiatric facility by her husband Bill. Taneko is very angry, sobbing hysterically, and screaming at Bill for bringing her to the hospital instead of her doctor's office. Bill maintains that Taneko is a danger to herself because she has been depressed for several months and this morning threatened suicide.

Taneko is seeing a psychotherapist on a regular basis and feels that her depression is related to her father's death, which occurred nine months ago. Upon further assessment, the nurse learns that Taneko does not feel she is suicidal even though she made a statement to that effect earlier in the day. Taneko feels that she is being held against her will and wants to speak to an attorney. Bill is tired and frustrated. He does not want to take Taneko home because he does not feel that he can adequately take care of her.

1. Should Taneko be committed to the psychiatric facility or released? Defend your position.

2. One of Taneko's neighbors is a nurse working at the psychiatric facility where Bill took Taneko. What is the neighbor's responsibility, if any, toward Taneko now that she knows Taneko is a client there?

3. Even though Taneko is only being detained on a temporary basis, she has been placed on elopement precautions. Explain the rationale for elopement precautions.

4. How will Taneko's rights be affected if she decides to stay hospitalized and undergo treatment for her depression?

5. As a mental health professional, how can Taneko's nurse show she cares? How can this best be achieved?

6. Elaborate on why Taneko and Bill's situation creates an ethical dilemma.

For an additional Case Study, please refer to the Companion Web site for this book.

In spite of the fact that clients do not lose their legal rights, 44 states restrict voting rights for people with mental illness. This is further evidence of the stigma that remains part of American society. Many states prohibit voting by people who have been declared "incompetent." Twelve states prohibit voting by "idiots," "lunatics," or "the insane" without specifying how the condition is supposed to be determined. Six states have no voting restrictions: Colorado, Indiana, Kansas, Michigan, New Hampshire, and Pennsylvania. The National Alliance for the Mentally Ill (NAMI) has begun a campaign to educate representatives throughout the country on this denial of rights of citizenship (Carolla, 2000).

Clients must be informed of the potential risks of psychotropic medications and/or treatments. Competent adults have the right to refuse treatment, including medication. When clients' values are different than those of health professionals, the responsibility of the professional is to respect and facilitate clients' self-determination in regard to health care decisions.

If a client refuses and the physician believes it is essential for effective treatment, the physician may take the case to the courts for a decision (see Figure 6.1 ■).

REPORTING LAWS

All states make it mandatory for nurses to report suspected cases of child abuse or neglect. Failure to report these cases subjects the nurse to both criminal penalties and civil liability. Reporting protects the nurse from being sued by the parents or guardian. Many states have enacted adult abuse laws similar to the child abuse reporting laws. It is important that you know the laws for your state.

DUTY TO DISCLOSE/PROTECT

The **duty to disclose/protect** is the health care professional's obligation to warn identified individuals if a client has made a credible threat to kill them. In some states, the duty to disclose also includes threats against property. When a client threatens violence, mental health providers have a special responsibility to evalu-

provision of sufficient care for the client with the least restrictive methods in the least restrictive setting. (For more information about mental health care consumers' rights, see Chapter 10.)

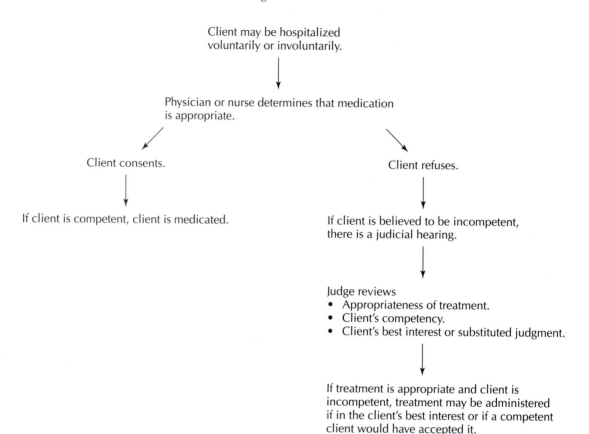

FIGURE 6.1 ■ Outcomes of client medication decisions.

SOURCE: Adapted from Applebaum, P. S. (1988). The right to refuse treatment with antipsychotic medications. *American Journal of Psychiatry, 145*(1), 145–146.

ate the person's dangerousness and to take appropriate actions to protect others from the danger. Studies show that almost half of the targets of clients' threats are family members, spouses, boyfriends, or girlfriends (McNiel, Binder, & Fulton, 1998).

The duty to disclose supersedes the client's right to confidentiality. The general rule is to warn identified persons and the local police of believable threats when the client is not confined to the hospital.

LEAVING AGAINST MEDICAL ADVICE (LAMA)

Clients, who have had a voluntary admission to a restrictive hospital setting, may wish to exercise their right to liberty and leave the facility. A client who is competent and who is no danger to self or others may not be prevented from leaving. If they are a danger to themselves or others, the staff must make a decision between safety and the right to refuse treatment. If necessary, commitment proceedings are initiated. Some of the more common reasons people seek discharge against medical advice include (McGihon, 1998):

- Family concerns, such as the care of young children or dependent elderly

- Financial reasons such as wanting to conserve lifetime benefits for mental health care

- A need to return to work

- Disagreement with staff that the length of hospitalization is necessary for treatment goals

- Uncomfortable withdrawal symptoms from substance abuse

Some clients simply walk out of the facility with no notification to staff. This is often called **elopement**, and the client may be either a voluntary admission or committed to the facility. When a client successfully elopes, the staff notifies the physician, the hospital administration, and the family. If it is determined that the client is dangerous to self or others, local police are informed of the situation. A hospital can be sued when clients who elope commit suicide, are injured or killed in accidents, or injure or kill others while away from the hospital. The liability is determined on the basis of two elements. The first element is how much the staff knew or should have known about the level of danger to self or others. The second element is the appropriateness of precautions taken to prevent LAMA in light of that knowledge.

If you are assigned to a locked unit, you should take some basic precautions. When entering or leaving the unit, look around and be aware of clients very near the door. These clients may slip out when the door is opened. If you leave the unit with other students, make sure that a client has not joined your group. When clients ask you to accompany them off the unit, check with the staff on each client's status for off-unit privileges.

OMNIBUS MENTAL ILLNESS RECOVERY ACT

The Omnibus Mental Illness Recovery Act is a new initiative targeted to state legislatures and state governments. It is designed to build a more comprehensive service-delivery system (Ross, 1999). The Act includes eight components and where further information is found in this text:

1. Increase in consumer and family-member participation in treatment planning (Chapter 3)
2. Health care coverage for mental illnesses the same as for medical illnesses (Chapter 3)
3. Access to new medications (Chapter 8)
4. Expansion of assertive community treatment programs (Chapter 4)
5. Work incentives for persons with severe mental illness (Chapter 4)
6. Reduction in the use of restraint and seclusion except for emergency safety situations (Chapter 10)
7. Reduction in the criminalization of mental illness (Chapter 6)
8. Increased access to permanent, safe, and affordable housing with appropriate community-based services (Chapter 3)

CLIENTS WITH LEGAL CHARGES

Some clients admitted to the psychiatric unit may have legal charges pending. You may have difficulty working with these clients when the behavior that resulted in the legal charges is in conflict with your personal values. Examples are a client admitted for severe depression with legal charges of sexually molesting his child and a client admitted to a substance abuse program who hit a pedestrian while driving under the influence. When ethical dilemmas arise, you must identify your feelings and seek peer or supervisor advice in managing the situation and avoiding punitive reactions. Confidentiality is extremely important in such circumstances. Clients must also be informed that the court may request their medical records and that staff members may be required to testify in court.

THE MENTALLY ILL IN CORRECTIONAL SETTINGS

The number of mentally ill people in correctional settings has increased over the past 30 years. Studies indicate that 10 to 18 percent of prison inmates suffer from a major mental disorder. With few long-term psychiatric facilities, many people who were previously cared for in state hospitals are now found in jails and prisons. The increase in numbers is also related to a lack of support in the community for the disabled mentally ill population. About one third of these individuals are homeless and victims of a cycle of mental hospitals, the street, and jail as a way of life over which they have no control. They may be jailed because no other agencies are available to respond to their psychiatric emergency. The jail has become the mental hospital that cannot say "no." Often, the crimes with which they are charged are misdemeanors resulting from their symptoms of mental illness, such as disorderly conduct, trespassing, camping out, and public intoxication. This *"criminalization"* of mental illness is one of the most disturbing trends in our nation and must be stopped. Under the 14th Amendment of the Constitution, mentally ill jail detainees have a right to mental health services. The reality is that psychiatric evaluation and intervention is haphazard at best. Mental health treatment is primarily centered on decreasing the symptoms through medications (Maeve, 2000).

The prison subculture makes those who are seriously mentally ill more vulnerable to abuse and victimization by both inmates and guards, since those who are mentally ill hold low status. Women prisoners remain sexually vulnerable to a largely male correctional force. Many mentally ill people suffer cruelty and abuse by other inmates, including torment, beatings, and rape. When an inmate needs someone to take the blame or punishment, the inmate who is mentally ill is easily manipulated into this position. Guards often place severely mentally ill prisoners in solitary confinement for misbehavior that is a product of their mental illness. Symptoms worsen with the prolonged social isolation, sensory deprivation, excessive use of force by guards, use of restraints as punishment, and inadequate medical care. Solitary confinement is no place for any prisoner, especially one who is seriously mentally ill (Teplin, Abram, & McClelland, 1997).

The suicide rate among jail inmates is eight times that of the U.S. population, with hanging being the most common method. The first 24 hours following the arrest is the period of highest risk as people with mental illness are put in cells and abandoned and ignored during an extremely stressful period. Adolescents may be especially vulnerable due to feelings of fear, humiliation, and isolation from their peer group. People charged with murder may be at highest risk due to a generalized impulsivity (Scheflen & Giltman, 1999).

At the present time Congress is examining strategies to create local mental health courts. These programs would provide supervision of offenders with mental illness or mental retardation who are charged with nonviolent crimes. It is hoped that there will be provision for life-skills training, housing placement, vocational training, education, job placement, health care, and relapse prevention for each participant. The goal of these programs would be to create alternatives to incarceration (Scheflen, 2000).

CARING: A PREREQUISITE TO ETHICAL BEHAVIOR

Caring is the essence of nursing and foundation for ethical behavior. People who are in a caring relationship are likely to behave in an ethical manner toward each other. Caring involves compassion and sensitivity to each person within the context of her or his entire life. Caring is being respectful of people's choices as to the best course of action to be taken. Caring is accepting people as they are and envisioning what they may become. Caring is honoring each person's wholeness of being—mind, body, emotions, and spirit.

NURSING ETHICS

Ethics refers to a system or morals or rules of behavior. It is the evaluation of right or wrong behaviors in any given culture. Ethics are the principles that govern human behavior. The term *ethics* is also used to describe the study of standards governing the practice of professional nurses. Nursing, like many disciplines, has identified guidelines for ethical behavior.

PRINCIPALISM

Nursing is a value-laden practice. We are required to make numerous ethical decisions every day. Traditionally, nurses have been taught ethics from the perspective of principalism. This is based on the belief that there are universal, objective principles that ought to govern the moral behavior of people. The principles are autonomy, beneficence, nonmaleficence, and justice. Autonomy is the right to make decisions for oneself. Beneficence is the performance of good acts that benefit others, in contrast to nonmaleficence, which is not acting in a way that would cause harm to self or others. The principle of justice states that people should be treated equally and people should be recognized for responsible behavior. The problem with the perspective of principalism is that socioeconomic and cultural contexts are completely ignored. They are also far too abstract to have any practical application in clinical practice (Artnak & Dimmitt, 1996; McGee, 1996).

VALUES

Caring for clients whose values and lifestyles are similar to ours does not challenge us to make the choice to accept the client's inherent worth. As our society becomes more ethnically diverse and multicultural in character, the potential for rising ethical conflicts increases. When values and lifestyles are dissimilar, we are challenged to make caring, ethical decisions. Consider how each of the following clients might pose an ethical dilemma when admitted to a mental health care facility: a known drug pusher; a mother who has killed her baby through physical abuse; a teenager who has sexually molested his sister; an adult daughter who has physically abused her elderly father; an accused rapist. As nurses, we must be able to respect the humanness of every client in spite of differences in values and lifestyles.

COMPETENT CARE

The expectation that nurses will deliver competent care is fundamental to the notion of professional nursing practice. This is evidenced by the American Nurses Association's Nursing Code of Ethics described in Box 6.1. Competence is both "knowing what" and "knowing how." It is not a permanent state achieved when you get your nursing license but rather a continuing process of improving and refining your skills and knowledge. Competence is both education and attitude. Education is the academic program you are enrolled in and continuing education throughout your years of practice. Attitude includes being open to criticism by colleagues and a willingness to admit to lack of knowledge or error when appropriate. Competence is the recognition of one's limitations as well as one's strengths and skills. With the explosion of scientific information, competent nurses must stay current with developments in their areas of practice (Weis & Schank, 2000). The ANA Code of Ethics can be viewed online by accessing the American Nurses Association's Web site, which can be accessed through a resource link on the Companion Web site for this book.

RESEARCH

An ethical dimension exists in mental illness as it relates to clients and their participation in nursing

---

BOX 6.1

ANA Code of Ethics for Nurses

1. The nurse, in all professional relationships, practices with compassion and respect for the inherent dignity, worth, and uniqueness of every individual, unrestricted by considerations of social or economic status, personal attributes, or the nature of health problems.

2. The nurse's primary commitment is to the patient, whether an individual, family, group, or community.

3. The nurse promotes, advocates for, and strives to protect the health, safety, and rights of the patient.

4. The nurse is responsible and accountable for individual nursing practice and determines the appropriate delegation of tasks consistent with the nurse's obligation to provide optimum patient care.

5. The nurse owes the same duties to self as to others, including the responsibility to preserve integrity and safety, to maintain competence, and to continue personal and professional growth.

6. The nurse participates in establishing, maintaining, and improving health care environments and conditions of employment conducive to the provision of quality health care and consistent with the values of the profession through individual and collective action.

7. The nurse participates in the advancement of the profession through contributions to practice, education, administration, and knowledge development.

8. The nurse collaborates with other health professionals and the public in promoting community, national, and international efforts to meet health needs.

9. The profession of nursing, as represented by associations and their members, is responsible for articulating nursing values, for maintaining the integrity of the profession and its practice, and for shaping social policy.

SOURCE: Reprinted with permission from American Nurses Association. Code of Ethics for Nurses with Interpretive Statements, © 2001 American Nurses Publishing, American Nurses Foundation/American Nurses Association, Washington, DC.

research. This is especially true for people with the more debilitating mental illnesses such as schizophrenia and bipolar disorder. When problems with cognition, emotion, motivation, and memory are combined with symptoms such as delusions and hallucinations, these impairments might well limit clients' abilities to understand, appreciate, and reason about the choices they have in regard to research.

Clients who are considering participation in research, along with their caregiving family members, must be fully aware of what the protocols involve, what risks they will face, what options they have, and who they should contact with questions or issues as they arise. We must not mistakenly assume that impaired capacities necessarily imply that potential research subjects cannot give informed consent. What is often the case is that individuals may have a harder time grasping the content of the disclosure. Approaches to this problem include repetitive disclosure of information, group sessions to have questions answered, and the involvement of family members.

Research involving people with mental disorders is essential if we are to better understand the underlying causes of these illnesses, how individuals and families cope, and which interventions are most effective. There are also rewards for individuals participating in nursing research. Rewards may include the pride that comes from altruistic behavior, the hope that they themselves might benefit from the results of the study at some point in the future, and the more immediate possibility that they may have access through the study to therapeutic approaches that would not otherwise be available to them (Flynn, 1998; Roberts, Warner, & Brody, 2000).

The challenge is to continue to work with volunteers who have mental disorders to discover and develop better nursing interventions while at the same time doing all we can to protect the rights and well-being of those who participate in research.

ETHICS OF CARE

Nursing is based on an ethics of care. We use many perspectives in the process of ethical decision making, which can be summarized in four categories: medical indications, client preferences, quality of life, and contextual factors. *Medical indications* include the diagnosis, prognosis, and treatment options with probable outcomes. *Client preferences* relate to the individuals' values and goals for life in general and their advance directives when they are acutely ill. *Quality of life* involves clients' perceptions about what their life is like and what they would like it to be. *Contextual factors* include social and environmental details about the problem and how these affect treatment options (Artnak & Dimmitt, 1996).

The nursing profession places a high value on client autonomy and the client's right to participate in treatment planning and implementation, as reflected in the Nursing Code of Ethics. This code implies that one of the primary functions of the nurse is to be an advocate for the client's wishes. At times, you will function much in the same way as an advance directive. The Patient Self-Determination Act became federal law in 1990. This law states that clients have a right to participate in their own care. In addition, health care professionals are required to inform clients of the right to accept or refuse medical care, including medications.

Ethics is more a process than a set of answers. At the heart of every ethical dilemma is the potential for conflict—conflict within ourselves, conflict between nurse and client, or conflict among professionals. We must confront difficult ethical problems and arrive at options that best support the client's own values and wishes.

CHAPTER REVIEW

COMMUNITY RESOURCES

Links to these Web sites can be accessed on the Companion Web site for this book.

Commission on Mental and Physical Disability Law
American Bar Association
740 15th St. NW
Washington, DC 20005
202-662-1570
www.abanet.org/disability

International Society of Psychiatric-Mental Health Nurses
1211 Locust St.
Philadelphia, PA 19107
800-826-2950
www.ispn-psych.org

Judge David L. Bazelon Center for Mental Health Law
1101 15th St. NW, Suite 1212
Washington, DC 20005-5002
202-467-5730
www.bazelon.org

KEY CONCEPTS

Introduction

- Whenever possible, client autonomy and liberty must be ensured by treatment in the least restrictive setting and by active client participation in treatment decisions.

Types of Admission

- Voluntary admission occurs when a client consents to confinement in the hospital and signs a document indicating as much.

- Commitment, or involuntary admission, may be implemented on the basis of dangerousness to self or others. Some states also have the criterion of prevention of significant physical or mental deterioration for involuntary admission.

- Adult clients can be held temporarily on an emergency basis until there is a court hearing determining the need for commitment.

- Commitment is for a specified period of time. At the end of this time, the client must be discharged or the court must be petitioned again for continued hospitalization.

- Clients can initiate advance directives to guide families and caregivers in making decisions when they are unable to make them for themselves.

Competency

- Competency is a legal determination that a client can make reasonable judgments and decisions about treatment and other significant areas of personal life.

- An adult is considered competent unless a court rules him or her incompetent. In such cases, a guardian is appointed to make decisions on that person's behalf.

- Clients who are committed are still capable of participating in health care decisions.

Confidentiality

- Adherence to the principle of confidentiality is extremely important in the practice of psychiatric nursing.

- There are federal rules regarding chemical dependence confidentiality. Staff members are not allowed to disclose any admission or discharge information.

- Some states require written consent before HIV tests may be performed. States have laws regarding when HIV test results or the diagnosis of AIDS may be disclosed.

Informed Consent

- Informed consent is a client's right not to be touched or treated without consent. Clients must be given enough information to make a decision, must be able to understand the information, and must communicate their decision to others.

- In an emergency situation with no time to obtain consent without endangering health or safety, a client may be treated without legal liability.

Client Rights

- Clients do not lose their constitutional or legal rights when they are admitted to the hospital to treat a mental disorder.

- Clients have the right to refuse psychotropic medications.

- If the court finds the client to be incompetent and medications are in the client's best interest, the judge may order the client to take the medications.

KEY CONCEPTS *(continued)*

Reporting Laws

■ All states make it mandatory for nurses to report suspected cases of child abuse or neglect. Some states have enacted similar adult abuse laws.

Duty to Disclose/Protect

■ The duty to disclose is the health care professional's obligation to warn identified individuals if a client has made a credible threat to kill them.

Leaving Against Medical Advice (LAMA)

■ Staff members must take precautions to prevent LAMA, or elopement, from the unit by those clients who are dangerous to self or others.

Omnibus Mental Illness Recovery Act

■ This Act is a new initiative targeted to state legislatures to build a more comprehensive service-delivery program.

Clients with Legal Charges

■ Clients who have legal charges pending against them must be informed that the court may request their medical records.

The Mentally Ill in Correctional Settings

■ Criminalization of mental illness is one of the most disturbing trends in our nation and must be stopped.

■ Clients with mental disorders may be jailed because their symptoms are mistaken for criminal behavior or there may be no other agencies available to respond to their psychiatric emergency.

■ Clients with mental disorders who are imprisoned are vulnerable to abuse and victimization by other inmates and correction officers.

■ The suicide rate among jail inmates is eight times that of the U.S. population.

■ Congress is examining strategies to create alternatives to incarceration for people who have been charged with nonviolent crimes and who are mentally ill.

Caring: A Prerequisite to Ethical Behavior

■ Caring behaviors include attentive listening; providing comfort, honesty, patience, and responsibility; providing adequate information, touch, sensitivity, and respect; and calling the client by name.

Nursing Ethics

■ Nurses are required to make numerous ethical decisions every day. Client differences in values and lifestyles often present nurses with an ethical dilemma when clients are admitted to a mental health care facility.

■ Competent care involves knowing what and how to do things, being open to criticism, and a willingness to admit to lack of knowledge or error when appropriate.

■ The perspective of principalism in ethics ignores the socioeconomic and cultural contexts and is too abstract to have practical application in clinical practice.

■ Nursing is based on an ethics of care, including medical indications, client preferences, quality of life, and contextual factors.

■ Clients who are considering participation in nursing research must be fully aware of what the protocols involve, what risks they will face, what options they have, and who they should contact with questions or issues as they arise.

■ The challenge is to continue to work with volunteers who have mental disorders to discover and develop better nursing interventions while at the same time doing all we can to protect the rights and well-being of those who participate in research.

EXPLORE *MediaLink*

■ Interactive resources, including animations, for this chapter can be found on the Companion Web site at *http://www.prenhall.com/fontaine.* Click on Chapter 6 and select the activities for this chapter.

■ For NCLEX review questions and an audio glossary, access the accompanying CD-ROM in this book.

REFERENCES

American Nurses Association. (2001). *Code for nurses with interpretative statements.* Washington, DC: Author.

Artnak, K. E., & Dimmitt, J. H. (1996). Choosing a framework for ethical analysis in advanced practice settings. *Archives of Psychiatric Nursing, 10*(1), 16–23.

Carolla, B. (2000). The last frontier? *NAMI Advocate, 21*(3), 11–12.

Carpenter, W. T. (1999). The challenge to psychiatry as society's agent for mental illness treatment and research. *American Journal of Psychiatry, 156*(9), 1307–1310.

Clark, N., & Bowers, L. (2000). Psychiatric nursing and compulsory psychiatric care. *Journal of Advanced Nursing, 31*(2), 389–394.

Flynn, L. (1998). Research and ethics must go hand in hand. *Decade of the Brain, 9*(3), 1–3.

Gardner, W., Lidz, C. W., Hoge, S. K., Monahan, J., Eisenberg, M. M., Bennett, N. S., et al. (1999). Patients' revisions of their beliefs about the need for hospitalization. *American Journal of Psychiatry, 156*(9), 1385–1391.

Lidz, C. W., Mulvey, E. P., Hoge, S. K., Kirsch, B. L., Monahan, J., Eisenberg, M. M., et al. (1998). Factual sources of psychiatric patients' perceptions of coercion in the hospital admission process. *American Journal of Psychiatry, 155*(9), 1254–1260.

Maeve, M. K. (2000). Speaking unavoidable truths: Understanding early childhood sexual and physical violence among women in prison. *Issues in Mental Health Nursing, 21*(5), 473–498.

McGee, G. (1996). Waiting for Godot: Where is the philosophy of nursing? *Journal of Psychosocial Nursing, 34*(6), 43–44.

McGihon, N. N. (1998). Discharges against medical advice: Provider accountability and psychiatric patients' rights. *Journal of Psychosocial Nursing, 36*(1), 22–27.

McNiel, D. E., Binder, R. L., & Fulton, F. M. (1998). Management of threats of violence under California's duty-to-protect statute. *American Journal of Psychiatry, 155*(8), 1097–1101.

Roberts, L. W., Warner, T. D., & Brody, J. L. (2000). Perspectives of patients with schizo-phrenia and psychiatrists regarding ethically important aspects of research participation. *American Journal of Psychiatry, 157*(1), 67–74.

Ross, E. C. (1999). Nutural reinforcement: NAMI's omnibus recovery state initiative and federal policy agenda. *NAMI Advocate, 20*(5), 5.

Scheflen, K. (2000). Mental health court bills introduced in Congress. *NAMI Advocate, 21*(3), 13.

Scheflen, K., & Giltman, L. (1999). Innovative approaches to jail diversion. *NAMI Advocate, 21*(1), 17–18.

Teplin, L. A., Abram, K. M., & McClelland, G. M. (1997). Psychiatric disorders among women in jail. *Decade of the Brain, 8*(2), 8–10.

Watson, T. L., Bowers, W. A., & Andersen, A. E. (2000). Involuntary treatment of eating disorders. *American Journal of Psychiatry, 157*(11), 1806–1810.

Weis, D., & Schank, M. J. (2000). An instrument to measure professional nursing values. *Journal of Nursing Scholarship, 32*(2), 201–204.

PART TWO

Foundations of Neurology

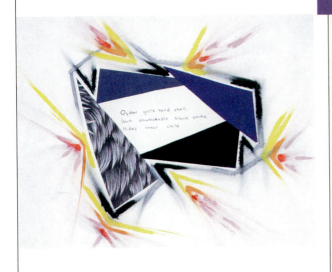

Oyster girl's hard shell.
Dark uncrackable black shield.
Hides inner child.

—Kate, Age 19

CHAPTER 7

Neurobiology and Behavior

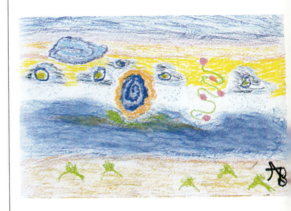

OBJECTIVES

After reading this chapter, you will be able to:

- DESCRIBE basic brain development.
- DISCUSS selected functions of the brain.
- RELATE brain function to major brain structures.
- EXPLAIN basic neurophysiology.
- DISCUSS nutritional neuroscience.
- IDENTIFY the role of neuroanatomy and neurophysiology in brain dysfunction.

*F*ree-floating Connections

—*Anthony, Age 17*

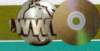

MediaLink

CD-ROM
- *Audio Glossary*
- *NCLEX Review*

Animations
- *Neurosynapse*
- *Reuptake Inhibitor*
- *PET and SPECT Scans*
- *Agonist/antagonist*
- *Cytochrome Oxidase*

Companion Web site
www.prenhall.com/fontaine
- *Critical Thinking*
- *More NCLEX Review*
- *Case Study*
- *Care Map Activity*
- *Links to Resources*

The human brain is among the most complicated objects in the universe. It is a dynamic ecosystem that adapts to internal and external environments and responds to use or disuse. The brain has 100 billion neurons, 1,000 billion other cells, multiple levels of organization, and thousands of genes that construct it and permit it to function properly. Each neuron may have from 1 to 10,000 synaptic connections to other neurons. No brain is perfect, no two brains are alike, and each individual's brain is continually changing.

The *mind* is a property of brain activity, that is, it is a process, not a thing. Psychophysiological processes such as perception, thinking, emotion, memory, motivation, behavior, and conscious experience reflect the activation of complex networks of neurons throughout the brain (Ratey, 2001).

Historically, lack of understanding of brain function led to separating mental disorders from other serious illnesses and to stigmatizing those who were suffering. Problems were blamed on childhood trauma or bad parenting. Mental disorders are now understood as brain deficits, and neuropsychiatric science is focusing on the etiology and treatment of these mental disorders. Biological psychiatry encompasses neuroanatomy, neurophysiology, neurochemistry, neurogenetics, neuroimmunology, neuropsychology, neuroendocrinology, neuroimaging, and neurocomputational sciences. Researchers hope to learn how the brains of those affected by mental disorders are different from the brains of those who are not. We still have a long way to go in understanding how they occur, but we do know that mental disorders, like strokes and brain tumors, are serious brain disorders.

What this means for you, as a nursing student, is that in addition to principles from nursing, sociology, and psychology, nursing care of clients with mental disorders also includes principles from the biological sciences.

DEVELOPMENT OF THE BRAIN

GENES AND ENVIRONMENT

Mental health and mental illness both involve complex interactions of genes and environments from conception through the end of life. *Genes* give direction for initial development and provide the broad outline of development. Although they are the basic building blocks, genes do not determine destiny. The term *environment* refers to the multiple factors that turn genes on or off, causing cells to differentiate, divide, sprout new connections, or strengthen others. For a given nerve cell, these "environments" may be the number, rate, and firing patterns of neighboring neurons; hormonal factors within the brain; stress hormones passed within the mother's breast milk; trauma to specific nerve cells; and events and experiences perceived by the brain. For the developing brain, environment refers to factors ranging from obstetric complications, intrauterine infections, and early nutrition to exposure to stressful life experiences such as community violence. As our knowledge increases, we have learned that some disorders such as autism are disorders of brain development, while others such as posttraumatic stress disorder results from traumatic experiences that affect the brain's structure and function.

Genes and environment interact continually from the moment of conception to death. In some situations genes are more important, and in others environment is more important. Our brain changes every second of our lives in response to everything we perceive, think, feel, and do (Ratey, 2001). (Genetics are covered in more detail in Chapter 1.)

FETAL AND INFANT BRAIN DEVELOPMENT

Fetal brain development is a highly regulated process under the control of a large number of genes, many of which remain to be discovered. It proceeds in a sequence of steps, and each step is strongly dependent on those that precede it.

During the third and fourth week after fertilization, the *neural tube* develops, which will give rise to the brain and spinal cord. The first major step in the development of the brain is the generation of a huge number of nerve cells. Complications during this period are usually fatal to the fetus.

The second major step occurs during the second trimester as these cells migrate and differentiate. After a cell is born, it *migrates* to where it is genetically programmed to go. Nerve cells destined for the brain migrate over considerable distances, following guides provided by other cells. When the cell gets to its predetermined location, it starts to *differentiate* and *communicate* with other neurons. This process continues until a person is about eight years old. Consequences of deficient cell migration and differentiation can be devastating. Trauma or disruption during this process affects a neuron's ability to communicate with other neurons. Problems in neuronal communication ultimately affect overall brain function. At present, we cannot predict deficits in a structure before the structure develops. For example, higher-level cognitive functions, such as planning and predicting, generally develop around the age of 16. If the frontal lobe structures of the brain are even slightly damaged, the deficit will not be apparent until that developmental stage (Smock, 1999).

The third major step, the *brain growth spurt*, begins in the third trimester, reaches peak acceleration prior to full term, and continues at a gradually decreasing rate until around the age of two. The infant's brain contains twice as many neurons as the adult brain but there are relatively few synapses. Synapses develop in the context of experiences with caregivers, and synaptic density peaks during childhood, followed by a decline of 30 to 40 percent during adolescence to reach adult levels, which remain relatively stable (Grigsby & Stevens, 2000).

As the brain ages, weak or unused neurons are *pruned* away. This means the environment in early years can have an incredible impact. In many cases there is a window of time during which a person must have a particular experience in order to keep particular neurons. For example, an infant born with cataracts will not have her or his vision neurons stimulated. If the problem is not corrected by 6 months of age, the vision neurons are eliminated since they are not being used. In this situation, the child will never gain sight, even when the cataracts are removed (Ratey, 2001).

The newborn infant has an incompletely developed central nervous system. There are as many as 12 growth spurts between birth and the early twenties when brain development is finally completed. Adult function is determined by intact neuroanatomy and neurophysiology and by the brain's ability to repair itself—**neuroplasticity.** The brain is extraordinarily plastic, which means that it spends much of its life improving itself, refining structures, and responding to internal and external changes. Neuroplasticity illustrates the unity of our internal and external worlds and the interaction of nature and nurture. Dendrites grow and retract, synapses may increase or decrease in number, the release of neurotransmitters changes, and receptors may alter their shape (see Figure 7.1 ■). Research has demonstrated that even in old age, new synaptic connections are formed. Recent research has discovered that, in a few specific regions, such as the hippocampus, neutrons are actually regenerated. This gives us hope that in the future we will learn how the brain regenerates itself and repairs damage caused by aging, disease, or trauma (Black, 2001; Ratey, 2001).

GENDER DIFFERENCES

Scientists have found convincing evidence that the brains of women and men are different in overall size, size of certain brain structures, cerebral blood flow, and glucose metabolism. In the XY fetus, the testes secrete testosterone, which masculinizes the reproductive tract and the brain of male fetuses. The female fetal brain is

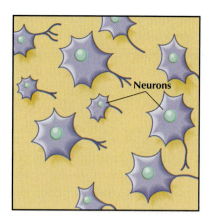

A At birth, the infant's brain has a complete set of neurons but not very many synaptic connections.

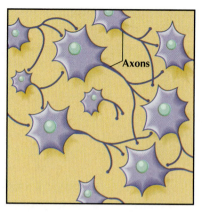

B During the first year, the axons grow longer, the dentrites increase in number, and a surplus of new connections is formed.

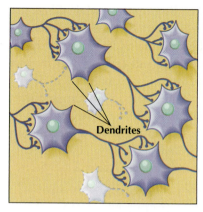

C Over the next few years, active connections are strengthened, while unused connections atrophy.

FIGURE 7.1 ■ The developing brain. At birth, the infant's brain has a complete set of neurons but relatively few synaptic connections.

SOURCE: Kassin, S. (2001). *Psychology* (3rd ed.). Upper Saddle River, NJ: Prentice Hall.

not exposed to testosterone and develops in a female pattern. These disparities may help to explain *gender-related differences* in behavior. A consistent finding is that men perform better than women in spatial and motor targeting tasks, whereas women have greater verbal fluency and fine motor skills than men do. The same emotion might trigger a man to fight and a woman to react with words, facial expressions, and gestures. Women are more vulnerable to mood disorders and Alzheimer's disease while men are more vulnerable to schizophrenia. Thus, it is recognized that the adult brain has been shaped in part by its hormonal environment (Kimura, 1999; Seeman, 1997).

AGING

Until recently it was thought that brain cells die off by the millions throughout life, resulting in a poorly functioning brain in old age. New research shows that although the cells function less efficiently, there is not a devastating loss of function in *healthy aging brains*. The reductions in brain dopamine (DA) activity that occur as part of aging are associated with changes in motor activity and cognitive changes in the speed of processing information and memory retrieval. Aging causes a slowdown in the communication network of the brain

rather than a massive death of brain cells (Backman et al., 2000; Volkow et al., 2000).

Some of the normal changes of aging can be slowed down through active use of your brain. Intellectual activity stimulates brain cells to develop new dendrites, creating millions of new synapses between neurons. The brain is like a muscle—using it leads to growth, while disuse causes atrophy. Education appears to make brains more resistant to deterioration and Alzheimer's disease (Carper, 2000).

BRAIN REPAIR

Throughout life, all cells, including brain cells, are bombarded by attacks from unstable chemicals called *oxygen free radicals*. As the body goes through its normal processes and oxygen is used to provide cellular fuel, some of the oxygen molecules lose one of their pair of electrons. When this happens, the formerly stable oxygen molecules become dangerous free radicals that try to stabilize themselves by stealing another electron from stable molecules, thus damaging them and creating more free radicals. All organs and tissues are subject to damage from free radicals, but the brain is extremely vulnerable because it uses so much oxygen in producing vast amounts of energy to fire millions of neurons. In addition, as enzymes in the brain synthesize neurotransmitters, more oxygen free radicals are formed.

Free radicals are normally kept under control through the production of **antioxidants**, enzymes that act as free radical scavengers to search out and neutralize dangerous free radicals (Fontaine, 2000). These antioxidants are vitamin E, vitamin C, glutathione, coenzyme Q10, and lipoic acid. An antioxidant donates an electron to a free radical, thus neutralizing it. As a result, the antioxidant itself becomes unstable but harmless. Antioxidants work together as a team when another antioxidant donates an electron needed for rehabilitating the first one, ensuring continued survival of the antioxidants. One family of enzymes, called SOD (superoxide dismutase) is thought to be deficient in amyotrophic lateral sclerosis (Lou Gehrig's disease) (Black, 2001; Carper, 2000).

Antioxidants manage to repair at least 99 percent of the free radical damage to cells. The amount of permanent brain damage depends on the strength of the antioxidant defenses. As we age we produce more free radicals and fewer antioxidants. The more free radical damage, the more likely we are to age prematurely and experience chronic diseases. Many people believe the best way to avoid these age-related changes is to boost the intake of antioxidants (Black, 2001; Carper, 2000).

Research suggests that regular *physical exercise* makes our bodies more adept at delivering oxygen and nutrients to the brain. Your brain is a hungry machine that makes up just 2 percent of your body weight but consumes 20 percent of your total oxygen and glucose stores. It functions best when arteries are kept clear, which is more likely to happen with exercise. Ultimately, genetics and lifestyle have a significant impact on the aging process of the entire body, including the brain (Carper, 2000).

NEUROANATOMY

The brain is regionally specialized; that is, different regions do different things. This is in contrast to functionally homogeneous organs like the liver in which any section can more or less substitute for another. Every area of the brain is directly or indirectly interconnected with every other area.

The most abundant cells in the brain are the *glial cells*. There are 10 glial cells for every neuron. They are embedded in a matrix that contains growth factors, sugars, and proteins. There are four types of glial cells: astrocytes, oligodendroglia, ependyma, and microglia. Astrocytes regulate groups of neurons by controlling the concentration of neurotransmitters and ions. They even release their own neurotransmitters, causing dramatic changes in nearby neurons. Astrocytes are also responsible for the blood–brain barrier. Oligodendroglia coat the axon with a fatty substance called *myelin*, which protects the axon and controls the speed of impulses in the axon. The ependymal cells produce cerebrospinal fluid, and the microglial cells are responsible for phagocytosis (Minton & Hickey, 1999; Ratey, 2001).

There are as many as 100 billion individual *neurons.* Each neuron has a small, rounded body with short, dense branches called dendrites and a single long nerve fiber called an axon. Dendrites are the way neurons get information, and axons are the way neurons pass on information. Dendrites are covered with receptors that receive incoming signals from other neurons. **Receptors** are proteins in the cell membrane that combine with a hormone, chemical transmitter, or a drug to alter the function of the cell. The synapse is the space between the end of the axon of one cell to the dendrites of other cells. Each neuron may have a direct synaptic connection with as many as 10,000 other neurons. All neurons, directly or indirectly, talk to each other, relay information, and network in ways we are only beginning to understand. There are at least 50 different kinds of neurons varying in lengths and branching patterns of dendrites and axons. Even then, no two cells are alike. From day to day, some synaptic connections are not likely to remain exactly the same. Some will have retracted their dendrites or axons; others will have extended new ones; and certain others will have died, depending on the individual's experiences. It is through strengthening or weakening these connections that most development and learning occurs. This is part of neuroplasticity previously discussed (Edelman & Tononi, 2000).

Individual cells are effective only in a group working together toward a single goal. *Ganglia* are dense collections of nerve cells with common functions. Ganglia may have as few as 50 neurons or as many as 10,000 neurons. There may be as many as 100 million ganglia in the brain.

Nerve tracts are groups of nerve fibers carrying signals to and from the same area. The two main nerve tracts are the corpus callosum and the cingulate gyrus.

The *corpus callosum* is composed of 200 million nerve fibers that connect the left and right cerebral hemispheres and relays sensory information between the two. The *cingulate gyrus*, part of the limbic system, encircles the hippocampus and other limbic structures. The cingulate gyrus is the main information highway of emotion. It integrates emotions with thinking in order to send a coherent message to the hypothalamus (Grigsby & Stevens, 2000).

The brain is divided into three main areas: the brain stem, the cerebellum, and the cerebrum. They are all interconnected and work as an integrated unit.

BRAIN STEM

The brain stem, consisting of the midbrain, pons, and medulla, forms the stalk from which the cerebral hemispheres and the cerebellum sprout (see Figure 7.2 ■). The brain stem is the location of those functions vital to sustaining life. Such functions include the central processing of respiration, heart rate, balance, and blood pressure. It is the part of the brain that is most important to life. A person can survive damage to the cerebrum and cerebellum, but damage to the brain stem usually means rapid death. The brain stem is also the home of the 12 *cranial nerves*, which carry sensory and motor information to and from higher brain regions.

Three tiny structures in the brain stem—the raphe nuclei, the locus coeruleus, and the substantia nigra—are the focus of great interest to neuroscientists. The *raphe nuclei* are the primary source for serotonin (5-HT) in the brain and spinal cord. Clusters of serotonergic neurons lie along the midline of the brain stem, from the midbrain to the medulla, and project to all levels of the brain. The *locus coeruleus*, located in the pons and with connections to almost every part of the brain, is the primary source of norepinephrine. Stimulation of the locus coeruleus creates an instant fear response in humans and animals. The locus coeruleus and the raphe nuclei are part of the *reticular activating system* (*RAS*). The RAS controls both inhibitory and excitatory functions by receiving impulses from all over the body and relaying them to the cortex. It is the central structure in the brain responsible for arousal, wakefulness, consciousness, sleep regulation, and learning. It may influence whether our behavior is aggressive or passive. The relationship between RAS dysfunction and mental disorders is not well understood at this time (Dilts, 2001; Smock, 1999).

The *substantia nigra* is a major source of dopamine for the brain. It projects axons to the striatum, which is

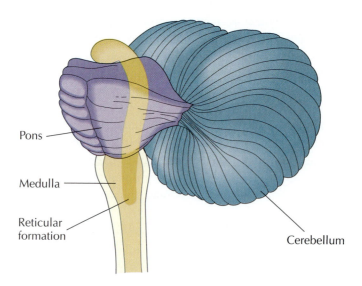

FIGURE 7.2 ■ The brain stem. The brain stem is the most primitive structure of the brain. Resting atop the spinal cord, it contains the medulla, pons, and reticular formation and is attached to the cerebellum.

SOURCE: Kassin, S. (2001). *Psychology* (3rd ed.). Upper Saddle River, NJ: Prentice Hall.

involved in the initiation of voluntary movement. This area of the brain appears black because cells contain the pigment melanin, which is an end product of the breakdown of DA. Degeneration of the DA cells in the substantia nigra produces the motor disorders of Parkinson's disease. Many antipsychotic medications are potent DA receptor blockers, resulting in side effects such as movement disorders (Dilts, 2001; Smock, 1999).

CEREBELLUM

The cerebellum, which wraps around the brain stem, has a unique appearance and is composed of several lobes. The cerebellum helps coordinate the planning, timing, and patterning of skeletal muscle contractions during movement. It is the cerebellum that enables us to grasp a glass on the first try and walk in an upright manner. It maintains our posture and equilibrium by receiving input about balance from the inner ear. The cerebellum is responsible for the storage, retrieval, and use of procedural memory. Procedural memory impairments include difficulty performing tasks that are normally habitual, such as brushing teeth and getting dressed.

Just as the cerebellum coordinates physical movement, it also coordinates the movement of thoughts. It plays a role in our ability to visualize our favorite beach or plan the sequence of an argument. It has recently been discovered that the cerebellum also sets the timing and rhythm of brain function. It does this by delaying or speeding up the coordination of stimuli, memories, and thoughts (Ratey, 2001).

CEREBRUM

The cerebrum, sitting on top of and surrounding the brain stem, makes up 80 percent of the weight of the brain. The cerebrum is divided into two hemispheres—right and left. Each of the hemispheres has separate and unique functions. Yet if one hemisphere is damaged, the other hemisphere seems to be able to take on some of its functions.

Each hemisphere is divided into the *cortex* (the highly convoluted matter on the outside) and the *subcortical structures* (buried within). In fresh tissue, the outer surface of the cortex appears gray due to the presence of mostly cell bodies and dendrites, hence the term *gray matter*. Underneath the gray matter, the tissue appears white due to the presence of large numbers of axons covered in myelin, hence the term *white matter*.

The cortex is further divided into four lobes: frontal, parietal, temporal, and occipital (see Figure 7.3 ■). The subcortical structures include the limbic system and the basal ganglia.

Frontal Lobe

The frontal lobe is the site of our ability to think and plan, and is partially responsible for executive functions, discussed later in this chapter. The frontal lobe regulates emotions and behavior and stability of the personality and inhibits primitive emotional responses. The *ventromedial cortex* is the section of the frontal lobe that is responsible for the emotional component of decision making, especially in the context of interpersonal relationships. Feelings are an important part of decision making, in that feelings point us in the right direction. It is our "gut" feelings that distinguish us from inanimate computers in the decision-making process. Other functions of the frontal lobe include general motor ability and the motor aspects of spoken and written speech.

Parietal Lobe

The parietal lobe is the site of the sensory functions of touch, taste, and temperature and the perception of pain. Additional sensory functions include receptive speech and the ability to envision written words (e.g., to read the word *tree* and visualize a tree).

A significant function of the parietal lobe is **proprioception**, the ability to know where our body is in time and space (position sense). An example of disordered proprioception sometimes reported by people with mental disorders is the inability to see in three dimensions. This impairment may contribute to difficulty dressing, eating, and drinking in an organized manner.

The parietal lobe also regulates the ability to evaluate muscular activity. This lobe may control a person's capacity to sit motionless for hours or to hold a single body part in one position for long periods of time. Another function of the parietal lobe is the ability to associate the memory of primary sensory experiences with more complex memories. Dysregulation of this function may result in repeating the same mistake over and over.

Temporal Lobe

The temporal lobe is the site of the complex processes of memory, judgment, and learning. It processes the world of sight and sound into meaningful informa-

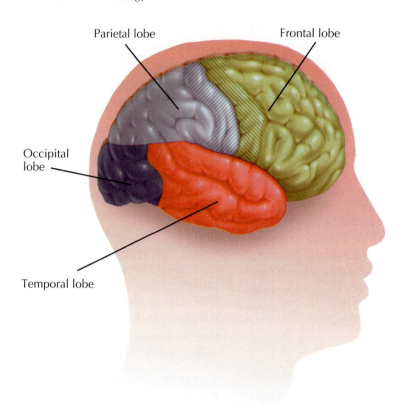

FIGURE 7.3 ■ The four lobes of the cerebral cortex. Deep fissures in the cortex separate these areas or lobes.

SOURCE: Morris, C. G., & Maisto, A. A. (2001). *Understanding psychology* (5th ed.). Upper Saddle River, NJ: Prentice Hall.

tion. The temporal lobe is the site for abnormal perceptions (illusions) and auditory hallucinations. Déjà vu (the sensation of having been somewhere before when you have not been there) and jamais vu (not recognizing familiar places) result from disturbances in the temporal lobe.

The dominant side, usually the left, is involved in understanding and processing language, complex memory, and emotional stability. Increased or decreased activity may contribute to labile moods, intense violent thoughts, aggression, and homicidal or suicidal behavior. Abnormal activity in the nondominant side leads to social skill problems and the inability to recognize facial expression (Amen, 2001; Black, 2001).

The temporal lobe connects with the limbic system to allow for memory and the expression of emotions. Another temporal lobe function is gender identity, the sense of being female or male. Do not confuse gender identity with sexual orientation, the site of which is

deep inside the brain in the anterior hypothalamus (Kimura, 1999).

Occipital Lobe

Unlike the other lobes, which have multiple functions, the occipital lobe has only one function—vision. It is responsible for sight and the ability to understand written words. It is also involved in producing visual hallucinations.

Limbic System

The limbic system is often referred to as "the emotional brain." Emotional responses such as anger, fear, anxiety, pleasure, sorrow, and sexual feelings are generated in the limbic system but are interpreted in the frontal lobe. The limbic system is the reward center of the brain, which is what motivates us to do something or learn something so we feel satisfied. Another function of the limbic system is the interpretation of our most basic and primitive sense: the sense of smell. The limbic system is thought to be the site of olfactory hallucinations. The ability to interpret sensations from the internal organs, referred to as visceral reflexes, also resides in this region.

The limbic system consists of portions of the frontal, parietal, and temporal lobes that form a continuous band of cortex in a ringlike formation around the top of the brain stem. Other structures of the limbic system are the amygdala, the hippocampus, the cingulate gyrus, the nucleus accumbens, the thalamus, and the hypothalamus (see Figure 7.4 ■).

The *amygdala* coordinates the actions of the autonomic nervous system and the endocrine system and is involved in the control of emotions. It is essential to nurturing behavior and fear conditioning. When something scares or upsets us, the amygdala stamps that moment in memory. From then on, when something seems to resemble that original moment of distress, the amygdala recognizes the similarity and dic-

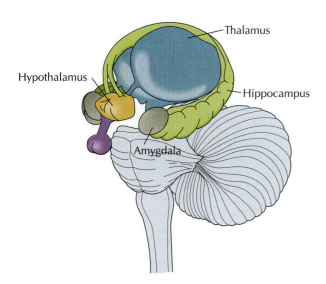

FIGURE 7.4 ■ The limbic system. Just above the inner core, yet surrounded by the cerebral cortex, the limbic system plays a role in motivation, emotion, and memory. As shown, this system is composed of many structures, including the thalamus, amygdala, hippocampus, and hypothalamus.

SOURCE: Kassin, S. (2001). *Psychology* (3rd ed.). Upper Saddle River, NJ: Prentice Hall.

tates our response in a few 100ths of a second, even before the stimulus reaches the cognitive centers of our brains. Dysfunction in the amygdala contributes to inappropriate rage and fear, anxiety, posttraumatic stress disorder (PTSD), and attention deficit/hyperactivity disorder (ADHD) (Ratey, 2001).

The *hippocampus* is the critical information-processing station between the parts of the brain that receive sensory experiences and the parts of the brain that translate these experiences into action. It channels sensory input to the appropriate brain area and regulates the resulting motor output pathways.

The hippocampus is intricately involved in regulation of the immune system and in collation of memories stored in other parts of the brain. Damage or incomplete formation of the hippocampus results in declarative memory impairment. People with hippocampal dysfunction appear to resist learning and may be perceived as lazy or unmotivated, when in fact they are unable to recall previously learned information (Dilts, 2001).

The *cingulate gyrus* has a role in regulating stress through changes in the autonomic nervous system. It receives more input from the thalamus than any other cortical region. It is also responsible for regulating the emotional content of physical pain. The cingulate gyrus is the executive organizer by directing our attention and deciding what information gets into the frontal lobes. It is also the link between motivation and behavior.

The *nucleus accumbens* is the reward center of the brain. When there are abnormally low DA receptors in this area, the person has a decreased ability to experience pleasure. Much attention has focused on the nucleus accumbens as the site of action of cocaine, amphetamines, nicotine, marijuana, alcohol, chocolate, and carbohydrates. Levels of DA in the nucleus accumbens are also increased through high-risk behaviors. High-risk behaviors demand increased attention and concentration for long periods of time, which forces an increase in the release of DA. This understanding has led to the identification of a new syndrome—the **reward deficiency syndrome**. The decreased ability to experience pleasure drives the person to seek external forms of gratification through the use of substances, pathological gambling, or other high-risk behaviors (Ratey, 2001).

The *thalamus* enables us to have impressions of agreeableness or disagreeableness in response to sensations. It monitors sensory input and acts as a relay station in processing nearly all sensory and motor information coming from the spinal cord, brain stem, and cerebellum. Pain sensations travel from the spinal cord through the brain stem to the thalamus, which then sends the pain signals to the parietal lobe. Dysfunction within the thalamus makes it difficult for people to sense or interpret pain. The thalamus is thought to regulate levels of awareness and emotional aspects of sensory experiences by exerting a wide variety of effects on the cortex (Smock, 1999).

Thalamic dysfunction is involved in obsessive–compulsive disorder, schizophrenia, and the mood disorders, and contributes to the similarity in symptoms experienced by people diagnosed with various mental disorders.

The *hypothalamus* is a neuroendocrine (neurons that produce hormones) group of nuclei that is vital to homeostasis. As an integration center, the hypothalamus converts thinking and feeling into hormones, causing physical changes throughout the body via the autonomic nervous system. With the *pituitary gland*, the hypothalamus helps regulate the autonomic nervous system by assisting with the vital functions of water balance, blood pressure, sleep, appetite, temperature, and carbohydrate and fat metabolism. When a person perceives a stressful event, the hypothalamus–pituitary–adrenal (HPA) axis responds. The hypothalamus increases production of corticotropin-releasing factor (CRF) which stimulates the pituitary gland to release adrenocorticotropic hormone (ACTH), which enters the general circulation and travels to the adrenal cortex where, within a few minutes, it stimulates cortisol release. Cortisol acts throughout the body to mobilize energy reserves in an effort to manage stress. Cortisol, which readily crosses the blood–brain barrier, interacts with specific receptors in the hypothalamus and other parts of the brain, completing the feedback cycle.

Dysregulation of the hypothalamus can lead to excessive thirst and insatiable hunger. The hypothalamus may be involved in anorexia nervosa and bulimia nervosa. As one of the main concentration sites of the neurotransmitter dopamine, the hypothalamus is implicated in many of the common side effects of psychotropic medications that influence dopamine transmission.

The *suprachiasmatic* nuclei (SCN) in the hypothalamus are responsible for circadian rhythms, discussed later in this chapter. Almost all the neurons in the SCN

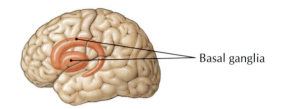

FIGURE 7.5 ■ Location of the basal ganglia.

SOURCE: Smock, T. K. (1999). *Physiological psychology: A neuroscience approach.* Upper Saddle River, NJ: Prentice Hall.

use gamma-aminobutyric acid (GABA) as their primary neurotransmitter. It is not yet clear how the SCN sets the timing of many important behaviors.

Basal Ganglia

The basal ganglia are areas of brain nuclei that lie in the center of each cerebral hemisphere deep in the temporal lobe (see Figure 7.5 ■). The basal ganglia consist of the caudate, the putamen, and the globus pallidus. The caudate and putamen together are called the *striatum*, which has an important role in the control of movement. The main stimuli to the basal ganglia come from the amygdala, hippocampus, thalamus, and cortex. The basal ganglia participate in many higher brain functions in concert with the cerebral cortex. The purpose of the basal ganglia is to organize complex patterns of thought and movement under the influence of emotional tone (see Table 7.1 ■) for brain structures, functions, and dysfunctions.

VENTRICLES

There are two large ventricles on either side of the cerebral hemispheres called the lateral ventricles. A smaller one in the center is called the third ventricle, and in the brain stem a fourth ventricle that communicates with the central canal of the spinal cord. The fluid in the ventricles is called cerebrospinal fluid (CSF), which circulates slowly through the brain and cord, cushioning the brain from physical shocks. CSF has an excretory function and regulates the chemical environment of the central nervous system. It also acts as a channel for chemical communication within the brain. Neurochemicals secreted by nearby neurons cross into the CSF, circulate, and cross back into the brain at any given point, facilitating communication between different areas of the brain (Smock, 1999).

TABLE 7.1

Major Brain Structures: Functions and Dysfunctions

Structure	Functions	Effects of Dysfunction
Frontal lobe	Ability to think and plan	Difficulty with abstract thinking, attention, concentration; lack of motivation
	Insight	Inability for self-evaluation
	Stability of personality	Instability of personality
	Inhibition of primitive emotional responses	Labile affect, irritability; impulsiveness; inappropriate behavior
	Motor aspects of written speech	Unintelligible and illogical writing
	Motor aspects of spoken speech	Words are garbled and difficult to understand
Parietal lobe	Receiving and identifying sensory information	Inability to recognize sensations such as pain, touch, temperature; inability to sense pain from an uncomfortable body position
	Memory association	Inability to learn from past
	Proprioception	Inability to recognize the body in relation to the environment
		Difficulty dressing, eating, etc. in an organized manner
	Sensory speech	Inability to recognize spoken or written words
Temporal lobe	Hearing	Auditory hallucinations
	Complex memory	Memory impairment; difficulty learning
	Emotion	Difficulty recognizing own emotions and controlling sexual and aggressive drives
	Gender identity	Confusion about masculinity and femininity
	Production of speech	Types of aphasia
	Analysis of speech	Difficulty attaching meaning to spoken words
Occipital lobe	Vision	Visual hallucinations; loss of visual memory
	Visual speech	Inability to understand the meaning of written words
Limbic system	Regulation of emotional responses	Excessive emotional responses; inability to recognize own emotions; decreased ability of cognition to affect emotions
	Interpretation of smell	Olfactory hallucinations; inability to interpret smell
	Memory collation	Difficulty with declarative memory

(continued)

TABLE 7.1

Major Brain Structures: Functions and Dysfunctions *(continued)*

Structure	Functions	Effects of Dysfunction
Limbic system *(continued)*	Memory collation *(continued)*	Working and long-term memory problems; difficulty learning
	Impressions of agreeableness or disagreeableness of sensations	Hypersensitivity or hyposensitivity to pain
	Regulation of autonomic nervous system	Increased thirst; insatiable hunger
Reticular activating system (RAS)	Receiving of impulses from entire body and relaying to cortex	Sedation and loss of consciousness; difficulty controlling aggression; may contribute to passivity
Cerebellum	Coordination of skeletal muscles during movement	Difficulty learning motor skills; problems regulating the force and range of movements
	Maintenance of equilibrium	Problems with balance
	Maintenance of posture	Difficulty walking upright
	Procedural memory	Difficulty performing tasks
	Reward center	Decreased ability to experience pleasure
		Reward deficiency syndrome

BLOOD–BRAIN BARRIER

The blood–brain barrier is a membrane between circulating blood and the brain. Unlike capillaries throughout the rest of the body, brain capillary pores are specialized and do not allow free movement of substances. This permeability barrier serves to protect the brain. The first function is to import critical nutrients and hormones, while exporting metabolic waste products. The second function is to protect the brain against foreign circulating chemicals, thereby protecting it from exposure to potential toxins (Black, 2001).

NEUROPHYSIOLOGY

Our knowledge of brain physiology at present is incredibly incomplete in many areas. Our current technology used to examine brain function still has many limitations. It is likely that whatever models we have today will be replaced by more advanced models as our understanding expands.

We are all subject to fluctuations in brain chemistry. The structures of the brain depend on hundreds of chemicals—glucose, vitamins, minerals, amino acids, and neurotransmitters—to carry out their functions. As our brain chemistry fluctuates, we all experience episodic problems with speech patterns, memory recall, spontaneous decision making, and any or all of the executive functions. People who experience more severe disruptions in brain chemistry may exhibit symptoms of mental disorders.

Interestingly, during rapid eye movement (REM) sleep, each of us experiences "symptoms" of mental illness. Thinking about your own experiences may help you understand clients' experiences. Box 7.1 describes what happens when we sleep.

NEUROTRANSMISSION

Neurotransmission is the electrochemical process that allows nerve signals to pass from one cell to another at the synapse, the microscopic area where two neurons meet. As the impulse travels through the axon of a neu-

BOX 7.1

How the Brain Goes Out of Its Mind

Every 80–90 minutes, during REM sleep, we become completely psychotic.

Experience	Psychiatric Label
We see things that are not there.	Hallucinations
We believe things that could not possibly be true.	Delusions, magical thinking
We become confused about times, places, and persons.	Disorientation
Scenes simply appear and thoughts come and go.	Attention deficit
We think we are awake even though we are doing and seeing impossible things.	Lack of insight
We experience wildly fluctuating emotions.	Labile affect
We invent implausible narratives.	Confabulation, loose association
We forget almost everything on awakening.	Amnesia

This nocturnal madness is not only normal but probably essential to our health. Deprived of REM sleep, we become anxious and irritable and have trouble concentrating. Understanding this normal delirium may help you become more empathetic with persons experiencing those same symptoms while awake.

SOURCES: Hobson, J. A. (1996). How the brain goes out of its mind. *Harvard Mental Health Letter, 12*(8), 3–5; and LaBerge, S., & Rheingold, H. (1990). *Exploring the world of lucid dreaming.* New York: Ballantine Books.

ron, storage vesicles release a small amount of stored neurotransmitters, which diffuse across the synapse and latch on to *receptor proteins* embedded in the postsynaptic, or second, neuron. Receptors are specific to one neurotransmitter much like a lock and key. No matter how much of a neurotransmitter is released, if it does not have a perfect fit, the receptors will not be activated. Binding of the neurotransmitter to the receptor triggers the activation of the second cell. Once the transmitter completes its function, the receptor releases it back into the synapse. At this point, one of two things happens: An enzyme deactivates the transmitter or *transporters* take the transmitter back into the presynaptic terminal (reuptake). Transporters allow the body to recycle previously used transmitters so they do not have to be replaced by biosynthesis (Smock, 1999) (see Figure 7.6 ■).

Neuromodulators are chemicals that alter the threshold to the flow of information but do not necessarily alter the nature of the signal. They act as filters, allowing information to be processed more or less.

The term **ligand** is used to describe any substance that binds to the receptors. Ligands can be subdi-

vided into two categories. **Agonists** bind to and activate the receptor and are described as having weak or strong potency. Agonists include neurotransmitters and hormones as well as drugs. **Antagonists** block the action of a neurotransmitter at its receptors. Once an antagonist occupies the receptor, agonists can no longer bind and neurotransmission is blocked (see Figure 7.7 ■).

Neurotransmitters may be deactivated or returned to the presynaptic terminal before they reach the receptors. The postsynaptic neuron can be temporarily deactivated so it fails to respond to the stimulus. Neurotransmitters can act together to enhance transmission of impulses while at other times they act as antagonists—with one neurotransmitter inhibiting the action of another. Other factors such as hydration, electrolyte balance, overall metabolic demand, and glial cell influences affect the readiness of the neuron to fire. As you can see, the process of neurotransmission is complicated with potential for errors at many points along the way (Grigsby & Stevens, 2000; Smock, 1999). See Box 7.2 for factors influencing the rate of neurotransmission.

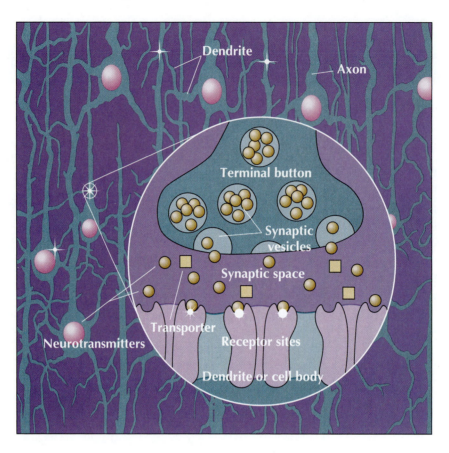

FIGURE 7.6 ■ Neurotransmission: How neurons communicate.

SOURCE: Morris, C. G., & Maisto, A. A. (2001). *Understanding psychology* (5th ed.). Upper Saddle River, NJ: Prentice Hall.

NEUROTRANSMITTERS

Neurotransmitters are the key information molecules of the brain. We currently know of at least 50 to 100 possible neurotransmitters representing diverse chemical *classes*, including the biogenic amines, amino acids, peptides, neurohormones, and gases. Neurotransmitters act, as the word implies, to transmit signals from one neuron to another. They can facilitate, activate, or inhibit postsynaptic neurons. Smaller molecule neurotransmitters, such as the biogenic amines, are usually *rapid acting* and generate the most dramatic responses in the brain. The larger and *slower-acting* molecules, such as the peptides, have less dramatic effects but cause more long-term alterations at the receptor sites by changing the number or sizes of the synapses. These effects can persist for days.

Neurons in different parts of the brain contain different neurotransmitters. Most neurons have numerous receptor types for a variety of neurotransmitters, enabling each neuron to receive many different signals.

In addition, there are several types of receptor sites for each neurotransmitter. For example, there are 5 dopamine receptor types and 18 serotonin receptor types.

It is difficult to fully appreciate the role of neurotransmitters; entire textbooks are devoted to each of them. Neurotransmitters do not operate in isolation. Much like a symphonic orchestra, they interact with each other and function as a group. It is believed that when dysfunctions occur with some neurotransmitters, others adapt and compensate for the dysfunction (Smock, 1999) (see Table 7.2 ■). You may want to review the principles of psychopharmacology in Chapter 8 after you read this section, as each category of medication affects one or more of the neurotransmitters.

Biogenic Amines

The biogenic amines are more often implicated in the psychobiology of mental disorders. There are six bio-

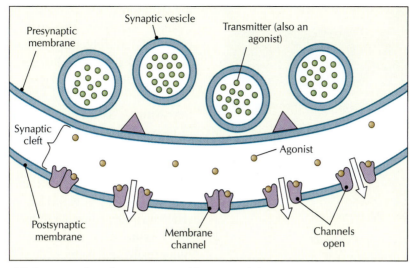

(A) Strong agonist activates receptors without transmission.

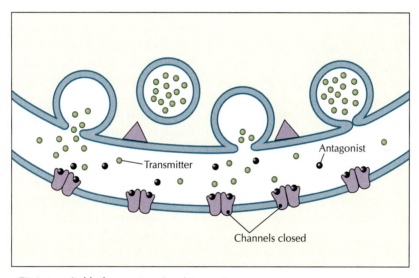

(B) Antagonist blocks receptors. Agonist cannot act.

FIGURE 7.7 ■ Ligands: agonists and antagonists. Agonists and antagonists bind to the same binding site as transmitter. An agonist has potency so it activates the cell biologically (A). Antagonists bind and have no potency (B). An antagonist produces its effect by blocking the binding site, preventing a transmitter from binding, and producing its biological effect.

SOURCE: Smock, T. K. (1999). *Physiological psychology: A neuroscience approach.* Upper Saddle River, NJ: Prentice Hall.

genic amine neurotransmitters: dopamine, serotonin, norepinephrine and epinephrine, acetylcholine, and histamine, which are synthesized in neurons. Dopamine, norepinephrine, and epinephrine are synthesized from the same dietary amino acid called *tyrosine*. Serotonin is synthesized from the dietary amino acid called *tryptophan*.

Dopamine   Dopamine (DA) is considered the grandparent of neurotransmitters. It is a catecholamine from which norepinephrine and epinephrine are metabolized. An excess or deficit amount of DA affects the levels of these other neurotransmitters.

DA plays an important role in motor activity, motivation, and reward. High levels of DA are reflected in sharper thinking, focused attention, and formation of long-term memory. It is often referred to as the "learning neurotransmitter."

DA also provides the motivation to act and find what you need for survival. When you perceive that you need something, DA directs your motor system to move your body to get it. DA is also what makes you smile and feel alert and energetic. It drives you to seek pleasure and rewards and takes you on an emotional high. DA is the *"gotta have it"* neurotransmitter, the facilitator, and the motivator. If DA reaches levels that are too high, hypomania or even mania can result (Volkow et al., 2000).

Dopamine deficiency interferes with learning, memory, and motivation. Antipsychotic drugs, used to treat hallucinations and delusions, block DA receptors, which decreases the ability to feel pleasure. People who are chronically deficient in DA (reward-deficient individuals) often engage in dopamine-boosting activities such as addictions from cigarettes to drug abuse to

hypersexuality. Other reward deficiency syndromes include attention deficit/hyperactivity disorder (ADHD) and Tourette's syndrome (see Chapter 17). Activities that provide instant reward become more important than long-term goals (Ratey, 2001).

Serotonin   Serotonin (5-HT) plays an important role in mood and emotional behavior. In contrast to DA, 5-HT is the soother, the constrainer, and the anti-impulsive neurotransmitter. 5-HT acts to balance DA. It decreases your focus and flow of information. It is what you need when you are feeling overwhelmed and prevents you from getting out of control from fear or worry. 5-HT calms us and elevates mood and self-esteem. Abnormally low levels of 5-HT result in decreased impulse control, aggression, and violence (Ratey, 2001).

5-HT is the *"got it"* neurotransmitter, allowing you to stop a particular behavior when you have achieved what you need. For example, when you are hungry DA drives you to search for food and 5-HT lets you know when you have had enough to eat. Without 5-HT, you would be unable to stop eating once you found food.

5-HT is quickly becoming the most widely researched neurotransmitter because of its broad range of functions. 5-HT tends to control the activity of other neurotransmitters and is the key player in all brain functions related to circadian rhythms. It is synthesized from the dietary amino acid tryptophan.

A significant research finding relevant to mental health nursing is that isolation reduces 5-HT levels. This finding helps to explain some of the devastating effects of seclusion on many clients. The converse is also true. Spending time in the company of people who are trusted can raise 5-HT levels. Cocaine, alcohol, and nicotine are known to reduce 5-HT levels. Newer antidepressants are selective inhibitors of 5-HT reuptake, keeping more 5-HT available in the synapse (Ratey, 2001).

Norepinephrine and Epinephrine   Norepinephrine (NE) and epinephrine (E) are derived from dopamine and are the adrenaline of the brain. Although NE accounts for only 1 percent of all available neurotransmitter content, we are very sensitive to even the smallest fluctuations. NE and E function similarly to DA, with a role in regulation of mood, memory, cognition, energy, and appetite.

TABLE 7.2

Neurotransmitters: Functions and Dysfunctions

Neurotransmitter	Functions	Effects of Excess	Effects of Deficit
Dopamine (DA)	Abstract thinking, decision making Pleasure and reward system Integration of thoughts and emotions Increase in sex drive, facilitation of orgasm	Mild: Enhanced creativity and problem solving; ability to generalize situations; good spatial ability; premature ejaculation Severe: Disorganized thinking, loose associations; disabling compulsions; tics; stereotypic behaviors	Mild: Poor impulse control; poor spatial ability; inability to think abstractly; no joy, no anticipation of pleasure Severe: Parkinson's disease; endocrine changes; movement disorders
Norepinephrine (NE) Epinephrine (E)	Alertness, ability to focus attention, ability to be oriented Necessary for learning and memory Primes nervous system for fight or flight	Hyperalertness; anxiety, panic Paranoia Loss of appetite Increased sensation-seeking behaviors	Dullness, low energy Depression
Serotonin (5-HT)	Inhibition of activity; calmness, contentedness Regulation of temperature of sleep cycle Pain perception Precursor to melatonin, which plays a role in circadian rhythms	Sedation; decreased anxiety Increased sleep Decreased sex drive; decreased orgasms Indecision Craving for sweets and carbohydrates If greatly increased, may have hallucinations	Irritability, hostility; increased aggression Decreased impulse control; increased suicidal tendencies Insomnia Increased sex drive
Acetylcholine (ACh)	Preparation for action; stimulation of parasympathetic system Emotional regulation Social play, exploration Control of muscle tone by balance with DA	Self-consciousness, excessive inhibition; anxiety Somatic complaints Depression	Lack of inhibition; euphoria Poor short-term memory Antisocial behaviors Parkinson's disease
GABA	Calmness, contentedness Reduction of aggression	Sedation Impaired recent memory Anticonvulsant	Irritability Lack of coordination Seizures

Acetylcholine

Acetylcholine (ACh) is found in abundance in the brain and is the "guardian angel" of the parasympathetic nervous system. ACh continually strives to keep the sympathetic nervous system in check. DA and ACh function in relative balance. ACh is thought to greatly influence learning and memory; it may also be involved in mood and sleep disorders. Other effects include emotional regulation, social play, exploration, thermoregulation, water intake, and motor function.

There are two types of ACh receptors: nicotinic and muscarinic. The medication succinylcholine (Anectine) is a nicotinic receptor antagonist that is given to clients receiving electroconvulsive therapy to induce muscle relaxation and prevent injury-producing muscle contractions. Blockage of the muscarinic receptors results in the anticholinergic side effects of many of the psychotropic drugs (Keltner, 2000).

ACh and glutamate also act on the glia and increase the production of *nerve growth factor (NGF)*. NGF accelerates nerve fiber growth necessary for synapse formation and also strengthens synapses (Black, 2001).

Histamine

Little is known about the functions of histamine as a neurotransmitter. We do know that histamine is involved in allergic reactions and may be involved in the medication side effects of sedation and hypotension. Recent research has suggested that histamine plays a role in sexual behavior (Pert, 1997).

Amino Acids

The major amino acid neurotransmitters are GABA, glutamate, and glycine. The major excitatory amino acid neurotransmitters are glutamate and aspartate. Glycine and aspartate appear to be particularly active in the spinal cord.

Gamma-Aminobutyric Acid

Gamma-amino-butyric acid (GABA) is the principal inhibitory neurotransmitter and is present in 25 to 40 percent of the synapses. GABA regulates anxiety and influences muscular coordination. Deficiencies can cause a high level of tension and anxiety, a lack of coordination, and expression of epileptic seizures. GABA may play a role in cognition, memory, and aggressive behavior. It is also one of the neurotransmitters involved in antianxiety-agent dependence. Antianxiety agents partially fill the receptor sites normally filled by GABA, and the normal production of GABA is reduced. Over time, the brain becomes reliant on the exogenous antianxiety agents to fill the receptor sites, and dependency results.

Glutamate

Glutamate (glu) is one of the most abundant neurotransmitters; it is stored in large quantities, and is the main excitatory neurotransmitter. Glu excites neurons and makes them fire. Without glu, our brain neurons could not communicate. Glu is important to learning and memory as well as to the development and strengthening of synapses. Blockage of glu receptors stimulates symptoms of schizophrenia (Brown, 2001).

Too much glu in the brain can lead to a number of brain diseases and even death. Glu-induced cell death is seen in stroke, epilepsy, brain damage due to hypoglycemia, brain trauma, Alzheimer's disease, and amyotrophic lateral sclerosis. Damage to neurons releases toxic levels of glu, which rapidly kill neurons by overexciting them, a process called **excitotoxicity**. The administration of glu antagonists appears to prevent cell death. The same process seems to occur in situations of uncontrolled neuron firing such as during repeated seizures. The process is less clear in Alzheimer's disease in which destruction of certain brain areas is responsible for the devastating memory loss. When the same brain area is treated with excitotoxins in animals, they exhibit characteristic memory deficits and plaques and tangles (Black, 2001).

Neuropeptides

Neuropeptides include substance P, neurotensin, L-tryptophan (L-T), neuropeptide Y (NPY), vasoactive intestinal polypeptide (VIP), galanin, and cholecystokinin (CCK). These neurotransmitters were discovered only recently and their functions are just being understood. Neuropeptides are large molecules stored in and released from secretory granules in axon terminals. Since peptides are often found in the same neuron with other neurotransmitters, they may serve as modulators for other transmitters, the neuroendocrine system, and the autonomic system.

Galanin can affect memory, mood, learning, epilepsy, and weight. Too little may lead to increased pain and seizures. Too much may cause memory loss, depression, and obesity. Researchers are hopeful that galanin may be the foundation for the next era of psychotropic drugs.

Neurohormones

Hormones are chemical substances produced by cells within an organ or gland.

Hormones are manufactured and stored in the cells. When the cells receive the appropriate signal, usually from the nervous system, they release an appropriate amount of the stored hormone into the circulatory system. Neurohormones are those hormones that act as neurotransmitters or modify the actions of neurotransmitters. Neurohormone examples that relate to mental disorders are endorphin and enkephalin, dehydroepiandrosterone (DHEA), oxytocin, vasopressin, phenylethylamine (PEA), and estrogen.

Endorphin and Enkephalin. Endorphin and enkephalin are opioids that are produced in the brain from a complex chain of amino acids. They play a significant role in our ability to experience pleasure and help protect us from pain perception. Being touched and stroked by another person increases the amount of endorphin in our brain. Endorphin also increases when we smile and when we think positive thoughts. We may smile because we are experiencing a surge of endorphin or we may get a surge of endorphin when we smile.

DHEA. There is more DHEA in our bodies than any other hormone. It could be called the parent of all hormones because most of our other hormones are derived from it. Although most of our DHEA is produced by the adrenals, our brain can make its own. DHEA improves cognition, protects the immune system, decreases cholesterol, promotes bone growth, and serves as an antidepressant. As the precursor of pheromones, it influences who we find attractive and who is attracted to us. DHEA serves as a natural aphrodisiac and increases in the brain during orgasm (Crenshaw, 1996).

Oxytocin. Oxytocin is secreted from the pituitary gland and travels to receptor sites in various parts of the brain as well as to the reproductive tract. It increases DA, 5-HT, estrogen, testosterone, prolactin, and vasopressin. Oxytocin promotes touching and is instrumental in the bonding between mates and between parents and children. It decreases cognition and impairs memory (Ratey, 2001).

Vasopressin. Vasopressin balances the influence of oxytocin. It improves cognition through enhancing attention and alertness while reducing emotional extremes. One benefit of vasopressin is its influence on how we think. It focuses us on the present moment and helps us pay attention to what we are doing. It is an antidote for both anxiety and depression. Increased levels of vasopressin may be related to higher levels of aggression. Serotonin may be a balancing factor by inhibiting vasopressin-induced anger by stopping its release in the hypothalamus (Ratey, 2001).

PEA. PEA is a natural form of amphetamine produced in our brain and fluctuates according to our thoughts, feelings, and experiences. It is believed that PEA is our "hormone of love," rising to high levels during romantic times in our lives and possibly involved in love at first sight. Low levels of PEA have been associated with depression, and high levels may contribute to psychotic symptoms (Pert, 1997).

Estrogen

Estrogen maintains and restores memory in the brain. It appears to work by increasing the activity of ACh and by stimulating the growth of dendrites and synapses, thus improving communication. Estrogen also serves as an antioxidant, destroying destructive free radicals.

Gases

In the brain, *nitric oxide (NO)* is formed in the neurons in response to the release of other neurotransmitters. As a gas, it cannot, however, be stored in the synaptic vesicles. There are no receptors for NO, and it appears to work by diffusion into neighboring cells. NO is critical for penile erections and may also play a role in learning and memory (Snyder & Ferris, 2000).

Little is known about the role of carbon monoxide (CO) as a neurotransmitter. It may be involved in the regulation of olfactory neurons. It appears to be the neurotransmitter mediating ejaculation (Snyder & Ferris, 2000).

CYCLIC PATTERNS

The daily lives of all living things are filled with various changes that take place in cyclic patterns. **Circadian rhythms** are regular fluctuations of a variety of physiological factors over 24 hours. These include adrenal, thyroid, and growth hormone–secreting patterns, as well as temperature, sleep, arousal, energy, appetite, and motor activity patterns. *Ultradian rhythms* are regular fluctuations shorter than 24 hours and repeat more than once a day. An example of an ultradian rhythm is the 90-minute REM/non-REM sleep cycle. *Infradian rhythms* are regular fluctuations over periods longer than 24 hours, such as the menstrual cycle.

The biological "clock," or internal pacemaker is located in the suprachiasmatic nuclei in the hypothalamus. Neurons in the SCN are sensitive to light, which coordinates sleeping and waking with light–dark cycles. It is not yet clear how the SCN sets the timing of so many important behaviors.

Rhythms may be desynchronized by external or internal factors. An example of external desynchronization is jet lag, in which rapid time zone changes result in decreased energy level and ability to concentrate, as well as mood variations. In some individuals, internal desynchronization may result in depression. The tendency toward internal desynchronization is probably inherited, but stresses, lifestyle, and normal aging also influence it.

FUNCTIONS OF THE BRAIN

The brain is the site of all nonconscious and conscious processing. Most of the brain's work is done *nonconsciously*, that is, by automatic selection of perceptual, cognitive, and behavioral routines that are appropriate to the situation. This type of processing is fast and efficient, which is critically important. The lowest levels of the brain are specialized for the quick and automatic handling of routine tasks, such as reflexes, eye movements, and basic perceptions that do not require deliberate processing. Simple tasks like talking and walking become automatic early in childhood. Nonconscious processing allows you to devote your limited *conscious processing* capacity to higher-level activities such as self-monitoring, planning, and organizing your actions. This awareness of yourself and the outside world

CRITICAL THINKING

You have been attending a medication group at a community mental health center as part of your clinical rotation. The group meets weekly to assist clients who are taking medications for a variety of psychiatric illnesses. There are eight clients in the group, and a nurse leads the group. You are enjoying the group, but you feel overwhelmed with all the different medications and you are trying to connect what you know about neurobiology and behavior to the medications and the client behavior and communication that you observe in the group.

You ask the nurse leader if you can meet with her to discuss some of your questions. She agrees that it would be a good idea and that she would have some questions for you to think about too. Before you meet with her, you think about the group and the clients. Medications that have been discussed in the group are antipsychotics and antidepressants. Based on the group discussions, you know that the clients are experiencing or have experienced the following symptoms: illusions, hallucinations, violent thoughts, lack of motivation, stress, and obsessive–compulsive symptoms. Some clients appear to have problems understanding metaphors and focus on facts and use literal interpretations. You read in the records that some of the clients

have loose association, but you are not sure if you have observed it. One client uses very rapid speech, and you cannot seem to interrupt her.

1. What is the relationship between genes and the environment and mental illness?

2. The nurse discusses the importance of understanding brain function and symptoms to better appreciate the effect that medications have on clients. What is the relationship of the following symptoms to brain function: illusions, hallucinations, violent thoughts, lack of motivation, stress, and obsessive–compulsive symptoms?

3. What is the importance of neurotransmission to the effect of biochemical treatment?

4. Compare and contrast the neurotransmitters dopamine and serotonin.

5. The nurse tells you that it is important to understand client behavior, cognition, and language. What are some data that indicate these clients have problems with cognition and language?

For an additional Case Study, please refer to the Companion Web site for this book.

occurs at higher brain levels. In a well-functioning brain, nonconscious and conscious processes work in tandem (Grigsby & Stevens, 2000).

The brain relies on complex feedback and feedforward systems for the regulation of activity. **Feedback** dynamics allows for a modification of a behavior while it is in progress. For example, your toddler has just stepped into the busy street. In running toward your child, you assimilate perceptual input—obstacles in your way, how close the cars are to the child—as you are running. **Feedforward** is the prediction of what is about to occur without waiting for feedback. Thus, behavior—running toward child—is begun before you fully understand the situation. Feedback and feedforward work together. Feedback provides more precise control of behavior but also requires more processing, which is slower. Feedforward quickly takes the person to the needed area or initiates the necessary response (Grigsby & Stevens, 2000).

EXECUTIVE FUNCTIONS

Executive functions of the brain are complex cognitive abilities that include interpreting, analyzing, sorting, and retrieving information about our internal and external environments. It also includes our ability to plan ahead and problem solve. *Insight* is the ability to observe ourselves and come to an understanding of our motivation for our behavior. You will find that some of your clients lack insight; that is, they have little or no ability to observe their own behavior or determine if it is appropriate for the situation. The ability to *regulate behavior* is another executive function. This allows us to stop purposeless or inappropriate behavior as well as to initiate and complete goal-directed activity. Problems in regulating behavior result in either distractibility or apathy. Clients who are *distractible* find it difficult or impossible to inhibit their responses to a wide range of internal and external stimuli and are unable to focus their attention. Clients who are *apathetic* are unable to start or follow through with even simple self-care activities without being told to do so.

MEMORY

Learning is the gathering of new knowledge, and **memory** is the retention of that knowledge for future use. Memory is not static but changes over time and involves a variety of brain systems. Without memory,

you would be unable to read this sentence or find your way to school tomorrow or recognize your family members. Memory provides the foundation for learning throughout life. Every thought we have, every word we speak, our very sense of self and our sense of connectedness to others, we owe to our memory, to the ability of our brains to record and store our experiences. It is why the loss of memory due to Alzheimer's disease or accidents is so profound.

Memory is not static but changes over time and involves a variety of brain systems. Two types of memory exist: *working* or *short-term memory* and long-term memory. Working memory, lasting minutes to hours, causes temporary changes in the function of neurons. Working memory allows us to ignore distractions so that we can make sense out of what we experience at any given moment. It also allows us to make judgments, anticipate consequences, and take responsibility.

It is only if the stimulation is strong and repetitive that *long-term memory* is activated (see Figure 7.8 ■). So yes, it would pay to read this chapter more than once before the exam! In general, events that cause us great joy or pain are easier to recall. Bits and pieces of a single memory are stored in different neuronal groups all around the brain. It is thought that the hippocampus brings these pieces together when it is time to recall that memory. Rather than storing memories, the hippocampus collates memories (Ratey, 2001).

The REM stage of sleep is important to human memory. Brain wave activity in the hippocampus during REM sleep consolidates our experiences into long-term memory. This is evidenced by experiments interrupting either REM sleep or non-REM sleep 60 times a night. When REM sleep is interrupted, there is a complete block of learning, while interruption of non-REM sleep appears to have no effect on learning. Thus, it is believed that REM sleep is critical for organizing the pieces for long-term memory (Ratey, 2001).

Our memories are more imperfect and suggestible than we like to think. The act of imagining an event makes it familiar to us, and this familiarity later gets mistakenly "remembered" as a past experience. We must keep in mind that memory is vulnerable to the power of suggestion and that we cannot take our memory as truth (Ratey, 2001).

Long-term memory is divided into two types: declarative and procedural memory. *Declarative memory* is

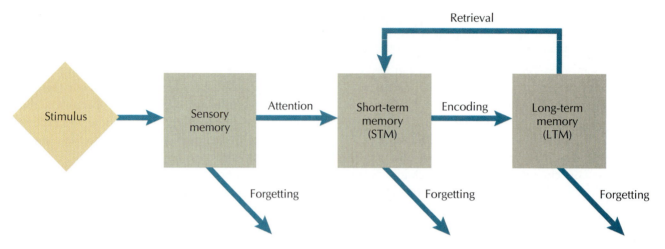

FIGURE 7.8 ■ An information-processing model of memory. Many stimuli register in sensory memory. Those that are noticed are briefly stored in short-term memory, and those that are encoded are transferred to a more permanent facility. As shown, forgetting may be caused by failures of attention, encoding, or retrieval.

SOURCE: Kassin, S. (2001). *Psychology* (3rd ed.). Upper Saddle River, NJ: Prentice Hall.

memory for people and facts, is consciously accessible, and can be verbally expressed (can be declared). The hippocampus and the medial temporal lobes are the seat of declarative memory. But the process of capturing and recalling information spreads throughout the brain, often in milliseconds. Each memory seems to be a compilation of tiny bits of information stored in a vast network of different cells. Just the simple ability to recall a phone number is believed to involve the activation of several thousand neurons throughout the brain. *Procedural memory* (knowing how) does not require conscious awareness and involves the memory of motor skills and procedures, such as riding a bicycle or typing a paper. The basal ganglia are involved in procedural memory (Smock, 1999).

COGNITION AND LANGUAGE

People with mental disorders may have noticeable problems in the form and content of their thinking and speech. *Abstract thinking* is the ability to generalize information, make predictions, build on prior memory, and evaluate the consequences of decisions. In the absence of abstract thought, thinking becomes concrete. It is also the ability to appreciate nuances in meaning and use metaphors and allegories. *Concrete thinking* is characterized by a focus on facts and details, a literal interpreta-

tion of messages, and an inability to generalize. Concrete thinking is a significant problem in people with mental disorders because it results in impulsiveness, instant need gratification, egocentricity, and an inability to follow a multiple-stage command. When there is no apparent relationship between thoughts, the person is said to have *loose association*. A person appears to have *illogical thinking* when expressed ideas are inconsistent, irrational, or self-contradictory. Some people exhibit *tangential speech* when thoughts veer from the main idea and never get back to it. *Circumstantial speech* occurs when the person includes many unnecessary and insignificant details before arriving at the main idea. A person is said to have *pressured speech* when her or his speech is rapid, tense, strained, and difficult to interrupt.

Language functions are distributed throughout the brain more than previously thought. The sound of a word may be in one area and the meaning of that word may be in another area. Language is primarily in the left hemisphere in 90 percent of the population, in the right hemisphere in 5 percent of the population, and split evenly in 5 percent of the population. The emotional aspect of language is located in the right hemisphere for most of us. The left inferior frontal cortex is involved in the production of audible speech and also

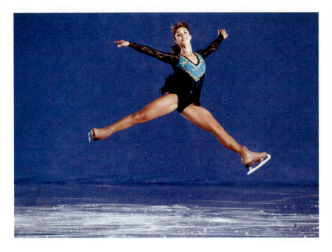
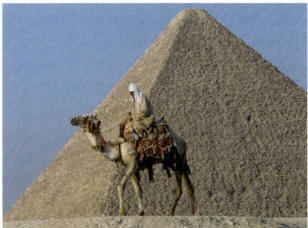

PHOTO 7.1 ■ There are two types of long-term memory. Procedural memory contains our knowledge of various skills, such as how to figure skate. Declarative memory contains our knowledge of facts, for example, what a pyramid is or where it can be found.

SOURCE: William R. Sallaz/Duomo Photography Incorporated; Kathleen Campbell/Getty Images, Inc.

where we engage in *self-talk*. Self-talk is part of problem solving as we think of solutions, consider consequences, and make decisions. Self-talk is indispensable for the development of empathy, understanding, and cooperation, which are basic to human social interaction (Ratey, 2001).

EMOTION

Emotions are the result of multiple brain and body systems working together. When an emotional stimulus enters the brain, it goes through two pathways. One pathway is for a body reaction via the limbic system. The stimulus goes to the amygdala for motor responses, the anterior cingulate for autonomic nervous system responses, the hypothalamus for endocrine responses, and the brain stem for heart rate and breathing responses. The other pathway is to the cerebral cortex where a cognitive assessment is made. For example, when we see a growling dog (stimulus), our body prepares for fight or flight and we begin to run away (body reaction) even before our brain registers that we are afraid (cognitive assessment) (see Figure 7.9 ■).

There are four basic emotions: fear, anger, sadness, and joy, although some researchers would add surprise, disgust, and guilt. All other emotions are combinations of these four. A new theory suggests that people have an inborn set point for mood, similar to the set point

for weight. This means that we have a steady, overall sense of happiness or sadness. Although our mood may change with life circumstances, it will inevitably return to our base level (Ratey, 2001).

Fear is the fastest physical reaction possible as the body is flooded with adrenaline. As just described, the most rapid pathway is through the limbic system, which provides a fast but less accurate assessment of the danger. The pathway to the frontal cortex is slower but provides a more accurate assessment of the danger.

It is important that all social animals, including humans, be able to control their *anger* and aggression. When the frontal lobes are underactive and executive function is compromised, anger may turn to aggression. We need frontal lobe activity to restrict impulses.

Sadness ranges from feeling "blue" to uncontrollable crying. Sadness gives us an opportunity to take a "time-out" to regroup and process what we are experiencing. Sadness may also be motivation to change. When we are feeling sad, there is increased activity in the left amygdala and right frontal cortex as well as decreased activity in the right amygdala and left frontal cortex. When we are sad for long periods of time, our store of neurotransmitters is depleted and we enter a state of depression or emotional numbness.

Joy is its own incentive. DA and endorphins play an important role in the nucleus accumbens. One of the

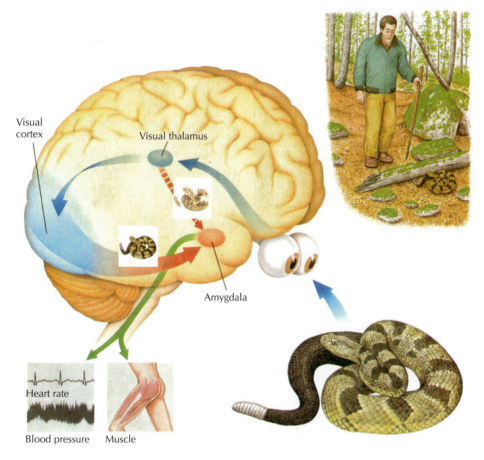

FIGURE 7.9 ■ Pathway of fear without "thought."

SOURCE: Kassin, S. (2001). *Psychology* (3rd ed.). Upper Saddle River, NJ: Prentice Hall.

side effects of medications that block DA is a sense of unhappiness and lack of motivation. When DA levels are too high, euphoric, disorganized, and psychotic behavior may be seen.

MOTIVATION

Motivation is not an emotion per se, but ties emotion to action. Motivation is what creates and guides our goal-directed behavior. It is what drives us to act. The cingulate gyrus, part of the limbic system, is our link between motivation and behavior. Outputs to the basal ganglia cause a motor reaction, outputs to the brain stem lead to physiological arousal, and outputs to the hippocampus contribute to memory formation. *Apathy* is considered a disorder of motivation or a malfunction of the motivation circuits of the brain. Increasing levels of DA in the limbic system may improve the sense of apathy (Ratey, 2001).

PSYCHONEUROIMMUNOLOGY

Psychoneuroimmunology is the study of relationships between environment, the hormonal system, immune system, and the central nervous system. Examples are damaging effects of chronic stress on the central nervous system, the body's defense against external infection, and aberrant cell division.

Stress is a term that includes a wide rage of environmental events that affect a person as well as a person's reactions to a stressful life event. *Acute stressors* are minor disturbances that often are insignificant in terms of general health. Acute stressors may affect health, however, when people are already "at risk" because of high chronic or severe stress such as chronic pain, chronic job stress, or severe relationship difficulties. In this situation, a moderate acute stressor can change the balance and contribute to illness. *Chronic stressors* may affect health. The effect of daily repeating stress is more pronounced than the effect of a major life event such as death or divorce. More important than the number of daily stressors, is the person's sense of control over stressors in terms of immune response (Heijnen, 2000).

The *immune system* is a surveillance system that protects the body. The immune system responds to a person's internal and external environments. It must distinguish between normal cells and malignant cells, as well as identify and destroy foreign and disease-causing organisms.

Cytokines are the chemical messengers of the immune system. They coordinate antibody and T-cell immune interactions. They include interferons, lymphokines, and interleukins. *Interferons* are formed when cells are exposed to a virus and prevent the spread of the virus to other cells. *Lymphokines* attract macrophages to the site of infection or inflammation and prepare them for attack. *Interleukins* have a variety of activities and they are named for their specific activity. *Proinflammatory interleukins* supplement the immune response to help increase the elimination of pathogens and resolve the inflammatory process. *Anti-inflammatory interleukins* inhibit the immune response by suppressing macrophage and natural killer T-cell functions. *Hematopoietic interleukins* promote the proliferation of blood cells, particularly bone marrow stem cells, B cells, and eosinophils. Because cytokines are closely associated with neurotransmitters and because stress stimulates cytokine production, researchers are beginning to investigate a possible role for cytokines in major mental disorders such as depression, schizophrenia, and Alzheimer's disease (Keller, 2000; Kronfol & Remick, 2000).

The central nervous system and the immune system work as an integrated whole to maintain a state of healthy balance within the body. Dysregulation in one induces change in the other. The pathways of communication are the autonomic nervous system and the neuroendocrine system. The autonomic nervous system innervates all the immune tissue and releases transmitters that activate the immune system. The other communication pathway involves hormone production by the hypothalamus and pituitary gland. These hormones are capable of altering the function of virtually every type of immune cell. The release of many of these hormones is significantly related to thoughts and feelings. Each thought and feeling has a chemical consequence within the brain relating to the production of neurotransmitters and neurohormones by the limbic system (Kronfol & Remick, 2000).

Cognitive and sociocultural stimuli are among the most potent factors in activating the biological responses to stress. An example is the effect of bereavement on a person's health. After the death of a spouse, the surviving spouse's risk of death is especially high during the first six months. This increased risk is thought to be related to a depressed immune system.

NUTRITIONAL NEUROSCIENCE

Nutritional neuroscience is a new research area regarding ways to keep the brain functioning at a peak level with supplements, diet, and other lifestyle changes.

Glucose is needed for neurotransmitter synthesis and secretion. Other necessary nutrients are amino acids, vitamins, minerals, and essential fatty acids. For example, brain cells need tryptophan to create 5-HT and choline to synthesize ACh. B vitamins are necessary for synthesis of 5-HT and GABA, and copper and tyrosine are needed for DA synthesis. Carnitine promotes cognition, magnesium is involved in sleep, and vitamin C is needed to cope with stress. Cholesterol is necessary to make myelin that surrounds and protects nerve fibers. Rapidly lowered cholesterol levels have been associated with depression, anxiety, panic disorder, violence, and suicide. Memory loss, confusion, depression, and other mental problems in the elderly, once thought to be part of normal aging, can result from a poor diet (Ratey, 2001).

Omega-3-type fish oil is necessary to keep your brain in top shape. It is made up of two specific fatty acids: DHA (docosahexaenoic acid) and EPA (eicosapentaenoic acid). DHA maintains pliability of neurons and increases supplies of ACh. The precursor to DHA is alpha-linolenic acid found in green leafy vegetables, flax seed, canola oil, walnuts, Brazil nuts, seaweed, and algae. Even if you ate enough of these foods, you would still need already-formed DHA found in omega-3-rich seafood. Replenishing EPA has improved brain function, especially in people who have schizophrenia. EPA can also be transformed to DHA in your brain (Carper, 2000).

Antioxidants are critically important for optimal brain function, as discussed earlier in the chapter. It is often necessary to take antioxidant vitamins such as vitamin A, thiamine, folic acid, vitamin C, vitamin E, and coenzyme Q10 in supplemental form, as most Western diets do not contain high enough levels.

Vitamin A acts as an antioxidant and is closely related to the carotenoids including beta-carotene, alpha-carotene, lycopene, lutein, and xeazanthin. These are found in deeply colored fruits and vegetables. Flavonoids, found in citrus fruits and berries, are also antioxidants. Nutrients with the highest levels of antioxidants are prunes, raisins, blueberries, blackberries, garlic, kale, cranberries, strawberries, spinach, raspberries, and tomatoes, as well as black and green tea and red wine. Vitamin C is an antioxidant that is required for tissue growth and repair. It also aids in the production of interferon, which enhances immunity. Vitamin E inhibits the oxidation of lipids and the formation of free radicals. It also aids in the utilization of vitamin A. Coenzyme Q10 may be an even more powerful antioxidant than vitamin E. It has also been used to improve mental function in people with schizophrenia and Alzheimer's disease (Balch & Balch, 1997; Fontaine, 2000).

DYSREGULATION

The ability to function and problem solve in everyday life depends on how the brain functions and processes information. Dysregulation of the brain, regardless of the cause, results in disruption of the ability to process information. There are four main causes of brain dysregulation: anatomical abnormalities or damage, lack of oxygen and/or glucose, electrolyte imbalance, and neurotransmitter dysfunction (see Table 7.3 ■). It is important that you understand the current information in biological psychiatry in order to respond to the client as a bio-psycho-social-spiritual being.

It is essential that you understand the contribution of neurobiology to mental illness. For example, it is important that you teach clients and families about neurotransmitter imbalances and the rationale for biochemical treatment (medications). It is hoped that when society recognizes that mental disorders are brain diseases, the current level of stigma will decrease or go away.

TABLE 7.3

Causes of Brain Dysregulation

Cause	Source	Clinical Implications
Anatomical abnormalities	Trauma Brain tumors Problems in brain development	Difficulty in information processing and coping with daily life stressors
Lack of oxygen and/or glucose	Blood flow to brain slowed Lack of oxygen in blood Insufficient food intake	Symptoms of dementia, delirium, and schizophrenia
Alteration in electrolytes	Insufficient food intake Disordered electrolyte balance	Behavior may be stuporous or manic Hallucinations and delusions may occur Anxiety may be experienced
Neurotransmitter dysfunction	Substance abuse Diets high in sugar and fat Genetic influence	Symptoms of depression, bipolar disorder, schizophrenia, and panic disorder. Difficulty in information processing and coping with daily life stressors

CHAPTER REVIEW

COMMUNITY RESOURCES

Links to these Web sites can be accessed on the Companion Web site for this book.

Centre for Clinical Research in Neuropsychiatry
Graylands Hospital
John XXIII Ave.
Mt. Claremont, Western Australia 60101
08-9347-6429
www.ccrn.uwa.edu

Dana Alliance for Brain Initiatives
745 Fifth Ave., Suite 700
New York, NY 10151
212-223-4040
www.dana.org

Society for Neuroscience
11 Dupont Circle NW
Washington, DC 20036
202-462-6688
www.sfn.org

KEY CONCEPTS

Introduction

- The human brain is a dynamic ecosystem that adapts to internal and external environments and responds to use or disuse.
- The mind is a property of brain activity; that is, it is a process, not a thing.

Development of the Brain

- Brain development results from constant interaction between genetic and environmental factors such as firing patterns of neighboring neurons, hormones, trauma, and life experiences.
- The process of cell migration and differentiating continues until a person is about eight years old.
- As the brain ages, weak or unused neurons are pruned away.
- The brain's ability to improve itself, refine structures, and respond to internal and external changes is called neuroplasticity.
- There are gender differences in brain anatomy, which may help explain gender-related differences in behavior.
- Aging causes a slowdown in the communication network of the brain, but there is not a massive death of brain cells as previously believed.
- The brain is extremely vulnerable to damage from oxygen free radicals because it uses so much oxygen.
- Antioxidants are free radical scavengers that search out and neutralize dangerous free radicals.
- Physical exercise makes our bodies more adept at delivering oxygen and nutrients to the brain.

Neuroanatomy

- Glial cells regulate groups of neurons by controlling the concentration of neurotransmitters and ions and by releasing their own neurotransmitters. Other types of glial cells coat axons with myelin, which controls the speed of impulses.
- Each neuron may have a direct connection with as many as 10,000 other neurons. There are at least 50 different kinds of neurons varying in lengths and branching patterns of dendrites and axons.
- Neuronal groups are dense collections of nerve cells with common functions.
- Nerve tracts are groups of nerve fibers carrying signals to and from the same area.
- The corpus callosum is a large body of nerve fibers connecting the left and right hemispheres.
- The cingulate gyrus, part of the limbic system, integrates emotions with thinking to send a coherent message to the hypothalamus.
- The brain stem is the location of functions necessary to life such as respiration, heart rate, blood pressure, and balance. It is also the home of the 12 cranial nerves.
- The reticular activating system (RAS) in the brain stem receives impulses from the entire body and relays them to the cortex. It is responsible for our state of arousal, consciousness, and sleep regulation.
- The cerebellum coordinates skeletal muscles during movement and maintains equilibrium and posture. It is responsible for procedural memory and sets the timing and rhythm of brain function.

- The cerebral hemispheres are the sites of perceptual, cognitive, and higher motor functions, as well as emotion and memory.

- The frontal lobe is the site of the ability to think and plan, control movement, and develop insight. It regulates the motor aspects of written and spoken speech, maintains the stability of the personality, inhibits primitive emotional responses, and regulates emotions and behavior.

- The parietal lobe is the site of receiving and identifying sensory information, memory association, proprioception, and sensory speech.

- The temporal lobe is the site of hearing, complex memory, emotions, sexual identity, and the production and understanding of speech.

- The occipital lobe is the site of vision and the ability to understand written words.

- The limbic system is the site of regulation of emotional responses (amygdala), interpretation of smell, declarative memory storage (hippocampus), stress regulator (cingulate gyrus), the reward center (nucleus accumbens), impressions of agreeableness or disagreeableness of sensations (thalamus), and it helps to regulate the autonomic nervous system (hypothalamus and pituitary gland).

- The purpose of the basal ganglia is to organize complex patterns of thought and movement under the influence of emotional tone.

- The blood–brain barrier imports critical nutrients, exports metabolic waste products, and protects the brain against the influx of toxins.

Neurophysiology

- In neurotransmission, a cell releases neurotransmitters that diffuse across the synapse and activate the second cell by latching onto its receptors; after a transmitter fulfills its function, the receptor releases it back into the synapse, where it is either deactivated by an enzyme or transported back into the presynaptic terminal (reuptake).

- Neuromodulators are chemicals that alter the threshold to the flow of information.

- Receptor antagonists are substances that block receptor sites, thereby inhibiting neurotransmission.

- Receptor agonists are substances other than the receptor's specific neurotransmitter that are capable of stimulating the receptor.

- Substances the body makes are called endogenous and those that enter from outside the body are called exogenous.

- There are diverse chemical classes of neurotransmitters, including biogenic amines, amino acids, peptides, neurohormones, and gases.

- Dopamine (DA) greatly influences thought processing, abstract thinking, muscular coordination, emotional responses, memory, and coping abilities; it makes you feel alert and energetic and takes you on an emotional high.

- Serotonin (5-HT) is primarily an inhibitory neurotransmitter. It is anti-impulsive, provides a sense of calmness, and acts to balance DA.

- Norepinephrine (NE) and epinephrine (E) play a role in mood, memory and cognitive functions, energy, and appetite.

- Acetylcholine (ACh) is involved in the parasympathetic nervous system and has an effect on mood, sleep, and memory.

- Gamma-aminobutyric acid (GABA) is an inhibitory neurotransmitter that regulates anxiety and influences muscular coordination. It may play a role in aggressive behavior.

- Endorphin and enkephalin are neurohormones that allow us to experience pleasure and help protect us from pain.

- Most other hormones are derived from dehydroepiandrosterone (DHEA); DHEA improves cognition, protects the immune system, and serves as an antidepressant.

- Oxytocin promotes touching and is instrumental in the bonding process; it decreases cognition and impairs memory.

- Vasopressin improves cognition by enhancing attention and alertness.

- Phenylethylamine (PEA) is a natural form of amphetamine in our brain; low levels may contribute to depression and high levels may contribute to psychotic symptoms.

- Estrogen maintains and restores memory in the brain.

- Nitric oxide may play a role in learning and memory.

- Circadian rhythms are regular fluctuations of a variety of physiological factors over 24 hours, ultradian rhythms are shorter than 24 hours, and infradian rhythms are longer than 24 hours.

Functions of the Brain

- Unconscious brain function is the automatic selection of routines appropriate to the situation. This type of processing is fast and efficient.

- Conscious brain functions are higher-level activities such as self-monitoring, planning, and organizing activity.

- Feedback dynamics allows for modification of behavior while it is in progress. Though it is slower, it provides more precise control of behavior.

- Feedforward is the prediction of what is about to occur without waiting for feedback.

- Executive functions of the brain include insight, the ability to plan ahead and problem solve, and the ability to regulate one's own behavior.

- Working or short term memory allows us to ignore distractions, make judgments, anticipate consequences, and take responsibility.

- Only if the stimulus is strong and repetitive does working memory convert to long-term memory.

- Rapid eye movement (REM) sleep is critical for organizing memory into long-term storage.

- Declarative memory is memory for people and facts, is consciously accessible, and can be verbally expressed.

- Procedural memory is the memory of motor skills: the behavioral expression of memory.

- Abstract thinking is the ability to generalize information, make predictions, build on prior memory, and evaluate the consequences of decisions.

- Concrete thinking is the literal interpretation of messages and an inability to generalize.

- Loose association is thinking in which there is no apparent relationship between thoughts.

- Illogical thinking is characterized by inconsistent, irrational, or self-contradictory ideas.

- In tangential speech, thoughts veer from the main idea and never get back to it.

- In circumstantial speech, the person includes many unnecessary and insignificant details before arriving at the main idea.

- Pressured speech is tense, strained, and difficult to interrupt.

- Emotions are the result of multiple brain and body systems working together.

- Fear is the emotion with the fastest physical reaction possible.

- When frontal lobes are underactive and executive function is compromised, anger may turn to aggression.

- When we are sad for prolonged periods of time, our store of neurotransmitters is depleted and we enter a state of depression.

- DA and endorphins play a role in the reward center of our brain—the nucleus accumbens.

- The cingulate gyrus is our link between motivation and behavior.

Psychoneuroimmunology

- Cytokines are the chemical messengers of the immune system which coordinate antibody and T-cell immune interactions. They include interferons, lymphokines, and interleukins.

- The central nervous system and the immune system work as an integrated whole to maintain a state of healthy balance within the body.

Nutritional Neuroscience

- Omega-3-type fish oil contains DHA and EPA, which maintains pliability of neurons, increases ACh, and improves brain function.

- Antioxidants include vitamin A, thiamine, flavonoids, folic acid, vitamin C, vitamin E, and coenzyme Q10.

Dysregulation

- Dysregulation of the brain results in disruption of the ability to process information.

EXPLORE *MediaLink*

- Interactive resources, including animations, for this chapter can be found on the Companion Web site at *http://www.prenhall.com/fontaine*. Click on Chapter 7 and select the activities for this chapter.

- For NCLEX review questions and an audio glossary, access the accompanying CD-ROM in this book.

REFERENCES

Amen, D. G. (2001). *Healing ADD.* New York: Putnam.

Backman, L., Ginovart, N., Dixon, R. A., Wahlin, T. R., Wahlin, A., & Halldin, C. (2000). Age-related cognitive deficits mediated by changes in the striatal dopamine system. *American Journal of Psychiatry, 157*(4), 635–637.

Balch, J. F., & Balch, P. A. (1997). *Prescription for nutritional healing* (2nd ed.). Garden City Park, NY: Avery Publishing.

Black, I. B. (2001). *Life, death, and the changing brain.* New York: McGraw-Hill.

Brown, A. (2001). Young investigators in 2001. *National Alliance for Research on Schizophrenia and Affective Disorders, 13*(1), 7–32.

Carper, J. (2000). *Your miracle brain.* New York: HarperCollins.

Crenshaw, T. L. (1996). *The alchemy of love and lust.* New York: GP Putnam's Sons.

Dilts, S. L. (2001). *Model of the mind.* York, PA: WellSpan Health System.

Edelman, G. M., & Tononi, G. (2000). *A universe of consciousness: How matter becomes imagination.* New York: Basic Books.

Fontaine, K. L. (2000). *Healing practices: Alternative therapies for nursing.* Upper Saddle River, NJ: Prentice Hall.

Grigsby, J., & Stevens, D. (2000). *Neurodynamics of personality.* New York: Guilford Press.

Heijnen, C. J. (2000). Psychoneuroimmunology: Perseptives of an immunologist. In K. Goodkin & A. P. Visser (Eds.), *Psychoneuroimmunology: Stress, mental disorders and health* (pp. 395–405). Washington, DC: American Psychiatric Press.

Keller, S. E. (2000). Stress, depression, immunity and health. In K. Goodkin & A. P. Visser (Eds.), *Psychoneuroimmunology: Stress, mental disorders and health* (pp. 1–25). Washington, DC: American Psychiatric Press.

Keltner, N. L. (2000). Neuroreceptor function and psychopharmacologic response. *Issues in Mental Health Nursing, 21*(1), 31–50.

Kimura, D. (1999). *Sex and cognition.* Cambridge, MA: MIT Press.

Kronfol, Z., & Remick, D. G. (2000). Cytokines and the brain: Implications for clinical psychiatry. *American Journal of Psychiatry, 157*(5), 683–694.

Minton, M. S., & Hickey, J. V. (1999). A primer of neuroanatomy and neurophysiology. *Nursing Clinics of North America, 34*(3), 555–572.

Pert, C. B. (1997). *The molecules of emotion.* New York: Scribner.

Ratey, J. J. (2001). *A user's guide to the brain.* New York: Pantheon Books.

Seeman, M. V. (1997). Psychopathology in women and men: Focus on female hormones. *American Journal of Psychiatry, 154*(12), 1641–1647.

Smock, T. K. (1999). *Physiological psychology: A neuroscience approach.* Upper Saddle River, NJ: Prentice Hall.

Snyder, S. H., & Ferris, C. D. (2000). Novel neurotransmitters and their neuropsychiatric relevance. *American Journal of Psychiatry, 157*(11), 1738–1751.

Volkow, N. D., Logan, J., Fowler, J. S., Wang, G., Gur, R. C., Wonq, C., et al. (2000). Association between age-related decline in brain dopamine activity and impairment in frontal and cingulated metabolism. *American Journal of Psychiatry, 157*(1), 75–80.

Psychopharmacology

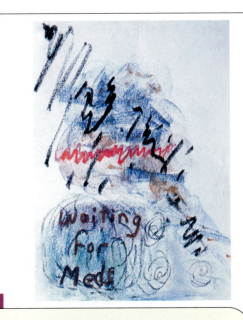

OBJECTIVES

After reading this chapter, you will be able to:

- DESCRIBE the physiological and therapeutic effects of psychotropic medications.
- DISCUSS the side effects and toxic effects of psychotropic medications.
- DISCUSS the use of psychotropic medications with special populations.
- DESCRIBE the process of client medication teaching.

MediaLink

CD-ROM
- *Audio Glossary*
- *NCLEX Review*

Videos
  Tardive Dyskinesia
- *Mouth*
- *Trunk*
- *Ambulation*
  Extrapyramidal Side Effects
- *Tremor—hands and arms*
- *Grasping tremor*
- *Lateral tremor*
- *Akathisia—legs*
- *Akinesia and pill rolling*
- *Bradykinesia—shuffling gait*
- *Dystonia—blepharospasm, cervical torticollis*

Companion Web site www.prenhall.com/fontaine
- *Critical Thinking*
- *More NCLEX Review*
- *Case Study*
- *Care Map Activity*
- *Links to Resources*

M *ajor source of irritability*

—*Brian, Age 19*

More psychotropic medications are available these days than ever before. The good news is that there are more options and more people have found medications that work better and help them lead more fulfilling lives. However, more choices can complicate things. The challenge is to find the most effective medications and use them in ways that maximize the chance of success.

INTRODUCTORY CONCEPTS

PHARMACOKINETICS

The way the body handles medications is referred to as **pharmacokinetics**. This includes the absorption, distribution, metabolism, and excretion of drugs. These processes determine the concentration of medications in the blood. *Absorption* refers to the way in which the drug passes from dosage form to available molecules. The fastest rate of absorption is intravenous (IV), followed by intramuscular (IM), subcutaneous (SC), and oral. *Distribution* is the process by which the drug is transported to various sites in the body. Many psychiatric drugs bind with transport proteins and only the unbound drugs are active and capable of crossing the blood–brain barrier. Changes in the concentration of drug-binding proteins are very important to the effectiveness of medications.

The primary site of *metabolism* is in the liver. Metabolism is critical to therapeutic blood levels and is affected by environmental and genetic factors. Environmental factors include stress, social support, personality styles, compliance, and prescribing patterns, all of which may influence the way individuals respond to medications. Genetic differences in the drug-metabolizing enzymes are responsible for ethnic variations in therapeutic response (Ruiz, 2000).

The *CYP* enzyme system (cytochrome P450) is the main pathway of drug metabolism. The three CYP enzymes of interest in psychiatry are *CYP2D6* (the enzyme that metabolizes most of the antipsychotic and antidepressant drugs), *CYP2C19* (the enzyme that metabolizes benzodiazepines and some antidepressants), and *CYP3A4* (the enzyme that metabolizes mood stabilizers, benzodiazepines, calcium channel blockers, and antidepressants). There are significant genetic variations or mutations that inactivate, impair, or accelerate the function of these enzymes. The interaction of genetics and ethnicity is discussed later in this chapter. Other factors that affect the function of these enzymes include toxins, other medications, sex hormones, tobacco, alcohol, and caffeine. Depending on enzyme activity, some people are slow metabolizers of medications and tend to have higher blood levels, more severe side effects, and a potential for toxicity. Those who are superextensive metabolizers have very low blood levels with typical doses and may even be thought to be noncompliant with their medications. As a nurse, you have a role in monitoring effectiveness of medications. It is important that you consider the role of environmental factors and genetic factors in assessing objective and subjective responses (Ruiz, 2000).

Excretion of most medications is through the kidney although some drugs are secreted through the bile, feces, skin evaporation, and via the lungs. The *half-life* of a medication is the time required for half of the drug to be eliminated. This is an important consideration in determining the proper amount and frequency of dose of the drug to be administered. The estimated half-life of medications is based on normal liver and kidney function. Drugs with a short half-life are given in more frequent doses than are those with a long half-life.

Potency refers to the strength of a medication. It is the power to produce the desired effects per milligram of the drug. Drugs that are low-potency need higher doses to create the desired effect. High-potency medications have lower dosage levels and thus the dosage range provides you with information regarding potency.

PHARMACODYNAMICS

Pharmacodynamics refers to drug action at the cellular level. Psychotropic medications act on cell receptors and turn postsynaptic cellular functions on or off. Medications act as either agonists or antagonists. As you recall from Chapter 7, an agonist stimulates receptor actions and antagonists prevent cellular response.

SMOKING, ALCOHOL, HYDRATION, AND NUTRITION

It is important that you assess clients for any of their usual habits that may impact the effectiveness of their medications. *Smoking* has a direct impact on liver enzymes, blood flow, and nicotine receptors in the central nervous system. Smoking increases the rate of metabolism of antidepressants and antianxiety agents, contributing to a need for higher doses. The combination of nicotine and antipsychotics puts the individual at higher risk for tardive dyskinesia. Nicotine decreases the therapeutic effect of Inderal (propranolol). Cocaine causes vasoconstriction, which is further enhanced by the use of nicotine (Turkoski, Lance, & Bonfiglio, 2000).

Excessive *alcohol* affects liver and kidney function, thus impacting metabolism and excretion of medications. Alcohol also has an additive effect with drugs that depress the central nervous system.

Poor *hydration* lessens blood flow to the kidney, decreasing the excretion rate. Poor *nutrition* may result in less protein available for binding drugs. A recent discovery finds that *grapefruit* may cause potentially serious interactions when taken with a number of drugs. A

compound specific to grapefruit has the ability to block CYP3A4, which metabolizes medications, resulting in increased blood levels of Serzone (nefazodone), Xanax (alprazolam), and the calcium channel blockers used to stabilize mood (Lin & Smith, 2000; Margolis, 1998).

Disease states can change all aspects of pharmacokinetics. For example, cirrhosis impairs enzyme metabolism of drugs, as does abnormal thyroid function. Circulatory problems impact absorption, distribution, and excretion, and kidney disease decreases excretion of medications (Turkoski, Lance, & Bonfiglio, 2000).

OFF-LABEL USE

Many medications that are on the market have not been officially approved by the Food and Drug Administration (FDA) for a variety of disorders. For example, some antidepressants (FDA approved for depression) are used to treat some of the anxiety disorders (off-label use). For some medications, the off-label use is supported by data from studies, while in other situations off-label use is supported by anecdotal reports. As we learn more about neuropsychiatry, we will better understand how a variety of medications are effective in a number of disorders.

PSYCHOTROPIC MEDICATIONS

Psychotropic medications are medications that affect cognitive function, emotions, and behavior. They are categorized into classes: antipsychotic, antidepressant, mood-stabilizing, antianxiety, and stimulant medications. They may be used alone or in combination with one another.

ANTIPSYCHOTIC MEDICATIONS

PHYSIOLOGICAL EFFECTS

Symptoms of severe mental illness are classified as positive and negative. To make sense of this, you must understand that positive does not mean good and negative does not mean bad. Rather, positive symptoms are added behaviors that are not normally seen in mentally healthy adults, such as hallucinations, delusions, or loose associations. Positive symptoms are thought to result from an excess of dopamine (DA) or from hypersensitive DA receptors and are usually responsive to medication. Negative symptoms are the absence of behaviors that are normally seen in mentally healthy adults, such as social withdrawal, minimal self-care, concrete thinking, and flat affect. (See Chapter 14 for further description of positive and negative symptoms.) Until recently, negative symptoms have been less responsive to treatment with antipsychotic medications. Antipsychotic medications act by blocking the overreactive DA receptors or by decreasing the amount of available DA (Nyberg, Eriksson, Oxenstierna, Halldin, & Farde, 1999).

THERAPEUTIC EFFECTS

The therapeutic purpose of antipsychotic medications is to decrease as many of the psychotic symptoms as possible. This action allows clients to assume more control over their lives. With reduced symptoms, they can participate more effectively in other forms of treatment.

Initially, clients take or receive their medication in divided doses, two to four times a day, which decreases the occurrence of side effects. It usually takes two to four weeks before the client shows a significant response to the medication. Once the client's symptoms are under control, the dosage may be changed to once a day. Once maintenance on a particular drug is established, the client is kept on the lowest possible dosage.

Conventional Antipsychotics

Conventional antipsychotic medications (Table 8.1 ■) are generally more successful at relieving the positive symptoms of mental illness than negative symptoms and cognitive dysfunction. It may take two to four weeks to see clinical improvement from these medications. Although no evidence suggests the superiority of any one conventional antipsychotic agent, some people respond better to one drug than another. Choosing which medication to use with individual clients also depends on its side effects. For example, one client may respond well to haloperidol but have dangerous episodes of hypotension, while another client may do well on haloperidol with little or no side effects. Approximately 15 to 25 percent of clients with schizophrenia experience little clinical improvement with conventional antipsychotic medication. People with treatment-resistant schizophrenia remain highly symp-

tomatic and require extensive periods of hospitalization. Half of the people will get one or more side effects and, in response, many will discontinue their medication (Conley et al., 1998).

Newer Antipsychotics

New-generation or newer antipsychotic medications offer promise to many people with chronic psychotic disorders. Sixty percent of those who do not respond to conventional antipsychotics will have significant clinical improvement with these newer medications. Newer agents are characterized by:

■ Effectiveness in eliminating negative as well as positive symptoms

■ Effectiveness for many people who are not responsive to conventional agents

■ Effectiveness for people who also experience depressive symptoms

■ A significantly lower incidence of extrapyramidal side effects (EPSs), which increases compliance

On the basis of effectiveness, safety, and low side effects, newer antipsychotic agents should be considered the preferred option, especially in first-episode psychosis (Breier et al., 1999; Sanger et al., 1999).

Risperdal (risperidone) and Zyprexa (olanzapine) have been found to be effective for persons with oppositional defiant disorder, conduct disorder, and rage disorder, although these are off-label uses. The FDA has approved Zyprexa (olanzapine) for the short-term treatment of acute manic episodes associated with bipolar disorder.

Geodon (ziprasidone) is an newer antipsychotic for which both an oral and a rapid-acting intramuscular form has been developed. The IM form is used for the control and short-term management of clients who are acutely psychotic and agitated. Effect is apparent within one hour after injection without being profoundly sedating. Geodon is also effective for decreasing the anger associated with bipolar disorder. It may be used to treat social withdrawal for persons with autistic disorder or Asperger's syndrome. Zomaril (iloperidone) and Abilitat (aripiprazole) are currently in Phase III trials and thus far demonstrate good effectiveness against the positive and negative symptoms with very low side effects (see Table 8.1 for a list of newer antipsychotics).

TABLE 8.1

Antipsychotic Medications

Class	Generic Name	Trade Name	Adult Dosage (mg/day)
Newer antipsychotics	Aripiprazole*	Abilitat	15–30
	Clozapine	Clozaril	300–900
	Olanzapine	Zyprexa	5–20
	Quetiapine	Seroquel	150–750
	Risperidone	Risperdal	4–16
	Sertindole	Serlect	12–24
	Ziprasidone	Geodon	40–160
Phenothiazines	Acetophenazine	Tindal	40–120
	Chlorpromazine	Thorazine	30–800
	Fluphenazine	Prolixin, Permitil	1–40
	Mesoridazine	Serentil	75–300
	Perphenazine	Trilafon	8–64
	Thioridazine	Mellaril	150–800
	Trifluoperazine	Stelazine, Suptazine	15–20
	Triflupromazine	Vesprin	60–150
Thioxanthenes	Chlorprothixene	Taractan	75–600
	Thiothixene	Navane	6–120
Butyrophenones	Haloperidol	Haldol	1–50
Dibenzoxazepine	Loxapine	Loxitane	10–160
Dihydroindolone	Molindone	Moban	15–225
Diphenylbatylperidine	Pimozide	Orap	1–10

* Awaiting FDA approval.

SIDE EFFECTS
Conventional Antipsychotics

Conventional antipsychotic medications provide relief from the symptoms of severe mental illness for many people, but side effects are common. Some are bothersome (e.g., dry mouth), some affect mood (e.g., akathisia), some are disfiguring (e.g., tardive dyskinesia), some are frightening (e.g., dystonia), and others are dangerous (e.g., neuroleptic malignant syndrome). These adverse effects interfere with function, reduce the quality of life, and contribute to clients' stopping their medication.

The most common side effects of conventional antipsychotic medications include anticholinergic effects, photosensitivity, weight gain, sexual difficulties, and extrapyramidal side effects.

Anticholinergic side effects occur when the medication blocks the acetylcholine receptors, resulting in the inhibition of the transmission of parasympathetic nerve impulses. These side effects are more bothersome than anything else and include dry mouth, blurry vision, trouble urinating, constipation, memory difficulties, and confusion.

Photosensitivity is the increased sensitivity of the skin to sunlight. Relatively brief exposure to sunlight may cause edema, rashes, or severe burns. Clients need to be cautioned to wear protective clothing and use high-potency sunscreen to avoid this complication.

The amount of *weight gain* varies by medication because of differing degrees of action of the various neurotransmitters. The degree of weight gain also increases with length of time of administration. It is believed that the weight gain is associated with a medication-induced rise in the level of leptin, a hormone involved in weight regulation (Kraus, Amsterdam, Quitkin, & Reimherr, 1999). Weight gain may cause clients to discontinue their medications, which may predispose them to relapse. The medications with the highest weight gain are thioridazine (Mellaril) and chlorpromazine (Thorazine).

Interference with *sexual function* is very common. Some of the side effects are direct; that is, they are the result of chemical action of the medication. These include decreased sex drive, erection difficulties, ejaculation irregularities, and decreased ability to achieve orgasm. Indirect sexual side effects are related to other side effects such as anticholinergic effects, sedation, changes in energy, weight gain, or body image. Thus, individuals may avoid sexual interaction because of fatigue, dry mucous membranes, indigestion, dizziness, tremors, or self-image. Sexual side effects are one of the most important factors influencing medication compliance.

Smooth body movements and body posture depend on a critical ratio of DA to acetylcholine (ACh) in the brain. When medications block DA receptors, they lower this ratio, and **extrapyramidal side effects (EPSs)** occur. EPSs include akinesia, akathisia, parkinsonism, dystonia, oculogyric crisis, and tardive dyskinesia. **Akinesia** is muscular weakness or a partial loss of muscular movement. **Akathisia** is the inability to sit or stand still, along with an intense feeling of anxiety. This side effect usually begins within the first 60 days of treatment and persists as long as the client is on medication. It is extremely distressing to people and is a frequent cause of medication noncompliance. Akathisia is less responsive to treatment than are parkinsonism and dystonia. Medications to counteract akathisia are Inderal (propranolol), Benadryl (diphenhydramine), and Cogentin (benztropine).

Parkinsonism is evidenced in clients' stooped posture and shuffling gait. Their faces resemble masks, and they may drool. They experience tremors and pill-rolling motions of the thumb and fingers at rest. This reaction is likely to begin within the first 30 days of treatment and occurs throughout the use of the medication.

Dystonia has an abrupt onset, with frightening muscle spasms in the head and neck. *Oculogyric crisis* and *laryngospasm* are terms used to describe acute dystonic reactions in specific body regions. In oculogyric crisis, the person's eyes roll up and sideways and are held in a fixed position for minutes or several hours. In laryngospasm, there is a spasmodic closure of the larynx. These reactions usually occur within the first five days of therapy or when dosage is significantly increased. Episodes are more likely to occur during the afternoon and evening than during the night and morning. Treatment is IM Cogentin (benztropine) or IM Benadryl (diphenhydramine).

Tardive dyskinesia, a form of EPS, occurs in 20 to 40 percent of clients who take conventional antipsychotic medications for over two years. Females and older people are at higher risk for tardive dyskinesia. Many of the cases are mild, but the disorder can be socially disfiguring. Symptoms include frowning, blinking, grimacing, puckering, blowing, smacking, licking, chewing, tongue protrusion, and spastic facial distortions. Abnormal movements of the arms and legs include rapid, purposeless, irregular movements; tremors; and foot tapping. Body symptoms include dramatic movements of the neck and shoulders and rocking, twisting pelvic gyrations and thrusts. Because tardive dyskinesia is often irreversible, the goal is prevention. If symptoms begin to appear, the medication is reduced or the person is switched to a newer antipsychotic medication (Tsai et al., 1998; van Harten et al., 1998).

Neuroleptic malignant syndrome (NMS) is a potentially fatal side effect related to sympathetic nervous system hyperactivity. It affects 1 to 2 percent of clients who take conventional antipsychotic medication. The risk is higher when clients are on two or more of these medications and/or suffering from organic brain disease. Symptoms of NMS develop suddenly and include muscle rigidity and respiratory problems. Hyperpyrexia ranges from 101°F to 107°F (38°C to 41.6°C). During the next two to three days, clients develop tachycardia, hypertension, respiratory problems, diaphoresis, urinary incontinence, confusion, and delirium. The mortality rate with NMS is 14 to 30 percent; it is estimated that 1,000 to 4,000 people die every year. There is no specific treatment for NMS other than discontinuation of the medication and supportive measures in the intensive care setting. Parlodel (bromocriptine) may be of some help in halting the DA blockage. Muscle relaxants such as Dantrium (dantrolene) may lessen the rigidity (Gurrera, 1999).

Recently concerns have been raised about antipsychotic medications associated with *QT prolongation* in cardiac conduction. QT prolongation may be associated with palpitations, dizziness, and lightheadedness. In some cases it may progress to ventricular fibrillation and sudden death. Females are at higher risk because of normally longer QT intervals. Risk for the elderly is higher due to an increased risk for coronary disease and the use of multiple medications. The antipsychotics with the most risk include Mellaril (thioridazine) and Serentil (mesoridazine). Geodon (ziprasidone) prolongs the QT interval, but there is no current evidence that this leads to sudden death (Turkoski, Lance, & Bonfiglio, 2000).

Because of the side effects, many people do not like the way their bodies feel when taking conventional antipsychotic medication. Identifying and managing side effects may help people stay on the medication and maintain a higher level of functioning, thus avoiding acute hospitalization. Some people will stop taking their medication and relapse, while others relapse first and, as a result of their symptoms, stop taking their medication.

Newer Antipsychotics

Among the newer antipsychotics, Clozaril (clozapine) has the most significant side effect in that about 0.5 percent of those taking this drug develop agranulocytosis. This carries a 40 percent fatality rate, usually from an overwhelming infection. Monitoring white blood counts (WBCs) weekly for the first six months, and then every other week, is required to administer this drug safely. It is desirable that the WBCs stay above 3,500 cells/cm (Henderson et al., 2000).

Because there is less DA receptor action, newer antipsychotic agents have fewer EPSs, making them more tolerable to clients. Weight gain is a considerable problem as with the conventional antipsychotic agents. Medications that cause the most weight gain are Clozaril (clozapine), Zyprexa (olanzapine), Serlect (sertindole), and Risperdal (risperidone), in decreasing order. Geodon (ziprasidone) and Moban (molindone) cause little or no weight gain. Other side effects of newer antipsychotic medications include sedation, hypersalivation, nervousness, headache, and dizziness. Neuroleptic malignant syndrome is less likely but remains a possibility (Allison et al, 1999; Hasan & Buckley, 1998).

TOXICITY AND OVERDOSE

The primary symptom of overdose is central nervous system (CNS) depression, which may extend to the point of coma. Other symptoms include agitation and restlessness, seizures, fever, EPSs, arrhythmias, and hypotension. Caring for a client who has overdosed includes monitoring vital signs, especially of cardiac function; maintaining a patent airway; and gastric lavage. Antiparkinsonian medications may be given for EPSs. Valium (diazepam) may be given for seizures.

ADMINISTRATION

Administration of antipsychotic medications is oral, in liquid or pill form, or by injection. Long-acting injectable medications such as Prolixin (fluphenazine) Decanoate and Haldol (haloperidol) Decanoate are often used to treat clients with schizophrenia. These medications are administered IM once every two to six weeks, a helpful regimen for clients who have difficulty remembering to take medications daily.

The FDA has approved an injectable form of Zyprexa (olanzapine) to treat agitation in schizophrenia, mania, and dementia. Consumers with these disorders who require injectable medication from the start of their treatment can now begin treatment with a newer antipsychotic rather than having to rely on a conventional antipsychotic.

TABLE 8.2

Adjunctive Medications for EPSs

Class	Generic Name	Trade Name	Adult Dosage (mg/day)
Anticholinergic	Amantadine	Symmetrel	100–300
	Benztropine	Cogentin	1–6
	Biperiden	Akineton	2–8
	Diphenhydramine	Benadryl	50–300
	Ethopropacine	Parsidol	50–200
	Orphenadrine	Disipal, Norlex	50–300
	Procyclidine	Kemadrin	5–30
	Trihexyphenidyl	Artane	6–10
Specialized agents	Bromocriptine	Parlodel	5–50
	Dantrolene	Dantrium	60–600
	Propranolol	Inderal	30–120
	Pindolol	Visken	10–60

ADJUNCTIVE MEDICATIONS FOR EPSs

A number of medications may be used to lessen the EPS effects of the conventional antipsychotics. Some of these medications reduce ACh, thereby restoring the DA:ACh ratio (see Table 8.2 ■ for a list of these medications). Symmetrel (amantadine) is an antiviral medication that also works as an antidyskinetic by stimulating the release of DA.

Anticholinergic agents should be used with caution in people who have difficulty urinating or have an enlarged prostate; glaucoma; myasthenia gravis; or cardiovascular, kidney, or liver disease. Side effects include blurry vision, dizziness, orthostatic hypotension, and drowsiness. Clients may find sunglasses are necessary if their eyes become more sensitive to light. Decreased sweating may result in a rise in body temperature. Symptoms of overdose include unsteadiness; seizures; severe drowsiness; severe dryness of the mouth, nose, and throat; tachycardia; shortness of breath; hallucinations; and coma.

ANTIDEPRESSANT MEDICATIONS

PHYSIOLOGICAL EFFECTS

The neurotransmitters involved in depression are dopamine (DA), serotonin (5-HT), norepinephrine (NE), and acetylcholine (ACh). It is believed that during a depressive episode, there is a functional deficiency of these neurotransmitters or hyposensitive receptors. Antidepressant medications increase the amount of available neurotransmitters by inhibiting neurotransmitter reuptake, by inhibiting monoamine oxidase (MAO), by blocking certain receptors, or by modulating the effect of neurotransmitters.

THERAPEUTIC EFFECTS

Antidepressant medications can be classified as older-generation agents, the tricyclics, tetracyclics, and monoamine oxidase inhibitors (MAOIs); and the new-generation agents, the selective dopamine–

norepinephrine reuptake inhibitors (DNRIs), selective serotonin reuptake inhibitors (SSRIs), the serotonin–norepinephrine reuptake inhibitors (SNRIs), the serotonin modulators, and the norepinephrine–serotonin modulators. The new-generation medications have dramatically changed the treatment of depression, with more effective action and fewer side effects.

Because depressions are heterogeneous in terms of which neurotransmitters are depleted, different people respond differently to various antidepressants. At times, a period of trial and error is necessary to determine which medication is most effective. The therapeutic purpose of antidepressants is to decrease as many of the depressive symptoms as possible, thereby enabling clients to participate more effectively in other forms of treatment. Maintenance continues until clients are free of symptoms for four months to one year. Then the drugs are slowly discontinued.

Antidepressants do not cause dependence, tolerance, addiction, or withdrawal. It takes an average of 10 to 14 days for the beginning effect of most antidepressants, and the full effect may not be apparent for two to four weeks. Approximately 30 percent of clients do not respond after a trial of four to six weeks. At that point, the health care provider may try a different antidepressant or augment with other medications.

Eldepryl (selegiline), a patch-delivered MAOI, shows dramatic improvement within one week. The quick results are seen because patches send drugs on a direct route to the blood and the brain, while pills are diluted as they pass through the liver. At the present time, it is FDA approved only for Parkinson's disease. It is in clinical trials for major depression (see Table 8.3 ■ for a list of antidepressant medications).

A significant number of clients improve when 600 mg of lithium is added to the antidepressant treatment. Other clients improve when triiodothyronine (T_3) is administered daily. For clients who are delusional or severely agitated, antipsychotic medication may be indicated (Nierenberg et al., 2000).

Zyban (bupropion) is used in smoking cessation programs. It is thought that DA counters the craving associated with nicotine withdrawal (Keltner, 2000). Sarafem (fluoxetine) is the same medication as Prozac and has been FDA approved for the treatment of premenstrual dysphoric disorder. Studies show that women's mood improved and they had fewer physical complaints. Zoloft (sertraline) is the first drug to receive FDA approval for the treatment of posttraumatic stress disorder. It is also used for panic disorder and obsessive–compulsive disorder.

Antidepressants currently in clinical trials include Edronax, Vestra (reboxetine), flesinoxan, and duloxetine.

SIDE EFFECTS

Anticholinergic side effects occur when the medication blocks the ACh receptors, resulting in the inhibition of the transmission of parasympathetic nerve impulses. These side effects are more bothersome than dangerous and include dry mouth, blurry vision, trouble urinating, constipation, memory difficulties, and confusion. The SSRIs, SDNIs, SNRIs, and the modulators have fewer anticholinergic effects. There are additional problems with the anticholinergic properties of these medications for the older person. If the client has dentures, an extremely dry mouth can lead to gingival erosion. If the older male client has prostatic enlargement, the anticholinergic effect of urinary retention can cause very serious problems. Anticholinergic properties can also intensify unsuspected glaucoma, resulting in increased intraocular pressure. Antidepressant medications may also cause orthostatic hypotension, resulting in a higher risk of dizzy spells and falls. Relatively brief exposure to sunlight may cause edema, rashes, or severe burns. Clients need to be cautioned to wear protective clothing and use high-potency sunscreen to avoid this side effect.

Some of the most troublesome and most frequently overlooked side effects are *sexual difficulties*. Men and women may experience desire disorders and painful intercourse. Women may have orgasmic problems and decreased lubrication. Men may have difficulty with erections, inhibited ejaculation, and decreased ejaculatory volume. Sexual problems more commonly occur after six weeks of treatment.

Weight gain is a significant problem with these medications and can contribute to poor body image and avoidance of sexual activity. Prozac (fluoxetine) is associated with modest weight loss during treatment. Medications with the least sexual side effects and the least weight gain (0 to 10 pounds) are Norpramin (desipramine) and Pamelor (nortriptyline). Those with the most significant sexual side effects and the greatest weight gain (5 to 40 pounds) include Elavil (amitriptyline), Adapin (doxepin), Sinequan (doxepin), and

TABLE 8.3

Antidepressant Medications

Class	Generic Name	Trade Name	Adult Dosage (mg/day)
Dopamine–norepinephrine reuptake inhibitor (DNRI)	Bupropion	Wellbutrin, Zyban	100–450
Selective serotonin reuptake inhibitor (SSRI)	Citalopram	Celexa	20–60
	Fluoxetine	Prozac, Sarafem	20–80
	Fluvoxamine	Luvox	50–300
	Paroxetine	Paxil	50–200
	Reboxetine*	Edronax	
	Sertraline	Zoloft	50–200
Serotonin–norepinephrine inhibitor (SNRI)	Venlafaxine	Effexor, Effexor XR	75–375
Serotonin modulators	Nefazodone	Serzone	150–300
	Trazodone	Desyrel	50–600
Norepinephrine–serotonin modulator	Mirtazapine	Remeron	15–45
Tricyclic	Amitriptyline	Elavil, Endep	50–300
	Clomipramine	Anafranil	75–250
	Desipramine	Norpramin, Petrofrane	50–300
	Doxepin	Adapin, Sinequan	50–300
	Imipramine	Tofranil	50–300
	Nortriptyline	Aventyl, Pamelor	50–200
	Protriptyline	Vivactil	10–60
	Trimipramine	Surmontil	50–300
Tetracyclic	Amoxapine	Ascendin	50–400
	Maprotiline	Ludiomil	50–225
MAOI	Isocarboxazid	Marplan	10–30
	Phenelzine	Nardil	45–90
	Tranylcypromine	Parnate	30–60
	Selegiline	Eldepryl	Patch

*Awaiting FDA approval.

Anafranil (clomipramine). Wellbutrin (bupropion) has no negative sexual side effects. SSRIs have been used to treat rapid ejaculation, but the value may be complicated by decreased desire. Men who experience erectile difficulties may find that Viagra (sildenafil) helps them stay on the antidepressant medication (Leiblum & Rosen, 2000).

MAOIs decrease the amount of monoamine oxidase in the liver, which breaks down the essential amino acids tyramine and tryptophan. If a person eats food that is rich in these substances while taking a MAOI, he or she risks a *hypertensive crisis*. The first sign of a hypertensive crisis is a sudden and severe headache, followed by neck stiffness, nausea, vomiting, sweating, and tachycardia. Death can result from circulatory collapse or intracranial bleeding. Box 8.1 lists the foods and medications clients must avoid while taking an MAOI. Because of Eldepryl's (selegiline) unique properties, food interactions are not a problem and there are no dietary restrictions. Individuals may experience some skin irritation from the patch.

BOX 8.1

Foods to Avoid with MAOIs

Absolutely Restricted

- Aged cheeses
- Aged and cured meats
- Dried or pickled fish
- Liver
- Flavor cubes or meat extracts
- Bananas
- Broad bean pods
- Sauerkraut
- Soy sauce and other soy condiments
- Draft beer
- Vitamins with Brewer's yeast

Consume in Moderation

- Red or white wine (no more than two 4-oz glasses per day)
- Bottled or canned beer, including nonalcoholic (no more than two 12-oz servings per day)
- Chocolate
- Yogurt (4 ounces per day)

SOURCE: Adapted from Roach, S. S., & Scherer, J. C. (2000). *Clinical pharmacology* (6th ed.). Philadelphia: Lippincott.

The SSRIs and SNRIs increase the availability of 5-HT, which relieves depression but can also cause the hyperserotonergic state known as the **serotonin syndrome (SS)**. This syndrome is more likely to occur when these agents are used in combination with MAOIs, lithium, and St. John's wort. Serotonin syndrome develops very quickly and is characterized by:

- Mental changes such as agitation, confusion, or hypomania
- Altered muscle tone such as hyperreflexia, rigidity, twitching, or tremor
- Autonomic changes such as hyper- or hypotension, tachycardia, or diaphoresis
- CNS changes such as discoordination, coma, or seizures
- Hyperthermia with temperatures as high as 101°F to 107°F (30°C to 41.6°C)

Treatment of serotonin syndrome is supportive, which includes controlling hyperthermia with antipyretics and cooling devices. Muscle rigidity and twitching can be treated with Klonopin (clonazepam), Cogentin (benztropine), and Ativan (lorazepam). Anticonvulsants are used for seizures secondary to serotonin syndrome (Turkoski, Lance, & Bonfiglio, 2000).

TOXICITY AND OVERDOSE

Symptoms of toxicity include confusion, disturbed concentration, agitation, irritability, hallucinations, seizures, dilated pupils, delirium, hypotension or hypertension, hyperactive reflexes, tachycardia, arrhythmia, respiratory depression, coma, kidney failure, and cardiac arrest. Caring for a client who has overdosed includes monitoring vital signs, especially of cardiac function, and maintaining a patent airway. Vomiting is induced if the client is alert, while gastric lavage is initiated for the client who is stuporous. Following this procedure, activated charcoal may be administered to minimize absorption. Antilirium (physostigmine) 1 to 3 mg may be given IV to counteract the toxic effects. Valium (diazepam) may be administered for seizures and vasopressors or lidocaine for cardiovascular effects (Turkoski et al., 2000).

If MAOIs and other antidepressants are administered together, serious reactions may occur. Symptoms include hyperthermia, severe agitation, delirium, and coma. Two to five weeks should elapse between the use of MAOIs and other antidepressants.

ADMINISTRATION

Administration of antidepressant medications is primarily oral. It usually takes two to four weeks to reach therapeutic levels, at which point the client is able to notice a reduction in symptoms. Other people may actually see changes in energy and mood before the client experiences an improvement. It is important to educate clients about this fact so that they do not become frustrated and stop taking the medication before it becomes effective.

Eldepryl (selegiline) is the only antidepressant in a skin patch. At the present time, it is not known whether all antidepressants can be administered through a patch-delivery system. Individuals who are stabilized on 20 mg daily of Prozac (fluoxetine), may consider Prozac Weekly, the first available once-a-week medication for depression.

MOOD-STABILIZING MEDICATIONS

PHYSIOLOGICAL EFFECTS

The mood stabilizers include a small group of diverse medications that are useful in stabilizing clients' affect. Lithium is the best known and most often prescribed mood stabilizer. In recent years, several anticonvulsant medications have been added to this category: Tegretol (carbamazepine), Depakene and Depakote (valproate), and Klonopin (clonazepam). Calcium channel blockers (Calan and Isoptin [verapamil]) are increasingly being used with success in manic disorders either alone or in combination with other mood stabilizers. Antihypertensives (Catapres [clonidine] and Tenex [guanfacine]) help in controlling rage attacks (Table 8.4 ■ lists the mood-stabilizing medications).

Lithium

Lithium has been found to potentiate the therapeutic effects of antidepressants. In the body, lithium substitutes for sodium, calcium, potassium, and magnesium. It also interacts with DA, NE, and 5-HT. Lithium affects a complex biological system called the phosphatidyl inositol cycle inside many cells. This cycle is referred to as a "second messenger" system that relays and amplifies signals. It is thought that this system may be overactive in both mania and depression, and lithium serves to inhibit the activity of this pathway (Roach & Scherer, 2000).

Anticonvulsants/Calcium Channel Blockers/Antihypertensives

It is thought that Tegretol (carbamazepine) reduces the rate of impulse transmission and that Depakote (valproate) increases levels of the inhibitory neurotransmitter gamma-aminobutyric acid (GABA). Increasing GABA activity seems to have an antimanic, antipanic, and antianxiety effect. Manic episodes may be triggered by persistent low-level stimulation of the brain. The anticonvulsants may be effective in that they block this persistent stimulation. Clients with an acute manic episode have been found to have increased levels of intracellular calcium, which decrease when lithium is administered. Calcium channel blockers have been found to be effective in the treatment of bipolar disorder and seem to work best in people who also respond to lithium. Two antihypertensives, Catapres (clonidine) and Tenex (guanfacine) have been found to stabilize mood in some individuals. The molecular action is unclear but it is thought that clonidine binds to the hypothalamic receptors thus affecting the hypothalamus–pituitary–adrenal axis (Papolos & Papolos, 1999).

THERAPEUTIC EFFECTS

For clients with problems such as bipolar disorder, major depression, schizoaffective disorder, treatment-resistant schizophrenia, alcohol and opiate withdrawal, rage outbursts, and other problems concerning the regulation of mood, mood-stabilizing medications have been found to be helpful.

The antimanic effectiveness of lithium is 70 to 80 percent; some people seem to be resistant to it and others cannot tolerate the side effects. Because it takes one to three weeks to control symptoms, antipsychotic medications or benzodiazepines are given initially for more immediate relief. Lithium reduces the frequency, duration, and intensity of both manic and depressive episodes and is the drug of choice for long-term treatment of bipolar disorder. Those individuals who are considered to be "rapid cyclers" (those who have four or more bipolar cycles in a one-year period) may not do as well on lithium as they do on other mood stabilizers.

TABLE 8.4

Mood-Stabilizing Medications

Class	Generic Name	Trade Name	Adult Dosage (mg/day)
Lithium	Lithium carbonate	Eskalith, Lithane, Lithobid	900–2,400, acute
			300–1,200, maintenance
	Lithium citrate	Cibalith-S	900–2,400, acute
			300–1,200, maintenance
Anticonvulsants			
	Carbamazepine	Tegretol	200–1,400
	Clonazepam	Klonopin	1.5–20
	Gabapentin	Neurontin	900–1,800
	Lamotrigine	Lamictal	200
	Tiagabine	Gabitril	32
	Topiramate	Topamax	100–400
	Valproate	Depakote, Depakene	750–1,000
Calcium Channel Blockers			
	Isradipine	DynaCirc	5
	Nimodipine	Nimotop	90–360
	Verapamil	Calan, Isoptin	120–480
Antihypertensives			
	Clonidine	Catapres	0.1–0.6
	Guanfacine	Tenex	1–3

Depakote (valproate) has a 57 percent response rate. It may improve a person's response to lithium. Valproate may be especially useful in rapid-cycling bipolar disorder and in treating the mood disorders associated with organic syndromes. Klonopin (clonazepam) is a benzodiazepine that is also an anticonvulsant. Its use is typically in addition to lithium, the combination of which lengthens the periods of remission. It has a more rapid onset than the other anticonvulsants, which may take two to three weeks to be effective.

Tegretol (carbamazepine) has a favorable response rate in about 60 percent of clients and is most often used with persons who are unable to take lithium. If given in combination, it may also increase the effectiveness of lithium. Tegretol (carbamazepine) also has antiaggressive properties, which makes it useful for people with frequent rage attacks.

Neurontin (gabapentin), Lamictal (lamotrigine), Topamax (topiramate), Gabitril (tiagabine), and Zonegran (zonisamide) are anticonvulsant medications that are often effective for controlling rapid-cycling bipolar disorder and for some people with social phobia. Neurontin and Lamictal are not to be given to children under the age of 16.

Calcium channel blockers are involved in cellular electrical activity and neurotransmitter release as well as regulation of circadian rhythms. This group of drugs, which includes Calan and Isoptin (verapamil), Nimotop (nimodipine), and DynaCirc (isradipine) has recently been established as mood stabilizers. It is unlikely that you will see Nimotop (nimodipine) prescribed because it is extremely expensive and must be taken three to four times a day, one to two hours before or after meals.

Catapres (clonidine) and Tenex (guanfacine) are antihypertensive agents that seem to be helpful for persons with rage attacks, tic disorders, attention deficit/hyperactivity disorder, and for pervasive developmental disorders. They are also used for opioid and alcohol withdrawal syndromes (Roach & Scherer, 2000).

SIDE EFFECTS

Lithium is nonsedating and nonaddictive. The early side effects of lithium often disappear after four weeks. These side effects include lack of spontaneity, memory problems, difficulty concentrating, nausea, vomiting, diarrhea, a metallic taste in the mouth, and hand tremors. Weight gain and a worsening of acne often persist throughout treatment.

The side effects of Tegretol (carbamazepine) are primarily related to the CNS and include drowsiness, dizziness, blurred or double vision, ataxia (unsteady or staggered gait), and nystagmus (involuntary rolling of the eyes). They often disappear over time and are less likely to occur when dosage is gradually increased. Women taking oral contraceptives should understand that Tegretol interferes with the contraceptive ability of the pills and they may experience breakthrough bleeding and false-positive pregnancy tests.

Likewise, the side effects of Depakote (valproate) tend to occur early in treatment and include sedation, tremor, ataxia, and gastrointestinal effects. Weight gain tends to persist throughout treatment, and clients may stop taking their medication as a result. Low doses of Topamax (topiramate) may counteract the extreme hunger associated with Depakote.

Lamictal (lamotrigine), Topamax (topiramate), Gabitril (tiagabine) and Neurontin (gabapentin) have few side effects except for some fatigue, dizziness, ataxia, and tremor. They cause no weight gain, and Topamax actually causes weight loss.

Lamictal (lamotrigine) may cause a rash within the first eight weeks of treatment. If this occurs, the primary health care provider must be notified immediately since the rash may be associated with a life-threatening syndrome known as **Stevens–Johnson syndrome**. This is a severe and sometimes fatal allergic reaction that attacks the skin, mucous membranes, lungs, and kidneys. Stevens–Johnson syndrome can be caused by sulfa drugs, penicillin, Dilantin (phenytoin), and Lamictal, especially when Lamictal is combined with Depakote (Brown & Weaver, 1998; Calabrese et al., 1999).

The most common side effects of calcium channel blockers are due to excessive vasodilation and include dizziness, hypotension, headaches, facial flushing, and nausea. Clients need to be cautioned not to eat or drink grapefruit because it inhibits an enzyme in the intestines that breaks down calcium channel blockers and can lead to toxic blood levels.

Children and adults who are taking Catapres (clonidine) or Tenex (guanfacine) should never stop the drug abruptly. A gradual weaning over two to four days is necessary to prevent rebound high blood pressure. Side effects of the antihypertensives include agitation, depression, dizziness, drowsiness, orthostatic hypotension, decreased sex drive, and difficulty with erections. Blood pressure should be monitored frequently.

TOXICITY AND OVERDOSE

There is a fine line between therapeutic levels and toxic levels of lithium. The kidneys excrete both lithium and sodium. If there is a low sodium level in the body, lithium will be retained in its place, which could result in toxicity. Therefore, a normal sodium balance is needed to ensure a therapeutic lithium level. Lithium can rapidly rise to toxic levels whenever there is a severe loss of fluids such as that caused by fevers, vomiting and diarrhea, or excessive sweating. Other causes of toxicity include excessive intake (deliberate or accidental) and reduced excretion of lithium (resulting from kidney disease and low salt intake).

At the beginning of lithium treatment, blood levels are monitored at least three times a week. Blood needs to be drawn about 12 hours after the last lithium dose and before the person takes the next dose. Because the initial side effects are similar to signs of toxicity, it is impossible to know clinically what is happening in the body. After the side effects disappear and the drug has stabilized in the body, blood levels typically are obtained every three to four months. If symptoms occur during this maintenance period, you can be sure they are signs of toxicity. Box 8.2 lists the signs of lithium toxicity. Caring for a client who is toxic includes monitoring vital signs, maintaining a patent airway, and administering intravenous fluids (adding NaCl if hyponatremic). Severe toxicity is treated with hemodialysis (Bauer et al., 2000).

Symptoms of toxicity with Tegretol (carbamazepine) include seizures, hypotension, arrhythmia, respiratory depression, and coma. Depakote (valproate)

overdose can cause severe coma and death. There is no specific treatment other than monitoring vital signs, maintaining a patent airway, and decreasing absorption by the use of activated charcoal. Narcan (naloxone) may be used to reverse the coma (Masters, 1996).

Symptoms of toxicity with Catapres (clonidine) and Tenex (guanfacine) include hypotension, bradycardia, lethargy, irritability, weakness, and hypoventilation.

ADMINISTRATION

The administration of lithium is oral, in capsule or liquid form. There is some speculation that the liquid form is absorbed more quickly and is therefore more beneficial when initiating the medication. Some capsules are in slow-release or controlled-release forms. Lithium is usually administered in divided doses, and the ultimate dosage is determined by the reduction of symptoms and blood lithium levels.

Both carbamazepine and valproate are available in tablet and liquid forms. They are given in divided doses, beginning with low dosage and a gradual increase. The ultimate dosage is determined by the reduction of symptoms, blood levels, and side effects. Calcium channel blockers are increased gradually over several days, during which clients are monitored for hypotension and bradycardia.

Catapres (clonidine) given orally is likely to cause significant drowsiness. A steady dose via a patch is less likely to be a problem. For those who experience skin sensitivity to the patch or want to swim, clonidine cream (0.1 mg/0.1 mL) is available. To avoid another person receiving the medication, the client should be the one to rub the cream into the skin.

BOX 8.2

Signs of Lithium Toxicity

Mild (serum level about 1.5 mEq/L)

- Slight apathy, lethargy, drowsiness
- Decreased concentration
- Mild muscular weakness, slight muscle twitching
- Coarse hand tremors
- Mild ataxia

Moderate (serum level about 1.5–2.5 mEq/L)

- Severe diarrhea
- Nausea and vomiting
- Mild to moderate ataxia
- Moderate apathy, lethargy, drowsiness
- Slurred speech
- Tinnitus (ringing in the ears)
- Blurred vision
- Irregular tremor
- Muscle weakness

Severe (serum level above 2.5 mEq/L)

- Nystagmus
- Dysarthria (speech difficulty due to impairment of the tongue)
- Deep tendon hyperreflexia
- Visual or tactile hallucinations
- Oliguria or anuria
- Confusion
- Seizures
- Coma or death

ANTIANXIETY MEDICATIONS

PHYSIOLOGICAL EFFECTS
Benzodiazepines

Benzodiazepine antianxiety medications act on the limbic system and the reticular activating system (RAS). They produce a calming effect by potentiating the effects of GABA, one of the inhibitory neurotransmitters. CNS depression can range from mild sedation to coma. Other physiological effects include skeletal muscle relaxation and anticonvulsant properties.

CRITICAL THINKING

Mrs. Salazar is a 67-year-old client who is being placed on Prozac (fluoxetine), an SSRI, for depression. The nurse teaches Mrs. Salazar and her daughter that:

■ They may not notice an improvement in Mrs. Salazar's depression for two to four weeks.

■ Side effects such as dry mouth, blurred vision, insomnia, rapid heartbeat, or sexual dysfunction can occur.

■ Prozac can cause significant weight gain and hypertension. The nurse advises Mrs. Salazar to reduce her salt intake and maintain a low-calorie, low-fat diet.

■ Toxicity to the drug is uncommon but can occur; therefore, confusion, irritability, or seizures should be reported to the physician immediately.

Upon completion of teaching Mrs. Salazar and her daughter about the drug, the nurse turns and leaves the room.

1. How would you explain the actions of a serotonin reuptake inhibitor to Mrs. Salazar and her daughter?

2. How will Mrs. Salazar know if the SSRI is being effective?

3. Based on your understanding of these drugs, evaluate the nurse's teaching session with Mrs. Salazar and her daughter.

4. What aspects of teaching should be different for Mrs. Salazar than for younger clients on the same drug?

5. What is the best explanation for including Mrs. Salazar's daughter in the teaching session?

For an additional Case Study, please refer to the Companion Web site for this book.

Azaspirones

Azaspirone antianxiety medications do not bind at GABA receptors but rather balance 5-HT activity by stimulating the 5-HT receptors. These medications do not tranquilize and sedate and may have mild antidepressant effects. Typically, it takes one to two weeks for the level of anxiety to decrease.

THERAPEUTIC EFFECTS

Although antianxiety medications will not eliminate all the symptoms of anxiety, they will decrease the level of anxiety, thereby enabling clients to function more effectively. These medications are used for anxiety symptoms, anxiety disorders, acute alcohol withdrawal, and convulsive disorders.

Individual benzodiazepines differ in potency, speed in crossing the blood–brain barrier, and degree of receptor binding. High-potency and short-acting benzodiazepines include Xanax (alprazolam), Ativan (lorazepam), Paxipam (halazepam), and Serax (oxazepam). Low-potency and long-acting benzodiazepines include Tranxene (clorazepate), Valium (diazepam), and Librium (chlordiazepoxide) (Table 8.5 ■ lists the various antianxiety medications).

SIDE EFFECTS
Benzodiazepines

Side effects of benzodiazepines are primarily related to the general sedative effects and include drowsiness, fatigue, dizziness, and psychomotor impairment. Sedation usually disappears within one to two weeks of treatment. These medications potentiate the effects of alcohol on the CNS, leading to severe CNS depression. Consuming alcohol while taking benzodiazepines can lead to fatal consequences. When administered intravenously, there is a potential for cardiovascular collapse and respiratory depression. There is a potential for addiction and abuse in vulnerable client populations. Benzodiazepines may improve sexual aversion, vaginismus, and rapid ejaculation.

Azaspirones

BuSpar (buspirone) has no potential for dependence and does not potentiate the effects of alcohol on the CNS. It is the drug of choice for clients who are prone to substance abuse or for those who require long-term treatment with antianxiety medications. Its side effects include drowsiness, dizziness, headache, and nervousness. This drug does not negatively affect sex drive or arousal; in fact, sexual desire is often enhanced. It may improve delayed ejaculation and may worsen rapid ejaculation (Crenshaw & Goldberg, 1996).

TOXICITY AND OVERDOSE

Symptoms of toxicity include euphoria, relaxation, slurred speech, disorientation, unsteady gait, and

TABLE 8.5

Antianxiety Medications

Class	Generic Name	Trade Name	Adult Dosage (mg/day)
Benzodiazepines	Alprazolam	Xanax	0.75–4.0
	Chlordiazepoxide	Librium	15–100
	Clonazepam	Klonopin	5–20
	Clorazepate	Tranxene	15–60
	Diazepam	Valium	6–40
	Halazepam	Paxipam	60–160
	Hydroxyzine	Atarax, Vistaril	200–400
	Lorazepam	Ativan	4–12
	Oxazepam	Serax	30–120
	Prazepam	Centrax	10–60
Azaspirones	Buspirone	BuSpar	15–60
Metathizanone	Chlormezanone	Trancopal	300–800

impaired judgment. Symptoms of overdose include respiratory depression, cold and clammy skin, hypotension, weak and rapid pulse, dilated pupils, and coma. Caring for a client who has overdosed includes monitoring vital signs, especially of cardiac function, and maintaining a patent airway. If the client is alert, vomiting is induced, while gastric lavage is initiated for the client who is stuporous. Following this procedure, activated charcoal may be administered to minimize absorption. Forced diuresis may increase elimination of the medication.

Romazicon (flumazenil) is the antidote for overdose and can reverse sedation, respiratory depression, and coma within two minutes. Doses may need to be repeated. The initial dose is 0.2 mg IV, followed by 0.3 mg one minute later and then as necessary to counteract the overdose symptoms (Turkoski et al., 2000).

ADMINISTRATION

All the antianxiety medications may be taken orally. Antacids interfere with the absorption of these medications and should not be taken until several hours later. Atarax and Vistaril (hydroxyzine) may also be administered IM. Librium (chlordiazepoxide), Valium (diazepam), and Ativan (lorazepam) may be administered IM and IV.

Benzodiazepines should not be discontinued abruptly after three to four months of therapy because of the risk of severe withdrawal symptoms, which include seizures, abdominal and other muscular cramps, vomiting, and insomnia. These medications must be gradually reduced very carefully.

CENTRAL NERVOUS SYSTEM STIMULANTS

CNS stimulants are used in the management of attention deficit/hyperactivity disorder (ADHD) and Tourette's disorder (see Table 8.6 ■ for these medications). These medications increase the ability to focus attention by blocking out irrelevant thoughts and impulses. CNS

TABLE 8.6

Medications to Treat ADHD and Tourette's Disorder

Generic Name	Trade Name	Dosage
CNS Stimulants		
Dextroamphetamine	Dexedrine	5–15 mg every 4–6 hours
	Adderall	5–30 mg every 4–6 hours
Methylphenidate	Ritalin	0.3–0.8 mg/kg BID or TID
Modafinil	Provigil	200–400 mg once a day
Pemoline	Cylert	maximum dose 112.5 mg once a day
Mood Stabilizers/Antihypertensives		
Clonidine	Catapres	0.1–0.6 mg per day
		Available in patch
Guanfacine	Tenex	1–3 mg per day
Antidepressants		
Bupropion	Wellbutrin	100–450 mg per day
Antidyskinetic		
Pergolide	Permax	50–500 µg per day
Antispastic		
Tizanidine	Zanaflex	8 mg every 6–8 hours

stimulants lead to significant improvement in 70 to 75 percent of cases. The use of CNS stimulants can be compared to the use of glasses for those who are nearsighted (myopic). Glasses allow the child to see the board in the front of the classroom, and CNS stimulants focus attention. You would never say to a myopic child, "You don't need your glasses. Just concentrate and you can read the material on the board." And yet, we often tell children with ADHD to "just concentrate" and do the work. For most of these children, it is impossible without medication. See Box 8.3 for therapeutic effects of CNS stimulants.

The advantage of Ritalin (methylphenidate) and Dexedrine (dextroamphetamine) is that effectiveness is almost immediate, whereas the same effect with Cylert (pemoline) may take six to eight weeks. Clients are cautioned not to eat or drink citrus products within one hour of taking Dexadrine (dextroamphetamine) because citrus interferes with absorption of the drug. Individuals taking CNS stimulants should avoid caffeine and products with ephedrine (e.g., cough medicine) as these will increase the sense of jitteriness. Common side effects include pallor, a pinched facial expression, dark hollows under the eyes, anorexia, insomnia, headache, and dryness of the mouth.

Atomoxetine is a new drug under study. If approved for use, it will be the first nonstimulant medication for ADHD. Initial studies demonstrate a decrease in symptoms and improved social and family functioning.

BOX 8.3

Therapeutic Effects of CNS Stimulants

Increases

- Attention
- Accuracy
- Concentration
- Coordination
- Learning
- Memory
- On-task behavior

Decreases

- Aggression
- Daydreaming
- Defiance
- Distractability
- Destructiveness
- Hyperactivity
- Lying
- Oppositional defiant disorder

SPECIAL POPULATIONS AND PSYCHOPHARMACOLOGICAL TREATMENT

Certain groups of clients present a challenge to nurses when psychotropic medications are part of their treatment. These groups include older adults, pregnant women, children, medically complex clients, those who are psychiatrically disabled, and culturally diverse clients.

OLDER ADULTS

The physiological changes of aging affect the use of psychotropic medications. Absorption of medication is influenced by a decrease in gastric emptying time, a reduction in blood flow to the gastrointestinal (GI) system, and a decrease in GI motility. Once through the GI system, most psychotropic medications bind to albumin. Albumin levels decrease with aging, and there is more free-floating medication in the bloodstream, thereby contributing to increased sedation in older adults. At the same time, adipose tissue increases by 10 to 50 percent over the age of 65. Medications such as the long-acting benzodiazepines, which are stored in adipose tissue, are thus available for longer periods of time. Changes in liver metabolism contribute to slower metabolism of medications, which prolongs elimination and leads to increased toxicity. The renal filtration rate may decrease by 50 percent by age 70, which also contributes to increased toxicity. Aging reduces the amount of NE, 5-HT, DA, ACh, and GABA in the central nervous system, leading to increased receptor sensitivity. The result is a change in responsiveness to medications (Brown & Lempa, 1997).

Older adults are more sensitive than younger adults to the side effects of antipsychotic medications. This is important information since 25 to 45 percent of geriatric nursing home residents are given these medications. Increased sedation may lead to confusion and agitation. Orthostatic hypotension increases the risk of falls and fractures. Older people are likely to have more severe EPSs, especially a higher risk of tardive dyskinesia. Drugs with high potency and low dosage are particularly successful in small doses (Jeste et al., 1999).

Older adults are also more sensitive to antidepressant side effects. The anticholinergic effects may increase symptoms of prostatic hypertrophy, blurred vision, and constipation. The anticholinergic properties of these medications may lead to short-term memory problems, disorientation, and impaired cognition. These side effects may be mistaken for organic brain disease (pseudodementia).

The new generation of antidepressants, the SSRIs and SNRIs, are especially useful for treating depression in older people. The response time between initiation of the medication and relief of depressive symptoms is much shorter than with tricyclic antidepressants. The most commonly used are Prozac (fluoxetine) for people experiencing psychomotor retardation, and Zoloft (sertraline) for those experiencing anxiety.

Because the production of MAO increases with age, MAOIs may be more effective for older clients. Another benefit to older people is the absence of anticholinergic side effects. There is, however, a higher risk of hypotension, which may be a contributing factor in falls. The disadvantage of this group of medications is the strict dietary limitations. The nutritional options of many older clients are limited because of their finances; they may find it difficult to follow the severely restricted diet.

Because the metabolism of antianxiety medications slows with aging, medications that are metabolized quickly are more frequently prescribed. Older clients are more sensitive to the side effects of sedation, which may contribute to confusion and agitation. Other effects in older adults include unsteadiness, slowed reaction time, increased forgetfulness, and decreased concentration (see Table 8.7 ■ for medications and dosage for older adults).

PREGNANT WOMEN

The benefits and dangers of the use of antidepressants must be carefully considered for women who are pregnant, breast-feeding, or trying to conceive. Tricyclic antidepressants and the new-generation antidepressants do not have any significant increase in birth defects. The low concentrations in breast milk allow for breast-feeding when on antidepressants. MAOIs

may cause birth defects and contribute to complications during delivery. Lithium should be avoided during the first trimester of pregnancy. The newer antipsychotics do not appear to cause birth defects. However, it is recommended that the dose be lowered as much as possible a few days before birth to avoid withdrawal symptoms in the infant. Women should be discouraged from breast-feeding while they are taking psychotropic medications because these medications pass into breast milk (Stowe et al., 2000).

CHILDREN

Psychotropic medications may be prescribed for children with mental, behavioral, or emotional symptoms when the potential benefits of treatment outweigh the risks. Some problems are so serious and persistent that

TABLE 8.7

Medications for Older Adults

Class	Generic Name	Trade Name	Older Adult Dosage (mg/day)
Antipsychotic			
	Fluphenazine	Prolixin, Permitil	0.25–6.0
	Haloperidol	Haldol	0.25–6.0
	Risperidone	Risperdal	4–16
	Thiothixene	Navane	4–20
	Trifluoperazine	Stelazine, Suptazine	4–20
Antidepressant			
	Desipramine	Norpramin, Petrofrane	25–150
	Paroxetine	Paxil	10
	Phenelzine	Nardil	7.5–30.0
	Tranylcypromine	Parnate	10–40
	Venlafaxine	Effexor	75–375
Antianxiety			
	Alprazolam	Xanax	0.125–2.0
	Lorazepam	Ativan	0.5–2
	Oxazepam	Serax	10–30

they would have significant negative consequences if the child went untreated. The safety and efficacy of most psychotropic medications have not yet been studied in young children. Treatment of children with these medications is off-label use.

When medications are used, they should not be the only intervention. Other interventions include family therapy, family support services, and behavior management techniques.

Children tend to have a faster absorption rate compared to adults. Children also metabolize medications more quickly than adults do. This increased efficiency in absorption and metabolism indicates that it is more appropriate to administer smaller multiple doses through the day rather than larger, less frequent doses. Dosages for children are based on the child's tolerance of side effects. Other considerations include effects on growth retardation, school performance problems, lower cognitive test scores, and reproductive risks that extend beyond treatment.

Teenagers are very concerned with their body image. Many psychotropic medications cause significant weight gain, which is especially problematic for teens. Medications can also become the focus for power struggles between parents and teens. As a nurse, you can help parents establish new "ground rules" so adolescents can begin to assume responsibility for their own medications (Papolos & Papolos, 1999).

MEDICALLY COMPLEX CLIENTS

Medically complex clients are those who have an underlying medical problem with or without a preexisting psychiatric disorder. For instance, the development of delirium or acute confusional states occurs in some 10 to 30 percent of hospitalized clients. As many as 51 percent of postoperative clients develop delirium and up to 80 percent of people with terminal illnesses develop delirium near death (Trzepacz, Breitbart, Franklin, Levenson, & Martini, 1999). The cause may be environmental (ICU psychosis), medication toxicity, or underlying pathophysiology of the illness. The essential part of diagnosis and treatment of these clients is determining the underlying cause of the symptoms. If the cause is medical, such as pneumonia, Parkinson's disease, or undiagnosed infections, then treating the underlying disorder will eliminate the psychiatric symptoms.

Clients with chronic illnesses may suffer from major depression. Depression may result from hyper-

thyroidism, hypothyroidism, diabetes, or acquired immune deficiency syndrome (AIDS). Medications such as antihypertensives, antiarthritics, sedatives, and cardiovascular medications may also cause depression. The treatment of choice is a trial of antidepressant therapy. Clients with a history of cardiac problems may be more difficult to treat with tricyclic antidepressants because these medications may trigger further arrhythmias. The SSRIs are better tolerated and less likely to produce cardiovascular side effects (Nelson et al., 1999).

Clients with both a medical illness and psychiatric symptoms must be monitored for multidrug interactions. Americans over the age of 64 use 30 percent of the prescription drugs sold, along with an unknown number of over-the-counter (OTC) medications (Margolis, 1998). These data point to the problem of polypharmacy, especially in the older adult population—but more importantly, to the increased likelihood of multidrug interaction, which is potentially life threatening. Assess the functional level and baseline cognitive abilities of clients to determine whether they are able to learn or retain information about their medications. Obtain a complete listing of the medications. Do not simply ask what medications clients are taking; have them bring in medications and describe their administration. Consult a pharmacist to determine whether any drug may interact adversely with others.

PSYCHIATRICALLY DISABLED CLIENTS

Despite advances in medical science, some clients remain psychiatrically disabled. The symptoms these clients suffer from are usually debilitating and interfere dramatically with their ability to function in daily life. Their capacity to learn or retain new information is often impaired. Assessing cognitive skills is important in designing appropriate teaching strategies. Determine what medications have been effective in the past and how well the client was able to remain on the medication. Identifying supportive people in the client's environment, as well as community resources, can be helpful for medication compliance.

CULTURALLY DIVERSE CLIENTS

Ethnopharmacology, the study of the interaction of drugs, culture, and ethnicity, is a topic only recently studied. Within a few years of discovering medications for people with mental disorders, the drugs were introduced throughout the world. Most of the studies regarding safety, efficacy, and dosage involved young, Euro-American males. Ethnic variations were not a primary consideration. More recently, researchers examining the benefits of drug treatment and toxicity have found that these are not the same for all groups of people. High metabolism of a medication may contribute to ineffective treatment, while low metabolism may increase side effects or lead to toxicity. Recognizing the ethnic differences in response to drugs promotes giving culturally competent care.

Remember that people grouped together as Asians, Hispanics, or Arabs are in fact very diverse ethnic, cultural, and linguistic groups. Thus, many variations will be found within each of these groups. The CYP enzymes involved in the metabolism of medications have many mutations from which some generalizations can be made. Those who tend to be *slow metabolizers* are Asians, Africans, African Americans, Hispanics from the Caribbean, Mexicans, and some Spaniards. Individuals with these heritages must be closely monitored for increased sensitivity, increased side effects, and increased toxicity. They often need lower doses of psychotropic drugs. Asian Americans may be at increased risk for acute dystonic reactions when taking antipsychotics. In one study, 50 percent of Asian Americans developed acute dystonic reaction within the first two weeks of Haldol (haloperidol) administration compared with 28 percent of Euro-Americans (Pi & Gray, 2000; Mendoza & Smith, 2000).

Rapid metabolizers include Ethiopians, Arabs, and some Spaniards. These individuals often need extremely high doses of medications to achieve therapeutic levels (Ruiz, 2000).

Cultural assessment should be taken prior to negotiating a treatment plan that includes medication. This assessment should identify client beliefs about the causes of mental illness, home remedies, spiritual treatments, and attitudes toward health care professionals. Personal beliefs about medication will influence compliance. For example, if the client believes in the "magic" of medication, he or she may take extra pills, thinking that more is better. For those who believe that taking medicine is a sign of weakness, the medication may not be taken at all. The health-belief model of clients and families is one of the significant reasons why people stop taking medications. Other reasons include financial burden and horrendous side effects (Lin & Smith, 2000).

Health care providers prescribing medications bring their own values, priorities, modes of thinking, and belief systems into the client–provider relationship. Unfortunately, that has resulted in significant differences in diagnosis and treatment for ethnic minorities in the United States. For example, African Americans are more likely to receive antipsychotics and higher doses of medications across all diagnostic categories with more adverse consequences. Since African Americans are often slow metabolizers, they tend to respond more quickly to antipsychotics, tricyclic antidepressants, and lithium than Euro-Americans do. It is often safer to use SSRIs, newer antipsychotics, and mood stabilizers other than lithium (Lawson, 2000).

NURSING INTERVENTIONS

Box 8.4 lists the nursing interventions classifications (NIC) that are appropriate for medication management and client/family education (McCloskey & Bulechek, 1996).

BOX 8.4

Nursing Interventions Classification

DOMAIN: Physiological: Complex

Class: Drug Management
Intervention: Medication Management: Facilitation of safe and effective use of prescription and over-the-counter drugs

Class: Thermoregulation
Intervention: Temperature Regulation: Attaining and/or maintaining body temperature within a normal range

DOMAIN: Behavioral

Class: Patient Education
Interventions: Teaching: Prescribed Medication: Preparing a patient to safely take prescribed medications and monitor for their effects

SOURCE: McCloskey, J. C., & Bulechek, G. M. (1996). *Nursing interventions classification (NIC)* (2nd ed.). St. Louis, MO: Mosby.

PHYSIOLOGICAL: COMPLEX: DRUG MANAGEMENT
Medication Management

Part of psychiatric nursing is the administration and management of psychotropic drugs. Proper medication management can often make a tremendous difference in a consumer's life. Adult clients have many of their own ideas about medications and do have the right to refuse treatment. The word *noncompliance* has negative connotations such as disobeying or being defiant. However, it is still the commonly used term among health care professionals. It is up to us, as nurses, to ensure that compliance means mutually agreed-upon goals and outcomes rather than simply clients obeying orders. It is not just people with mental disorders that struggle with this issue. People with diabetes, hypertension, chronic lung disease, and other illnesses have compliance problems also. If we are to understand people's refusal to take medications, we have to find out their reasons, which are many and often intermixed. Compliance problems are often related to errors due to the illness and side effects. (Table 8.8 ■ provides information clients should receive regarding the consequences of medication interactions.)

TABLE 8.8
Medication Interactions: Client Teaching

If you take this . . .	And this . . .	This could happen:
Lithium	Antidepressants	May increase the risk of manic relapse in people with rapid-cycling bipolar disorder
Lithium	Diuretics	Retention of lithium and consequent toxicity
Lithium	Nonsteroidal anti-inflammatory drugs (NSAIDs)	May raise lithium levels with consequent toxicity
Lithium	Angiotensin-converting enzyme (ACE) inhibitors	May raise lithium levels with consequent toxicity
Lithium	Xanthines	May lower lithium levels
Anticonvulsants	Benzodiazepines	Decreased antianxiety levels
MAOIs	Tricyclics, SSRIs	Severe agitation, nausea, confusion
MAOIs	Narcotic pain relievers	Reactions may include extreme restlessness, confusion, seizures, coma
MAOIs	OTC decongestants, cough medicines that contain pseudoephedrine or phenylpropanolamine	Hypertensive crisis
MAOIs	Lamictal (lamotrigine)	Dizziness, headache, double vision, nausea, unsteadiness
Calcium channel blockers; Serzone; Xanax	Grapefruit	Increased drug levels and potential for toxicity
Ritalin (methylphenidate)	Antihistamines	Decreases effect of Ritalin
Ritalin (methylphenidate)	Drugs with ephedrine, caffeine	Increased jitteriness
Dexedrine (dextroamphetamine)	Citrus products within one hour of medication	Interferes with absorption of medication

A common error due to one's mental disorder is believing that one is not ill. Awareness of illness, or insight, seems to be affected by both biological and psychological factors. Arguing or threatening clients is useless. Saying something like, "If you don't take your meds, you'll end up in the hospital" has a blaming sound to it. It may be better to say, "Most of the time, if people stop their meds, they end up in the hospital." Threatening clients is unethical and is heard in such statements as, "If you don't take your meds, you cannot have your cigarettes today." Forgetfulness or memory loss may be other errors related to a mental disorder. You need to plan strategies for helping these clients remember to take their medications. A container designed to hold morning, noon, evening, and nighttime dosages for an entire week is often very helpful in reminding people of their medications. Some people wear watches that can be set with an alarm signal whenever medications are due to be taken. If one strategy isn't effective, try another strategy until the client is successful.

Intolerance of side effects is another factor in noncompliance. When a side effect becomes severe, it is no longer a side effect—it becomes the primary effect of the medication. The more severe the side effect, the more people cannot feel the positive effect of the drug. As new drugs are developed with reduced side effects and increased effectiveness, clients will be able to manage their medications more easily.

In order to assist your clients with proper medication management, encourage them to ask questions and do their own research for further information and self-education. One useful Web site for drug information is *http://www.nlm.nih.gov/medlineplus/druginformation*. Such data can be viewed on the National Institute of Health Web site, which can be accessed through a resource link on the Companion Web site for this book.

PHYSIOLOGICAL: COMPLEX: THERMOREGULATION
Temperature Regulation

When thinking about heat exhaustion or heatstroke, we generally imagine those at risk to be people with chronic medical problems, especially older individuals. However, many psychotropic medications make clients more susceptible to heat-related illnesses (see Table

8.9 ■). Other factors increasing the risk for heat exhaustion or heatstroke are obesity, self-care deficits, inadequate living conditions, and difficulty in recognizing signs and symptoms of heat-related illnesses. You can help clients plan ahead by providing written and verbal information about the increased risk for heatstroke. Clients should be taught to maintain an adequate fluid intake while avoiding caffeinated drinks, which tend to increase heart rate. During the day, clients can plan to spend time in an air-conditioned building such as a library, a mall, mental health centers, or cooling centers. Cool baths or showers and loose, light clothing are also beneficial.

BEHAVIORAL: PATIENT EDUCATION
Teaching: Prescribed Medication

Successful treatment depends to a great extent on clients' understanding of the treatment and their participation in making the best treatment decisions for themselves. Medication teaching is an important consideration for any client taking psychotropic medications. Clients and families must be actively involved in either individual or group teaching sessions. See Box 8.5 for medication teaching plans.

CLIENT AND FAMILY PARTICIPATION

Consumers of mental health care have the right to make decisions about taking medications. As a nurse, your role is to help clients and families understand how to make such decisions. Some of the influences on this decision-making process are:

■ Client's and family's relationships with health care professionals; the freedom to ask questions or the fear of disapproval

■ The severity of the illness and symptoms

■ The positive and negative personal experiences clients have had with medications

■ The convenience of taking the medication as it fits into the person's lifestyle

■ Group support and suggestions for managing side effects

■ The media (magazine articles, newspaper and television reports)

TABLE 8.9

Medications/Drugs and Heat-Related Illnesses

Medication/Drug	Increased Risk Through:
Antipsychotics	Altered sweat production, impaired temperature regulation, impaired thirst recognition, weight gain
Anticholinergics	Altered sweat production
Tricyclics	Altered sweat production, weight gain
SSRIs	Increased heat production, inhibited heat loss
MAOIs	Weight gain
Lithium	Increased heat production, inhibited heat loss, fluid loss through increased urination
Beta blockers	Dehydration through increased sweating
Smoking	Respiratory conditions such as asthma or emphysema impair oxygen exchange, which inhibits heat loss
Alcohol	Excess fluid loss through increased urination
Stimulants	Increased metabolic requirements

SOURCES: Batscha, C. L. (1997). Heat stroke: Keeping your clients cool in the summer. *Journal of Psychosocial Nursing, 35*(7), 12–17; and Hermesh, H., et al. (2000). Heat intolerance in patients with chronic schizophrenia maintained with antipsychotic drugs. *American Journal of Psychiatry, 157*(8), 1327–1329.

Other influences that affect the decision include the number of medications prescribed, health benefits, financial concerns, and social support systems available in the community.

An important topic for discussion is that of side effects. Most repeat hospitalizations occur because clients stop taking their medications in response to disturbing side effects such as weight gain and sexual dysfunction. They may need help in reporting their concerns and fears so they can be more active mental health care consumers.

Teach clients the purpose of their medications, how to take them (timing, with food or alone, actions to take if doses are missed), potential side effects, and when to call the doctor. Combine verbal and written instructions. Use pictures for those clients who are unable to read English.

MEDICATION TEACHING GROUPS

Medication teaching groups are successful with most clients. Talking with others and helping others with similar disabilities provides emotional support and reinforces medication information. The groups use role playing, audiovisual tools, lectures, and discussion. Crane, Kirby, and Kooperman (1996) describe the various functions of medication groups:

- Providing information about medications
- Helping clients discuss and manage fears about medications
- Increasing client understanding of mental disorders and the role of medications
- Expanding client participation in the treatment planning process
- Helping clients become accountable for their decision making

Nurses are often asked to provide clients and families with information on medications. The nurse provides information and then elicits reactions and comments from the group members. Knowledge about medications helps clients develop their own coping strategies.

BOX 8.5

Medication Teaching

General Considerations

- Carry at all times a card or other identification listing the names of the medications you are taking.
- If you are taking your medication several times a day and you forget to take a dose, do the following: If within one to two hours of the missed time, take the medication; if more than two hours after the missed dose, skip the dose and take the next dose at the regularly scheduled time.
- Do not stop taking the medication abruptly; this might produce withdrawal symptoms.
- Do not take nonprescription medication without approval from your primary health care provider.
- If you experience drowsiness or dizziness, do not drive or operate dangerous machinery.
- Limit your intake of caffeine.
- If you experience sexual difficulties, discuss these with your primary health care provider. A different medication may or may not be helpful.
- If you experience a dry mouth, take frequent sips of water, chew sugarless gum, or suck on ice chips or hard candy. Frequent brushing of your teeth is also helpful. You may need to use an artificial saliva preparation.
- If you experience constipation, increase your fluid intake if it is low, increase your consumption of vegetables and fiber, and increase your exercise. You may find bulk laxatives such as Metamucil, Surfak, or Colace to be helpful.
- If weight gain becomes a problem, increase your exercise and decrease your caloric intake.

Antipsychotic Medications

- Rise slowly from a sitting or lying position to prevent a sudden drop in blood pressure.
- When outdoors, always use a sunscreen, wear protective clothing, and limit your exposure to the sun. You can become badly sunburned in a very short period of time.
- Call your primary health care provider immediately if you experience a sore throat, high fever, or mouth or skin sores or rashes.

Antidepressants

- The effect of the medications may not be felt for four weeks.

- Rise slowly from a sitting or lying position to prevent a sudden drop in blood pressure.
- When outdoors, always use a sunscreen, wear protective clothing, and limit your exposure to the sun. You can become badly sunburned in a very short period of time.
- These medications decrease the seizure threshold, making you more prone to have a seizure. Because alcohol and some drugs also lower the seizure threshold, do not use these substances while taking this medication.

Lithium

- Daily fluid intake should range from 2,500 to 3,000 mL/day.
- Avoid heavy intake of caffeine, which increases urine output.
- Maintain normal dietary sodium levels.
- Report any sudden weight gain and/or edema to your primary health care provider.
- Immediately report any sign of toxicity: persistent nausea and vomiting, severe diarrhea, ataxia (lack of muscle coordination), blurred vision, or ringing in the ears.
- Blood drawn to measure lithium levels should be drawn 12 hours after the last dose.
- Use the following medications very cautiously and only under medical supervision:
  - Aminophylline, sodium bicarbonate: wash lithium out of the body
  - Muscle relaxants: lithium increases their effect
  - Nonsteroidal anti-inflammatory drugs: increase the risk of lithium toxicity
  - Thiazide diuretics: increase the risk of lithium toxicity

Antianxiety Agents

- Do not use alcohol or any drugs that depress the central nervous system. Taken in combination, they can be fatal.
- Report any restlessness or spastic movements to your primary health care provider.
- Do not stop taking the drug abruptly. Severe withdrawal reactions may occur such as anxiety, depression, insomnia, vomiting, sweating, convulsions, and delirium.

FAMILY SUPPORT

To achieve the best outcome, family members and/or significant others must be viewed as potential allies and resources for rehabilitation. Family members can be a significant support to the client and can, when educated, help with symptom monitoring, decision making regarding medications, and avoiding relapses. Families are a significant resource for the care and long-term management of their relatives if they are given practical support and information. Begin teaching family members in your initial contact with them. Help them express their feelings about living with the person who has the disorder. Identify the strengths the family brings to the living situation. Support the family in developing ways to maintain the client at the highest level of functioning.

Family education is accomplished in both individual and group sessions. The functions of medication groups, as described above, also apply to the family. Each family member must weigh the costs and benefits of any and all medications. Support their right to participate in these treatment decisions by functioning as a client advocate in the clinical setting.

CHAPTER REVIEW

BOOKS FOR CLIENTS AND FAMILIES

Chavis, L. M. (2001). *Ask your pharmacist.* New York: St. Martins Press.

Griffith, H. W. (2000). *Complete guide to prescription & nonprescription drugs.* New York: Perigee Book.

2002 Drug hand book (2002). San Francisco: Blanchard & Loeb.

KEY CONCEPTS

Introduction

■ Psychotropic medications affect cognitive function, emotions, and behavior. They are categorized into five classes: antipsychotic, antidepressant, mood-stabilizing, antianxiety, and stimulant medications.

Antipsychotic Medications

■ Conventional antipsychotic medications are more effective in diminishing the positive characteristics (hallucinations, delusions, loose association, inappropriate affect) than in diminishing the negative characteristics (withdrawal, minimal self-care, concrete thinking, flat affect) of severe mental illness. Newer antipsychotic agents decrease both positive and negative symptoms.

■ By reducing symptoms, medication enables clients to assume more control over their lives and participate more effectively in other forms of treatment.

■ The IM form of Geodon (ziprasidone) or Zyprexa (olanzapine) is used for the control and short-term management of clients who are acutely psychotic and agitated. Effect is apparent within one hour after injection.

■ Extrapyramidal side effects (EPSs) are caused by an imbalance of DA and ACh and are more frequently associated with high-potency medications. Newer antipsychotics have the lowest incidence of EPSs.

■ Types of EPS include akinesia, akathisia, parkinsonism, dystonia, oculogyric crisis, and tardive dyskinesia.

■ Neuroleptic malignant syndrome is a potentially fatal side effect. Symptoms develop suddenly and include muscle rigidity, respiratory problems, hyperpyrexia, tachycardia, hypertension, confusion, and delirium.

■ Side effects such as weight gain, and sexual dysfunction cause a high percentage of clients to stop taking their medication.

Adjunctive Medications for EPSs

■ Anticholinergic medications and several specialized agents lessen the EPS effects by restoring the DA:ACh ratio.

Antidepressant Medications

■ Antidepressant medications increase the amount of available neurotransmitters by inhibiting reuptake, inhibiting monoamine oxidase (MAO), by blocking receptors, or by modulating the effect of neurotransmitters.

■ Side effects of antidepressants include anticholinergic effects, photosensitivity, sexual difficulties, and weight gain.

■ If a person eats food rich in tyramine and tryptophan while taking an MAOI (MAO inhibitor), he or she risks a hypertensive crisis, which may be fatal.

■ Serotonin syndrome is a potentially fatal side effect. Symptoms develop quickly and include mental changes, hyperreflexia, muscle rigidity, tachycardia, hyperthermia, coma, and seizures.

Mood-Stabilizing Medications

■ Mood-stabilizing medications include lithium, anticonvulsants, calcium channel blockers, and antihypertensives.

■ Mood stabilizers are effective for clients with bipolar disorder, major depression, schizoaffective disorder, treatment-resistant schizophrenia, alcohol withdrawal, and other problems concerning the regulation of mood. They are most effective as antimanic medications.

■ Catapres (clonidine) and Tenex (guanfacine) are antihypertensives that seem to be helpful for people with rage attacks, tic disorders, ADHD, and pervasive developmental disorders.

■ There is a fine line between therapeutic levels and toxic levels of lithium. Older people are more susceptible to toxicity.

■ Stevens–Johnson syndrome is a severe and sometimes fatal allergic reaction that attacks the skin, mucous membranes, lungs, and kidneys.

■ Toxicity with Tegretol and Depakene/Depakote can cause coma and even death.

Antianxiety Medications

■ Benzodiazepines potentiate the effects of GABA in the limbic system and the reticular activating system.

■ Azaspirones attach to 5-HT and DA receptors.

■ Side effects of benzodiazepines include sedation, potentiation of the effects of alcohol, and chemical dependence.

■ BuSpar (buspirone) is the drug of choice for clients who are prone to substance abuse or those who require long-term treatment.

■ Symptoms of toxicity are primarily CNS effects. Symptoms of overdose include respiratory depression, cold and clammy skin, hypotension, weak and rapid pulse, dilated pupils, and coma.

■ All the antianxiety medications may be taken orally. Atarax and Vistaril may also be administered IM. Librium, Valium, and Ativan may be administered IM and IV.

■ Benzodiazepines should not be discontinued abruptly because of the risk of severe withdrawal symptoms.

Central Nervous System Stimulants

■ These medications increase the ability to focus attention by blocking out irrelevant thoughts and impulses.

Special Populations and Psychopharmacological Treatment

■ Older adults are more sensitive than younger adults to the side effects of many medications. Increased sedation may lead to confusion and agitation. Orthostatic hypotension increases the risk of falls and fractures.

■ Older adult clients are more likely to have severe EPSs and anticholinergic side effects.

■ The benefits and dangers of psychotropic drugs must be carefully considered for women who are pregnant, breast-feeding, or trying to conceive.

■ Children absorb and metabolize medications more quickly than adults and should be given smaller multiple doses throughout the day.

■ Medically complex clients who experience medical problems and psychiatric symptoms must be assessed for the underlying cause, such as environmental causes, medication toxicity, or underlying pathophysiology of the illness.

■ Clients must be assessed for multidrug interactions; many people take several medications at once.

Nursing Interventions

■ Compliance problems are often related to errors due to the illness, side effects, and lack of education.

■ Variables that influence a client's decision whether or not to take medication include the media, relationships with health care professionals, severity of the illness, personal experiences, group support and suggestions, the number of medications, health benefits, financial concerns, and social support systems in the community.

■ Clients must be taught the purpose of their medications, how to take them, potential side effects, and situations in which to call the physician.

■ Medication teaching groups provide information, help manage fears, increase understanding of mental disorders and the role of medications, expand client participation in treatment planning, and help clients become accountable for decision making.

■ To achieve the best possible outcome, families and significant others must be included in medication teaching.

EXPLORE *MediaLink*

■ Interactive resources, including animations and videos, for this chapter can be found on the Companion Web site at *http://www.prenhall.com/fontaine*. Click on Chapter 8 and select the activities for this chapter.

■ For NCLEX review questions and an audio glossary, access the accompanying CD-ROM in this book.

REFERENCES

Allison, D. B., Mentore, J. L., Heo, M., Chandler, L. P., Cappelleri, J. C., Infante, M. C., et al. (1999). Antipsychotic-induced weight gain: A comprehensive research synthesis. *American Journal of Psychiatry, 156*(11), 1686–1696.

Bauer, M., Bschor, T., Kunz, D., Berghofer, A., Strohle, A., & Muller-Oerlinghausen, B., (2000). Double-blind, placebo-controlled trial of the use of lithium to augment antidepressant medication in continuation treatment of unipolar major depression. *American Journal of Psychiatry, 157*(9), 1429–1435.

Breier, A. F., Malhotra, A. K., Su, T., Pinals, D. A., Elman, I., Adler, C. M., et al. (1999). Clozapine and risperidone in chronic schizophrenia. *American Journal of Psychiatry, 156*(2), 294–299.

Brown, A., & Lempa, M. (1997). Late life depression. *NARSAD Newsletter, 9*(3), 10–15.

Brown, A., & Weaver, R. (1998). Promising new medications in development. *NARSAD Newsletter, 10*(2), 24–31.

Calabrese, J. R., Bowden, C. L., McElroy, S. L., Cookson, J., Andersen, J., Keck, P. E., et al. (1999). Spectrum of activity of lamotrigine in treatment—refractory bipolar disorder. *American Journal of Psychiatry, 156*(7), 1019–1023.

Conley, R. R., Tamminga, C. A., Bartko, J. J., Richardson, C., Peszke, M., Lingle, J., et al. (1998). Olanzapine compared with chlorpromazine in treatment-resistant schizophrenia. *American Journal of Psychiatry, 155*(7), 914–920.

Crane, K., Kirby, B., & Kooperman, D. (1996). Patient compliance for psychotropic medications. *Journal of Psychosocial Nursing, 34*(1), 8–15.

Crenshaw, T. L., & Goldberg, J. (1996). *Sexual pharmacology*. New York: Norton.

Gurrera, R. J. (1999). Sympathoadrenal hyperactivity and the etiology of neuroleptic malignant syndrome. *American Journal of Psychiatry, 156*(2), 169–180.

Hasan, S., & Buckley, P. (1998). Novel antipsychotics and the neuroleptic malignant syndrome. *American Journal of Psychiatry, 155*(8), 1113–1116.

Henderson, D. C., Cagliero, E., Gray, C., Nasrallah, R. A., Hayden, D. C., Schoenfeld, D. A., et al. (2000). Clozapine, diabetes mellitus, weight gain, and lipid abnormalities. *American Journal of Psychiatry, 157*(6), 975–981.

Jeste, D. V., Laero, J., Palmer, B., Rockwell, E., Harris, J., Caligiuri, M. P., et al. (1999). Incidence of tardive dyskinesia in early stages of low-dose treatment with typical

neuroleptics in older patients. *American Journal of Psychiatry, 156*(2), 309–311.

Keltner, N. L. (2000). Mechanisms of antidepressant action. *Perspectives in Psychiatric Care, 36*(2), 69–71.

Kraus, T., Amsterdam, J. D., Quitkin, F. M., & Reimherr, F. W. (1999). Body weight and leptin plasma levels during treatment with antipsychotic drugs. *American Journal of Psychiatry, 156*(2), 312–314.

Lawson, W. B. (2000). Issues in pharmacotherapy for African Americans. In P. Ruiz (Ed.), *Ethnicity and psychopharmacology* (pp. 37–53). Washington, DC: American Psychiatric Press.

Leiblum, S. R., & Rosen, R. C. (2000). *Principles and practice of sex therapy* (3rd ed.). New York: Guilford Press.

Lin, K. M., & Smith, M. W. (2000). Psychopharmacotherapy in context of culture and ethnicity. In P. Ruiz (Ed.), *Ethnicity and psychopharmacology* (pp. 1–36). Washington, DC: American Psychiatric Press.

Margolis, S. (1998). *The Johns Hopkins complete home encyclopedia of drugs*. New York: Medletter Associates.

McCloskey, J. C., & Bulechek, G. M. (1996). *Nursing interventions classification (NIC)* (2nd ed.). St. Louis, MO: Mosby.

REFERENCES *(continued)*

Masters, J. C. (1996). When lithium does not help. *Geriatric Nursing, 17*(2), 75–78.

Mendoza, R., & Smith, M. W. (2000). The Hispanic response to psychotropic medications. In P. Ruiz (Ed.), *Ethnicity and psychopharmacology* (pp. 55–89). Washington, DC: American Psychiatric Press.

Nelson, J. C., Kennedy, J. S., Pollock, B. G., Thode, F., Narayan, M., Nobler, M. S., et al. (1999). Treatment of major depression with nortriptyline and paroxetine in patients with ischemic heart disease. *American Journal of Psychiatry, 156*(7), 1024–1028.

Nierenberg, A. A., Farabaugh, A. H., Alpert, J. E., Gordon, J., Worthington, J. J., Rosenbaum, J. F., et al. (2000). Timing of onset of antidepressant response with fluoxetine treatment. *American Journal of Psychiatry, 157*(9), 1423–1428.

Nyberg, S., Eriksson, B., Oxenstierna, G., Halldin, C., & Farde, L. (1999). Suggested minimal effective dose of risperidone based on PET-measured D2 and 5-HT 2A receptor occupancy in schizophrenic patients.

American Journal of Psychiatry, 156(6), 869–884.

Papolos, D., & Papolos, J. (1999). *The bipolar child*. New York: Broadway Books.

Pi, E. H., & Gray, G. E. (2000). Ethnopsychopharmacology for Asians. In P. Ruiz (Ed.), *Ethnicity and psychopharmacology* (pp. 91–113). Washington, DC: American Psychiatric Press.

Roach, S. S., & Scherer, J. C. (2000). *Clinical pharmacology* (6th ed.). Philadelphia: Lippincott.

Ruiz, P. (2000). Foreword. In P. Ruiz (Ed.), *Ethnicity and psychopharmacology* (pp. xv–xx). Washington, DC: American Psychiatric Press.

Sanger, T. M., Lieberman, J. A., Tohen, M., Grundy, S., Beasley, C., & Tollefson, G. D. (1999). Olanzapine versus haloperidol treatment in first-episode psychosis. *American Journal of Psychiatry, 156*(1), 79–87.

Stowe, Z. N., Cohen, L. S., Hostetter, A., Ritchie, J. C., Owens, M. J., & Nemeroff, C. B.

(2000). Paroxetine in human breast milk and nursing infants. *American Journal of Psychiatry, 157*(2), 185–189.

Trzepacz, P., Breitbart, W., Franklin, J., Levenson, J., & Martini, D. R. (1999). Practice guideline for the treatment of patients with delirium. *American Psychiatric Association Practice Guidelines, 156*(5), 1–20.

Tsai, G., Goff, D. C., Chang, R. W., Flood, J., Baer, L., & Coyle, J. T. (1998). Markers of glutamatergic neurotransmission and oxidative stress associated with tardive dyskinesia. *American Journal of Psychiatry, 155*(9), 1207–1212.

Turkoski, B. B., Lance, B. R., & Bonfiglio, M. F. (2000). *Drug information handbook for advanced practice nursing* (2nd ed.). Hudson, OH: Lexi-Comp.

Van Harten, P. N., Hoek, H. W., Matroos, G. E., Koeter, M., & Kahn, R. S. (1998). Intermittent neuroleptic treatment and risk for tardive dyskinesia. *American Journal of Psychiatry, 155*(4), 565–567.

PART THREE

Therapeutic Approaches

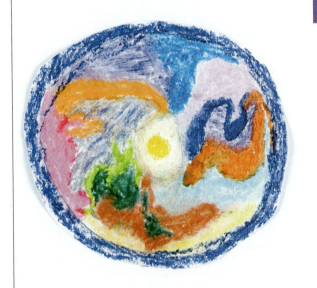

My mandala is all forced on my soul—the yellow-whitish burning fire of my life. The blue on the outside is my spirituality that I have all around in my life. Orange is for integrity, power, and strength. Brown is for earth and the colors of life with green. Gray is for confusion as I deal with that throughout my life. Pink is for love and happiness. Neon green is for humor that cures a broken soul. Purple is for comfort and manageability.

—Anthony, Age 17

CHAPTER 9

Cross-Diagnosis Behaviors

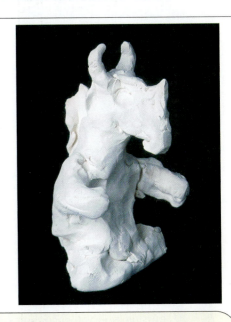

OBJECTIVES

After reading this chapter, you will be able to:

- IDENTIFY behaviors that are common to a number of mental disorders.
- DIFFERENTIATE the types of hallucinations.
- DISTINGUISH between the types of delusions.
- DESCRIBE the functions of self-mutilating behaviors.
- IDENTIFY signs of escalating aggression.
- INTERVENE with clients who are experiencing hallucinations, delusions, self-mutilating behavior, and aggression.

M y anger is like a dragon. I'm trying to find a way to control the dragon. I'm trying to find the triggers to my anger. If I don't, it will get out of control and I'll either end up in jail or dead.

—Terrance, Age 12

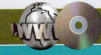

MediaLink

During your clinical rotation in mental health nursing, you will encounter certain common problems. These problems occur in a variety of settings, including inpatient units, residential care programs, outpatient settings, and the home. Not necessarily related to a specific disorder, these problems may be symptoms of a number of mental disorders. Since these problems are not limited to a specific disorder, they are referred to as **cross-diagnosis behaviors**.

Hallucinations and delusions often accompany **psychosis**, a state in which a person is unable to comprehend reality and has difficulty communicating and relating to others. Psychosis is a nonspecific indicator for severe mental illness and is usually characterized by hallucinations, delusions, and/or gross disorganization of thought or behavior. Hallucinations may trigger violent episodes if voices command the person to hurt himself or others. Delusions may lead to dangerous situations such as jumping from high places because of the belief that one can fly.

Violence against oneself, such as self-mutilation, and aggression against others are two problems needing immediate intervention. These behaviors are often impulsive. **Impulsivity** is the failure to resist an impulse or urge or to respond after a period of reflection. Impulsive behavior is related to low levels of serotonin (5-HT), hyperactivity of the limbic system, and/or inadequate control by the cortex. Any verbal or nonverbal force meant to harm or abuse another person is referred to as **aggression** (Krakowski, 2000).

CLIENTS EXPERIENCING HALLUCINATIONS

A **hallucination** is the occurrence of a sight, sound, touch, smell, or taste without any external stimulus to the sensory organs. The experience is real to the person. These perceptual changes are often an early symptom in mental disorders. **Illusions** are simply one or more of your five senses playing tricks on you. They are a sensory misperception of environmental stimuli. An example of an illusion is looking at a cord on the floor and thinking you are seeing a snake. A common illusion is seeing heat rising from highway pavement and believing there is a large pool of water on the pavement.

Although hallucinations are most commonly associated with schizophrenic disorders, only 70 percent of clients with schizophrenia experience them. Hallucinations also occur in the manic phase of bipolar disorder, severe depression, substance dependence, and substance withdrawal. Hallucinations represent a complex interaction between brain physiology, environmental stimuli, and the person's perception of the world. Studies have shown that 90 percent of people who experience hallucinations also experience delusions (Hoffman, Rapaport, Mazure, & Quinlan, 2000; Papolos & Papolos, 1999).

TYPES OF HALLUCINATIONS

Auditory hallucinations, which account for 70 percent of hallucinations, are thought to be caused by dysfunction in the language centers of the cerebral cortex, located in the temporal lobes of the brain. These sounds can fluctuate from a simple noise or voice to a voice talking about the client, to a voice talking about what the client is thinking, to complete conversations between two or more people. The majority of people say the hallucinations are distressing to them. The voices may make derogatory remarks and try to get them to do or say something that is potentially harmful to themselves or others (Hoffman & McClashan, 1997).

Visual hallucinations are thought to be caused by dysfunction in the occipital lobes of the brain. They can fluctuate from flashes of light or geometric figures to cartoon figures to elaborate and complex scenes or visions. Visual hallucinations are often accompanied by auditory hallucinations.

Gustatory and *olfactory hallucinations* typically consist of putrid, foul, and rancid tastes or smells of a repulsive nature. *Tactile hallucinations* involve the sense of touch. People may verbalize feeling electrical sensations coming from the ground or inanimate objects or feel like "they are being touched by others" when there is no one around. *Kinesthetic hallucinations* involve the feeling of body processes such as blood pulsing through the veins, food digesting, or urine forming. These types of hallucinations are typically associated with organic changes such as those that occur in a stroke, brain tumor, seizures, substance dependence, and substance withdrawal (Papolos & Papolos, 1999).

A *command hallucination* is a special type of auditory hallucination that is potentially dangerous. Occasionally, the command can be to do something useful, such as calling the doctor. More typically, the voice orders the person to do something that is frightening and may cause harm, such as cutting off a body part or striking out at someone. Fear from command hallucinations can also cause dangerous behavior, such as jumping out a window to escape a person who is trying to intervene.

ASSESSMENT

Hallucinations are as real to the person having them as your dreams are to you. They are symptoms that need to be assessed in the same manner as any other symptoms. Left unattended, hallucinations will continue and may escalate. Talking about one's hallucinations is a reassuring and self-validating experience. Such a discussion can take place only in an atmosphere of genuine interest and concern.

Ask yourself: How can I tell if my client is actually experiencing hallucinations? Behaviors often perceived as inappropriate may be a response to hallucinations. These behaviors include inappropriate laughter, conversations with an unseen person, difficulty paying attention to the task at hand, and a slow verbal response. In the case of severe hallucinations, the person may be unable to respond to anything in the external environment (see Table 9.1 ■).

Hallucinations serve as a useful indicator in the ongoing assessment of a client's level of functioning. It is important to identify hallucinations as a *symptom* of psychosis. They can interfere with activities of daily living (ADLs) to the point of complete withdrawal, depending on the level of intrusiveness. Assessment of the level of functioning provides direction for nursing interventions.

INTERVENTIONS

Intervening with clients experiencing hallucinations requires patience and the ability to spend time with them. Clients consistently report the following three interventions to be most helpful during the acute phase of hallucinations:

1. Having someone with them
2. Hearing a real person talk
3. Being able to see the person who is talking

Clients experiencing hallucinations have no voluntary control over the neurobiologic dysfunction that is causing the hallucinations. Hallucinations cannot be simply willed or talked away. It is crucial that you *stay with clients* during this intense and often frightening experience. Isolating clients during this time of sensory confusion often exacerbates the hallucinations. Remain nearby, because having a real person to talk and listen to will help them return to reality.

When you *talk to clients*, you may need to talk slightly louder than usual, but use very short and simple phrases. Maintain friendly eye contact, and use their preferred name. If the hallucinations are being caused by abnormalities in the temporal lobes, clients may not be able to hear you but will see that your mouth is moving and have a sense that you are real. Perceiving that someone real is talking and calling them by name validates that they are alive. Even if they may not be able to respond to you, they are aware of your presence.

Ask the client to describe what is happening. Talking about the hallucination gives the person permission not to continue to try and hide the experience. Look around the immediate area and *identify* any possible environmental *triggers*. Objects that are reflective or cause glare, such as television screens, photographs behind glass, and fluorescent lights, can contribute to visual hallucinations.

Encourage the client to *describe feelings* related to the hallucinations. If asked, simply point out that you

TABLE 9.1

Hallucinations and Client Behaviors

Sense	Observable Client Behaviors
Auditory	■ Moving eyes back and forth as if looking for someone ■ Listening intently to a person who is not speaking ■ Engaging in conversation with an invisible person ■ Grinning or laughter that seems inappropriate ■ Slowed verbal responses as if preoccupied
Visual	■ Suddenly appearing startled, frightened, or terrified by another person or object or by no apparent stimulus ■ Suddenly running into another room
Olfactory	■ Wrinkling nose as if smelling something horrible ■ Smelling parts of the body ■ Smelling the air while walking toward another person ■ Responding to an odor with terror
Gustatory	■ Spitting out food or beverage ■ Refusing to eat, drink, or take medications
Tactile	■ Slapping self as if putting out a fire ■ Trying to brush invisible things, like bugs, off the body ■ Jumping up and down on the floor as if avoiding pain or other stimuli to feet
Kinesthetic	■ Verbalizing and/or obsessing about body processes ■ Refusing to complete a task that may require a part of the body the client believes is not working

SOURCE: Adapted from Moller, M. D., Rice, M. J., & Murphy, M. F. (1998). *Psychiatric protocols for family nurse practitioners.* Philadelphia, PA: Saunders.

are not experiencing the hallucination. Do not argue about what is or is not occurring. The client is usually seeking validation and may be grateful to learn that you are not experiencing the same phenomenon.

Teaching clients self-management techniques will assist those who experience ongoing hallucinations to cope better. These strategies involve focusing, reducing anxiety, and distraction. Box 9.1 provides detailed information to include in the psychoeducation process.

BOX 9.1

Hallucinations and Self-Help Strategies

Self-Monitor
■ Keep a journal of when each hallucination occurred and what was happening at the time.
■ Develop a list of what makes a hallucination better or worse.

Read Aloud/Talk with Someone
■ Speaking may reduce the loudness, clarity, and duration of auditory hallucinations.
■ Reality orientation may reduce fear associated with hallucinations.

Increase Physiological Arousal Level
■ Walking or jogging may distract from hallucinations.
■ Doing housework or yard work may distract from hallucinations.

Decrease Physiological Arousal Level
■ Listening to music or a relaxation tape with headphones decreases anxiety and shifts attention away from hallucinations.
■ Wearing earplugs may decrease environmental triggers.

Talk Back to/Ignore the Voices
■ Responding to the voices may make them go away.
■ Saying "stop and go away" aloud is a thought-stopping technique to reduce auditory hallucinations.
■ Naming environmental objects aloud may block the auditory input of the voices.

Participate in Structured Activities
■ Hallucinations decrease in situations with more structure such as playing games, participating in groups, etc.

SOURCES: Biccheri, R., Trygstad, L., Kanas, N., & Dowling, G. (1997). Symptom management of auditory hallucinations in schizophrenia. *Journal of Psychosocial Nursing, 35*(12), 20–28; and Sayer, J., Ritter, S., & Gournay, K. (2000). Beliefs about voices and their effects on coping strategies. *Journal of Advanced Nursing, 31*(5), 1199–1205.

CLIENTS EXPERIENCING DELUSIONS

Delusions are false beliefs that cannot be changed by logical reasoning or evidence; they result from misunderstanding reality. These thoughts are so firmly fixed that providing evidence to the contrary does nothing to change the false belief. It is important to realize that a delusion does not always last. It may be fixed in the person's mind only for a few weeks or months or may fluctuate over time. Many clients have reported relief when they realized the belief was a delusion and not a reality.

Delusions can be a single thought, or they can pervade the person's entire cognitive process. When there is an extensively developed central delusional theme from which conclusions are deduced, the delusions are called *systematized*. Of people experiencing delusions, 90 percent have concurrent hallucinations.

Delusions are believed to be caused by dysfunction in the information-processing circuits within and between the brain's two hemispheres. Studies demonstrate a positive correlation between the degree of reality distortion and activity in the medial temporal and ventral limbic areas. Delusions occur in schizophrenia, delusional disorder, depression with psychotic features, bipolar disorder, anorexia, obsessive–compulsive disorder, body dysmorphic disorder, hypochondriasis, and dementia. As with hallucinations, the severity of delusions can be a valuable indicator in monitoring the course of a mental disorder (Blackwood et al., 2001).

TYPES OF DELUSIONS

There are a number of delusional types. *Grandiosity*, also known as *delusions of grandeur*, is an exaggerated sense of importance or self-worth. It is often accompanied by beliefs of magical thinking, when a person believes that thinking about a possible occurrence can make it happen. *Delusions of control* occur when the person believes that feelings, impulses, thoughts, or actions are not one's own but are being imposed by some external force. *Erotomanic delusions* are beliefs that a person, usually someone famous and of higher status, is in love with her/him. *Somatic delusions* occur when people believe something abnormal and dangerous is happening to their bodies. *Ideas of reference* are remarks or actions by someone else that in no way refer to the person but that are interpreted as related to her or him. *Thought broadcasting* occurs when people believe that others can hear their thoughts. *Thought withdrawal* is the belief that others are able to remove thoughts from one's mind. *Thought insertion* is the belief that others are able to put thoughts into one's mind (see Table 9.2 ■).

Religious delusions involve false beliefs with religious or spiritual themes. Religious ideas that may appear to be delusional in one culture may be commonly held in another. It is important that you be able to distinguish religious beliefs and experiences from delusional psychotic symptoms. Delusions in psychotic episodes:

- Are more intense than usual experiences in their religious community
- Are often terrifying for the person
- Involve obsessional preoccupation with the delusion
- Are associated with deterioration of self-care and social skills
- Often involve special messages from religious figures

Delusions of persecution involve beliefs that someone is trying to harm the person and are preoccupying, obtrusive, and distressing to them. The danger is that

TABLE 9.2

Types of Delusions

Delusion	Example
Grandiosity (delusions of grandeur)	"I've been a member of the President's cabinet since the Kennedy years. No president can do without me. If it weren't for me, we would probably be in World War IV by now."
Persecution	"The CIA and the FBI are both out to get me. I am constantly being followed. One of the other patients in here is really a CIA agent and is here to spy on me."
Control	"I have this wire in my head, and my family controls me with it. They make me wake up and make me go to sleep. They control everything I say. I can't do anything on my own."
Religious	"As long as I wear these 10 religious medals and keep all these pictures of Jesus pinned to my clothes, nothing bad can happen to me. No one can hurt me as long as I do this."
Erotomanic	"Julia Roberts is really my wife. We got married last week. She adores me and will be here soon to visit."
Sin and guilt	"I know I often hurt my parents' feelings when I was growing up. That's why I can't ever keep a job. When I get a job and start doing good, I have to quit it to make up for my bad behavior."
Somatic	"My esophagus is being torn apart. I have this rat in my stomach, and sometimes he comes all the way up to my throat. He's eating away at my esophagus. Look in my throat now—you can probably see the rat."
Ideas of reference	"People on TV last night told me I was in charge of saving the environment. That's why I'm telling everyone to stop using their cars. It's my job because that's what they told me last night."
Thought broadcasting	"I'm afraid to think anything. I know you can read my mind and know exactly what I'm thinking."
Thought withdrawal	"I can't tell you what I'm thinking. Somebody just stole my thoughts."
Thought insertion	"You think what I'm telling you is what I'm thinking, but it isn't. My father keeps putting all these thoughts in my head. They are not my thoughts."

clients will act on their delusional beliefs, harming others in an attempt to protect themselves. People with persecutory delusions are hypervigilant to threat-related stimuli. When things are going well for them, they are convinced it is their own doing. When things go badly, they are convinced that it is the fault of other people who are "out to get them." They are preoccupied with the intentions of others. It is hypothesized that excessive amygdala activity underlies persecutory delusions since the amygdala is important in the processing of threatening stimuli and the social meaning of that stimuli (Blackwood et al., 2001).

ASSESSMENT

Delusions are as real to the person having them as your thoughts are to you. They are symptoms that need to be assessed in the same manner as any other symptoms. Ask yourself: How can I tell if my client is experiencing delusions? Behaviors often perceived as inappropriate may be a response to delusional thoughts. The kinds of assessment questions appropriate for delusional clients are:

- What kinds of thoughts bother you the most?
- Do you feel that anyone is trying to harm you?
- Do you feel that anyone is controlling you?
- Do you believe that you are someone very important?
- Have you ever thought you have special powers that other people do not have?
- Do you think about religion a lot?
- Do you believe that you are very guilty for something you have done?
- Do you think anything abnormal is happening to your body?
- Do you think people are talking about you often?
- Do you believe others can hear your thoughts?
- Do you believe others can take away your thoughts?
- Do you believe others can put thoughts into your head?
- Do you have thoughts of harming yourself? Harming others?

Delusions serve as a useful indicator in the ongoing assessment of a client's level of functioning. It is impor-

tant to identify delusions as a symptom of psychosis. Assessment of the level of functioning provides direction for nursing interventions.

INTERVENTIONS

Delusions are often very frightening. *Providing an opportunity to discuss delusions* may lessen the fear. Provide comfort and *reassurance of safety.* After listening and reassuring, refocus the conversation to another topic to provide distraction from the troubling thoughts. If possible, help the client identify situations in which it is socially unacceptable to discuss delusions to prevent further public rejection and social isolation.

It is important that you *monitor delusions for content.* Identifying beliefs that may be self-harmful or harmful to others is necessary to protect the client and others from behaviors that may be harmful. Encourage clients to verbalize delusions to caregivers before impulsively acting on them.

If asked, simply point out that the *delusion is not your experience.* Always present reality, but do it gently, without implying that the client is wrong. Do not attempt to reason, argue, or challenge the delusion since that would put the client on the defensive. Do not attempt to logically explain the delusion. Only the client understands the logic behind the delusional content.

Identify triggers of the delusion. Focus on the underlying feelings since unexpressed feelings can trigger delusions. Once triggers have been identified, assist the client in problem solving ways to avoid or eliminate stressors that precipitate delusions.

Teach coping techniques that reinforce and focus on reality. Talk about real people and real events. Recreational and diversional activities that require attention and skill provide temporary relief from disturbing delusions.

CLIENTS WHO SELF-MUTILATE

Self-mutilation is the deliberate destruction of body tissue without conscious intent of suicide. Other terms used to describe self-mutilation include deliberate self-harm, self-injurious behavior, and aggression against the self. Understanding this behavior, recognizing the warning signs, and managing ongoing risk is an important challenge to mental health nurses.

Females are more likely than males to self-mutilate, usually beginning in adolescence. Self-mutilation affects people of all ethnic backgrounds in the United States. Every year as many as 2 million Americans deliberately cut, burn, or hurt themselves in other ways, which is 30 times the rate of suicide attempts (Strong, 1998).

Self-mutilative behavior may occur once or sporadically, or it may become repetitive. The behavior occurs in an estimated 24 to 40 percent of mental health clients. It is a symptom associated with childhood sexual and physical abuse, borderline personality disorder, eating disorders, cognitive impairment disorders, obsessive–compulsive disorder, posttraumatic stress disorder, dissociative identity disorder, and mental impairment. Self-mutilation may occur in response to delusions, command hallucinations, and substance abuse or dependence (Strong, 1998).

Juan goes to a specialized school for emotionally handicapped students. One of the ways he "copes" with stress is through self-mutilation. One morning at breakfast he got into a verbal confrontation with a peer that escalated into a pushing match. Juan threw his breakfast tray at the other boy, who then started hitting Juan. They were separated by staff and went to the classroom for school activities. The teacher noticed that Juan was exhibiting increasing signs of anxiety and could not concentrate on school work. Juan began to stare into space and started rubbing the inside of his eyelids with his finger, which progressed to using the sharp end of a pencil on his inner eyelids. The teacher sat down directly in front of Juan and talked to him in a low, calm voice. Within a short period of time, Juan was able to leave his dissociative state and stop his self-mutilative behavior.

FORMS OF SELF-MUTILATION

People who self-mutilate often use multiple methods of self-harm. The most common forms are *superficial* to *moderate* self-mutilation behaviors, including skin cutting, skin carving (words, designs, symbols), skin burning, severe skin scratching, needle sticking, self-hitting, tearing out hair, inserting dangerous objects into the vagina or rectum, ingesting sharp objects, bone breaking, and interfering with wound healing. Occasionally, *severe* acts of self-mutilation occur, such as eye enucleation, castration, and amputation of fingers, toes, or limbs. Psychosis is a major factor in severe self-mutilation often related to delusions and command hallucinations.

Stereotypic self-mutilation occurs in fixed patterns that are often rhythmic, such as head banging and finger biting. This behavior occurs most often in people who are institutionalized for mental impairment (Green, Knysz, & Tsuang, 2000). Box 9.2 describes the stages of self-mutilation.

BOX 9.2

Stages of Self-Mutilation

Stage 1: Precipitating Event
- This may include events such as the loss of a significant relationship or the perception or threat of an imminent loss.

Stage 2: Intensification of Feelings
- Unpleasant feelings such as anxiety, anger, helplessness, hopelessness, emptiness, and despair increase to high levels.

Stage 3: Attempts to Cope
- Client tries to delay the act of self-inflicted violence.

Stage 4: Action
- Client "gives in" to internal demand to self-mutilate.
- Acts of self-mutilation occur in private; unless medical attention is required, the behavior is often not discovered.

Stage 5: Aftermath
- Client may experience feelings of relief from tension or feelings of shame, guilt, or sense of failure.

SOURCES: Faye, P. (1995). Addictive characteristics of the behavior of self-mutilation. *Journal of Psychosocial Nursing, 33*(6), 36–39; and Strong, M. (1998). *A bright red scream: Self-mutilation and the language of pain.* New York: Viking.

Biological studies have found that the neurotransmitters dopamine (DA) and serotonin (5-HT) influence self-mutilative behavior. Both DA and 5-HT dysfunction are related to impulsive and aggressive behaviors. Dysphoria may be lessened as endorphins are released in response to the physical pain (Strong, 1998).

ASSESSMENT

Self-mutilating behavior is generally impulsive, and the onset is often linked to a stressful situation. As one client described her experience: "I thought I needed to be punished, that I was bad. I'd cut myself and get relief. I got relief from seeing my own blood; it was like my feelings were flowing out." Self-mutilation has great meaning, often hidden from others, for those who do it. One of the purposes of client assessment is to understand the unique meaning of the behavior for each client. Only when the meaning is understood can nursing interventions be designed. Some of the many possible meanings of or reasons for self-mutilation are:

- Ending a dissociative experience
- Reorienting from flashbacks
- Reenacting childhood trauma
- Reconnecting to a feeling of being real and alive
- Seeking distraction from emotional pain
- Feeling something other than despair
- Releasing tension or rage
- Punishing oneself
- Requesting nurturance
- Crying for help
- Feeling powerful and in control
- Manipulating others

INTERVENTIONS

It is very important to establish a *trusting relationship* with clients who self-mutilate. They have probably experienced much criticism and little understanding regarding their self-injurious behavior. Victims often have been told that they should just stop the behavior and have been scolded for not being competent enough. Under these conditions, the failure to stop the self-harm leads to even greater shame and concealment.

People who self-mutilate respond best to a *nonjudgmental* and accepting attitude, a caring approach, and the setting of limits to minimize the potential for phys-

ical injury. It is also understandable that staff members may react with frustration and even guilt when clients choose to harm themselves despite well-planned interventions and a caring approach (Loughrey, 1997).

There are three basic goals in helping clients manage their self-harmful behavior. The first goal is to *encourage communication* about self-injury, since clients are often secretive and shameful about the behavior. Supportive listening may help them communicate and thus feel less isolated. The second goal is to *improve the related quality of life*, such as through reducing their shame and isolation, decreasing their self-criticism, and ensuring that they receive adequate medical attention. Your ability to respond without blame or shame may help clients begin the process of self-healing. The third goal is to *diminish or extinguish the use of self-mutilation* as a coping tool. As clients grow in their understanding of their own experiences, they will improve their ability to manage, live with, or cease their behavior.

Box 9.3 describes appropriate nursing interventions when intervening with people who self-mutilate. Finding alternatives to self-harming behaviors is a critical step for people who wish to stop hurting themselves. Sometimes this means learning new skills in the areas of problem solving or relaxation and anxiety reduction. *Teaching* clients alternative coping skills is an appropriate intervention. Box 9.4 lists noninjurious alternatives clients may wish to consider.

CLIENTS WHO ARE AGGRESSIVE

Physical aggression and destruction of property are among the most severe and frightening client behaviors, occurring in treatment settings as well as in the home. Violence is often directed at family members, friends, and acquaintances and may result in physical injuries. When violence occurs in treatment settings, professionals and/or other clients are often the victims. Aggression affects every person in the environment in which it occurs. A violent client may be injured directly from the aggressive behavior or during a restraining procedure. Other clients and staff members may be purposefully or accidentally injured. Studies show that nurses are threatened, verbally abused, and physically assaulted at higher rates than other professionals. Out-of-control behavior frightens everyone,

BOX 9.3

Behavior Management: Self-Harm

Identify the Functions of the Behavior

■ In a nonjudgmental manner, ask "How does this help you?" or "What does this do for you?" This will increase clients' self-understanding and decrease feelings of shame.

Identify the Triggers

■ Have clients keep a journal describing the stressors preceding the behavior, situations in which the behavior occurs, and the effect on others.

Use Behavioral Contracts

■ Contracts focus on the fact that clients are responsible for their own behavior and they have to live with the consequences of their behavior.
■ Contracts include a clear understanding of treatment goals and mutual expectations of behavioral change.

SOURCES: McCloskey, J. C., & Bulechek, G. M. (1996). *Nursing interventions classification (NIC)* (2nd ed.). St. Louis, MO: Mosby; and Strong, M. (1998). *A bright red scream: Self-mutilation and the language of pain*. New York: Viking.

BOX 9.4

Alternatives to Self-Mutilation

Nonharmful Symbolic Enactments

■ Draw the "blood" or "cuts" on paper.
■ "Injure" a toy or stuffed animal.
■ Make marks with red marker or crayon on your skin.

Physical Awareness

■ Breathe slowly and mentally scan each part of the body.
■ Stroke your arm or leg, place ice on your skin, snap a rubber band on your wrist.

Distraction

■ Promise yourself to wait 5 to 10 minutes before self-injuring.
■ Read a book, watch a video, go to a movie.

Interpersonal Contact

■ Call a friend; talk about the impulse toward self-harm.
■ Call a support group member.

Physical Activity, Tension Reduction

■ Exercise, dance, play a physical game.

Art and Writing Activities

■ Draw the feeling or the memory.
■ Write about your feelings; write a letter to a significant person.

Expressive Anger Activities

■ Pound a tennis racket on a bed; pound pillows.
■ Break old dishes or glasses in safe ways; throw ice cubes; smash aluminum cans.

SOURCES: Loughrey, L. (1997). Patient self-mutilation: When nursing becomes a nightmare. *Journal of Psychosocial Nursing, 35*(4), 30–34; and Strong, M. (1998). *A bright red scream: Self-mutilation and the language of pain*. New York: Viking.

and violence disrupts the unit or home environment (Carlsson, Dahlberg, & Drew, 2000).

Aggressive behavior is a complex phenomenon that may occur in clients with schizophrenia, mood disorders, borderline personality disorder, conduct disorder, and substance use disorders. Aggression may be related to a lower level of activity in the frontal cortex and an underactive executive system. The end result is a lack of inhibition messages and an inability to moderate aggressive thoughts and behaviors. When an individual learns that acting on aggressive impulses brings a kind of relief, they can get "addicted" to aggression as a way to solve problems and relieve frustrations. This makes it very difficult for the person to control angry outbursts, even when they want to (Ratey, 2001; Stanley et al., 2000).

TRIGGERS TO AGGRESSION

Violence may be a consequence of poor frustration tolerance, ineffective individual coping, impulsivity, and real or imagined threats to the person's territory, body space, or life. In residential and day programs and inpatient settings, aggression and violence have been related to staff provocation. Violence occurs at a higher rate in settings where staff has an authoritarian or controlling approach to clients. Telling clients what they can or cannot do, detaining them against their will, and forcing them to take medication contribute to staff–client conflicts. When these actions are used with people who are used to controlling their environment through aggression and violence, one can predict an escalation of violent behavior.

Curtis, age 17, lives in a residential setting for severely emotionally handicapped adolescents. He was physically and emotionally abused as a child, and his family environment is very chaotic. He has a cyclical pattern of aggressive and passive behaviors. Curtis had talked to his mother by phone earlier in the day. At the time he was supposed to be in group therapy, he was in the kitchen with the staff. The staff told him to leave the kitchen and go to the group room. Curtis refused. As they repeated their directions, he began to posture aggressively, stare without blinking, and refused to move. More staff members were called to the kitchen to defuse the situation. One staff member took the lead and began talking to Curtis in a calm, nonthreatening manner, while the other staff members remained in the background. The staff member helped him identify his feelings of abandonment that resurfaced following the phone conversation with his mother. After a period of time, the intervention was successful and Curtis was able to join the group for the remainder of the therapy session.

It is believed that the increase in violence is related to increased substance abuse by people with mental disorders. Tardiff (1997) describes the relationship of violence to substance use:

- Direct effect of the substance on the brain—especially crack cocaine, which is associated with irritability, impulsiveness, and paranoid delusional thinking
- Exposure to a dangerous environment, such as drug dealing and crack houses
- Activities, such as robbery and prostitution, through which money is obtained for drugs

ASSESSMENT

Aggressive behavior can range from slaps, pushes, or shoves in play or in irritation to serious attempts to hurt another person. The threat of imminent violence is very frightening to staff, other clients, and indeed, to the aggressive person him- or herself. The best predictor of future violence in a client is a *history of violent behavior*. In assessing for the potential, keep in mind the following situations in which violence is more likely to occur:

- First one or two days after admission: Person may not be completely evaluated and treatment may not have begun
- Auditory hallucinations: Telling person to strike out
- Visual hallucinations: Protecting self from what is being seen
- Tactile hallucinations: Disengage self from what is being felt
- Delusions: May perceive violence as the only option; may believe they are fighting for their life
- Affective dysfunction: Motivated by fear, frustration, or rage
- Poor impulse control: In response to limit setting by caregivers
- Drugs or alcohol: Intoxication can contribute to aggressive behavior
- Secondary gains: Motivated by power and control
- Environmental cues: Violence may be reinforced through encouragement by peer group
- Poor impulse control: Overreact to intrusions or insults from other clients
- Alzheimer's disease: Aggression usually unplanned and reactive; often during ADLs
- General medical problems triggering aggression: Hypoglycemia, acute febrile illness, temporal lobe epilepsy, head trauma

It is important that you continually assess for ongoing signs of escalation of aggressive behavior. If you assess accurately and respond early and appropriately, you may be able to halt the progression of aggressive behavior (see Table 9.3 ■).

Warning signs of aggression include (Shea, 1998):

- Speaking more quickly with subtly angry tone of voice

TABLE 9.3

Phases of Aggression

Phase 1	**Triggering Phase**
Feeling	Anxiety
Behavior	Agitation, pacing, avoidance of contact
Nurse's response	Identify triggering factors, decrease anxiety, problem solve if possible
Phase 2	**Transition Phase**
Feeling	Anger
Behavior	Increased agitation
Nurse's response	Do not match anger with anger; keep talking; set limits and give directions; negotiate compromise; explore consequences; get help
Phase 3	**Crisis**
Feeling	Increased anger and aggression
Behavior	Agitation, threatening gestures, invasion of personal space; profanity; shouting
Nurse's response	Continue phase 2 interventions; increase personal space; warn (do not threaten) of consequences; try to maintain communication
Phase 4	**Destructive Behavior**
Feeling	Rage
Behavior	Assault; destruction
Nurse's response	Protect other clients; escape; physical restraint
Phase 5	**Descent Phase**
Feeling	Aggression
Behavior	Stopping of overtly destructive behavior; reduction in level of arousal
Nurse's response	Remain vigilant as new violent behavior is still possible; avoid retaliation or revenge
Phase 6	**Transition Phase**
Feeling	Anger
Behavior	Agitation, pacing
Nurse's response	Resume focus on problem solving

SOURCE: Adapted from Leadbetter, D., & Paterson, B. (1995). De-escalating aggressive behaviour. In B. Kidd & C. Stark (Eds.), *Management of violence and aggression in health care* (pp. 49–84). London: Gaskell.

- Sarcastic comments or challenges such as "You think you're a big shot, don't you!"
- Pacing, refusing to sit down
- Rapid and jerky gestures
- Lengthy, intense staring
- Threatening gestures such as vigorously pointing a finger at the nurse
- Clenching fists, raising of closed fist, pounding fist into opposite palm

INTERVENTIONS
Prevention

It is much better for all people involved to prevent out-of-control behavior than to manage it. In some instances, no matter what preventative actions are undertaken, aggression will erupt. The goal is to decrease the likelihood of this happening.

An effective intervention is to teach *nonviolent coping strategies*. This is done at a time when the client is not angry or tense. Assist the client in identifying the source of the anger or frustration. Following that, you can help identify the function that anger, frustration, and rage serve for the client. Teach the client to develop appropriate methods to express feelings such as assertiveness and "I" feeling statements. Together you can plan strategies to prevent inappropriate expression of anger. Some clients may find physical outlets helpful, such as vigorous exercise, lifting weights, strenuous cleaning or gardening, throwing light foam balls, or other nondestructive physical activities. Others may find time-outs help decrease feelings of hostility. You may also role play potentially frustrating situations at a time when the client is feeling calm and in control.

A *behavioral contract* is often a very effective way to prevent violence. It is one way to present the rules of the milieu and help the client become engaged in the treatment process. Understanding that there are consequences, perhaps legal consequences, to violent acts may help clients gain control of their impulses. The contract also enables clients to feel like they have some input into the treatment plan and thus responsibility for carrying out the plan (Bernay & Elverson, 2000).

Shortly after Curtis's violent episode, an intervention and contract was initiated. He had to reflect on and respond in writing to these topics:

1. Reflect on the facts of the situation.

2. Identify what he was feeling at the time.

3. List alternative behaviors that he could have chosen.

4. Identify consequences, such as loss of privileges, for skipping group therapy.

Interpersonal Skills

The way that you interact, as a nurse, may decrease or increase violent behavior. A *calm*, professional, confident *approach* often diffuses hostility. In an impending aggressive situation, it is important that you not lose sight of the client as a unique individual with unique needs and one who is deserving of respect. Acknowledging that you are trying to understand the situation helps individuals respond without violence. When people are treated with dignity, they often deescalate their aggression.

The cultural background of the client is also a consideration. Concepts of respect and disrespect vary, as do boundaries, personal space, and gender roles. You must understand these cultural variations so that you do not unwittingly behave in some way that would offend or threaten a client from a different culture (Bernay & Elverson, 2000).

Nonverbal Communication Skills

Your nonverbal behavior is very important when interacting with clients who are aggressive. Aggression is a two-person process. Your nonverbal behavior may inadvertently escalate an already agitated client. Approach the client in a *nonauthoritarian manner*. Stand in front at an angle, give enough interpersonal space, and do not attempt to touch the person. Maintain normal eye contact. Prolonged eye contact is perceived as aggressive and avoidance of eye contact implies fear or lack of interest. Avoid using threatening body language such as clenched fists, hands on hips, or arms crossed. If the client says "Get away from me!", move away in a slow manner that is respectful of the communication but not a sign of fear.

Verbal Communication Skills

The immediate goal is to gain some time and help the person regain self-control. At all times, be aware of how your verbal messages are delivered, that is, the tone, loudness, and pitch of your voice. Your voice should be normal, unhurried, and assertive. Do not speak in an authoritarian manner or make antagonistic remarks that would likely escalate the hostility. Use clear, appropriate language and short sentences in a nonthreatening manner. Do not overreact or talk too much. Paraphrase what you hear the client saying.

Telling people what they can do is more effective than stating what is not allowed. "Put the chair by the table" may work better than "Don't pick that chair up." Telling people what they cannot do may set up power struggles. Losing control can be equally as frightening to clients as to staff. Another approach is to give clients choices. "There are two quieter places you may go to: your room or the deck. Which one would you like?" Each time a choice is given, the person will pause and consider the option. Each pause decreases the amount of energy behind the anger. Giving choices also helps people to feel they have some control in the situation.

Talking down is another effective approach. For the time being, agree with what the client is saying. Avoid arguing so that you do not get stuck on the content of the client's communication. At this point, it does not matter if all nurses are uncaring, whether you should go jump in the lake, or who your ancestors are. None of that matters. What matters is that you deescalate the person by not arguing and not giving the person a reason to continue to be angry. Continue to speak in a soft voice and give the person choices.

Medications may be necessary to help people regain control of themselves. The use of medications to prevent psychosis and/or violent behavior is covered in Chapter 8. Geodon (ziprasidone) is a new atypical antipsychotic agent that can be given IM (intramuscularly) for the control and short-term management of clients who are acutely psychotic and agitated. It produces less sedation than other medications and the effect is within one hour. IM Haldol (haloperidol) is effective in controlling aggressive behavior usually within 30 minutes. IM Ativan (lorazepam) is frequently used for the immediate control of psychotic disruptive behavior. It may also be given at the same time as Haldol to decrease the side effects of akathisia and acute dystonias. Unfortunately, this means two injections since Ativan (lorazepam) cannot be mixed in the same syringe with any other medication (Crowner, 2000; Dorevitch, Katz, Zemishlany, Aizenberg, & Weizman, 1999).

Seclusion and Restraints

Some clients find it helpful to go to the "quiet room" when they feel they are going to lose control. This should be a room under close staff supervision where the person can be comfortable and away from other clients.

In rare instances, when medications and other interventions may not work rapidly enough to protect clients and staff, seclusion or restraints may be necessary. Familiarize yourself with the state laws regarding their use. Most clients experience restraint as traumatic, dehumanizing, or humiliating. Use of restraints requires physical force that increases the risk of injury to the client and staff. Use of physical force with clients reinforces their perception that violence is a valid method of gaining control. It also reinforces the client's self-image as a tough person and increases the likelihood of future violent confrontations. Unfortunately, these methods do not teach clients coping skills to help them avoid using aggression in the future. Because clients often view restraints as punishment, this method fosters distrust of, and malice toward, staff members (Oberleitner, 2000). (See Chapter 10 for further discussion on problems regarding the use of restraints.)

Critical Incident Review

After a serious assault, staff are angry and apprehensive, the aggressive client is humiliated, angry, and fearful, and other clients who witnessed the event are intimidated and terrified. After everyone's safety is assured, all staff participate in a critical incident review. The goal of this review is to understand what happened prior to the assault and during the assault. There is a discussion of measures that were taken to calm the client and ensure everyone's safety. Precipitants to the hostility are identified, as well as client behaviors that indicated escalating aggression. Any necessary revisions to the treatment plan will be made. The main questions are: "What did we do to deescalate the behavior?", "Was the person treated with respect?", and "How can we help this person learn nonviolent means of coping with stress?"

Cross-diagnosis behaviors occur in a variety of settings among clients with a variety of mental disorders. Recognition that these problematic behaviors are not limited to a specific diagnosis allows you to respond to the individual with the problem rather than be limited by the diagnostic category.

CRITICAL THINKING

You are a staff nurse working the day shift on an acute care psychiatric unit that has 20 beds. During morning report you learn that there have been three new admissions since yesterday. The unit has 18 clients at this time. Because a client's first day on the unit is an important one for assessment and treatment, you know that it is important to listen to the report on the new clients. You have been assigned to one of the clients, Mr. Rodriguez. The nurse giving the report discusses Mr. Rodriguez's first evening and night on the unit. He was admitted via the emergency room after being picked up by police in a restaurant. He became abusive to a waitress, threw dishes, and was not "making any sense" according to the police. He has a long history of mental illness and lives alone. In the last few days he has failed to show up for work at a warehouse. Admitting diagnosis is schizophrenia, paranoid type.

The second new patient is a 25-year-old woman, Ms. Wilson, who was admitted for an overdose of aspirin. Her physical condition is stable. This is her first known suicide attempt. During the evening she was pleasant with staff, and she was on suicide precaution to ensure her safety. She was cooperative.

The third admission was a 40-year-old man, Mr. Jackson, whose admitting diagnosis is bipolar disorder. On admission he seemed pleasant with staff and clients; however, at 10 P.M. he argued with another client in the lounge and then attempted to hit that client. Staff restrained Mr. Jackson and administered Geodon (ziprasidone) 80 mg IM at 10:15 P.M. He exhibited no additional escalation during the night. Presently, he is quietly eating breakfast.

As you consider your day, you know you will need to gather more assessment data on Mr. Rodriguez. You have also been assigned to work with Ms. Wilson during the time that her nurse will be off the unit at a required training session. The third new admission, Mr. Jackson, is not your assigned client; however, as a nurse on the unit you need to be aware of all of the clients in a therapeutic milieu.

1. Mr. Rodriguez has a history of auditory hallucinations. In your assessment, what are three possible causes of his escalation the night before?

2. What data might you need to support the possible causes of Mr. Rodriguez's recent behavior?

3. If you decide that Mr. Rodriguez is experiencing auditory hallucinations, what interventions might you use?

4. As you enter Ms. Wilson's room to introduce yourself and explain why her nurse will be off the unit most of the day, you notice that she has several small burn areas on her right forearm. These were not mentioned in her medical record; however, you remember that she was admitted from the emergency department at 1 A.M. Maybe these marks were noticed on her admission to the unit and recorded in the medical record as they should have been, but they were not mentioned in the report. When you ask her about the marks, she responds with "Oh, sometimes I accidentally burn myself with my cigarette." You say, "How does that happen?" She smiles at you and says, "Well, maybe it really isn't an accident." What does this data suggest to you? Based on what you know about this type of behavior, what is the relationship between the behavior and the client's feelings?

5. As you round the corner in the hallway, you hear Mr. Jackson arguing with another staff member about the requirement to attend a meeting. The staff member tells Mr. Jackson he has no choice. What concerns you about Mr. Jackson at this time, and why might triggers be something for you to consider as you approach the client and staff member?

6. Considering that you have two clients on the unit who have exhibited escalating behavior in the past 24 hours, either outside the hospital or on the unit, what are several interventions that you think would be important for the staff to consider at this time?

7. Why might the staff have administered Geodon (ziprasidone) to Mr. Wilson last night instead of Haldol (haloperidol) and Ativan (lorazepam)?

For an additional Case Study, please refer to the Companion Web site for this book.

CHAPTER REVIEW

COMMUNITY RESOURCES

A link to this Web site can be accessed on the Companion Web site for this book.

National Alliance for the Mentally Ill (NAMI)
200 N. Glebe Rd., Suite 1015
Arlington, VA 22203-3754
800-950-6264
www.nami.org

BOOKS FOR CLIENTS AND FAMILIES

McKay, M., & Rogers, P. (2000). *The anger control workbook.* Oakland, CA: New Harbinger.

Sutton, J. (1999). *Healing the hurt within: Understand and relieve the suffering behind self-destructive behavior.* Oxford: Pathways.

Williams, R., & Williams, V. (1993). *Anger kills: Seventeen strategies for controlling the hostility that can harm your health.* New York: HarperCollins.

KEY CONCEPTS

Introduction

- Common clinical problems, such as hallucinations, delusions, self-mutilating behavior, and aggression, are symptoms of a number of mental disorders, such as schizophrenia, mood disorders, substance use disorders, anorexia, obsessive–compulsive disorder, borderline personality disorder, conduct disorder, body dysmorphic disorder, hypochondriasis, and dementia, as well as strokes, head injuries, temporal lobe epilepsy, and hypoglycemia.

Clients Experiencing Hallucinations

- A hallucination is the occurrence of a sight, sound, touch, smell, or taste without any external stimulus to the corresponding sensory organ. The experience is real to the person.

- An illusion is a sensory misperception of a real environmental stimulus.

- Auditory hallucinations are caused by dysfunction in the language centers of the cerebral cortex, located in the temporal lobes.

- Visual hallucinations are caused by dysfunction in the occipital lobes.

- Gustatory, olfactory, tactile, and kinesthetic hallucinations are associated with organic changes such as those that occur in a stroke, a brain tumor, seizures, substance dependence, and substance withdrawal.

- A command hallucination is potentially dangerous because the voice may order the person to cause harm to self or others.

- Left unattended, hallucinations will continue and may escalate.

- Cues that a client is hallucinating include inappropriate laughter, conversations with an unseen person, difficulty paying attention to the task at hand, and a slow verbal response.

- If the hallucinations are severe, the person may be unable to respond to anything in the environment.

- Hallucinations can serve as an indicator in the course of a mental disorder.

- The levels of intensity of the hallucination correspond to levels of anxiety.

- Level I hallucinations are accompanied by moderate anxiety, and the hallucination is comforting. If the anxiety does not escalate, the hallucination is within conscious control.

■ Level II hallucinations are accompanied by severe anxiety, and the hallucination becomes condemning. There is less control over the experience, and the person may withdraw from others to avoid embarrassment.

■ Level III hallucinations are accompanied by severe anxiety, and the hallucination is controlling. The person gives in to the experience and may feel lonely if the hallucination stops.

■ Level IV hallucinations are accompanied by panic-level anxiety, and the hallucination is conquering. There may be command hallucinations with a potential for danger, and the person may be filled with terror.

■ Clients report that it is most helpful to have someone with them, to hear a real person talk, to see the person who is talking, and to be touched while they are experiencing hallucinations.

■ Self-help strategies include self-monitoring, reading aloud/talking with someone; increasing or decreasing physiological arousal level, talking back to or ignoring the voices, and participating in structured activities.

Clients Experiencing Delusions

■ Delusions are false beliefs that cannot be changed by logical reasoning or evidence. They may have a central theme and be systematized or may extend to many areas and be nonsystematized.

■ Types of delusions are grandeur; persecution; control; religious; erotomanic; somatic; ideas of reference; and thought broadcasting, withdrawal, and insertion.

■ Intervening with clients experiencing delusions includes providing the opportunity to discuss the delusions, monitoring for content, pointing out your different experience, identifying triggers, and teaching coping techniques.

Clients Who Self-Mutilate

■ Self-mutilation is the deliberate destruction of body tissue without conscious intent of suicide. It is a symptom that is associated with many mental disorders.

■ The most common forms of self-mutilation are superficial to moderate behaviors.

■ Dopamine (DA) and serotonin (5-HT) dysfunction and the release of endorphins may influence self-mutilative behavior.

■ Some of the many meanings of or reasons for self-mutilation are ending dissociation, reorienting from flashbacks, reenactment of childhood trauma, reconnecting to feeling real, seeking distraction from emotional pain, releasing tension or rage, punishing oneself, requesting nurturance, cry for help, feeling powerful, and manipulating others.

■ Stages of self-mutilation are precipitating event, intensification of feelings, attempts to cope, action, and aftermath.

■ Goals in helping clients manage their behavior are to encourage communication, improve the quality of life, and diminish or extinguish the use of self-mutilation.

■ Help clients identify the functions and the triggers to self-mutilate; develop behavioral contracts to help clients regain control.

■ Alternatives to self-harm include symbolic enactments, physical awareness, distraction, interpersonal contact, physical activity, art and writing activities, and expressive anger activities.

Clients Who Are Aggressive

■ The best predictor of future violence in a client is a history of violent behavior.

■ The increase in violence is related to increased substance abuse; factors include the direct effect of the drug on the brain, exposure to dangerous environments, and illegal activities to obtain drugs.

■ Violence occurs at higher rates in settings where staff has an authoritarian or controlling approach to clients.

■ Warning signs of aggression include speaking quickly in angry tone of voice, sarcastic comments or challenges, pacing, rapid and jerky gestures, intense staring, and threatening gestures.

■ Nursing interventions aimed at prevention of aggression include teaching nonviolent coping strategies such as assertiveness, physical outlets, and behavioral contracts.

■ When people are treated with dignity, they often deescalate their aggression.

■ Nursing interventions include giving the person enough personal space, maintaining normal eye contact, and avoiding threatening body language.

■ Telling clients what they can do, giving them choices, and talking them down are appropriate interventions for the client who is aggressive.

■ Zeldox (ziprasidone), Haldol (haloperidol), and/or Ativan (lorazepam) may be used to control aggressive behavior.

■ Seclusion and restraints may be used to manage an aggressive client, but these can lead to further injury and do not teach the client coping skills for avoiding aggression in the future.

■ The goal of a critical incident review is to understand what happened prior to the assault and during the assault.

EXPLORE *MediaLink*

■ Interactive resources, including animations, for this chapter can be found on the Companion Web site at *http://www.prenhall.com/fontaine*. Click on Chapter 9 and select the activities for this chapter.

■ For NCLEX review questions and an audio glossary, access the accompanying CD-ROM in this book.

REFERENCES

Bernay, L. J., & Elverson, D. J. (2000). Managing acutely violent inpatients. In M. L. Crowner (Ed.), *Understanding and treating violent psychiatric patients* (pp. 49–68). Washington, DC: American Psychiatric Press.

Blackwood, N. J., Howard, R. J., Bentall, R. P., & Murray, R. M., et al. (2001). Cognitive neuropsychiatric models of persecutory delusions. *American Journal of Psychiatry, 158*(4), 527–539.

Carlsson, G., Dahlberg, K̊., & Drew, N. (2000). Encountering violence and aggression in mental health nursing: A phenomenological study of tacit caring knowledge. *Issues in Mental Health Nursing, 21*(5), 533–545.

Crowner, M. L. (2000). A brief guide to the assessment and pharmacological treatment of violent adult psychiatric inpatients. In M. L. Crowner (Ed.), *Understanding and treating violent psychiatric patients* (pp. 3–19). Washington, DC: American Psychiatric Press.

Dorevitch, A., Katz, N., Zemishlany, Z., Aizenberg, D., & Weizman, A. (1999). Intramuscular flunitrazepam versus intramuscular haloperidol in the emergency treatment of aggressive psychotic behavior. *American Journal of Psychiatry, 156*(1), 142–144.

Green, C. A., Knysz, W., & Tsuang, M. T. (2000). A homeless person with bipolar disorder and a history of serious self-mutilation. *American Journal of Psychiatry, 157*(9), 1392–1397.

Hoffman, R. E., Rapaport, J., Mazure, C. M., & Guinlan, D. M. (2000). Selective speech perception alterations in schizophrenic patients reporting hallucinated "voices." *American Journal of Psychiatry, 156*(3), 393–399.

Hoffman, R. E., & McClashan, T. H. (1997). Synaptic elimination, neurodevelopment, and the mechanism of hallucinated "voices" in schizophrenia. *American Journal of Psychiatry, 154*(12), 1683–1689.

Krakowski, M. (2000). Impulse control: Integrative aspects. In M. L. Crowner (Ed.), *Understanding and treating violent psychiatric patients* (pp. 147–165). Washington, DC: American Psychiatric Press.

Loughrey, L. (1997). Patient self-mutilation: When nursing becomes a nightmare. *Journal of Psychosocial Nursing, 35*(4), 30–34.

Oberleitner, L. L. (2000). Aversiveness of traditional psychiatric patient restriction. *Archives of Psychiatric Nursing, 14*(2), 93–97.

Papolos, D., & Papolos, J. (1999). *The bipolar child.* New York: Broadway Books.

Ratey, J. J. (2001). *A user's guide to the brain.* New York: Pantheon Books.

Shea, S. C. (1998). *Psychiatric interviewing: The art of understanding.* Philadelphia: Saunders.

Stanley, B., Molcho, A., Stanley, M., Winchel, R., Gameroff, M. J., Parsons, B., et al. (2000). Association of aggressive behavior with altered serotonergic function in patients who are not suicidal. *American Journal of Psychiatry, 157*(4), 609–614.

Strong, M. (1998). A bright red scream: Self-multilation and the language of pain. New York: Viking.

Tardiff, K., Mohr, P., Saito, T., & Volauka, J. (1997). Violence by patients admitted to a private psychiatric hospital. *American Journal of Psychiatry, 154*(1), 88–93.

CHAPTER 10

Treatment Modalities

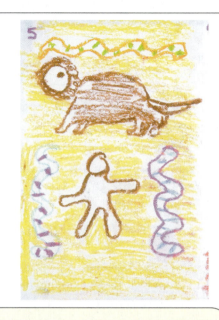

OBJECTIVES

After reading this chapter, you will be able to:

- DISCUSS consumer-sensitive health care goals and programs.

- DIFFERENTIATE the various professional roles in the mental health care setting.

- IDENTIFY the principles of milieu, individual therapy, crisis intervention, group, and family therapy in the clinical setting.

- PROVIDE basic care for clients receiving electroconvulsive therapy.

- OFFER social skills training and physical exercise for appropriate clients.

- PROVIDE psychoeducation for all clients.

- DESCRIBE the philosophy of self-help groups including 12-step programs.

- EXPLAIN how complementary/alternative therapies are used in mental health care.

*D*anger in the jungle

—Sandy, Age 32
Young mother who lost her child in a motor vehicle accident—she was driving.

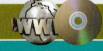

MediaLink

CD-ROM
- *Audio Glossary*
- *NCLEX Review*

Companion Web site www.prenhall.com/fontaine
- *Critical Thinking*
- *More NCLEX Review*
- *Case Study*
- *Care Map Activity*
- *Links to Resources*

MENTAL HEALTH CARE CONSUMERS

For decades, people with mental disorders were shut away in psychiatric institutions and effectively barred from demanding better treatment while their families were blamed and shamed into silence. That is now changing. People with mental disorders and their families are fighting for **civil rights protection** and more government services. According to the National Institute of Mental Health (*Mental Health*, 1999), one in three adult Americans meets the criteria for a mental disorder at some point during his or her lifetime. **Consumers**, those people who utilize mental health services, are children, adolescents, adults, and older adults, and they come from all segments of society. They need a wide variety of services: individual therapy,

crisis intervention, family therapy, group therapy, residential services, short-term or long-term inpatient services, rehabilitative services, partial-hospitalization programs, and home care programs (see Figure 10.1 ■). Such data can also be viewed on the NIMH Web site, which can be accessed through a resource link on the Companion Web site for this book.

Increasingly, psychiatric nurses are supporting *consumer-sensitive health care goals* and programs. Mental health care should be consumer-centered, based on and responsive to the needs of the consumers rather than of the mental health system or the needs of the professionals. Consumers have the right to the fullest possible control over their own lives and should be actively involved in treatment-planning decisions, including selecting the services and therapies they want and need, the setting of care, and who will provide the care. Consumers have the right to humane treatment; to personal privacy; to be free from excessive medication, physical restraint, and isolation; to exercise the right to refuse treatment; and to be free from retaliation. Box 10.1 provides a list of mental health care consumers' rights, as established by Congress.

You will meet mental health consumers in a variety of clinical settings—in emergency rooms, in the general hospital, in clinics, in homes, and in shelters. Even if psychiatric nursing is not your specialty, there are standards of care that all nurses are expected to provide. You must be able to relate to these clients in a therapeutic manner and foster a caring relationship.

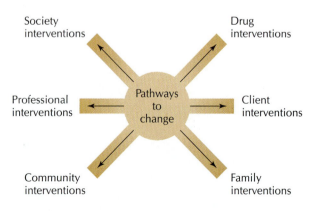

FIGURE 10.1 ■ Pathways to change.

Mental Health Care Consumers' Rights

1. Right to appropriate treatment supportive of a person's personal liberty.

2. Right to an individualized, written treatment plan and its appropriate periodic review and reassessment.

3. Right to ongoing participation in the treatment plan and a reasonable explanation of the plan.

4. Right not to receive treatment, except in an emergency situation.

5. Right not to participate in experimentation without informed, voluntary, written consent.

6. Right to freedom from restraint or seclusion.

7. Right to a humane treatment environment.

8. Right to confidentiality of records.

9. Right of access to one's mental health care records.

10. Right of access to telephone, mail, and visitors.

11. Right to be informed of these rights.

12. Right to assert grievances based on the infringement of these rights.

13. Right of access to a qualified advocate to protect these rights.

14. Right to exercise these rights without reprisal.

15. Right to referral to other mental health services on discharge.

SOURCE: Adapted from Mental Health Systems Act Report, 1980.

You must be able to provide basic mental health nursing care and collaborate with a variety of professionals.

A variety of treatment options are available to consumers. The choice may be dictated by the setting of care, as in milieu therapy, or by the people involved, as in family therapy. Consumers often participate in several therapies during the course of their mental disorder. This chapter describes the more common treatment modalities.

MENTAL HEALTH CARE PROFESSIONALS

Many different professional groups provide services to clients experiencing mental health problems. All professional groups are educated according to the philosophical and theoretical beliefs of their particular discipline, which gives them specific skills. In reality, the functions and responsibilities of the various professionals often overlap. Professionals from the various disciplines work together in what is referred to as the multidisciplinary team.

NURSES

"Psychiatric–mental health nursing is the diagnosis and treatment of human responses to actual or potential mental health problems. Psychiatric–mental health nursing is a specialized area of nursing practice, employing the wide range of explanatory theories of, and research on, human behavior as its science, and purposeful use of self as its art" (*Scope and Standards of Psychiatric–Mental Health Nursing Practice*, 2000, p. 10).

Working with individuals, families, groups, and communities, nurses gather assessment data for the purpose of diagnosing, planning, implementing, and evaluating nursing care. Because they spend more time with clients than any other staff members do, they often have the most information about a client's day-to-day level of functioning. With this knowledge base, nurses act as the liaison between other members of the multidisciplinary team.

Nursing also assumes responsibility for the physiological integrity of clients. Aside from psychiatrists, nurses are the only other members of the team who have the education and skill to perform physiological assessments. While other team members may not understand the significance of physical problems, nurses are expected to identify potential or actual problems and follow up with the appropriate action.

Client education about health is another area of expertise nurses bring to the psychiatric setting. Empowering clients with knowledge about their illness and prescribed treatments is very important.

Nurses assume a wide variety of roles within the mental health care system. Specific roles are determined by educational level and specialized preparation. Nurses with a bachelor's or associate degree, practice at the *basic level* as staff nurses, case managers, and nurse managers. Practice includes health promotion, intake screening and evaluation, case management, milieu therapy, promotion of self-care activities, psychobiological interventions, health teaching, counseling, crisis care, and psychiatric rehabilitation (*Scope and Standards of Psychiatric–Mental Health Nursing Practice*, 2000). (See Chapter 1 for additional information on the standards of care.)

Advanced practice registered nurses (APRNs) with a doctorate or master's degree in mental health nursing are found in all settings, from private practices, home health care, schools, community centers, and acute care hospitals to prisons. They focus on health promotion, illness prevention, education, and counseling. APRNs are well educated in individual and group therapy and may have taken advanced preparation in such other areas as family therapy, sex therapy, and/or substance abuse therapy. They also have prescriptive authority, provide consultation, and design and implement research activities. Since January 1998, APRNs are directly reimbursed for services provided to Medicare recipients at 85 percent of the physician rate. This provision allows more clients to receive quality primary care at a lower cost (Mohit, 2000; Sullivan-Marx & Maislin, 2000).

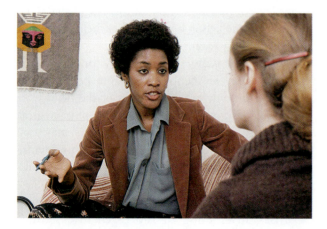

PHOTO 10.1 ■ Psychiatric–mental health nurses perform a wide variety of roles as staff nurse, educator, case manager, nurse manager, therapist, and researcher.

SOURCE: Michael Heron/Heron Photography.

PSYCHIATRISTS

Psychiatrists are physicians who have completed a residency program in psychiatry. They are able to admit clients to the inpatient setting and order the necessary diagnostic and laboratory tests. Psychiatrists are responsible for diagnosing mental disorders and prescribing medications and other somatic therapies. Some are well educated in psychotherapy, and others focus more heavily on the biochemical causes of mental illness. Subspecialties within psychiatry include psychiatrists who work with children and adolescents, those who work with older adults, and those who work with special types of problems such as eating disorders, substance abuse, and crisis situations.

PSYCHOLOGISTS

Psychologists practice in all areas of the mental health care system. People with a bachelor's degree in psychology are frequently hired as mental health technicians in inpatient and residential settings. Those with a master's degree in psychology are often employed in community mental health centers. Those with a doctorate in psychology (clinical psychologists) usually maintain a private practice or contract their services to an agency.

Most clinical psychologists are educated in psychotherapy and conduct individual, couple, family, and group sessions. One of the characteristics that distinguishes them from other professionals is their expertise in psychological testing. Psychologists administer and interpret all psychological tests that aid in the diagnosis and treatment of clients. Some common tests include the Minnesota Multiphasic Personality Inventory-2 (MMPI-2), Psychological Screening Inventory (PSI), Sentence Completion Test, Thematic Apperception Test (TAT), and the Rorschach test.

PSYCHIATRIC SOCIAL WORKERS

Psychiatric social workers have earned a master's degree in social work. They are found on inpatient units, in community mental health centers, and in private practice. Many states require the presence of a psychiatric social worker to perform social histories and arrange placement for clients. These trained professionals are the best informed about referral resources for clients. Many are educated in psychotherapy and provide individual, couple, family, and group sessions. People with a bachelor's degree in social work may be hired as mental health technicians for inpatients or as case managers for outpatients.

OCCUPATIONAL THERAPISTS

Occupational therapists have either a bachelor's or a master's degree in occupational therapy. Usually employed on inpatient units or in partial-hospitalization programs, they are responsible for providing activities that help clients increase their attention span, improve their motor skills, expand their socialization skills, and improve their ability to perform activities of daily living (ADLs). Through goal-directed activities, occupational therapists create situations in which clients can feel a sense of accomplishment.

RECREATIONAL THERAPISTS

Recreational therapists usually have a bachelor's degree. They are responsible for providing group diversional activities that allow clients to engage in appropriate social and physical functions on inpatient units or in partial-hospitalization programs.

SPECIALISTS

The mental health care system often includes therapists with specialized expertise. These specialists may be skilled in the use of dance, art, music, and play to help clients communicate their thoughts, feelings, and needs in creative ways. Pastoral counselors and healers from various cultural and religious groups are also part of the multidisciplinary team in many clinical settings.

COLLABORATION

Nurses collaborate with consumers and families of mental health care. **Collaboration** involves people who have mental illnesses, their family members, and professionals, all of whom are working together to improve quality of life and achieve the highest level of functioning. Nurses help clients acquire new knowledge and skills for basic living, learning, and working in the community and in developing new resources for success. Consumers must be treated with dignity and respect. They have the same needs, aspirations, rights, and responsibilities as other people. They have the right to access the opportunities and supports everyone needs as well as a variety of mental health services (Rogers, 1996).

The current challenge to all mental health care professionals is to learn how to collaborate with other professionals in order to ensure the best possible care for all clients. We must give up our "What's in it for me?" attitude. It is necessary to develop cooperative relationships based on trust, communication, and commitment to quality care. Building on each other's ideas and goals will help all of us develop new strategies for mental health care delivery.

MILIEU THERAPY

In its earliest conception, milieu was a word that described a scientifically planned community. Research efforts focused on defining the types of environments that would be most therapeutic for specifically diagnosed psychiatric clients. The work of Cummings and Cummings (1962) suggested that the environment (milieu) itself might be a strong force in bringing about changes in client behavior.

Kraft (1966) defined the idea of **milieu** more precisely as a therapeutic community in which the entire social structure of the unit or residence is designed to be part of the helping process. Kraft's idea of a therapeutic community emphasized the social and interpersonal interactions that become the therapeutic tools influencing change in client behavior. This view differed somewhat from the pure idea of milieu therapy, in which the emphasis was on "manipulation" of the environment to effect therapeutic change.

Hildegard Peplau (1952), the mother of psychiatric nursing theory, described the roles of the nurse in the therapeutic milieu. Peplau also described the *therapeutic use of self*, that is, using one's personhood to provide psychiatric nursing care. Within the nurse–client relationship, nurses use their personalities, beliefs, values, feelings, cognitions, and perceptions as they implement holistic nursing practice. (These roles are discussed in detail in Chapter 1.)

Milieu therapy has certain basic goals, whether the setting is a group home, a community center, a day program, or an inpatient unit. These goals include an emphasis on:

- Clients as responsible people
- Group and social interaction
- Clients' rights to choose and participate in a variety of treatments
- Informality of relationships with health care professionals

CHARACTERISTICS OF THE THERAPEUTIC MILIEU

Clear Communication

Communication between all people in the milieu is open, honest, and appropriate. Clients are encouraged to express their thoughts and feelings without retaliation, and staff members have a responsibility to hear what clients are saying without feeling threatened. Communication skills are role-modeled by staff members, helping clients learn the positive effects of therapeutic communication. Respect for the dignity of each person in the milieu is emphasized through the communication process.

Safe Environment

Policies, procedures, and rules of the residence, center, or unit are designed to ensure the safety of all members of the therapeutic milieu. All members of the community are informed of the rules. Structures and controls are provided for clients who are confused, anxious, suicidal, homicidal, or out of control to assure their safety as well as the safety of those around them.

Activity Schedule with Therapeutic Goals

In short-term acute care settings, clients will usually be at different levels of functioning. In most therapeutic communities, clients will be assigned to specific groups for activities. This assignment usually depends on the client's level of functioning at the time of admission and is changed as the client's level of functioning improves. Level of functioning can be determined by asking questions such as:

- Does the client have some insight into the illness? Little insight? No insight?
- How well does the client understand the goals of treatment? Well? Only slightly? Not at all?
- Is the client in contact with reality?
- How motivated is the client?

It is common to see high-functioning groups, moderate-functioning groups, and low-functioning groups in the same setting. Activities are then planned to meet the individual needs, interests, and skills of clients in that group.

Group activities are balanced to provide clients with different types of experiences. We all need balance between work, sleep, and play—a fact that is frequently overlooked in the psychiatric setting. Even a well-functioning person would have difficulty with six hours of intense therapy in one day. Therefore, the activity schedule is varied, with daily therapeutic community meetings, group therapy, ADL training, some type of physical activity such as sports or movement therapy, art therapy, play therapy, medication teaching and other educational groups, reality orientation groups, periods of rest and relaxation, time for one-to-one interactions, free time, and mealtime.

Support Network

Clients will begin to feel a sense of support from the therapeutic community or milieu. Through the process of group therapy and other support groups, clients begin to feel a sense of commonality with other clients. Clients often value treatment that helps them feel some control over crisis and a sense of social connectedness. One of the greatest benefits of the therapeutic community is that it is one of the few places where clients may feel safe, secure, and supported.

Because in many settings nurses spend more time with clients than do any other staff members, they often have the most influence on the effectiveness of the milieu. As a nurse, you can help establish the milieu as an open, confirming, and dignified place for people to be ill and to get well. Individuals who are psychiatrically disabled have problems relating to others. When clients have been conditioned to a life of loneliness and stigma, you may find it takes a great deal of time to establish the trusting relationship necessary for successful treatment. As nurses, we are healers, and through the milieu we create an atmosphere of nurturance and protection that removes the pressure to "cure" and allows the sometimes, slow process of healing to take place.

INDIVIDUAL PSYCHOTHERAPY

Individual psychotherapy is a reciprocal agreement between client and therapist to enter into a therapeutic relationship. It is performed by a variety of health care professionals such as advanced practice registered nurses, psychiatrists, psychologists, and psychiatric social workers. The goals of psychotherapy are to help clients:

- Clarify perceptions
- Identify feelings
- Make connections between thoughts, feelings, and events
- Gain insight

The process can also help clients develop better coping strategies such as problem solving, stress reduction, and crisis management. For some clients, it is an opportunity to feel supported in their struggle to overcome symptoms or interpersonal problems. Some individual therapies deal with specific issues, such as sex therapy or eating disorders. Certain therapies are short term, such as crisis intervention, and the goals are met relatively quickly. Others, such as psychoanalysis, are long term because they deal with deep-rooted anxieties or problems. There are many different models of individual psychotherapy—for example, cognitive therapy, intrapersonal therapy, humanistic therapy, and existential therapy—as well as models that combine several approaches.

As a student nurse, you will be doing individual counseling in your one-to-one relationships with clients. The details of the phases, goals, and process of this professional relationship are covered in Chapter 1.

CRISIS INTERVENTION

There are many definitions of crisis, most of which concur that a *crisis* is a turning point in a person's life—a point at which usual resources and coping skills are no longer effective. Two symbols in the Chinese language communicate the meaning of crisis: the symbol for *danger* and the symbol for *opportunity*. This text views crisis as both a danger and an opportunity.

Throughout life, people experience events to which they must respond. Many of these events are expected life changes that are anticipated at particular ages—changes such as graduation, employment, marriage, and parenthood. Depending on individual circumstances, these expected life changes may evoke crisis states referred to as *maturational crises*. Because of individual differences, not all people choose or have the opportunity to experience all the expected life changes. Unexpected life changes—such as divorce, serious illness, or death—may result in *situational crises*. It is only when the expected or unexpected event is per-

ceived subjectively as a threat to need fulfillment, safety, or a meaningful existence that the person enters a maturational or situational crisis state. The inability to maintain emotional equilibrium is an important feature of a crisis. This state of disequilibrium usually lasts four to six weeks. Typically, the high level of anxiety during this short period forces the individual to do one of the following:

- Adapt and return to the previous level of functioning
- Develop more constructive coping skills
- Decompensate to a lower level of functioning

It is during this time that people are most receptive to professional intervention. A thorough assessment of supports and previous coping behaviors includes an evaluation of the client's self-destructive feelings and behavior. If there is considerable threat to client safety, inpatient intervention may be necessary (see Table 10.1 ■).

The primary goal of **crisis intervention** is to assist the client to resolve the immediate problem and regain emotional equilibrium. The minimum goal of intervention is to help clients adapt and return to the precrisis level of functioning. The maximum goal is to help clients develop more constructive coping skills and move on to a higher level of functioning. Assisting the client in crisis resolution will, hopefully, lead to better use of coping mechanisms when dealing with future stressful life events.

Your role as a nurse in crisis intervention is one of active participation in solving the problem. It is important to point out that you do *not* take over and make decisions for clients unless they are suicidal or homicidal. The primary point of crisis intervention is self-help on the part of the client, with assistance from the nurse.

There are behavioral, affective, spiritual, cognitive, and psychosocial skills that people can draw on or learn so they can adapt to a crisis state. The relative importance of these skills varies with each person and each crisis. Most likely, they are used in various combinations, with the effectiveness of specific skills depending on the specific event.

Behavioral skills involve seeking information as the first step in the problem-solving process. As a nurse, you help the individual identify alternative ways of

TABLE 10.1

Crisis Assessment

Individual Assessment

1. What is the most significant stress/problem occurring in your life right now?

2. For whom is this a problem? You? Family members? Employer? Community?

3. How long has this been a problem?

4. Is this a temporary or permanent problem?

5. What does this problem mean to you?

6. What are the factors that cause this problem to continue?

7. Have you had similar stresses/problems in the past?

8. What other stresses do you have in your life?

9. How are you managing your usual life roles (partner, parent, homemaker, worker, student, etc.)?

10. In what way has your life changed as a result of this problem?

11. Are you feeling like you want to harm yourself or others?

12. Describe how you have managed problems in the past.

13. What have you done to try and solve the problem so far?

14. What happened when you tried this?

15. Describe possible resources (e.g., family, friends, employer, teacher, financial, spiritual).

16. What are your expectations and hopes concerning this problem?

17. What is the most you hope for when this problem is resolved?

18. What is the least you will settle for to resolve this problem?

19. What part of the overall problem is most important to deal with first?

Family Assessment

1. How do you perceive the current problem?

2. In what way has the problem affected your roles in the family?

3. How has your lifestyle changed since this problem began?

4. Describe communication within the family before this current problem.

5. Describe communication within the family since the problem began.

6. How does the family typically manage problems?

7. What has the family done to try and solve the problem so far?

8. What happened when you tried this?

9. How well do you believe the family is coping at this time?

TABLE 10.1

Crisis Assessment *(continued)*

Family Assessment (continued)

10. Describe possible resources (e.g., extended family, friends, financial).

11. What are your expectations and hopes concerning this problem?

12. Which part of the overall problem is most important to deal with first?

Community Assessment

1. What are the special demands of the client's community?

2. What are the living conditions of the neighborhood?

3. Are recreational centers available?

4. Are there affordable child care services available?

5. Is there a community mental health center?

6. What support groups are available in the community?

7. What are the possible funding resources?

resolving the crisis and predict probable consequences for each of the alternatives. The next step is choosing an alternative and taking concrete action. The final step is an evaluation of the consequences, and, if necessary, a return to finding solutions. (See Chapter 2 for more detail on the problem-solving process.) During the crisis state the client is more receptive to trying a variety of coping behaviors to decrease anxiety. You must remember to continually reinforce the client's strengths by reviewing the crisis event, the coping effectiveness, and new methods of problem solving that have been learned.

Beth has come to your mental health center seeking crisis intervention. Jill, her partner of five years, has abruptly left her saying that she (Jill) could not take Beth's passivity any more. For example, Jill told Beth that she never had a personal opinion about anything, never made an independent decision, and never voiced her preference for social activities. As you work through the problem-solving process with Beth, you want to keep in mind that assertiveness training might be an option for Beth to consider. If she does not list this as a possible new coping strategy, you may want to suggest it.

Affective skills focus on managing the feelings provoked by the event and maintaining a reasonable balance. Venting feelings by talking, crying, or even screaming allows for emotional discharge of anger, despair, and frustration. The ability to identify and discuss one's feelings is an adaptive skill. To be able to tolerate ambiguity and maintain some hope is very helpful during a crisis period.

Spiritual skills help the individual find meaning in and understand the personal significance of an unexpected event. Finding meaning is an ongoing issue during and after the crisis period. The result of the search is dependent on the individual's spirituality or philosophy of life. Some people may find this by living for causes beyond themselves. Others believe in divine purpose, in which they find a great source of consolation.

Cognitive skills help the individual in coping temporarily and in long-term resolution of the crisis. Denial may be temporarily effective. To prevent feeling overwhelmed, individuals may deny the unexpected event or its possible consequences. Another cognitive skill is the ability to redefine the unexpected event. In this instance, the person accepts the basic reality of the event but reshapes the situation into something favorable. For example, the individual might focus on the potential positive outcomes or compare herself or himself with those less fortunate. The goal of adaptive cognitive skills is to maintain a satisfactory self-image and a sense of competence and mastery.

Psychosocial skills enable a person in crisis to maintain relationships with family and friends throughout and after the crisis period. The person must be open to accepting the comfort and support offered by others. Family and friends may be sources of information that will enable the person to make wise decisions. Not to be overlooked are community resources such as hot lines, mental health centers, support groups, and self-help groups.

In addition to behavioral, affective, spiritual, cognitive, and psychosocial skills, there are other factors influencing the outcome of unexpected events. Demographic and personal factors influence how a person defines and resolves these crises. These factors include age, gender, ethnicity, economic resources, spiritual resources, and past experiences. Factors specific to the event also influence the outcome. Tasks and coping skills vary among biologic, psychologic, environmental,

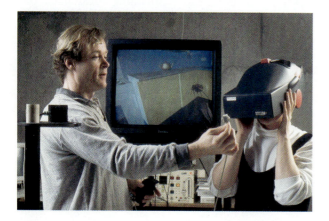

PHOTO 10.2 ■ Some cognitive behavior therapists are experimenting with using virtual reality for exposure therapy.

SOURCE: Mary Levin/University of Washington Photography.

and social crisis events. The more control a person has over these factors, the more adaptive she or he is likely to be. Successful resolution of crisis leads to growth and an increased ability to cope in the future. Failure to resolve the issues contributes to decreased adaptation and perhaps problems in the future.

GROUPS

There are many different kinds of groups with a variety of purposes. In your professional career, you most likely will have the opportunity to lead many different kinds of groups.

TASK GROUPS

Task groups are designed to carry out a particular type of task and are product oriented. It is called a task group because its purpose is very specific. This kind of group usually meets one or just a few times and ends when the task is completed. The emphasis is on problem solving and decision making. Staff meetings, case conferences, and planning sessions are examples of task groups. Consumer task groups might plan and prepare a community meal or draw up a list of responsibilities and privileges for the clinical setting. The nurse's role in the task group is to keep the group on task and to facilitate appropriate interaction.

PSYCHOEDUCATION GROUPS

Psychoeducation groups teach members about a specific topic. Often, nurses are asked to provide clients and families with information on various topics. The nurse provides information and then elicits reactions and comments from the members. Knowledge about the disorder and treatment helps family members provide for the needs of the client, develop their own coping strategies, and develop a collaborative relationship with professionals and other families.

Psychoeducation includes information about the etiology, treatment, and prognosis of the mental disorder. Clients and families are taught stressors associated with relapse, setting of realistic expectations, stress management, communication skills, and problem-solving skills. When families' educational needs are met, they have an increased ability to cope, understand, and deal with their loved one's illness. (See Chapter 2 for more information on psychoeducation.)

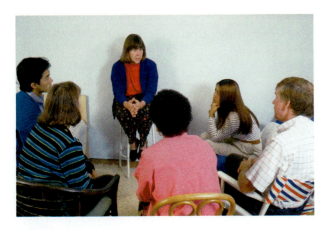

PHOTO 10.3 ■ Group therapy gives clients the opportunity to meet with and learn from other people who have similar problems.

SOURCE: Mary Kate Denny/PhotoEdit.

GROUP THERAPY

Therapeutic groups provide support to the members as they work through their problems. **Group therapy** is a beneficial experience in which the group members and group therapist help people with psychological, cognitive, behavioral, or spiritual dysfunctions through a process of change. Groups can be held in an inpatient unit, an outpatient clinic, a community mental health center, or a variety of other settings.

Yalom (1995) identified mechanisms of change within a group and called them *curative factors* of group therapy. These factors provide a rationale for a variety of group interventions (see Table 10.2 ■).

Yalom also identified two concepts basic to group therapy: the group as a social microcosm and the here-and-now quality. *Social microcosm* refers to the concept that group members eventually behave in the therapy group in the same way they behave with their families and friends. The group becomes a living example of how each member relates to others outside the group. The therapist's task is to help members recognize dysfunctional ways of relating to others. As group members interact with one another and discuss this process, individuals engage in self-reflection leading to affective, behavioral, cognitive, and spiritual changes. The *here-and-now* concept refers to the present moment of group experience. Although past and future have some importance, changes can be made only in the present

time. People who get stuck in the past ruminate over what was and what might have been. Others spend a great deal of time worrying about the future. The therapist's task is to keep the focus in the present time by discussing what happens and why it happens.

Nurses function as group therapists in many different settings, establishing the type of group that is appropriate for the desired outcomes. A single nurse leader may lead groups, or two co-therapists may share the leadership. Initially, the members are strangers, and the leader, as the unifying force, helps the members in their attempts to relate to one another. Some of the important tasks of the group leader include (Yalom, 1995):

- Encouraging members to remain in the group
- Helping the group develop a sense of cohesiveness
- Establishing a code of behavior and norms with the group

Throughout the therapeutic process, the nurse leader assumes two basic roles (Ballinger & Yalom, 1995):

1. *Technical expert.* Using a variety of nondirective or directive approaches, the leader moves the group in a desirable direction. The leader may give explicit directions for conduct or imply suggestions.

2. *Model-setting participant.* The leader shapes behavior by the example set in personal behavior within the group. The leader molds the group in a health-oriented direction by encouraging adaptive behavior. Through encouraging frank expression of feelings, the leader sets a model in which responsibility and restraint temper honesty with concern for others' feelings and defenses. By modeling the leader's responses, the group members work toward improving interpersonal skills.

Group therapy can be effective with both *children* and *adolescents*. In working with young children, the size of the group is usually limited to five. Age and attention span determine the length of the group session. Group therapy with children is usually activity oriented, for example, daily goal setting, art projects, music or movement therapy, and play therapy.

Because adolescents can reason and talk about their behavior, thoughts, and feelings, group therapy is a verbal process rather than the activity process used with children. Peers, as a source of support, feedback,

TABLE 10.2

Curative Factors of Group Therapy

Factor	Description
Instillation of hope	As clients observe other members farther along in the therapeutic process, they begin to feel a sense of hope for themselves.
Universality	Through interaction with other group members, clients realize they are not alone in their problems or pain.
Imparting of information	Teaching and suggestions usually come from the group leader but may also be generated by the group members.
Altruism	Through the group process, clients recognize that they have something to give to the other group members.
Corrective recapitulation of the primary family group	Many clients have a history of dysfunctional family relationships. The therapy group is often like a family, and clients can learn more functional patterns of communication, interaction, and behavior.
Development of socializing techniques	Development of social skills takes place in groups. Group members give feedback about maladaptive social behavior. Clients learn more appropriate ways of socializing with others.
Imitative behavior	Clients often model their behavior after the leader or other group members. This trial process enables them to discover what behaviors work well for them as individuals.
Interpersonal learning	Through the group process, clients learn the positive benefits of good interpersonal relationships. Emotional healing takes place through this process.
Existential factors	The group provides opportunities for clients to explore the meaning of their life and their place in the world.
Catharsis	Clients learn how to express their own feelings in a goal-directed way, speak openly about what is bothering them, and express strong feelings about other members in a responsible way.
Group cohesiveness	Cohesiveness occurs when members feel a sense of belonging.

SOURCE: Adapted from Ballinger, B., & Yalom, I. D. (1995). *The theory and practice of group psychotherapy* (4th ed.). New York: Basic Books.

and information, are very important in teenagers' lives. Group therapy with adolescents is often more productive than individual sessions.

There is often a parallel group for the *parents* of children and adolescents so that the entire family can receive treatment simultaneously. Such a group enables the parents to support each other, learn growth and developmental stages, gain an awareness of their contribution to family dynamics, increase parenting skills, and explore their own needs and problems.

SUPPORT GROUPS

As a nurse, you frequently refer clients and their families to support groups, which are very important for consumers of mental health care. In this type of group, members share thoughts and feelings and help one another examine issues and concerns. The characteristics of support groups include:

■ Clients define own needs.

■ Members have equal power.

- Groups may or may not be autonomous from mental health professionals.

- Attendance is totally voluntary.

- Groups may be responsive to a special population such as bilingual, eating disorders, domestic violence, or those defined by racial, gender, or sexual identity.

Support groups function to educate community members, to help family and friends support the individual, and to act as a crisis support, a source of referrals, and an advocate to help people get their needs met through the health care system. Because people who are psychiatrically disabled often have a very restricted social network or are even socially isolated, the interpersonal contact of support groups is vitally important. These groups contribute to an increased self-esteem, a sense of identity, increased dignity, and improved self-responsibility.

Online support groups are becoming more popular. Some support groups offer a variety of services such as chat rooms, reference materials, "ask an expert," and assessment services and referrals. Other online support groups limit their offerings to online support for people with similar concerns. The advantages of online support groups include 24-hour-a-day service from anywhere in the world; a high level of anonymity, which protects confidentiality; and a reasonable cost. While more women participate in face-to-face support groups, equal numbers of men and women participate in online support groups. A disadvantage for those who are socially isolated is the lack of face-to-face human interaction. Since nonverbal communication is extremely important in communicating with others, the lack of these cues makes the nuances of communication more difficult to understand. In addition, some vulnerable individuals may become addicted to online support groups (Finfgeld, 2000).

TWELVE-STEP PROGRAMS

In the United States, an estimated 3.5 million people attend 12-step programs annually. **Twelve-step programs** are fundamentally a spiritual plan for recovery. The first one, Alcoholics Anonymous (AA), originated in Akron, Ohio, in 1935, and the first edition of the "Big Book" was published in 1939 and continues today as the principle guideline for AA. Today, worldwide AA membership is estimated at 2 million scattered across 100 countries. Other 12-step programs emerged in the 1950s and 1960s, including Al-Anon, Narcotics Anonymous, Cocaine Anonymous, Adult Children of Alcoholics, Emotions Anonymous, Gamblers Anonymous, Overeaters Anonymous, and Sex Addicts Anonymous (Tonigan, Toscova, & Connors, 1999).

The 12-step program consists of prescribed beliefs, values, and behaviors. The sequential plan for recovery is stated in 12 steps, as described in Box 10.2. Step work is considered to be a lifelong process and is usually accomplished with the aid of a sponsor. Twelve-step fellowship includes the activities of the organization such as helping others, building relationships among members, and the sharing of joys and hardships (Tonigan et al., 1999).

The only requirement for membership is the sincere desire to change the target behavior. Any interested person can attend open meetings. Closed meetings are reserved only for the members. Some 12-step groups cater to demographic subsets such as women, men, adolescents, gays or lesbians, nurses, and so on. There are four common meeting formats:

1. *Open discussion.* Individuals are asked to share thoughts and feelings regarding a general topic introduced at the beginning of the meeting.

2. *Speaker meetings.* One to three members talk for the entire meeting, usually about what life was like before membership, what happened to facilitate membership, and what life is like now as the result of membership.

3. *Big Book or 12-by-12 meetings.* Often called step meetings, the primary focus is on the meaning and practice of the 12 steps.

4. *Birthday meetings.* Once a month members recognize specified periods of continuous abstinence. Thirty-, 60-, and 90-day intervals are recognized as well as 6-, 9-, and 12-month birthdays. Thereafter, birthdays are celebrated annually.

FAMILY THERAPY

Family therapy is a specialized area of study, and becoming a family therapist requires extensive preparation. In **family therapy**, the family system is treated as a unit, and the focus is on family dynamics. The goal is to help families cope, improve their communication and interpersonal skills, establish boundaries, and moderate family cohesion and flexibility. Families strive to maintain balance and harmony. When change

BOX 10.2

The 12 Steps of Alcoholics Anonymous

We

1. Admitted we were powerless over alcohol, that our lives had become unmanageable.

2. Came to believe that a Power greater than ourselves could restore us to sanity.

3. Made a decision to turn our will and our lives over to the care of God as we understood Him.

4. Made a searching and fearless moral inventory of ourselves.

5. Admitted to God, to ourselves, and to another human being the exact nature of our wrongs.

6. Were entirely ready to have God remove all these defects of character.

7. Humbly asked Him to remove our shortcomings.

8. Made a list of all persons we had harmed and became willing to make amends to them all.

9. Made direct amends to such people wherever possible, except when to do so would injure them or others.

10. Continued to take personal inventory and when we were wrong promptly admitted it.

11. Sought through prayer and meditation to improve our conscious contact with God as we understood Him, praying only for knowledge of His will for us and the power to carry that out.

12. Having had a spiritual awakening as the result of these steps, we tried to carry this message to alcoholics and to practice these principles in all our affairs.

SOURCE: The Twelve Steps are reprinted with permission of Alcoholics Anonymous World Services, Inc. (A.A.W.S.) Permission to reprint the Twelve Steps does not mean that A.A.W.S. has reviewed or approves the contents of this publication, or that A.A.W.S. necessarily agrees with the views expressed herein. A.A. is a program of recovery from alcoholism <u>only</u>—use of the Twelve Steps in connection with programs and activities which are patterned after A.A., but which address other problems, or in any other non-A.A. context, does not imply otherwise.

families that they invest their energies in maintaining the status quo. The result is that they seem more interested in enabling the illness of one of its members than in supporting changes that will improve health.

One of the problems with family therapy is that the Euro-American, middle-class, heterosexual family ideal has been used as the yardstick for determining "normal family function." This traditional stance has ignored families from other cultures, social classes, or family structures—all of whom may have very different values. Currently, family therapists are committing to not "pathologize" that which is different. Using multicultural theory, they take a more investigative approach and help family members define their own unique culture and values (Griffin & Greene, 1999).

Family therapy is recommended when the nurse or family determines that the family system is impaired because of the presence of a psychosocial problem or mental disorder in one or more family members. Schools, courts, or health care providers may identify impairment of family functioning. All family members must feel that they are part of the problem-solving and decision-making processes and that their personal welfare is always considered. Some advanced practice nurses are providing home-based family therapy. This allows the nurse–therapist to observe the family in the natural setting of the home. Comfort with one's own

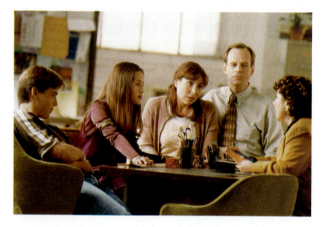

PHOTO 10.4 ■ Family therapy includes at least two or perhaps more or all family members in treatment. Family therapists strive to improve mental health by altering family relationships.

SOURCE: Bruce Ayres/Getty Images, Inc.

affects this balanced state, families must use their internal and external resources to adapt. Competent families seem to adapt more efficiently than dysfunctional families. Change is so frightening or alien to some

environment encourages family members' participation. In addition, the therapist becomes a guest; therefore a measure of control remains with the family. Direct observation illuminates family dynamics rather quickly and can effectively guide nursing interventions (Mohit, 2000).

Family therapy is often the preferred approach when a child or adolescent is the identified client. Family therapists help family members look at a number of issues. They assess the family hierarchy, which defines power relationships among the members. They identify subsystems—groups of people within the family who join together to perform various functions—such as the parental or sibling subsystem. Therapists identify and discuss boundaries, which define the degree of emotional closeness among family members and subsystems (Selekman, 2000).

The overall goals of family therapy are to:

- Develop better parenting and nurturing skills
- Reinstate generational boundaries in the family hierarchy
- Assist adults to become more involved with each other
- Decrease family reactions to symptoms to prevent inadvertent reinforcement of the problems

Although most nurses are not family therapists, this is not to say that nurses in the mental health care system will not intervene with families at all. It is very likely that nurses in both inpatient and outpatient settings will have a great deal of contact with the families of their clients. Family members are usually not in formal family therapy and have contact only with the nurse who assumes the responsibility of working with the family and client.

When nurses work with families informally, they assess for a number of factors, including:

- Relationships between individual members of the family
- Roles assumed by various members of the family
- Family communication patterns
- Achievement of the developmental tasks of the family
- Normal coping strategies used by the family
- Family support systems
- Sociocultural norms and values of the family

Disagreements and conflicts in family relationships are normal. The problem is not that people disagree, but that they do not know how to resolve their differences. Teaching families general principles for resolving conflict is a helpful nursing intervention. Box 10.3 lists eight steps to resolve family disagreements. See Chapter 3 for more in-depth information about families.

BEHAVIORAL THERAPY

Behavioral therapy is based on the principle that all behavior has specific consequences. Behavior is changed by conditioning—a process of reinforcement, punishment, and extinction. Consequences that lead to an increase in a particular behavior are referred to as *reinforcement*. Positive reinforcement is providing a reward for the desired behavior, such as an allowance for the completion of household responsibilities. Negative reinforcement is the removal of a negative stimulus to increase the chances that the desired behavior will occur. An example of negative reinforcement would be ignoring a child who holds his breath in the midst of a temper tantrum in an effort to frighten the parents. Consequences that lead to a decrease in undesirable behavior are referred to as *punishment*. Positive punishment is the addition of a negative consequence if the undesirable behavior occurs; for example, the child who does not complete her schoolwork gets a demerit and has to stay after school. Negative punishment is the removal of a positive reward if the undesirable behavior occurs; for example, the child who does not complete her schoolwork is unable to attend the next field trip with her class. *Extinction* refers to the progressive weakening of an undesirable behavior through repeated nonreinforcement of the behavior.

Most behavioral therapists believe that reinforcement procedures are more desirable than punishment procedures. There is no doubt that punishment is effective and is sometimes necessary when the behavior is dangerous. But behavior that is changed through reinforcement is a more desirable clinical outcome than behavior changed through punishment.

Behavioral therapy is not a set of techniques that are followed for every client. Rather, the plan is tailored to the person's assets, deficits, values, culture, and environmental resources. Clients are expected to be active par-

Eight Steps to Resolve Family Disagreements

1. **Stay calm.** When people are calm, they think much more clearly. Calmness is difficult to maintain when people call each other names, become sarcastic, or drag up past injustices. Do not try to solve problems when members are very angry.

2. **Express commitment to the relationship.** Arguments often leave people feeling like enemies rather than members of a caring family unit. It is important to defuse that by saying, "I love you. Let's work together to work this problem out."

3. **Identify areas of agreement or success.** Teach people to look for similarities in their viewpoint or find positive characteristics in the other person. Family members often get stuck on arguing about one small point and overlook that they agree on many other points.

4. **Identify the specific problem.** It is difficult to resolve problems when arguments keep escalating with the addition of more and more problems.

5. **Express the desired outcome.** Family members should clearly state what they want to happen so that everybody is clear about each other's goals.

6. **Listen carefully to the other person's concerns.** Each person needs to hear what the other is saying. If necessary, have them repeat the essence of what they heard to show that they understand. Problems cannot be solved if individuals are planning what they are going to say next, rather than listening carefully to what is being said to them.

7. **Seek solutions that benefit the relationship.** Teach family members to brainstorm possible solutions and how to look for ways to compromise and meet everyone's needs.

8. **Assess the outcome.** Teach family members to analyze the solution before it is implemented. Has everyone felt respected and heard? Is everyone at least partially satisfied with the solution? If so, the conflict has probably been resolved successfully.

ticipants, and therapists plan learning experiences designed to modify maladaptive behavior patterns.

Intervention focuses on changing those behaviors that have the most detrimental effect on the client. The nurse takes an active role in the process of helping clients identify learned behaviors that can be changed. There must be a plan, which is made clear to everyone working with the client, that identifies the goals of treatment and the behavioral consequences. Reinforcement is used to effect change, and if punishment procedures are necessary, clients are consistently assured that painful responses are reversible. As with many of the other therapies, nurses are in an ideal position to evaluate client response to treatment. Because they spend a great deal of time with clients, nurses can see developing patterns of behavioral change.

PLAY THERAPY

Play therapy is the purposeful use of play to provide information for assessment and subsequent interventions. Play therapy is especially helpful for children under 12 because their developmental level makes them less able to verbalize thoughts and feelings. You must establish objectives for the use of play, as well as consider the age and needs of the child. Play therapy may be a one-to-one session, or it may be used with a group of children. The limits, discussed prior to the session, are that children are not allowed to hurt themselves or others, and they must not destroy any property. Within those limits, children are allowed to express any feelings and act out any of their experiences.

A typical play therapy room is equipped with a variety of toys and objects, including dolls of various sizes, shapes, and colors; a doll house; puppets; stuffed animals; clay; a sandbox; a sink for water play; toy cars and trucks; toy airplanes; blocks; soft balls; punching toys; soft foam bats; and magic markers or crayons. As you observe and interact with the children, you learn about family dynamics, conflicts, and traumas, as well as positive experiences and people in their lives. Play therapy allows you to develop a sense of how each child perceives and experiences the world.

The overall goals of play therapy are to:

- Establish rapport with children
- Reveal the feelings that children are unable to verbalize

- Enable children to act out feelings of anxiety or tension in a constructive manner
- Understand children's relationships and interactions with significant others in their lives
- Teach children adaptive socialization skills

Sand play is often used with children. It is a nondirective form of play therapy in which the child is allowed to "play out" emotions and/or distressful situations in a sand box or sand tray. Being more directive, you can ask children to create a picture of anything they would like to and to put some toy animals or people in the scene. You then ask them to tell you about the picture, what is happening in the picture, how the people/animals feel, and what they would say if they could talk. You may wish to take a picture of the creation for future reference. Children need to be told that other children use the sand to express their feelings and so, when they return, they will have a fresh box to express themselves. Otherwise, they will expect you to keep their "scene" exactly as they left it.

ART THERAPY

Art therapy—the use of painting, drawing, sculpting, or other media—is a way for children and adults to express what is contained in the unconscious. You may ask them to draw or paint a picture themselves or tell you how to draw something. You may ask them to draw their family, draw themselves, draw feelings, draw what happened, draw a hero or an imaginary helper, or draw a nightmare. Art allows questions to be raised naturally. As clients are engaged in creative art, you should observe them. Are they timid? Worried about making mistakes? Bold? Haphazard? Anxious or relaxed? Is the style small and neat or messy and careless? Art therapy provides information on how people perceive themselves and others and how they interact with significant others in their lives.

BIOLOGICAL THERAPIES

ELECTROCONVULSIVE THERAPY

Electroconvulsive therapy (ECT) produces a deliberate, artificially induced grand mal seizure of the brain lasting about a minute. No one is sure exactly why ECT works and what the seizure does to the brain. It is thought that the treatment enhances dopamine (DA) sensitivity, reduces uptake of serotonin (5-HT), increases the amount of gamma-aminobutyric acid (GABA), and activates the systems in the brain that use norepinephrine (NE). ECT also increases slow-wave activity, reduces regional cerebral blood flow and glucose metabolism, and increases the blood–brain permeability. It is also thought to reduce brain activity in the prefrontal cortex (Nobler et al., 2001; Papolos & Papolos, 1999).

ECT may lead to shorter and less costly inpatient care. Even though it is a safe and effective treatment, the use of ECT varies widely and depends on geographic location, with some areas in the United States not using the treatment at all. In addition, socioeconomically disadvantaged clients do not have equal access to ECT. Groups associated with a decreased probability of receiving ECT include African Americans, Latinos, those who live in a poor area, those with Medicaid payment, and those who lack health insurance. ECT is rarely available in state and county hospitals (Olfson, Marcus, Sackeim, Thompson, & Pincus, 1998).

The most common indications for ECT are major depressive disorder and bipolar I disorder, depressed. It is indicated for clients in the following situations:

- Failure to respond to medications
- Severe symptoms, such as severe psychosis or dangerously suicidal or homicidal behaviors
- Adverse reactions to psychotropic medications
- Medical conditions, such as heart disease or glaucoma, that could be worsened by psychotropic medications
- Previous successful response to ECT
- Client preference

ECT is sometimes employed in the treatment of people with schizophrenia. It is primarily used in clients experiencing catatonia, those who have predominant affective symptoms, those who have had a previous successful response to ECT, and those who do not respond to medications. Because of concurrent medical conditions, poor tolerance of psychotropic medications, and marked disability with depression, ECT is often the treatment of choice in older clients.

Even the oldest clients tolerate ECT as well as younger clients. Several studies have shown that ECT is a safe and effective treatment for adolescents with catatonic or psychotic symptoms of depression. ECT is safe in all trimesters of pregnancy and may be less harmful to the fetus than psychotropic medications (Cohen et al., 2000; Tew et al., 1999).

ECT is usually given as a series of 6 to 12 treatments administered three times a week. Before a client is given ECT, a complete history is taken, along with physical and neurological exams. There are several contraindications for ECT: brain tumor, recent cerebrovascular accident (CVA), subdural hematoma, recent myocardial infarction (MI), congestive heart failure, angina pectoris, retinal detachment, acute or chronic respiratory disease, and current use of cocaine or heavy use of alcohol (Olfson et al., 1998).

The client should ingest nothing by mouth for at least eight hours prior to the treatment. Thirty minutes prior to the treatment, the client is given 1 mg atropine sulfate IM to control secretions and to prevent bradycardia, which sometimes occurs with ECT. A short-acting barbiturate is administered intravenously as a general anesthetic. Succinylcholine chloride (Anectine) is injected to induce muscle relaxation and prevent the full-body muscular response to the grand mal seizure. The client is preoxygenated with 95 to 100 percent oxygen before treatment, and oxygen is provided until the client awakens. Electrodes are placed on either one side of the temple or on both sides, through which a very small current of electricity is delivered. Side effects are more severe or persistent with the use of bilateral as opposed to right unilateral electrode placement. The client usually awakens 10 to 15 minutes after the procedure. Upon awakening, clients may experience a headache, some muscle aches, confusion, and disorientation, which usually disappear within an hour (Table 10.3 ■ describes nursing care for clients receiving ECT).

Memory is often affected by ECT—both memory of past events and newly learned information. Within six to nine months, the ability to learn new material returns to normal. Memory for past events also returns, except for the days prior to and during the course of ECT treatment (Bailine et al., 2000).

TRANSCRANIAL MAGNETIC STIMULATION

Transcranial magnetic stimulation (TMS) is a fairly new biological treatment. It is based on the principle of mutual induction, that is, that electrical energy can be converted into magnetic fields and magnetic fields can be converted into electrical energy. TMS is the use of a magnetic field that passes through the skull, which causes cells in the cerebral cortex to fire. TMS shows promise in improving mental disorders as a noninvasive tool and is being evaluated for treatment response in schizophrenia, depression, bipolar disorder, and obsessive–compulsive and other anxiety disorders (George & Belmaker, 2000).

The client sits in a lounge chair and a small but powerful, coiled electromagnet is placed on the scalp.

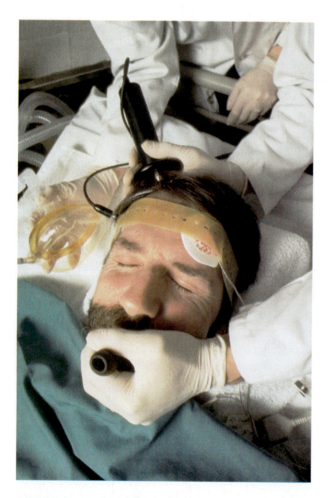

PHOTO 10.5 ■ A physician prepares a patient for unilateral electroconvulsive therapy (ECT).

SOURCE: W&D McIntyre/Photo Researchers, Inc.

TABLE 10.3

Nursing Care for Clients Receiving ECT

Nursing Diagnosis	Interventions
Knowledge deficit	Teach client and family about treatment and side effects. Allow client and family time to verbalize their understanding of the procedure. Document teaching.
Anxiety	Assure client that no pain will be experienced. Stay with client before and after treatment.
Altered thought processes	Reassure client that memory deficits and confusion are reversible. Reorient client as needed.

The client usually wears ear protection because of the noise of the machine. Forty stimulations are given in two seconds and this is repeated twenty times. As there is no pain or discomfort, no anesthesia is necessary. The most dangerous side effect is the induction of epileptic seizures. There are no other known lasting side effects in adults (George & Belmaker, 2000).

TMS is contraindicated in clients with increased intracranial pressure, brain tumors, recent CVAs, meningitis, encephalitis, severe head trauma, untreated epilepsy, and current use of cocaine or heavy alcohol use.

LIGHT THERAPY

Light therapy, or phototherapy, is often the treatment of choice for seasonal affective disorder (SAD), which appears to be directly related to the amount of light a person is exposed to. Light has an inhibiting effect on the production of melatonin, a hormone that affects mood, sensations of fatigue, and sleepiness.

Clients are exposed to very bright (10,000 lux) full-spectrum fluorescent lamps for 30 minutes for a minimum of five days. Light therapy is done in the home, and clients often read or watch TV during the painless treatment. It is thought that the bright light suppresses the production of melatonin and normalizes the disturbance in circadian rhythms. Light therapy may also be used prophylactically with clients susceptible to SAD (Kogan & Guilford, 1998).

Temporary eye or vision problems and headaches are experienced by about 20 percent of clients receiving light therapy. To prevent insomnia, the treatment is done in the morning or by 5:00 P.M. at the latest.

SLEEP DEPRIVATION

A biological treatment for depression is sleep deprivation. This may be total, for 36 hours, or partial, with the person being awakened after 1:30 A.M. and kept awake until the next evening. During this time, clients may be alone, in a group, or participating in activities. Some improve steadily after only one night of sleep deprivation. Others respond better if the deprivation is conducted once a week for several weeks. Merely advancing the sleep period to begin at 5:00 P.M. and end at 12:00 midnight for two to three weeks leads to an improvement of depression in 75 percent of clients (Berger, Small, Forsell, Winblad, & Backman, 1997).

SECLUSION AND RESTRAINT

Seclusion is the removal of a client from the general milieu into a single room, with or without a locked door. Restraint is physical restriction of movement; the most common form is to restrain arms and legs (four-point) or arms, legs, and waist (five-point) on a specially designed bed. The use of involuntary seclusion or mechanical or human restraints is justified only as an emergency safety measure to imminent danger to oneself or others and only after less restrictive methods have been deemed inadequate to prevent injury. Seclusion and restraints are not treatment interventions but security measures, and these are extreme measures that are very controversial in mental health care.

Tragically, seclusion and restraint are sometimes imposed for *staff convenience* to control individual behavior without having to use adequate staffing or clinical interventions. They may also be used for *coercion* to force a client to comply with the staff's wishes. And they have been used as *retaliation* to punish or penalize clients. None of these are legitimate reasons to impose seclusion or restraints.

Studies show that seclusion and restraint lead to feelings of fear, anger, anxiety, humiliation, depression, and helplessness. Clients perceive this as punishment, a form of torture, and of little therapeutic value. To some clients, these experiences are as devastating as physical abuse or rape. In these situations, nurses become perpetrators and are consequently feared by clients (Kennedy & Mohr, 2001).

In addition to negative feelings, clients in seclusion and restraints experience problems with sensory deprivation similar to prison inmates in solitary confinement. Problems include a hypersensitivity to external stimuli and hallucinations. A tragic consequence of restraints is accidental death from asphyxiation, strangulation, or cardiac arrest (Meehan, Vermeer, & Windsor, 2000; Mohr & Mohr, 2000).

Many states have strict guidelines for the use of seclusion and restraints, and many hospitals have instituted "no-seclusion" policies. The Health Care Financing Administration (HCFA), which finances and regulates Medicare and Medicaid, and the Joint Commission on Accreditation of Healthcare Organizations (JCAHO) have revised their standards regarding seclusion and restraint. The changes are geared toward staff education and changes in the milieu, with the goal of preventing the need for these aversive measures. Both agencies require that there be a high risk of harm to others, with seclusion and restraint being a last-resort, emergency measure (Kozub & Skidmore, 2001). Such data can also be viewed on the JCAHO Web site, which can be accessed through a resource link on the Companion Web site for this book. 🌐

Research shows that seclusion and restraints are related to milieu factors such as overcrowding, high noise level, staffing shortage, and an authoritarian attitude of the staff. Progressive institutions have made changes in the milieu to prevent or deescalate agitation and violence in clients. These changes include (Oberleitner, 2000):

■ High staff: client ratios

■ Less rigid rules and regulations

■ Decreased noise related to less overcrowding

■ Improved recreational activities and facilities

■ One-to-one care during a psychological crisis

■ Staff education regarding alternative interventions

■ Medications

■ Behavioral system to reward positive behavior

Chapter 6 covers triggers to aggression, assessment, prevention, and nonviolent interventions using interpersonal skills, nonverbal communication skills, and verbal communication skills.

PSYCHOSOCIAL NURSING INTERVENTIONS

SOCIAL SKILLS TRAINING

Individuals who are psychiatrically disabled often benefit from social skills training. Community treatment focuses primarily on the teaching of basic coping skills necessary to live as autonomously as possible in the community. Inadequate social and vocational skills may force clients to remain in institutional settings. Social skills training to overcome disabilities is repetitive and lengthy and is measured in months or years. Clients must also have opportunities and encouragement to practice the skills in real life and reinforcement for the use of the skills in community life.

Social skills training can be done in individual or group sessions. Clients have individualized behavioral goals to guide them as they empower themselves to adapt to community living. Steps in teaching social skills are:

1. Provide a rationale for learning the skill.
2. Break the skill into component steps.
3. Model the skill through role playing.
4. Review with clients what they observed in the role play.
5. Role play with clients to practice the skill.
6. Provide positive feedback about components that were performed well.
7. Provide corrective feedback on how the skill could be done better.
8. Help clients role play the skill with other clients.
9. Encourage clients to practice the skill at home/work.

Activities of Daily Living Skills

Activities of daily living (ADLs) skills include grooming and personal hygiene, room upkeep, laundry upkeep, cooking, shopping, eating at restaurants, budgeting, use of public transportation, and time management. Clients who are severely disabled benefit from being taught in their own setting. For instance, laundry upkeep is most effectively taught in the client's neighborhood laundromat; cooking, on his or her own stove; and room cleaning, in his or her own home. The inability to perform several of these basic ADLs for a length of time can create enormous frustration and stress, which may contribute to relapse.

Vocational Skills

Psychiatrically disabled clients may lack not only specific work skills, but also job-seeking abilities and good work habits. Being persistently unemployed contributes to feelings of inadequacy and low self-esteem. Clients may need support in locating positions, filling out applications, role-playing interviews, and learning job expectations and behaviors. Some community mental health centers provide job coaches if necessary; these coaches work alongside clients on the job until they can gradually be self-sufficient in the job.

Leisure Time Skills

Some clients lack either the interest or the necessary skills to fill their free time in a satisfying manner. When clients spend the majority of their free time in solitary television viewing, they are susceptible to increasing withdrawal, with accompanying loneliness and depression often leading to gradual decompensation. Clients are encouraged to find leisure and social activities that are enjoyable and involve interaction with others. Discover what are meaningful activities for each individual as well as their preferences for activities. Help them choose activities consistent with their physical, psychological, and social capabilities. Focus on skills they have rather than on deficits. Discuss with clients the scheduling of specific periods for leisure activity into their daily routine. As with ADLs, leisure-time activities should be carried out in the client's own neighborhood. Teach clients about available community resources for leisure activities (YMCA, YWCA, community center, local bowling alley, swimming pool, gym), support groups, and religious expression.

Interpersonal Skills

Without basic interpersonal skills, it is difficult to implement many of the activities just mentioned or to maintain a state of well-being. Clients need to learn how to interact appropriately with family members, friends, or strangers and at work and school. They must be able to identify and express their own feelings and respect and listen to those of others. Some will need assistance with *conversational skills* such as initiating conversations, asking questions, making appropriate self-disclosures, and ending conversations gracefully. *Assertiveness training* is appropriate for clients who are either passive or aggressive in their style of relating to others. Clients may need to learn *conflict resolution* skills, which involves learning compromise and negotiation skills so that conflicts with others can be worked out in a satisfactory manner. The most important process for clients to learn is how to *solve problems*. As they become increasingly skilled at problem solving, they will expand their social skills and enhance the quality of their lives. (See Chapter 2 for information on teaching problem solving.)

SELF-ESTEEM INTERVENTIONS

Self-esteem involves two components: the cognitive judgment of one's abilities or appearance and the emotional reaction to that judgment. People with high self-esteem have more positive evaluations of themselves, while those who have low self-esteem have more negative self-evaluation. Before the age of 6 or 7, young children are not able to accurately rate their own abilities. For example, young children will say they are very capable of doing almost any activity you can name. After age 6 or 7, children become more aware of their abilities and rate themselves in terms of academic performance, physical abilities, physical appearance, and social relationships. A person's self-esteem becomes fairly well established by middle childhood (Nida & Pierce, 2000).

Mental disorders often have a devastating effect on individuals' self-esteem. Negative social, educational, and vocational experiences influence how clients see themselves and their "problems." Carrying the burden of low self-esteem can hinder a sense of well-being and even contribute to relapse.

Clients improve their self-esteem when they feel good about themselves, know their good points, are satisfied with themselves, and forgive themselves. They also feel better about themselves when they take care of themselves, take calculated risks, accept failures, and learn from their mistakes. Box 10.4 lists ideas for discussion with clients who wish to improve their self-esteem. Additional nursing interventions regarding self-esteem issues are presented in Chapters 11 through 18.

REMINISCENCE THERAPY

Reminiscence is a guided recollection in which older clients are encouraged to remember the past and share their memories with family, peers, or staff. Reminiscence focuses on strengths and does not encourage people to dwell on losses. It can raise self-esteem and help people gain self-awareness and self-understanding, adapt to stress, and see their part in the larger historical and cultural context. Reminiscence therapy establishes group cohesiveness and increases social intimacy (Nussbaum, Pecchioni, Robinson, & Thompson, 2000).

BOX 10.4

Self-Esteem for All

1. Be patient, kind, and understanding with yourself.
2. Acknowledge your strengths.
3. Accept compliments.
4. Do not accept put-downs.
5. Set achievable realistic goals and work to accomplish them.
6. Visualize change. Imagine the person you want to become six months from now.
7. Take time to be pleased when you achieve something good. Reward yourself for your successes.
8. Don't blame yourself out of all proportion if something doesn't go the way you had planned.
9. Take up a new hobby or interest, join a new group, or try volunteering.
10. Counteract negative thoughts with positive thoughts.
11. Think of yourself as a lovable and capable person.

When conducting reminiscence therapy, choose a comfortable setting and set aside adequate time. Encourage verbal expression of feelings of past events. Comment on the feelings that accompany the memories in an empathic manner. Use direct questions to refocus back to life events if clients digress. Encourage clients to write about past events such as traditional values, wisdom, and lessons learned (McCloskey & Bulechek, 1996).

By encouraging older adults to tell you about their lives, you can learn about where they have been and where they would like to go. In listening, you will learn about hope, grief, achievement, and loss. It is a way that you can communicate caring while helping them maintain their sense of identity.

PHYSICAL EXERCISE

People who are psychiatrically disabled tend to have high rates of physical illness, poor general fitness, poor cardiovascular fitness, obesity, and low energy. Often, their main activities are sedentary, such as TV, listening to music, or reading. The physical benefits of exercise are well known in regard to heart disease, diabetes, colon cancer, sleep, and bone density. Exercise increases the number and density of blood vessels in the motor cortex and cerebellum. Exercise that involves learning complex movements, such as dance, basketball, or T'ai Chi, strengthens the neural networks in our brain (Ratey, 2001).

There have been a few studies on the psychological benefits of exercise. These studies show that there is less depression and anxiety, and better self-esteem when both the well and client population engage in exercise. Exercise also appears to have a positive effect on self-concept, mastery, self-sufficiency, body image, cognitive processing, and attention to the here-and-now (Ratey, 2001).

In the United States, 65 percent of 10- to 17-year-olds participate in exercise. That number drastically drops to only 15 percent of 18- to 64-year-olds. That means that the vast majority of our clients would benefit from an exercise program. Some nurses become more active with their clients by walking with clients during the one-to-one session. Other nurses and clients spend 30 minutes of the 90-minute group therapy time walking or running together (Hays, 1999).

Clients should have a health clearance before beginning an exercise program. You must also assess the

CRITICAL THINKING

You are having your rotation at the local community mental health center. Your instructor explains that this center offers a variety of services to members of the community. It provides emergency psychiatric services and has an ambulatory care crisis intervention service for clients in crisis. The ambulatory care center also offers short treatment services and social rehabilitation to clients with long-term problems. There are two acute care units where clients remain for short periods of time. One focuses on psychiatric clients and the other on substance abuse problems. During your rotation you will have the opportunity to have experience in several of the community mental health center's service areas.

1. Your first assignment is in the acute care psychiatric unit. You are told that electroconvulsive therapy (ECT) is done on the unit. As you observe one of the nurses in a meeting with family members of a 65-year-old woman, the family asks the nurse to explain how ECT works. What would you tell the family?

2. The unit has a therapeutic milieu. In your last class you discussed mental health consumers and consumer-sensitive health care goals. What is the relationship between therapeutic milieu with consumers and consumer-sensitive health care goals?

3. Your next assignment is with one of the nurses who covers the emergency services. She explains that some days are slower than others and that some of the clients are referred to the crisis intervention service. A 50-year-old woman comes into the emer-

gency services crying, unable to sleep for the past 2 days. The client says that her husband has left her and her three children. She is referred to crisis intervention. How does the primary goal of crisis intervention relate to the woman's crisis and the assessment?

4. You sit in on a team meeting in the ambulatory care service. The topic is the assignment of clients to the groups that are offered by the service. The service offers a group to learn how to do simple household budgeting, a group on stress management, and an evening 12-step group for recovering alcoholics, as well as several groups for therapy. The staff is focusing on the first three groups. What factors and criteria might you hear the team discuss as they consider what clients are appropriate for these groups?

5. The team also discusses the need to develop several new modalities. Two are discussed: interpersonal relationship skills and self-esteem development. How are these related?

6. When you were on the acute care unit, you heard staff discussing the increase in the number of incidents in which seclusion and restraints were used. You listen to them and remember that you saw one of these incidents. What is your personal opinion of the use of seclusion and restraints?

For an additional Case Study, please refer to the Companion Web site for this book.

---

client's readiness for exercise. It may be difficult for people suffering from depression to summon the energy to exercise. They often say, "I'll exercise when I feel better." An appropriate response on your part would be, "You'll feel better when you exercise." Often, people are more consistent if they have an exercise partner, perhaps a friend or family member.

Clients who are on psychotropic medications should begin with a low intensity of exercise. Side effects such as muscle rigidity, dehydration, muscle weakness, fatigue, and impaired coordination should be considered when designing the program. Help clients monitor short- and long-term benefits with regard to mood, energy, well-being, and weight control. If clients are to maintain an exercise program, the

activity must be enjoyable and there must be positive reinforcement.

COMPLEMENTARY/ ALTERNATIVE THERAPIES

Complementary/alternative therapies is an umbrella term for hundreds of therapies drawn from all over the world. Many forms have been handed down over thousands of years, both orally and as written records. These are based on the medical systems of ancient peoples, including Egyptians, Chinese, Asian Indians, Greeks, and Native Peoples. Others, such as osteopathy and chiropractic, evolved in the United States over

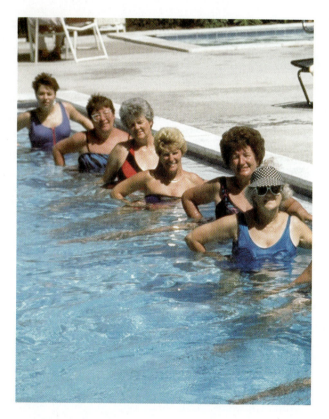

PHOTO 10.6 ■ People who exercise experience less depression and anxiety. Exercise also has a positive effect on self-concept, mastery, self-sufficiency, body image, and cognitive processing.

SOURCE: Dennis MacDonald/PhotoEdit.

the past two centuries. Still others, such as some of the mind–body and bioelectromagnetic approaches, are on the frontier of scientific knowledge and understanding.

As nursing begins the twenty-first century, it is advancing beyond the Western biomedical model to incorporate many healing tools used by our Asian, Latino, Native People, African, and European ancestors. We are rapidly rediscovering that these ancient principles and practices have significant therapeutic value. Consumers do not wish to abandon conventional medicine, but they do want to have a range of options available to them, including herbs, nutrition, manual healing methods, mind–body techniques, and spiritual approaches. Some healing practices, such as exercise, nutrition, meditation, and massage promote

health, manage stress, and prevent disease. Others, such as herbs or homeopathic remedies, address specific illnesses. Many other healing practices do both.

Studies show that more than one third of Americans use alternative treatments in a given year. Among people with mental disorders, the use is even more common. Forty-three percent of individuals with anxiety attacks and 41 percent of adults with severe depression utilize alternative therapies. Most of them also continue to use conventional health care (Kessler, Walters, & Forthofer, 2001; Unutzer, 2000).

Ethnocentrism, the assumption that one's own cultural or ethnic group is superior to others, has often prevented Western health care practitioners from learning "new" ways to promote health and prevent chronic illness. With consumer demand for a broader range of options, we must open our minds to the idea that other cultures and countries have valid ways of preventing and curing disease that could be good for Western societies. Although the information may be new to us, many of these traditions are hundreds or even thousands of years old and have long been part of the medical mainstream in other cultures.

Nursing is in a unique position to take a leadership role in integrating alternative healing methods into Western health care systems. We have historically used our hands, heart, and head in more natural and traditional healing interactions. As nurses, by virtue of our education and relationships with clients, we can help consumers assert their right to choose their own healing journey and the quality of their life and death experiences (Fontaine, 2000).

This section of the chapter provides an extremely brief definition of the more common forms of alternative therapies. In Chapters 11 through 18 you will find more information on alternative therapies for the specific mental disorders. If you wish to explore alternative practices in more depth, from a nursing perspective, I encourage you to use my text, *Healing Practices: Alternative Therapies for Nursing.*

ACUPUNCTURE

Acupuncture, acupressure, Jin Shin Jyutsu, Jin Shin Do, and reflexology are different forms of the same practice of stimulating points on the body to balance the body's life energy. Frequently, these practices are part of a holistic approach to wellness and are combined with diet, herbs, mind–body techniques, and spiritual therapies.

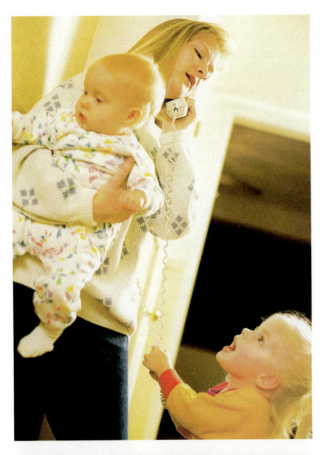

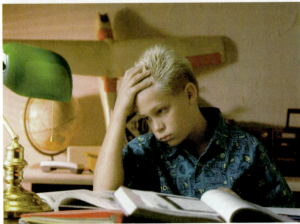

PHOTO 10.7 ■ Stress is a part of everyday life. Stress cannot be avoided, but some ways of coping with life's challenges are more effective than others.

SOURCE: Chris Lowe/Index Stock Imagery, Inc.; Superstock, Inc.

When the flow of energy becomes blocked or congested, people experience discomfort or pain on a physical level, may feel frustrated or irritable on an emotional level, and may experience a sense of vulnerability or lack of purpose in life on a spiritual level. The goal of care is to recognize and manage the disruption before illness or disease occurs. Pressure point practitioners bring balance to the body's energies, which promotes optimal health and well-being, and facilitates people's own healing capacity.

ANIMAL-ASSISTED THERAPY

Animal-assisted therapy is the use of specifically selected animals as a treatment modality in health and human service settings. Accredited professionals guide the human–animal interaction toward specific, individualized therapeutic goals. A variety of goals can be addressed: cognitive goals such as improved memory or verbal expression; emotional goals such as increased self-esteem and motivation; social goals such as building rapport and improved socialization skills; and physical goals such as balance and mobility.

For many people, interacting with a pet is less stressful than interacting with other people. In comparison to people, animals are nonjudgmental and accepting. This unconditional support system can be accessed at any time of day or night when one lives with a pet. Loneliness, lack of companionship, and lack of social support are major risk factors for depression and suicide that can be offset by the presence of a loved pet. Animals also facilitate socializing within the neighborhood by getting owners out of the house and providing a topic of conversation. Even sitting and looking at fish in an aquarium relaxes and relieves anxiety for many people. Children with short attention spans are able to sustain attention longer when interacting with animals (Hart, 2000).

AROMATHERAPY

Aromatherapy is the therapeutic use of essential oils in which the odor or fragrance plays an important part. It is an offshoot of herbal medicine, with the basis of action the same as that of modern pharmacology. The chemicals found in the essential oils are absorbed into the body, resulting in physiological or psychological benefit. Essential oils are extracted from plants and are massaged into the skin, inhaled, placed in baths, used as compresses, or mixed into ointments. Different oils may calm, stimulate, improve sleep, change eating habits, or boost the immune system. Some oils cause the brain to release enkephalins that decrease the perception of pain and increase the sense of well-being (Ratey, 2001). Oils you will find used in the mental health field include:

- *Anxiety*: Basil, bergamot, chamomile, green apple, lemon balm, neroli, and orange
- *Depression*: Bergamot, geranium, jasmine, lemon balm, rose, and ylang ylang
- *Insomnia*: Chamomile, clary sage, lavender, marjoram, neroli, and vetiver
- *Memory/mental function*: Basil, ginger, rosemary, thyme
- *Alertness*: Peppermint

Essential oils are quite potent and can irritate the skin, so they should be diluted with a carrier oil before being used on the skin. Carrier oils contain vitamins, proteins, and minerals that provide added nutrients to the body. Carrier oils include apricot kernel oil, sunflower oil, soy oil, sweet almond oil, grapeseed oil, sesame oil, avocado oil, jojoba, and wheat-germ oil.

AYURVEDA

The Indian system of medicine, Ayurveda, is at least 2,500 years old. Illness is viewed as a state of imbalance among the body's systems. Ayurveda emphasizes the interdependence of the health of the individual and the quality of societal life. Mentally healthy people have good memory, comprehension, intelligence, and reasoning ability. Emotionally healthy people experience evenly balanced emotional states and a sense of well-being or happiness. Physically healthy people have abundant energy with proper functioning of the senses, digestion, and elimination. From a spiritual perspective, healthy people have a sense of aliveness and richness if life, are developing in the direction of their full potential, and are in good relationships with themselves, other people, and the larger cosmos.

Nutritional counseling, massage, natural medicines, meditations, yoga, and other modalities are used to treat many disorders. This ancient system has adapted to modern science and technology, including biomedical science and quantum physics.

TRADITIONAL CHINESE MEDICINE

Traditional Chinese Medicine (TCM) has developed over 3,000 years and seeks to balance the flow of qi,

the energy or life force of a person. In TCM the mind, body, spirit, and emotions are never separated. Thus, the heart is not just a blood pump; it also influences one's capacity for joy, one's sense of purpose in life, and one's connectedness with others. The kidneys filtrate fluids, but they also manage one's capacity for fear, one's will and motivation, and one's faith in life. The lungs breathe in air and breathe out waste products, but they also regulate one's capacity to grieve, as well as one's acknowledgment of self and others. The liver cleanses the body, and it also influences one's feeling of anger as well as that of vision and creativity. The stomach has a part in digestion of food and influences one's ability to be thoughtful, kind, and nurturing as well. These are just a few of the mind–body connections that TCM practitioners recognize.

Practitioners are trained to use a variety of ancient and modern therapeutic methods, including acupuncture, herbal medicine, massage, heat therapy, Qigong, T'ai Chi, and nutritional and lifestyle counseling.

CHIROPRACTIC

Chiropractic is the third largest independent health profession in the Western world after conventional medicine and dentistry. It is based on the premise that the spine is literally the backbone of human health. Misalignments of the vertebrae or loss of mobility in the facet joints caused by poor posture or trauma result in pressure on the spinal cord, which may lead to diminished function and illness. Three primary clinical goals guide chiropractic intervention: reduce or eliminate pain; correct the spinal dysfunction; and preventative maintenance to assure the problem does not recur.

CURANDERISMO

Curanderismo is a cultural healing tradition found in Latin America and among many Latinos in the United States. Although it is a traditional healing system, it utilizes Western biomedical beliefs, treatments, and practices. Three levels of care are practiced among curanderos and curanderas: the material level, the spiritual level, and the mental level. Healers have the gift for working at only one of these levels. Healers working at the mental level have the ability to transmit, channel, and focus mental vibrations in a way that directly affects a person's mental or physical condition. When working with mental conditions, they send vibration into the person's mind to manipulate energies and modify behavior.

HERBAL MEDICINE

Herbal medicine is used by 80 percent of the world's population. Even though only a tiny fraction of plants have been studied for medicinal benefits, plant-derived products are used regularly by conventional health care providers. Twenty-five percent of all prescription drugs sold in the United States are derived from plants. Because herbs are marketed as "natural" or promoted as foods, consumers may assume incorrectly that herbs are safe and without side effects. It is important that you remember that natural remedies be approached with respect and that you teach people that though herbs are generally much safer than prescription drugs, if abused or overused they can cause harm. Herbs you will find used in the mental health field include:

- *Anxiety*: Chamomile and kava kava
- *Depression*: St. John's Wort and SAMe
- *Mood swings*: Ginseng
- *Insomnia*: Catnip, hops, lemon balm, melatonin passion flower, or valerian
- *Memory*: Ginkgo
- *Alcohol or drug withdrawal*: Chamomile, evening primrose oil, ginseng, and valerian

Herbs are drugs and you need to treat them with respect. The vast majority of herbal medicines present no danger. Some can, however, cause serious side effects if taken in excess or, for some, if taken over a prolonged period of time. Herbs can also interact with drugs and caution should be used when combining herbs with prescription and over-the-counter (OTC) medications. For example, St. John's Wort should not be combined with antidepressants as their effects may increase. St. John's Wort reduces the effectiveness of birth control pills, HIV treatment medications, and the asthma medication theophylline. Kava kava should not be mixed with antianxiety medication and some anithypertensives. It is important that people investigate herb–drug interactions before using herbs as an alternative therapy.

HOMEOPATHY

Practitioners use infinitesimal doses of natural substances, called remedies. If taken in large amounts, these natural compounds will produce symptoms of the disease. In the doses used by homeopaths; however, these remedies stimulate a person's self-healing capacity. Homeopaths also believe that it is necessary to have adequate nutrition, exercise, rest, good hygiene, and a healthy environment to adapt and maintain homeostasis. In other words, health is the ability of people to adapt their equilibrium in response to internal and external change. Remedies you will find used in the mental health field include pulsatilla (windflower) for insomnia and for people who are highly emotional, weepy, impressionable, easily influenced, fearful of abandonment, and worried about what others think of them; and ignatia (St. Ignatius bean) and arsenicum album (arsenic) for anxiety.

HYPNOTHERAPY AND GUIDED IMAGERY

Hypnosis and guided imagery are states of attentive and focused concentration during which people are highly responsive to suggestion. Therapists help people learn methods to take advantage of the mind–body–spirit connection through the medium of relaxation and imagination. Hypnosis and imagery cannot make people do anything against their will. These therapies can be used to help people gain self-control, improve self-esteem, and become more autonomous. People who are imprisoned by negative beliefs see themselves as hopeless, helpless victims. With hypnosis or guided imagery, they can learn how to substitute positive, empowering messages. These procedures are unsuitable for people with active psychosis or somatic delusions. It is generally considered that these individuals are often bombarded with too many images already and are unable to differentiate between voluntary and involuntary images.

KINESIOLOGY/APPLIED KINESIOLOGY

Applied kinesiology is both a diagnostic method and a treatment modality using energy, lymphatic, neurovascular, and muscle systems. Well-being and health are determined by the nature of the flow of energy within and without the body. Disease and pain occur when energy is blocked, fixed, or unbalanced. When someone's thoughts and emotions are out of alignment with the energy necessary to meet a life challenge, an energy imbalance results. It is believed that people are responsible for their own health and that they can take simple steps to improve and maintain their level of wellness.

MASSAGE THERAPY

Massage therapy, the scientific manipulation of the soft tissues of the body, is a healing art, an act of physical caring, and a way of communicating without words. The goal of massage therapy is to achieve or increase health and well-being and to help people heal themselves. On the mental level, massage therapy induces a relaxed state of alertness; reduces mental stress, thus clearing the mind; and increases one's capacity for clearer thinking. On the emotional level, massage therapy satisfies the need for caring and nurturing touch, increases feelings of well-being, decreases mild depression, enhances self-image, reduces levels of anxiety, and increases awareness of the mind–body connection.

Massage has been used with psychiatrically disabled individuals as an adjunct to conventional psychiatric interventions. Clients are given an executive massage, done with the client fully dressed and seated on a massage chair. The head, neck, back, arms, and legs are massaged for 10 to 20 minutes per session. Hilliard's study (1995) found that massage was an effective stress reducer for inpatient and outpatient clients who sought safe touch and relaxation resulting in a sense of emotional well-being. Massage is also effective in decreasing agitation in persons with Alzheimer's disease (Ratey, 2001).

MEDITATION

Meditation is a general term for a wide range of practices that involve relaxing the body and easing the mind. Meditation is a process that anyone can use to calm down, cope with stress, and, for those with spiritual inclinations, feel as one with God or the universe. Meditation can be practiced individually or in groups and is easy to learn. It requires no change in belief system and is compatible with most religious practices. People who meditate say that they have clearer minds and sharper thoughts. The brain seems to clear itself so that new ideas and beliefs become available. This clearer mind may be accompanied by a cognitive restructuring in which people interpret life events in a more positive, more realistic fashion. Meditation's residual effects—improved stress-coping abilities—are a protection against daily stress and anxiety.

NATIVE AMERICAN HEALING

Spirituality and medicine are inseparable in Native American tradition. Medicine women and men see themselves as channels through which the Great Power helps others achieve well-being in mind, body, and spirit. The only healer is the One who created all things. Medicine people consider that they have certain knowledge to put things together to help the sick person heal and that knowledge has to be dispensed in a certain way, often through ritual or ceremony. The healer enters into the healing relationship with love and compassion. The two individuals experience a joining or merging as this process unfolds. This merger symbolizes the cementing together of people and the Divine Spirit.

Health is viewed as a balance or harmony of mind and body. The goal is to be in harmony with all things, which means first being in harmony with oneself. It is believed that most illness begins in the head and people must get rid of ideas that predispose illness. If the mind is negative, the body will be drained, making it more vulnerable. When people open up to the universe, learn what is good for them, and find ways to be happier, they can begin to work toward a longer and healthier life.

NATUROPATHY

Naturopathy is a primary health care system emphasizing the curative power of nature, working to restore and support the body's own healing ability using nutrition, herbs, homeopathic remedies, and Chinese medicine. It involves a 4-year course of study past the bachelor's degree, much like conventional medical school.

PRAYER

Prayer is most often defined simply as a form of communication and fellowship with the Deity or Creator. The universality of prayer is evidenced in all cultures having some form of prayer. Life-affirming beliefs and philosophies nourish people. They meditate and say prayers that elicit physiological calm and a sense of peacefulness, both of which contribute to longer survival.

RHEIKI

Rheiki is an ancient Tibetan healing system that uses light hand placements to channel healing energies to the client. It is commonly used to treat distress and acute and chronic health problems, and to achieve spiritual focus.

SPIRITUAL/SHAMANIC HEALING

A shaman is a woman or man who enters an altered state of consciousness, at will, to contact and utilize another type of reality to acquire knowledge and power

and to help other people. Shamans use ancient techniques to achieve and maintain well-being and healing for themselves and members of their communities, serving as a link between the world of matter and spirit. Shamanism is not a belief system. Rather, it is a broad umbrella covering ancient, indigenous, and holistic healing practices worldwide.

T'AI CHI

T'ai Chi and Qigong are Chinese practices consisting of breathing and mental exercises combined with body movements. They are easy and nontiring exercises that contain sets of moves designed to gather qi or energy. Most people spend 30 minutes a day doing the exercises and another 30 minutes in meditation. Practitioners discover how to generate more energy and conserve what they have in order to maintain health or treat illness. The benefits of T'ai Chi are seen in conditions such as hypertension, osteoporosis, and arthritis. T'ai Chi can decrease stress and fatigue, improve mood, and increase energy. It is especially helpful in improving balance in older adults, which decreases the risk of falls (Fontaine, 2000).

THERAPEUTIC TOUCH

Popularized by nursing professor Dolores Krieger in the 1970s, Therapeutic Touch is practiced by registered nurses and others to relieve pain and stress. It is believed that people must, and do, heal themselves. Healing environments are created when nurses enter into caring moments with clients in which the nurse becomes a resource for clients to self-heal. The nurse assesses where the person's energy field is weak or congested and then uses her or his hands to direct energy into the field to balance it. Indications include irritability and anxiety; lethargy, fatigue, and depression; premenstrual syndrome; nausea and vomiting, chemotherapy and radiation sickness; wound and bone healing; and acute musculoskeletal problems such as sprains and muscle spasms. Therapeutic Touch produces a sense of well-being and relaxation for both the nurse and the client.

YOGA

Yoga has been practiced for thousands of years in India, where it is a way of life that includes ethical models for behavior and mental and physical exercises aimed at producing spiritual enlightenment. It is a method for life that can complement and enhance any system of religion, or it can be practiced completely apart from religion. The Western approach to yoga tends to be more fitness oriented with the goal of managing stress, learning to relax, and increasing vitality and well-being. A typical yoga session lasts 20 minutes to an hour. Some people spend 30 minutes doing the poses and another 30 minutes doing breathing practices and meditations. Others spend the majority of the time doing poses and end with a short meditation or relaxation procedure. Even for those who are stiff and out of shape, sick, or weak, sets of easy exercises can help to loosen the joints and stimulate circulation. If practiced regularly, these simple exercises alone make a great difference in people's health and well-being.

Nursing and alternative therapies share the focus on what is unique about the individual and her or his role in healing. The individual is always at the center of treatment interventions, with the emphasis on growth toward health. Health promotion is a lifelong process that focuses on optimal development of our physical, emotional, mental, and spiritual selves.

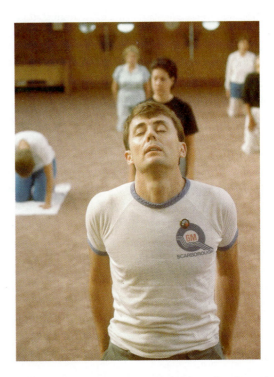

PHOTO 10.8 ■ Yoga is one form of relaxation training.

SOURCE: Stu Rosner/Stock Boston.

CHAPTER REVIEW

COMMUNITY RESOURCES

Links to these Web sites can be accessed on the Companion Web site for this book.

American Association of Pastoral Counselors
9504-A Lee Highway
Fairfax, VA 22031-2303
703-385-6967
www.aapc.org

American Group Psychotherapy Association
25 East 21st St., Sixth Floor
New York, NY 10010
212-477-2677
www.agpa.org

American Massage Therapy Association
820 Davis Street, Suite 100
Evanston, IL 60201-4444
847-864-0123
www.amta.org

Beck Institute for Cognitive Therapy and Research
GSB Building
City Line and Belmost Ave., Suite 700
Bala Cynwyd, PA 19004-1610
610-664-3020
www.beckinstitute.org

National Center for Complementary and Alternative Medicine
www.altmed.od.nih.gov/nccam

KEY CONCEPTS

Mental Health Care Consumers

- Consumers of mental health care come from all segments of society and are in need of a wide variety of services. Consumers must participate in the selection of services and therapies, the setting of care, and the selection of the care provider.

Mental Health Care Professionals

- Nurses with a bachelor's or associate's degree practice at the basic level as staff nurses, case managers, and nurse managers.

- Advanced practice registered nurses have a master's or doctorate degree, practice in a variety of settings, have prescriptive authority, provide consultation, and design and implement research activities.

- Nurses use the nursing process in providing care to clients. They also act as liaisons between other members of the multidisciplinary team, assume responsibility for the physiological integrity of clients, and implement client education about health.

- Psychiatrists are physicians who admit clients to inpatient settings, order diagnostic tests, and prescribe medications and other somatic therapies.

- Psychologists specialize in the administration and interpretation of psychological tests and conduct individual, couple, family, and group sessions.

- Psychiatric social workers are the most knowledgeable professionals about referral resources for clients. Many are also educated in psychotherapy.

- Occupational therapists provide clients with those types of activities that help increase their attention span, improve their motor skills, expand their socialization skills, and improve their ability to perform activities of daily living (ADLs).

- Recreational therapists provide healthy diversional activities in groups.

- Therapists with specialized expertise include those educated in the use of dance, art, music, and play to help clients communicate their thoughts, feelings, and needs in creative ways.

- Nurses collaborate with consumers, family members, and other professionals, all of whom are working together to help clients improve their quality of life and achieve the highest level of functioning.

Milieu Therapy

- Milieu refers to the therapeutic community in which the entire social structure of the unit or residence is designed to be part of the helping process. The goals are to provide a physically and emotionally safe environment, to provide activities that orient and socialize clients, and to provide opportunities for learning and healing.

Individual Psychotherapy

■ The goals of individual psychotherapy are to help clients gain insight; clarify perceptions; identify feelings; make connections between thoughts, feelings, and events; and develop better coping strategies such as problem solving, stress reduction, and crisis management.

Crisis Intervention

■ When maturational or situational events are perceived as a threat to need fulfillment, safety, or a meaningful existence, a crisis state is created.

■ The inability to maintain emotional equilibrium is an important feature of a crisis. The primary goal of crisis intervention is to assist the client to resolve the immediate problem and regain emotional equilibrium.

■ Clients in crisis need to draw on or learn the following skills: problem-solving, identifying and discussing feelings, finding meaning in the event, redefining the event, developing a sense of competence, and maintaining relationships.

Groups

■ There are many types of groups. Task groups are designed to carry out a particular type of task, psychoeducation groups teach members about a specific topic, group therapy helps people work through their dysfunctions, and support groups help members manage issues and concerns, and 12-step groups, which are spiritual and sequential, plan for recovery of addictions.

■ The curative factors of group therapy are the instillation of hope, universality, the imparting of information, altruism, the corrective recapitulation of the primary family group, the development of socializing techniques, imitative behavior, interpersonal learning, existential factors, catharsis, and group cohesiveness.

■ Social microcosm refers to the concept that group members eventually behave in the therapy group the same way they behave with family and friends.

■ It is possible to make changes only in the present time, which is referred to as the here-and-now concept.

■ Group therapy gives children and adolescents the opportunity to learn to talk openly about themselves, practice active listening, give and receive feedback, learn to help others, and learn new ways of relating to others.

■ Parents may be involved in a parallel group to learn growth and development stages, give and receive support, increase parenting skills, and explore their own needs and problems.

Family Therapy

■ Family therapy is indicated when the nurse determines that the family system is impaired because of the presence of a psychosocial problem or mental disorder in one or more family members. It is also the preferred approach when a child or adolescent is the identified patient. Intervention focuses on helping families cope and improve their communication and interpersonal skills.

■ Teaching families how to resolve conflict is a helpful nursing intervention.

Behavioral Therapy

■ Behavioral therapy is based on the principle that all behavior has specific consequences. Behavior is changed through the process of conditioning, which includes reinforcement, punishment, and extinction.

Play Therapy

■ Play therapy is used to establish rapport with children, reveal feelings they are unable to verbalize, enable them to act out their feelings in a constructive manner, understand their relationships and interactions with others, and teach adaptive socialization skills.

Art Therapy

■ Art therapy is a way for people to express what is contained in the unconscious.

Biological Therapies

■ Depression is the most common indication for ECT. It may also be used with older adult clients, adolescents, pregnant women, or those with manic symptoms. Contraindications include brain tumor, recent CVA, subdural hematoma, recent MI, congestive heart failure, angina pectoris, retinal detachment, acute or chronic respiratory disease, and current use of cocaine or heavy use of alcohol.

■ Transcranial magnetic stimulation shows promise in treating people with schizophrenia, depression, bipolar disorder, and anxiety disorders.

■ Light therapy is the treatment of choice for seasonal affective disorder.

■ Sleep deprivation is effective for some people who experience depression.

■ Seclusion and restraints are extreme measures that clients perceive as dehumanizing, degrading, and punishing. Staff may resort to these measures when the milieu is nontherapeutic.

Psychosocial Nursing Interventions

■ Social skills training helps clients live as autonomously as possible in the community.

■ Social skills training includes ADLs, vocational skills, and leisure time skills. Interpersonal skills include conversational skills, assertiveness training, conflict resolution, and problem solving.

KEY CONCEPTS *(continued)*

- Self-esteem interventions help people feel good about themselves, acknowledge their good points, and take care of themselves.

- Reminiscence therapy helps older adults to gain self-awareness, adapt to stress, and improve self-esteem.

- Physical exercise decreases anxiety and depression. Exercise also improves self-concept, body image, and cognitive processing.

- Clients who are taking psychotropic medications should begin exercise at a low intensity because of the drug side effects.

Complementary/Alternative Therapies

- Nursing is in a unique position to take a leadership role in integrating alternative healing methods into Western health care systems since we have historically used our hands, heart, and head in more natural and traditional healing interactions.

- The flow of energy is a concept found in many alternative therapies. Illness and disease occur when energy is blocked, fixed, or unbalanced.

- Health is viewed as a balance or harmony of mind, body, and spirit.

- People must, and do, heal themselves. Healers provide support and guidance.

EXPLORE *MediaLink*

- Interactive resources, including animations, for this chapter can be found on the Companion Web site at *http://www.prenhall.com/fontaine.* Click on Chapter 10 and select the activities for this chapter.

- For NCLEX review questions and an audio glossary, access the accompanying CD-ROM in this book.

REFERENCES

Bailine, S. H., Rifkin, A., Kayne, E., Selzer, J. A., Vital-Herne, J., Blieka, M., et al. (2000). Comparison of bifrontal and bitemporal ECT for major depression. *American Journal of Psychiatry, 157*(1), 121–123.

Ballinger, B., & Yalom, I. D. (1995). The theory and practice of group psychotherapy (4th ed) New York: Basic Books.

Berger, M., Small, B. J., Forsell, Y., Winblad, B., & Backman, L. (1997). Sleep deprivation combined with consecutive sleep phase advance as a fast-acting therapy in depression. *American Journal of Psychiatry, 154*(6), 870–872.

Cohen, D., Taieb, O., Flament, M., Benoit, N., Chevret, S., Corcos, M., et al. (2000). Absence of cognitive impairment at long-term follow-up in adolescents treated with ECT for severe mood disorder. *American Journal of Psychiatry, 157*(3), 460–462.

Cummings, J., & Cummings, E. (1962). *Ego and milieu.* New York: Atherton Press.

Finfgeld, D. L. (2000). Therapeutic groups online: The good, the bad, and the unknown. *Issues in Mental Health Nursing, 21*(3), 241–255.

Fontaine, K. L. (2000). *Healing practices: Alternative therapies for nursing.* Upper Saddle River, NJ: Prentice Hall.

George, M. S., & Belmaker, R. H. (2000). Historical overview. In M. S. George & R. H. Belmaker (Eds.), *Transcranial magnetic stimulation in neuropsychiatry* (pp. 1–12). Washington, DC: American Psychiatric Press.

Griffin, W. A., & Greene, S. M. (1999). *Models of family therapy.* Philadelphia: Brunner/Mazel.

Hart, L. A. (2000). Psychosocial benefits of animal companionship. In A. H. Fine (Ed.),

Handbook on animal-assisted therapy (pp. 59–78). San Diego, CA: Academic Press.

Hays, K. F. (1999). *Working it out: Using exercise in psychotherapy.* Washington, DC: American Psychological Association.

Hilliard, D. (1995). Massage for the seriously mentally ill. *Journal of Psychosocial Nursing, 33*(7), 29–30.

Kennedy, S. S., & Mohr, W. K. (2001). A prolegomenon on restraint of children: Implicating constitutional rights. *American Journal of Orthopsychiatry, 71*(1), 26–37.

Kessler, R. C., Walters, E. E., & Forthofer, M. S. (2001). The use of complementary and alternative therapies to treat anxiety and depression in the United States. *American Journal of Psychiatry, 158*(2), 289–294.

Kogan, A. O., & Guilford, P. M. (1998). Side effects of short-term 10,000-lux light therapy.

REFERENCES *(continued)*

American Journal of Psychiatry, 155(2), 293–294.

Kozub, M. L., & Skidmore, R. (2001). Seclusion and restraint: Understanding recent changes. *Journal of Psychosocial Nursing, 39*(3), 25–31.

Kraft, A. (1966). The therapeutic community. In S. Arieti (Ed.), *American Handbook of Psychiatry, Vol. 2.* New York: Basic Books.

McCloskey, J. C., & Bulechek, G. M. (Eds). (1996). *Nursing interventions classification* (2nd ed.). St. Louis, MO: Mosby.

Meehan, T., Vermeer, C., & Windsor, C. (2000). Patients' perceptions of seclusion: A qualitative investigation. *Journal of Advanced Nursing, 31*(2), 370–377.

Mental Health: A Report of the Surgeon General—Executive Summary. (1999). Rockville, MD: U.S. Department of Health and Human Services. Center for Mental Health Services. National Institutes of Health, National Institute of Mental Health.

Mohit, D. (2000). Psychiatric home care and family therapy: A window of opportunity for the psychiatric clinical nurse specialist. *Archives of Psychiatric Nursing, 14*(3), 127–133.

Mohr, W. K., & Mohr, B. D. (2000). Mechanisms of injury and death proximal to restraint use. *Archives of Psychiatric Nursing, 14*(6), 285–295.

Nida, R. E., & Pierce, S. (2000). Children's social and emotional development. In C. E. Bailey (Ed.), *Children in therapy: Using the family as a resource* (pp. 428–474). New York: Norton.

Nobler, M. S., Fisher, I. A., Zarate, C., Kikinis, R., Jolesz, F. A., McCarley, R. W., et al. (2001). Decreased regional brain metabolism after ECT. *American Journal of Psychiatry, 158*(2), 305–307.

Nussbaum, J. F., Pecchioni, L. L., Robinson, J. D., & Thompson, T. L. (2000). *Communication and aging* (2nd ed.). Mahwah, NJ: Erlbaum.

Oberleitner, L. L. (2000). Aversiveness of traditional psychiatric patient restriction. *Archives of Psychiatric Nursing, 14*(2), 93–97.

Olfson, M., Marcas, S., Sackeim, H. A., Thompson, J., & Pincus, H. A. (1998). Use of ECT for the inpatient treatment of recurrent major depression. *American Journal of Psychiatry, 155*(1), 22–29.

Papolos, D., & Papolos, J. (1999). *The bipolar child.* New York: Broadway Books.

Peplau, H. (1952). *Interpersonal relations in nursing.* New York: Putman.

Ratey, J. J. (2001). *A user's guide to the brain.* New York: Pantheon Books.

Rogers, S. (1996). National clearinghouse serves mental health consumer movement.

Journal of Psychosocial Nursing, 34(9), 22–25.

Scope and standards of psychiatric–mental health nursing practice. (2000). Washington, DC: Amercian Nurses Association.

Selekman, M. D. (2000). Solution-oriented brief family therapy with children. In C. E. Bailey (Ed.), *Children in therapy: Using the family as a resource* (pp. 20–45). New York: Norton.

Sullivan-Marx, E. M., & Maislin, G. (2000). Comparison of nurse practitioner and family physician relative work values. *Journal of Nursing Scholarship, 32*(1), 71–76.

Tew, J. D., Mulsant, B. H., Haskett, R. F., Prudic, J., Thase, M. E., Crowe, R. R., et al. (1999). Acute efficacy of ECT in the treatment of major depression in the old-old. *American Journal of Psychiatry, 156*(12), 1865–1871.

Tonigan, J. S., Toscova, R. T., & Connors, G. J. (1999). Spirituality and the 12-step programs. In W. R. Miller (Ed.), *Integrating spirituality into treatment* (pp. 122–135). Washington, DC: American Psychological Association.

Unutzer, J. (2000). Mental disorders and the use of alternative medicine: Results from a national survey. *American Journal of Psychiatry, 157*(11), 1851–1857.

PART FOUR

Mental Disorders

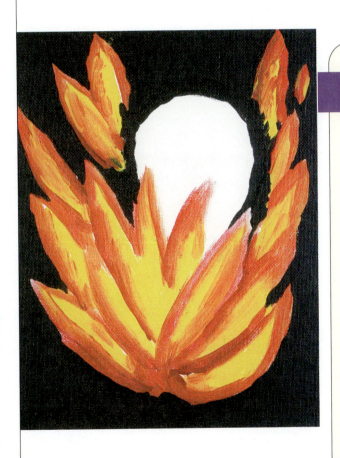

*T*his is where I see myself now. A face with no identity surrounded by a head of darkness, consumed by a fire turning my soul into ashes.

Brenda, Age 25

Anxiety Disorders

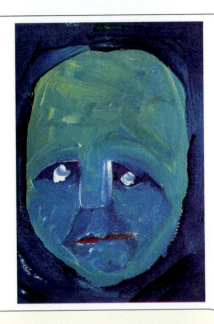

OBJECTIVES

After reading this chapter, you will be able to:

- FORMULATE examples of conscious and unconscious attempts to manage anxiety.

- DISTINGUISH between the different characteristics of the various anxiety disorders.

- DIFFERENTIATE concomitant disorders from the primary anxiety disorder.

- DESCRIBE the alterations in neurobiology occurring in the anxiety disorders.

- APPLY the nursing process when intervening with clients experiencing anxiety disorders.

*A*nxiety/Depression

dying inside
invisible to others

reaching out
with arms not there

trying to find hope
in a dim light dying

hope in anything
to keep breathing

Heather, Age 30

MediaLink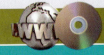

CD-ROM
- *Audio Glossary*
- *NCLEX Review*

Companion Web site www.prenhall.com/fontaine
- *Critical Thinking*
- *More NCLEX Review*
- *Case Study*
- *Care Map Activity*
- *Links to Resources*

KEY TERMS

tinction is made, fear is a feeling that arises from a concrete, real danger, whereas anxiety is a feeling that arises from an ambiguous, unspecific cause or that is disproportionate to the danger.

Anxiety is a common human emotion. It is a biologically mediated response to stress and change. Anxiety helps us mobilize our protective resources necessary for adaptation. When anxiety loses its link with precipitating circumstances or becomes excessive or maladaptive, a person is said to be experiencing an anxiety disorder.

Since September 11, 2001, many Americans have experienced an unfamiliar level of anxiety related to the terrorists acts on the World Trade Center and the Pentagon. For the first time in our lives, we feel vulnerable in our homes, in our cities, and in our country. We had to give up the illusion that we are untouchable. As we gave up our unrealistic expectation of security, we moved into a time of uncertainty and for many, a time of diffuse anxiety. Many of those directly impacted by the attacks—survivors, family members, rescuers, and health care professionals—experienced acute stress disorder and some developed posttraumatic stress disorder. Both of these disorders are presented in this chapter.

In terms of the "normal" or nonviolent world, you, like other people, probably are anxious about certain aspects of your life. When you began the study of nursing, you were introduced to a new and foreign subculture—that of health care professionals and institutions. Your first few days in the clinical setting were likely highly anxious times, as you were uncertain about your skills and insecure in your role as a nursing student. As your skills increased and your professional role became more comfortable, your level of anxiety decreased. Now, as you begin your experience in mental health nursing, your anxiety once again increases as you struggle with new skills and new professional roles. You are probably skeptical of your ability to intervene with clients and are uncertain about what is expected of you in this role. Some of you not only have to adapt to the health care subculture but also are adapting to a different larger culture because of geographical relocation or becoming part of a more culturally diverse group of people. Since too much anxiety interferes with learning, for both you and the clients, finding effective coping mechanisms is necessary for optimal education.

In addition to understanding the meaning of anxiety, it is important to know its process and characteris-

Anxiety is an uncomfortable feeling that occurs in response to the fear of being hurt or losing something valued. Some professionals distinguish between fear and anxiety. When this dis-

tics, as well as the defenses against anxiety. Consciously and unconsciously, people try to protect themselves from the emotional pain of anxiety. Conscious attempts are referred to as **coping mechanisms**, which may be effective or ineffective. *Ineffective coping behaviors* may be such things as becoming involved in physical fights, abusing substances, social withdrawal, or addictive behaviors.

People often effectively use physical activity—walking, jogging, competitive sports, swimming, strenuous housecleaning—to counteract the tension associated with anxiety. *Effective cognitive coping behavior* includes realistically reviewing strengths and limitations, determining short- and long-term goals (both individual and family), and formulating a plan of action to confront the anxiety-producing situation. Effective affective coping behavior may include expressing emotions (laughter, words, tears) or seeking support from family, friends, or professionals. Stress-reduction techniques may also be used, such as meditation, progressive relaxation, visualization, and biofeedback. Effective coping mechanisms contribute to a person's sense of competence and self-esteem.

Unconscious attempts to manage anxiety are referred to as **defense mechanisms**. They often prevent people from being sensitive to anxiety and therefore interfere with self-awareness. When they allow for gratification in acceptable ways, defense mechanisms may be adaptive; however, when the anxiety is not reduced to manageable levels, the defenses become maladaptive. (See Chapter 1 for examples of defense mechanisms.)

The consistent use of certain defenses leads to the development of *personality traits* and characteristic behaviors. How a person manages anxiety and which defense mechanisms are used are more behaviorally formative than the source of the anxiety. Consider the basic human need to be loved and cared for by another person. The anxiety produced by fear of the loss of love may result in a variety of behaviors. One person may be driven to constantly look for love and affirmation by engaging in frequent one-night sexual encounters. Another person may seek out and develop a warm, intimate relationship. A third person may be so frightened of not finding love and so fearful of rejection that he or she avoids relationships to decrease the anxiety. The management of defenses can become so time consuming that little energy remains for other aspects of living.

It is estimated that 27 million adults suffer from anxiety disorders at some point in their lives, making these disorders the single largest mental health problem in the United States. Essentially all anxiety disorders are twice as common in women as in men. Only 25 percent of sufferers receive psychiatric intervention; the remaining 75 percent use other health care services or go untreated. Without relief, anxiety disorders can dramatically reduce productivity and significantly diminish the quality of life (Mendlowicz & Stein, 2000).

Clients with varying levels of anxiety are found in all types of clinical facilities, from community clinics to medical–surgical settings to intensive care units. In a person who has the added stress of an acute or chronic physical illness, the anxiety disorder may be especially pronounced. Included with the anxiety disorders in this chapter are the dissociative disorders, somatoform disorders, factitious disorder, and malingering. All of these disorders are presented in the same chapter because anxiety is the underlying theme in each disorder. The DSM-IV-TR feature lists the categories and different types of disorders presented in this chapter.

KNOWLEDGE BASE

This section describes the various categories of disorders that develop in response to anxiety. At times, it may be difficult to determine which disorder the person is experiencing, as the symptoms often cut across the various disorders. This should not be a great problem for you since your focus, as a nurse, is on clients' responses to their illnesses.

ANXIETY DISORDERS

Generalized Anxiety Disorder

Generalized anxiety disorder (GAD) is a chronic disorder characterized by persistent anxiety but without phobias or panic attacks. Affecting more than 5 percent of the population, it usually begins in childhood or adolescence but may begin in one's twenties. It can be triggered by stress or come out of nowhere. Most sufferers worry excessively about everyday concerns such as whether or not the boss thinks they are doing a good job, or how they are going to pay the bills. In more severe cases, a victim may become preoccupied with catastrophic thoughts and visions. Other symp-

DSM-IV-TR CLASSIFICATIONS

Anxiety Disorders

Generalized Anxiety Disorder

Panic Disorder: with or without agoraphobia

Phobic Disorders: Specific, Social, Agoraphobia

Obsessive–Compulsive Disorder

Posttraumatic Stress Disorder

Acute Stress Disorder

Dissociative Disorders

Dissociative Amnesia

Dissociative Fugue

Depersonalization Disorder

Dissociative Identity Disorder

Somatoform Disorders

Somatization Disorder

Conversion Disorder

Pain Disorder

Hypochondriasis

Body Dysmorphic Disorder

Factitious Disorder

Malingering

SOURCE: Reprinted with permission from the *Diagnostic and Statistical Manual of Mental Disorders, Fourth Edition, Text Revision.* Copyright 2000 American Psychiatric Association.

toms include overall fatigue, muscular tension, restlessness, irritability, difficulty concentrating, and sleep disturbance (see Table 11.1 ■). This unremitting stress and tension can suppress the immune system, which makes one more susceptible to disease (Mendlowicz & Stein, 2000).

Panic Disorder

Panic attack is the highest level of anxiety, characterized by disorganized thinking, feelings of terror and helplessness, and nonpurposeful behavior. It may occur in a variety of anxiety disorders. In this intense experience, people believe they are about to die, lose control, or "go crazy." See Table 11.1 for symptoms of the panic level of anxiety. Some studies suggest that

occasional panic attacks occur in 35 percent of the U.S. population. These episodes are usually associated with public speaking, interpersonal conflict, exams, or other situations of high stress (American Psychiatric Association [APA], 2000).

Panic disorder, which affects more than 1.5 million Americans, is diagnosed when there are recurrent panic attacks. It usually develops between 15 and 24 years of age with one third to one half of individuals also having agoraphobia. Typically, the onset of panic attacks is sudden and unexpected, with intense symptoms lasting from a few minutes to an hour. The episodes involve intense fear and a premonition of doom, which is accompanied by a variety of symptoms (see Table 11.1).

Although panic attacks are an essential feature of panic disorder, other psychiatric symptoms include widespread catastrophic thinking, phobic avoidance, anxiety, depression, and obsessions (McNally, 2001).

The frequency of panic attack varies widely among persons with panic disorder, as do symptom clusters. Some people experience primarily respiratory symptoms, some primarily cardiovascular symptoms, and others are more overwhelmed by cognitive symptoms. Many people with panic disorder believe they are suffering from heart or lung disease, which may lead to avoiding exercise due to their fear that it could precipitate a heart attack (APA, 2000).

A rating scale for the severity of the symptoms provides direction for the multidisciplinary team in helping people with panic disorders improve their quality of life (see Table 11.2 ■).

Dowoyne has been experiencing panic attacks for the past six months. He feels very stressed at work because his new boss is "riding everyone." The same boss recently fired his girlfriend. He describes his panic attacks as a combination of dizziness, trembling, sweating, gasping for breath, and severe pounding of his heart. When the panic subsides, he feels exhausted, as if he has survived a traumatic experience. It has become very stressful for him to commute to work on the train because he fears having an attack in front of everyone. Dowoyne is seriously considering changing jobs so he won't have to take the train.

TABLE 11.1

Physiological Characteristics According to Levels of Anxiety

Anxiety Level	Physiological Response
Mild	Slightly elevated heart rate and blood pressure
	Feels safe and comfortable
	Perceptual field increased
	Ability to learn increased
Moderate	Occasional shortness of breath
	Mild gastric symptoms such as "butterflies" in the stomach
	Facial twitches, trembling lips
	Selective inattention
	Narrowing of the perceptual field
Severe	Frequent shortness of breath
	Increased heart rate, possible premature contractions
	Elevated blood pressure
	Dry mouth, upset stomach, anorexia, diarrhea, or constipation
	Body trembling, fearful facial expression, tense muscles, restlessness, exaggerated startle response, inability to relax, difficulty falling asleep
	Extremely narrowed perceptual field
	Difficulty problem solving or organizing
Panic	Shortness of breath, choking or smothering sensation, sweating
	Hypotension, dizziness, chest pain or pressure, palpitations, chills or hot flashes
	Nausea
	Agitation, poor motor coordination, involuntary movements, entire body trembling, facial expression of terror
	Feeling of losing control, fear of dying
	Completely disrupted perceptual field

A variation of panic disorder is *nocturnal panic.* Panic attacks awaken the person and usually occur within one to four hours after falling asleep, usually during non-REM sleep. No one knows the cause of nocturnal panic, although some believe it may be related to sleep apnea. Panic is further discussed later in the chapter along with agoraphobia, since the two disorders often occur together.

Phobic Disorders

Phobic disorders are behavioral patterns that develop as a defense against anxiety. They develop as a way of

TABLE 11.2

Psychiatric Rating Scale: Levels of Severity for Panic Disorder

Level	Description
6	At least one panic episode per day
5	At least one panic episode per week but less than one per day
4	Persistent fear of panic
3	Limited-symptom panic
2	Sometimes feels on the verge of an attack but is able to control it
1	None of the above

SOURCE: Adapted from Yonkers, K. A., Zlotnick, C., Allsworth, J., Warshaw, M., Shea, T., & Keller, M. B. (1998). Is the course of panic disorder the same in women and men? *American Journal of Psychiatry, 155*(5), 596–602.

objectifying underlying anxiety, displacing it to something concrete that can then be identified and avoided. Other features common to these disorders include fear of losing control, fear of appearing inadequate, defense against threats to self-esteem, and perfectionistic standards of behavior.

Almost all people try to avoid physical dangers. If this avoidance is generalized to situations other than realistic danger, it is called a *phobia*. It is estimated that 20 to 45 percent of the general population have some mild form of phobic behavior. However, phobic disorders occur in only 5 to 15 percent of the population (Paris, 1999). There are many phobic disorders, but they all have four features in common:

1. Unreasonable behavioral response
2. Persistent fears
3. Avoidance behavior
4. Disabling behavior

Although the feared object or situation may or may not be symbolic of the underlying anxiety, the *primary fear* in all phobic disorders is the fear of losing control.

A *specific phobia* is a fear of only one object or situation; it can arise after a single unpleasant experience. The most common phobias are of old dangers such as closed spaces, heights, snakes, and spiders. Very seldom are people phobic about current dangers such as guns,

knives, and speeding cars. Phobias usually begin early in life and are experienced as often by men as by women. People with specific phobias experience anticipatory anxiety; that is, they become anxious even thinking about the feared object or situation. A specific

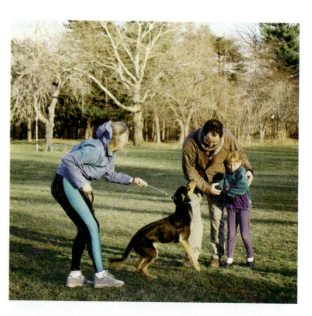

PHOTO 11.1 ■ People with specific phobias experience high levels of anxiety when confronted with the feared situation or object.

SOURCE: Innervisions.

phobia is not disabling unless the feared object or situation cannot be avoided.

Since a rattlesnake bit Carlos five years ago, he has developed a specific phobia of snakes. Normally, his phobia causes no disability because he lives in a large urban area. However, the phobia has prevented him from participating in certain leisure activities such as hiking and camping.

Janelle has a specific phobia of being in an elevator with other people. Her phobia is mildly disabling because she must use the stairs almost all the time. Her vocational opportunities are somewhat limited because she is unable to work on the upper floors of a high-rise office building.

Social phobias are fears of most social situations and affect more than one in eight people. They are characterized by the fear of situations in which an individual fears humiliation or embarrassment when under the scrutiny of others. Unlike shyness, social phobia makes victims literally sick with fear. Social phobias may take many forms, such as meeting new people, attending social gatherings, talking to people in authority, stage fright, fear of public speaking, using public bathrooms, eating in public, and being observed at work. Many people with social phobia fear and avoid a wide variety of situations resulting in negative social, vocational, and financial consequences and functional impairment. Despite the availability of effective treatments for social phobias, most adults in the United States do not receive mental health care for their symptoms. They are often ashamed of their symptoms and fear what professionals may think or say about them (APA, 2000).

When Asela wakes up in the morning, she begins to dread who she is going to have to say hello to that day. Although she is able to work, she is so anxious about eating or talking in public that she avoids lunching with friends, dating, chatting with co-workers, or even answering the phone. She is not able to use a public bathroom if any other woman is present in the facility. She orders all of her clothing by catalog because she is unable to interact with salespeople.

Agoraphobia, the most common and serious phobic disorder, is a fear of being away from home and of being alone in public places when assistance might be needed and where escape might be difficult. A person with agoraphobia will avoid groups of people, whether on busy streets or in crowded stores, on public transportation or at town beaches, at concerts or in movie theaters. Places where the person might become trapped, such as in tunnels or on elevators, are also sometimes avoided.

Agoraphobia is often triggered by severe stress. Moving, changing jobs, relationship problems, or the death of a loved one may precipitate it. The two peak times for the onset are between ages 15 and 20 and then again between ages 30 and 40. Some people may experience a brief period of agoraphobia, which then disappears, never to recur. If it persists for more than a year, the disorder tends to be chronic, with periods of partial remission and relapse (Paris, 1999).

BEHAVIORAL CHARACTERISTICS

The dominant behavioral characteristic of people with phobic disorders is *avoidance*. Fearing loss of control, they avoid the phobic object or situation that increases their level of anxiety. They dread the next encounter and develop elaborate strategies intended to avoid it. If the person demonstrates minor rechecking or ritualistic behavior, avoidance may take on an obsessive–compulsive aspect. Even when they know their fears are irrational, they still try to avoid the object or situation. If it cannot be avoided easily, the behavior may interfere with overall functioning and even lifestyle.

People who suffer from disabling agoraphobia are excessively *dependent* because their avoidance behavior dominates all activities. They may even be so panic-stricken outside the home that they become housebound (see Table 11.3 ■).

Edith, who lives in a large urban area, developed agoraphobia 10 years ago during a time of severe marital distress. In the beginning, she merely avoided large crowds of people. She then began to fear leaving her neighborhood.

(continued)

TABLE 11.3

Psychiatric Rating Scale: Levels of Severity for Agoraphobia

Level	Description
6	Severe avoidance resulting in near or total restriction to home or inability to leave home unaccompanied
5	Avoidance resulting in constricted lifestyle or fear endured with great anxiety (e.g., able to leave house alone but unable to go more than a few miles unaccompanied)
4	Some avoidance and relatively normal lifestyle (e.g., travels unaccompanied when necessary, such as to work or to shop, but otherwise avoids traveling alone)
3	Moderate anxiety when in a phobic situation but no avoidance
2	Slight anxiety in a phobic situation (or anticipation of the situation) but no avoidance
1	None of the above

SOURCE: Adapted from Yonkers, K. A., Zlotnick, C., Allsworth, J., Warshaw, M., Shea, T., & Keller, M. B. (1998). Is the course of panic disorder the same in women and men? *American Journal of Psychiatry, 155*(5), 596–602.

Five years ago, she became housebound and experienced panic attacks if she attempted to leave her home. Two years ago, her phobia progressed to the point that she cannot leave her living room couch. She now needs a great deal of assistance in the activities of daily living. Her husband and a cleaning woman provide for her basic needs. She is alert and continues to manage all the household finances and any other activities that can be accomplished from her couch.

AFFECTIVE CHARACTERISTICS

For people suffering from phobic disorders, *fear* predominates. Mainly, there is fear of the object or situation. There are also fears of exposure, which could result in being laughed at and humiliated, and fear of being abandoned during a phobic episode.

When confronted with the feared object or situation, phobic people feel panic, which may include a feeling of impending doom. Panic in itself is often accompanied by additional fears, such as losing control, causing a scene, collapsing, having a heart attack, dying, losing one's memory, and going crazy. Having once experienced an unexpected attack of panic, they begin to fear the attack will happen again. Because

these attacks are so terrifying, the fear of another attack becomes the major stress in their lives. This *fear of fear*, which is extreme anticipatory anxiety, may become the dominant affective experience, particularly for people with agoraphobia (APA, 2000).

COGNITIVE CHARACTERISTICS

The behavioral and affective characteristics of people with phobic disorders are *ego-dystonic*. Although sufferers recognize that their responses are unreasonable and their thoughts irrational, they are unable to explain them or rid themselves of them. They are consumed with thoughts of anticipatory anxiety and have negative expectations of the future. Phobic people develop low self-esteem and describe themselves as inadequate and as failures. They believe they are in great need of support and encouragement from others. They begin to define themselves as helpless and dependent and often despair of ever getting better. They may even begin to believe they are mentally ill and fear ending up in an institution for the rest of their lives.

In an attempt to localize anxiety, phobic people often use *defenses* that allow them to remain relatively free of anxiety as long as the feared object or situation is avoided. Defenses—such as repression, displacement, symbolization, and avoidance—can also keep the original source of anxiety out of conscious awareness. In agoraphobia, however, defense mechanisms are not adequate to keep anxiety out of conscious awareness. People with agoraphobia live in terror of future panic attacks, and anticipatory anxiety is a constant state.

Ever since they were married, Mike has been emotionally abusive to Velda, telling her what a worthless wife, a terrible housekeeper, and an unimaginative lover she is. Velda has now developed a phobic fear of dirt, germs, and contamination. This phobia so dominates her life that whenever Mike comes home, she immediately scrubs the floor where he has walked because "you can't tell where he has been or what dirt or germs he is bringing in on his shoes." Because the anxiety caused by Mike's abuse and his threats to abandon her was too painful to confront, repression *was used to force her fears out of conscious awareness. Since repression is never completely successful by itself, the anxiety became* displaced *from her inadequacies in the relationship and transferred to dirt, germs, and contamination. Constant cleaning then became* symbolic *of her fears and threatened self-esteem, over which she had more control than her husband's behavior.*

SOCIAL CHARACTERISTICS

The impact of agoraphobia on the family system is usually severe and may cause considerable disruption to family patterns of behavior. People with agoraphobia are often unable to leave home, which means they cannot be employed outside the home, cannot go out with friends, and cannot attend their children's school or sports activities. Thus, though appearing weak, they actually have a great deal of power to control family and friends through their dependency and helplessness.

Advantages from or rewards for being ill are referred to as **secondary gains**. The secondary gains of agoraphobia are the relinquishing of responsibilities, the satisfying of dependency needs that cannot be met directly, and the power to control others. Weakness as a form of control cannot work without another's cooperation. The secondary gains for the partner may be in fulfilling nurturing needs or being the main support of the family.

Obsessive–Compulsive Disorder

Obsessions are unwanted, repetitive thoughts that lead to feelings of fear, anxiety, or guilt, such as the thought of killing someone or of being contaminated with germs. **Compulsions** are behaviors or thoughts used to decrease the fear or guilt associated with obsessions. Behaviors might involve hoarding objects or frequent washing of hands. Examples of cognitive compulsions or thoughts might be silently counting or repeatedly thinking a sequence of words. When obsessive–compulsive thoughts and behaviors dominate a person's life, the person is described as having **obsessive–compulsive disorder (OCD)**. OCD affects approximately 3 percent of the U.S. population (APA, 2000). Males usually develop this disorder at a younger age (6 to 15 years) than females (20 to 29 years).

The degree of interference in the lives of OCD sufferers can range from slight to incapacitating. Often, there is significant interference with home, school, work, and interpersonal functioning. Once begun, OCD usually runs a lifelong course, waxing and waning in severity, but seldom stopping spontaneously. About 10 percent are disabled by this illness. Rapoport (1989) describes the severity in terms of time involved in the compulsive behavior:

- *Mild*: Less than one hour a day
- *Moderate*: One to three hours a day
- *Severe*: Three to eight hours a day
- *Extreme*: Nearly constant

Some people believe that OCD is really a spectrum disorder, that is, not one disorder but several that exhibit repetitive, unwanted behavior. These disorders include compulsive shopping; compulsive gambling; other compulsions related to television, computers, and pornography; substance abuse; nail biting; hair pulling; autism; anorexia and bulimia; somatization disorders; paraphilias; stuttering; and tic disorders. The validity of this hypothesis has not yet been proven.

BEHAVIORAL CHARACTERISTICS

Almost all people have experienced a mild form of obsessive–compulsive behavior known as *folie du doute*, consisting of thoughts of uncertainty and *compulsions to check* a previous behavior. Some common forms are setting the alarm clock and checking it before being able to sleep, turning off an appliance and then returning to make sure it is off, and locking the door and then checking to be sure it is locked. People are bothered by uncertainty and have such thoughts as "Are you sure you locked the door?" There is a feeling of subjective compulsion: "You better check to make sure you locked the door." But there is often a resistance to the compulsion: "You don't have to check the door because you know you locked it." The obsessive thoughts continue and anxiety increases until the compulsive behavior is performed.

Jeanine's mother always worried that the house would be set on fire if she forgot to unplug the iron. Now an adult, Jeanine always checks three times that she unplugged the iron before she leaves the laundry room. Her obsessive thoughts focus on the house burning down with her two children in it. Returning to check the iron reduces her fear to manageable levels. If she resists the urge to perform the compulsion, her anxiety mounts until she is forced to check the iron.

People with OCD often display *consuming*, and at times bizarre, *behavior*. Obsessive–compulsive disorder sufferers describe their behavior as being forced from within. They say, "I have to. I don't want to, but I have to." Of the women, 90 percent are compulsive cleaners who have an unreasonable fear of contamination and avoid contact with anything thought to be unclean. They may spend many hours each day washing themselves and cleaning their environment. Cleaning rituals and avoidance of contamination decrease their anxiety and reestablish some sense of safety and control. With increased public awareness of AIDS, one third of people with OCD now cite the fear of AIDS to explain their washing behavior.

Jay feels a drop in his eye as he looks up while passing a building and cannot dismiss the thought that someone with AIDS has spit out of a window. To reassure himself, he proceeds to knock on the door of every office on that side of the building, asking if anyone there has spit out the window.

Male OCD sufferers are more likely to experience *compulsive checking* behavior, which is often associated with "magical" thinking. They hope to prevent an imagined future disaster by compulsive checking, even though they may recognize it to be irrational.

Other examples of obsessive behavior are arranging and rearranging objects, counting, hoarding, seeking order and precision, and repeating activities such as going in and out of a doorway. The *ritualistic behavior* may become so severe that the person may not be able to work or socialize. Professional help may not be sought until the individual is unable to meet basic needs, or when the family can no longer tolerate the symptoms (Mendlowicz & Stein, 2000). See Box 11.1 for types of obsessions and compulsions.

BOX 11.1

Types of Obsessions and Compulsions

Obsessions: Unwanted, Repetitive Thoughts

- Fear of dirt, germs, contamination
- Fear of something dreadful happening
- Constant doubting
- Somatic concerns
- Aggressive and/or sexual thoughts
- Religious ideation

Compulsions: Behaviors or Thoughts Used to Decrease Fear or Guilt Associated with Obsessions

- Grooming, such as washing hands, showering, bathing, brushing teeth
- Cleaning personal space
- Repeating movements, such as going in and out of doorways, getting in and out of chairs, touching objects
- Checking, such as doors, locks, appliances, written work
- Counting silently or out loud
- Hoarding
- Frequent confession (of anything)
- The need to ask others for reassurance
- The need to have objects in fixed and symmetrical positions

Two years after Betty had moved in, her two-bedroom condo was so cluttered with junk mail, newspapers, unfinished craft projects, old clothes, and broken gadgets that the only spot to sit was on one side of the bed. When Betty finally asked a friend for help, he spent 14 hours throwing out her junk—which she reclaimed from the dumpster as soon as he left. She feared that something dreadful would happen if she threw those things away.

AFFECTIVE CHARACTERISTICS

People with OCD often experience a great deal of *shame* about their uncontrollable and irrational behavior, and they may try to hide it. They may be consumed with fears of being discovered. OCD sufferers respond to anxiety by feeling tense, inadequate, and ineffective. To alleviate the anxiety, *control* is all-important. They fear that if they do not act on their compulsion, something terrible will happen. Thus, in most cases, compulsions serve to temporarily reduce anxiety. But the behavior itself can create further anxiety. The affective distress may range from mild anxiety to almost constant anxiety about thoughts and behaviors. Obsessive–compulsive people often experience *hopelessness* that their situation will never improve. They may also develop phobias when faced with situations in which they can no longer maintain control.

COGNITIVE CHARACTERISTICS

Traditionally, it has been thought that OCD is egodystonic because many sufferers feel tormented by their symptoms. These people recognize the senselessness of much of their behavior and want to resist it. The drive to engage in the behavior is overpowering, however, and they often feel extreme distress about their actions. A smaller number have limited recognition of their behavior, and a few are unable to see their behavior as senseless.

The most common *preoccupations* involve dirt; safety; and violent, sexual, or blasphemous thoughts. There may be magical thinking, false beliefs, superstitions, or religious ideation, the content of which is culturally determined. They say, "No matter how hard I try, I cannot get these thoughts out of my mind."

Ramona has persistent thoughts such as: What if the smell of gasoline gets in my lungs? What if I breathe it in when I am pumping gas and get lung cancer? What if my cat licks the gasoline off my hands? What if she gets sick? What if she dies? What if she spreads it to my mom? What if I die?

OCD sufferers are consumed with constant *doubts*, which lead to difficulty with concentration and mental exhaustion. They doubt everything related to their particular compulsion and cannot be reassured by what they see, feel, smell, touch, or taste. Their OCD symptoms make them very slow in solving problems but do not interfere with accuracy in problem solving.

Yvette is a 27-year-old mechanical engineer. Her obsessive–compulsive behavior has been increasing during the past five years, and she is now in danger of losing her job because of decreased productivity. She checks and rechecks every project she is assigned to the degree that she is unable to complete any project. She is able to identify when a project is completed, but her fear of making a mistake drives her to continue to recheck her work and avoid handing it in to her supervisor. She recognizes her behavior is unrealistic and will likely result in the loss of her job.

SOCIAL CHARACTERISTICS

OCD is a devastating illness that alters the lives of both clients and their family members. OCD symptoms are all-encompassing and involve family members and the home itself. Relationships are often strained and at times destroyed. Family members find themselves manipulated into enabling behavior in order to keep the peace and often end up bitter and resentful. Nearly all affected children involve their parents, and sometimes siblings, in their rituals (Mendlowicz & Stein, 2000).

Posttraumatic Stress Disorder

People exposed to extremely dangerous and life-threatening situations may develop **posttraumatic stress disorder (PTSD)**. Only a minority of people exposed to extreme stress develop PTSD. Those more vulnerable to the disorder include people with low social support systems, preexisting mental disorders, childhood physical or sexual abuse, childhood separation from parents, and family instability (McNally, 2001).

Symptoms of PTSD usually begin within the first three months after the trauma, although there may be a delay of months, or in some cases even years, before symptoms appear. Any time a trauma occurs, the potential to develop PTSD exists. In severe trauma, a person confronts extreme helplessness and terror in the face of possible annihilation. Ordinary coping behaviors are ineffective, action is of no avail, and the person can neither resist nor escape. For example, rape, child sexual abuse, and battering involve the use of force by the perpetrator. Whether it is a sudden shock or a repetitive torment, the stress of the assault is inescapable and the end result is often PTSD. Disaster workers are also at risk of PTSD thought to be related to the exposure to violent death, severely mutilated bodies, the impact of life-threatening situations, and physically demanding activities.

It is important to understand that PTSD sufferers are normal people who have experienced abnormal events such as terrorist attacks, physical or sexual assault, hostage situations, natural disasters, and military combat (Woods, 2000). Chapters 21, 22, and 23 discuss domestic violence, sexual violence, and community violence, respectively.

Traumatic events may result in two categories of symptoms: undercontrol and overcontrol. Those with *undercontrol* relive the event and are diagnosed as having PTSD. Those with *overcontrol* experience denial and amnesia and are diagnosed as having one of the dissociative disorders. Thus, PTSD and the dissociative disorders may have similar precipitating causes.

BEHAVIORAL CHARACTERISTICS

People with PTSD often exhibit a *hyperalertness* resulting from their need to constantly search the environment for danger. Increasing anxiety can cause unpredictably *aggressive* or *bizarre behavior*. PTSD sufferers may resort to abusing drugs or alcohol in an effort to decrease this anticipatory anxiety. They may also behave as if the original trauma were actually recurring. Thus, they may try to defend themselves against a past enemy who is perceived to be in the present. Triggering events create a continuous cycle of reminders. Examples

are the anniversary of the crime or event; holidays and family events, especially if a perpetrator is involved; tastes, touches, and smells; and media coverage such as articles, talk shows, and movies. Many of these people develop a phobic avoidance of the triggers that remind them of the original trauma. *Avoidance* may become so all-encompassing that a socially isolated lifestyle develops (Goenjian et al., 2000).

Holly was robbed and beaten at gunpoint on a Sunday evening as she put her car in her garage. A few days later, she tried to return to work. "I tried to walk to the corner to take the bus and was terrified to walk just half a block for fear I would be assaulted again. When I came home from work, I was terrified again to walk the half block and I cried all the way home. I was afraid to come out of the house after that and would ask family and friends to come and get me when I had to go somewhere. I felt like a prisoner."

AFFECTIVE CHARACTERISTICS

People suffering from PTSD experience *chronic tension*. They are often irritable and feel edgy, jittery, tense, and restless. They commonly experience labile affective responses to the environment. Anxiety is frequent and ranges from moderate anxiety to panic. When triggers remind them of the original trauma, the original feelings are experienced with the same intensity.

Guilt is another common affective characteristic of PTSD. When the traumatic event entailed the death of others, the guilt stems from the person's having survived when others did not. If the person is a war veteran, he may feel guilty about the acts he was forced to commit to survive the combat experience.

In addition to anxiety, tension, irritability, aggression, and guilt, there can be a *numbing* of other *emotions*. Often, people with PTSD discover they can no longer appreciate previously enjoyed activities. Feeling detached from others, they are unable to be intimate or tender. Obviously, this difficulty contributes to relationship problems.

COGNITIVE CHARACTERISTICS

A sudden, life-threatening trauma often causes people to reevaluate themselves and their experiences. In the face of imminent death, the fantasy of personal immortality is exploded. Confrontation with severe injury or death results in long-lasting changes in a person's thinking patterns.

Memory may be affected by trauma. Memory of the traumatic event may be erased by amnesia, which may vary from a few minutes to months or even years. Some may have intermittent memories about the trauma that range from quick flashes to entire recollections of the event. Although this experience is distressing, it may be tolerable if the memories are infrequent. In contrast to amnesia, some people experience memories that return in the form of unpredictable and uncontrollable *flashbacks*. These memories can be so intrusive and persistent that people become obsessed by them. In a sense, victims of trauma live with ghosts and are haunted by their past. Recurring nightmares, in which the person reexperiences the event, are also common. A person may become preoccupied with thoughts of the trauma recurring. All these cognitive changes contribute to the development of an external locus of control, and PTSD sufferers feel themselves to be at the mercy of the environment.

Jeanmarc, 35 years old, has a home decorating business. Three months ago he was stabbed in the back by a client while working in her home. The attack was unprovoked, and Jeanmarc did not attempt to defend himself for fear of hurting the woman and thus ending up in prison. His attacker lives in his neighborhood and is now out on bail. He states that since the incident he has been preoccupied with death. His sleep has deteriorated to two to three hours a night, and he has terrible nightmares. Other symptoms include decreased appetite, a 20-pound weight loss, decreased concentration, listlessness, decreased sex drive, headaches, and diarrhea. Prior to the event, he lived by himself in an apartment. Since the attack, he has moved in with his sister and her three children. His relationships with both his sister and his girlfriend are strained due to his recurrent symptoms.

Another cognitive characteristic that may accompany PTSD is *self-devaluation*. For some, the sense of

self is shattered, while for others it is not allowed to develop at all. Repetitive childhood trauma interferes with the developmental organization of the personality. Being treated like an object results in feelings of dehumanization. A rape survivor may be influenced by cultural myths and begin to believe she was responsible for the act of violence committed against her. Survivors of disasters often feel guilty, believing that other, more capable people deserved to live more than they do. Upon returning from Vietnam, many veterans were assailed by society's reproach and indifference. This devaluation became a part of the self-image of many veterans.

SOCIAL CHARACTERISTICS

Family members of people with PTSD have a great deal of anxiety. One of the defenses for coping with the traumatic event is the numbing of emotions, or emotional anesthesia. Because of the PTSD sufferer's feelings of detachment, alienation, and doubts about an ability to trust and love, interpersonal relationships are strained to the limit. Loss of the ability to communicate feelings makes relationship problems inevitable. Outbursts of anger and aggression further alienate family and friends.

Acute Stress Disorder

Many people who experience or witness an extreme traumatic stressor develop **acute stress disorder**. During or shortly after the trauma, these individuals may feel numb and emotionally nonresponsive, have a decreased awareness of their environment, and may experience amnesia for part or all of the event. Like PTSD sufferers, they often experience recurrent images and flashbacks, which contribute to the avoidance of stimuli that remind them of the trauma. These events cause significant distress and impair activities of daily living. Acute stress disorder begins within a month of the traumatic event, lasts at least two days, and goes away within four weeks. If symptoms persist beyond four weeks, the person is given the diagnosis of PTSD.

Dissociative Disorders

Dissociation is defined in the *Diagnostic and Statistical Manual of Mental Disorders* (4th ed., Text Revision) (DSM-IV-TR) (APA, 2000) as a disruption in the usually integrated functions of consciousness, memory, identity, and perception of the environment. Dissociative symptoms exist along a continuum ranging from common experiences such as daydreaming and lapses in attention to a pathological failure to integrate thoughts, feelings, and actions.

Dissociative disorders are characterized by an alteration in conscious awareness of behavior, affect, thoughts, and memories, and an alteration in identity, particularly in the consistency of personality. The alteration in identity may be identity loss or the presence of more than one identity. Regardless of the type of dissociative disorder, all sufferers at times demonstrate behavior totally different from their usual behavior. Dissociative disorders are often precipitated by a traumatic event, such as a disaster, rape, or war (Simeon et al., 2001).

Dissociative Amnesia
Dissociative amnesia, memory loss not caused by an organic problem, is usually related to an acute, precipitating traumatic event. The most common type is *localized amnesia*, in which memory loss occurs for a specific time related to the trauma. *Selective amnesia* is localized for a specific time, with partial memory of events during that time. The least common types of psychogenic amnesia are *generalized amnesia*, a complete loss of memory of one's past, and *continuous amnesia*, in which memory loss begins at a particular point in time and continues to the present.

Yuki's firstborn child died of sudden infant death syndrome three months ago. Although she remembers arriving in the emergency department with her baby, she continues to have no memory of finding him in his crib, calling the paramedics, or hearing the doctor telling her that her baby was dead.

Dissociative Fugue
Dissociative fugue is a rare dissociative disorder in which people, while either maintaining their identity or adopting a new identity, wander or take unexpected trips. The disorder is often precipitated by subacute, chronic stress. The episode may last several hours or several days. During the fugue state, these people may appear either normal or disoriented and confused; they usually behave in ways inconsistent with their normal personality and values. The fugue state often ends abruptly, and there is either partial or complete amnesia for that period. Both dissociative amnesia and dissociative fugue are most commonly seen during war and in the aftermath of disasters.

Depersonalization Disorder
Depersonalization disorder is characterized by persistent or recurrent feelings of being detached from one's body or thoughts. People describe feeling like robots, being an outside observer of their bodies or thoughts, or feeling like they are living in a dream. They remain oriented to reality in that they know they are not really robots or living in a dream. The incidence and prevalence of this disorder are unknown, as it is one of the least studied dissociative conditions. It is thought to result from emotional abuse in childhood; the more severe the abuse, the more severe the symptoms. Depersonalization disorder usually begins in adolescence and is often not responsive to either therapy or medication (Guralnik, Schmeidler, & Simeon, 2000; Simeon, Guralnik, Schmeidler, Sirof, & Knutelska, 2001; Simeon et al., 2000).

Dissociative Identity Disorder
Dissociative identity disorder (DID), formerly multiple personality disorder, is the most severe form of dissociative disorders. This diagnosis is given when at least two personalities exist in the same person. Each personality, or "alter," is integrated and complex; that is, each has its own memory, value structure, behavioral pattern, and primary affective expression. The host personality, which is the original personality, has at best only a partial awareness of the other alters. People with DID suffer from an alteration in conscious awareness of their total being.

Efrain has been working for several years with Judith in outpatient therapy. Over a period of time he has been introduced to the following personalities within her "family" system:

Judith—35 years old, married, one son; very traditional, good housekeeper, attends church regularly, dresses in a careful and "proper" manner; good at art, draws with right hand. Role in the "family" is to be responsible.

Little Judy—5 years old; gentle, shy, playful; likes to draw "pretty" pictures, draws with her left hand. Role in the "family" is to serve as a distraction when there is too much pain and fear.

Mary—14 years old; assertive and outgoing; does not attend church, doesn't like housework, prefers to wear blue jeans and T-shirts; very knowledgeable about drugs; assumes large gaps of missing time related to drug use. Role in the "family" is the "party animal," able to have fun and play with peers.

Sue—15 years old; has a chip-on-the-shoulder, I-don't-care attitude; out only at night; sees self as totally separate from the "family"; plans to use men as she has been used. Role in the "family" is to try to understand sexuality, express anger for entire family.

Gail—powerful and wise; knows all the personalities and is known by all the others; position of trust in the "family"; role is as a spiritual guide to everyone.

Sometimes Judith finds herself at one of Mary's parties, wearing blue jeans and a sweatshirt. At times Mary finds herself sitting in church wearing a dress; both Judith and Mary are horrified by these experiences.

Recent reports agree that the origin of DID is severe, sadistic, often sexual, child abuse. The abusive incidents are repeated over time and inconsistently alternate with expressions of care and concern from the abuser. Another factor may be the secrecy and denial associated with this form of abuse. Subjectively, the child lives in a fragmented reality, and social support is limited because traumatization occurs through exactly the persons on whom the child is dependent (Draijer & Langeland, 1999).

In DID, the defense mechanisms of *repression* and *dissociation* are used to manage the anxiety, rage, and helplessness the child experiences in response to severe abuse. The only way for these people to survive the pain of the trauma is to eliminate it from conscious awareness. Dissociation is accomplished by self-hypnosis, which correlates with the onset of the abuse. This soon becomes the dominant method of managing severe stress, and people with DID are able to quickly and spontaneously enter hypnotic trances. What is a life-saving process in childhood becomes a self-destructive tool in adulthood.

Somatoform Disorders

The **somatoform disorders**—somatization, conversion, pain disorder, hypochondriasis, and body dys-

morphic disorder—all involve physical symptoms for which no underlying organic basis exists.

Somatization Disorder People diagnosed with a **somatization disorder** have multiple physical complaints involving a variety of body systems. This is a chronic disorder that usually begins in the teenage years and is identified more often in women than in men. Men may express symptoms of the disorder less dramatically, or perhaps physicians have been less likely to perceive men as having multiple unexplained somatic symptoms.

Conversion Disorder A **conversion disorder**, characterized by sensorimotor symptoms, can appear at any age but typically begins and ends abruptly. It is usually precipitated by a severe trauma such as war. Sensory symptoms range from paresthesia and anesthesia to blindness and deafness. Motor symptoms range from tics to seizures to paralysis. A person with a conversion disorder has only one symptom, whereas a person with a somatization disorder has several.

Pain Disorder Pain that cannot be explained organically is the primary symptom of a **pain disorder**. Unconscious conflict and anxiety are believed to be the basis for the pain. The pain may severely disrupt the person's life, and inadvertent substance abuse may occur.

Hypochondriasis People with **hypochondriasis** believe they have a serious disease involving one or several body systems, despite all medical evidence to the contrary, or they are terrified of contracting certain diseases. These people are extremely sensitive to internal sensations, which they misinterpret as evidence of disease. This disorder usually begins in midlife or late in life and affects women and men equally (APA, 2000).

Body Dysmorphic Disorder **Body dysmorphic disorder** is a serious chronic and often disabling condition. The prevalence is not well known since it is believed that people underreport their symptoms because of shame. Body dysmorphic disorder is a preoccupation with an imagined or slight defect in physical appearance. The most common concerns involve the face—facial skin, nose, and hair. As with those suffering from eating disorders, there is a lot of concern with bodily appearance. The disorder is probably related to OCD in that their thoughts are intrusive and they compulsively check their body appearance. They may avoid social and work activities because of embar-

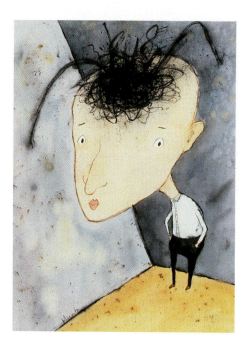

ILLUSTRATION 11.1 ■ Body dysmorphic disorder is characterized by a preoccupation with some imagined defect in appearance.

SOURCE: Robbie Marantz/Getty Images, Inc.

rassment, leading to social isolation. They experience feelings of low self-esteem, shame, and worthlessness, which may lead to suicidal thoughts and attempts (APA, 2000; Grant, Kim, & Crow, 2001).

Conversion disorders are rare, but the other somatoform disorders are frequently seen in community settings, health care offices, and acute care units. These three disorders account for a large portion of the medical expense in the United States. It is estimated that 4 to 18 percent of all physician visits are made by the "worried well." People with these disorders truly suffer, however; they must not be discounted as malingerers or manipulators. As a nurse, you can often provide a long-term caring relationship, which may be the most important intervention in preventing needless tests, medications, and surgeries. When people with somatoform disorders feel that no one is listening to or caring for them, they often go from one health care professional to another, duplicating tests and medical interventions. By being knowledgeable and sensitive, you can protect these clients by maintaining them within one health care system.

BEHAVIORAL CHARACTERISTICS

Typically, clients experiencing somatoform disorders purchase many OTC medications to reduce their symptoms or pain. Inadvertent *drug abuse* may result when medications are prescribed for long periods by a variety of physicians. Dependence on pain relievers or antianxiety agents is a common complication of these disorders.

These clients frequently discuss their symptoms and disease processes. Many adapt their behavior patterns and lifestyle to the disorder. Adaptation can range from a minor restriction of activities to the role of a complete invalid.

In the past year, Dorothy has been seen by eight health care providers, including her family physician, a cardiologist, an internist, an orthopedist, a chiropractor, a proctologist, and a cancer diagnostician. After extensive and repeated testing, no evidence of organic disease was found. Dorothy continues to complain about the incompetence of these people and is in the process of finding new health care providers.

AFFECTIVE CHARACTERISTICS

The primary gain in somatoform disorders is the *reduction of conflict and anxiety*. People with these disorders are usually unable to express anger directly out of fear of abandonment and loss of love. They actively avoid situations in which others will become angry with them. As a result, there is an unconscious use of physical symptoms to manage the anxiety caused by conflicting issues.

When they fail to get relief from the physical symptoms, these clients experience more anxiety. It may be manifested by obsessions about the physical illness, depression, or phobic avoidance of activities associated with the spread of disease.

Some people with conversion disorders exhibit *la belle indifference*, a relative lack of concern for their physical symptoms. People showing a sudden onset of symptoms, even severe ones like paralysis or blindness, sometimes seem nonchalant about their condition. This reaction usually occurs in people who do not want to be noticed by others. But others with conversion disorders may be very verbal about their distress over the sudden appearance of symptoms. This reaction is more likely to occur in people with a high need for attention and sympathy.

COGNITIVE CHARACTERISTICS

Somatoform disorder sufferers are *obsessively interested in bodily processes* and diseases. Almost all their attention is focused on the discomfort they are experiencing. So obsessed are they with their bodies that they are constantly aware of very small physical changes and discomforts that would go unnoticed by others. In hypochondriasis, these changes are regarded as concrete evidence of an active disease process. They are highly resistant to reassurance from health care providers. Information, education, and explanation only temporarily lessen their disease fears.

Ray is convinced that he has AIDS in spite of all negative diagnostic tests. He is not reassured by the fact that he is at low risk because of having been in a monogamous relationship for 20 years, has never used intravenous drugs, and has never had a blood transfusion. He is hyperalert to all slight variations in bodily function and regards these normal variations as evidence of AIDS.

Denial is the major defense mechanism in clients with somatoform disorders. Initially, these clients deny the source of anxiety and conflict, and the energy is transformed into physical complaints. Along with physical symptoms is a denial that there could be any psychological component to the physical symptoms. If confronted with the possibility of a psychological cause, clients often change health care providers in an effort to maintain their system of denial. Rarely will they follow through on referrals for psychotherapy.

SOCIAL CHARACTERISTICS

The media are a contributing factor in somatoform disorders. Magazines, radio, and television bombard us with advertisements for "cures" for every imaginable physical problem. In addition, there has recently been an emphasis on staying healthy—an emphasis that, at times, seems like a morbid preoccupation with death. Another form of the somatoform disorders is an obsessive, unrealistic fear of contracting HIV, the virus that

causes AIDS. Low-risk individuals with a somatoform disorder are terrified they may have AIDS. With such intense media attention, it is hardly surprising that people become obsessed with bodily processes.

Any one of the somatoform disorders may completely disrupt a person's life. Sufferers may need to change their vocation to one more adaptable to their physical symptoms. Others may be unable to work in any capacity, either inside or outside the home. The chronic nature of these disorders often places a severe financial and emotional strain on the family. Physician, diagnostic, and hospital expenses may place the family in debt. The emotional drain on both client and family leads to increased stress and interpersonal conflict, especially when there is no physical improvement. This increased level of conflict contributes to the continuation of the disorder, and a vicious cycle is established.

Factitious Disorder

Individuals are diagnosed with **factitious disorder** when they intentionally simulate or produce physical or psychological symptoms in order to assume the sick role. *Subjective* complaints may concern feeling unwell or the presence of pain. They may ingest psychoactive substances to produce symptoms such as restlessness, insomnia, or hallucinations. Examples of falsified *objective* signs are hematuria (by ingesting anticoagulants), fever (manipulating a thermometer), self-inflicted conditions (injecting toxic substances such as poisons, own urine or feces; creating bruises, lesions, or other injuries consistent with illness), or an exaggeration of a preexisting condition (feigning a hypoglycemic attack with a history of diabetes). They may present with predominantly physical complaints, predominantly psychological complaints, or with combined complaints. The most severe and chronic form of this disorder is referred to as *Munchausen's syndrome.* (See Chapter 21 for Munchausen's syndrome by proxy as a form of child abuse.)

People with factitious disorder usually present in a dramatic manner but are extremely vague and inconsistent during the medical history. When extensive workups demonstrate no underlying pathology, they may complain of other problems and new symptoms. The only motivation for the behavior is to assume the sick role and gain attention. Factitious disorder usually consists of intermittent episodes with an onset in early adulthood (APA, 2000).

Malingering

Malingering is similar to factitious disorder in that the individual intentionally produces false physical or psychological symptoms. Unlike factitious disorder, the motivation in malingering is external incentives such as getting sick leave from work, obtaining financial compensation, evading criminal prosecution, or obtaining drugs.

CULTURE-SPECIFIC CHARACTERISTICS

While anxiety may be a universal emotion, the context in which it is experienced, the meaning it is given, and the responses to it are strongly influenced by cultural beliefs and practices. Cross-cultural studies have found significant differences in the expression of anxiety. These include differences in the type of specific fears as well as the associated behavioral, affective, and cognitive characteristics. In some cultures, anxiety is expressed predominantly through somatic symptoms, in others through cognitive or affective symptoms. It is important to consider the cultural context when assessing clients for anxiety disorders (see Figure 11.1 ■). (See Chapter 5 for culture-bound syndromes related to anxiety.)

AGE-SPECIFIC CHARACTERISTICS
Children

It is common for children to experience anxiety. This experience is usually temporary and requires no professional intervention. Infants fear loud and sudden noises, loss of support, and heights. Very young children fear strangers, being left alone, and the dark; preschoolers fear separation from caregivers, imaginary creatures, animals, and the dark. Anxiety about physical safety and storms are common among young school-age children. During the middle-school years, the focus of anxiety changes to academic, social, and health-related issues. This focus continues into adolescence (see Table 11.4 ■).

Developmentally appropriate fears and anxieties must be distinguished from those that are inappropriate and/or pathological. Anxiety disorders are the most

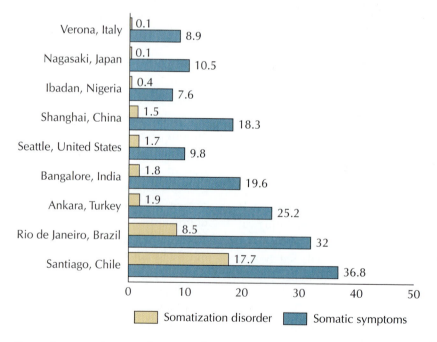

FIGURE 11.1 ■ Prevalence of somatization disorder and somatic symptoms in different countries. Somatization is *not* more common in nonindustrialized countries, contrary to common assumptions. (*Note*: Somatization disorder was based on ICD-10 diagnosis; somatic symptoms included a minimum of four for men and six for women.)

SOURCE: Reprinted with permission; rights held by APA. Gureje, O., Simon, G. E., Usrun, T. B., & Goldberg, D. P. (1997). Somatization in cross-cultural perspective: A World Health Organization study in primary care. *American Journal of Psychiatry, 154,* 989–995.

TABLE 11.4

Anxiety Disorders in Children and Adolescents

Disorder	Age	Description
Obsessive–compulsive disorder (OCD)	As young as 2; mean age 10 years	Most common behaviors are washing and cleaning, followed by checking, counting, repeating, touching and straightening, and hoarding. Fears include contamination, harm to self, and harm to familiar person. Many are embarrassed and secretive, and the disorder is often unrecognized.
Posttraumatic stress disorder (PTSD)	Related to traumatic event	Traumatic events prior to age 11 are three times more likely to result in PTSD. Younger children may repeatedly act out specific themes of the trauma. Some engage in high motor activity in effort to keep minds off recurring thoughts.
Generalized anxiety disorder (GAD)	5–17 years	Formerly referred to as overanxious disorder of childhood. Affects about 3–15% of children and adolescents. Variety of worries such as future events, performance, personal safety, and the social environment. Often have somatic complaints. Self-conscious and excessive need for reassurance from others. Perfectionistic, eager to please, hypermature.
Specific phobia	Childhood, adolescence	Common phobias include heights, small animals, doctors, dentists, darkness, noises, and thunder and lightning. Behaviors include screaming, crying, or running to loved one for safety. There is a common belief that confrontation with phobic stimulus will result in personal harm.
Social phobia	As young as 8; early to mid-adolescence	Persistent fear of one or more situations such as formal speaking, eating in front of others, going to parties, writing in front of others, using public restrooms, speaking to authority figures. Fear is of criticism or failure. Sixty percent of distressing events occur at school.

SOURCES: American Psychiatric Association. (2000). *Diagnostic and statistical manual of mental disorders* (4th ed., Text Revision). Washington, DC: Author; and Malcarne, V. L., & Hansdottir, I. (2001). Vulnerability to anxiety disorders in children and adolescence. In R. E. Ingram & J. M. Price (Eds.), *Vulnerability to psychopathology* (pp. 271–303). New York: Guilford Press.

prevalent form of mental disorders in children. Some anxiety disorders are specified as Axis I disorders as Other Disorders of Infancy, Childhood, or Adolescence. Other anxiety disorders of children and adolescents are described under the adult disorders. Estimates for the presence of any anxiety disorder range from 6 to 18 percent. Anxiety disorders are three to four times higher in children who also suffer from depression and two to three times higher in children with oppositional or conduct disorders. Preadolescent girls and boys experience the same rate of anxiety disorders. This changes, however, in puberty when rates of anxiety in girls are higher than those in boys (Byrne, 2000; Malcarne & Hansdottir, 2001).

Characteristics of anxiety in children and adolescents include fears, worries, uneasiness, apprehension, restlessness, decreased concentration, self-doubt, decreased school performance, dizziness, lightheadedness, shortness of breath, nausea and vomiting, headaches, and stomachaches. Between 10 and 30 percent of schoolchildren experience anxiety severe enough to impair academic achievement. Highly anxious adolescents engage in more problem behavior, are more disliked by peers, have poorer self-concepts, and have lower school achievement when compared to less anxious teens. Individuals who experience anxiety disorders in childhood or adolescence are at a significantly higher risk for a recurrent anxiety disorder in young adulthood. It must also be noted that many anxious children do not develop anxiety disorders as adults (Byrne, 2000).

Separation Anxiety Disorder   A mild form of separation anxiety is fairly common in young children. Most children fear losing their parents. Separation anxiety disorder may develop at any age, although it is more common in children than in adolescents, and onset can be as early as age 2 to 3 years, with the peak onset between 7 and 9 years. The child may follow the parent around the house, needing to be in close proximity at all times. Their worries may focus on separation themes such as being kidnapped or killed, or the parents being killed. The school-age child may refuse to go to school, although not all refusals are due to separation anxiety. Physiological manifestations include

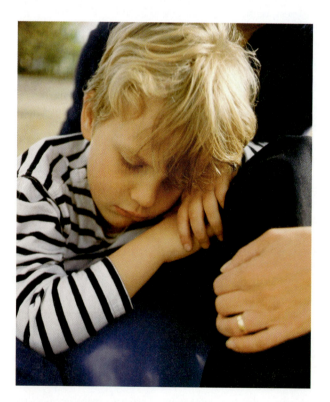

PHOTO 11.2 ■ Some children are overly dependent on parents.

SOURCE: Mel Curtis/Getty Images, Inc./PhotoDisc, Inc.

nausea, vomiting, stomachache, and sore throat. Older children may have palpitations, respiratory distress, and dizziness (APA, 2000; Way, Hayward, Levin, & Sondheimer, 1999).

Separation anxiety disorder may have either an acute or an insidious onset. Many children recover without any further problems, while others may have periodic exacerbations. Some may have symptoms into adulthood, especially when attachments are threatened or disrupted.

Selective Mutism   Selective mutism, a form of social phobia, is the steady failure to speak in specific social situations in which speaking is expected. The onset is usually between 3 and 6 years and occurs more frequently among girls. The extent to which the child speaks varies greatly. Some children speak loudly and freely at home but never say a word at school. Some speak to strangers in public, while others do not. Some are unable to speak to others face to face but may be able to speak to these same individuals on the phone. As is obvious, this disability interferes with education and social relationships. The majority of the children "outgrow" the disorder, although it may persist for several years (APA, 2000).

Reactive Attachment Disorder   Reactive attachment disorder is associated with grossly pathological care resulting from parental inexperience, extreme poverty, or prolonged institutionalization of the child. Not all children in these circumstances develop this disorder. The primary characteristic of this disorder is developmentally inappropriate social interactions. There are two subtypes: inhibited and disinhibited. Children suffering from the inhibited subtype do not initiate social contact nor do they appropriately interact with others. Those with the disinhibited subtype have few social boundaries and become quickly attached to multiple individuals. The course of the disorder appears to be related to the severity and duration of the pathological care as well as the effectiveness of a corrective supportive environment (APA, 2000).

Generalized Anxiety Disorder   In children and adolescents with GAD, anxieties often concern school performance, athletic performance, and catastrophes such as war, massive bombings, earthquakes, tornadoes, or hurricanes. They typically seek approval and frequent reassurance from adults. They may obsessively redo work out of a drive for perfectionism (APA, 2000).

Panic Disorder   Panic disorder occurs in children and, more commonly, adolescents. It often is preceded by or is comorbid with separation anxiety disorder. Panic disorder is often accompanied by a variety of specific phobias including fear of the dark, monsters, kidnappers, bugs, small animals, heights, and open or closed-in spaces. These specific phobias may be common triggers for panic and thus are responsible for many of the avoidance behaviors seen in children and adolescents with panic disorder (APA Practice Guidelines, 1998; D'Alli, 2000).

Social Phobia   Behavioral inhibition refers to the tendency among some young children to respond to unfamiliar people and situations with wariness and avoidance. This is considered to be an early temperamental precursor of later anxiety disorders. Children with behavioral inhibition are shy and fearful as toddlers; shy with strangers and timid in unfamiliar situations as preschoolers; and cautious, quiet, and introverted at school age. Those diagnosed with social phobia may fail to achieve in school, refuse to go to school, or avoid age-appropriate social activities. The terms *school phobia* and *school refusal* are often used to refer to children with social phobia (Fish, Jensen, Reichert, & Wainman-Sauda, 2000).

Obsessive–Compulsive Disorder   There are two peak onset ages for OCD, with one peak around age 10 and another during young adulthood. It is unknown at this time if these are different subtypes of the disorder. Juvenile-onset OCD has a stronger family genetic transmission, affects more boys than girls, has a higher incidence of tics and neurological symptoms, and is less responsive to treatment. As with adults, OCD is characterized by repetitive, ritualistic behaviors and thoughts. Children with OCD may be misdiagnosed with learning disabilities when the compelling need to count or check interferes with homework and testing (Henin et al., 2001).

Posttraumatic Stress Disorder   Children who experience natural disasters, war, unexpected personal tragedies, and ongoing interpersonal violence are at risk for developing PTSD. Urban children and adolescents experience a distressingly high rate of trauma. Forty percent of urban adolescents report having experienced or witnessed frightening violent events. About 25 percent of these individuals develop PTSD (Silva et al., 2000; Way et al., 1999). See Chapter 23 for a complete discussion of community violence.

Older Adults

Anxiety symptoms and disorders are among the most common psychiatric illnesses experienced by older adults. Panic attacks and phobic disorder often begin earlier in life and continue on in the older years, especially when those affected have received no treatment. People who develop late-onset panic attacks, after age 55, have less avoidance behavior than those with early-onset panic attacks. Phobias remain quite common in later life (APA Practice Guidelines, 1998).

Anxiety can be manifested in various ways, including somatic complaints, rigid patterns of behavior, fatigue, hostility, and confusion. Sleep disturbances are common in persons with anxiety. Many have difficulty in getting to sleep and staying asleep, and have poor quality of sleep.

Anxiety is often associated with medical illness. The symptoms of cardiovascular disease, such as angina pectoris and myocardial infarction, may simulate panic attacks. Medications such as cold and allergy drugs, amphetamines, bronchodilators, and some calcium channel blockers may produce anxiety-like symptoms. Akathisia, a side effect of antipsychotic agents, is often indistinguishable from anxiety. Alcohol withdrawal and sedative/hypnotic withdrawal produce high levels of anxiety. There is a high prevalence of anxiety disorders in persons with Parkinson's disease. In addition, the medications used to treat Parkinson's disease may themselves cause anxiety. People suffering from dementing disorders often experience concomitant anxiety. See Chapters 18 and 19 for further information.

PHYSIOLOGICAL CHARACTERISTICS

Healthy people can usually adapt to anxiety for brief periods of time. However, when the cause is unknown, the intensity severe, or the duration chronic, normal physiological mechanisms no longer function efficiently. Refer back to Table 11.1 for the physiological characteristics of anxiety.

In *mild anxiety*, people experience an agreeable, perhaps even a pleasant, increase in tension. Mild anxiety helps people deal constructively with stress. This level of anxiety also motivates learning and produces creativity.

In *moderate anxiety*, a person remains alert but the perceptual field narrows. The focus is on the immediate concerns while blocking out extraneous sensory stimuli—a process called *selective inattention*. They may also experience a twitch in the eyelid, trembling lips, and mild gastric symptoms.

As anxiety increases to the *severe* level, the survival response of fight or flight begins. Starting in the cerebral cortex, this response is mediated through the body's nervous system and endocrine system. The sympathetic nervous system and the response of the adrenal glands lead to changes throughout the body. Heart rate increases and blood pressure rises to send more blood to the muscles. There may be frequent episodes of shortness of breath. The pupils dilate, the person may sweat, and the hands may feel cold and clammy. Some body trembling, a fearful facial expression, tense muscles, restlessness, and an exaggerated startle response may all be noticeable. There is an increased blood glucose level due to increased glycogenolysis. The moderately anxious person may verbalize subjective experiences such as a dry mouth, upset stomach, anorexia, tension headache, stiff neck, fatigue, inability to relax, and difficulty falling asleep. There may also be urinary urgency and frequency as well as either diarrhea or constipation. Sexual dysfunction may include painful intercourse, erectile disorder, orgasmic difficulties, lack of satisfaction, or a decrease in sexual desire.

When anxiety continues to the *panic level*, the body becomes so stressed it can neither adapt effectively nor organize for fight or flight. At this level of anxiety, the person is helpless to care for or defend the self. As blood returns to the major organs from the muscles, the person may become pale. Hypotension, which causes the person to feel faint, may also occur. Other signs are a quavering voice, agitation, poor motor coordination, involuntary movements, and body trembling. The facial expression is one of terror, with dilated pupils. A person feeling panic may complain of dizziness, lightheadedness, a sense of unreality, and, at times, nausea. Some of the most frightening symptoms of the panic level of anxiety are chest pain or pressure, palpitations, shortness of breath, a choking or smothering sensation, and fear of imminent death. Each person tends to experience the physiological sensations in a pattern that repeats itself with every episode of anxiety. Some people are primarily aware of internal organ reactions, whereas others primarily exhibit symptoms of muscular tension. Still others experience both visceral and muscular responses.

Medical conditions that may cause *secondary anxiety* or produce symptoms mimicking panic include hypoglycemia, hyperthyroidism, hypoparathyroidism, Cushing's syndrome, pheochromocytoma, pernicious anemia, hypoxia, hyperventilation, audiovestibular system disturbance, paroxysmal atrial tachycardia, caffeinism, and withdrawal from alcohol or benzodiazepines.

People with panic disorder, including agoraphobia, have a significantly higher incidence of mitral valve prolapse (MVP) than the general population: 57 percent compared to 5 to 7 percent. The exact relationship between MVP and panic is unclear. The symptoms of MVP—particularly tachycardia, palpitations, and shortness of breath—are similar to the symptoms of panic levels of anxiety. People predisposed to panic attacks often interpret the sensations of MVP as increased anxiety. The interpretation or expectation then evokes panic (Martin-Santos et al., 1998).

Individuals with panic disorder frequently have significantly higher cholesterol levels compared to control groups. It is thought that chronic anxiety, like stress, increases blood cholesterol (Wakefield & Pallister, 1997).

People with somatization disorders have multiple physical symptoms involving a variety of body systems. These symptoms may be vague and undefined, and they do not follow a particular disease pattern.

Pain is the primary symptom in pain disorder. The pain is severe and prolonged and usually does not follow the nerve-conduction pathways of the body.

Conversion disorder symptoms can occur in any of the sensory or motor systems of the body. The person may become suddenly blind or deaf. Loss of speech may range from persistent laryngitis to total muteness. Body parts may tingle or feel numb. Motor symptoms range from spasms or tics to paralysis of hands, arms, or legs.

In hypochondriasis, symptoms may be limited to one or several body systems. The most frequent symptoms appear in the head and neck. These include dizziness, loss of hearing, hearing one's own heartbeat, a lump in the throat, and chronic coughing. Symptoms in the abdomen and chest are common, including indigestion, bowel disorders, palpitations, skipped or rapid heartbeats, and pain in the left side of the chest. Some people may also have skin discomfort, insomnia, and sexual problems.

CONCOMITANT DISORDERS

There is a high correlation between anxiety disorders and *substance abuse*. As many as 50 to 60 percent of those who abuse substances also have one of the anxiety disorders. Typically, severe anxiety precedes the onset of the substance abuse, although for some the abuse precedes the anxiety. Believing that alcohol decreases anxiety, people with anxiety disorders often self-medicate in an effort to feel better. In fact, alcohol actually increases anxiety. The combination of increased anxiety, addiction, and continued self-medication contributes to an ever-increasing self-destructive cycle (Kushner, Sher, & Erickson, 1999).

Frequently, *depression* follows the onset of an anxiety disorder. It is thought that depression and anxiety disorders share a common biological predisposition, which may be activated by stress. Co-morbidity between anxiety disorders and major depression is associated with more impairment than either anxiety or depression alone and predicts poorer outcomes. The depression may be a response to feelings of loss of control, hopelessness, helplessness, decreased self-esteem, and severe restrictions on lifestyle. Suicide can be a lethal complication. Of those suffering from panic attacks, 20 percent make suicide attempts (Mendlowicz & Stein, 2000; Silverstone & Salinas, 2001).

Children with anxiety disorders often struggle with depression, attention deficit disorders, oppositional behaviors, and peer deficits. The child who is anxious is less likely to have friends or even be able to develop relationships with peers. It is possible that feeling anxious and alone leads to depression. Some behaviors of anxious children, such as fidgeting and distractibility, are also criteria for attention deficit disorder. Anxious children often exhibit oppositional behavior such as tantrums, refusal to do things, and arguing with authority. See Chapter 17 for more information on these spectrum disorders.

CAUSATIVE THEORIES

No single theory can adequately explain the cause and maintenance of any of the anxiety disorders. They are best understood as a complex interaction of situational and constitutional factors.

Genetics

It appears that some component of anxiety runs in families, although the exact role of *genetic predisposition* is unknown at this time. It is thought that a general "anxiety proneness" may be genetically transmitted. People with a high sensitivity to anxiety report more subjective anxiety and more intense physical symptoms. They are more likely to experience anticipatory anxiety (McNally, 2001).

It is believed that multiple genes are involved in anxiety disorders. First-degree relatives of persons with panic disorder have a 3- to 21-fold higher lifetime risk of panic disorder. Relatives of persons with social phobia have a 10 times greater risk of social phobia. Twin studies suggest that there is a significant heritable component in both panic disorder and generalized anxiety disorder with the concordance rate of 35 percent for monozygotic twins and only 6 to 12 percent for dizygotic twins (Biederman et al., 2001; Smoller & Tsuang, 1998; Stein et al., 1998).

Research in obsessive–compulsive disorder is now focusing on *genetic factors*. In this disorder, children and adults experience identical symptoms, whereas in most of the other mental disorders, children's symptoms are quite different from those of adults. In addition, 50 percent of adults with OCD state that their symptoms began when they were children; only 5 percent of adults with other mental disorders report childhood onset. In 39 percent of women with OCD who also have children, the onset of the disorder occurred during pregnancy. Of OCD sufferers, 20 percent have a first-degree relative with the same problem. Father–son combinations are the most common in these families. It is unlikely that the behavior is learned within the family, given the high level of secrecy. In addition, children and parents may have very different rituals; for example, the parent may engage in checking rituals, whereas the child may engage in washing rituals (Pauls, 1995).

Neurobiologic Theory

The neurobiologic factors involved in the anxiety disorders include dysregulation of neurochemical and neuroendocrine processes and alterations in central nervous system structure.

Women are more prone than men to essentially all anxiety disorders. Simple phobia is twice as common in women as in men. The lifetime prevalence of social phobia is about 2 percent in the general population, and 70 percent of those affected are women. Uncomplicated panic disorder occurs at a gender ratio of 20 to 8. Agoraphobia with or without panic attacks is found in nearly 8 percent of women versus 3 percent of men. Generalized anxiety disorder is twice as common in women as in men. Almost twice as many women as men suffer from posttraumatic stress disorder. Because women complain of premenstrual and postpartum exacerbations of anxiety and panic states, *hormonal fluctuations* are being considered as possible contributors to understanding the difference between the genders in anxiety disorders. Progesterone and estrogen act as agonists at the GABA (benzodiazepine) receptor. It is possible that cyclic withdrawal of these hormones makes women more sensitive to stress and anxiety (Seeman, 1997).

Some believe anxious individuals have an overly responsive autonomic nervous system related to a *dysfunction* of *serotonin* (5-HT) and *norepinephrine* (NE) neurotransmission. A hyperactive autonomic nervous system may be responsible for the characteristics of high levels of anxiety such as impulsiveness, agitation, restlessness, sleep and cognitive disturbances, and aggression. People with panic disorder and PTSD suffer from an *abnormally sensitive fear network* that includes the amygdala, hippocampus, and other brain stem areas. The oversensitivity means that the brain is instantly hyperaroused by fearful stimuli, with the cortex so overwhelmed that it is unable to focus. Whether this abnormality reflects altered blood flow, a change in neuronal activity, or an unusual input or output from the area is not known at this time (Gorman et al., 2000; Ratey, 2001).

Panic attacks often occur in areas such as restaurants, elevators, cars, and planes, where there is an *increased concentration* of people and *carbon dioxide* (CO_2). Fresh air has a CO_2 level of 300 parts per million (ppm). In cars, the CO_2 level reaches 750 ppm, and in elevators and planes as high as 900 ppm. As CO_2 increases in the brain, neurons in the brain stem activate and send signals to the locus coeruleus, which increases the release of norepinephrine (NE), leading to the fight-or-flight response. Stimulants that alter NE transmission (including caffeine, cocaine, and amphetamines) can precipitate panic attacks. It is believed that some biological vulnerability is present, which—when combined with certain psychological,

social, and environmental events—leads to the development of panic disorder (Kent et al., 2001).

Social phobia may be associated with *decreased dopamine* (DA) transmission related to a reduced number of DA synapses. High DA transmission leads to increased activity, novelty seeking, and exploratory behavior, all of which are the opposite of symptoms of social phobia (Schneier et al., 2000).

Positron-emission tomography (PET) scans and magnetic resonance imaging (MRIs) provide evidence of *neurological deficit* in many individuals suffering from OCD. The abnormality apparently lies in a pathway that links the frontal lobes of the cerebral cortex with the basal ganglia. Heightened activity in the cortex may reflect obsessional thinking, while compulsions may originate in the basal ganglia where body movements are planned and executed (Antai-Otong, 2000; Henin et al., 2001).

There appear to be biological changes in PTSD that illustrate the influence of psychological events on neurobiology. When high levels of adrenaline and other stress hormones are circulating, *memory traces* are deeply imprinted. These are then reactivated as if the traumatic event were actually occurring. Traumatic nightmares can occur in stages of sleep in which people do not ordinarily dream. Thus, traumatic memories appear to be based in altered neurophysiological organization. People with PTSD tend to have low levels of the stress hormone cortisol, but have an overabundance of epinephrine and norepinephrine, which could be why they continue to feel anxious after the trauma. In addition, they tend to have higher-than-usual levels of corticotropin-releasing factor (CRF), which switches on the stress response and may explain why people with PTSD startle so easily (Bremner et al., 2000; National Institute of Mental Health [NIMH], 2000).

Little is known about the biology of depersonalization disorder. PET scans demonstrate higher-than-normal glucose metabolism in portions of the *sensory cortex* in the temporal, parietal, and occipital lobes. Normally, it is in these areas where visual and somatosensory information is integrated to provide an intact well-integrated body image (Simeon et al., 2000).

Intrapersonal Theory

Intrapersonal theorists view anxiety disorders as a reaction to anticipated future danger based on past experiences such as separation, loss of love, and guilt. The resulting anxiety is pushed out of conscious awareness by the use of *defense mechanisms* such as repression, projection, displacement, or symbolization. As stress increases, the defenses become increasingly inefficient, symptoms develop, and the person engages in repeated self-defeating behavior.

In dissociative disorders, stressful life events are disowned and kept out of conscious awareness by *amnesia*. For example, a young girl who is abused physically and sexually by her father remains dependent on her family system. The perpetrator is a trusted parent, and the other parent is incapable of protecting or rescuing her from the situation. The trauma of abuse leaves the child terrified, depressed, angry, and filled with shame and guilt. Dissociating the abuse and denying the events enable the child to remain in the family with the least amount of pain.

People suffering from anxiety disorders often have an *external locus of control*. They regard life events as out of their control, occurring by luck, chance, or fate. When stressful events occur, they attribute the feeling of anxiety not to themselves but to external sources, which then can be phobically avoided.

Adaptation to stress and anxiety depends to some extent on *personality traits*, which determine how one views stress and also the coping activities that follow. For example, individuals with negative expectations may have less successful coping strategies when confronted with high levels of anxiety. Other people fear anxiety-related sensations and believe that these sensations have harmful consequences. For example, a person may fear that the sensation of palpitations indicates a heart attack. According to *expectancy theory*, such a person may become anxious whenever this symptom is experienced and may tend to avoid activities or places that are believed to bring it on.

The tendency to react to stressful situations with somatic complaints may be part of an *avoidant coping style*. The original source of anxiety is unrecognized, and the discomfort is experienced as physical symptoms or disorders. Somatoform disorders may also be unconscious expressions of anger in those unable to communicate such feelings directly. Because physical distress provides an acceptable excuse for avoiding certain activities and situations, people may unconsciously use physical limitations to *rationalize* their inadequacies.

Interpersonal Theory

Interpersonal theorists believe people with anxiety disorders become anxious when they sense or fear disapproval from significant others. They may feel trapped in unpleasant circumstances, believing they are unable to leave the situation. Fearing abandonment, they are unable to behave assertively during conflict. Thus, the anxiety experienced during *interpersonal conflict* is displaced onto the immediate surroundings, thereby allowing them to deny the interpersonal problem. Obsessive–compulsive or phobic behavior protects the self and the relationship during interactions with significant others.

Interpersonal theories focus on the *secondary gains* for people suffering from somatoform disorders. For those with a high degree of dependency, physical symptoms may receive a great deal of attention and support from significant others. The sympathy and nurturing these people receive may be a major factor in maintaining the disorders. The attention from others may be viewed as seeking reassurance of care and love or, since sick or weak people are often in a position of power, as an unconscious attempt to gain power and control.

Cognitive Theory

Cognitive theorists believe symptoms develop from ideas and thoughts. On the basis of limited events, people with anxiety disorders magnify the significance of the past and overgeneralize to the future. They become preoccupied with impending disaster and self-defeating statements. These *cognitive expectations* then determine reactions to and behavior in various situations (Wakefield & Pallister, 1997).

Cognitive theory explains phobic disorders in a three-part sequence:

1. Phobic people have negative thoughts that increase anxiety and actually precede the feeling of fear in the phobic situation. Phobic people also have irrational thinking and unrealistic expectations about what might occur if the phobic situation is encountered.

2. These anticipatory thoughts and feelings enhance the physiological arousal level even before the phobic situation is encountered.

3. The physiological arousal level is misinterpreted. Although thought to be caused by an external

object or situation, the arousal is caused by the negative thoughts and *irrational expectations*. This mislabeling of feelings causes phobic people to displace the feelings onto objects or situations that can be avoided.

Learning Theory

Phobias may be *learned* from significant others. If a child observes a parent experiencing anxiety in certain situations, the child may learn that anxiety is the appropriate response. For example, if the mother has a phobic avoidance of elevators, the child soon learns to fear entering an elevator. A child can also learn parental fears through information given by the parent. A father may talk about the dangers of going outside when it is dark, and the child may develop agoraphobia during the nighttime.

People who develop dissociative disorders often consider themselves passive and helpless. They are fearful of others' anger and aggressive behavior. Unable to behave assertively or aggressively, they learn to cope by escaping or avoiding the anxiety-producing situations. Thus, they learn to avoid pain through *amnesia* or the development of dissociative identities.

Behavioral Theory

Closely related to learning theory is the behavioral theory of how phobic disorders develop. Behavioral theorists believe phobias are *conditioned, learned responses*. Classical conditioning occurs when a stimulus results in anxiety or pain. The person then develops a fear of that particular stimulus. An example is a person who fears all dogs after being bitten by one dog. The learning component of behavioral theory states that the avoidance of the phobic object or situation is negatively reinforced by a decrease in anxiety. Because the person experiences less anxiety when avoiding the object or situation, avoidance becomes a habitual response.

Behavioral theorists view OCD as learned responses to anticipatory anxiety. It is thought that these individuals always expect bad things to happen and worry constantly. The compulsive behaviors and thoughts are maladaptive attempts to reduce anxiety.

According to behavioral theory, the somatoform disorders are learned somatic responses. It is thought that these individuals are unable to deal directly with stress and habitually respond to stress with physical sensations or symptoms.

Feminist Theory

Feminist theory has been used to explain the disproportionate number of women who experience agoraphobia. These theorists believe women have been reinforced to behave *dependently, passively,* and *submissively*. This behavior often results in adult women who are unable to assume responsibility for themselves and who view themselves as incompetent and helpless. Often, the symptoms are reinforced by family members who also have been socialized to expect women to be helpless and dependent. Thus, the pattern of withdrawal can continue until the woman is completely homebound.

PSYCHOPHARMACOLOGICAL INTERVENTIONS

Medications are often used on a short-term basis to help people manage anxiety disorders (see Table 11.5 ■).

In GAD, the therapeutic goal in using antianxiety agents is to limit unpleasant symptoms to help the person return to a high level of functioning. Effexor (venlafaxine), a selective norepinephrine reuptake inhibitor (SNRI) antidepressant has Food and Drug Administration (FDA) approval for GAD. Another medication choice is the nonbenzodiazepine antianxiety agent BuSpar (buspirone), which is more effective than the benzodiazepines in managing GAD. BuSpar blocks 5-HT receptors and causes minimal sedation. This medication is better than the benzodiazepines for the addiction-prone person because dosage increases result in a general sense of feeling ill. In addition, BuSpar reacts only minimally with alcohol, since it interacts very little with other central nervous system (CNS) depressants. However, clients should be cautioned not to expect an immediate effect.

Because anxiety may be related to a dysregulation of 5-HT and NE, tricyclic antidepressants have been used in the medical treatment of GAD. Tofranil (imipramine) has been found to be the most effective medication in this group.

Selective serotonin reuptake inhibitors (SSRIs) are rapidly becoming the first-line medication treatment for panic disorder. The goal of treatment is to reduce the intensity and frequency of panic attacks, decrease anticipatory anxiety, and treat the associated depression.

TABLE 11.5

Medications Commonly Used to Treat Anxiety Disorders

Generic Name	Trade Name	Disorders
Antianxiety Agents		
Buspirone	BuSpar	GAD, panic disorder, agoraphobia, PTSD
Alprazolam	Xanax	PTSD
Tricyclic Antidepressants		
Imipramine	Tofranil	GAD, agoraphobia
Selective Serotonin Reuptake Inhibitors (SSRIs)		
Citalopram	Celexa	Panic disorder, OCD,
Fluoxetine	Prozac	body dysmorphic disorder,
Fluvoxamine	Luvox	social phobia, PTSD
Paroxetine	Paxil	
Sertraline	Zoloft	
Venlafaxine	Effexor	
Monoamine Oxidase Inhibitors (MAOIs)		
Phenelzine	Nardil	Social phobia, agoraphobia
Beta Blockers		
Atenolol	Tenormin	Social phobia (given before the event), PTSD
Propranolol	Inderal	

Typically, it takes 4 weeks before a therapeutic response occurs, but some people will not experience full response for 8 to 12 weeks. Combining an antidepressant with an antianxiety agent provides for rapid stabilization of panic symptoms (Goddard et al., 2001; Gorman, 2000).

Social phobias severe enough to interfere with social and occupational functioning may be treated with Paxil (paroxetine), an FDA-approved antidepressant for social phobias. Paxil does not eliminate the anxiety entirely but controls it enough that other interventions are more effective.

Social phobias severe enough to interfere with occupational functioning may be treated with a beta blocker, either Inderal (propranolol) or Tenormin (atenolol). Beta blockers are particularly effective in situations in which cardiovascular symptoms of anxiety are disruptive to the individual. Because they do not

cross the blood–brain barrier, beta blockers have no effect on neurotransmission, nor do they produce loss of fine motor control (Stein et al., 1999).

The following SSRIs are often effective in the treatment of OCD: Prozac (fluoxetine), Zoloft (sertraline), Luvox (fluvoxamine), and Paxil (paroxetine). Of people suffering from OCD, 70 to 80 percent respond to these medications (Greist, 1999).

Probably the most useful drugs for people with PTSD are the antidepressants, which not only relieve depression but also improve sleep and suppress intrusive thoughts, jumpiness, and explosive anger. Zoloft (sertraline) is the only FDA-approved drug for PTSD. The beta blockers Inderal (propranolol) and Tenormin (atenolol) may reduce the restlessness and anxiety by depressing the sympathetic nervous system (Davidson et al., 2001). See Chapter 8 for more in-depth information on these medications.

MULTIDISCIPLINARY INTERVENTIONS

Medications play an important role in medical interventions, but intrapersonal and interpersonal aspects must also be treated. Clients and their families need to cope with various aspects of anxiety, learn to take control of their lives, and manage family stress. All of these are accomplished through a blending of techniques and the use of individual, family, and group psychotherapy.

The most effective behavioral intervention technique is *exposure and response prevention.* Clients are exposed, in reality or in their mind, to feared situations or objects and try to refrain from or delay their usual phobic or ritualistic response. Virtual reality programs safely simulate the object or situation most feared. Gradually, the unwanted response disappears. *Stress inoculation training* involves rehearsing other coping skills and testing these skills under stressful situations. While this process provides fairly immediate relief from anxiety, it must be practiced over a period of time for long-term effect. This is often referred to as a desensitization process.

Florean has a strong fear of contamination. Whenever she touches any surface that she thinks might be contaminated, she washes her hands for five minutes. With the help of her therapist, Florean has planned a program in which she will touch a wastebasket several times and stop herself from washing her hands until one minute has passed. The goal is to refrain from handwashing for longer and longer periods of time. After that goal has been reached, Florean will work on reducing the length of time she spends washing her hands until the behavior is largely under her control.

Individual psychotherapy and hypnosis are used to uncover the abuse and trauma of DID. Nonverbal therapies, such as play therapy, art therapy, and occupational therapy, and journal writing are also extensively used. One goal is to help the client discover that the various personalities are real and distinct but are not separate individuals. The client learns that all the personalities belong to each other and that they are all parts of the same person and same body. Hypnosis helps the personalities come to know each other, communicate with each other, and share skills.

ALTERNATIVE THERAPIES

There are several *herbs* that are used for the treatment of anxiety disorders. Chamomile can be infused by pouring hot water over the herb, steeped for three to five minutes, and strained before drinking. Honey or lemon may be added to taste. Chamomile can also be purchased as a tincture with a dosage of 1 teaspoon three times a day. Chamomile, a member of the ragweed family, should not be used by people who have ragweed allergy (Muskin, 2000).

Kava kava, a South Pacific herb, contains alphapyrones, a recently discovered class of potent skeletal muscle relaxants. It is unknown at this time if kava affects the GABA (benzodiazepine) receptors. The dose is 70 to 100 mg, three times a day. Kava kava should not be taken with St. John's wort, any antianxiety medications, any antidepressants, or with alcohol as its effects may be increased.

Essential oils influence health on physical, mental, and emotional levels. The basis of action is thought to be the same as modern pharmacology, using smaller doses. The purity and authenticity of essential oils is critical to their effectiveness. Oils that are diluted, adulterated, or synthetic should not be used for aromatherapy. Essential oils are quite potent and can irritate the skin, so they should be diluted with a carrier oil before being used on the skin. Oils used to decrease anxiety include chamomile, green apple, lemon balm, neroli, and orange. Oils to improve sleep include chamomile, clary sage, lavender, marjoram, neroli, and vetiver.

Homeopathic remedies are believed to stimulate a person's self-healing capacity. Pulsatilla (windflower) is helpful for people who are highly emotional, weepy, fearful of abandonment, and worried about what others think of them. Ignatia (St. Ignatius bean) is helpful for those experiencing anxiety.

Massage has been used with people having anxiety disorders as an adjunct to conventional psychiatric interventions. Clients are given an executive massage, done with the client fully dressed and seated on a massage chair. The head, neck, back, arms, and legs are massaged for 10 to 20 minutes per session.

Therapeutic Touch (TT) works in conjunction with other medical or therapeutic techniques to alleviate anxiety and irritability. It has been found to significantly reduce "state anxiety" in some clients and to reduce stress in both children and adults. TT has also

CRITICAL THINKING

You are working on a medical unit in a large teaching hospital. It is a very busy unit, but the nurse manager is very aware of the needs of the clients on the unit, including their psychological needs. In fact, this is one of the reasons you decided to take your first job as a nurse on this unit. In the past week, there have been several complex clients on the unit. Mr. Grenstein was transferred from the coronary care unit following a myocardial infarction (MI). This was his first MI. At the age of 50, he had had no significant health history. Mr. Grenstein is irritable, is unable to sleep for more than four hours at night, and complains of periods of shortness of breath. On assessment, he is sweating and appears tense. After careful assessment, it is determined that he is not experiencing further cardiac problems.

Another patient, Mrs. Smithville, was admitted with a diagnosis of pneumonia. She has a history of asthma. Her family explained that Mrs. Smithville, who is 70 years old, became ill two days ago with a high fever; however, they said that they were concerned about her before the pneumonia. She was unusually tense, unable to concentrate for long periods of time, and felt the need to move around. Prior to the pneumonia, Mrs. Smithville was prescribed new medications for her asthma, Poventil (albuterol) and Slo-Bid (theophylline). Mrs. Smithville's daughter said that she was not sure that her mother was taking the medication as prescribed as she ran out of the medications before the dates on the prescriptions.

It is not unusual to have clients on the unit with multiple problems, and the nurse manager has called for a meeting to discuss some of these client problems and how the staff can better meet the needs of their clients.

1. Mr. Grenstein's anxiety is discussed in the meeting. Based on the data provided, what level of anxiety might he be experiencing? Explain the physiological symptoms of this level. Why would they be of concern with this particular client?

2. One staff member brings up her concern about the need to assess anxiety and depression. What might you add to the conversation about concomitant disorders, particularly anxiety and depression?

3. One staff member has recently attended a seminar on anxiety, and he discusses the need to understand GAD and also coping and defense mechanisms. Compare and contrast coping and defense mechanisms. How do they relate to GAD?

4. Considering the comments from Mrs. Smithville's daughter and Mrs. Smithville's diagnoses and history, what is important about Mrs. Smithville's new medications for asthma?

5. The discussion then moves to the nursing care for these two clients. What might be some nursing diagnoses and related interventions for Mr. Grenstein related to his anxiety?

For an additional Case Study, please refer to the Companion Web site for this book.

---

been found to reduce anxiety levels for people who are hospitalized for medical–surgical problems (Engle & Graney, 2000; Gerber, 2000).

Yoga is tailored to the individual and can be done with great benefit at the beginner level as well as the most advanced level. Attention is paid to how the body feels and what it is doing. Every movement is made gently and slowly. Every yoga session ends with a few minutes of complete and total relaxation. The psychiatric benefits of yoga include increasing brain endorphins, enkephalins, and serotonin; and to promote relaxation, and manage stress. In PTSD due to sexual and physical abuse, yoga postures should be used with extreme caution because they may stimulate flashbacks to the traumatic situation (Muskin, 2000).

If practiced regularly, even 15 minutes twice a day, *meditation* produces widespread positive effects on physical and psychological functioning. The autonomic nervous system responds with a decrease in heart rate, lower blood pressure, decreased respiratory rate and oxygen consumption, and a lower arousal threshold. All of this is helpful in reducing levels of general anxiety and worry. There are as many ways to meditate as there are people. When people say they have tried meditation and cannot do it, they just have not found the right practice for them. One may want to sit, one do repetitive prayers, one swim or run, one walk, and one do yoga or T'ai Chi. Encourage clients to explore a variety of techniques and develop the habit of meditation on a daily basis.

NURSING PROCESS

Assessment

Assess the client using the knowledge base provided in this chapter. Because of the shame and secrecy surrounding anxiety disorders, clients may not reveal symptoms unless you ask direct, specific questions. An organized scheme of focused assessment ensures that all areas—behavioral, affective, cognitive, and social characteristics—are assessed. As always, assessment questions must be modified to the individual client's cognitive, developmental, educational, and language abilities. See the Focused Nursing Assessment feature on the following pages.

You will see the majority of clients suffering from anxiety disorders in community settings, clinics, physicians' offices, emergency departments, and medical–surgical units. Because these clients often have complicated and detailed medical histories, careful physiological assessment is necessary. Remember that, at any given time, a client with an anxiety disorder may develop an organic illness. Thus, continual physiological assessment is a necessary component of your nursing care.

The physiological assessment must differentiate anxiety responses from various organic conditions that have similar symptoms. The most common conditions are hypoglycemia, hyperthyroidism, hypoparathyroidism, pheochromocytoma, and mitral valve prolapse. Similar symptoms may also occur during withdrawal from barbiturates and antianxiety agents and with the use of cocaine. High levels of caffeine, amphetamines, theophyllines, beta agonists, steroids, and decongestants may also be initially confused with anxiety disorders. Anxiety will frequently be seen as another symptom in people who have been diagnosed with schizophrenia, a mood disorder, or an eating disorder.

Children can be assessed through verbal interaction, nonverbal observations, and parental or teacher reports. Young children may not have the language skills to describe their thoughts and feelings, but they are often able to communicate through play, sand trays, and art. Nonverbal assessments should be consistent with the child's developmental level.

Diagnosis

The next step in the nursing process is to analyze and synthesize the assessment data to form nursing diag-

noses. You must consider the client's level of anxiety as well as the behavioral, affective, cognitive, and physiological responses to the anxiety. Other considerations are the client's self-evaluation, degree of insight, positive coping behavior, defense mechanisms, and the family/friendship systems. See the Nursing Diagnoses with NOC & NIC feature on pages 302–303 for examples of diagnoses for clients with anxiety disorders.

Outcome Identification and Goals

Based on the assessment data, you select outcomes appropriate to the nursing diagnoses. The most common outcomes are found in the Nursing Diagnoses with NOC & NIC feature.

Once you have established outcomes, you and the client mutually identify goals for change. Client goals are specific behavioral prescriptions that you, the client, and significant others identify as realistic and attainable. The following are examples of goals that may be pertinent to those with anxiety disorders:

- Verbalize feeling less anxiety
- Verbalize less tension and restlessness
- Experience fewer episodes of panic
- Report less time in obsessive–compulsive behaviors
- Verbalize less shame about the disorder
- Develop effective coping behaviors
- Utilize support systems when anxious
- Report fewer dissociative episodes
- Verbalize fewer somatic complaints
- Describe a state of spiritual well-being

Nursing Interventions

Nursing diagnoses give direction for the development of goals and outcome criteria, which help focus your nursing care. If possible, involve the client in developing the plan of care. If the client wants something quite different from what you expect, the nursing care plan

Behavior Assessment	Affective Assessment	Cognitive Assessment	Social Assessment
Obsessive–Compulsive Disorder			
What kinds of objects or situations do you feel a need to check or recheck frequently? How much time during a day do you spend on checking activities? Describe any movements you are forced to repeat. What kinds of things do you count, silently or out loud?	Describe how you experience the feeling of anxiety. What happens to you when you feel out of control in situations? Describe your relationships with significant others. How do these others relate to you? What are your greatest fears in life?	Describe the qualities you like about yourself. Describe the qualities you do not like about yourself. What are your thoughts about your compulsive behavior? Would you like to decrease the need for your compulsive behavior? How much time a day do you spend doubting what you have done?	In what way do habits or thoughts get in the way of work? Social life? Personal life? Describe situations in which you feel close to and warm with your family members. In what ways do you feel dependent on your family?
Phobic Disorders			
What situations or objects do you try to avoid in life? Describe what you do to avoid these situations or objects. To what degree do these fears interfere with your daily routines? Are your social or work activities limited to a prescribed geographic area? How often and in what circumstances are you able to leave home?	What are your greatest fears in life? Do you fear others laughing at you? Being humiliated? Being abandoned by others? Being alone in an unfamiliar situation? What feelings do you experience when you are confronted with the situation or object that you fear? What else happens to you at this time? To what degree do you fear having future panic attacks?	Do you dislike being controlled by your fears? What does the future look like for you? Describe the qualities you like about yourself. Describe the qualities you do not like about yourself. How much support do you need from others to cope with life? How helpless and dependent on others do you feel?	Who is able to support you in avoiding your feared situations or objects? Describe how family living patterns have changed around your fears. Under what circumstances are you able to socialize with friends?
Posttraumatic Stress Disorder			
Under what circumstances do you experience outbursts of aggressive behavior? In what ways have you been reexperiencing the original trauma?	How much time during a day do you feel tense or irritable? Have you been experiencing panic attacks? Describe the guilt you have been experiencing in relation to the original trauma.	Describe difficulties you have had with concentration. Describe difficulties you have had with your memory.	In what ways do your family members and friends tell you that you are distant or cold in your relationships with them? Describe your communication patterns with family members and friends.

Behavior Assessment	Affective Assessment	Cognitive Assessment	Social Assessment

Posttraumatic Stress Disorder *(continued)*

Behavior Assessment	Affective Assessment	Cognitive Assessment	Social Assessment
In what ways do you attempt to avoid situations or activities that may remind you of the original trauma? How frequently do you participate in social activities? Have you had any employment difficulties since the original trauma?	What types of activities do you enjoy doing? What are sources of pleasure for you in your life? Describe relationships in which you feel emotionally close to other people.	How often, in a day, do you have recurrent thoughts about the original trauma? Do you feel you have control over these thoughts? Describe any nightmares you have. Describe the qualities you like about yourself. Describe the qualities you do not like about yourself.	Describe what happens when you lose control of your anger. How is violence handled within your family system? Are you experiencing relationship difficulties?

Dissociative Identity Disorder*

Behavior Assessment	Affective Assessment	Cognitive Assessment	Social Assessment
Does the client have widely varying behavior patterns, such as at times being submissive and quiet and at other times loud and outspoken? Does the client have different styles of dressing that correspond to a change in behavior? Are vocational or leisure skills inconsistent; that is, are these skills apparent at some times and not at other times?	Does the client experience anxiety about "lost" time? In what ways is the client passive and submissive? In what ways is the client angry and aggressive?	Describe the frequency of amnesic periods. Under what circumstances does this amnesia seem to appear? Are there times when the client can remember specific events and other times when there is amnesia for the same events?	Do family members describe the client as having different personalities? How has the family tried to manage the situation thus far? Is there a known history of child abuse for the client? Describe the client's relationship to his or her parents as a child.

Somatoform Disorders

Behavior Assessment	Affective Assessment	Cognitive Assessment	Social Assessment
What OTC medications are you currently taking? How effective are they? What prescription medications are you currently taking? How effective are they? What medications have you taken in the past? What results were obtained with them? Who have you consulted professionally for your illness in the past five years? What diagnostic procedures have been performed? What surgeries have you had in your lifetime?	In what situations do you experience feelings of anger? In what situations do you experience feelings of anxiety? In what way do you share your feelings with others? How do you respond when others become angry with you?	How often, in a day, are you aware of your physical symptoms? How aware are you of bodily sensations? Do you believe you have a serious illness? Has this illness been confirmed by a health care provider? Describe your level of concern for your physical health.	How is your family managing with your illness? Who is supportive to you in this illness? Who cares for you when you are unable to care for yourself? How has your illness affected the family's financial situation?

Since the client is unaware of changes in personalities, the assessment data are based on your observations and family reporting.

will not be appropriate; in fact, the client will likely sabotage it. The overall goal is to help the client improve the response to anxiety and develop more constructive behavior to manage anxiety. Some agencies develop critical pathways for treatment planning and evaluation. See Critical Pathway for a Client with Panic Disorder feature on pages 304–305 for a sample critical pathway.

Behavioral: Psychological Comfort Promotion

Anxiety Reduction

Clients who are extremely anxious or in a panic state of anxiety respond best to a *calm, direct approach*. Stay with clients to promote safety and reduce fear. Provide reassurance that you will stay with them and that this attack will go away. Speak slowly in a gentle voice and use short simple sentences, as highly anxious people have great difficulty focusing or concentrating. Examples are: "I will stay," "Sit down," or "I will help." Loosen any tight clothing to ease the sensation of choking. Tell clients to take slow, deep breaths, and breathe with the client to demonstrate and to gradually slow down the breathing. Direct them to imagine inhaling and exhaling through the soles of the feet. During a panic attack, people feel disconnected from the environment, and this imagery helps people feel grounded and therefore safer. If possible, move to a quieter room in the home, clinic, or hospital.

Clients who have a phobia experience anxiety when confronted with the feared object or situation. Help them *express the fears* that interfere with their lives while presenting a nonjudgmental attitude. Encourage clients to search for, confront, and relieve the source of the original anxiety. Together, you can *rehearse* various *coping behaviors* that increase their sense of control. They may picture the event step by step, picture themselves coping effectively, and practice relaxation techniques during this process. This visualization helps them move in the direction of their expectations. Visualizing effective coping reinforces their self-image as a person capable of dealing with fear, while relaxation training reduces the physical sensations that provoke anxiety and panic.

Distraction techniques are also useful tools because they allow the person to remain in control when experiencing moderate levels of anxiety. Examples of distraction techniques are listening to music, reading a book, talking to a close friend, and playing a game.

Positive imagery allows the person to focus away from the anxiety-producing stimulus and onto a positive image that feels safe. Examples are picturing sitting quietly on a beach, being held by a trusted person, and playing with a pet. Counting backward by threes also provides a distraction from the sensations of anxiety.

Many anxiety-disordered clients find *journal keeping* extremely helpful. Making entries one or several times a day is a useful way to keep track of thoughts, feelings, and memories. This self-monitoring technique helps them identify events preceding, during, and after anxiety occurs. They are encouraged to write down effective coping strategies that they will be able to refer to during a future time of anxiety. For clients with OCD, journal keeping often helps them begin to identify anxiety cues and to initiate anxiety-reducing techniques before the anxiety becomes overwhelming. Clients with DID might find journal keeping to be less threatening than sharing the same details verbally with you. Talking about the abuse is usually a later step. Because several personalities often write, the journal becomes one way the personalities can communicate and cooperate with one another. Some DID units have a journal group in which clients talk about self-discovery through writing.

Clients who have a somatization disorder benefit from *set limits* on the amount of time they talk about their physical complaints. Encourage them to recognize and discuss their fears rather than to somatize their feelings. Avoid implying that physical symptoms are imaginary because anxiety would increase if the client did not feel believed.

Calming Technique

Calming techniques such as *muscle relaxation* and *deep breathing* are useful for managing the physiological dimensions of anxiety. Deep breathing replaces the shallow breathing that highly anxious people adopt unconsciously, and prevents hyperventilation. The goal is to provide clients with a skill response so that they can experience anxiety without feeling overwhelmed. In addition to focusing on and relaxing specific muscle groups, teach clients to take a deep breath through the nose, inhaling to the count of five, and then exhaling to the count of five. Progressive relaxation should be practiced twice a day for 20 minutes. It will be several weeks before clients experience significant benefit. Even fairly young children can be taught this technique. Children often enjoy this exercise, and it helps

NURSING DIAGNOSES with NOC & NIC

Clients with Anxiety Disorders

DIAGNOSIS	OUTCOMES	INTERVENTIONS
Anxiety, mild, related to threat to self-concept due to fear of being out of control	**Anxiety Control**: Personal actions to eliminate or reduce feelings of apprehension and tension from an unidentifiable source	Anxiety Reduction Simple Guided Imagery Cognitive Restructuring Nutritional Counseling Exercise Promotion Massage Acupressure
Ineffective breathing pattern related to choking or smothering sensations, shortness of breath, and hyperventilation associated with the panic level of anxiety	**Anxiety Control**	Calming Technique
Sensory-perceptual alteration related to decreased perceptual field during panic level of anxiety	**Anxiety Control**	Calming Technique
Alteration in thought processes related to difficulty in concentrating and concrete thinking during panic level of anxiety	**Concentration**: Ability to focus on a specific stimulus	Calming Technique
Ineffective individual coping related to being consumed with obsessive and/or compulsive behavior	**Coping**: Actions to manage stressors that tax an individual's resources	Emotional Support Cognitive Restructuring

them recognize when their bodies are tightening up. Eventually, they learn how to cope with stress by breathing deep and then shaking it off.

Other calming techniques you can teach clients involve changing their sensory experiences or getting involved in activities. Some people like to take a walk or read a book; others like to hold on to a pillow or rub a worry stone; and others find that talking to a friend or singing a song calms them down. They can say positive affirmations aloud such as: "I am calm and happy," "My breathing is slow and even," "I am very relaxed."

DIAGNOSIS	OUTCOMES	INTERVENTIONS
Alteration in family process related to detachment and inability to express feelings, or to struggle for power and control	**Family Coping:** Family actions to manage stressors that tax family resources	Family Integrity Promotion
Fear related to confrontation with feared object or situation	**Fear Control:** Personal actions to eliminate or reduce disabling feelings of alarm aroused by an identifiable source	Anxiety Reduction Security Enhancement Cognitive Restructuring
Social isolation related to fear of leaving neighborhood or home or to physical symptoms and disability	**Social Support:** Perceived availability and actual provision of reliable assistance from other persons	Support System Enhancement Socialization Enhancement
Spiritual distress related to a view of the world and people as threatening following a severe traumatic event	**Spiritual Well-Being:** Personal expressions of connectedness with self, others, higher power, all life, nature, and the universe that transcend and empower the self	Spiritual Support

SOURCES: Johnson, M., Maas, M., & Moorhead, S. (2000). *Nursing outcomes classification (NOC)* (2nd ed.). St. Louis, MO: Mosby; McCloskey, J. C., & Bulechek, G. M. (1996). *Nursing interventions classification (NIC)* (2nd ed.). St. Louis, MO: Mosby; and North American Nursing Diagnosis Association (1999). *Nursing diagnoses, definitions and classification 1999–2000.* Philadelphia: Author

Simple Guided Imagery

Simple guided imagery is the purposeful use of imagination to achieve relaxation and/or direct attention away from undesirable sensations. It is not appropriate to use if anxiety is at the severe or panic level. Instruct individuals to assume a comfortable position and close their eyes. Make suggestions that induce relaxation such as describing peaceful images or slow, gentle breathing. Ask clients to imagine something they would like to have happen, such as no fear response when confronted with their phobic situation. Ask them to imagine that it has already happened and have

CRITICAL PATHWAY for a CLIENT with PANIC DISORDER

Outpatient Treatment

Expected length of treatment 8 weeks	Date _____ Weeks 1–2	Date _____ Weeks 3–6	Date _____ Weeks 7–8
Weekly outcomes	Client will: • Identify initial goals for therapy. • Contract for ongoing treatment. • Participate in treatment plan. • Begin to identify sources of anxiety/panic.	Client will: • Identify ongoing goals for therapy. • Maintain contract for ongoing therapy. • Participate in treatment plan. • Identify strategies to manage anxiety and panic.	Client will: • Describe ongoing strategies to manage panic disorder. • Demonstrate ability to cope with ongoing feelings of panic. • Describe strategies to cope with an inability to cope with stressors.
Assessments, tests, and treatments	Psychosocial assessment. Explore factors that precipitate panic attacks.	Psychosocial assessment. Assess recent history of anxiety and panic attacks. Explore contributing factors. Discuss effectiveness of cognitive restructuring strategies.	Psychosocial assessment. Assess recent history of anxiety and panic attacks. Explore contributing factors. Discuss effectiveness of cognitive restructuring strategies.
Knowledge deficit	Orient client to therapy program. Assess learning needs of client. Review initial plan of care. Assess understanding of teaching. Discuss the etiology and management of anxiety and panic disorders. Discuss the physical symptoms of panic and the importance of understanding the meaning of anxiety and panic disorders. Instruct client to maintain journal of anxiety and panic attacks.	Review therapy program and treatment objectives. Review journal of recent panic attacks. Assist client to identify the early signs of anxiety and panic attacks. Discuss strategies to cope with early signs and symptoms of panic attacks, including talking or activity. Discuss additional strategies to cope with panic attacks, including expressing anger, positive self-talk, or guided imagery. Teach principles of cognitive restructuring and practice during session. Teach relaxation techniques and practice during session. Discuss use of exercise to alleviate anxiety/panic. Assist client to explore problem-solving strategies. Assess understanding of teaching.	Review plan of care. Review principles of cognitive restructuring. Assess understanding of teaching.
Diet	Nutritional assessment	Encourage a well-balanced diet from all food groups.	Encourage a well-balanced diet from all food groups.

	Date _____ Weeks 1–2 *continued*	Date _____ Weeks 3–6 *continued*	Date _____ Weeks 7–8 *continued*
Diet (*continued*)	Encourage well-balanced diet from all food groups. Contract with client to avoid stimulants.	Encourage the avoidance of stimulants.	Encourage the avoidance of stimulants.
Activity	Discuss the importance of regular aerobic exercise. Contract for regular exercise program. Assess sleep patterns. Discuss strategies to provide sleep-enhancing atmosphere for 45 min prior to sleep.	Review ability to begin and continue exercise program. Maintain contract for regular exercise program. Encourage client to practice relaxation response. Discuss effectiveness of sleep-enhancing strategies.	Review ability to continue exercise program. Maintain contract for regular exercise programs. Discuss effectiveness of sleep-enhancing strategies.
Psychosocial	Approach with nonjudgmental and accepting manner. Observe and monitor behavior. Assist client to understand relationship of unexpressed feelings to anxiety and panic experience. Encourage client to express feelings, thoughts, ideas, and beliefs.	Approach with nonjudgmental and accepting manner. Observe and monitor behavior. Encourage client to express feelings, thoughts, ideas, and beliefs. Provide positive feedback for efforts to incorporate coping strategies into daily life. Assist client to understand relationship of feelings to panic. Assist client to realistically identify strengths and limitations. Explore ways of reframing limitations in a positive manner. Assist client to practice and implement effective coping strategies. Assist client to identify potentially stressful situations and role-play coping strategies.	Approach with nonjudgmental and accepting manner. Encourage client to review strategies to manage anxiety and panic.
Medications	Identify target symptoms.	Assess target symptoms. Assess need for medications and refer as indicated. Administer meds as ordered.	Assess target symptoms. Administer meds as ordered.
Consults and discharge plan	Family assessment Establish objectives of therapy with client	Review with client progress toward therapy objectives.	Review with client progress toward therapy objectives. Make appropriate referrals to support groups.

them picture the situation as clearly as possible with themselves in the picture. Next, have them surround this image with a pink bubble. Then have them let go of the bubble and watch the bubble float off into the universe and become one with the higher power of the universe. If clients desire, tape this guided imagery so they can practice it at home. Plan follow-up sessions to assess the results of the imagery.

Guided imagery can also be used as a behavioral rehearsal for anxiety-producing situations. It is a "safe" way to practice new cognitive and behavioral responses.

Behavioral: Coping Assistance
Emotional Support

Clients need reassurance and encouragement during times of stress. Assist clients in distinguishing between feelings such as anxiety, frustration, guilt, and hostility. Discuss ways to *express feelings appropriately* in order to provide more effective options for managing them. Help clients recognize that suppressing feelings requires energy, which is depleting. If clients fear that direct verbal expression of negative feelings leads to rejection from others, suggest that they problem-solve to find safe physical outlets for their negative feelings, such as exercise, working out in the gym, or pounding clay.

Clients who have a lifestyle of helplessness feel powerless in many areas of their lives. Do not force them into situations they cannot handle, but instead support their defenses as long as necessary to protect themselves. Do not try to reason away helpless behavior, since helplessness serves to control anxiety. Provide only as much assistance as is needed to help them gradually *gain control* over their lives. Explore beliefs that support a helpless mode of behavior, taking into consideration cultural values and patterns. *Identify secondary gains* such as decreased responsibility and increased dependency, and problem-solve ways to meet needs in a more adaptive fashion. As clients gain insight, they will be better able to modify their behavior.

Clients who experience compulsive or ritualistic behavior need support and encouragement in managing their daily lives. Often, clients are aware that their behavior is pointless but are unable to make changes in these activities. Help clients *problem-solve* ways in which they can modify their environment and per-

sonal schedules so that rituals can be included into daily routine. *Safety measures* may need to be implemented, such as plenty of dry towels and hand lotion for those who compulsively wash their hands. Explore the relationship between obsessive behavior and anxiety reduction, and problem-solve to find other behaviors that are more effective in managing anxiety. One such behavior may be daily schedule planning, which helps people feel in control of what happens to them. Clients who are obsessed with work and routines need help planning and scheduling hobbies and pleasurable activities during leisure time.

Security Enhancement

Some people experience a moderate level of anxiety in response to fears of being out of control. You can begin to help by having clients identify one anxiety-producing situation. Problem solving will be more effective when it is focused on a manageable single situation. Discuss clients' thoughts regarding control issues as well as their negative anticipatory thoughts. Teach them to redefine the sensations of anxiety as sensations of excitement, since they will be less disabled if their expectations are positive. Help them *analyze their fears* of losing control and make the connection between these fears and their increased anxiety. Talk over the possibility of the potential loss of control in this specific situation in order to differentiate between fantasy and the reality of the fear. Review how anxiety has been handled in the past and what behaviors were most effective. Teach *relaxation techniques* and explain that one cannot be relaxed and anxious at the same time. These skills will facilitate clients' sense of control over anxiety and life events.

Spiritual Support

People who experience severe traumatic events often suffer from spiritual distress because the world has become threatening. Explore clients' perceived lack of control over life events. Encourage them to *search for meaning* in the trauma to further their reestablishing a purpose in life. To increase their feelings of connectedness to others, help them identify *interpersonal support systems*. Be available to listen to their feelings; this allows them to vent rather than suppress their emotions. If appropriate, refer them to a religious counselor of their choice and support their use of meditation, prayer, or other religious traditions and rituals.

Support System Enhancement

Support systems are an essential component of managing anxiety disorders. *Group therapy* and self-help *support groups* are often effective treatment approaches, particularly for clients with phobic disorders and PTSD. Groups of people with similar problems provide an environment in which each person can establish trust and share with others. In group therapy, where instillation of hope, interpersonal learning, and universality are emphasized, more significant improvement is often seen than in individual therapy. Within the group, members are able to identify with others' feelings of anger, fear, guilt, and isolation. This identification increases the participation of, and resulting support for, each person.

Support groups are very helpful for family members. Information they receive about the disorders helps them understand that the client is not to blame for the problem. In addition, groups focus on stress management, the problem-solving process, adaptive coping measures, and ways to mobilize other resources (see Community Resources at the end of this chapter).

Behavioral: Cognitive Therapy

Cognitive Restructuring

Cognitive intervention techniques concentrate on teaching people to change their maladaptive beliefs, self-statements, and phobic imagery that contribute to anxiety disorders. In *guided self-dialog*, clients are taught to think certain thoughts before acting, such as "I will get on the elevator and go to the second floor successfully." In a technique known as *thought stopping*, they are taught to say "stop" to obsessional thoughts. Some clients work on changing irrational ways of thinking, such as "Thinking is the same as acting" or "There is a right and wrong on every situation."

Clients who worry a great deal can be taught to *control their worrying thoughts*. The process begins with identifying the thoughts, which are often so automatic that they are no longer aware of them. They can then choose to either counter the thoughts or challenge the thoughts. Countering the thoughts involves distraction, which prevents the buildup of anxiety. This might be engaging in a vigorous physical activity or mental activity such as reciting poetry. Some people find that refocusing and concentrating on some aspect in the environment, such as counting the number of items on a shelf, is helpful.

Challenging the thoughts is a process of identifying which thoughts are unrealistic, exaggerated, and catastrophic. Examples are: "Yesterday was terrible; today is likely to be awful too," "I stammered during my speech so I have ruined my daughter's wedding and she won't forgive me," and "My son is late—he's had an accident." Teach clients to identify that negative thoughts are not facts, and to identify what part of the thoughts is unrealistic or improbable. These thoughts can be transformed into: "Yesterday was terrible; no, parts of it were good and although parts were uncomfortable, I coped." "I stammered during my speech, but this is not the end of the world. Many people get nervous when speaking in public," and "My son is late; maybe he got held up in traffic."

A cognitive restructuring technique with anxious children is to separate the fearful part of the child from the calm and nonanxious part of the child. Because children have become accustomed to viewing themselves as constantly fearful, they ignore the times that they are successful and brave. You can provide opportunities for success. Praise and reinforce their behavior whenever possible. Focusing on positive characteristics and behaviors is often more helpful than focusing on limitations. Ask clients to draw up a list of all their strengths, for example: I am honest, I am a good friend, I can throw a ball, I can skip rope, I am a good big brother, and so on. You and your client can discuss this list and discover ways to use these characteristics in a positive manner.

Behavioral: Communication Enhancement

Socialization Enhancement

Clients may have relationship difficulties and will benefit from *social skills training*. In a group setting, they can learn how to be less self-absorbed, pay attention to others' feelings and thoughts, and be considerate of others. People who have learned to behave passively and dependently often benefit from assertiveness training. Others have had limited practice with communication skills and need to be taught appropriate ways to communicate. They are encouraged to express their feelings directly and say what they mean. Both assertiveness and communication skills are best learned within a group format to allow for practice and feedback. (See Chapter 10 for detailed information on social skills training.)

Social skills training is beneficial for anxious children and adolescents. The goal of social skills training is to increase the ability to negotiate stressful interpersonal situations with parents, teachers, peers, and others. Improving interpersonal skills helps alter negative self-perceptions.

Family: Life Span Care

Family Integrity Promotion

Relationship or *family therapy* is appropriate in many cases. Family members may need help defining and clarifying their relationships. Some fear losing themselves in a close relationship, so they interact with distance and alienation. Others get caught in a pattern of excessive dependency and must discover how this type of helplessness actually establishes a position of power within the family.

Often, family members have secondary gains that meet individual needs such as nurturing or control but that interfere with the growth and development of the family system. They must understand how the illness may, in fact, perpetuate existing family dynamics. They must learn how to restore and maintain balance without the presence of an anxiety disorder. Family members often need help labeling feelings and sharing them with one another. You can teach the use of "I" language to express thoughts and feelings, such as "I think . . ." or "I feel. . ." "I" statements help people assume responsibility for their own feelings rather than blaming others with "you" statements, such as "You make me feel. . . ." or "You never do anything right."

Physiological: Basic: Nutrition Support

Nutritional Counseling

Nutritional interventions include teaching clients about balanced diets, how to shop wisely, and how to cook simple meals. Because caffeine, chocolate, and alcohol may increase anxiety, strongly encourage them to stay away from these substances.

L-tryptophan (TRY) is an amino acid that is essential for the production of both 5-HT and niacin. If clients increase their intake of niacin, TRY will be forced to produce more 5-HT. Available in time-release capsules, it should not be taken by those suffering from peptic ulcer, liver impairment, diabetes, or gout. Vitamin B_6 is necessary for the conversion of TRY to 5-HT. It is important for clients to recognize that vitamin B_6 is depleted from the body by the use of antidepressants, birth control pills, and antihypertensive agents. Clients may need to supplement their vita-

min B_6 intake (50 mg, three times a day with meals) in these cases (Balch & Balch, 1997).

Calcium (2,000 mg daily) and magnesium (600 to 1,000 mg daily) help to relieve anxiety and tension. Vitamin B_1 (50 mg, three times a day with meals) and vitamin C (5,000 to 10,000 mg daily, in divided doses) are known to decrease anxiety. Zinc (not to exceed a total of 100 mg from all supplements) has a calming effect on the central nervous system.

Physiological: Basic: Activity and Exercise Management

Exercise Promotion

Exercise has an overall relaxing effect on the body and may be used to manage anxiety. Discuss with clients the benefits of exercise and design a program that fits their lifestyle. Assist clients to prepare and maintain a

---

Complementary/Alternative Therapies

How to Help Clients Decrease Anxiety

The next time you feel anxious, try this procedure to decrease your anxiety:

1. Hold your frontal eminences on your forehead either with the first two fingers of your hands—the right and the left at the same time—or place the palm of your hand flat on your forehead.

2. While applying light pressure, in your mind go over exactly what you are thinking and how you are feeling. Continue holding these points and going over what is bothering you for a few minutes or until you feel the anxiety becoming less strong.

3. Let go with your hands and look around you. Mentally review the issue again. If anxiety is still there or has changed to other stressful feelings (frustration or anger, for example), go back and begin the process again. After a further few minutes, release the pressure and check your feelings about the situation again.

Hopefully your mind feels clearer and the anxiety no longer has the same stressful impact.

SOURCE: Fontaine, K. L. (2000). *Healing practices: Alternative therapies for nursing.* Upper Saddle River, NJ: Prentice Hall.

CLINICAL INTERACTIONS

A Client with Obsessive–Compulsive Disorder

Detra, age 23, lives with her parents and has recently become obsessed with thoughts of her parents' deaths. She has developed several compulsions to manage the associated anxiety. When walking outside, she must never step on a crack in the sidewalk, and she silently repeats to herself over and over again: "Step on a crack, break your mother's back." She also fears that if she does not keep the house clean enough, her parents will get sick and die. She usually spends at least eight hours a day cleaning their two-bedroom apartment. She insists that the windows and doors remain closed to prevent contamination and allows no one into the apartment other than immediate family members. Lately, she has begun to use a magnifying glass to see if she has missed cleaning any fingerprints off the tables and chairs. In the interaction, you will see evidence of:

■ Ego-dystonic feelings about the obsession
■ A desire to resist the obsession
■ Shame about the uncontrollable behavior
■ Temporary relief of anxiety by compulsive behavior

NURSE: It sounds like you have a lot of worries.

DETRA: Yeah.

NURSE: Your mother said you worry about the family a lot. Is that true?

DETRA: Yeah.

NURSE: Are you worried about your parents right now?

DETRA: No, not if I don't think about it.

NURSE: Well, when you're worried about your parents, does anything help?

DETRA: Yeah. [Pauses, looks embarrassed.] It's really stupid. I clean the apartment over and over all day long.

NURSE: You are constantly cleaning. Does that help?

DETRA: Sort of, but it's stupid.

NURSE: What do you mean, stupid?

DETRA: Just stupid. I wish I could quit thinking about it.

NURSE: Do you have other worries you wish you could quit thinking about?

DETRA: Yeah.

NURSE: Tell me about one of your other worries that you think is kind of stupid.

DETRA: I worry about dirt and germs coming in through the windows and doors.

NURSE: Do you do anything when you have these worries?

DETRA: I go around the apartment and keep checking that all the windows and doors are sealed. I search to see if there is any way germs can get in.

NURSE: When you check the windows and doors, that helps your worry about germs?

DETRA: Yeah. That's stupid, isn't it?

NURSE: Well, it sounds like you have a problem, but I don't think you're stupid.

---

progress graph/chart to motivate their adherence to the exercise program.

Physiological: Basic: Physical Comfort Promotion

Massage

Clients who are anxious may benefit from hand and foot massage. Essential oils can be combined with carrier oils and help clients relax and decrease their levels of anxiety. In the psychiatric setting, you may integrate executive massages for those clients who wish to use massage as a stress reducer. Debbie Hilliard (1995), a Clinical Nurse Specialist and a Certified Massage Practitioner, has utilized massage with people experiencing persistent mental illness. She found that while massage was not suitable for all clients, the majority who sought the treatment reported subjective relief from anxiety and tension. See the text *Healing Practices: Alternative Therapies for Nursing* (Fontaine, 2000) for details on hand and foot massage.

Acupressure

Acupressure is the application of firm, sustained pressure to special points on the body to decrease pain and produce relaxation. You can teach clients about a number of pressure points as you advocate self-help. Teach clients several finger holds to improve their general level of well-being. Explain that they should gently hold the appropriate finger on either hand while imaging the negative emotions melting away and an easing of symptoms:

- *Thumb*: Corresponds to worry and anxiety
- *Index finger*: Corresponds to fear
- *Ring finger*: Corresponds to fear of rejection
- *Little finger*: Corresponds to insecurity and nervousness

Evaluation

To complete the nursing process, you evaluate clients' responses to nursing interventions based on the outcomes you selected. You determine the appropriate intervals for measurement and document the condition of clients according to each individual's status. Johnson, Maas, and Moorhead (2000) is the resource for identifying measurement scales and specific indicators for each outcome.

Anxiety Control

Individuals demonstrating improved anxiety control plan and implement effective coping strategies. They rehearse and use techniques such as slow, deep breathing, muscle relaxation, guided imagery, distraction techniques, and a quiet environment to manage their feelings of anxiety. They utilize journal writing as a self-monitoring technique.

Concentration

As signs and symptoms of anxiety disorders abate, clients are able to ignore environmental distractions. They are able to control their worrying thoughts to limit distraction from internal cues.

Coping

Clients differentiate effective from ineffective coping patterns. They use the process of guided self-dialog to think through situations before responding to them.

Family Coping

Family members define and clarify relationships within the family system. They identify and replace secondary gains. They label feelings and share them with one another.

Fear Control

Clients identify unrealistic, exaggerated, and catastrophic thoughts. They analyze their fear of losing control and the reality of that fear. They transform these thoughts to more realistic ideas. They verbalize feelings appropriately.

Memory

Clients who achieve successful memory control experience an increased length of time between flashbacks and decreased duration of flashbacks.

Social Support

Clients and families utilize group therapy and self-help support groups in managing their anxiety disorder. They verbalize increased trust of others and a feeling of empathy for group members. Clients behave more assertively and communicate more directly. They are able to effectively negotiate stressful interpersonal situations.

Spiritual Well-Being

Individuals with adequate spiritual well-being express a sense of hope and of meaning and purpose in life. They participate in spiritual experiences such as meditation, prayer, worship, song, and/or spiritual reading. They express feelings of serenity and a connectedness with others.*

To build a care plan for a client with an anxiety disorder, go to the Companion Web site for this book.

---

*These selected outcome indicators are from Johnson, M., Maas, M., & Moorhead, S. (2000). *Nursing outcomes classification* (*NOC*) (2nd ed.). St. Louis, MO: Mosby.

CHAPTER REVIEW

COMMUNITY RESOURCES

Links to these Web sites can be accessed on the Companion Web site for this book.

Agoraphobics Building Independent Lives (ABIL)
3805 Cutshaw Ave., Suite 415
Richmond, VA 23230
804-353-3964
E-mail: *abil1996@aol.com*
www.anxietysupport.org

Anxiety Disorders Association of America
11900 Parklawn Dr., Suite 100
Rockville, MD 20852
301-231-9350
www.adaa.org

National Center for Posttraumatic Stress Disorder
215 Main St.
White River Junction, VT 05009
802-296-5132
www.ncptsd.org

Obsessive Compulsive Foundation, Inc.
337 Notch Hill Road
North Branford, CT 06471
203-315-2190
www.ocfoundation.org

Veteran Outreach Program
Disabled American Veterans
807 Maine Ave. SW
Washington, DC 20024
www.v-o-p.org

BOOKS FOR CLIENTS AND FAMILIES

Allen, J. G. (1995). *Coping with trauma.* Washington, DC: APA Press.

Chansky, T. D. (2000). *Freeing your child from obsessive–compulsive disorder.* New York: Times Books.

Gentry, M. (1997). *After the accident: Triumph over trauma.* New York: Tinker Press.

Granoff, M. D., & Lee, A. (1996). *Help! I think I'm dying!: Panic attacks and phobias.* New York: Mind Matters.

Hyman, B. M., & Pedrick, C. (1999). *The OCD workbook: Your guide to breaking free from obsessive–compulsive disorder.* Oakland, CA: New Harbinger.

Penzel, F. (2000). *Obsessive–compulsive disorder: A complete guide to getting well and staying well.* New York: Oxford University Press.

KEY CONCEPTS

Introduction

- Anxiety disorders are the single largest mental health problem in the United States and are twice as common in women as in men.

- Coping mechanisms are conscious attempts to control anxiety, which, if effective, contribute to a person's sense of competence and self-esteem.

- Defense mechanisms are unconscious attempts to manage anxiety, attempts that may or may not be successful.

Knowledge Base
Anxiety Disorders

- Generalized anxiety disorder (GAD) is a chronic disorder characterized by persistent anxiety without phobias or panic attacks. Symptoms include excessive worrying, fatigue, muscular tension, irritability, difficulty concentrating, and sleep disturbance.

- Panic attacks, the highest level of anxiety, are characterized by disorganized thinking, feelings of terror and helplessness, and nonpurposeful behavior.

- Panic disorder is characterized by sudden and unexpected panic attacks, catastrophic thinking, phobic avoidance, anxiety, depression, and obsessions. It may or may not be accompanied by agoraphobia.

- People with phobic disorders suffer from persistent, unreasonable fears that result in avoidance behavior, which is often disabling. When confronted with the feared object or situation, the person panics.

- Agoraphobia is characterized by fear of being away from home and of being alone in public places when assistance might be needed.

- The major defense mechanisms present in phobias are repression, displacement, symbolization, and avoidance.

- Obsessive–compulsive disorder (OCD) is characterized by unwanted, repetitive thoughts and behaviors. Behavior is often time consuming and bizarre.

- Posttraumatic stress disorder (PTSD) is characterized by a constant anticipation of danger and a phobic avoidance of triggers that remind the person of the original trauma. Other characteristics include irritability, aggression, flashbacks, and self-devaluation.

- Acute stress disorder is a short-term response to an extreme trauma. If it persists longer than one month, the client is given the diagnosis of PTSD.

Dissociative Disorders

- Dissociative disorders are characterized by an alteration in conscious awareness of behavior, affect, thoughts, and memories, and an alteration in identity, particularly in the consistency of personality.

- People with a dissociative disorder block the thoughts and feelings associated with a severe trauma from conscious awareness. This may take the form of amnesia, fugue, depersonalization, or identity disorder (DID).

Somatoform Disorders

- The somatoform disorders involve physical symptoms for which no organic basis exists. Denial is used to transform anxiety into physical symptoms. The disorders include somatization disorder, conversion disorder, pain disorder, hypochondriasis, and body dysmorphic disorder.

Factitious Disorder

- Factitious disorder is diagnosed when a person intentionally simulates or produces physical or psychological symptoms in order to assume the sick role. The most severe and chronic form is referred to as Munchausen's syndrome.

Malingering

- Seeking external incentives such as sick leave or financial compensation is the motivation behind malingering.

Sociocultural Characteristics

- Advantages from or rewards for being ill are referred to as secondary gains.

- People with anxiety disorders may have a profound effect on their family systems. They may control their family through dependency and helplessness or through detachment and emotional distance. Secondary gains may perpetuate the disorder.

- The meaning of anxiety and the responses to it are strongly influenced by cultural beliefs and practices.

Childhood and Adolescence

- The anxiety disorders of childhood and adolescence are separation anxiety disorder, selective mutism, reactive attachment disorder, GAD, panic disorder, social phobia, OCD, and PTSD.

Physiological Characteristics

- Mild anxiety helps people deal constructively with stress.

- Moderately anxious people focus on immediate concerns and may experience mild gastric symptoms or trembling lips.

- Signs of severe anxiety include increased heart rate and blood pressure, shortness of breath, sweating, trembling, restlessness, fatigue, tension headache, and stiff neck.

- Signs of panic include hypotension, agitation, poor motor coordination, nonpurposeful behavior, dizziness, chest pain, palpitations, a choking sensation, and a feeling of terror.

Concomitant Disorders

- There is a high correlation between anxiety disorders and substance abuse, depression, and suicide. Anxious children often exhibit oppositional behavior.

Causative Theories

- Factors that contribute to the development of anxiety disorders include genetic predisposition, altered neurobiology, inefficient defense mechanisms, problems with interpersonal relationships, cognitive expectations, learned avoidance responses, and rigid gender-role expectations.

Multidisciplinary Interventions

- A variety of antianxiety agents and antidepressants may be used for treatment, along with individual, family, and group psychotherapy.

- Alternative therapies include herbs, essential oils, homeopathic remedies, massage, Therapeutic Touch, yoga, and meditation.

Nursing Interventions

Assessment

- You will be assessing the majority of clients with anxiety disorders in community settings, clinics, offices, emergency departments, and medical–surgical units.

Diagnosis

- Most of the nursing diagnoses in this chapter apply to many individuals regardless of the specific medical diagnostic category. It is through understanding the issues and problems most significant for each client that care plans are developed and implemented.

Intervention

- Techniques for reducing anxiety include muscle relaxation, deep breathing, physical exercise, and distraction techniques.

- Stay with the person experiencing a panic state and speak slowly in short, simple sentences.

- Journal keeping is an effective way for clients to keep track of their thoughts, feelings, and memories.

- Calming techniques include deep breathing, muscle relaxation, changing sensory experiences, doing activities, and positive affirmations.

- Help clients identify secondary gains and find more adaptive ways to meet those needs.

- Aid clients in the search for meaning in life, connecting with others, and developing a support system.

- Cognitive interventions include guided self-dialog, thought stopping, and changing irrational ways of thinking.

- Many clients benefit from social skills training, assertiveness training, and communication skills training.

- Relationship or family therapy is appropriate in many cases, as the entire family system suffers from the effects of anxiety disorders.

- Nutritional interventions include teaching clients to increase their intake of niacin and vitamin B_6, which are necessary for the production of 5-HT.

Evaluation

- The nursing process is dynamic, and an evaluation of outcomes leads to further assessment and modification of the plan of care.

EXPLORE *MediaLink*

- Interactive resources, including animations, for this chapter can be found on the Companion Web site at *http://www.prenhall.com/fontaine*. Click on Chapter 11 and select the activities for this chapter.

- For NCLEX review questions and an audio glossary, access the accompanying CD-ROM in this book.

REFERENCES

American Psychiatric Association. (2000). *Diagnostic and statistical manual of mental disorders* (4th ed., Text Revision). Washington, DC: Author.

American Psychological Association Practice Guidelines. (1998). *Practice guideline for the treatment of patients with panic disorder.* Washington, DC: American Psychiatric Association.

Antai-Otong, D. (2000). The neurobiology of anxiety disorders: Implications for psychiatric nursing practice. *Issues in Mental Health Nursing, 21,* 71–89.

Balch, J. F., & Balch, P. A. (1997). *Prescription for nutritional healing* (2nd ed.). Garden City Park, NY: Avery.

Biederman, J., Faraone, S. V., Hirshfeld-Becker, D. R., Friedman, D., Robin, J. A., & Rosenbaum, J. F. (2001). Patterns of psychopathology and dysfunction in high-risk children of parents with panic disorder and major depression. *American Journal of Psychiatry, 158*(1), 49–57.

Bremner, J. D., Innis, R. B., Southwick, S. M., Staib, L., Zoghbi, S., & Charney, D. S. (2000). Decreased benzodiazepine receptor binding in prefrontal cortex in combat-related post-traumatic stress disorder. *American Journal of Psychiatry, 157*(7), 1120–1126.

Byrne, B. (2000). Relationships between anxiety, fear, self-esteem, and coping strategies in adolescence. *Adolescence, 35*(137), 201–215.

D'Alli, R. (2000). Childhood anxiety disorder. *Medscape Mental Health, 5*(5), 1–6.

Davidson, J., Pearlstein, T., Londborg, P., Brady, K. T., Rothbaum, B., Bell, J., et al. (2001). Efficacy of sertraline in preventing relapse of posttraumatic stress disorder. *American Journal of Psychiatry, 158*(12), 1974–1981.

REFERENCES (continued)

Draijer, N., & Langeland, W. (1999). Childhood trauma and perceived parental dysfunction in the etiology of dissociative symptoms in psychiatric inpatients. *American Journal of Psychiatry, 156*(3), 379–385.

Engle, V. F., & Graney, M. J. (2000). Biobehavioral effects of Therapeutic Touch. *Journal of Nursing Scholarship, 32*(3), 287–293.

Fish, L. S., Jensen, M., Reichert, T., & Wainman-Sauda, J. (2000). Anxious children and their families. In C. E. Bailey (Ed.), *Children in therapy* (pp. 192–214). New York: Norton.

Fontaine, K. L. (2000). *Healing practices: Alternative therapies for nursing.* Upper Saddle River, NJ: Prentice Hall.

Gerber, R. (2000). *Vibrational medicine for the 21st century.* New York: Eagle Brook.

Goddard, A. W., Rickels, K., DeMartinis, N., Garcia-Espana, F., Greenblatt, D. J., Mandos, L. A., & Rynn, M. (2001). Early coadministration of clonazepam with sertraline for panic disorder. *Archives of General Psychiatry, 58,* 681–686.

Goenjian, A. K., Steinberg, A. M., Najasian, L. M., Fairbanks, L. A., Tashjian, M., & Pynoos, R. S. (2000). Prospective study of posttraumatic stress, anxiety, and depressive reactions after earthquake and political violence. *American Journal of Psychiatry, 157*(6), 911–916.

Gorman, J. M., Kent, J. M., Sullivan, G. M., & Coplan, J. D. (2000). Neuroanatomical hypothesis of panic disorder, revised. *American Journal of Psychiatry, 157*(4), 493–504.

Grant, J. E., Kim, S. W., & Crow, S. J. (2001). Prevalence and clinical features of body dysmorphic disorder in adolescent and adult psychiatric inpatients. *Journal of Clinical Psychiatry, 62,* 517–522.

Greist, J. (1999). Obsessive–compulsive disorder. *NAMI Advocate, 21*(1), 8.

Guralnik, O., Schmeidler, J., & Simeon, D. (2000). Feeling unreal: Cognitive processes in depersonalization. *American Journal of Psychiatry, 157*(1), 103–109.

Henin, A., Savage, C. R., Rauch, S. L., Deckersbach, T., Wilhelm, S., Baer, L., et al. (2001). Is age at symptom onset associated with severity of memory impairment in adults with obsessive–compulsive disorder?

American Journal of Psychiatry, 158(1), 137–142.

Hillard, D. (1995). Massage for the seriously mentally ill. *Journal of Psychosocial Nursing, 33*(7), 29–30.

Johnson, M., Maas, M., & Moorhead, S. (2000). *Nursing outcomes classification (NOC)* (2nd ed.). St. Louis, MO: Mosby.

Kent, J. M., Papp, L. A., Martinez, J. M., Browne, S. T., Coplan, J. D., Klein, D., et al. (2001). Specificity of panic response to CO_2 inhalation in panic disorder. *American Journal of Psychiatry, 158*(1), 58–67.

Kushner, M. G., Sher, K. J., & Erickson, D. J. (1999). Prospective analysis of the relation between DSM-III anxiety disorders and alcohol use disorders. *American Journal of Psychiatry, 156*(5), 723–732.

Martin-Santos, R., Bulbena, A., Porta, M., Gago, J., Molina, R., & Duro, J. C. (1998). Association between joint hypermobility syndrome and panic disorder. *American Journal of Psychiatry, 155*(11), 1578–1583.

McNally, R. J. (2001). Vulnerability to anxiety disorders in adulthood. In R. E. Ingram & J. M. Price (Eds.), *Vulnerability to psychopathology* (pp. 304–321). New York: Guilford Press.

Mendlowicz, M. V., & Stein, M. B. (2000). Quality of life in individuals with anxiety disorders. *American Journal of Psychiatry, 157*(5), 669–682.

Muskin, P. R. (2000). *Complementary and alternative medicine and psychiatry.* Washington, DC: American Psychiatric Press.

National Institute of Mental Health. (2000). Anxiety disorders research at the National Institute of Mental Health. *www.nimh.nih.gov/publicat/anxresfact.cfm.*

Paris, J. (1999). *Nature and nurture in psychiatry.* Washington, DC: American Psychiatric Press.

Pauls, D. L. (1995). A family study of obsessive–compulsive disorder. *American Journal of Psychiatry, 152*(1), 76–84.

Rapoport, J. L. (1989). *The boy who couldn't stop washing.* Washington, DC: Dutton.

Ratey, J. J. (2001). *A user's guide to the brain.* New York: Pantheon Books.

Schneier, F. R., Liebowitz, M. R., Abi-Dargham, A., Zea-Ponce, Y., Lin, S. H., & Laruelle, M. (2000). Low dopamine D_2 receptor binding potential in social phobia.

American Journal of Psychiatry, 157(3), 457–458.

Seeman, M. V. (1997). Psychopathology in women and men: Focus on female hormones. *American Journal of Psychiatry, 154*(12), 1641–1646.

Silva, R. R., Alpert, M., Munoz, D. M., Singh, S., Matzner, F., & Dummit, S. (2000). Stress and vulnerability to posttraumatic stress disorder in children and adolescents. *American Journal of Psychiatry, 157*(8), 1229–1235.

Silverstone, P. H., & Salinas, E. (2001). Efficacy of venlafaxine extended release in patients with major depressive disorder and comorbid generalized anxiety disorder. *Journal of Clinical Psychiatry, 62,* 523–529.

Simeon, D., Guralnik, O., Schmeidlen, J., Sirof, B., & Knutelska, M. (2001). The role of childhood interpersonal trauma in depersonalization disorder. *American Journal of Psychiatry, 158*(7), 1027–1033.

Simeon, D., Guralnik, D., Hazlett, E. A., Spiegel-Cohen, J., Hollander, E., & Buchsbaum, M. S. (2000). Feeling unreal: A PET study of depersonalization disorder. *American Journal of Psychiatry, 157*(11), 1782–1788.

Smoller, J. W., & Tsuang, M. T. (1998). Panic and phobic anxiety: Defining phenotypes for genetic studies. *American Journal of Psychiatry, 155*(9), 1152–1162.

Stein, M. B., Chartier, M. J., Hazen, A. L., Kozak, M. V., Tancer, M. E., et al. (1998). A direct-interview family study of generalized social phobia. *American Journal of Psychiatry, 155*(1), 90–97.

Stein, M. B., Fyer, A. J., Davidson, J. R. T., Pollack, M. H., & Wiita, B. (1999). Fluvoxamine treatment of social phobia. *American Journal of Psychiatry, 156*(5), 756–760.

Wakefield, M., & Pallister, R. (1997). Cognitive-behavioral approaches to panic disorder. *Journal of Psychosocial Nursing, 35*(3), 12–20.

Way, W. W., Hayward, A. R., Levin, M. J., & Sondheimer, J. M. (1999). *Current pediatric diagnosis & treatment* (14th ed.). Stamford, CT: Appleton & Lange.

Woods, S. J. (2000). Prevalence and patterns of posttraumatic stress disorder in abused and postabused women. *Issues in Mental Health Nursing, 21*(3), 309–324.

Eating Disorders

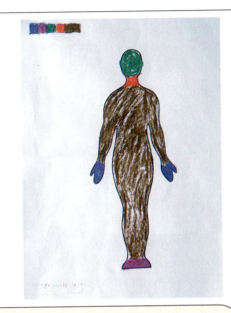

OBJECTIVES

After reading this chapter, you will be able to:

- DESCRIBE the eating patterns of persons with obesities, Prader–Willi syndrome, anorexia, and bulimia.

- DISCUSS the causative theories of eating disorders.

- ASSESS clients from physical, psychological, and sociocultural perspectives.

- PLAN overall goals in the care of eating-disordered clients.

- INDIVIDUALIZE standard interventions to specific clients.

- EVALUATE and modify the plan of care for clients with eating disorders.

I felt fine doing this. I am very uncomfortable with my body and always have been. I hate pretty much everything about myself.

—Jeanne, Age 30

Color scale 1–5 represents comfortability with self. Brown #5 = most uncomfortable.

MediaLink

CD-ROM
- *Audio Glossary*
- *NCLEX Review*

Companion Web site www.prenhall.com/fontaine
- *Critical Thinking*
- *More NCLEX Review*
- *Case Study*
- *Care Map Activity*
- *Links to Resources*

ANOREXIA NERVOSA AND BULIMIA NERVOSA

Anorexia nervosa and bulimia nervosa are not single diseases but syndromes with multiple predisposing factors and a variety of characteristics. Although the most obvious symptom is the eating problem, these disorders are not simply a matter of eating too much or too little. It is because of the complex interaction of biological, psychological, developmental, familial, and sociocultural factors that certain people develop eating disorders.

There is no clear-cut distinction between the two disorders, and they have many features in common. The traditional division of anorexia and bulimia is still appropriate until more is known about eating disor-ders. Body weight may be a significant distinguishing characteristic; people with anorexia are severely under-weight and people with bulimia are at normal or near-normal weight. About 30 percent of people with bulimia have a history of anorexia. In addition, 47 per-cent of those with anorexia exhibit bulimic behaviors. Conversion from anorexia to bulimia may be a way of moving from a "visible" to an "invisible" eating disor-der in an effort to deceive family, friends, and health care providers. Thus, the two disorders can occur in the same person, or the person can revert from one dis-order to the other. There are far more similarities than differences between anorexia and bulimia (American Psychiatric Association [APA], 2000b; White, 2000). However, to help you understand the differences, the disorders have been separated in this chapter (see DSM-IV-TR feature).

People with anorexia nervosa lose weight by dra-matically decreasing their food intake and sharply increasing their amount of physical exercise. Individu-als with bulimia nervosa develop cycles of binge eat-ing followed by purging. The severity of the disorder is determined by the frequency of the binge–purge cycles.

Determining the incidence of anorexia and bulimia is difficult because of the variety of definitions that exist. Certainly, the frequency of these disorders has been increasing, but the increase may be partly due to increased reporting. Ninety percent of women and 25 percent of men diet at some time in their lives. Estimates are that clinical eating disorders affect 8 to 20 percent of the population. They are more com-monly seen among females, with estimates of the male–female ratio ranging from 1:6 to 1:10, although 19 to 30 percent of younger people with anorexia are

DSM-IV-TR CLASSIFICATIONS

Anorexia Nervosa

Bulimia Nervosa

Eating Disorder NOS (not otherwise specified)

SOURCE: Reprinted with permission from the *Diagnostic and Statistical Manual of Mental Disorders, Fourth Edition, Text Revision.* Copyright 2000 American Psychiatric Association.

male. The estimate may be low since primary health care providers are less likely to diagnose an eating disorder in a male than in a female. The disorders usually develop during adolescence: age 13 to 17 for anorexia and age 17 to 23 for bulimia. The age of onset has been dropping in recent years, and we now see children as young as age 7 with anorexia. Anywhere from 30 to 70 percent of people with anorexia develop chronic symptoms (APA, 2000; Boskind-White & White, 2000; Grogan, 1999; Keel, Leon, & Fulkerson, 2001).

Eating disorders are more common among competitive athletes than the general age-matched population. Female athletes are especially at risk in sports that emphasize a thin body such as gymnastics, ballet, figure skating, and distance running. Males in sports such as bodybuilding and wrestling are also at greater risk. Parents and coaches may support problematic eating behavior in a misguided effort to increase their competitive edge. Other groups at risk include dancers and models.

You will encounter people with eating disorders in a number of clinical settings. In schools, camps, community health care settings, pediatric units, medical–surgical units, and intensive care units, you must be aware of the characteristics of eating disorders so you can provide prompt attention to those in need. More young women 15 to 24 years old die from anorexia than all other causes combined. They have a suicide rate that is much higher than the general population. With a mortality rate as high as 22 percent, it is extremely risky to underestimate the seriousness of eating disorders (Boskind-White & White, 2000; Levenkron, 2000).

BINGE EATING DISORDER

The bulimic pattern is different from **binge eating disorder**, which is often associated with obesity. This is a proposed new category that needs further study before inclusion into the *Diagnostic and Statistical Manual of Mental Disorders* (4th ed., Text Revision) (DSM-IV-TR) (APA, 2000a). The obese who overeat tend to follow one of two patterns, neither of which includes purging the body after excessive food intake. The first pattern is overeating in response to a number of feelings such as anxiety or depression. Some binge eat in response to losing control over a weight-loss diet. Although these people lose weight in weight-control programs, they regain it after going off the diet. People with this eating pattern say that their eating and/or weight interfere with their relationships and their self-esteem. Women are more likely to have this eating pattern than are men.

The second pattern is overeating because of the enjoyment of food. Seldom attempting to diet, these people have no sense of loss of control. They are more accepting of their body size and understand it to be the result of their enjoyment of eating.

NOCTURNAL SLEEP-RELATED EATING DISORDER

Nocturnal sleep-related eating disorder is a newly recognized form of binge eating. It is characterized by sleepwalking and sleep eating. Safety becomes a problem when individuals actually prepare meals while asleep, resulting in burns or even a fire. Some sufferers discover bruises and lacerations from bumping into walls or furniture while sleepwalking. Upon awakening, the individual may have no recall or may have vague recall of the nighttime behavior. This eating disorder is found in both those individuals of normal weight and those who are overweight. Some may also experience a daytime eating disorder such as anorexia or bulimia (Montgomery & Haynes, 2001).

OBESITIES

Obesities are the most common form of malnourishment in the United States. Using the body mass index, it is estimated that 55 percent of adults in the United States are overweight, and about one half of these are considered obese. Since the mental health of obese people is comparable to that of the general population, obesity is not considered a mental disorder. The only similarity between obesity and anorexia and bulimia is dissatisfaction with body size and shape. Therefore, a brief overview is presented here, and you are encouraged to consult other resources, books and journals, for a more comprehensive description (Devlin, Yanovski, & Wilson, 2000).

Obesity is thought to result from a variety of combinations of psychosocial and physiological factors. There is no universal cause and therefore no single treatment approach. There are many ways of becoming and staying obese.

A variety of psychosocial factors may contribute to the development and maintenance of obesity. Eating habits are primarily learned *patterns of behavior* in response to both hunger (a physiological sensation) and appetite (social and psychological cues). Some people manage negative feelings—such as anxiety, anger, and loneliness—by overeating. Others may view eating as a reward. These patterns may have been learned in childhood if parents used food as a way to decrease stress or reward good behavior. Because social events are frequently associated with food, some people make a connection between pleasure and eating—a connection that may predispose them to overeating.

Many researchers believe *physiological factors* are more significant than psychosocial factors. More than 200 genes that contribute to appetite, hunger, satiety, metabolism, fat storage, and activity tendencies have been identified. Recently, a gene for obesity, ob, and its protein product, leptin, were discovered. Leptin is produced in fat cells and travels to the brain, where it decreases appetite and increases metabolic rate. Adoption, twin, and family studies note that obesity has a strong inheritable component, with about 30 to 70 percent of variability in body weight or fat mass being genetically determined (Devlin et al., 2000).

In both obese and nonobese people, the amount of *body fat* seems to be precisely regulated and maintained. This explains the difficulty most people have in changing the amount of their body fat. There is frequently no clear difference between the amount of food eaten by obese people and by nonobese people. The belief that all obese people overeat is inaccurate and underlies many of our culture's negative stereotypes about obesity.

Weight gain is among the most problematic *side effects* of psychotropic medications and is one of the most frequent reasons for individuals discontinuing their medications. Weight gain is a side effect for all the antipsychotic agents, lithium and other mood stabilizers, and many of the antidepressants.

Some people are blatantly hostile toward overweight people. It is no longer acceptable to stigmatize people on the basis of race or ethnic origin and therefore obesity remains one of the last socially acceptable forms of *prejudice*. Because of the high level of prejudice against obese people in America, the social consequences of being overweight can be severe. Obese individuals may suffer from job discrimination because employers assume they are less healthy, less diligent, and less intelligent than their thinner peers. In stores, obese customers may be treated with less respect and less consid-

eration. When obese people eat in public, they are often given disapproving looks and comments from thinner people. Frequent exposure to such treatment increases feelings of hurt and failure. Being bombarded with antifat values further increases the obese person's level of self-disgust. Health care professionals add to this discrimination by viewing obesity not only as a health hazard but also as an indication of emotional disturbance. In fact, it is the internalization of the culture's hatred and rejection, rather than body weight and size, that contributes to psychological problems.

People who are 35 percent or more above ideal body weight are at high risk for developing a number of *medical conditions*. These include diabetes mellitus, hypertension, cardiovascular disease, hyperlipidemia, gallbladder disease, arthritis, and complications of pregnancy. The risk of mortality is higher for women than men and higher for the young than the old (Goldfein, Devlin, & Spitzer, 2000).

Obesities are among the easiest to recognize and the most difficult to treat of medical conditions. A wide variety of treatment approaches have been tried. In all the approaches, there is a general tendency to regain lost weight. At this point, preventing obesity is more effective than treating it.

PRADER–WILLI SYNDROME

Prader–Willi syndrome (PWS) is a congenital disorder of the 15th chromosome with an estimated prevalence of 1 in 15,000. PWS not only causes an unrelenting feeling of hunger, but low muscle tone, short stature, incomplete sexual development, mild to severe mental retardation, and behavioral problems. By age two or three, the child's appetite becomes insatiable and there is a rapid and excessive weight gain. The physiologically driven eating behavior is not under the individual's cognitive control. The person cannot decide "not to eat." Compounding the excessive appetite is decreased calorie utilization in those with PWS due to low muscle mass and inactivity. Their calorie needs are about 60 percent of other persons. Access to food must be rigidly enforced if they are not to become morbidly obese. Restricting food intake must extend out of the home and into school, work, and community settings. Hoarding food and stealing money to buy food are very common problems for this group of individuals. Morbid obesity may lead to serious medical consequences, including cardiovascular diseases, diabetes mellitus, sleep disturbances, and respiratory compromise. These are the most common causes of premature death among those suffering from PWS (Basic Facts About PWS, 2000; Martin et al., 1998).

Behavioral problems can lead to curtailed psychosocial development and poor social functioning. Symptoms may include temper tantrums, oppositional behavior and stubbornness, labile emotions, and obsessive thinking or compulsive behaviors such as skin-picking. Some individuals compulsively engage in rectal digging, which often causes embarrassment to them and their families. Rectal digging has potential risks ranging from fecal contamination to rectal bleeding and sphincter problems. Treatment is growth hormone that increases muscle tone and enhances growth. For those who are depressed or anxious, antidepressants are often prescribed (Martin et al., 1998).

KNOWLEDGE BASE

BEHAVIORAL CHARACTERISTICS
Anorexia

Anorexic young women have a desperate need to please others. Their self-worth depends on responses from others, rather than on their own self-approval. Thus, their behavior is often *overcompliant*; they always try to meet the expectations of others in order to be accepted. They may overachieve in academic and extracurricular activities, but these accomplishments are usually an attempt to please parents rather than a source of self-satisfaction.

To control themselves and their environment, they develop rigid rules. Such rigidity often develops into *obsessive rituals*, particularly concerning eating and exercise. Cutting all food into a predetermined size or number of pieces, chewing all food a certain number of times, allowing only certain combinations of food in a meal, accomplishing a fixed number of exercise routines, and having an inflexible pattern of exercises are rituals common to anorexic people. These rules and rituals help keep anxiety beyond conscious awareness. If the rituals are disrupted, the anxiety becomes intolerable. Paradoxically, all these efforts to stay in control lead to out-of-control behaviors (Levenkron, 2000).

Many people with anorexia are hyperactive and discover that *overexercise* is a way to increase their weight

loss. Solitary running tends to be the exercise of choice and there are often obsessional qualities to it. For example, they feel that before they can eat, they have to earn calories by exercising. Conversely, if they overeat, they feel they have to punish themselves with excessive exercise. Excessive exercise signifies the triumph of will over the body and is a possible indication of poor prognosis in recovery (Hays, 1999).

Hopeless, helpless, and ineffective is how people with anorexia often feel. Because of being overcompliant with their parents, they believe they have always been controlled by others. Their *refusal to eat* may be an attempt to assert themselves and gain some control within the family. As weight is lost, they are rewarded with praise, admiration, and envy from their peers, which reinforces the restricted eating pattern.

Phobias in people with anorexia are common. Initially, the fear is of weight gain, but it develops into a *secondary food phobia*. The mechanism of phobic avoidance in anorexic people is different from that in others. In nonanorexic people, the phobia has an external stimulus, such as an animal or object, a place or situation. Avoidance prevents the escalation of anxiety, but the person receives no pleasure in the process. In people with anorexia, the phobia has an internal stimulus: the fear of being fat. Avoidance of food provides a feeling of control and a sense of pleasure when weight is lost.

Inez is a high school junior who has lost 35 pounds (15.9 kg) in the past year and now weighs 90 pounds (40.9 kg). She typically goes two to three days without eating. She has a rigid, 2½-hour exercise routine, which she does before and after school. She tries to avoid sitting still, since she believes this will cause weight gain. When her parents force her to eat, she focuses on her superstitious number of seven; that is, she will eat only seven peas or seven kernels of corn or drink seven tiny sips of milk. She chews everything seven times and must complete her meal in seven minutes.

Bulimia

Unlike those with anorexia, people who begin their eating disorder with a bulimic pattern are often *overweight* before the onset of the disorder. They often learn this maladaptive pattern of weight control from peers who have used purging as a method of losing weight. This sort of bulimia may go undetected for years because often there is no significant weight loss. For both males and females, the behavior rapidly becomes both impulsive and compulsive, and the frequency and severity of the eating disorder tend to increase.

Amy states that when she was 15 years old, she weighed 140 pounds (63.6 kg). One of her friends said to her, "I see you're working on a stomach there." She describes that incident as the beginning of her bulimic behavior.

There is a *cyclic behavioral pattern* in bulimia. It begins with skipping meals sporadically and overstrict *dieting* or fasting. In an effort to refrain from eating, the person may use amphetamines, which can lead to extreme hunger, fatigue, and low blood glucose levels. The next part of the cycle is a period of *binge eating*, in which the person ingests huge amounts of food (about 3,500 kcal) within a short time (about one hour). Binges can last up to eight hours, with consumption of 12,000 kcal. Binge eating usually occurs when the person is alone and at home, and is most frequent during the evening. The cycle may occur once or twice a month for some and as often as five or ten times a day for others. The binge part of the cycle may be triggered by the ingestion of certain foods, but this is not consistent for everyone. Although eating binges may involve any kind of food, they usually consist of junk foods, fast foods, and high-calorie foods.

The final part of the cycle is *purging* the body of the ingested food. After excessive eating, people with bulimia force themselves to vomit. They often abuse laxatives and diuretics in an attempt to purge their bodies of the food. Some use as many as 50 to 100 laxatives per day. In rare cases, they may resort to syrup of ipecac to induce vomiting. Purging becomes a purification rite and a means of regaining self-control. Some describe it as feeling "completely fresh and clean again."

After the purging, the cycle begins all over again, with a return to strict dieting or fasting. Some people with bulimia eat highly nutritious meals when not binging/purging in an effort to repair harm done to the body.

Binge eating and purging begin as a way to eat and stay slim. Before long, the behavior becomes a response to stress and a way to cope with negative feelings such as anger, anxiety, and depression. For some, it is poor impulse control, and for others it is an expression of rebellion against family members.

People with bulimia may engage in *sporadic excessive exercise*, but they usually do not develop compulsive exercise routines. They are more likely to abuse street drugs to decrease their appetite and alcohol to reduce their anxiety. Since their binges are often expensive, costing as much as $100 per day, they may resort to *stealing* food or money to buy the food. The binge/purge cycle can become so consuming that activities and relationships are disrupted. To keep the secret, the person often resorts to excuses and lies (Boskind-White & White, 2000).

Akera, 23 years old, is a senior nursing student whose bulimia has been carefully hidden from family, friends, and teachers for the past three years. During a typical day after school, she stops at the local grocery store to buy two pounds of cookies, which she consumes on the way to the ice cream store. There she buys a gallon of ice cream. She eats that quickly and continues on to a fast-food restaurant, where she has three cheeseburgers, fries, and two milkshakes. Before she goes home, she stops at the drugstore, buys a pack of gum, and steals a box of laxatives so the clerks won't suspect she has an eating disorder. As soon as Akera arrives home, she forces herself to vomit and then takes the entire package of laxatives. This cycle repeats itself at home during the evening, when she eats any available food.

AFFECTIVE CHARACTERISTICS
Anorexia

People with anorexia are often beset by *fears*; some fear becoming mature and assuming adult responsibilities. Because of their need to please others with high levels of achievement, some fear they are not doing well enough. Almost all have an extreme terror of weight gain and fat. A paradoxical response occurs when this fear actually increases as body weight decreases. If weight gain (real or imagined) occurs, anxiety surfaces to the conscious level and is perceived as a threat to the entire being. People with anorexia also fear a loss of control. Although this fear is usually related to losing control over eating, it may extend to other physiological processes such as sleeping, urination, and bowel functioning. The steady loss of weight becomes symbolic of mastery over self and environment. However, if they lose control and eat more than they believe to be appropriate, they experience severe guilt (Levenkron, 2000).

Bulimia

Because of their need for acceptance and approval, people with bulimia repress feelings of frustration and anger toward others. *Repressing feelings* and avoiding conflict protect them from rejection. As the ability to identify feelings decreases, they often confuse negative emotions with sensations of being hungry. Food then becomes a source of comfort and a way to defend against anger and frustration. Life is often viewed as tragic and *hopeless*. Talents and interests are abandoned and their lives are devoid of fun, humor, or genuine self-pleasure (Boskind-White & White, 2000).

Like people with anorexia, people with bulimia experience multiple *fears*. They fear a loss of control, not only over their eating but also over their emotions. They are extremely fearful of weight gain and, with real or perceived changes in their weight, they feel panic. Motivating much of their behavior is fear of rejection.

The binge–purge cycle can be understood from the affective perspective as well as the behavioral perspective. *Anxiety* increases to a high level, at which point the person engages in binge eating to decrease the anxiety. Afterward, the person experiences *guilt* and self-disgust because of the loss of control. Guilt and disgust increase the anxiety, and purging, through vomiting and other methods, is then used to decrease this anxiety. Because this behavior is an indirect and ineffective way to manage anxiety, the levels rebuild, and the cycle starts anew. Some are able to talk about their feelings of helplessness, hopelessness, and worthlessness, while others do not seem to have the language to talk about their feelings.

Andrea, a 19-year-old college student, lives at home with her parents and younger brother.

She has just been admitted to the eating disorders unit. She states that the only reason she has been admitted is because "my mother says I'm not eating right. She has been on me forever. She told me if I didn't eat I would have to get out of the home. I came in here so she would leave me alone." Andrea is angry with her mother for treating her like a baby on the one hand and threatening her with abandonment on the other.

COGNITIVE CHARACTERISTICS
Anorexia

The desire to be thin and the behavioral control over eating are ego-syntonic in the anorexic client. **Ego-syntonic behavior** is behavior that agrees with one's thoughts, desires, and values. Anorexic people regard their obsessions with food and eating as conventional behavior. The major defense mechanism for defining the behavior in an ego-syntonic manner is *denial*: denial of sensations of hunger, denial of physical exhaustion, and denial of any disorder or illness.

People with anorexia experience **cognitive distortions** that are similar to those experienced by sufferers of mental disorders. These cognitive distortions are considered errors in thinking that continue even when there is obvious contradictory evidence. Cognitive distortions involve food, body image, loss of control, and achievement. One type of distortion is **selective abstraction**, or focusing on certain information while ignoring contradictory information. Another distortion is **overgeneralization**, in which the person takes information or an impression from one event and attaches it to a wide variety of situations. Using such words as *always, never, everybody,* and *nobody* indicates that the client is overgeneralizing. Anorexic people also have a tendency toward **magnification**, attributing a high level of importance to unpleasant occurrences. Through **personalization**, or **ideas of reference**, they believe that what occurs in the environment is related to them, even when no obvious relationship exists. There is also a tendency for **superstitious thinking**, in which the person believes that some unrelated action will magically influence a course of events. A further distortion is **dichotomous thinking**, an all-or-none type of reasoning that interferes with people's realistic perceptions of themselves. Dichotomous thinking involves opposite and mutually exclusive categories such as eating or not eating, all good or all bad, and celibacy or promiscuity (see Table 12.1 ■).

Rachael, 18, has been diagnosed with anorexia. She does not believe that her 5 foot 9 inch frame is underweight at 102 pounds (46.3 kg). Rachael believes she will look better when she reaches 85 pounds (38.6 kg). She says that when she goes to college, she wants to be active in student government and that fat people are never elected. Her superstitious thinking relates to white clothing, which she feels decreases her hunger.

Body image is an integration of people's perceptions, thoughts, and feelings about their own body. *Perceptions* involve how big or small they estimate their body to be. *Thoughts* include an evaluation of body attractiveness, and *feelings* are the emotional association with their body shape and size. Body image is a psychological phenomenon (see Figure 12.1 ■), but it is significantly affected by social factors. By age 13, 53

percent of girls in the United States are unhappy with their bodies and consider themselves to be fat. By age 18, that number jumps up to 78 percent. As men's bodies become more exposed by the media, men are becoming more dissatisfied with their bodies. In one study of 548 men, 43 percent reported that they were dissatisfied with their overall appearance, 63 percent were dissatisfied with their abdomen, and 52 percent were unhappy with their weight. What we are discovering is that men are just as unhappy as women about their bodies (Boskind-White & White, 2000; Pope, Phillips, & Olivardia, 2000).

People suffering from anorexia experience *a severely distorted body image* that often reaches delusional proportions. Incapable of seeing that their bodies are emaciated, they continue to perceive themselves as fat. Some perceive their total body as obese, whereas others focus on a particular part of the body as fat, such as their hips, stomach, thighs, or face. While others see these people as starving and disappearing, they view themselves as strong and in the process of creating a whole new person.

Anorexic individuals believe they are in charge of their lives and in complete control. They believe their

TABLE 12.1
Examples of Cognitive Distortions

Distortion	Example
Selective abstraction	"I'm still too fat—look at how big my hands and feet are."
Overgeneralization	"You don't see fat people on television. Therefore, you have to be thin to be successful at anything in life."
Magnification	"If I gain two pounds, I know everyone will notice it."
Personalization	"Jim and Bob were talking and laughing together today. I'm sure they were talking about how fat I am."
Superstitious thinking	"If I wear all white, I'll lose weight faster." "Sitting still will cause my weight to go up rapidly."
Dichotomous thinking	"If I gain even one pound, that means I am totally out of control and I might as well gain 50 pounds." "If I eat one thing, I will just keep eating until I weigh 300 pounds." "If I'm not thin, I'm fat."

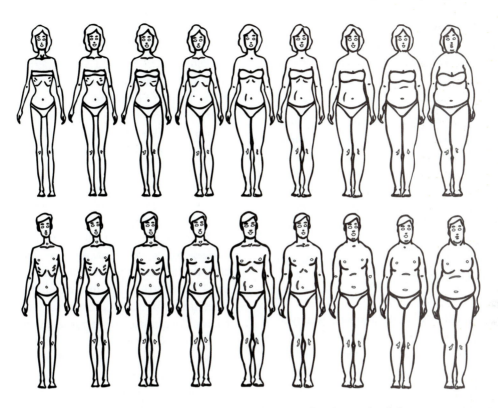

FIGURE 12.1 ■ Ideal body image—Which image do you think is ideal for your sex? And which comes closest to your body? This task is commonly used to assess whether a person has a positive or negative body image.

SOURCE: Kassin, S. (2001). *Psychology* (3rd ed.). Upper Saddle River, NJ: Prentice Hall.

peers are jealous of their willpower and thinness, which gives them an additional sense of power. The disorder becomes an issue of *autonomy* because no one can make them eat or make them gain weight. They think of food not as a necessity for survival but as something that threatens survival. Cognitively, fat represents need and loss of control; thinness represents strength and control. These people are frequently secretive about their behavior. The secrecy is not viewed as manipulative but rather protective. From their point of view, anorexia is the solution, not the problem.

Anorexia contributes to distorted perceptions of internal physical sensations, a distortion referred to as **alexithymia**. Hunger is not recognized as hunger. When they eat a small amount of food, they often complain of feeling too full. There is also a decreased internal perception of fatigue, so they often push their bodies to physical extremes. Even after long and strenuous exercise, they seem unaware of any sensations of fatigue.

Young people with anorexia are overly concerned with how others view them. Many are convinced that other people have more insight into who they are than they do themselves. This *self-depreciation* and fear of self-definition contribute to beliefs and fears of being controlled by others. Feeling they have no power in their interpersonal relationships, they attempt to please and placate significant others whom they perceive to be more powerful.

People with anorexia develop *perfectionistic standards* for their behavior and moralistic guidelines about all aspects of life. Their decision-making ability is hampered by their need to make absolutely correct decisions. They are in such dread of losing control that they impose extremes of discipline on themselves. During the times they are able to maintain control, their perfectionistic behavior and dichotomous thinking lead them to believe they are better than other people. However, these standards of behavior become self-defeating when they fail to achieve them consistently.

Another part of perfectionism is the ability to exceed other's expectations. They develop an identity as a person who can survive and flourish with little food (Finelli, 2001).

Kunjali, a 35-year-old woman, developed anorexia at age 12. She claims that life without an eating disorder would be a life without an identity. She believes she has not been "successful" as an anorexic because she has never reached an extremely low weight. She believes that truly successful anorexics die of starvation and that somehow they should be respected for their accomplishment. She believes that she has "failed" as an anorexic.

While it is unclear whether anorexia is a type of obsessive–compulsive disorder, anorexic people typically exhibit *obsessive–compulsive symptoms*. They spend a great deal of time obsessing about their weight and their bodies. They are preoccupied with thinking about food. Often, they develop complex rituals around food preparation, even though they refuse to eat the final product. Even after long-term weight recovery, their obsessions and compulsions continue (Levenkron, 2000).

Bulimia

In contrast to people with anorexia, bulimic individuals are troubled by their behavioral characteristics. They experience **ego-dystonic behavior**, behavior that does not conform to the person's thoughts, wishes, and values. Another facet of ego-dystonic symptoms is that one feels the symptoms are beyond personal control. The person feels compelled to binge, purge, and fast; helpless to stop the behavior; and full of self-disgust for continuing the pattern.

Although bulimic people are not pleased with their body shape and size, they usually do not experience the delusional distortions of anorexic people. There is a direct correlation between the frequency and severity of the disorder and the degree of perceived distortion of body size. Many were overweight before the disorder, so there is an *obsessional concern* about not regaining the lost weight. It is difficult for them to think of anything other than food. Since they eat in response to hunger, appetite, and thoughts of food, the obsessions

also involve getting rid of the food ingested in an effort to counteract the caloric effects of binge eating.

People with bulimia also experience the *cognitive distortions* discussed for anorexic people. They tend to relate their problems to weight or overeating. Their fantasy is that if they could only be thin and not overeat, all other problems would be solved. Another example of this all-or-none thinking is the belief that one bite will automatically lead to binge eating. The person may say, "As long as I have eaten one cookie, I have failed, so I might as well eat the entire package."

Bulimic people are *perfectionistic* in their personal standards of behavior. Even with their typically high level of professional achievement, they are extremely self-critical and often feel incompetent and inadequate. They set unrealistic standards of weight control and feel like failures when unable to maintain these standards. The thought of failure is a contributing factor to the binge phase of the cycle. Following the purge phase, they promise themselves to be more steadfast and disciplined with their diet. Because these resolutions are unrealistic, they set themselves up for another failure (Pope, Phillips, & Olivardia, 2000). Characteristics of people with anorexia and bulimia are listed in Table 12.2 ■.

Bill, who suffers from bulimia, states: "If I see another guy my age at the gym with perfectly defined abs, it really ruins my day."

SOCIAL CHARACTERISTICS

Women's bodies, much more so than men's, have always been perceived as unfinished and in need of revamping to make them conform to the cultural standards of beauty. From Chinese women with bound feet in the 12th and 13th centuries, to corsets in the 19th century, to binding breasts in the early 20th century, to today's lean, physically fit, and surgically altered body, women have tried to change their bodies to "look good."

In American society, *female attractiveness* is strongly equated with thinness. Models, actresses, and the media glamorize extreme thinness, which is then equated with success and happiness. This cultural obsession for an extremely thin female body has led to widespread prejudice against overweight people. This prejudice has a significant impact on overall self-esteem and self-acceptance. Self-worth is enhanced for

TABLE 12.2

Characteristics of Eating Disorders

Characteristic	People with Anorexia	People with Bulimia
Self-evaluation	Are dependent on response from others; are self-depreciating	Are self-critical; view themselves as incompetent
Decision making	Need to make perfect decisions	Need to make perfect decisions
Rituals	Are obsessive in eating and exercise	Perpetuate the binge/purge/fast cycle
Sense of control	Create a sense of control and achievement by refusing to eat	Set unrealistic standards for own behavior; feel out of control
Phobia	Initially fear weight gain; develop food phobia	None specific
Exercise	Have obsessive routines	Exercise sporadically
Fears	Fear not being perfect, weight gain, fat, loss of control	Fear loss of control, weight gain, rejection
Guilt	Experience guilt when they eat more than they believe appropriate	Experience guilt when they binge eat and purge
Defense mechanisms	Deny hunger, exhaustion, disease	Do not deny hunger
Insight into illness	Are ego-syntonic; do not believe they have a disorder; see anorexia as the solution, not the problem	Are ego-dystonic; are disgusted with self but helpless to change
Cognitive distortions	Practice selective abstraction, overgeneralization, magnification, personalization, dichotomous thinking	Practice selective abstraction, overgeneralization, magnification, personalization, dichotomous thinking
Body image	Experience delusional distortion	See themselves as slightly larger
Relationships	Attempt to please and placate others	Experience conflicts between dependency and autonomy
Social isolation	Tend to isolate themselves to protect against rejection; tend to be more introverted	Need privacy for binge eating and purging; tend to be extroverted
Weight loss	Experience 25–50% weight loss	Maintain normal weight or experience slight weight loss
Death	Results usually from starvation, when body proteins are depleted to half the normal levels	Often results from hypokalemia, a deficiency of potassium (leading cause), and suicide (second most frequent cause)

those who are judged attractive and diminished for those deemed unattractive (Grogan, 1999).

Box 12.1 lists the cultural values that are extremely harmful to all women, whether overweight, normal weight, or underweight.

Magazines marketed for adolescent women often present diet and weight control as the solutions for adolescent crises and contain 90 percent more articles and advertisements promoting dieting as compared to magazines read by young men. Thus, the body

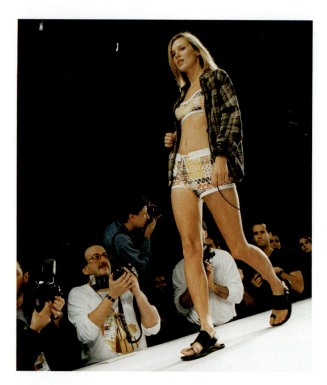

PHOTO 12.1A ■ Images of women in advertising and the popular media often equate thinness with beauty, success, and happiness.

SOURCE: Ron Frehm/AP/Wide World Photos.

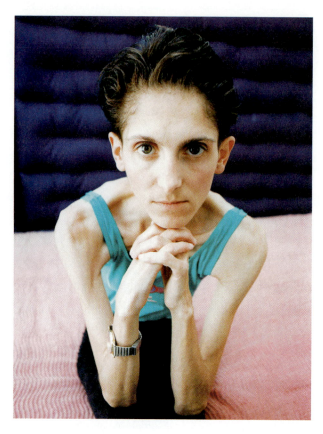

PHOTO 12.1B ■ Caraline, 28 years old, told a reporter, "I'm not telling you how much I weigh because I'm ashamed I don't weigh less." She later died of complications due to anorexia nervosa.

SOURCE: Express Newspapers/Getty Images, Inc.

becomes the central focus of existence, and self-esteem becomes dependent on the ability to control weight and food intake. This *preoccupation with body image* continues throughout women's lives. In fact, dieting and concerns about weight have become so pervasive that they are now the norm for American women.

Fear of fat is a constant companion. Young girls are often rewarded for their attempts at weight control. Peers, family members, coaches, dance teachers, and others may actively support the attainment or maintenance of low body weight. Those who go on to develop eating disorders may have internalized an exaggerated version of the cultural ideal, the basis of which is that women define their value and worth in terms of being attractive to and obtaining love from men. No wonder eating disorders occur when women have grown up in a culture that is fat phobic, where they may have been ridiculed for being overweight or may have participated in ridiculing others. Discovering that thin girls frequently have more friends, go on more dates, and receive higher grades in school, they believe they can win approval, parental love, and social recognition by a frantic pursuit of thinness.

Young women with anorexia usually find that severe dieting does not produce the reward of being sought after by young men. In response to this real or perceived rejection, they feel even more unattractive and undesirable. To protect themselves, they begin to lose interest in social activities and *withdraw* from their peers. Dating is minimal or nonexistent, and they purport to have no interest in sexual activities. High scholastic achievement may be an attempt to compensate for the lack of peer relationships (Ghizzani & Montomoli, 2000).

The ideal of *male attractiveness* in American society has been changing and has contributed to an increase in eating disorders among men. Magazines targeted for a predominantly male audience tend to focus on body-

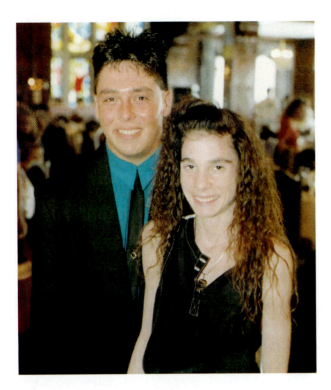

PHOTO 12.1C ■ Olympic-class gymnast Christy Heinrich with her boyfriend in 1993. After a 3-year struggle with anorexia nervosa, she died of multiple organ failure in 1994. She weighed less than 50 pounds at the time.

SOURCE: AP/Wide World Photos.

building, weight lifting, or muscle toning. The "ideal" male body is one with well-developed muscles on the chest, arms, and shoulders with a slim waist and hips. This ideal is becoming more and more difficult for the average boy or man to attain. Little boys are being taught to value their self-esteem on being strong and athletic. Their action toys have washboard abdominal muscles, and their heroes are members of the World Wrestling Federation (WWF). Men with eating disorders have an overwhelming fear of fatness and a desire to maintain a masculine appearance or shape. It is not uncommon to see males with eating disorders use anabolic steroids to improve muscle tone and build strength (Pope et al., 2000).

Research has demonstrated that a disproportionately high number of men with eating disorders are gay or bisexual. Much like expectations for women, within the gay male culture there are strong pressures on men to be physically attractive, thin, and youthful looking, especially among gay men whose social life is centered on the "gay scene"—clubbing, drinking, and the like. Being less likely to be satisfied with their body weight and shape, gay men have an increased risk for developing anorexia or bulimia (Alexander, 1996; Grogan, 1999; Woodside et al., 2001).

People with bulimia experience shame and guilt about their behavior and may *withdraw socially* to hide it. They also need privacy for binge eating and purging, which contributes further to their isolation. The more isolated they become, the more the behavior tends to escalate, as food is used to fill the void and provide a source of comfort. Generally, they do not become as socially isolated as those do with anorexia. Although they are sexually active, they have difficulty enjoying sex because of fears relating to loss of control. Feeling inadequate and incompetent, they may fear the intimacy of a long-term relationship.

BOX 12.1

Cultural Values Harmful to All Women

Thinness equals power and control, and fat equals helplessness and lack of self-control. Those who are fat are viewed as helpless people who are weak-willed, nonachieving, and out of control. What often goes unrecognized, however, is the fact that it's the compulsion for thinness that is out of control.

Thinness equals beauty, and fat equals ugliness. Thinness is the most important aspect of physical attractiveness, and fat women are considered to be sexually unattractive.

Thinness equals happiness, and fat equals unhappiness. The main determining factor of joy in life becomes tied to body size and shape. A slim body is seen as the only way to achieve a happy life.

Thinness equals goodness, and fat equals immorality. The message is that those who diet and are thin are good, whereas those who eat normally are fat and bad. Because fat is considered a moral issue, discrimination is accepted as an appropriate response.

Thinness equals fitness, and fat equals laziness. The fitness movement has perpetuated the glorification of thinness as the cultural ideal. Those people who are overweight or even normal weight are considered lazy and have only themselves to blame for their body size.

CULTURE-SPECIFIC CHARACTERISTICS

There is considerable evidence that eating disorders occur predominantly in industrialized, developed countries and that they occur less often in traditional societies. For example, Native Canadians (Ojibway-Cree) tend to show a preference for heavier body types compared to the Euro-Canadian population. The incidence is changing, however, as cultures around the world become more Westernized. In a sense, anorexia and bulimia could be considered to be culture-reactive syndromes in the Western world (Keel et al., 2001).

A surprising influence in a girl's vulnerability may be her ethnic background. Recent studies have found, for instance, that African American women's perceptions of beauty are less media driven than those of Euro-American women. Dieting is less rampant, as are unhealthy weight management practices, and African American teens may be more accepting of the way they look. African American women and men are more positive about higher weights in women than are Euro-American women and men. African American women who are obese have a more positive body image than their Euro-American counterparts.

Typically, Asian American and Latino women have been less likely to describe themselves as fat, less dissatisfied with their body size, and less likely to diet. Recent research, however, indicates that a cultural shift is occurring. Asian American and Latino women are becoming less satisfied with their bodies, and cultural media are currently presenting thin ideal body sizes for women, similar to those presented in the Anglo media (Grogan, 1999).

Women in other cultures experience behaviors and symptoms that superficially appear to be similar but may not be identical in the causes or meanings of the disorder. Arab women in Qatar experience a culture-bound syndrome characterized by nausea, poor appetite, breathing difficulty, palpitations, faintness, and fatigue. The majority of these victims are either unmarried or have fertility problems. The disorder is rooted in the cultural belief that the value of women is based on their husbands and the children they have. As women become more educated and are exposed to Western media, they discover the different female–male relationships of more developed nations. Thus, they find themselves caught between traditional cultural values and new values and role expectations. Women in Zar cults in North Africa and parts of Asia experience a culture-bound syndrome called *Zars*, which is possession by spirits. Symptoms include anorexia, nausea, depression, anxiety, headaches, and fertility problems (Silverstein & Perlick, 1995).

PHYSIOLOGICAL CHARACTERISTICS

There are many physiological effects of starvation and purging of the body. *Electrolyte imbalance* may cause muscle weakness, seizures, arrhythmias, and even death, with hypokalemia being the most critical electrolyte abnormality. There are several ways hypokalemia develops. With vomiting, there is some loss of potassium itself. Perhaps more important is metabolic alkalosis, which results from the loss of stomach acid through vomiting. This, in turn, causes a shift of potassium from the extracellular space into the cells, thereby lowering the serum potassium level. In addition, laxative abuse causes loss of potassium through the lower GI system (Boskind-White & White, 2000).

Decreased blood volume results in lowered blood pressure and postural hypotension. Lessened sympathetic nervous system activity is reflected in symptoms such as hypotension, bradycardia, and hypothermia. Elevated blood urea nitrogen (BUN) indicates decreased blood flow to the kidneys, which predisposes these individuals to edema. Cardiovascular changes include a decrease in cardiac chamber dimensions and thinning of the heart muscle wall. With underoxygenation of the heart muscle and bradycardia, cardiac output is decreased.

Gastrointestinal complications such as constipation, cathartic colon, and laxative dependence may develop. When food is in short supply, gastric emptying slows to improve the efficiency of nutrient absorption. This also delays the expenditure of energy required for digestion, absorption, and storage. Frequent vomiting can lead to esophagitis, with scarring and stricture. Changes in the epithelial lining of the esophagus have the potential to advance to cancer. If perforation or rupture of the esophagus occurs, there is a 20 percent mortality rate even with immediate treatment. Gastric rupture, fortunately a fairly rare occurrence, carries a mortality rate of 85 percent. Repeated vomiting decreases tooth enamel, causing dental caries and tooth loss. There may be a chronic sore throat, and salivary glands are usually swollen and tender. Some people with bulimia may demonstrate **Russell's sign**, a callus on the back of the hand, formed by repeated trauma from the teeth when forcing vomiting (Boskind-White & White, 2000).

Amenorrhea is an extremely common occurrence in females with anorexia, and irregular menses are frequently associated with bulimia. Although the exact mechanism is unclear, menstrual problems are thought to be related to the degree of stress the person is experiencing, the percentage of body fat lost, and altered hypothalamic function. There are also abnormalities in the secretion of luteinizing hormone and follicle-stimulating hormone, resulting in low estrogen and progesterone levels. With low estrogen levels, these young women are at higher risk for *osteoporosis*. In a similar fashion, testosterone levels drop in male sufferers. In an adaptive effort to limit energy expenditure and conserve protein, thyroid hormone levels drop. People with anorexia develop lanugo hair on their body, reflecting their state of starvation. Lanugo is the soft, downy hair covering a fetus beginning in the fifth month of gestation and which is almost entirely shed by the ninth month (Levenkron, 2000).

People with anorexia usually experience a *weight loss* of 25 percent, but a loss as high as 50 percent is possible. People with bulimia do not reach such low levels of weight and may, in fact, remain at normal weight. Since a large food intake speeds up the gastric emptying rate, a significant number of calories are absorbed before the purging begins.

The physiological effects of malnutrition and vomiting are widespread throughout the body. In some cases, death occurs as a result of these disruptions. See Boxes 12.2 and 12.3 for an overview of the physical complications of eating disorders.

CONCOMITANT DISORDERS

The most frequently observed disorder is *depression*. In some cases, this may be the result of abnormal eating and weight loss. In other cases, the depression is the primary disorder to which the eating disorder is a

---

BOX 12.2

Physical Complications of Anorexia

Organ System	Signs and Symptoms
Whole body	Weakness; malnutrition; low weight; low body fat
Central nervous system	Apathy; poor concentration; cognitive impairment; depression; irritable mood
Cardiovascular system	Palpitations; irregular pulse; dizziness; hypotension; shortness of breath; chest pain; peripheral vasoconstriction with cold extremities; decrease in cardiac chamber dimensions; thinning of heart muscle walls
Skeletal	Bone pain with exercise; arrested skeletal growth; osteoporosis
Muscular	Weakness; muscle wasting
Reproductive	Loss of menses or primary amenorrhea; arrested sexual development; decreased sex drive; pregnancy and neonatal complications
Endocrine, metabolic	Low body temperature; fatigue; electrolyte abnormalities; low thyroid levels; elevated serum cortisol; dehydration
Hematologic	Anemia; neutropenia; low erythrocyte sedimentation rate
Gastrointestinal	Abdominal pain; distention and bloating with meals; delayed gastric emptying; constipation; abnormal bowel sounds
Urinary	Low glomerular filtration rate; elevated BUN; pitting edema; kidney failure
Skin	Presence of lanugo hair on body

SOURCES: American Psychiatric Association (2000). *Practicing guideline for the treatment of patients with eating disorders* (2nd ed.). Washington, DC: Author; Levenkron, S. (2000). *Anatomy of anorexia.* New York: Norton; and White, J. H. (2000). Symptom development in bulimia nervosa: A comparison of women with and without a history of anorexia nervosa. *Archives of Psychiatric Nursing, 14*(2), 81–92.

Physical Complications of Bulimia

Organ System	Signs and Symptoms
Whole body	Weakness; malnutrition; average body weight
Central nervous system	Irritability; depression
Cardiovascular system	Palpitations; arrhythmias
Reproductive	Fertility problems; irregular menses
Endocrine, metabolic	Hypokalemia; hypochloremic alkalosis (vomiting); hypomagnesemia and hypophosphatemia (laxative abuse)
Gastrointestinal	Abdominal pain; gastritis; esophagitis; perforation of the esophagus; increased rate of pancreatitis; constipation; bowel irregularities
Oropharyngeal	Dental decay; chronic sore throat; swollen salivary glands
Skin	Scarring on back of hand (Russell's sign)

SOURCES: American Psychiatric Association (2000). *Practice guideline for the treatment of patients with eating disorders* (2nd ed.). Washington, DC: Author; Boskind-White, M., & White, W. C. (2000). *Bulimia/anorexia* (3rd ed.). New York: Norton. White, J. H. (2000). Symptom development in bulimia nervosa: A comparison of women with and without a history of anorexia nervosa. *Archives of Psychiatric Nursing, 14*(2), 81–92.

response. And for other people, the depression and eating disorder are both primary disorders (APA, 2000b; White, 2000).

There is a high prevalence of several *anxiety disorders* associated with eating disorders. *Social phobias* may occur in people with eating disorders, possibly in response to others' awareness of their abnormal eating behaviors. *Obsessive–compulsive symptoms* are common, especially among people with anorexia. Obsessive–compulsive symptoms often continue even after weight is restored in anorexia. *Panic attacks* are likely when anorexic people are prohibited from exercising their usual behavior patterns. It is unclear whether these are primary disorders or are secondary to the eating disorders (Ranson, Kaye, Weltzin, Rao, & Matsunaga, 1999).

Eating-disordered people often *abuse substances*. In some, this may be an effort to self-medicate the symptoms of anxiety or depression. Others may abuse substances, such as cocaine, in an effort to decrease their appetite. Eating disorders share many features with problem drinking. Both begin with a decrease in anxiety in response to the behavior (drinking or not eating). Eventually both groups of people lose control over the behavior and continue on a path of self-destruction. There is a compulsive need to engage in

the behavior with considerable distress if the behavior is disrupted. Denial is the central defense mechanism of both disorders, and both have a chronic course with frequent relapses (APA, 2000b; Woodside et al., 2001).

CAUSATIVE THEORIES

The causes of eating disorders are multiple in individuals and across a variety of people. Fatness and thinness are outcomes of biological, psychological, and social processes. Weight is determined by the balance between energy intake and expenditure, and this balance is the product of many influences. Having a knowledge base about the major theories will help you understand individual clients from a composite perspective.

Genetics

Family risk studies demonstrate that relatives of eating-disordered clients are four to five times more likely to develop an eating disorder. It appears that in anorexia, the more severe the disorder, the more likely a strong genetic predisposition. Twin studies for anorexia show that the concordance rate for monozygotic twins is 55 to 71 percent and for dizygotic twins, 0 to 32 percent. These data suggest that there may be a *genetic predisposition* to anorexia. Concordance rates for bulimia range from 23 to 83 percent for monozygotic twins and 0 to 27 percent for dizygotic twins. Some studies report a higher rate among first-degree relatives while others do not (Bellodi et al., 2001; Paris, 1999; Strober, Freeman, Lampert, Diamond, & Kaye, 2000).

Neurobiologic Theory

Recent studies indicate that *neurotransmitter dysregulation* may be involved in eating disorders, particularly serotonin (5-HT). Being full of food to the point of satisfaction is referred to as *satiety*. Normally, a low level of 5-HT decreases a person's satiety and thereby increases food intake. In contrast, a high level of 5-HT increases satiety and thereby decreases food intake. Carbohydrates (CHOs) are involved in the synthesis of 5-HT by increasing tryptophan, the precursor of 5-HT. The neurotransmitter hypothesis of bulimia is that the recurrent binge episodes may result from a deficiency in 5-HT and low satiety levels. Since people with bulimia tend to binge on high-CHO foods, this may be a reflection of the body's adaptive attempt to increase 5-HT levels. The neurotransmitter hypothesis of anorexia is that decreased food intake is related to excess 5-HT and increased satiety (Kaye et al., 2001; Smock, 1999).

Other neurotransmitters affect eating behavior. Norepinephrine (NE) and neuropeptide Y (NPY) increase eating behavior while dopamine (DA) suppresses food intake. DA agonists such as amphetamines and cocaine are known appetite suppressants (Smock, 1999).

Endogenous opioids, such as endorphins, are associated with food intake and mood. Opioids increase food intake and enhance positive mood states; therefore, insufficient levels cause decreased food intake and depressed mood. It has been found that underweight people have significantly lower levels of endorphins compared to healthy volunteers. When the person's weight is returned to normal levels, the endorphin level is also within normal limits (Smock, 1999).

Intrapersonal Theory

Intrapersonal theorists believe that people at higher risk for eating disorders are those who have low self-esteem, experience significant adolescent turmoil, and who have difficulty with identity formation. Personality characteristics of people with anorexia are anxiety intolerance, a lack of personal effectiveness and self-

direction, and difficulty achieving the maturational tasks of adolescence. People with bulimia are described in terms of affective instability and poor impulse control.

Motivation for losing weight is viewed in terms of how the people see themselves relating to others. For some, the motivation is an attempt to create closeness by gaining attention from parents, siblings, and friends. Others are motivated to create distance by avoiding identification with a disliked parent. The third possible motive is deliberate action against people, using eating behavior to express anger and control parental behavior. The intense concern over food says, "This is an area in which I am in control and can defy the demands of others," while at the same time saying, "I am only a little child who has to be looked after" (Boskind-White & White, 2000).

Impulsive personality traits are characteristic of many people suffering from bulimia. The loss of control and the inability to stop binging once it starts is the typical bulimic pattern. This impulsivity resembles other addictive disorders (Paris, 1999).

Cognitive Theory

Cognitive theorists believe that cognitive distortions and dysfunctional thoughts such as dichotomous thinking and catastrophizing (exaggerating failures in one's life) contribute to disordered eating patterns. The extreme belief is: "It is absolutely essential that I be thin." This belief leads to dieting, avoidant behavior, and increased isolation, which in turn cause a lack of responsiveness to alternative cognitive input. Given the cultural emphasis on thinness, there is a sense of gratification, self-control, mastery, and approval of or concern from others.

Behavioral Theory

Behavioral theorists are concerned with what the disordered behavior accomplishes rather than why the behavior occurs. Eating disorders are considered phobias. In this context, anxiety rises with eating and decreases with fasting or purging. Anxiety reduction is the reinforcer for both anorexia and bulimia.

Family Theory

Most family theorists believe family issues are not specific to eating disorders. The family is viewed more as an enabler of the disorder than as a primary causative factor. Some eating-disordered people are survivors of childhood or adolescent sexual abuse, which may or may not have occurred within the family or extended family system. (Sexual abuse is discussed further in Chapter 22.)

As the result of anorexia, some families become enmeshed; that is, the boundaries between the members are weak, interactions are intense, dependency on one another is high, and autonomy is minimal. Everybody is involved in each member's concerns, and there is minimal privacy. The enmeshed family system becomes overprotective of the child, and the entire family system becomes preoccupied with food, eating, and rituals involving meals. In contrast, current research indicates that families of people with bulimia are less enmeshed than those of anorexic people. Family members tend to be isolated from one another, and eating behavior may be an attempt to decrease feelings of loneliness and boredom (Levenkron, 2000).

Many families of those with eating disorders have difficulty with conflict resolution. An ethical or religious value against disagreements within the family supports the avoidance of conflict. When problems are denied for the sake of family harmony, they cannot be resolved, and growth of the family system is inhibited. The anorexic child may protect and maintain the family unit. In some family systems, the parents avoid conflict with each other by uniting in a common concern for the child's welfare. In other family systems, the issues of marital conflict are converted into disagreements over how the anorexic child should be managed. In both systems, the marital problems are camouflaged in an effort to prevent the disruption of the family unit. (See Chapter 3 for more details on family dynamics.)

Many families of clients with eating disorders are achievement and performance oriented, with high ambitions for the success of all members. In these families, body shape is related to success, and priorities are established for physical appearance and fitness. The family's focus on professional achievement as well as on food, diet, exercise, and weight control may become obsessional.

Feminist Theory

From the feminist perspective, eating disorders arise out of a conflict between female development and traditional developmental theories. Western culture has viewed male development as the norm, and autonomy as the opposite of dependency. For women, the oppo-

site of dependency is isolation. Conflict arises when women believe they must become autonomous and minimize relationships in order to be recognized as mature adults. For some, this conflict is acted out in self-destructive eating behavior (Striegel-Moore, 1995).

Cultural stereotypes contribute to women's preoccupation with their bodies. Attractiveness is determined by how closely a woman's appearance matches the cultural ideal of thinness. Thus, identity and self-esteem are dependent on physical appearance. Being disgusted with one's flesh is the same as having an adversarial relationship with the body—a relationship that often results in eating disorders.

PSYCHOPHARMACOLOGICAL INTERVENTIONS

Medications, primarily antidepressants, are used to reduce the frequency of disturbed eating behaviors such as binge eating and vomiting. In addition, medications are used to ease symptoms that may accompany eating disorders such as depression, anxiety, obsessions, or impulse control problems.

So far, medications seem to be more effective in treating bulimia than anorexia. The tricyclic antidepressant Tofranil (imipramine) produces a 50 to 75 percent reduction in the frequency of binge eating and reduces the preoccupation with food, as well as anxiety and depressive symptoms. Another tricyclic antidepressant, Norpramine (desipramine), appears to decrease binge eating in those who do not have current symptoms of depression. Tricyclic antidepressants are started at very low doses (10 to 25 mg/day) and over a period of three to four weeks are increased to 3 mg/kg of body weight. Prozac (fluoxetine) and Zoloft (sertraline), selective serotonin reuptake inhibitors (SSRIs), are also effective for these clients, when given at the higher dose of 50 to 60 mg per day. Typically, the medication is continued until six months following the disappearance of symptoms. In some studies, lithium has been used alone or in conjunction with tricyclic antidepressants. Caution must be taken, however, when prescribing lithium for a client who is purging. Vomiting will decrease intracellular potassium, and lithium may exacerbate this effect. Overemphasis on pharmacological treatment of bulimia is dangerous and demeaning to people as it may become an attempt to medicate away a psychosocial disorder (APA, 2000b; Devlin et al., 2000; Walsh et al., 2000).

MULTIDISCIPLINARY INTERVENTIONS

The current therapeutic approach for eating disorders relies on a combination of psychological, behavioral, and nutritional techniques often provided in an inpatient or intensive outpatient setting. If the anorexic client is evaluated as highly endangered, as assessed by weight, current rate of weight loss, nutritional status, organ functioning, and cardiac health, she or he may be admitted to an acute care medical facility. Medical treatment may include a feeding schedule, potassium supplements, and bed rest. Tube feeding and parenteral nutrition are avoided unless absolutely necessary because they do not help clients assume responsibility for their own health.

Psychological treatment may include individual therapy, group work, family therapy, cognitive therapy, and systematic desensitization. Behavior therapists view bulimia as attempts to change or control painful emotional states through binge eating and purging. Consumers are taught skills to replace their dysfunctional behaviors. The majority of centers that treat clients with eating disorders also use cognitive behavior therapy to change the disordered eating pattern (Safer, Telch, & Agras, 2001).

When people have incorporated their eating disorder into their identities, therapy can be a threat. Unlike many clients with other mental disorders who wish to be free of their symptoms, people with eating disorders are often very reluctant to give up the drive for thinness or low weight. They may also believe that there is a positive stigma to having an eating disorder—such as being a member of the "eating disorder club." Their lives can become filled with support groups, and they continually discuss their obsessions regarding food, weight, and shape. Groups of people with eating disorders can become competitive: Who is the thinnest? Who ate the least? Who exercised the most? Understanding the function that the eating disorder serves in terms of creating an identity is essential in treatment planning.

ALTERNATIVE THERAPIES

Clients with eating disorders should take vitamin and mineral complexes. They are usually taken in very high doses because they are passed through the gastrointestinal tract rapidly and are poorly assimilated. The multivitamin complex should contain (Balch & Balch, 1997):

Natural beta-carotene	25,000 IU daily	
Vitamin A	10,000 IU daily	
Calcium	1,500 mg daily	
Copper	3 mg daily	
Magnesium	1,000 mg daily	
Potassium	99 mg daily	
Selenium	200 µg daily	
Zinc	80 mg daily	Do not exceed a total of 100 mg daily from all supplements.

Clients who are vomiting or using laxatives should take acidophilus, which replaces the "friendly" bacteria lost through purging. Acidophilus should be taken on an empty stomach so that it passes quickly to the small intestine. The following herbs may be used as appetite stimulants: gingerroot, ginseng, gotu kola, and peppermint. Clients should not use ginseng if they are hypertensive.

NURSING PROCESS

Assessment

A focused nursing assessment, which includes a physiological assessment, should be completed for clients with eating disorders (see the Focused Nursing Assessment feature). You must be on the alert for medical emergencies such as acute cardiac failure, acute gastric dilatation, esophageal bleeding, and massive peripheral edema.

Clients with bulimia may welcome the opportunity to talk about their disorder with a caring, nonjudgmental nurse. Moreover, learning that they are not alone in having bulimia may relieve some of their anxiety and distress. Clients with anorexia, on the other hand, may not be as willing to talk about their disorder. Client denial of problems or illness may interfere with your ability to obtain an accurate nursing assessment. A supportive and caring approach is necessary to establish rapport with these clients.

Behavior Assessment	Affective Assessment	Cognitive Assessment
What type of eating patterns do you have?	Describe any of the following fears: gaining weight, being fat, rejection by others, losing control over eating.	Do you believe your eating pattern is in any way unusual?
Do you have rules for eating, such as places to eat? Combination of foods? Number of pieces of food? Number of times to chew food?	What kinds of situations make you feel guilty? Ashamed? Anxious? Frustrated? Helpless?	Do you have any desire to alter your eating behavior?
What time of day do you usually binge? Where do you do this? How often? How long does it last? Foods that trigger a binge? Favorite foods to eat on a binge?	What are your feelings when you eat more than your diet allows?	Describe your body to me. Describe what an attractive person looks like. What would your life be like if you were as thin as you wished?
After binge eating, how do you rid your body of the food? Vomit? Laxatives? Diuretics?		What will happen if you gain weight?
How much time do you spend exercising each day?		
How does the use of alcohol or drugs help you cope with your problems?		

In general, nursing assessment includes a detailed analysis of eating patterns and weight fluctuations, methods of weight control, food avoided and the reasons they are avoided, and the occurrence and frequency of binge eating and purging. In addition, you explore the individual's and family's beliefs about nutrition and attitudes toward eating, exercise, and appearance. Side effects of steroid abuse may include several psychiatric symptoms such as hallucinations, manic symptoms, and depression. Other mental disorders that must be taken into consideration include depression, anxiety disorders, and substance abuse. If left untreated, these comorbid conditions can significantly reduce treatment effectiveness.

Nurses who work with adolescent and young adult athletes, particularly those athletes participating in the at-risk sports, must be alert to early symptoms of eating disorders. Simple screening questions about weight, possible dissatisfaction with appearance, exercise routine, and nutritional intake on the day before evaluation may help identify a person who is developing an eating disorder.

Diagnosis

After analyzing and synthesizing the client assessment data, you develop nursing diagnoses. The client's level of malnourishment must be identified because, in some cases, death could be imminent. The client's binge eating and/or purging patterns must be identified, as well as her or his fears, cognitive distortions, and relation-

Social Assessment

How often do you socialize with friends? What activities do you do together?

How close are the members of your family?

What are the family rules about disagreements?

Describe your family's standards for physical fitness and appearance.

How do other members of the family control their weight?

Physiological Assessment

Weight
What is your present weight?

What is the most you have ever weighed?

What is the least you have ever weighed?

Endocrine
Are you having menstrual periods?

Describe your usual cycle to me.

Cardiovascular
Do you get dizzy when you stand up from a lying position?

Have you experienced any heart palpitations? Irregular heartbeat?

Are you having any problems with your ankles and feet swelling? Your fingers?

Gastrointestinal
Have you had an increase in the number of dental caries?

Have you lost any teeth?

Do you have frequent sore throats?

Do you experience heartburn?

Do you have problems with constipation?

Neurological
Have you experienced any seizures or convulsions?

---

ships with family and friends. See the Nursing Diagnoses with NOC & NIC feature for examples of nursing diagnoses for clients with eating disorders.

Outcome Identification and Goals

Based on the assessment data, you select outcomes appropriate to the nursing diagnoses. The most common outcomes are found in the Nursing Diagnoses with NOC & NIC feature.

Once you have established outcomes, you and the client mutually identify goals for change. Client goals are specific behavioral prescriptions that you, the client, and significant others identify as realistic and attainable. The following are examples of goals appropriate to people with eating disorders:

- Verbalizes increased satisfaction with self
- Demonstrates more flexible daily routines
- Exercises appropriately
- Decreases frequency of binge eating and purging
- Verbalizes fewer fears
- Achieves target weight
- Identifies secondary gains
- Verbalizes fewer cognitive distortions
- Family problem-solves together

Nursing Interventions

In response to the unrelenting demand of the cultural ideal, fat has become a feminist issue. It is time for

NURSING DIAGNOSES with NOC & NIC

Clients with Eating Disorders

DIAGNOSIS	OUTCOMES	INTERVENTIONS
Altered nutrition: Less than body requirements related to reduced intake; purging	**Nutritional Status:** Extent to which nutrients are available to meet metabolic needs	Eating Disorders Management
Anxiety related to fears of gaining weight and losing control	**Anxiety Control:** Personal actions to eliminate or reduce feelings of apprehension and tension from an unidentifiable source	Eating Disorders Management
Altered thought process related to dichotomous thinking, overgeneralization, personalization, obsessions, and superstitious thinking	**Distorted Thought Control:** Self-restraint of disruption in perception, thought processes, and thought content	Cognitive Restructuring
Body image disturbance related to delusional perception of body in anorexia	**Distorted Thought Control:** Self-restraint of disruption in perception, thought processes, and thought content	Cognitive Restructuring
Impaired social interaction related to withdrawal from peer group and fears of rejection	**Social Involvement:** Frequency of an individual's social interactions with persons, groups, or organizations	Eating Disorders Management
Powerlessness related to having no control over bulimic pattern	**Impulse Control:** Self-restraint of compulsive or impulsive behaviors	Eating Disorders Management
Altered family processes related to enabling disordered eating or enmeshed family system	**Family Functioning:** Ability of the family to meet the needs of its members through developmental transitions	Family Involvement

SOURCES: Johnson, M., Maas, M., & Moorhead, S. (2000). *Nursing outcomes classification (NOC)* (2nd ed.). St. Louis, MO: Mosby; and McCloskey, J. C., & Bulechek, G. M. (1996). *Nursing interventions classification (NIC)* (2nd ed.). St. Louis, MO: Mosby. North American Nursing Diagnosis Association (1999). *Nursing diagnoses, definitions and classification 1999–2000*. Philadelphia: Author

nursing to challenge the cultural ideal and respond appropriately to people suffering from eating disorders. Nurses must become leaders in fostering a humane approach to body size.

Because we, as nurses, are products of our culture, we have probably internalized the prejudice against fat. Before intervening with clients, we must rethink our values and rid ourselves of unrealistic ideals. When working with overweight clients, we must understand that they do not necessarily have more emotional problems than people of normal weight. Their emotional problems are most likely a result of prejudice and stigma and the cultural pressure to lose weight. Decreasing the stigma as well as the internalized disgust will greatly benefit overweight clients. We must be careful not to perpetuate the misconception that losing weight will solve all other problems in life. A thin body is neither a magical cure nor a guarantee for living happily ever after.

You can actively challenge idealized cultural values by eliminating all negative references to overweight people in verbal and written communications. You can support people of average weight and express concern for people who are severely underweight. You can speak up about the potential life-threatening aspects of dieting behavior. You can help expand the standard of feminine beauty. We can teach our daughters how to defend against cultural pressures for weight loss and how to love, respect, and celebrate their bodies. We can teach our sons that women are not ornaments or sex objects, teach them to respect and appreciate women who have many qualities and many sizes and shapes. Finally, we must help all clients view themselves as competent people who have many talents and traits—creativity, humor, empathy, warmth, and wisdom. All of us must work together to eliminate the depreciation of women and instead celebrate womanhood.

Most clients will be seen in an outpatient setting. Inpatient care is necessary when clients are in life-threatening circumstances related to starvation, are at risk for suicide, or are experiencing extreme social isolation. It is a challenge to develop a therapeutic alliance with eating-disordered clients. They often resist interventions and are angry about being in treatment. You should use a kind, firm, and consistent approach and work toward a collaborative relationship. It is sometimes difficult to maintain the balance between setting clear limits on behaviors and helping these clients grow in autonomy. The ultimate goal is to have them take responsibility for their own behavior. See the Nursing Diagnosis with NOC & NIC feature for clients with eating disorders.

Physiological: Basic

Nutritional Support

Eating Disorders Management People with anorexia or bulimia have multiple anxieties, most of which get translated into fears of weight gain and loss of control. Help them *identify underlying fears*, such as a fear of rejection, that have been transformed into a fear of gaining weight. Those with bulimia typically confuse negative emotions as sensations of hunger and binge eat as a source of comfort. Help them label a variety of negative feelings and begin to distinguish these from hunger pangs. The fear of weight gain can be all-consuming. In fact, encouraging them to gain weight asks them to do the very thing of which they are most frightened. The term *weight restoration* may be more acceptable because the term *weight gain* often creates an instant phobic response. Provide repeated assurance that they will not be allowed to become fat.

It is important that a *target weight* be identified. This is usually set at 90 percent of the average weight for the person's age and height. Identifying a reasonable target weight reassures clients that they will not be forced to become overweight. It is best to choose a weight range of four to six pounds rather than a single target weight, since this helps clients learn to accept a certain amount of normal weight fluctuation. Clients should be weighed only once or twice a week to decrease the amount of time spent in obsessing about weight. Be alert to techniques of artificially increasing weight, such as concealing heavy objects in clothing or drinking large amounts of water.

Negotiate with clients a reasonable *contract* that states how much to eat for each meal and snack. The contract usually begins with a moderate amount, such as 1,000 to 1,500 kcal per day, which is gradually increased. Begin with a diet low in fats and milk products, since starvation has led to an insufficiency of the bowel enzymes necessary for digestion of these foods. The sensation of bloating may lessen if the calories are spread across six meals a day. A food diary is often helpful to both clients and staff. Clients are to keep the diary with them at all times and record all food eaten as well as any binge eating and purging. They are also to include notation of their thoughts and feelings associated with eating or not eating.

There are a number of ways you can assist people to decrease binge eating. Talk over the difference between emotions and sensations of hunger, since misinterpretation of emotions contributes to binge eating. Through the *food diary*, have them analyze which particular foods trigger binge eating. Review situations that precede binge eating, and explore alternative coping behaviors. Insight into high-risk situations will help clients gain control of binges. Encourage delay in responding to the urge to binge by trying alternative behaviors such as talking to a teacher or counselor, calling a friend, or using relaxation techniques. The delay interrupts the habitual cycle of behavior. Confer with clients on ways to *avoid privacy* at the usual time of binges, since most binge eating occurs in isolation. Being with other people decreases opportunities to binge eat. Other methods of inhibiting binge-eating behavior include avoiding fast-food restaurants, formulating a list of "safe" foods, and shopping for food with a friend. Teach clients to eat three to six meals a day, since this interrupts the fasting part of the cycle. They should include a carbohydrate at each meal, since deprivation may trigger binge eating.

Another nursing intervention is to *discourage purging activities*. Discuss how purging is used to manage negative feelings. When clients make the connection between purging and anxiety, guilt, and self-disgust; they may be able to identify healthier behaviors. Clients who typically purge after meals are not allowed to use the bathroom unsupervised for two hours after eating. Since anxiety often escalates in relation to eating and the prevention of purging, one-to-one support is often necessary before, during, and after meals. Clients are encouraged to talk to staff, parents, and friends when they feel the urge to vomit and thus increase their control over impulsive behavior.

Physical activity should be adapted to the client's food intake and with consideration of bone mineral density and cardiac function. For the severely underweight person, *exercise* should be restricted and always carefully supervised. The focus is on helping clients assume responsibility for themselves as they move from the destructive use of exercise to healthy exercise.

Behavioral: Cognitive Therapy
Cognitive Restructuring

Suggest that clients write a list of the pros and cons of their eating disorder. Often, they have been warned of the dangers of their disorder but have never identified the benefits. Treatment will not be successful if they do not compensate for the loss of these benefits. To this end, you should help clients identify *secondary gains*, that is, the ultimate purpose the disorder serves. There are many possible purposes, and accurate identification will lead to effective interventions. For some, the purpose is the

attainment of the ideal body, with thoughts that this will protect them from all future pain. For others, eating disorders are a way of gaining a sense of control, as well as individuating and separating from parents. Eating disorders may develop in response to competition with siblings for parental attention. For some, it is a response to depressive feelings. Superimposed on the teenage crisis of identity, eating disorders may represent a regression to a younger and safer time in life.

To plan nursing interventions that will help these clients meet their needs in constructive and healthy ways, it is vital that secondary gains of the disorder be identified. If the secondary gain of the eating disorder is a sense of being in control of oneself, point out to clients that the binge/purge cycle that began as a method of control is now out of control. As clients develop insight into the paradox of the behavior, they can begin to explore alternative behaviors for maintaining control. As they learn to identify their own pleasurable activities, ways to spend their leisure time, and vocational interests, they increase their ability to define and control themselves, while decreasing their feelings of powerlessness. Increased self-acceptance decreases dependency on others.

To facilitate movement from a negative and distorted body image, clients keep a *body image diary* in which they record situations that provoke concerns over their appearance, their body image beliefs, and the effect of these on their mood and behavior. Cognitive interventions involve the identification of multiple automatic thoughts linking weight to self-worth. As they recognize their maladaptive thoughts, they can begin to reframe those thoughts in positive affirmations or distract themselves by focusing on more pleasing aspects of their appearance.

See the Complementary/Alternative Therapies feature on teaching clients how to alter negative cognitions.

It is important that clients consider sociocultural factors and body image issues. Topics include the pressures for women to be thin, the consequences of evaluating oneself largely in terms of weight, and how the female body is used in advertising and in the media. It is important that they see themselves as *being in control* rather than as passive sex objects valued mainly for appearance.

Several interventions are effective for clients who believe that achieving an ideal body will solve all problems in life. Point out the cognitive process of overgen-

Complementary/Alternative Therapies

How to Help Clients Alter Negative Cognitions

Often, we endure such runs of negative thoughts that we are unaware of the process until we have been "beating ourselves up" for 10 to 15 minutes. To become more aware of this habitual process and to counter with positive thoughts, try this procedure:

■ When you become aware of your thoughts, tap your left finger on a firm surface for every negative thought. When your finger becomes quite sore, you will have another level of awareness of your negativity.

■ Negative thoughts can be countered with positive ones. When you catch yourself thinking and feeling a negative thought, such as how fat your body is or how inadequate you are, **STOP.**

■ Look for and substitute a positive thought or feeling in the place of the one you removed, such as how lovely your hair looks or how well you have succeeded at something.

■ Now listen to yourself saying the positive phrase out loud.

■ Continue in this way, adding other phrases and wishes for yourself.

SOURCE: Fontaine, K. L. (2000). *Healing practices: Alternative therapies for nursing.* Upper Saddle River, NJ: Prentice Hall.

eralization in developing the belief that all life's problems will be solved if enough weight is lost. You can help clients identify how losing weight is symbolic of other problems, and begin to separate interpersonal problems from physical problems. After you and the client generate a list of problems together, the problems can be prioritized and tackled one by one.

Family: Life Span Care

Family Involvement

Education for the client and family about eating disorders is another primary concern for nurses. The general public has many misconceptions that interfere with effective treatment. Both families and clients need to be made aware of the seriousness of the disorders and the potential complications if left untreated. Accurate information will assist families in solving problems together, rather than blaming one another for the onset of the disorder. Be prepared to answer questions honestly and admit limitations of your own knowledge. Give clients and family members a list of self-help groups to support them throughout the long-term treatment process (see Community Resources feature at the end of the chapter). Teach clients who are taking antidepressants all you can about their medication.

The family needs to let the *client take responsibility* for her or his own eating behavior. Conflict about food is likely to be counterproductive. On the other hand, families must not ignore evidence that relapse is occurring. Psychoeducation may include discussions on family cohesion, the degree of emotional bonding that occurs within a family. At one end of the continuum of cohesion is the family system that is disengaged; that is, the family members are isolated and alienated from one another. At the other end of the continuum is the enmeshed family system in which the members are immersed in and absorbed by one another. Eating disorders often lead to an enmeshed family system as everyone becomes concerned and involved with the eating behavior of one family member. The family may also develop rigid rules and expectations for the identified client. Since the most adaptive family systems function between the two extremes of disengaged and enmeshed, families may need help in problem-solving ways to achieve a healthy balance. Increasing the autonomy of young people may decrease the use of food as a passive–aggressive adolescent rebellion and increase feelings of self-control.

Evaluation

To complete the nursing process, you evaluate clients' responses to nursing interventions based on the outcomes you selected. You determine the appropriate intervals for measurement and document the condition of clients according to each individual's status. Johnson, Maas, and Moorhead (2000) is the resource for identifying measurement scales and specific indicators for each outcome.

Nutritional Status

Clients with anorexia agree to and maintain a contract for how much to eat for each meal and snack. They eat small frequent meals and exercise no more than 30

CRITICAL THINKING

Ann is a school nurse for a large high school in a suburban area. She took this job a year ago and is still learning about school nursing and adolescent health issues. Sometimes just trying to communicate with the students is a challenge for her. One particular student has become a concern over the last few weeks. Ann noticed the student, Marie, in the hallway. She was very thin—too thin from what Ann could tell from her brief observation of Marie. Later the same day, Ann was in the teachers' lounge having a cup of coffee. Ann learned early on that this is often a place that teachers will talk about students who might be having problems, many of them health related. On this day, several teachers are discussing Marie. Her English teacher comments that Marie is an excellent student, is extremely organized, never turns in late assignments, and is extremely polite. However, she does not take criticism well. The gym teacher notes that Marie has been on the track team, and she becomes very upset when she fails to meet her own running goals. Lately, the gym teacher has noticed that Marie is out on the track running alone very early in the morning, always at the same time. Ann is sitting in the lounge and thinking, "I am hearing valuable assessment data and something is wrong with Marie." Several days later, Ann enters the cooking classroom where a popular elective on cooking is taught. Ann notices that Marie is in the class. The teacher mentions Marie to Ann. Marie is very involved in the class and the details of the recipes; however, Marie will not eat anything cooked in the class. The teacher sees this as unusual as this is the part the students love. She says to Ann, "What adolescent doesn't love to eat?"

A week later, Ann gets a stat call from the principal's office to get to the second floor where a student is apparently having a seizure. She finds that the student is

Marie. She goes with Marie in the ambulance to the hospital. On admission to the hospital and after further evaluation, it is determined that Marie has anorexia nervosa. She returns to school a month later. Ann begins to read up on anorexia and consults a psychiatric nurse practitioner to gain a better understanding of Marie's problems.

1. Identify the critical data that Ann had about Marie from the school environment that might support the diagnosis of anorexia nervosa.

2. Ann is also told that Marie has an anxiety disorder. Marie has been told and has agreed to a plan to decrease the amount of running that she has been doing. What might Ann expect Marie's response to be to this intervention given Marie's anxiety? Considering the symptoms, what might be some interventions?

3. Ann meets with Marie, and Marie makes several comments about the way people look and how she looks. Why would you expect these comments from Marie?

4. Marie's seizure was a serious problem. What is the importance of a thorough physiological assessment for clients with anorexia nervosa? What should be included in the assessment?

5. Ann begins to wonder if there are other students with eating disorders in the high school. She suspects that there are and wants to provide some support services for them. What are some key questions that Ann might ask students to screen for eating disorders?

6. What aspects of eating disorders management would be appropriate for Marie?

For an additional Case Study, please refer to the Companion Web site for this book.

minutes a day. Eating-disordered clients maintain a food journal regarding eating, binge eating, purging, and triggers to abnormal eating patterns. They identify their thoughts and feelings associated with eating and not eating. They utilize friends and family for support when they feel the urge to starve, binge, or purge, and the frequency of these episodes decreases.

Anxiety Control

Clients with eating disorders identify underlying fears and negative emotions. They verbalize an understand-

ing of what began as "control" is now "out of control." Those with bulimia verbalize the connection between purging and anxiety, guilt, and self-disgust. They acknowledge the appropriateness of setting a target weight and verbalize an increased tolerance for anxiety as weight gain occurs.

Distorted Thought Control

Clients keep a body image diary and reframe maladaptive thoughts into positive affirmations. They identify the consequences of evaluating one's worth in terms of

CLINICAL INTERACTIONS | A Client with Anorexia

Lorna, 23 years old, entered the eating disorders unit at the urging of her husband and physician. Lorna and her husband would like to start a family, and she has been told that her eating disorder (anorexia) would be very dangerous to a fetus. She weighed 95 pounds (43 kg) when she was admitted, and now, 3 weeks later, weighs 102 pounds (46 kg). In the interaction, you will see evidence of:

- Denial
- Distorted body image
- Obsessions
- Fear of gaining weight

NURSE: You said that you still have difficulty believing you have a problem.

LORNA: Well, my doctor says I do, but it's just hard for me to see it.

NURSE: What do you see?

LORNA: I see a lot of fat.

NURSE: You see a lot of fat—on yourself? You mean, you look in the mirror and see yourself as fat?

LORNA: Yes. That's all I can see.

[Period of silence]

LORNA: All I think about is food. My mind is like a computer—it just keeps going on thinking about food.

NURSE: Do you feel trapped?

LORNA: Very trapped. It's like a habit. I just can't stop it. And now, here on the unit, we spend so much time talking about food and weight and everything. I think you are all as obsessed as I am.

NURSE: Do you think the staff are as out of control as you feel you are? That might be a scary thought.

LORNA: No, not really. I'm just so frustrated. Getting on the scale every few days is frightening. Seeing the numbers going up—I just want to stop it. I want to lose weight—go back to where I was. Yet I want a future, too. I want to have a baby, and part of me knows that I have to get healthier before I can get pregnant. So it's an immense conflict every single day.

NURSE: As painful as the conflict sounds, I also see some progress in you. When you first came to the unit, you believed there was nothing dangerous with your lack of eating. Now it sounds like you understand that your eating disorder is a real problem, especially in terms of becoming a mother.

LORNA: Yeah, I know. My husband's being very supportive. I just wish I didn't have to gain this weight in order to become pregnant.

---

body weight. They identify cognitive distortions that maintain eating disorders. They verbalize decreasing delusional thoughts regarding their body image. Clients acknowledge that they cannot be perfect and that it is acceptable to make mistakes.

Social Involvement

Clients socialize with peers and participate in extracurricular activities. They identify the benefits from interpersonal and intimate relationships.

Impulse Control

Triggers to binge eating are identified, and the cyclic pattern of bulimia occurs with less frequency. Clients avoid the use of alcohol or drugs to decrease their anxiety and appetite.

Family Functioning

Family members acknowledge the seriousness and potential complications of untreated eating disorders. They verbalize an understanding of clients' need to take responsibility for their own eating behavior. Clients discuss and maintain an appropriate family cohesion that is neither disengaged nor enmeshed.

To build a Care Plan for a client with an eating disorder, go to the Companion Web site for this book.

CHAPTER REVIEW

COMMUNITY RESOURCES

Links to these Web sites can be accessed on the Companion Web site for this book.

American Anorexia/Bulimia Association, Inc.
165 West 46th St., Suite 1180
New York, New York 10036
212-575-6200
www.aabainc.org

Anorexia and Bulimia Hotline
800-772-3390

Anorexia Nervosa and Related Eating Disorders, Inc.
P.O. Box 5102
Eugene, OR 97405
503-344-1144
www.anred.com

National Association of Anorexia Nervosa and Associated
    Disorders, Inc.
P.O. Box 7
Highland Park, IL 60035
847-831-3438
www.anad.org

National Eating Disorders Organization
6655 South Yale Ave.
Tulsa, OK 74136
918-481-4044
www.laureate.com

International Prader–Willi Syndrome Organization
Adalbert Stiffer Str.
8D-68259
Mannheim, Germany
49-621-799-2193
www.ipwso.org

Prader–Willi Syndrome Association
5700 Midnight Pass Road
Sarasota, FL 34242
800-926-4797
www.pwsausa.org
E-mail: *pwsausa@aol.com*

BOOKS FOR CLIENTS AND FAMILIES

Alpert, J. (1999). *I always start my diet on Monday.* Northfield, IL: Pearl.

Andersen, A., Cohn, L., & Holbrook, T. (2000). *Making weight: Men's conflicts with food, weight, shape, and appearance.* Carlsbad, CA: Gurze Books.

Gilbert, S. D., & Commerford, M. C. (2000). *The unofficial guide to managing eating disorders.* Foster City, CA: IDG Books.

Nash, J. D. (1999). *Binge no more: Your guide to overcoming disordered eating.* Oakland, CA: New Harbinger.

KEY CONCEPTS

Introduction
- People with anorexia lose weight by dramatically decreasing their food intake and sharply increasing their amount of physical exercise.
- People with bulimia remain at near-normal weight and develop a cycle of minimal food intake, followed by binge eating and then purging.
- The two disorders have many features in common, and a person can revert from one disorder to the other.

- Eating disorders are more common among competitive athletes than the general population.

Knowledge Base: Obesities
- Psychosocial factors contributing to the development of obesity include learned patterns of eating, overeating to manage negative feelings, and viewing food as a reward.
- Obesity has a strong inheritable component.
- Weight gain is among the most problematic side effects of psychotrophic medications and is one of the most fre-

quent reasons for individuals discontinuing their medication.

■ Obese people are no more prone to emotional problems than are people of normal weight. It is the internalization of the culture's hatred and rejection that contributes to the psychological problems of obese people.

■ Prader–Willi syndrome causes an unrelenting feeling of hunger that can never be satisfied. Access to food must be rigidly enforced if these individuals are not to become morbidly obese.

Knowledge Base Anorexia and Bulemia

■ Behaviors associated with anorexia and bulimia are compulsions and rituals about food and exercise, phobic responses to food, eating binges, purging, and the abuse of laxatives and diuretics.

■ Affective characteristics include multiple fears, dependency, guilt, and a high need for acceptance and approval from others.

■ Cognitive characteristics include selective abstraction, overgeneralization, magnification, personalization, superstitious thinking, dichotomous thinking, distorted body image, self-depreciation, and perfectionistic standards of behavior.

■ People suffering from anorexia experience a severely distorted body image.

■ The entire family system often becomes preoccupied with food, eating, and rituals involving meals.

■ In American society, thinness for women and a muscular build for men are equated with attractiveness, success, and happiness. This is a contributing factor to eating disorders.

■ Physiological characteristics include fluid and electrolyte imbalances, decreased blood volume, cardiac arrhythmias, elevated blood urea nitrogen (BUN), constipation, osteoporosis, esophagitis, potential rupture of the esophagus or stomach, tooth loss, swollen salivary glands, Russell's sign, menstrual problems, and weight loss.

■ Concomitant disorders include depression, social phobias, panic attacks, obsessive–compulsive symptoms, and substance abuse.

■ Neurobiological factors in the development of eating disorders include 5-HT dysregulation, low levels of endorphins, and a genetic predisposition.

■ Intrapersonal theorists consider low self-esteem, problems with identity formation, anxiety intolerance, and maturational problems to be factors in the development of eating disorders.

■ Cognitive theorists believe that cognitive distortions and dysfunctional thoughts contribute to disordered eating patterns.

■ The family system of a person with an eating disorder may be enmeshed. Family members may have difficulty with conflict resolution and have high ambitions for achievement and performance.

■ Feminist theorists consider that women's preoccupation with their bodies results from the cultural ideal of thinness, and that their identity and self-esteem depend on physical appearance.

■ Antidepressant medication is more helpful in treating bulimia than anorexia.

Nursing Interventions

Assessment

■ Eating disorders cause multiple physical complications. Accurate physical assessment may prevent death.

■ The client's level of malnourishment must be identified, as well as binge eating and/or purging patterns, fear, cognitive distortions, and relationships with family and friends.

Diagnosis

■ Examples of nursing diagnoses are altered nutrition, anxiety, body image disturbance, powerlessness, and altered family processes.

Interventions

■ Help clients discuss their fears related to weight gain and loss of control.

■ Clients contract for the amount of food to be eaten in a day; a target weight is established, usually at 90 percent of average weight for the client's age and height.

■ Contract for a reasonable intake, beginning with 1,000 to 1,500 kcal per day.

■ Help clients identify situations that precede a binge and explore alternative coping behaviors. Discussion also focuses on how purging is used to cope with feelings.

■ Clients may find it helpful to keep a food diary and a body image diary.

■ Secondary gains must be identified in order to design interventions that will help clients meet these needs in constructive and healthy ways.

■ The family needs to let the client take responsibility for her or his own eating behavior.

■ Nurses must be leaders in actively challenging idealized cultural values in an effort to help women accept and value themselves as they are, and to prevent a continued increase in eating disorders.

Evaluation

■ It appears that people with bulimia are more responsive to treatment than people with anorexia, who often remain intensely preoccupied with weight and dieting.

EXPLORE *MediaLink*

- Interactive resources, including animations, for this chapter can be found on the Companion Web site at *http://www.prenhall.com/fontaine*. Click on Chapter 12 and select the activities for this chapter.

- For NCLEX review questions and an audio glossary, access the accompanying CD-ROM in this book.

REFERENCES

Agras, W. S. (2000). Outcome predictors for the cognitive behavior treatment of bulimia nervosa. *American Journal of Psychiatry, 157*(8), 1302–1308.

Alexander, C. J. (1996). *Gay and lesbian mental health: A sourcebook for practitioners.* New York: Harrington Park Press.

American Psychiatric Association (2000a). *Diagnostic and Statistical Manual of Mental Disorders* (4th ed., Text Revision). Washington, DC: Author.

American Psychiatric Association (2000b). *Practice guideline for the treatment of patients with eating disorders.* (2nd ed.). Washington, DC: Author.

Basic facts about PWS. (2000). *www.pwsausa.org/basicfac.htm.*

Balch, J. F., & Balch, P. A. (1997). *Prescription for nutritional healing* (2nd ed.). Garden City Park, NY: Avery.

Bellodi, L., Cavallini, M. C., Bertelli, S., Chiapparino, D., Riboldi, C., & Smeraldi, E. (2001). Morbidity risk for obsessive–compulsive spectrum disorders in first-degree relatives of patients with eating disorders. *American Journal of Psychiatry, 158*(4), 563–569.

Boskind-White, M., & White, W. C. (2000). *Bulimia/anorexia* (3rd ed.). New York: Norton.

Devlin, M. J., Yanovski, S. Z., & Wilson, G. T. (2000). Obesity: What mental health professionals need to know. *American Journal of Psychiatry, 157*(6), 854–866.

Finelli, L. A. (2001). Revisiting the identity issue in anorexia. *Journal of Psychosocial Nursing, 39*(8), 23–29.

Ghizzani, A., & Montomoli, M. (2000). Anorexia nervosa and sexuality in women. *Journal of Sex Education and Therapy, 25*(1), 80–88.

Goldfein, J. A., Devlin, M. J., & Spitzer, R. L. (2000). Cognitive behavioral therapy for the treatment of binge eating disorder. *American Journal of Psychiatry, 157*(7), 1051–1057.

Grogan, S. (1999). *Body image.* London: Routledge.

Hays, K. F. (1999). *Working it out: Using exercise in psychotherapy.* Washington, DC: American Psychological Association.

Johnson, M., Maas, M., & Moorhead, S. (2000). *Nursing outcomes classification (NOC)* (2nd ed.). St. Louis, MO: Mosby.

Kaye, W. H., Frank, G. K., Meltzer, C. C., Price, J. C., McConaha, C. W., Crossan, P. J., et al. (2001). Altered serotonin 2A receptor activity in women who have recovered from bulimia nervosa. *American Journal of Psychiatry, 158*(7), 1152–1155.

Keel, P. K., Leon, G. R., & Fulkerson, J. A. (2001). Vulnerability to eating disorders in childhood and adolescence. In R. E. Ingram & J. M. Price (Eds.), *Vulnerability to psychopathology* (pp. 389–411). New York: Guilford Press.

Levenkron, S. (2000). *Anatomy of anorexia.* New York: Norton.

Martin, A., State, M., Koenia, K., Schultz, R., Dykens, E. M., Cassidy, S. B., et al. (1998). Prader–Willi syndrome. *American Journal of Psychiatry, 155*(9), 1265–1273.

Montgomery, L., & Haynes, L. C. (2001). Nocturnal sleep-related eating disorder. *Journal of Psychosocial Nursing, 39*(8), 14–20.

Paris, J. (1999). *Nature and nurture in psychiatry.* Washington, DC: American Psychiatric Press.

Pope, H. G., Phillips, K. A., & Olivardia, R. (2000). *The Adonis complex.* New York: Free Press.

Ranson, K. M, Kaye, W. H., Weltzin, T. E., Rao, R., & Matsunaga, H. (1999).

Obsessive–compulsive disorder symptoms before and after recovery from bulimia nervosa. *American Journal of Psychiatry, 156*(11), 1703–1708.

Safer, D. L., Telch, C. F., & Agras, W. S. (2001). Dialectical behavior therapy for bulimia nervosa. *American Journal of Psychiatry, 158*(4), 632–635.

Silverstein, B., & Perlick, D. (1995). *The cost of competence.* Oxford, England: Oxford University Press.

Smock, T. K. (1999). *Physiological psychology: A neuroscience approach.* Upper Saddle River, NJ: Prentice Hall.

Striegel-Moore, R. H. (1995). A feminist perspective on the etiology of eating disorders. In K. D. Brownell & C. G. Fairburn (Eds.), *Eating disorders and obesity* (pp. 224–229). New York: Guilford Press.

Strober, M., Freeman, R., Lampert, C., Diamond, J., & Kaye, W. (2000). Controlled family study of anorexia nervosa and bulimia nervosa: Evidence of shared liability and transmission of partial syndromes. *American Journal of Psychiatry, 157*(3), 393–401.

Walsh, B. T., Agras, W. S., Devlin, M. J., Fairburn, C. G., Wilson, G. T., Kahn, C., et al. (2000). Fluoxetine for bulimia nervosa following poor response to psychotherapy. *American Journal of Psychiatry, 157*(8), 1332–1334.

White, J. H. (2000). Symptom development in bulimia nervosa: A comparison of women with and without a history of anorexia nervosa. *Archives of Psychiatric Nursing, 14*(2), 81–92.

Woodside, D. B., Garfinkel, P. E., Lin, E., Goering, P., Keplan, A. S., Goldbloom, D. S., et al. (2001). Comparisons of men with full or partial eating disorders, men without eating disorders, and women with eating disorders in the community. *American Journal of Psychiatry, 158*(4), 570–574.

CHAPTER 13

Mood Disorders

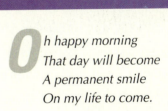

OBJECTIVES

After reading this chapter, you will be able to:

- COMPARE and contrast people who have unipolar disorder (major depression) with people who have bipolar disorder.

- ANALYZE the sociocultural factors that contribute to the incidence of depression.

- DISCUSS the impact of mood disorders on the family.

- EXPLAIN altered neurotransmission in people with mood disorders.

- ASSESS clients from physical, psychological, and sociocultural perspectives.

- PLAN overall goals in the care of clients with mood disorders.

- INDIVIDUALIZE standard interventions to specific clients.

- EVALUATE and modify the plan of care.

MediaLink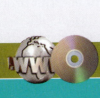

CD-ROM
- *Audio Glossary*
- *NCLEX Review*

Companion Web site www.prenhall.com/fontaine
- *Critical Thinking*
- *More NCLEX Review*
- *Case Study*
- *Care Map Activity*
- *Links to Resources*

Oh happy morning
That day will become
A permanent smile
On my life to come.

No depression here
But ever watchful I'll be
Sadness to go PERMANENTLY!

Absolute gladness
Happiness I want badly
Life FREE OF SADNESS!

—Rosalie, Age 57

Mood is defined as a sustained emotional state and how you subjectively feel. The way in which you communicate your mood to others is called affect. **Affect** is the immediate and observable emotional expression of mood, which you communicate verbally and nonverbally. *Verbal cues* we may use to describe our emotional state are words such as elation, happiness, pleasure, frustration, anger, or hostility. *Nonverbal cues* to feelings include facial expressions such as smiling, frowning, and looking blank; motor activities such as making hands into fists and pacing; and physiological responses such as profuse sweating and increased respirations. We may choose not to communicate verbally to another person, but it is almost impossible to prevent nonverbal expression of our feelings.

A variety of descriptors of affect are used to facilitate communication among health care professionals (see Table 13.1 ■). Affect and mood can be pictured along a continuum ranging from depression through normal to mania. The normal range of mood is stable and appropriate to the situation. People diagnosed with mood disorders experience disrupting disturbances at varying points along the continuum.

The mood disorders are characterized by changes in feelings ranging from severe depression to inordinate elation. They are best understood as syndromes with a core cluster of symptoms. At present, we do not know if depression is one disease with various levels of severity, or many diseases.

The two types of depressive disorders are major depression and dysthymic disorder. The medical diagnosis of **major depression** (also called **unipolar disorder**) is made when, along with a loss of interest in life, a person experiences a depressed mood that moves from mild to severe, with the severe phase lasting at least two weeks. It is twice as common among females as males. Major depression often has a chronic course with lengthy episodes or incomplete remission between episodes. Compared with people with chronic medical conditions, such as cardiovascular disease, pulmonary disease, and back problems, people with chronic depression are less successful in their social and occupational roles (Keller et al., 2000; Peden, Hall, Rayens, & Beebe, 2000).

Some people with major depression also experience delusions and hallucinations. When this occurs, it is referred to as *severe depression with psychotic features*, although in the future it may be listed as a distinct syndrome. Those who have psychotic symptoms in one episode are much more likely to exhibit psychotic features in future episodes. Some studies have found that people with psychotic depression have lower rates of recovery, more chronic symptoms, and higher rates of relapse (American Psychiatric Association [APA], 2000; Flint & Rifat, 1998).

Dysthymic disorder is a chronic disorder in which periods of depressed mood are interspersed with normal mood. With this disorder, people experience a depressed mood for most of the day more days than not for at least two years. Symptoms in dysthymic disorder tend to be less severe than those in major depressive disorder, and there are fewer physiological symptoms (disturbed sleep, altered appetite, and weight loss or gain). People with dysthymic disorder are at high risk of developing superimposed major depressive episodes (APA, 2000; Klein, Schwartz, Rose, & Leader, 2000).

TABLE 13.1

Descriptors of Affect

Affect	Definition	Behavioral Example
Appropriate	Mood is congruent with the immediate situation.	Juan cries when learning of the death of his father.
Inappropriate	Mood is not related to the immediate situation.	When Sue's husband tells her about his terrible pain, Sue begins to laugh out loud.
Stable	Mood is resistant to sudden changes when there is no provocation in the environment.	During a party, Dan smiles and laughs at the appropriate social interchanges.
Labile	Mood shifts suddenly in a way that cannot be understood in the context of the situation.	During a friendly game of checkers, Dorothy, who has been laughing, suddenly knocks the board off the table in anger. She then begins to laugh and wants to continue the game.
Elevated	Mood is one of euphoria not necessarily related to the immediate situation.	Sean bounces around the dayroom, laughing, singing, and telling other clients how wonderful everything is.
Depressed	Mood is one of despondency not necessarily related to the immediate situation.	Leo sits slumped in a chair with a sad facial expression, teary eyes, and minimal body movement.
Overreactive	Mood is appropriate to the situation but out of proportion to the immediate situation.	Karen screams and curses when her child spills a glass of milk on the kitchen floor.
Blunted	Mood is a dulled response to the immediate situation.	When Tom learns of his full-tuition scholarship, he responds with only a small smile.
Flat	There are no visible cues to the person's mood.	When Juanita is told about her best friend's death, she says "Oh" and does not give any indication of an emotional response.

The bipolar disorders are a group of mood disorders that include manic episodes, mixed episodes, depressed episodes, and cyclothymic disorder. The medical diagnosis of **bipolar disorder** (also called **manic–depressive disorder**) is given when a person's mood alternates between the extremes of depression and elation, with periods of normal mood in between the pathological phases. *Bipolar I disorder* is characterized by the occurrence of one or more manic episodes and one or more depressive episodes. *Bipolar II disorder* is on the less severe end of the continuum and is characterized by one or more hypomanic episodes and one or more depressive episodes. Bipolar disorder is equally common in women and men (APA, 2000).

Bipolar disorder with *rapid cycling* is defined as four or more episodes of illness within a 12-month period. Rapid cycling occurs in 10 to 20 percent of persons with bipolar disorder, with 70 to 90 percent of rapid cyclers being women. This form of the disorder tends to be more resistant to treatment than the non–rapid-cycling disorder (APA, 2000). Bipolar disorder is further clarified as:

- *Mixed*: The person has rapidly alternating moods.
- *Manic*: The person is presently in the manic phase.
- *Depressed*: The person is in the depressed phase but has a history of manic episodes.

Cyclothymic disorder is characterized by a mood range from moderate depression to hypomania, which

DSM-IV-TR CLASSIFICATIONS

Depressive Disorders

Major Depressive Disorder
Dysthymic Disorder
Depressive Disorder NOS

Bipolar Disorders

Bipolar I Disorder
Bipolar II Disorder
Cyclothymic Disorder
Bipolar Disorder NOS

Mood Disorder

Due to a general medical condition
Substance-induced mood disorder
Mood Disorder NOS

SOURCE: Reprinted with permission from the *Diagnostic and Statistical Manual of Mental Disorders, Fourth Edition, Text Revision.* Copyright 2000 American Psychiatric Association.

may or may not include periods of normal mood, lasting at least two years. Clients with cyclothymic disorder do not experience the severe symptoms that qualify for a diagnosis of manic disorder or major depressive disorder.

All of these disorders may be recurrent and are often chronic. More than 80 percent of individuals will have at least one recurrence (Hammen, 2001) (see Figure 13.1 ■). The DSM-IV-TR feature lists the categories and types of mood disorders presented in this chapter.

Schizoaffective disorder is diagnosed when clients suffer from symptoms that appear to be a mixture of schizophrenia and the mood disorders. The person experiences one or more of the following symptoms: delusions, hallucinations, disorganized speech, disorganized behavior, or negative symptoms (see Chapter 14 for more detailed discussion of these symptoms). In addition, the person experiences symptoms of the mood disorders: major depressive symptoms, manic symptoms, or mixed symptoms. Clients often have difficulty maintaining job or school functioning, experience problems with self-care, are socially isolated, and often suffer from suicidal ideation. The age of onset is typically late adolescence or early adulthood, and it is more common in women than in men (Brown & Weaver, 1998).

Major depression is 10 times more common than bipolar disorder. During any six-month period, approximately 10 million people in the United States are suffering

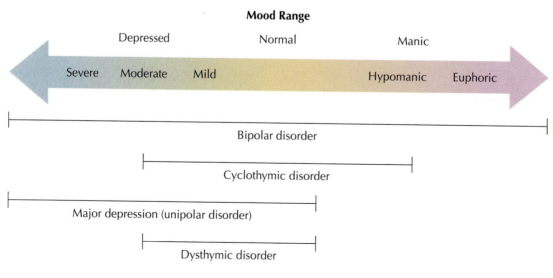

FIGURE 13.1 ■ Mood disorders and ranges.

from depression. It is thought that 8 to 12 percent of men and 18 to 25 percent of women will suffer a major depression in their lifetime. At least 50 percent of individuals experience recurrent episodes. Estimates are that only 25 to 50 percent of these individuals will seek and receive treatment. An untreated major depression may last six months to a year. The incidence of depression is increasing with each passing decade, and the age of onset is lowering into adolescence and even childhood (Hammen, 2001; Solomon et al., 2000).

Psychotic features, including delusions and hallucinations, are common in mood disorders. About 75 percent of people with mania and 14 percent of people with major depression have psychotic features. Symptoms typically reflect the extreme mood state at the time (i.e., grandiosity during mania and worthlessness during depression). Less than 40 percent of these individuals attain functional recovery as measured by independent living, occupational stability, and interpersonal relations (Tohen et al., 2000).

Men and women are equally at risk for bipolar disorder, which affects 1.2 percent of the adult population, although women are three times more likely to develop the rapid-cycling form of the illness. The disorder most commonly begins during adolescence but has often been underrecognized and misdiagnosed in this age group. Untreated, the depressive phase may last six to nine months and the manic phase two to six weeks. It is difficult to predict the course of the disorder; some may have only one episode every 10 years, while others may have several episodes a year. More than 20 percent of individuals experience a chronic course. Four or more episodes a year lead to the diagnosis of bipolar disorder, rapid cycling. People with bipolar II disorder have a higher frequency of episodes than those who have bipolar I disorder (Maj, Pirozzi, Formicola, & Tortorella, 1999; Preisig et al., 2000).

Although 10 to 15 percent of *pregnant women* meet criteria for depression, they often remain undiagnosed because the symptoms of depression are similar to the somatic changes of pregnancy. The prevalence of depression among pregnant adolescents is almost twice as high as among adult pregnant women and is more severe between the second and third trimesters. Untreated maternal depression is associated with poor prenatal care, preterm delivery, small infant size, postpartum depression, and maternal suicide (Szigethy & Ruiz, 2001).

Mood disorders in women after delivering a child are fairly common. Symptoms can be described along a continuum from postpartum blues to postpartum depression to the rare form, postpartum psychosis. *Postpartum blues* begin within the first 10 days postpartum and last a few days to two weeks with symptoms disappearing spontaneously. The mood may be unstable, accompanied by sadness, weepiness, irritability, anxiety, and fatigue. As many as 80 percent of new mothers may experience these symptoms, which are thought to be caused by hormonal fluctuations. Most of these women had not had previous emotional problems (Weinberg et al., 2001).

Postpartum depression is estimated to occur in 10 to 16 percent of new mothers, often beginning within three months of delivery but may strike at any time during the first year after having a child. Women with this disorder experience insomnia, loss of energy, inability to concentrate, anxiety, mood swings, periods of crying, and feelings of despair as they ruminate over perceived inadequacies as a mother. If depression is untreated, it will affect the ability to parent and to cope with stressful situations. These symptoms are more intense and longer lasting than those in postpartum blues. Any symptoms lasting longer than two weeks qualify as postpartum depression. Contributing factors are hormonal changes, family history of depression, feeling overwhelmed by parenting tasks, changes in family dynamics, and inadequate support. Those who develop postpartum depression are at an increased risk for depression after subsequent pregnancies (Bloch et al., 2000).

One woman in a thousand experiences a *postpartum psychosis*—a medical emergency. The incidence of relapse for women who have a diagnosed bipolar disorder is 25 to 40 percent during postpartum or 260 women per 1,000 deliveries. The symptoms usually occur between the first two to six weeks after delivery but may occur as early as 48 hours postpartum. Symptoms develop rapidly and include insomnia, hallucinations, agitation, and bizarre feelings or behavior. An inordinate concern with the baby's health, guilt about lack of love, and delusions about the infant's being dead or defective also may be present. The mother may deny having given birth or hear voices that command her to hurt the baby. In extreme cases, the mother may even kill the child and/or herself (Jones & Craddock, 2001; Straub et al., 1998).

Fathers also need to adjust during pregnancy and after childbirth, and there is evidence that some men experience depressive symptoms following the birth of their children. Comparisons of mothers and fathers show that they have similar levels of parenting-related stress and anxiety. Factors increasing the risk for depression include inexperience with child care, unemployment, relationship conflict with partner, and less emotional and social support from family and friends (Deater-Deckard, Pickering, Dunn, & Golding, 1998).

The high rate of mood disorders makes these disorders a major concern for nurses. Mood-disordered clients are found in the community and in all types of clinical settings and are not restricted to psychiatric settings. It is vital that you be alert to cues because one of the tragic results in untreated depression is suicide.

KNOWLEDGE BASE

People with mood disorders display a variety of characteristics involving changes in behavior, affect, cognition, and physiology. Mood disorders occur within a person's sociocultural context, and interactions with others are often disrupted. The particular combinations and severity of symptoms vary among affected individuals.

BEHAVIORAL CHARACTERISTICS

One of the changes in people with mood disorders is their level of *desire to participate in activities*. Initially, in depression, there is a decreased desire to engage in activities that do not bring immediate gratification. As the depression deepens, there is a further decrease in participation, and clients regard themselves as incompetent and inadequate. This further contributes to feelings of discouragement and, in severe depression, results in an inability to do anything, even the simplest activities of daily living (ADLs). If you suggest that clients attempt ADLs, they will often respond with something like "It's pointless to even try because I can't do it."

In the early stages of an elevated mood (hypomania), people with bipolar disorder increase their work productivity. This leads to positive feedback from employers and family members, which contributes to increased self-esteem around the issues of competency

and power. When they reach the manic end of the continuum, however, their productivity decreases because of a short attention span. People in a manic phase are interested in every available activity and are supremely confident of being able to accomplish them all perfectly. Poor judgment can result in reckless driving, spending sprees, and foolish business investments. Many clients have poor impulse control and have episodes of spending enormous amounts of money.

Jorge and Ava have been married for 12 years and are experiencing severe marital problems centering on financial issues. Jorge has had multiple episodes of bipolar disorder. Eighteen months ago they took a $10,000 home equity loan to pay off all the bills Jorge had run up during a manic phase. At that time they agreed that their credit cards would be used only for an emergency. Two weeks ago Ava needed to use the credit card to pay for some medication and found that the card was up to its limit of $5,000. During a confrontation with Jorge, Ava found out that he had received two new credit cards and had taken a cash advance of $5,000 on each card. He could not explain what he had done with the $15,000.

Interaction with others is altered in people with a mood disorder. In the beginning of a depressive episode, people may avoid social activities that are not highly interesting and stimulating. As the depression deepens, the tendency is to withdraw from most social interactions because they are too demanding and require too much effort. Depressed people say they feel lonely but also say they feel incapable of halting the process of withdrawal and isolation. Family and friends, frustrated with the withdrawal, often respond with criticism and anger, further contributing to isolation. In depression, people may experience more friction, tension, and conflict than usual when interacting with family and friends. Difficulty communicating often leads to disputes and hostility within the family. So painful can interactions become that some clients become silent as a way to decrease unpleasant interactions.

Ellen describes her interactions with her son in this way: "I have a 3-year-old son, and I want to be able to take care of him. I've been so short with him lately. I don't seem to have any patience with him, and I just don't have any energy. This isn't fair to him."

During manic episodes, people are unusually talkative and gregarious. Unable to control the impulse to interact with everyone in the environment, they are oblivious to the social convention of not interrupting a private discussion. While interacting with others, they may share intimate details of their lives with anyone who will listen. When their mood returns to its normal range, they are often embarrassed about what they have said to others.

A change in *affiliation needs* also occurs in the mood disorders. During a depressive episode, normally self-sufficient people experience an increase in dependency. This begins with a desire to have others participate in activities with them. As the depression progresses, they may seek advice and assistance in work responsibilities and leisure activities. Affiliation needs are frequently expressed as demands or through whining complaints. If these demands, unrealistic though they are, are rejected by others, depressed people view this as validation of their being unlovable and unwanted by family and friends. If, on the other hand, intense assistance is given to them, their dependency needs are reinforced, which contributes to a lack of self-confidence. In severe depression, people tenaciously cling to significant others. They no longer want advice only—they want total care and attention. If others leave them for even a short time, they may become maudlin about the significance and length of the separation. At this level, as the need to cling to others becomes incessant and extreme, agoraphobia may develop.

Those experiencing a shift in mood toward elation show a decreased need for affiliation. Neither seeking nor heeding advice, they view themselves as independent and completely self-sufficient. They have confidence in their ability to be self-sustaining while believing themselves to be indispensable to others.

AFFECTIVE CHARACTERISTICS

During depression, the mood begins with an intermittent sense of *sadness*. Statements are made such as "I feel down in the dumps." Stimulation from family and friends or other pleasurable experiences can sometimes elevate a person's mood. As depression deepens, people become more gloomy and dejected. You might hear such statements as "There is no joy in my life anymore" or "I feel really unhappy." In severe levels of depression, there is a sense of desolation. Depressed people despair over the past, present, and future; the misery is uninterrupted. A cue to the depth of the feeling might be something like "I'll always feel this awful; I'll never be any better."

Ghada describes her changes in this way: "I worry about what's going to happen to me. I mean, I didn't have this numbness a month ago. I could be lying here dying and not even know it. I just don't have any feeling anymore."

On the manic end of the continuum, there is an *unstable mood* state. Beginning with cheerfulness, it escalates toward euphoria. People in this state are exuberant, energetic, and excitable. You will hear statements such as "Everything is just wonderful" or "I feel so high and great." The instability of mood is observed when, with minimal environmental stimulus, the person suddenly becomes irritable, argumentative, openly hostile, and even combative. Arrogance contributes to an intolerance of criticism. As the stimulus is withdrawn, however, the person's mood returns to euphoric.

Guilt is another common affective experience on which depressed people focus. For some, the source of guilt is vague; for others, it is specific. Cues are such statements as "I have a loving wife and good children, a nice house, and no money problems. But I'm so unhappy. I shouldn't be feeling this way. It's terrible for me to be so miserable." Guilt sometimes occurs in people who blame themselves for all the difficulties in their life. Evidence of this is heard in "It's my fault I'm so depressed. If I had been a better wife, my husband would not have beaten me." Depressed people ruminate over incidents they feel guilty about, and it is difficult to change their focus of attention.

Mark is a 27-year-old client who has had multiple hospitalizations over the past nine years. He has just been readmitted for a suicide attempt. Three years ago his father had coronary artery *(continued)*

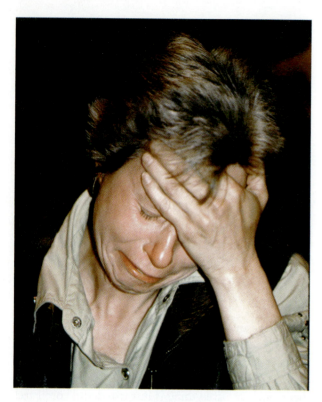

PHOTO 13.1 ■ The quality of a depressed mood is often different from the sadness that might arise from an event such as the loss of a loved one. Some depressed people say that they feel like they are drowning or suffocating.

SOURCE: Vincent DeWitt/Stock Boston.

bypass surgery and is doing very well. Mark's mother died two years ago from cancer. He talks about guilt in relation to both his parents. About his father he says: "Dad is very sick. I feel guilty about leaving him alone while I'm here in the hospital." About his mother he says: "I yelled at my mom the night before she died. Now I can't say I'm sorry. If I killed myself, I would be able to tell her I'm sorry." These two themes are continually repeated throughout the day.

During a manic episode, people are unable to experience any sense of guilt. Confronted with behavior that has hurt another person, they respond with indifference, laughter, or anger. The ability to experience guilt returns when their affect returns to a normal level.

Crying spells may occur during a depressive state. In mild and moderate depressions, people have an increased tendency to cry in situations that would not normally provoke tears. Where the cultural norm dictates that men ought not to shed tears, depressed men who cry may feel a sense of shame. In a severe depression, there is often a complete absence of crying, although there may be a desire to cry. Some people do not even have the energy to cry. The depth of despair is indicated by a comment such as "Why can't I cry? I want to, but the tears just won't come." During the manic state, sudden and unpredictable crying spells may occur. These may last only 20 to 30 seconds before a rapid return to a euphoric mood.

People's feelings of *gratification* are altered in mood disorders. In a mild depression, there is a narrowing of interest in pleasurable activities, and there may be a shift from active to passive participation. As the depression increases, people may resort to activities that result in immediate gratification such as excessive eating, drinking, or drug use. At this point, participation in normally pleasurable activities decreases. This is exhibited by remarks such as "I don't enjoy playing the piano anymore. It doesn't do anything for me. I just sit and watch TV all day" and "I can't seem to get interested in my stamp collection any more. I used to enjoy spending an hour a day working on it." In severe depression, people become **anhedonic**, that is, incapable of experiencing pleasure.

People who are manic, on the other hand, try to participate in every available pleasurable activity. Skillfulness is not a concern; they enjoy the activity regardless of the outcome. There is a constant need for fun, excitement, and stimulation.

Accompanying a depressive state is a loss of *emotional attachment*. It begins with decreased affection for family members and friends, along with dissatisfaction with these relationships. In a moderate depression, people often become indifferent to others and remarks are made such as "I don't even think about my wife or children. I just don't care anymore." As the depression intensifies, a severe disengagement from family members and a repudiation of all significant relationships may occur. Statements are heard such as "I hate teenagers. I hope I never see my kids again."

People in the manic state form intense emotional attachments very rapidly. They feel affectionate toward everyone in the environment and may "fall in love" in a matter of minutes and with a number of people. During a manic state, a person may think nothing of having simultaneous sexual relationships. Accompanying this is a preoccupation with sex, which others may find offensive.

> *Juanita, a nurse, is doing a nursing history admission on Sid, a 73-year-old man with bipolar disorder, manic phase. He is sexually preoccupied throughout the interview. When asked what his major strengths are, he replies, "Making love." When asked how he handles stress at home, the response is, "Making it with as many girls as I can."*

Alterations in the affective experience of people suffering from mood disorders are both broad and deep. In depression, there is an overall sense of *powerlessness* and *helplessness*, which are the precursors to feelings of *hopelessness*. People who are depressed feel that the future will never bring any changes in mood or any pleasure or loving relationships. In a manic state, there is little recognition that they have not always felt this *euphoric* and wonderful. They feel all powerful and in total control.

> *Rozell describes himself in this way: "I feel so good since I stopped taking my lithium. I'm not sick and I never needed it anyway. You know Susan, who just came into the group home yesterday? Well, we really hit it off and are thinking about getting married as soon as we can."*

PERCEPTUAL CHARACTERISTICS

Major depression can be accompanied by *psychotic symptoms*, often with depressive themes. Clients may hear voices telling them that they are bad or to kill themselves, or they may have *delusions* that they have a terminal illness or are responsible for some disaster. *Hallucinations* occur in 15 to 25 percent of people with mood disorders and may be the result of sleep deprivation. They may be reluctant to talk about their delusions and hallucinations if they realize that their thinking processes are not quite right (Flint & Rifat, 1998).

> *Sherry describes her hallucinations this way: "I'm hearing voices telling me to kill myself. I hear them all the time. I feel like I'm going crazy. The voices are getting clearer. They tell me to kill myself and I'll be at peace. Kill yourself and your problems will be solved."*

COGNITIVE CHARACTERISTICS

A person's thoughts about personal worth and value contribute to an overall sense of *self-esteem*. In the mood disorders, there is an alteration in the ability to self-evaluate objectively. In mild depression, people overreact to mistakes they may make and reproach themselves for minor errors. Their self-evaluation is flexible at this level because they are still able to recognize some positive attributes in themselves. As the depression worsens, however, people focus much of their attention on past, present, and future failures. A good deal of their thinking is self-deprecatory and self-accusatory. They blame themselves for feeling depressed and attribute the depression to a personal defect or inadequacy. This magnification of failures is called **catastrophizing**. Such negative thoughts make them feel more depressed, which causes further self-deprecation. These negative thoughts then make them feel more helpless, powerless, and depressed, which causes more self-deprecation. They believe the depression proves they are weak and inferior to others. Severely depressed people have a global negative view of themselves. One hears statements such as "I am completely incompetent" or "I am a total failure at everything."

People on the manic end of the continuum have an exaggerated self-concept. They have *grandiose beliefs* about their physical and intellectual talents. In any undertaking, there is a supreme sense of self-confidence. During manic episodes, they do not regard their behavior as inappropriate, nor do they realize their need for professional assistance.

> *Steve is telling Keasha, his nurse, about firing his divorce lawyer right before coming into the hospital.*
>
> **Steve:** *[Angry tone of voice] I didn't like how he was handling the case. I know what I want to*
> *(continued)*

happen with the divorce. I want to make sure my daughters are taken care of.

Keasha: *What was your lawyer doing to make you feel like he wasn't handling things right?*

Steve: *I don't know; it was just the way he did things. I could do much better. I already filed five motions before I came here. The paperwork is not a problem. I've always had this instinct about things like the law. I've always liked to read. What got me so angry is that the judge was against me because I'm handling my own case. She just doesn't know what a great job I can do.*

People's *expectations* of themselves, others, and the future are altered during mood disorders. Persistent negative expectations reinforce depressive behaviors. In the beginning of a depressive episode, people have a pessimistic view of outcomes, particularly in ambiguous situations. Often, they ignore positive experiences or misinterpret them as negative ones. This *overgeneralization* is a cognitive distortion. As the depression continues, the view of the here-and-now and the future becomes more gloomy still. *Dichotomous thinking* suggests that experiences will either be all good or, more likely, all bad. Statements are made such as "I can't do it," "I'll fail anyway," or "It won't do any good." In severe depression, the present and future are viewed as completely hopeless. Even simple goals are unachievable because of self-perceived inadequacies. They see no reason to make an effort, since life is not worth living and they might as well be dead. The inability to cope is evidence of an *external locus of control*.

Wendy is a severely depressed young woman. She verbalizes her negative expectations in this way: "Dr. Lee isn't doing anything. The antidepressants aren't working. I'm getting worse, and I won't get better this time. There is nothing anyone can do to help me and no one cares. I wish I could just die."

In contrast, people in a manic state have inordinate expectations of themselves, others, and the future. They become involved in activities without consider-

ing any possible negative outcomes. For instance, because of their certainty that every investment will be a wonderful success, they are open to abuse in business ventures. They often go on buying sprees without concern for the consequences of incurring great debt.

People's *decision-making* ability deteriorates in mood disorders. In mild depression, people show obsessiveness about making decisions. They need to look at every possible choice and potential result before deciding on a course of action. There is a high priority on doing "the right thing." They often seek advice and affirmation from others before making the decision. As the depression deepens, there is a decreased ability to concentrate on a subject long enough to formulate a decision. A person might stand in front of the closet for 20 minutes, trying to decide what clothes to wear. Planning meals, shopping, or concentrating on homework may be very difficult. In severe depression, people are incapable of making decisions. Because they cannot concentrate, they cannot recall information from the past to help them. Lack of concentration also interferes with their ability to compare alternatives and potential outcomes in the problem-solving process.

During manic episodes, people also have difficulty making decisions. Easily distracted by stimuli in the environment, they cannot concentrate long enough to go through the problem-solving process. Their short attention span causes them to respond impulsively to environmental stimuli. Because of their inability to think through the consequences of behavior before impulsively engaging in it, manic people often have poor judgment and self-control.

Mario and his wife Tanya have been fighting more as Mario's manic phase progresses. At the end of one day, Tanya refuses to take Mario over to the service station to pick up his car, which had been repaired. She says, "You have treated me badly all day. I won't take you to get your car. You can take the bus or ask a neighbor to take you." Thirty minutes later a stretch limousine with a chauffeur arrives in front of the house, and Mario gets in it. Tanya becomes very angry at Mario's lack of judgment and impulsive behavior—they simply cannot afford this extra expense.

Flow of thought is disrupted in people with mood disorders. In depression, there may be slowed speech, an inability to think of specific words, or an inability to complete sentences, referred to as *poverty of speech*. In severe depression, it may take the person several minutes to respond to a question and they may even be mute.

During manic episodes, *flight of ideas* is often present. The flow of thought is fragmented by any external stimuli. Thoughts come so quickly that there is not enough time to completely express one idea before another is stimulated. These thoughts may be connected by a theme or by alliteration or rhymes.

"I want to see my little niece. I haven't seen her yet. She's only 3 weeks old. Her name is Diamond. Do you like diamonds? I got my mother a necklace like that (pointing to the case manager's necklace) and earrings to match when I was 14 and I'm still paying on it. I insured it. I got life insurance. I'm completely insured. Even my fingernails are insured. I got in an accident. Someone hit me in the rear end. I got $10,000 for it because I was insured. It was my Dad's car. I'm going to call my Dad."

Geoff describes the police bringing him to the hospital in this way: "My neighbor and I rigged this up. We called about six police guys that we knew and an ambulance and set it up. We wanted to teach the kids about law and order. Everything is closed on holidays. No doctors, no pharmacies, no police. It's hard to get hold of anyone. No pharmacies are open. If you need something, you're in trouble. I don't like the medical profession, especially doctors. No, especially psychiatrists. They don't do anything. They give you medicine. You can fix yourself up. I know everything there is to know about medicine in the pharmacy. I don't need a doctor to tell me."

Thoughts about *body image* are also distorted in those clients with mood disorders. In a mild or moderate depression, distortion begins as an obsessional concern over physical appearance, with a focus on the disliked body parts. As the depression worsens, people believe they are unattractive and may actually erroneously perceive their body as being disfigured or deformed.

People in a manic state have exaggerated self-esteem, which may contribute to believing they look like well-known people or famous beauties. If others challenge this perception, they often respond with a great deal of anger.

Meg is 5 feet tall and weighs 150 pounds. She has long frizzy hair that is several shades of blonde and brown. She approaches the nurse and says, "Don't I look like Gwyneth Paltrow? Look at my hair; I just washed it. Isn't it a pretty shade of blonde? And look at me; I look just like her. I think I will go into the movies. Maybe I can make it as a Gwyneth look-alike."

Faulty perceptions of body image may escalate into *delusions*. Depressed people may experience *somatic delusions*, in which they believe themselves to be hopelessly ill or that part of the body has been infected or contaminated by outside agents. An example is the person who says, "I'm afraid I might have rabies because my friend spit in my throat. My sister has rabies because a wild rabid wolf pissed on her cocaine." Manic people may experience *delusions of grandeur* focusing on beliefs of being famous or *erotomanic delusions*, that is having personal relationships with prominent, well-known people. These delusions may include paranoid content.

Milan has a very large protruding ventral hernia that is very noticeable even when clothed. He states that he has had this for three or four years and that the doctors want him to get it repaired, which he refuses. He says: "I drain it at home. I can take care of it myself. I stand in the bathtub and I puncture it and white fluid comes out. After that brown fluid comes out— that's all the bacteria. It's not a hernia. It's fluid collecting there. I know having sex will make it go away."

People with mood disorders may experience *ambivalence about treatment*, which may be related to denial. They may minimize or deny the reality of a prior episode, their own behavior, and often the consequences of their behavior. People who deny that they have a serious disorder are not likely to seek treatment. Some clients may be reluctant to give up the experience of mania. The increased energy, euphoria, and heightened self-esteem may be very desirable and enjoyable.

Aida, 40 years old, lives in a group home. She states, "I was hospitalized 23 years ago because I wasn't having fun in school and I was overweight." She states she is in the group home because "I am the way I am and because I couldn't figure out why I was gaining weight. I think my gallbladder operation four years ago has something to do with it."

Loss of faith is a common experience during depressive episodes. People lose faith in their ability to ever again feel love for family members, in the possibility of their negative thoughts ever going away, and in their religion. Unable to find meaning in their illness, they feel a sense of injustice in life. This loss of faith contributes to an overwhelming sense of spiritual distress.

SOCIAL CHARACTERISTICS

As part of the depression, individuals have *dysfunctional interpersonal skills* that create negative interactions with other people. Excessive reassurance seeking, high dependency, and negative expectations often elicit rejection and negative responses in the social context. All of this increases the likelihood of more stressful events, which then maintain depressive symptoms and lead to further interpersonal problems.

The impact of mood disorders on the *family* must not be underestimated. Many families report that for several of their extended family and friends, mental illness is still associated with moral weakness or failure. This results in being treated differently or stigmatized. The family's frustration, confusion, and anger in response to the multiple changes in their loved ones are all understandable. Initially, family members may react with support and concern but in some families, when the depression does not improve, support changes to frustration and anger. A vicious cycle may be established. Increased conflict causes increased symptoms,

further rejection, and deepening depression. Other families may become overly solicitous and assume total care of the depressed person. Total care may contribute to increased symptoms because the person feels helpless and indebted to the family.

Nearly every family who has a loved one with bipolar disorder perceives the illness as a moderate to severe *caregiver burden*. About 33 percent of people with bipolar I disorder are unable to live independently. During manic episodes, a person's family may be subjected to bizarre, hostile, and even destructive behavior. Family members often call the police to protect themselves and their property. Untreated bipolar disorder can devastate individual and family life and often leads to a downward spiral in interpersonal, economic, and occupational functioning (Tohen et al., 2000).

There has been increasing awareness of the impact of *parental mood disorders* on children and adolescents. During an acute episode, youngsters must try to cope with parental behavior that is not easily understood. They may also experience repeated separations from the parent. Since both genetic and psychosocial influences are involved in the transmission of these disorders from parent to child, they are at higher risk for experiencing symptoms by the end of their adolescence.

Mood disorders often disrupt a couple's *sex life*. Depressed people lose interest in sexual activity, both autoerotic and with their partner. The depressed person often decreases initiation of sexual activity but continues to give and receive pleasure in the usual pattern. With deepening depression, further change in sexual activity is common. Some people, needing comfort, seek out the partner more frequently. Others may change their patterns by increasing sexual behavior that takes less energy such as cuddling or oral sex. In severe depression, most people experience a complete loss of sexual desire and fulfillment. The person and the partner must understand that these changes are symptoms of the depression, not necessarily a reflection of the relationship.

During a manic state, there is an exaggerated sexual desire, which is often acted out with a variety of partners. People's ethical and moral restraints on sexual activity do not function during the elevated mood state. Seductive behavior, frequency of activity, and number of partners may all increase. Families are often angry and hurt, and this may be the particular behavior that forces treatment or hospitalization. At the height of manic episodes, a paradoxic decrease in sexual behavior may occur. Because they may be constantly trying to seduce everyone in the environment, there is no time for consummating any of the relationships. When mood levels return to normal, they often feel embarrassed and guilty about their behavior.

CULTURE-SPECIFIC CHARACTERISTICS

The Global Burden of Disease study conducted by the World Health Organization recently assessed the extent of disability (measured by the number of work days lost) and mortality associated with noncommunicable disease in different countries (Lopez & Murray, 1998). The study concluded that depression is one of the most debilitating health problems in the world. Researchers predict that by the year 2020, depression will rank second after heart disease in terms of disease burden in the world (Kupfer, 1999).

Throughout the world, *women* experience more depression than do men. Certainly, there are cross-cultural similarities in the way women are socialized and in the inferior status that they experience in many societies. Psychosocial stressors, including multiple work and family responsibilities, poverty, sexual and physical abuse, gender discrimination, lack of social supports, and traumatic life experiences, may contribute to women's increased vulnerability to depression. In the United States and Canada, African American women are at higher risk for depression than Euro-American women are. Research suggests that additional risk factors include minority status, socioeconomic stress, and multiple roles (Schreiber, Stern, & Wilson, 2000; Takeuchi et al., 1998).

Appropriate *expressions of mood* are largely culturally determined. For example, situations in which people are expected to experience sadness, anger, loneliness, frustration, joy, or happiness are defined by the culture. The culture also determines how people are to behave when experiencing a variety of feelings. For example, cultural expectations of grieving individuals may be self-control and a "stiff upper lip" or may be loud mourning and ripping of clothing. Extreme pleasure may be expressed with a nod and a smile or may be expressed with loud laughter and exuberant behavior.

The Western interpretation of feelings is that emotions are intrapersonal. In contrast, in Micronesia, emotions are considered to be not within a person but rather between people. In some Middle Eastern,

African, Hispanic, and Chinese cultures, emotions are viewed and expressed in somatic (bodily) terms. The process by which psychological distress is experienced and communicated in the form of somatic symptoms is called **somatization**. Because these cultures are not subject to the mind–body dualism of Western thinking, psychological distress is viewed as arising from bodily imbalances (Parker, Gladstone, & Chee, 2001).

Emotions of dysphoria and depression have dramatically *different meaning and forms* of expression in different cultures. Many Americans view suffering as unexpected or unacceptable and perceive depression as something to overcome through personal striving. Latin American cultures associate suffering with a deep sense of tragedy. Shi'ite Muslims view suffering within a religious context of martyrdom, while Buddhist cultures view suffering as a positive feature of life. Throughout the entire world, most cases of depression are experienced and expressed in bodily terms such as fatigue, headaches, heart distress, dizziness, and so on. It is only in Western cultures that depression is considered to be a mental disorder (Silverstein & Perlick, 1995). When assessing clients from cultures different from your own, it is important to understand that the expression of depression is culturally determined.

African Americans and Latinos often look to family and their faith communities for help rather than seeking professional help. There is a strong fear of hospitalization and involuntary commitment, and both of those are more likely than for Euro-Americans. African Americans and Latinos who experience mood disorders are often misdiagnosed as having schizophrenia. As a result of this misdiagnosis, they may receive antipsychotic medication and no antidepressants. Thus, appropriate treatment is delayed resulting in poorer therapeutic response (Lawson, 2000).

AGE-SPECIFIC CHARACTERISTICS

The incidence of depression in children is often underestimated. The cultural norm is that childhood is a carefree and happy time and that there is no reason for children to be depressed. The reality, however, is that at least 2.5 percent of *children* and 8 percent of *adolescents* are depressed at any point in time. Furthermore, half of all adults with depression report onset before age 20. While the recovery rate from a single episode of major depression in young people is quite high, episodes are likely to recur (Lynch, Glod, & Fitzgerald, 2001).

In childhood, boys and girls appear to be at equal risk for depressive disorders; but during adolescence, girls are twice as likely as boys to develop depression. Children and adolescents who develop major depression are more likely to have a family history of the disorder than people with adult-onset depression. Twenty to forty percent of adolescents with major depression develop bipolar disorder within five years after the initial diagnosis. People with early-onset bipolar disorder (before the age of 21) are more likely to be male, have a more severe form of the disorder, and experience a more chronic course. The presence of substance abuse appears to lower the age at onset of bipolar disorder (Carlson, Bromet, & Sievers, 2000; Harrington, 2000).

Depression is often manifested through negativism, acting-out behaviors, and/or unexplained physical complaints. Symptoms are often related to the develop-mental levels. See Box 13.1 for problem behaviors associated with depression. Depressive disorders can have far reaching effects on the functioning and adjustment of young people. Children and teens have school difficulties related to an inability to concentrate and their grades often worsen. Lack of energy and irritability may interfere with their participation in school and leisure activities, leading to disruption in peer relationships.

In early-onset bipolar disorder, manic symptoms are similar to the externalizing symptoms associated with childhood disruptive disorders, especially attention deficit hyperactivity disorder and conduct disorder. (See Chapter 17 for further discussion on bipolar disorder and disruptive disorders.)

Depression is a common and troublesome mental disorder among *older adults*, who are at higher risk because of changes in self-concept and the multiple losses they have likely experienced. Many older people

---

BOX 13.1

Behaviors Associated with Depression

Infants
- When separated from parent, may have weepy and withdrawn behavior
- Frozen facial expression
- Weight loss
- Increased incidence of infections

1 to 3 Years
- Delays or regression in toileting, eating, sleeping, intellectual growth
- Increase in nightmares
- Loss of interest in playing
- May appear sad or expressionless
- Apathetic or more clingy

3 to 5 Years
- Loss of interest in newly acquired skills
- Nightmares with themes of annihilation
- Decreased socialization
- Tantrums
- Nonspecific somatic complaints
- Enuresis, encopresis, anorexia, or binge eating may occur
- May also experience separation anxiety
- Frequent negative self-statements and thoughts or impulses of self-harm

6 to 12 Years
- Depressed mood, irritable, aggressive
- Academic difficulties, absence from school
- Social isolation
- Blames self for bad things
- Decreased concentration
- Eating and sleeping disturbances
- Severe self-criticism and guilt
- Suicidal ideation and plans

Adolescents
- Intense mood swings
- Academic difficulties
- Argumentative and/or assaultive
- Substance abuse
- Involvement with law enforcement
- Risk taking or antisocial behavior
- Hypersomnia
- Very low self-esteem

SOURCES: Adapted from Kaslow, N. J., et al. (2000). A family perspective on assessing and treating childhood depression. In C. E. Bailey (Ed.), *Children in therapy* (pp. 215–241). New York: Norton; and Way, W. W., Hayward, A. R., Levin, M. J., & Sondheimer, J. M. (1999). *Current pediatric diagnosis and treatment* (14th ed.). Stamford, CT: Appleton & Lange.

have an increase in stressful life events at the very time when they may have limited resources for managing such difficult circumstances. The more that stressful life events occur, the more their sense of helplessness becomes reinforced. If they reach the point of believing they have no control, they lose the will and the energy to cope with life, and depression frequently results.

Although depression is common, it may not be recognized and is frequently undertreated because health care professionals mistakenly view it as a "natural" part of aging. The consequences of this ageism include poor quality of life, cognitive impairment, nursing home placement, and increased risk of death by suicide. Of the older people living in the United States, about 4 to 15 percent are significantly depressed. For those living in residential care, the rate of depression is 15 to 20 percent (Zubenko, Mulsant, Sweet, Pasternak, & Tu, 1997).

Some studies report that older adults experience symptoms of depression similar to those of younger adults. Other studies indicate that older people experience symptoms related to anxiety and somatic complaints rather than feelings of sadness. Several factors are associated with depression in old age, including disabilities in daily living, lack of social support, institutionalization, and declining health. It is associated with higher rates of mortality, suicide, and cognitive decline.

Older people with depression may exhibit signs of cognitive impairment leading to incorrect diagnoses of dementia. Symptoms include short-term memory problems, word-finding difficulty, confusion, and disorientation. Depression that simulates dementia is referred to as *pseudodementia*. This form of depression must be recognized and differentiated from irreversible dementia, and appropriate treatment measures must be implemented.

Bipolar disorder accounts for 5 to 10 percent of all mood disorders treated in the older population. Only a few of these individuals become ill for the first time after age 50. The cause of late-onset bipolar disorder is often a neurological disease. One common precipitant is a cerebrovascular accident in the right hemisphere affecting the limbic system. Other causes include hyperthyroidism; epilepsy; trauma; and degenerative, vascular, or neoplastic disease of the right hemisphere. Medications that produce manic symptoms include adrenal steroids, levodopa, antidepressants, bronchodilators, and decongestants (Robinson, 2000).

PHYSIOLOGICAL CHARACTERISTICS

People experience many physiological symptoms during episodes of the mood disorders. A change in *appetite* is not unusual. Many people lose their desire for food when depressed, and statements such as "Nothing tastes good to me" and "I can't eat, I feel like there is a big knot in my throat" are common. Others discover their appetites increase when they become depressed, and their eating patterns cause them to gain weight. Another pattern is for people to overeat and gain weight when mildly depressed and to lose their appetite and weight when severely depressed.

People in a manic state may not obtain sufficient food and fluid because they cannot remain still long enough to eat a meal. The consequences of a change in appetite depend on the severity of the reduction or increase in food and fluid intake. The changes could become life threatening.

Sleep patterns are disrupted in people with mood disorders and sleep dysregulation may precede the onset of a unipolar depression. During mild or moderate depression, people may sleep more than usual or they may awaken earlier than usual. In severe depression, people usually have difficulty falling asleep and may sleep for only a few hours a night. The person often awakens in the early morning and is unable to return to sleep. Moreover, they may obsess about their lack of sleep and believe they need much more sleep than they actually do. Remarks are made such as "I've had insomnia, so I haven't been able to sleep. I need sleep so badly. I'm tired all the time, but I just can't sleep." Their difficulty sleeping is demonstrated with changes in the rapid eye movement (REM) cycle of sleep. Nondepressed individuals have more REM activity toward the end of the sleep period, whereas depressed people have more REM activity in the beginning of the sleep period. Additionally, depressed people experience less slow-wave sleep throughout the night. These sleep changes may or may not be evident in depressed children, but they are apparent by adolescence (APA, 2000; Giles et al., 1998).

During a manic episode, people experience a dramatic decrease in their amount of sleep. Although they may sleep only one or two hours a night, they are full of energy throughout the day. They have great difficulty taking naps or relaxing during the day to compensate for their lack of sleep.

Another change characteristic of mood disorders is in *activity level*. It begins with people's tiring more easily and extends to their becoming fatigued with all activities. At the depth of depression, people say they are too tired to do anything, even basic ADLs. Some people who are depressed experience extremely slowed motor activity. They walk slowly with a trudging gait. When speaking, they use a minimum of gestures to illustrate their thoughts. The pitch of the voice is lowered, and there is little speech inflection. Others experience constant and nonpurposeful activity such as wringing the hands, picking at the skin, or agitated pacing.

In manic episodes, people experience hyperactivity without being aware of fatigue. They move constantly and have great difficulty remaining seated for more than a few minutes. When they are seated, constant swinging of the legs is typical. The voice is pitched higher and is much louder than normal. Dramatic arm and facial gestures accompany their speaking. Because they are unaware of fatigue, they are in danger of total physical exhaustion.

Bowel activity may be a problem in both unipolar and bipolar disorder. A marked decrease in food and fluid intake and decreased physical activity can result in constipation. Constipation in manic episodes is related to distractibility and therefore the ignoring of bodily signals or the inability to take the time to have a bowel movement.

Physical appearance is often indicative of an altered mood state. Depressed people may wear the same clothes for days without laundering them. Personal hygiene may be poor because they do not have the energy to brush their teeth, shower, or wash their hair. During a manic state, people may change clothes as often as every hour. Separates, such as skirts, pants, and tops, may clash and seem to be chosen for their brightness rather than for their coordination. Personal hygiene may become a problem if distractibility interferes with normal ADLs. Women who wear makeup and jewelry have extravagant tastes during an elevated mood state. Their cosmetics tend to be very bright and may be carelessly applied.

Pam has been diagnosed as having a bipolar disorder, manic phase. Since admission two days
ago, she has been averaging two hours of sleep a night. The rest of the nighttime hours are spent pacing hallways and talking to staff. She is in constant motion and brags about how energetic she is. Her clothing consists of startlingly bright miniskirts, low-cut sweaters, and high heels. Every few hours she reapplies her makeup to match each change of clothing.

Although peripheral *thyroid hormone levels* may be normal, 35 percent of people with depression experience central nervous system (CNS) thyroid dysfunction, which has a major effect on serotonin (5-HT), dopamine (DA), and gamma-aminobutyric acid (GABA). It is believed that people who are depressed have a lower level of transthyretin, a protein important for transporting thyroid hormones in the brain. Current or past hypothyroidism may be associated with rapid-cycling bipolar disorder (APA, 2000).

Major depression is also associated with hyperactivity of the hypothalamus–pituitary–adrenal (HPA) axis. This dysfunction results in higher levels of circulating *cortisol*. Clinical depression is also associated with decreases in all measures of lymphocyte function. It is believed that the circadian rhythm of lymphocytes is entrained to the CNS. The result is a suppressed *immune function* with a vulnerability to infections and diseases.

Depression is also a risk factor of *osteoporosis* in both women and men and carries an increased risk of fractures. Loss of bone density may be the result of neuroendocrine alterations during depression (Keller, 2000; Schweiger, Weber, Deuschle, & Heuser, 2000; Sullivan et al., 1999; Weiss, Longhurst, & Mazure, 1999). For a review of the behavioral, affective, cognitive, sociocultural, and physiological characteristics of people with mood disorders, see Table 13.2 ■.

CONCOMITANT DISORDERS

Severe depression and *anxiety disorders* frequently occur at the same time. Studies indicate that as many as 40 percent of those suffering from agoraphobia, 50 percent of those experiencing panic attacks, 44 percent of those with obsessive compulsive disorder, and 17 percent of those with generalized anxiety disorder are also clinically depressed. An estimated 85 percent of adults with depression experience significant symptoms of anxiety. Individuals with bipolar disorder are

TABLE 13.2

Characteristics of Mood Disorders

Characteristic	Depressed State	Manic State
Behavioral		
Desire to participate in activities	Decreased to absent	Interested in all activities; increase in high-risk behaviors
Interaction with others	Limited; client withdraws	Talkative, gregarious
Affiliation needs	Increased dependency	Independent, self-sufficient
Affective		
Mood	Despair, desolation	Unstable: euphoric and irritable
Guilt	High level	Unable to experience guilt
Crying spells	Frequent crying to inability to cry	May have brief episodes
Gratification	Loss of interest in pleasurable activities	Constantly seeking fun and excitement
Emotional attachments	Indifference to others	Forms intense attachments rapidly
Cognitive		
Self-evaluation	Focuses on failures; sees self as incompetent; catastrophizes and personalizes	Grandiose beliefs about self
Expectations	Believes present and future hopeless; overgeneralizes one experience or fact	Inordinate positive expectations; unable to see potential negative outcomes
Self-criticism	Harshly critical of self; is a perfectionist; anticipates disapproval from others	Approves of own behavior; irate if criticized by others
Concentration	Decreased	Decreased
Decision-making ability	Decreased ability or inability to make decisions	Difficulty due to distractibility and impulsiveness
Flow of thought	Decrease in rate and number of thoughts	Flight of ideas; can't be interrupted
Body image	Believes self unattractive or ugly	Believes self unusually beautiful
Delusions	Somatic delusions	Delusions of grandeur
Hallucinations	Occur in 15 to 25% of cases	Occur in 15 to 25% of cases
Sociocultural		
Sexual desire	Loss of desire	Increase in activity and partners
Physiological		
Appetite	Increased or decreased in mild and moderate depression; decreased in severe depression	Difficulty eating due to inability to sit still
Amount of sleep	Increased or decreased in mild and moderate depression; decreased in severe depression	Sleeps only one or two hours a night
Activity level	Impaired motor activity; loss of energy	Hyperactivity; high energy
Bowel activity	Constipation	Constipation
Physical appearance	Unkempt; poor hygiene	Bright clothing; frequently changes clothing

more likely to have concomitant panic disorder than the general population. People with both mood and anxiety disorders have fewer personal and social resources and demonstrate poorer overall functioning (Feske et al., 2000; Lenze et al., 2000; Zimmerman, McDermut, & Mattia, 2000).

The rate of co-morbidity between mood disorders and *substance-related disorders* is high. In some cases, the primary diagnosis is a mood disorder, with substance abuse being an attempt to self-medicate. In other situations, the substance-related disorder is the primary diagnosis. An example is the person who becomes depressed on withdrawal from amphetamines or cocaine. A third possibility is that the person has both disorders as primary. Research reports that major depression tends to come before alcohol problems in women, while the opposite is true for men. Unfortunately, the use of alcohol to relieve depression can also aggravate depression by causing other problems for the drinker and also by intensifying the level of depression. Twenty percent of all depressed adolescents have a comorbid substance abuse disorder. Approximately 60 percent of people with bipolar disorder also have a substance abuse disorder—the highest rate across all people with major psychiatric illnesses. In bipolar disorder, substance abuse may be a natural result of the impulsive, expansive lifestyle and poor judgment during a manic episode, which may worsen the course of bipolar disorder. Treatment for both disorders should be concurrent (Dixit & Crum, 2000; Martin & Cohen, 2000; McElroy et al., 2001).

Lauren, a 23-year-old woman was admitted last evening after taking 10 Benadryl (diphenhydramine) tablets. She denies that she was trying to commit suicide and states that she just "wanted to sleep forever" and that she often wants to "end the pain of feeling bad." Her parents say she has been depressed for several months. She says, "I think I need to change my friends—they tend to consume too much alcohol and they also seem depressed." She is currently on probation for a DUI and public intoxication.

Many individuals with *medical conditions* develop major depression during the course of their medical illness. Depression is a major risk factor for death for those with general medical illnesses. Research demonstrates that mortality is significantly higher among depressed inpatients than those who are not depressed. After a myocardial infarction, people with major depression are three times more likely to die within one year than are people without depression (Badger, McNiece, & Gagan, 2000).

People who have Parkinson's disease have a 30 to 50 percent chance of also having a major depression. Often, the mood symptoms precede the motor changes, which suggests that the depression is not merely a reaction to the physiological changes of Parkinson's disease. Compared to other people with depression, these individuals are less guilty but more pessimistic, and have higher anxiety levels, frequent suicide ideation, and more cognitive deficits (Levy & Cummings, 2000). See Chapter 19 for more detailed information.

Of people who have had a cerebral vascular accident, 20 to 50 percent experience depression with more symptoms of anxiety and cognitive impairment than is typical for people who become depressed after other medical diagnoses. Depression is more common with left hemisphere stroke, especially when located close to the frontal lobe. Other disorders contributing to depression include hypothyroidism, alcoholism, hypoglycemia, and multiple sclerosis (Robinson, 2000). See Chapter 19 for more detailed information.

It is vital that you be alert to cues for self-harm, since as many as 15 percent of people with mood disorders go on to commit suicide. Suicidal behavior and suicide prevention is covered in Chapter 20.

CAUSATIVE THEORIES

Multiple theories have been developed to explain the cause of mood disorders. Depression, like schizophrenia, is considered a spectrum disorder. At one end of the spectrum is an incapacitating illness such as a recurrent depression or bipolar disorder with psychosis. At the other end is a depressive personality characterized only by a pessimistic outlook on life or mood swings that are mild in nature. The majority of the cases falls somewhere in between these two extremes.

In understanding people with mood disorders, you must look at how factors interacted within the person's past and how they interact in present circumstances. A person may have a genetic predisposition to changes in neurotransmission. The actual changes may occur only if certain psychological mechanisms are present, and these mechanisms may operate only if particular social interactions occur. Many factors in both the individual and the environment increase or decrease the risk of mood disorders. Different forms of the illness could have different risk factors. In some forms, predisposition may have a stronger role, and in other forms, stressors may have a stronger role. By applying genetic, neurobiological, intrapersonal, learning, cognitive, social, and feminist theories, you approach the client from a holistic perspective.

Genetics

Some evidence suggests that people who experience mood disorders have a genetic predisposition. It is not yet clear what is inherited, neurobiological vulnerability, cognitive vulnerability, or social vulnerability. The inheritability of major depression is 40 to 50 percent. The more severe the depression is, the stronger the genetic link. The general population rate of recurrent unipolar depression is 8 percent. Children of depressed parents (top-down sampling as shown in Figure 13.2 ■) have twice the risk or about 16 percent over a lifetime. If both parents have depression, the risk rises to 75 percent. First-degree relatives of depressed children (bottom-up sampling as depicted in Figure 13.3 ■) also have a twofold greater risk of depression. Studies of the incidence in twins show that in 50 percent of monozygotic twins, both twins developed a unipolar depression, compared with only 19 percent of dizygotic twins (Berrettini, 2000; Ferro, Verdeli, Pierre, & Weissman, 2000; Paris, 1999; Sullivan, Neale, & Kendler, 2000).

Bipolar disorder has the greatest inheritability where about 70 percent of the risk appears to be inherited. Early onset of the disorder may be the result of a particularly strong genetic effect. Studies of the incidence in twins demonstrate that in 80 percent of monozygotic twins, both twins developed bipolar disorder, compared with only 25 percent of dizygotic twins. (Badner, Detera-Wadleigh, & Gershon, 2000; Sullivan et al., 2000).

Studies suggest that a complex mode of inheritance exists, rather than a single dominant gene. It is probably the individual mix of these multiple genes that determines differences such as age of onset, symptoms, severity, and course of the mood disorders.

Neurobiologic Theory

The *prefrontal cortex* has been the subject of increasing attention in research on mood disorders. Studies of depressed people have shown lower than normal activity, low glucose metabolism, and decreased blood flow in the anterior cingulate cortex. These abnormalities may be associated with abnormal processing of emotion. Neuroimaging findings in bipolar disorder include ventricular enlargement and smaller volumes in the right hippocampus, left amygdala, and temporal lobe (Brody, Saxena, & Stoessel, 2001).

The *neurotransmission hypothesis* is specifically concerned with the levels of serotonin (5-HT), dopamine (DA), norepinephrine (NE), and acetylcholine (ACh) in the central nervous system. It is believed that there is a functional deficiency of these neurotransmitters during a depressive episode and a functional excess during a manic episode (Garber & Flynn, 2001; Meltzer et al., 1999).

Most likely there are different combinations of problems with the neurotransmitter systems. Both DA and the balance between DA and ACh are responsible

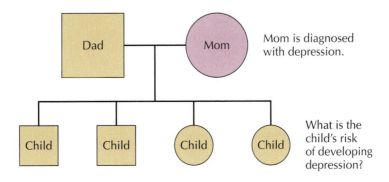

FIGURE 13.2 ■ Top-down sampling.

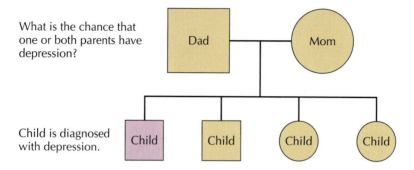

What is the chance that one or both parents have depression?

Dad

Mom

Child is diagnosed with depression.

Child · Child · Child · Child

FIGURE 13.3 ■ Bottom-up sampling.

for difficulties with motivation. ACh is implicated in the sleep disturbances of both bipolar and unipolar disorders. NE is important in motor arousal, movement, energy, concentration, and motivation. The principal neurotransmitter for mood states is 5-HT, which is associated with anxiety and aggression, especially self-destructive behavior. In addition, endogenous opioids are necessary to moderate sad moods. The interactions between these different neurotransmitters explain how clinical features tend to vary from client to client.

One way this imbalance may occur is through the action of the enzyme *monoamine oxidase (MAO)*, which is responsible for deactivating neurotransmitters after they have been released from the receptor sites. If there is an excess of MAO, neurotransmitter levels will be low, resulting in decreased impulse transmission. If levels are not sufficient to deactivate the neurotransmitters, they will accumulate at the synapse and increase the transmission of impulses.

This hypothesis may be one explanation for the higher incidence of depression in women and older people. Throughout life, women and older adults have consistently higher levels of MAO than do men and younger people. The result may be a functional decrease in the necessary neurotransmitters.

Another part of the hypothesis concerns the *sensitivity of the receptors* to the neurotransmitters. During depression, the receptors may be subsensitive, so that fewer impulses are transmitted. During the manic state, receptors may be supersensitive, resulting in an increase in the transmission of impulses. The sensitivity of the receptors is influenced by the thyroid hormone triiodothyronine (T_3). Thus, people with

hypothyroidism are at higher risk for a depressive episode, and those with hyperthyroidism are at higher risk for a manic episode (APA, 2000).

Continuing research into the relationship between *stress* and mood disorders indicates that the limbic system of the brain is the major site of stress adaptation. With stress, neurotransmitter production in the limbic system increases. When the stress becomes chronic or recurrent, the body can no longer adapt as efficiently, and a shortage of neurotransmitters results. During manic episodes, there appears to be a defective feedback mechanism in the limbic system. Even after the stressful event has been resolved, the limbic system continues to produce excessive neurotransmitters; the increased transmission of impulses continues. Different areas of the limbic system play a major role in the regulation of emotions such as fear, rage, excitement, and euphoria. The signs and symptoms of limbic dysfunction correlate to the characteristics seen in the mood disorders.

Another hypothesis involves **biological rhythms**. In some individuals, internal desynchronization may result in depression. The tendency toward internal desynchronization is probably inherited, but stresses, lifestyle, and normal aging also influence it. However, it is unclear whether changes in circadian rhythms cause mood disturbances or whether changes in mood alter circadian rhythms. (See Chapter 1 for a more detailed discussion of circadian rhythms.)

Some forms of mood disorders are related to the time of year and the amount of available sunlight. In **seasonal affective disorder (SAD)**, depression occurs annually during fall and winter, and normal mood or hypomania occurs in spring and summer. The depressive state appears to be directly related to the amount of light because symptoms disappear if the person is exposed to more sunlight. Light has an inhibiting effect on the production of melatonin, a hormone that affects mood, sensations of fatigue, and sleepiness. Seasonal light changes are not the only trigger. A change of living quarters, such as a move into a darker basement apartment or into a windowless office, can cause the disorder in some people.

The majority of SAD sufferers are women with a family history of mood disorders. Unlike major depression, in which symptoms for children and adults differ, children and adults with SAD exhibit similar symptoms: fatigue, decreased activity, irritability, sadness, crying, worrying, and decreased concentration. A symptom seen more frequently in SAD, compared to the other mood disorders, is increased appetite, carbohydrate craving, and weight gain (Glod & Baisden, 1999).

Secondary causes of depression may be related to a variety of medications and medical conditions. Medications implicated in secondary depression include antianxiety agents, antihypertensives, corticosteroids, estrogen/progesterone, and chemotherapeutic agents. Metabolic disorders that may cause depression include hyperthyroidism, hypothyroidism, Addison's disease, and vitamin B_{12} deficiency. Neurological disruptions include brain tumors or acute traumatic brain injury (especially in the frontal or basal ganglia areas), brain attack, Huntington's disease, multiple sclerosis, Parkinson's disease, and Alzheimer's disease (Levy & Cummings, 2000; Ratey, 2001).

Intrapersonal Theory

Intrapersonal theory focuses on the theme of loss, either real or symbolic. The loss may be of another person, a relationship, an object, self-esteem, or security. When grief concerning the loss is unrecognized or unresolved, depression may result. A normal feeling accompanying all losses is anger, a compensatory response to feelings of powerlessness. People who have been taught it is inappropriate to experience and express anger learn to repress it. The result is that anger is turned inward and against the self. Some theorists believe the repressed anger and aggression against the self are the cause of depressive episodes. Other theorists believe the cause of depression is an inability to achieve desired goals, the loss of these goals, and a feeling of lack of control in life.

People who are unusually sensitive to loss or abandonment issues are said to have dependent traits. People who are unusually sensitive to failure to achieve their goals are said to have self-critical traits. Both of these cognitive-personality features increase the likelihood that environmental stressors will lead to depression.

Learning Theory

Learning theory states that people learn to be depressed in response to an external locus of control, as they perceive themselves lacking control over their life experiences. Throughout life, depressed people experience little success in achieving gratification, and little positive reinforcement for their attempts to cope with negative incidents. These repeated failures teach them that what they do has no effect on the final outcome. The more that stressful life events occur, the more their sense of helplessness is reinforced. When people reach the point of believing they have no control, they no longer have the will or energy to cope with life, and a depressive state results.

Cognitive Theory

The cognitive schemas influence the way people with mood disorders experience themselves and others. Those who are depressed focus on negative messages in the environment and ignore positive experiences. These negative schemas contribute to a view of the self as incompetent, unworthy, and unlikable. All present experiences are viewed as negative, and there is no hope for the future (Zust, 2000). In the manic phase, people focus on positive messages in the environment and ignore negative experiences. These positive schemas contribute to a grandiose view of themselves. Everything that occurs is seen as positive, and the future holds no limits. When people get caught up in this process, a number of cognitive distortions may occur (see Table 1.5 in Chapter 1).

Social Theory

A variety of sociocultural conditions may contribute to a person's depressive feelings of powerlessness, hopelessness, and low self-esteem. Racism, classism, sexism, ageism, and homophobia are predominant sociocultural characteristics in the United States. Whatever way minorities are defined, they experience discrimination psychologically, educationally, vocationally, and economically. When one is the subject of cultural stereotypes in comments or jokes, it is difficult not to feel inadequate and shameful. When education has been substandard, one cannot expect to be successful without remedial work. When promotions are based on race, gender, age, or sexual orientation, it is difficult to feel hopeful about advancing in one's career. It is also difficult to combat the helplessness felt when one's financial compensation is clearly inadequate for the job being done.

There is a much higher rate of depression among women than among men. One of the contributing factors in Western society may be the stress of being a single parent. With the high divorce rate, there are increasing numbers of single parents, 85 percent of them are women. These women must deal with financial hardships, parenting problems, loneliness, and lack of a supportive adult relationship. A major predisposing factor for depression in women is having three or more children under the age of 14 living at home. When the children grow up and leave, the rate of depression decreases. This is contrary to the theory that depression results from the empty-nest syndrome. It appears that being responsible for children is a source of stress that contributes to depression (Paris, 1999).

Another sociocultural factor that may contribute to depression is the occurrence of stressful life events. Some events cause expansion of the family system: marriage, births, adoptions, other people moving into the home. Other events cause a reduction of the family system: children leaving, marital separations, divorce, death. Some life events involve a threat, as in job problems, difficulties with the police, and illness. Others can be emotionally exhausting, such as holidays, changing residences, and arguing with family and friends. Many people who experience major stressful events do not become depressed. However, for those who are vulnerable to depression, stressors may play a significant role in the exacerbation and course of the disorder (Weiss et al., 1999).

A number of factors influence the degree of stress that accompanies significant life events (see Figure 13.4 ■). The presence of a social support network can decrease the impact an event may have on a person. People who have developed adaptive coping patterns such as problem solving, direct communication, and use of resources are more likely to maintain their normal mood. Those who feel out of control, are unable

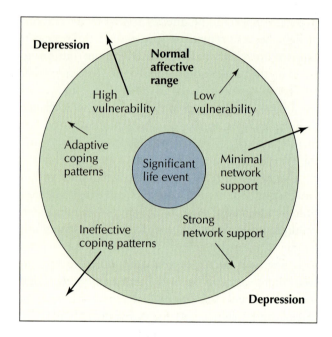

FIGURE 13.4 ■ The relationship between life events and depression.

to problem-solve, and ignore available resources are more apt to feel depressed. Thus, an individual's perception and interpretation of significant events may contribute to depression (Perraud, 2000a).

Feminist Theory

In the definition of mental health there has, in the past, been a double standard for women and men. A healthy woman has been described as acquiescent, subdued, dependent, and emotionally expressive. A healthy man, on the other hand, has been described as logical, rational, independent, aggressive, and unemotional. These stereotypes have had unfortunate consequences for both women and men. However, there is movement toward an androgynous definition of mental health. This perspective stresses positive human qualities such as assertiveness, self-reliance, sensitivity to others, intimacy, and open communication—qualities that legitimately belong in the repertoire of both women and men.

Gender socialization differences may be a factor in the higher rate of depression in women. It starts early, when many girls are encouraged to play with dolls and help take care of other children in the family. Girls are taught to be "nice," nonargumentative, and docile.

They become more concerned than boys about fitting in and backing down in the face of conflict. Gradually, they begin to question the worth of their abilities and opinions, which decreases self-esteem. Boys are socialized to be individualistic, to speak up, to raise their hands more in class. Gradually they begin to see themselves as autonomous individuals with good self-esteem.

Rigid expectations about gender roles continue to linger and contribute to higher rates of depression among women. Women who are full-time homemakers may develop no identity other than that of wife and mother. The tremendous duties of managing a household are often invisible to others and lack prestige. Positive feedback or positive reinforcement such as compliments, a paycheck, and retirement benefits are uncommon. And the position is continuous, 24 hours a day. Since one lives in the workplace, there is no stimulation from a change in the environment. Indeed, being a full-time homemaker is one of the most isolating professions in society today.

Women who are employed outside the home, in both professional and blue-collar positions, are less depressed than those who remain at home. This is true even for women who must assume the responsibility for two full-time jobs with minimal or no support from other family members. Employed women must often accept lower pay, inferior jobs, and fewer opportunities for career advancement. The legal system has been slow to redress employment discrimination, which increases women's frustration, anger, and distress. Thoughts of the future focus on the helplessness of their situations and contribute to depression.

Feminist theory can also be applied to the situation in which some older adults find themselves. In a society that places a premium on youth, older people feel useless, unimportant, incapable, and at times even repulsive. Role changes and losses may threaten their self-esteem. With aging, physiological changes may lead to a self-perception of being unfit, which then extends to further thoughts of being ineffectual and inferior. All these changes may contribute to despair about one's entire life and a sense of hopelessness about the limited future. Considering these effects, it is not surprising to find a higher rate of depression among older people. See Table 13.3 ■ for causative theories of mood disorders, with specific relevance to women and older adults.

PSYCHOPHARMACOLOGICAL INTERVENTIONS

The initial phase of medical intervention for clients with mood disorders begins with an in-depth assessment. The primary care provider must determine whether any drugs or medical conditions are contributing to or causing the depression.

Antidepressant and mood-stabilizing medications are often prescribed for clients with mood disorders. Because depressions are heterogeneous in terms of which neurotransmitters are depleted, different people respond differently to various antidepressants. At times, a period of trial and error is necessary to determine which medication is the most effective. Maintenance continues until clients are free of symptoms for four months to one year; then the drugs are slowly discontinued. See Chapter 8 for a detailed discussion of these medications.

Despite advances in treatment of mood disorder, there is still the problem of the delay of onset of therapeutic benefits. It takes an average of 10 to 14 days for the beginning effect of most antidepressants, and the full effect may not be apparent for four to six weeks. The addition of Inderal (pindolol), a beta-blocker, accelerates the onset of response to the selective serotonin reuptake inhibitors (SSRIs). Approximately 30 percent of clients do not respond to their antidepressant after a trial of four to six weeks. At that point, the primary care provider may try a different antidepressant or augment with other medications. A significant number of clients improve when 600 mg of lithium is added to the antidepressant treatment. Supplementation with triiodothyronine (T_3) can also improve the response rate. For the postmenopausal woman, the addition of estrogen may lessen the depressive symptoms.

For clients who are delusional or severely agitated, antipsychotic medication may be indicated. Individuals who experience psychotic manic episodes that are difficult to treat or have schizoaffective disorder may respond best to Zyprexa (olanzapine), which has been approved by the Food and Drug Administration (FDA) for treatment of acute manic episodes. Clients with bipolar disorder require a higher dose than those with schizophrenia. Risperdal (risperidone) combined with lithium provides more rapid mood stabilization than lithium alone (Keck, 2001; Tohen et al., 1999).

TABLE 13.3

Causative Theories of Mood Disorders

Theory	Main Points	Relevance to Women and Older Adults
Genetic	Increased sensitivity to chemical changes related to stress	
Neurobiologic	Impaired neurotransmission; limbic dysfunction	Higher levels of MAO in CNS in women and older people
Biologic rhythms	Internal desynchronization of circadian rhythms	
Sunlight	Decreased exposure to sunlight increases production of melatonin	Older people do not go outside as much during the winter months
Intrapersonal	Loss of person, object, self-esteem; hostility turned against the self; goals unachieved	Women are more dependent on others for self-esteem; older people suffer multiple losses
Learning	Lack of control over experiences; learned helplessness; failure to adapt	Expectation of women's dependency reinforces helplessness; older people have increased stress with decreased resources, which contributes to loss of control
Cognitive	Negative view of self, the present, and the future; focus on negative messages; cognitive errors	
Feminist	Internalization of cultural norms of behavior; rigid gender-role and age expectations	Women's identity may be limited to home-maker role; employment positions less prestigious; may hold two full-time jobs. Older people suffer from the cultural value on youth; many role changes and losses

To date, no psychotropic medication has been approved by the FDA for use during pregnancy. Tricyclic antidepressants and SSRIs have not generally been associated with a high risk of major birth defects. On the other hand, abrupt discontinuation of maintenance medications including antipsychotics, antidepressants, and mood stabilizers has been associated with a high, early relapse risk. The practice of abrupt discontinuation of these medications to minimize potential birth defects can place a woman and her fetus at risk due to impulsive or self-injurious behavior, substance abuse, or inattention to prenatal care. Untreated mood disorders during pregnancy have been associated with premature delivery, low birth weight, and lower Apgar ratings of neonatal status. Women who are breast-feeding and need antidepressant medication can usually take the SSRIs safely, although the infant should be monitored periodically. Taking medication immediately after breast-feeding minimizes the amount present in milk and maximizes clearance before the next feeding. Dosage should be as low as possible while still being clinically effective. Lithium and Tegretol (carbamazepine) are contraindicated while breast-feeding (Burt et al., 2001; Szigethy & Ruiz, 2001; Viguera et al., 2000).

Medication as a first-line course of treatment is considered for children and adolescents with severe symptoms that would prevent effective psychotherapy, those with psychosis, and those with chronic or recurrent episodes. The SSRIs are effective and safe for the short-term treatment of mood disorders in youth. The mood stabilizers Lamictal (lamotrigine) and Neurontin (gabapentin) should never be used in clients younger than 16 due to the risk of developing Stevens–Johnson syndrome (see Chapter 8). Carbamazepine and valproate are better choices for mood stabilization (Mohr, 2001).

The clinical response to antidepressant medications in older depressed clients is often delayed. The average time to easing of symptoms is 12 to 13 weeks. Studies show that while only 30 percent of older adults responded by week 6 of treatment, the number jumped to 55 percent at week 12. This suggests that longer treatment periods may be important to evaluate the effectiveness in older adults (Bondareff et al., 2000).

MULTIDISCIPLINARY INTERVENTIONS

Electroconvulsive therapy (ECT) may be useful for a variety of clients. ECT is a safer alternative for highly suicidal clients, those who suffer from psychotic depression, and those who are medically deteriorated. In addition it is a safe alternative for children and adolescents. ECT is safe in all trimesters of pregnancy and may be less harmful to the fetus than psychotropic medications. Clients who do not respond to medications or cannot tolerate the side effects often respond positively to ECT. Because of concurrent medication conditions, poor tolerance of the side effects of psychotropic medications, and marked disability with depression, ECT is often the treatment of choice in older clients (Papolos & Papolos, 1999). See Chapter 10 for more detailed information on ECT.

Another medical treatment for depression is *sleep deprivation*. Sleep deprivation is the only known intervention in depression that has proven benefits within 24 hours. It is beneficial for individuals ranging in age from adolescence through late life. It is believed that DA and 5-HT activity is altered in response to sleep deprivation. The deprivation may be total, for 36 hours, or partial, with the person being awakened after 1:30 A.M. and kept awake until the next evening. During this time, clients may be alone, in a group, or participating in activities. Some improve steadily after only one night of sleep deprivation. Sleep deprivation is inappropriate for people with rapid cycling bipolar disorder. For reasons that are unknown, these individuals have very delicate "internal clock" mechanisms, and disruption of these mechanisms by losing even a single night's sleep often results in a manic episode (Wu et al., 1999).

Phototherapy is often the treatment of choice for clients of any age who are experiencing SAD. Clients are exposed to very bright full-spectrum fluorescent lamps for 30 minutes a day. Clinical improvement is typically seen within three to five days. Phototherapy may be used prophylactically with clients susceptible to SAD. It is thought that the bright light suppresses the production of melatonin and normalizes the disturbance in circadian rhythms. See Chapter 10 for more information on phototherapy.

When one family member suffers from a mood disorder, there is frequently a detrimental effect on all family members. Families need information and support during this time, and *family therapy* is often very beneficial. Roles and relationships must be redefined during acute episodes and clients and families may need help with this process. If family interactions are dysfunctional, therapists may be able to assist in the development of healthier and more adaptive coping behaviors. Most family members want to be involved in treatment and believe that it is difficult to support the person with a mood disorder if they are excluded from the therapeutic process. Chapter 3 covers family issues, and Chapter 10 covers family therapy in more detail.

ALTERNATIVE THERAPIES

Depression, fatigue, insomnia, and anxiety are among the most commonly reported reasons for the use of alternative therapies in community surveys. The following are some alternative therapies used for mood disorders.

Transcranial Magnetic Stimulation

Transcranial magnetic stimulation (TMS) is the use of a magnetic field that passes through the skull, which causes cells in the cerebral cortex to fire. TMS in depression is the most-studied clinical application in psychiatry. The target area is the left prefrontal cortex which is the brain area thought to be disrupted in depression. The opposite lobe, the right prefrontal cortex, has therapeutic effects in manic episodes. TMS has a rapid onset of action of one to two weeks, which is faster than most psychotropic medications. ECT and TMS have the same effectiveness in depression without psychosis, while depression with psychosis is best treated with ECT. See Chapter 10 for more detailed information on TMS (Lisanby & Sackeim, 2000).

Vagus Nerve Stimulation

Vagus nerve stimulation (VNS) has been used successfully with hard-to-treat seizure disorders and has FDA approval for this use. Noticing an improvement in subjects' moods, researchers are now studying VNS for people suffering from treatment resistant depression. A cookie-size generator is surgically implanted in the chest under the skin that conveys electrical impulses via a connecting wire to the vagus nerve. The nerve is a leading provider of information from the heart and other organs to the brain; it also affects areas of the brain involved with mood. It provides continuous therapy for 8 to 12 years, which is the life of the implant's battery. Results of early studies show that 40 percent of subjects had up to a 50 percent improvement in symptoms (Perraud, 2000b).

Exercise

There have been numerous studies on the effect of exercise on depression. Short periods of vigorous aerobic exercise or longer periods of nonaerobic exercise, for at least several weeks, is most helpful in mild to moderate depression. Exercise raises levels of endorphins, which enhance one's feelings of well being. Exercise also increases levels of DA, 5-HT, and NE, which are related to feelings of reward, motivation, and attention (Ratey, 2001).

Yoga has been found to improve wellness and prevent disorders such as depression. The gentle nature of the exercises allows its use in almost any condition. People who practice yoga on a regular basis report improved life satisfaction, alertness, enthusiasm, and mental and physical energy, all of which are the opposite of the symptoms of depression (Becker, 2000).

St. John's Wort

St. John's Wort (hypericum perforatum) has been the most widely publicized alternative treatment for *mild to moderate depression*. A meta-analysis of 23 controlled trials with 1,757 outpatients found that St. John's Wort was almost three times more effective than placebo and comparable to standard antidepressants. The side effects of St. John's Wort in higher doses are similar to that of SSRIs. The dosage is 300 to 600 mg/day of 0.3 percent hypericin, the active component in St. John's Wort. It should *not* be combined with pre-

scription antidepressants. It may also interfere with the action of anticonvulsants. St. John's Wort has been found to reduce the effectiveness of birth control pills, HIV treatment medications, and the asthma medication, theophylline (Linde, 1996).

SAMe

A nutritional supplement called SAMe (pronounced "sammy") has been used by more than 1 million people in Europe, primarily for depression and arthritis. SAMe (S-adenosylmethionine), a compound made by every cell in the body, helps produce DA, 5-HT, and NE. Numerous trials have found SAMe to be effective in depression, postpartum depression, and postmenopausal depression. It may, however, worsen bipolar depression. Its rapid onset (10 to 12 days), low side effects (no weight gain or sexual dysfunction), and ability to boost antioxidants gives it many advantages in the treatment of depression. The dose is 800 to 1,600 mg/day and is best taken 30 minutes before meals. It has been successfully used as augmentation of all categories of antidepressants without adverse effects and there is no evidence that it interacts with other medications. Side effects are generally mild and temporary such as headaches, loose bowels, anxiety, and insomnia. Like tricyclic antidepressants, SAMe should be used with caution in people who have a history of cardiac arrhythmia. Infants normally have a three to four times naturally higher level of SAMe than do adults. Given this knowledge, the amount of SAMe passing to infants through breast milk may be inconsequential (Brown & Gerbarg, 2000).

Vitamin B$_{12}$

Vitamin B$_{12}$ is necessary for the production of DA, 5-HT, and NE as well as for the natural synthesis of SAMe. One study found that individuals with a significant vitamin B$_{12}$ deficiency were at twice the risk of depression than those who had normal levels. Depression itself could cause low levels through decreased appetite and resulting decreased food intake. In addition, many of the tricyclic antidepressants deplete the body of vitamin B$_{12}$.

Tyrosine

Tyrosine, an amino acid, is the precursor for DA and NE and as such, acts as a mood elevator. Supplemental tyrosine has been used in depression, stress reduction, anxiety, and chronic fatigue. People taking MAO inhibitors should not take any supplements containing tyrosine, as it may lead to a hypertensive crisis. Tyrosine combined with vitamin B_6 and vitamin C will provide better absorption.

Melatonin

Insomnia is a frequent complaint among people suffering from depression. Melatonin, a hormone secreted by the pineal gland, plays a critical role in the regulation of the day–night cycle. Studies have shown that melatonin is effective in inducing sleep and has no notable side effects. Slow-release melatonin combined with standard antidepressant treatment often improves the sleep pattern in depressed individuals.

DHEA

Dehydroepiandrosterone (DHEA) is a corticosteriod produced primarily in the adrenal glands. In addition to serving as a precursor to testosterone and estrogen, DHEA may be involved in regulating mood and one's sense of well being. The method of action is unclear but it may stimulate GABA receptors or increase 5-HT levels. It has been used alone or as an adjunct to antidepressants. Since there is little known about long-term risks, it is probably best used under medical supervision. The usual dose is up to 90 mg/day (Wolkowitz et al., 1999).

Omega-3 Fatty Acids

A number of studies have been done on the effects of omega-3 fatty acids from concentrated fish oils on mood disorders. Omega-3 fatty acids are thought to act on cells similar to lithium, block calcium channels as do the other mood stabilizers, and help regulate 5-HT. It appears to be antidepressant, antimanic, and a mood stabilizer. Research shows significantly low levels of omega-3 fatty acids in depression and the lower the levels, the more severe the depression.

Dr. Andrew Stoll (1999) found that doses of fish oil relieved symptoms in a group of 30 rapid-cycling bipolar clients. Sixty-five percent got better on fish oil compared to only 18% on placebo. The recommended dose is 5 grams per day, which is usually 7 or 8 capsules. The maximum dose is 15 grams daily. Taking the capsules at night and with orange juice cuts down on the fishy aftertaste.

Aromatherapy

Olfactory receptors are the only sensory pathways that open directly to the brain. Nerve cells relay this information directly to the limbic system, influencing emotions and behavior. Inhaling essential oils through the use of a diffuser or using essential oils in massage may be beneficial in relieving depressive symptoms. The following oils are the most helpful: bergamot, geranium, jasmine, lemon balm, rose, and ylang-ylang.

Acupuncture

Acupuncture is helpful in relieving feelings of depression and anxiety, most likely related to the rise in endorphin levels as a result of the treatment. Adding electrostimulation to acupuncture needles usually increases the effectiveness of the treatment. After only a single session, many people report a sense of well-being. It is unclear how helpful acupuncture is for bipolar disorder. Client response appears to be quite variable at the present time (Gerber, 2000).

Animal-Assisted Therapy

Companionship with animals is associated with people experiencing less depression and loneliness. Animals provide meaningful and substantial comfort for many individuals. Studies show elderly women, who are at higher risk for depression, who live alone to be in better emotional health if they lived with an animal. They were less lonely, more optimistic, and more interested in the future than those women who lived alone without a pet (Hart, 2000).

NURSING PROCESS

Assessment

Assessing clients with mood disorders is often done in segments of 15 to 20 minutes each. Those who are depressed do not have the energy to talk for longer

periods, and those who are in a manic phase are unable to concentrate and sit still for longer periods. You must exercise a great deal of patience when assessing these clients. Clients who are depressed may take a long time to answer your questions, and you may need to repeat them. If family members are present, discourage them from answering questions for the client who is responding slowly. Clients in a manic phase with flight of ideas must frequently be refocused on the topic at hand. Their elevated mood may interfere with their ability to give accurate information. See the Focused Nursing Assessment feature on the following pages. You may wish to use the Beck Depression Inventory (Table 13.4 ■). This is a self-rating scale that measures levels of depression.

At times your assessment will be focused toward differentiating between depression and grief (see Table 13.5 ■).

Be alert for nonverbal behaviors that may be a clue to depression. These include tearfulness, avoidance of eye contact, flat or blunted affect, and poor hygiene. Ask about a family history of mood disorders or other mental health problems, as well as the client's own history of mood disorders. Assess for concomitant disorders such as anxiety and substance abuse. Be aware that domestic violence or abuse may be a factor in a depressive episode.

Diagnosis

The next step in the nursing process is to analyze and synthesize the assessment data to form nursing diagnoses. You must consider the client's level of mood alteration as well as the behavioral, affective, cognitive, and physiological responses to their disorder. Another consideration is danger to self or others through suicide, homicide, or impulsive behavior. Nursing diagnoses in regard to priority physiological responses include exhaustion and inadequate intake. Consideration must be given to the areas in which the client has the most difficulty functioning such as ADLs, problem solving, and interpersonal relationships.

The Nursing Diagnoses with NOC & NIC feature contains those diagnoses most commonly identified for clients with mood disorders.

Outcome Identification and Goals

Once you have established diagnoses, you select outcomes appropriate to the nursing diagnoses. The most common outcomes are found in the Nursing Diagnoses with NOC & NIC feature.

Once you have established outcomes, you and the client mutually identify goals for change. Client goals are specific behavioral measures by which you, the client, and significant others identify as realistic and attainable. The following are examples of goals that may be pertinent to the client with a mood disorder:

- Remains safe
- Verbalizes decreasing suicidal ideation
- Establishes a routine schedule that balances exercise and quiet time
- Accomplishes ADLs
- Utilizes the problem-solving process
- Makes decisions that reflect good judgment
- Verbalizes logical thought processes
- Socializes with others
- Becomes a self-advocate
- Reports purpose and joy in life and a sense of connectedness to others

Nursing Interventions

Goals and outcome criteria help focus your nursing care. The overall goal is to help clients improve the response to mood disorders and develop effective coping behaviors. See the Nursing Diagnoses with NOC & NIC feature for an overview of interventions.

Safety: Crisis Management
Suicide Prevention

The first priority of care is *client safety*. Since as many as 15 percent of clients with mood disorders commit suicide, it is extremely important that you assess for suicide potential. Chapter 20 gives detailed information on assessment and interventions for clients who are suicidal.

Family members need to be taught the following: People who talk about suicide are at high risk; suicide attempts may follow the loss of an important person, position, or possession; social isolation and substance abuse increase the risk of a suicide attempt; suicide attempts may increase as the depression is beginning to improve, since thought patterns are still negative but the person now has enough energy to make the attempt; and getting one's "life in order" is a high-risk signal.

TABLE 13.4

Beck Depression Inventory

The Beck Depression Inventory is a self-rating scale that measures depression. The patient can complete the questionnaire in about 10 minutes. The total score provides an estimate of the degree of severity of the depressed mood. Add the raw scores. The mean scores can be interpreted as follows.

Total Score	Levels of Depression
1–10	Normal ups and downs
11–16	Mild mood disturbance
17–20	Borderline clinical depression
21–30	Moderate depression
31–40	Severe depression
Over 40	Extreme depression

(A persistent score of 17 or above indicates professional treatment might be necessary)

1. 0 I do not feel sad.
   1 I feel sad.
   2 I am sad all the time and I can't snap out of it.
   3 I am so sad or unhappy that I can't stand it.

2. 0 I am not particularly discouraged about the future.
   1 I feel discouraged about the future.
   2 I feel I have nothing to look forward to.
   3 I feel that the future is hopeless and that things cannot improve.

3. 0 I do not feel like a failure.
   1 I feel I have failed more than the average person.
   2 As I look back on my life, all I can see is a lot of failures.
   3 I feel I am a complete failure as a person.

4. 0 I get as much satisfaction out of things as I used to.
   1 I don't enjoy things the way I used to.
   2 I don't get real satisfaction out of anything anymore.
   3 I am dissatisfied or bored with everything.

5. 0 I don't feel particularly guilty.
   1 I feel guilty a good part of the time.
   2 I feel quite guilty most of the time.
   3 I feel guilty all of the time.

6. 0 I don't feel I am being punished.
   1 I feel I may be punished.
   2 I expect to be punished.
   3 I feel I am being punished.

7. 0 I don't feel disappointed in myself.
   1 I am disappointed in myself.
   2 I am disgusted with myself.
   3 I hate myself.

(continued)

TABLE 13.4

Beck Depression Inventory (continued)

8. 0 I don't feel I am worse than anybody else.
    1 I am critical of myself for any weaknesses or mistakes.
    2 I blame myself all the time for my faults.
    3 I blame myself for everything bad that happens.

9. 0 I don't have any thoughts of killing myself.
    1 I have thoughts of killing myself, but I would not carry them out.
    2 I would like to kill myself.
    3 I would kill myself if I had the chance.

10. 0 I don't cry any more than usual.
    1 I cry more now than usual.
    2 I cry all the time now.
    3 I used to be able to cry, but now I can't even though I want to.

11. 0 I am no more irritated by things than I ever am.
    1 I am slightly more irritated now than usual.
    2 I am quite annoyed or irritated a good deal of the time.
    3 I feel irritated all the time now.

12. 0 I have not lost interest in other people.
    1 I am less interested in other people than I used to be.
    2 I have lost most of any interest in other people.
    3 I have lost all of my interest in other people.

13. 0 I make decisions about as well as I ever could.
    1 I put off making decisions more than I used to.
    2 I have greater difficulty in making decisions than before.
    3 I can't make decisions at all anymore.

14. 0 I don't feel that I look any worse than I used to.
    1 I am worried that I am looking old or unattractive.
    2 I feel that there are permanent changes in my appearance that make me look unattractive.
    3 I believe that I look ugly.

15. 0 I can work about as well as before.
    1 I take an extra effort to get started doing something.
    2 I have to push myself very hard to do anything.
    3 I can't do any work at all.

16. 0 I can sleep as well as usual.
    1 I don't sleep as well as I used to.
    2 I wake up 1–2 hours earlier than I used to and cannot get back to sleep.
    3 I wake up several hours earlier than I used to and cannot get back to sleep.

17. 0 I don't get more tired than usual.
    1 I get tired more easily than I used to.
    2 I get tired from doing almost anything.
    3 I am too tired to do anything.

18. 0 My appetite is no worse than usual.
    1 My appetite is not as good as it used to be.
    2 My appetite is much worse now.
    3 I have no appetite at all anymore.

TABLE 13.4

Beck Depression Inventory (continued)

19. 0 I haven't lost much weight, if any, lately.
    1 I have lost more than 5 pounds.
    2 I have lost more than 10 pounds.
    3 I have lost more than 15 pounds.

20. 0 I am no more worried about my health than usual.
    1 I am worried about physical problems such as aches and pains, or upset stomach, or constipation.
    2 I am very worried about physical problems and it's hard to think of much else.
    3 I am so worried about my physical problems that I cannot think about anything else.

21. 0 I have not noticed any recent change in my interest in sex.
    1 I am less interested in sex than I used to be.
    2 I am much less interested in sex now.
    3 I have lost interest in sex completely.

SOURCE: Beck, A. T., Ward, C. H., Mendelson, M., Mock, J., & Erbaugh, J. (1961). Inventory for measuring depression. *Archives of General Psychiatry, 4,* 561–571.

TABLE 13.5

Differences Between Depression and Grief

Trait	Depression	Grief
Trigger	Specific trigger not necessary	Trigger usually loss or multiple losses
Active/passive	Passive behavior tends to keep them "stuck" in sadness	Actively feel their emotional pain and emptiness
Emotions	Generalized feeling of helplessness, hopelessness	Experience a range of emotions that are usually intense
Ability to laugh	Likely to be humorless and incapable of being happy or even temporarily cheered up; likely to resist support	Sometimes will be able to laugh and enjoy humor; more likely to accept support
Activities	Lack of interest in previously enjoyed activities	Can be persuaded to participate in activities, especially as they begin to heal
Self-esteem	Low self-esteem, low self-confidence; feels like a failure	Self-esteem usually remains intact; does not feel like a failure unless it relates directly to the loss
Feeling of failure	May dwell on past failures; catastrophize	Any self-blame or guilt relates directly to the loss; feelings resolve as they progress toward healing.

Behavior Assessment	Affective Assessment	Cognitive Assessment
How are you managing your work/household/school responsibilities?	How would you describe your overall mood?	What qualities do you like about yourself?
Has there been a change in your activity level?	Do you have mood swings?	What would you like to change about yourself?
Are you having difficulty doing basic activities of daily living?	What kinds of things make you feel guilty?	Give me an example of past success in your life.
What are your leisure activities?	How much time each day do you spend thinking about failure or guilt?	Overall, how would you evaluate your life in the past?
How much exercise are you getting?	How often do you cry?	What are your hopes for the future?
Do you enjoy doing things with other people?	What activities have given you pleasure in the past? In the present?	What does criticism or rejection by others mean to you?
	How have you used food, alcohol, or drugs to increase your pleasure?	Are you having difficulty concentrating?
		Does it seem as though your thoughts come slowly or quickly?
		Do you make decisions easily?

Safety: Risk Management

Hallucination Management

Hallucinations are frightening experiences, and most clients welcome opportunities to discuss them. It is critical that you monitor the hallucinations for content that is self-harmful, suicidal, or violent toward others. Encourage clients to express these feelings appropriately rather than act on the violent messages.

Encourage clients to *validate their perceptions* with people whom they trust, such as yourself or family members. If a client asks you to verify a hallucination, point out that you are not experiencing the same stimuli. Arguments about the validity of the hallucination should be avoided. If hallucinations are interfering with a conversation, try to refocus the client to the topic. If that is unsuccessful, focus the discussion on the underlying feelings, rather than the content of the hallucination. You may say something like: "That sounds like a very frightening experience." Some people find that participation in reality-based activities such as a game or cooking may distract from the hallucination. Others find that music may "drown out" the voices (McCloskey & Bulechek, 1996). Further information on nursing interventions for hallucinations is found in Chapter 9.

Behavioral: Behavioral Therapy

Behavior Management: Overactivity

Clients experiencing a manic episode may become exhausted when excessive levels of activity are combined with decreased awareness of fatigue. When intervening you must first get clients' attention by calling their name or lightly touching the arm. If the environment (a person or a situation) is overstimulating, you may need to redirect or remove the client to a *quieter area* to facilitate self-control. Clients experiencing hypomanic or manic episodes should avoid stimulating places such as bars or busy shopping malls. Limiting intake of caffeinated food and fluids may also facilitate self-control. Clients should establish a routine

Social Assessment

Who lives in your household?

With whom do you communicate most easily?

Who can you depend on in a crisis?

Who can depend on you in a crisis?

What roles and responsibilities do you assume in your family?

How do people seem to be treating you?

What kinds of losses have you sustained during the past year?

Cultural Assessment

What is your ethnic identity?

What is your religious affiliation?

What do you believe is the source of your problems?

What home remedies or alternative therapies have you tried to make yourself better?

Physiological Assessment

How is your appetite?

How much weight have you gained or lost? In what period of time?

Are you having difficulty sleeping?

Do you tire easily or have a high level of energy?

Has your partner commented on a change in your level of sexual desire?

---

schedule that includes a balance of structured time (activities such as work, writing, painting, or crafts) and quiet time and post this in a visible place.

If you are helping clients who are hyperactive to follow a procedure, give instructions or explanations in *simple, concrete language* and ask them to repeat what they heard before beginning the task. Allow clients to carry out one instruction before being given another and provide positive feedback for the completion of each step.

Manic episodes cause some people to become interested in every person and every activity in the environment. Thus, they may be very intrusive in other people's conversations and create socially awkward situations. You or family members need to *set limits* on intrusive or interruptive behaviors. Appropriate social roles and the appropriate expression of feelings need to be taught and reinforced (McCloskey & Bulechek, 1996). See the Complementary/Alternative Therapies feature for teaching clients how to slow down their behavior.

Complementary/Alternative Therapies

How to Help Clients Slow Down Their Behavior

This exercise is designed to decrease hyperactive behavior and induce a sense of peace and calm.

1. Gently close your eyes and focus all your attention on the flow of air as you breathe in and exhale.

2. After three to five breaths, imagine that you are breathing in peace and breathing out tension. Tell yourself that the clean, fresh air that you breathe in through your nose has the power to clear your mind of distracting thoughts. With every exhaled breath, you are releasing stress and tension.

3. Repeat this breathing cycle for 5 to 10 minutes.

NURSING DIAGNOSES with NOC & NIC

Clients with Mood Disorders

DIAGNOSIS	OUTCOMES	INTERVENTIONS
High risk for violence, self-directed related to a sense of hopelessness or to poor impulse control	**Suicide Self-Restraint:** Ability to refrain from gestures and attempts at killing self	Suicide Prevention
High risk for violence, directed at others related to unrealistic thoughts of being inadequate as a parent, delusions, or command hallucinations	**Impulse Control:** Self-restraint of compulsive or impulsive behavior	Impulse Control Training
Impaired verbal communication related to fragmented thought, flight of ideas, or slowed thought processes	**Communication Ability:** Ability to receive, interpret, and express spoken, written, and nonverbal messages	Active Listening
Decisional conflict related to inability to utilize the problem-solving process	**Decision Making:** Ability to choose between one or more alternatives	Coping Enhancement
Deficit in diversional activity related to lack of interest in any activities, inability to focus on an activity	**Depression Control:** Personal actions to minimize melancholy and maintain interest in life events	Socialization Enhancement Recreational Therapy Exercise Promotion Constipation Management
Altered thought process related to delusions, hallucinations, or cognitive distortions	**Distorted Thought Control:** Self-restraint of disruption in perception, thought processes, and thought content	Hallucination Management Cognitive Restructuring

Behavior Management: Sexual

Adult clients who are depressed often experience a diminished interest in sex. You should introduce the topic of sexuality with the client and partner, to enable them to share concerns. Ascertain what, if any, problems existed prior to the depression. *Teaching* includes explaining that sexual desire usually returns as the depression recedes. Understanding that lack of desire is a symptom of depression will decrease feelings of hurt, inadequacy, and guilt. Stress the importance of nonsexual expressions of affection, such as hugging and holding each other, as reassuring forms of communication.

DIAGNOSIS	OUTCOMES	INTERVENTIONS
Self-esteem disturbance related to inability to evaluate self objectively, catastrophizing, or grandiose beliefs about physical and intellectual characteristics	*Self-Esteem*: Personal judgment of self-worth	Guilt Work Self-Esteem Enhancement
Spiritual distress related to lack of connection with others, hopeless view of the future, and no sense of purpose in life	*Spiritual Well-Being*: Personal expressions of connectedness with self, others, higher power, all life, nature, and the universe that transcend and empower the self	Spiritual Support
Caregiver role strain related to stigma, frustration, and increased conflict	*Caregiver Well-Being*: Primary care provider's satisfaction with health and life circumstances	Caregiver Support Family Mobilization Family Therapy
Altered sexuality patterns related to no desire for sex or to sexually acting-out behavior	*Well-Being*: An individual's expressed satisfaction with health status	Behavioral Management: Sexual
Knowledge deficit related to disease process, treatment options, medications	*Knowledge*: Extent of understanding conveyed about a specific disease process	Teaching: Disease Process
Sleep pattern disturbance related to insomnia or hyperactivity	*Sleep*: Extent and pattern of natural periodic suspension of consciousness	Sleep Enhancement

SOURCES: Johnson, M., Maas, M., & Moorhead, S. (2000). *Nursing outcomes classification (NOC)* (2nd ed.). St. Louis, MO: Mosby; McCloskey, J. C., & Bulechek, G. M. (1996). *Nursing interventions classification (NIC)* (2nd ed.). St. Louis, MO: Mosby; and North American Nursing Diagnosis Association (1999). *Nursing diagnoses, definitions and classification 1999–2000*. Philadelphia: Author

If the lack of desire continues after the depression has lifted, suggest that the couple consider sex therapy.

Clients in a manic episode often exhibit an impulsive increase in their sexual activity. Family members must understand that such behavior is a symptom of the manic state, is not within the client's control, and is not an indication of a change in ethics and values. As much as possible, the client should be protected from sexual acting out until he or she is able to assume control over this behavior.

Complementary/Alternative Therapies

How to Help Clients Moderate Their Level of Depression

This exercise is designed to empower yourself with your thoughts by transforming negative thoughts and events through imagery. Do this every day prior to bedtime.

1. Mentally go through your day and decide what you could have changed that would have brought better results.

2. Imagine that change occurring. For example, if you didn't enjoy lunch with your friends, imagine that you had a good time at lunch. If you are unhappy about something you said to a loved one, imagine saying something more caring.

3. As you progress in this exercise, pay attention to how your thoughts, feelings, and behaviors are becoming more positive and less depressing.

Behavioral: Cognitive Therapy
Cognitive Restructuring

Assess clients for altered thought processes such as overgeneralization, dichotomous thinking, catastrophizing, or personalization. Help them *identify negative self-statements* by asking questions such as: "What do you say about yourself? Is that true? Have these thoughts increased with your depression?" This helps clients understand that negative thinking is part of the disorder and not necessarily fact. Point out examples of dysfunctional thinking as it occurs. Remind clients and families that depression is neither related to personal failure nor a sign of inferiority. See the Complementary/Alternative Therapies feature for teaching clients how to moderate their level of depression.

It is not unusual for people with bipolar disorder to deny the disorder and the need for treatment. Frequently this occurs at the onset but may recur throughout the course of the disorder. When treatment is initiated and they start to feel better, clients may again deny the illness and the need for medication.

Clients working toward self-management typically go through several cognitive phases. The *first phase* is the realization of a need. In other words, individuals must accept that they have a disorder in order to be motivated to seek information. *Phase two* is the process of seeking information. You may need to alert clients and families to reliable resources so they can obtain the information they desire. The *third phase* has been identified as being a critical juncture in treatment. The information they receive must be perceived as being applicable to themselves. If clients are to move on to self-management, they must also have the energy and the will to succeed in self-care. *Phase four* is the process of self-management. In this advanced phase, clients select useful self-management strategies, including problem-solving skills, and learn how to deal with and overcome barriers to self-management.

Behavioral: Communication Enhancement
Active Listening

People with mood disorders experience either slowed or racing thought processes, both of which result in problems with communication. You can assist these clients through active listening. To do this you must clear your mind of preoccupying personal concerns, eliminate environmental distractions, and focus completely on the interaction. *Listen* for clients' unexpressed messages and feelings as well as the overt content of the conversation. You must *clarify* the message through use of questions and feedback and finally verify your understanding of what was communicated.

People who are depressed may be unaware of your presence or interest if you are not easily visible. Therefore, it is important that you sit in a position that is in the client's direct line of vision. To decrease fragmentation of thought processes, introduce only *one topic or question* at a time. Since their thought processes are slowed down, give clients plenty of time to respond verbally. Jumping in and answering for clients gives the message that you view them as incapable and is a blow to their self-esteem. Assure clients that you will remain for a specific period of time even if they choose not to talk. Your acceptance of clients should not be dependent on their ability to communicate. If verbalization is difficult, suggest activities such as taking a 10-minute walk, looking at a magazine together, or doing a simple occupational therapy project.

People in the manic phase of bipolar disorder often experience flight of ideas. Since flight of ideas is partially in response to multiple stimuli in the environment, you should *decrease environmental stimuli* by suggesting that the two of you go to a quieter area. If you cannot follow what is being said, say you are having difficulty such as, "Your thoughts are coming too quickly for me to follow what you are trying to say." Ask the person to try to slow down the communication in an effort to help organize their thinking. You might say, "Let's talk about one thought at a time" or "Let's stay with this idea for a minute." Try to *identify the theme* of the client's flight of ideas to increase your comprehension of what the client is attempting to communicate. In order to promote successful communication, you should provide clients the opportunity to validate or correct your perception. You might say, "You seem to be mentioning your mother often. Are you having some concerns about her?"

Socialization Enhancement

People who are depressed often experience a decreased desire to interact with others, which results in social isolation. However, the more alone and isolated people are, the more depressed they feel. When people connect to and interact with others, they feel less lonely and their mood often begins to lift. In severe depression it may be necessary for either you or one family member to *participate* with the person in solitary activities in the beginning. As the mood lifts, more people and more activities may be planned into the day. Encourage clients and families to identify the benefits of social interaction, as this reinforces the positive change in behavior.

Peer counseling may be another activity to enhance clients' socialization. Peer counseling is a free, safe, and effective self-help tool that encourages expression of feelings. It puts clients in control of their own healing process. In a peer counseling session, two people agree to spend a certain amount of time together, dividing the time equally, paying attention to each other's issues, needs, and distresses. Judging, criticizing, and giving advice are not allowed.

Behavioral: Coping Assistance

Coping Enhancement

Nurses can enhance coping by teaching clients to utilize the *problem-solving process*. This process is presented in more detail in Chapter 2. Initially, you must evaluate clients' abilities to problem-solve while discouraging decision making under situations of severe stress or during the acute phase of a mood disorder. In this phase it is appropriate to give limited choices until their deci-

sion-making ability is improved. You might say something like, "Would you like to take your shower before or after breakfast?" To increase self-confidence and self-esteem, allow as much control in situations as clients are able to manage effectively. When clients talk about being overwhelmed by all the decisions that have to be made, have them narrow the focus to one decision at a time to decrease feelings of helplessness.

Together, you, clients, and families can *explore previous methods* of dealing with life problems and the success or failure of those past attempts. Next, help them identify appropriate short- and long-term *goals* while ensuring that these are broken down into small, manageable steps (outcomes). Clients and families next *choose* which *strategies* they wish to implement to solve the problem. Following the actual implementation, they *evaluate* the process on the basis of how well their outcomes were achieved and how close they have come to meeting their goals. The mere process of working on the problem, analyzing the options, and actively selecting a course of action provides clients with a sense of control, which counteracts their feelings of helplessness and powerlessness.

Other activities to encourage coping include exploring clients' previous achievements of success, encouraging clients to *identify their own strengths* and abilities, and facilitating the evaluation of their own behavior. You can help them problem-solve situations in which they can become more autonomous, especially through vocational, social, and community activities.

Many people with mood disorders feel they have lost control over their own lives, rights, and responsibilities, and have lost the ability and right to effectively advocate for themselves. Nursing activities designed to help clients *advocate for themselves* give them hope and self-esteem. The following steps are a guide to assisting clients in this process:

- Encourage them to believe in themselves.
- Inform them of their rights.
- Help them clarify what they need and want by setting clear goals.
- Provide them with accurate information, preferably in writing.
- Help them strategize by using the problem-solving process.
- Facilitate their identification of resources such as

friends, family, self-help groups, and advocacy organizations.

- Encourage them to identify the best person(s) to assist them with this problem.

- Foster effective communication so they can get their message across by suggestions such as: Be brief, stick to the point, don't get diverted, and state your concern and how you want things changed.

- Promote firmness and persistence so they can get what they need for themselves.

Another activity to enhance clients' coping abilities is through the development of *advance directives*. While not legally binding in all states, these plans assist families and caregivers who must make decisions for clients when they are unable to make them for themselves. Advance directives are initiated by the client, formulated between acute episodes, and include:

- Symptoms that indicate the person is not able to make decisions at this time

- The names and phone numbers of at least three people, including health care professionals, and family members who should make decisions in their behalf

- A listing of medications, other treatments, and treatment facilities—ranked as preferred, acceptable, and unacceptable—including reasons

Clients are encouraged to develop their own mental health file containing information about their diagnoses, medications, self-help strategies, and resources. The advance directives should be kept in this file and a copy should be given to each specific supporter or health care professional.

Guilt Work Facilitation

In the midst of a severe depression, many people experience feelings of guilt, often more perceived than real. You can help clients identify and express their painful feelings of guilt and explore the situations in which these feelings are experienced. Encourage them to identify how they behaved in those situations. Following these discussions, you can use *reality testing* to help clients identify possible irrational beliefs. Global statements about guilt and inadequacy contribute to low self-esteem. More realistic evaluation will help correct cognitive distortions.

Impulse Control Training

Cognitive disruptions for clients in the manic phase of bipolar disorder often result in impulsive behavior, which may or may not be dangerous to themselves or others. There are a number of actions you can take to assist clients in *impulse control training*. You want to help clients identify situations that require thoughtful action and then teach them to cue themselves to "stop and think" before acting impulsively. In addition, they should identify other courses of action and the potential benefits of each course of action. An example might be impulse buying. Clients may decide that every time they take out their wallet, they must "stop and think" if they really need the item they are about to purchase. They might choose to leave their credit cards and checkbooks at home as well. If absolutely necessary, they may elect to have another person control access to credit cards, checkbooks, ATMs, and cash disbursements. The benefits from these decisions are financial stability and self-management.

Mood Management

It is easier to help clients manage mood instability before the episode has cycled into a severe depression or a manic phase. The development and maintenance of an *early warning signs chart* facilitates this process by helping clients and families identify symptoms that indicate the beginning of a relapse. For example, many people report that fatigue, isolating behaviors, and indecision are early warning signs of depression. Insomnia, racing thoughts, and rapid speech may be signs of mania. Each evening before bedtime, clients can review the chart to see if any of these warning signs have appeared during the day. If they have, or if they recur for several days, they may need to take a preplanned action to alleviate the symptoms.

Recreation Therapy

People who are depressed often say they have no energy or motivation to participate in social activities, and they often forget to do the things they enjoy that make them feel better. In contrast, people experiencing a manic episode are interested in every activity, whether appropriate or not. Nursing activities include assisting clients to choose *recreational activities* that are consistent with their physical, emotional, and social capabilities. For clients in the acute phase of a mood disorder, it is most helpful to keep activities simple and short, thus ensuring success and boosting self-esteem. You will want to avoid activities requiring intense concentration since their attention span is insufficient for success. Clients with manic behavior will manage better with nonstimulating activities, thereby avoiding the escalation of their mood by competition or sensory stimulation.

In the nonacute phase of mood disorders, clients find it helpful to make a list of things they enjoy doing, which becomes an easy reference when they are having a harder time. The list might include going for a walk, listening to music, working in the garden, watching funny videos, or visiting with friends. Part of self-management is making the time to include one or more of these activities in a regular schedule.

Self-Esteem Enhancement

People suffering from depression often experience self-esteem disturbances related to criticism and negative self-evaluation. One nursing activity that may be helpful is *setting limits* on the amount of time clients spend discussing past failures, since rumination intensifies guilt and low self-esteem. Help clients identify the significance of culture, religion, race, gender, and age on self-esteem. Based on this, assist them in setting realistic goals to achieve higher self-esteem. From there you can move on to encouraging review of past achievements and present successes. Designing *positive self-statements* and repeating these aloud several times a day increases feelings of self-esteem. Determine clients' locus of control and encourage behaviors that foster an internal locus of control. Help them develop confidence in their own judgment by *conveying your confidence* in their ability to handle various situations and by helping them acknowledge positive responses from others.

Clients in manic episodes often experience grandiose views of themselves. Do not argue about their delusions, as that would place them in the position of having to defend their belief. If they are excessively preoccupied, *set limits* on the amount of time they can discuss their beliefs, such as, "We will talk about how good you feel about yourself for 5 minutes and then we will talk about something else for 15 minutes."

Spiritual Support

In the midst of depression, many people experience spiritual distress related to a lack of purpose or joy in life and feeling disconnected with others. Be open to their expressions of loneliness and powerlessness. Review their past joys and successes in life and help them identify "small" purposes of current life such as contributions to their family, value to friends, and goals for next month. Help them identify possible new functions or purposes in life to counteract the depressed feelings. Review with them the availability of supportive people, as those people will increase their sense of connectedness to others. For clients who are religious, use *spiritual resources* to decrease distress. Facilitate their use of meditations, prayer, and other religious traditions and rituals. For many people religious beliefs improve self-esteem, life satisfaction, and the ability to cope.

Behavioral: Patient Education

Teaching: Disease Process

People who are self-managers say that it is absolutely essential to learn everything they can about their particular diagnosis and possible treatment strategies. Education is part of taking responsibility for wellness and facilitates appropriate decision making. This educational process must be continuous to keep clients and families up-to-date with the latest findings about their disorder. Clients should be informed of the treatments available and how to evaluate potential benefits and risks when deciding on a particular treatment. More detailed information on client and family teaching is found in Chapter 2.

Some individuals may reject the information you provide. One reason may be that they believe that they know all about their disorder and have no need to learn anything else. Others may reject information because they are in total denial of having a disorder. Barriers to learning must be identified and managed if your teaching is to be effective.

Family: Life Span Care

Caregiver Support

Mood disorders affect not only the client but also family and friends. During acute episodes, clients may be very dependent and needy or may need firm direction and limit setting. You must consider all significant others to be recipients of your care. Help these caregivers acknowledge the client's dependency issues and assume appropriate responsibility. Managing depressed older clients at home may require outside services for a period of time. Be alert for family interaction problems related to the care of the client. Provide information about the client's condition in accordance with client preferences, remembering the issue of confidentiality. Inform caregivers of community resources and encourage them to participate in support groups. See the Community Resources and Books for Clients and Families features at the end of this chapter.

Family Mobilization

Family mobilization includes education, communication skills training, and problem-solving skills training. In mobilizing the family, you apply the same principles that you use with clients. Assess how the family's behavior affects the client and how the client's behavior affects the family. Discuss how family strengths and resources can be used to enhance the health status of the client and the family's ability to cope. Collaborate with families and clients in planning and implementing lifestyle changes.

Teach families and clients how to identify early signs and symptoms of manic or depressive episodes. Such identification can help ensure that treatment is begun as early as possible in the course of a relapse. Relapse prevention and early recognition are important concepts in self-management.

Family Therapy

When caring for families, observe interactional behaviors and verbal communications to assess for functional or dysfunctional patterns of behavior. For example, you might look for messages to children that they are bad or deficient, or that the world is a hostile place. Repeated messages such as "You're not good," "I wish you had never been born," and "This is an unfair world—I hate it" contribute to a negative and distorted way of viewing oneself and the world. Help the family determine areas of dissatisfaction and/or conflict and see whether they want to resolve these issues. The goal is to help family members identify and change behaviors that maintain depression and dependency within the family system. Because family therapy is a specialized area of nursing practice and requires additional education, you should collaborate closely with colleagues who possess advanced practice skills.

Physiological: Basic: Activity and Exercise Management

Exercise Promotion

Exercise is the least expensive and most available antidepressant. It is nature's way of increasing neurotransmitters and endorphins, thus decreasing feelings of sadness and tension. A daily walk or some other kind of enjoyable exercise makes most people feel better.

Teach clients to begin slowly and increase the intensity and length of the exercise gradually. Have them keep a record of their physical activities as a way to monitor their own behavior. Clients who are depressed may tell you that they will exercise when they feel better. Teach them that, in contrast, they will feel better when they exercise. Finding an "exercise buddy" may facilitate this aspect of self-management. Since cognitive distortions of dichotomous thinking or overgeneralization may sabotage an exercise plan, help clients set small realistic exercise goals. Encourage them to keep a 1 to 10 rating of mood before and after exercise, which will help them focus on the effectiveness of the program.

Physiological: Basic: Elimination Management

Constipation Management

You may need to institute measures to relieve constipation, which may result from decreased activity, reduced intake, side effects of antidepressant medications, or ignoring bodily signals. Baseline data are established by reviewing clients' normal patterns of bowel activity and having them keep a record of current patterns. In addition to exercise, nutritional measures such as increased fiber in the diet and adequate fluid intake are helpful.

Physiological: Basic: Nutritional Support

Nutritional Management

Clients with mood disorders may have inadequate nutrition related to anorexia or hyperactivity. Instead of three main meals a day, encourage them to eat *six small meals* which will increase gastric motility and decrease the sensations of bloating. If clients are living with others, encourage social interaction at meal times to increase the perception of eating as a pleasurable experience. Hyperactive clients will benefit from a quiet meal time environment since there would be fewer distractions. Hyperactive clients often prefer high calorie foods that can be eaten while walking or

CRITICAL THINKING

Mr. Gillepski has been admitted to the psychiatric acute care unit. His admitting diagnosis is major depression. His wife brought him to the emergency room after he threatened to shoot himself with his gun. He was admitted for observation and to obtain a better assessment of his problems. You have been assigned to him and are meeting him for the admission assessment. You know from the emergency room record that he has experienced one other episode of depression last year, and although he received no treatment, he seemed to improve. This information came from his wife.

You meet with Mr. Gillepski, and you note that he does not greet you and remains in his chair, barely looking up at you. He responds to all of your questions with short answers, and some questions he does not answer. At one point he comments, "I feel sad and not able to do anything. Nothing seems worthwhile. Not even my wife and she is important to me." He does say he cannot get work done and cannot make decisions. He will say little about past depression or what happened when he improved. He does not seem to concentrate for long on any of the topics during the assessment. When asked about family history of psychiatric illness, he tells you that his father had depression, and he remembers several family members who had "spells of being out of control."

You then meet with his wife when Mr. Gillepski is meeting with the psychiatrist. His wife tells you that she has been worried about her husband for two years. His behavior has been "erratic." You ask her to give you some examples of this behavior. "My husband has been an active and fun person most of his life. Two years ago, he seemed sort of out of control and very busy. He talked much more than usual, had trouble sleeping, and wanted to be very active socially. At times, especially when I would question him about his behavior, he would get very irritable. After a time,

he seemed to slow down and be more like himself. He then had this first episode of depression, at least I thought it was depression. He slept more and had limited energy. He told me he felt hopeless and not good. It was different for him. This lasted for a few months, and then he got better and was back to his old self, maybe a little too happy, but it was better than that depression." You ask her how she is feeling about all of this. "I am so confused and feel torn. Exhausted. Sometimes not knowing what husband I am going to confront, the depressed one or the one who wants to have a good time. Does this make sense to you?"

1. Based on the data that you now have, what alternative diagnosis might be considered for Mr. Gillepski? Compare and contrast the major issues of the alternative diagnosis with the diagnosis of major depression, his admitting diagnosis.

2. What additional assessment data would be important to obtain to support the alternative diagnosis?

3. Since the staff are trying to determine if Mr. Gillepski has depression or bipolar disorder, you need to think about issues related to both of these diagnoses. Compare and contrast the following in depression and bipolar disorder: self-esteem and grandiose beliefs and decision making.

4. Is genetics important in this case, and if so, how would it apply to Mr. Gillepski?

5. If Mr. Gillepski began to exhibit some of the symptoms of mania, such as overactivity and difficulty thinking and communicating, what nursing management would you need to consider?

6. How might you assist Mr. Gillepski with coping enhancement during depression?

For an additional Case Study, please refer to the Companion Web site for this book.

---

moving about. Intake must be sufficient to provide energy for their high activity level.

Dietary modifications are being explored as an adjunct to more traditional interventions. The neurotransmitters that are implicated in the neurobiology of mood disorders are synthesized from dietary proteins. Specific protein intake might be increased, depending on which neurotransmitter is depleted. Tryptophan is

the precursor of 5-HT and niacin. If the body has more than enough niacin, tryptophan will be forced to choose the 5-HT pathway. Vitamin B_6 might be depleted by the use of antidepressants, birth control pills, and antihypertensive agents. By increasing tryptophan in the diet as well as adding niacin and vitamin B_6, the 5-HT levels are increased. If the mood disorder involves decreased levels of NE or DA, the diet is increased in tyrosine. Choline is increased in the diet when higher levels of ACh are desired. This evolving field of *dietary pharmacology* will become more important as neurobiology continues to be explored.

Physiological: Basic: Self-Care Facilitation

Sleep Enhancement

Another nursing intervention is helping clients reestablish normal sleep patterns. People who are depressed or in a manic episode, experience insomnia and frequent awakening. Ask clients what measures to improve sleeping have been successful in the past and help them find ways to adjust the environment of their bedroom to promote sleep. Implementing natural sedative measures may improve sleeping patterns. These methods include increased physical activity during the day but not right before bedtime, decreased amount of daytime napping, relaxation techniques,

---

CLINICAL INTERACTIONS   A Client with Bipolar Disorder

Ken, age 36, has been in a partial hospitalization program for the past two months. Both of his parents are deceased, and his two siblings are uninvolved with him. His mood ranges from euphoria to irritability. He believes he is very handsome, intelligent, and superior to other people. He is often preoccupied with sexual topics. The nurse is meeting Ken for the first time. In the interaction, you will see evidence of:

- Ken's grandiose beliefs about himself
- His flight of ideas
- His labile moods

KEN: You would like to talk and help me?

NURSE: I would like to get to know you first.

KEN: You will find me really interesting. I am rich.

NURSE: I would like to know a little bit about who you are, Ken.

KEN: I was a chosen child.

NURSE: Can you help me understand what that means, to be a chosen child?

KEN: I was my parents' favorite child and they treated me special.

NURSE: What does "special" mean to you?

KEN: Love would come from my mother to me. Jesus is the love child. Did you know that?

NURSE: Ken, let's concentrate on you and your family. You were telling me that your mother loved you very much.

KEN: Yes, she showed me how to love, but she died and left me. She went away. My father died later when I was 26.

NURSE: How did your parents' deaths affect you?

KEN: I like women. There is no room for homosexuals. I'm a heterosexual.

NURSE: Ken, let's concentrate on the topic of you and your parents. How did you feel when your parents died?

KEN: My father was a big man.

NURSE: Your father was a strong figure to you?

KEN: Big man. He would slap my mother. [Acts out how his father would slap his mother; seems to be getting angry and aggressive]

NURSE: Ken, did that anger you when your father hit your mother? Can you tell me about those times?

KEN: My father would slap my mother and hit me here. [Jumps up and points to his backside and legs]

NURSE: That must have been painful. How did you feel when that happened?

KEN: He had to show me the way. Like God the Father.

NURSE: Ken, let's continue on with your childhood father.

KEN: I signed up for the army and went to Vietnam. I killed the evil people. [Angry tone and then starts laughing]

NURSE: You sound angry about having killed but yet you laugh.

KEN: I had to kill those liars. My brother and sister were jealous.

NURSE: Ken, I don't understand. Slow down. Let's talk about the jealousy.

KEN: I was chosen. My mother loved me [loudly]. I came home with shell shock. I have a tattoo on my nose and a fracture on my skull. I'm tired of talking. I'll see you later.

avoidance of caffeine, and a warm bath or a warm drink just before bed. When clients are unable to sleep, encourage them to get out of bed to read or watch television. Since nighttime often increases feelings of hopelessness, clients tend to spend sleepless periods ruminating over problems. Redirection to other activities minimizes concentrating on negative thoughts.

Evaluation

To complete the nursing process, you evaluate clients' responses to nursing interventions based on the outcomes you selected. You determine the appropriate intervals for measurement and document the condition of clients according to each individual's status. Johnson, Maas, and Moorhead (2000) is the resource for identifying measurement scales and specific indicators for each outcome.

Suicide Self-Restraint

Individuals who are suicidal develop a list of reasons to live or die and goals they hope to achieve with suicide. They develop a list of alternative solutions to their problems. They discuss their beliefs regarding death and the impact of suicide on family members. They participate in developing and maintaining a no-suicide contract. They formulate a written list of support systems and community resources. Clients remain safe.

Impulse Control

Clients identify situations that require thoughtful action and stop and think before acting impulsively. They plan alternative behaviors before particular situations arise. There is a decrease in the episodes of sexual acting-out behaviors.

Communication Ability

The incidence of flight of ideas decreases, and people in a manic state are increasingly able to communicate their feelings and thoughts. As depressive episodes lift, people have improved flow of thought and are thus able to communicate more clearly.

Decision Making

Individuals and families identify past successful methods of dealing with life problems. They formulate goals and strategies to solve current problems. Evaluation of their progress is based on how well they achieved their outcomes and goals. They verbalize an internal locus of control and a sense of empowerment.

Depression Control

Clients who experience recurring mood disorders develop a chart listing behaviors that indicate impending relapse. They implement preplanned actions to alleviate the symptoms.

Distorted Thought Control

Individuals identify cognitive distortions that are symptoms of mood disorders. They distinguish between recurring negative or grandiose thinking and reality-based thinking.

Self-Esteem

Clients with mood disorders choose leisure activities that are consistent with their physical, emotional, and social capabilities. They develop a list of pleasurable activities to which they can refer when necessary. Individuals verbalize previous achievements of success and identify their own strengths and abilities. They discuss situations in which they are more autonomous using vocational, social, and community resources. Individuals function as self-advocates and, with persistence, get what they need for themselves.

Spiritual Well-Being

Individuals with adequate spiritual well-being express a sense of hope and of meaning and purpose in life. They participate in spiritual experiences such as meditation, prayer, worship, song, and/or spiritual reading. They express feelings of serenity and a connectedness with others.*

Caregiver Well-Being

Family members acknowledge clients' dependency issues during acute episodes and assume appropriate responsibility. If relevant, they utilize respite services to maintain their own sense of well-being. They participate in self-help groups within the community.

Well-Being

In the time between acute episodes, clients develop advance directives to guide those who must make deci-

---

*These selected outcome indicators are from Johnson, M., Maas, M., & Moorhead, S. (2000). *Nursing outcomes classification (NOC)* (2nd ed.). St. Louis, MO: Mosby.

sions when they are unable to make them for themselves.

Knowledge of the Disease Process

Individuals and families acknowledge the reality of mood disorders. They seek and act on information obtained from reliable sources. Clients manage their disorder by identifying barriers to self-management and problem-solving solutions to these barriers. They develop their own mental health file with information about their diagnoses, medications, self-help strategies, and resources.

Sleep

Based on past experience and experimentation, clients identify natural sedative measures that improve sleeping patterns. Incidents of insomnia and frequent awakenings decrease.

To build a Care Plan for a client with a mood disorder, go to the Companion Web site for this book.

CHAPTER REVIEW

COMMUNITY RESOURCES

Links to these Web sites can be accessed on the Companion Web site for this book.

Bipolar Disorder Information Center
www.mhsource.com/bipolar

Depression After Delivery
91 E. Summerset St.
Raritan, NJ 08869
800-944-4773
www.depressionafterdelivery.com

National Depressive and Manic Depressive Association
730 North Franklin, Suite 501
Chicago, IL 60610
312-642-0049
www.ndmda.org

National Foundation for Depressive Illness
P.O. Box 2257
New York, NY 10116
800-239-1265
www.depression.org

National Organization for Seasonal Affective
   Disorder (NOSAD)
P.O. Box 40133
Washington, DC 20016
www.nami.org/helpline/sad

Postpartum Support International
927 North Kellogg Ave.
Santa Barbara, CA 93111
805-967-7636
www.postpartum.net

BOOKS FOR CLIENTS AND FAMILIES

Berger, D., & Berger, L. (1991). *We heard the angels of madness: A family guide to coping with manic depression.* New York: William Morrow.

Court, B. L., & Nelson, G. E. (1996). *Bipolar puzzle solution:*

A mental health client's perspective. Washington, DC: Taylor & Francis.

Davidson, J. R. T., & Connor, K. M. (2000). *Herbs for the mind.* New York: Guilford Press.

BOOKS FOR CLIENTS AND FAMILIES *(continued)*

Emery, G. (2000). *Overcoming depression: Client manual.* Oakland, CA: New Harbinger.

Fawcett, J., Golden, B., & Rosenfeld, N. (2000). *New hope for people with bipolar disorder.* Roseville, CA: Prima Health.

Halebsky, M. A. (1997). *Surviving the crisis of depression and bipolar illness: Layperson's guide to coping with mental illness beyond the time of crisis.* New York: Personal and Professional Growth.

Steel, D. (1998). *His bright light: The story of Nick Traina.* New York: Delacorte Press.

KEY CONCEPTS

Introduction

- The mood disorders are major depression (unipolar disorder), dysthymic disorder, bipolar disorder, cyclothymic disorder, and schizoaffective disorder.

- Affect is the verbal and nonverbal expression of one's internal feelings or mood. Descriptors are appropriate versus inappropriate, stable versus labile, elevated versus depressed, and overreactive versus blunted or flat.

- Postpartum mood changes range along a continuum from postpartum blues to postpartum depression to postpartum psychosis.

Knowledge Base

- People who are depressed withdraw from activities and other people; experience feelings of despair, guilt, loss of gratification, and loss of emotional attachments; and suffer from self-depreciation, negative expectations, cognitive distortions, and self-criticism. They also have difficulty making decisions and experience a retarded flow of thought.

- People who are in a manic phase engage in any available activity, are effusive in interactions with others, and form intense emotional attachments quickly. They experience feelings of euphoria but may become suddenly irritable. Thoughts focus on grandiose expectations for themselves, exaggerated accomplishments, and a positively distorted body image. Distractibility and flight of ideas interfere with decision making.

- Mood disorders may be accompanied by psychotic symptoms such as hallucinations and delusions.

- Families may be oversolicitous or may become frustrated when a family member is unable to change affect, behavior, or cognition. If the person is hostile and destructive, police may be called upon to intervene.

- The sex life of couples is often disrupted by mood disorders. People who are depressed have little interest in sex, and people who are manic are obsessed with sex.

- Appropriate expressions of mood are largely culturally determined.

- Throughout the world, most cases of depression are experienced and expressed in somatic terms.

- Symptoms of depression in children and adolescents reflect developmental stages.

- Bipolar disorder in young people is frequently misdiagnosed as ADHD, conduct disorder, or schizophrenia.

- Although depression is common, it may not be recognized in older adults and may be confused with dementia.

- Older adults with chronic medical problems may develop a secondary depression.

- Physiologically, people who are depressed experience loss of appetite, insomnia, decreased mobility, and constipation, while people in the manic phase experience hyperinsomnia, hyperactivity, and may not take the time to eat.

- Concomitant disorders include anxiety disorders and substance-related disorders.

- The inheritability of major depression is 40 to 50 percent and is 70 percent for bipolar disorder. The mix of multiple genes determines differences such as age of onset, symptoms, severity, and course of the mood disorders.

- In the mood disorders, there is a change in the amount of neurotransmitters or a change in the sensitivity of the receptors, thus altering the transmission of electrical impulses.

- The mood disorders may involve a desynchronization of circadian rhythm in some people.

- Seasonal affective disorder (SAD) is cyclic and related to the amount of available sunlight.

- Depression may be secondary to prescribed medications, metabolic disorders, and neurological disruptions.

- Repressed hostility, losses, unachieved goals, learned helplessness, and cognitive distortions contribute to mood disorders.

- Racism, classism, sexism, ageism, and homophobia contribute to depression by increasing feelings of powerlessness, hopelessness, and low self-esteem.

- People experiencing multiple significant life events along with minimal support networks and maladaptive coping patterns are at higher risk for developing a depressive disorder.

- Rigid expectations about gender roles and being isolated within the home may contribute to higher rates of depression among women. Role changes and losses may contribute to higher rates of depression among older adults.

- Antidepressants, mood stabilizers, antipsychotics, electroconvulsive therapy (ECT), sleep deprivation, and phototherapy may be used in the treatment of mood disorders.

- Alternative therapies include transcranial magnetic stimulation, vagus nerve stimulation, exercise, St. John's Wort, SAMe, vitamin B_{12}, tyrosine, melatonin, DHEA, omega-3 fatty acids, and aromatherapy.

The Nursing Process

Assessment

- Nursing assessment must often be conducted in segments of 15 to 20 minutes for clients who have little energy or for those who are hyperactive.

Diagnosis

- Some clients are a danger to themselves or others; therefore, High risk for violence is a priority nursing diagnosis. Other diagnoses include Impaired verbal communication, Decisional conflict, Deficit in diversional activity, Fatigue, Constipation, Altered thought processes, Self-esteem disturbance, Spiritual distress, Caregiver role strain, Altered sexuality patterns, Knowledge deficit, and Sleep pattern disturbance.

Nursing Interventions

- The first priority of care is client safety. Safety concerns include monitoring for suicide potential and management of hallucinations.

- Behavioral interventions include prevention of physical exhaustion, decreasing environmental stimuli, simple explanations, limit setting with intrusive behavior, and protection from impulsive sexual behavior.

- Cognitive interventions include helping clients identify negative self-statements and distorted thought processes.

- There are four phases for clients working toward self-management: realization of a need, seeking information, energy and will to move on the information; and the selection of useful self-management strategies.

- Assisting clients through the process of active listening means that you listen for unexpressed messages and feelings and validate your understanding with the client.

- When interacting with people who are depressed, introduce only one topic at a time, allow plenty of time for response, and provide other interactions if they are unable to converse.

- Decreasing environmental stimuli, identifying themes, and focusing on one topic at a time are helpful for clients who are experiencing flight of ideas.

- Help clients and families identify the benefits of social interaction.

- Peer counseling may enhance clients' socialization levels.

- Problem solving is a key nursing intervention. The mere process of working on the problem, analyzing the options, and actively selecting a course of action provides clients with a sense of control which counteracts their feelings of helplessness and powerlessness.

- Nursing activities should be designed to help clients advocate for themselves as a way of improving self-esteem and providing hope.

- Advanced directives, initiated by clients, helps families and caregivers make decision for clients when they are unable to make them for themselves.

- Use reality testing to help clients identify irrational beliefs regarding their sense of guilt.

- Impulse control training includes stop and think, identifying other options, discussing the potential benefits of options, and decision making process.

- Clients and families need to recognize the early warning signs of relapse so they can take preplanned action to alleviate the symptoms.

- Help clients choose recreational activities that are consistent with their capabilities. In the acute phase, keep activities short and simple.

- Set limits on the amount of time clients talk about their failures or their grandiose beliefs. Teach positive affirmations as a way to counteract negative self-talk.

- Help clients identify purpose in life, value to friends, short-term goals, and availability of supportive people. Use spiritual resources to decrease distress.

- For clients to become self-managers, it is essential they learn everything they can about their diagnosis and treatment strategies. Families must be included in this educational process.

- Provide information to the family about the client's condition in accordance with client preferences, remembering the issue of confidentiality.

- Discuss with the family how their strengths and resources can be used to enhance the health status of the client and the family's ability to cope.

- One goal of family intervention is to help family members identify and change behaviors that maintain depression and dependency within the family system.

- Exercise is a natural way to increase neurotransmitters and endorphins, thus decreasing feelings of sadness and tension.

- Clients with mood disorders often find six small meals a day are easier to tolerate than three large meals a day.

- Implementing natural sedative measures such as increased physical activity, decreased daytime napping, relaxation techniques, avoidance of caffeine may improve sleeping patterns.

Evaluation

- Evaluation is accomplished by determining the client's progress toward achieving the outcome criteria. Modification of the plan of care is based on evaluation data.

EXPLORE MediaLink

- Interactive resources, including animations, for this chapter can be found on the Companion Web site at *http://www.prenhall.com/fontaine.* Click on Chapter 13 and select the activities for this chapter.

- For NCLEX review questions and an audio glossary, access the accompanying CD-ROM in this book.

REFERENCES

American Psychiatric Association. (2000). *Diagnostic and statistical manual of mental disorders* (4th ed., Text Revision). Washington, DC: Author.

Badger, T. A., McNiece, C., & Gagan, M. J. (2000). Depression, service need, and use in vulnerable populations. *Archives of Psychiatric Nursing, 14*(4), 173–182.

Badner, J. A., Detera-Wadleight, S. D., & Gershon, E. S. (2000). Genetics of early-onset manic-depressive illness and schizophrenia. In J. L. Rapoport (Ed.), *Childhood onset of "adult" psychopathology* (pp 3–26). Washington, DC: American Psychiatric Press.

Becker, I. (2000). Uses of yoga in psychiatry and medicine. In P. R. Muskin (Ed.), *Complementary and alternative medicine and psychiatry* (pp. 107–146). Washington, DC: American Psychiatric Press.

Berrettini, W. H. (2000). Genetic influences on schizophrenia and bipolar disorder. *NARSAD Research Newsletter, 12*(1), 38–40.

Bloch, M., Schmidt, P. J., Danaceau, M., Murphy, J., Nieman, L., & Rubinow, D. R. (2000). Effects of gonadal steroids in women with a history of postpartum depression. *American Journal of Psychiatry, 157*(6), 924–930.

Bondareff, W., Alpert, M., Friedhoff, A. J., Richter, E. M., Clary, C., & Batzar, E. (2000). Comparison of sertraline and nortriptyline in the treatment of major depressive disorder in late life. *American Journal of Psychiatry, 157*(5), 729–736.

Brody, A. L., Saxena, S., & Stoessel, P. (2001). Regional brain metabolic changes in patients with major depression treated with either paroxetine or interpersonal therapy. *Archives of General Psychiatry, 158*(1), 631–640.

Brown, A., & Weaver, R. (1998). Schizoaffective disorder: Just a set of symptoms or a separate disease? *NARSAD Research Newsletter, 10*(4), 25–29.

Brown, R. P., & Gerbarg, P. L. (2000). Integrative psychopharmacology. In P. R. Muskin (Ed.), *Complementary and alternative medicine and psychiatry* (pp. 1–66). Washington, DC: American Psychiatric Press.

Burt, V. K., Suri, R., Altshuler, L., Stowe, Z., Hendrick, V. C., & Muntean, E. (2001). The use of psychotropic medications during breast-feeding. *American Journal of Psychiatry, 158*(7), 1001–1008.

Carlson, G. A., Bromet, E. J., & Sievers, S. (2000). Phenomenology and outcome of subjects with early- and adult-onset psychotic mania. *American Journal of Psychiatry, 157*(2), 213–219.

Deater-Deckard, K., Pickering, K., Dunn, J. F., & Golding, J. (1998). Family structure and depressive symptoms in men preceding and following the birth of a child. *American Journal of Psychiatry, 155*(6), 818–823.

REFERENCES (continued)

Dixit, A. R., & Crum, R. M. (2000). Prospective study of depression and the risk for heavy alcohol use in women. *American Journal of Psychiatry, 157*(5), 751–758.

Ferro, R., Verdeli, H., Pierre, F., & Weissman, M. M. (2000). Screening for depression in mothers bringing their offspring for evaluation or treatment of depression. *American Journal of Psychiatry, 157*(3), 375–379.

Feske, U., Frank, E., Mallinger, A. G., Houck, P. R., Fagiolini, A., Shear, M. K., et al. (2000). Anxiety as a correlate of response to the acute treatment of bipolar I disorder. *American Journal of Psychiatry, 157*(6), 956–962.

Flint, A. J., & Rifat, S. L. (1998). Two-year outcome of psychotic depression in late life. *American Journal of Psychiatry, 155*(2), 178–183.

Garber, J., & Flynn, C. (2001). Vulnerability to depression in childhood and adolescence. In R. E. Ingram & J. M. Price (Eds.), *Vulnerability to psychopathology* (pp. 175–225). New York: Guilford Press.

Gerber. R. (2000). *Vibrational medicine for the 21st century.* New York: Eagle Brook.

Giles, D. E., Kupfer, D. J., Rush, A. J., Koffwarg, H. P. (1998). Controlled comparison of electrophysiological sleep in families of probands with unipolar depression. *American Journal of Psychiatry, 155*(2), 192–199.

Glod, C. A., & Baisden, N. (1999). Seasonal affective disorder in children and adolescents. *Journal of the American Psychiatric Nurses Association, 5*(1), 29–33.

Hammen, C. (2001). Vulnerability and depression in adulthood. In R. E. Ingram & J. M. Price (Eds.), *Vulnerability to psychopathology* (pp. 226–257). New York: Guilford Press.

Harrington, R. (2000). Childhood depression. In J. L. Rapoport (Ed.), *Childhood onset of "adult" psychopathology* (pp. 223–243). Washington, DC: American Psychiatric Press.

Hart, L. A. (2000). Psychosocial benefits of animal companionship. In A. H. Fine (Ed.), *Handbook on animal-assisted therapy* (pp. 59–78). San Diego: Academic Press.

Johnson, M., Maas, M., & Moorhead, S. (2000). *Nursing outcomes classification (NOC)* (2nd ed.). St. Louis, MO: Mosby.

Jones, I., & Craddock, N. (2001). Familiality of the puerperal trigger in bipolar disorder. *American Journal of Psychiatry, 158*(6), 913–917.

Keck, P. E. (2001). New treatments for bipolar disorder. *NARSAD Research Newsletter, 13*(2), 6–7.

Keller, M. B., McCullough, J. P., Klein, D. N., Arnow, B., Dunner, D. L., Gelenberg, A. J., et al. (2000). A comparison of nefazodone, the cognitive behavioral-analysis system of psychotherapy, and their combination for the treatment of chronic depression. *New England Journal of Medicine, 342*(20), 1462–1470.

Keller, S. E. (2000). Stress, depression, immunity, and health. In K. Goodkin & A. P. Visser (Eds.), *Psychoneuroimmunology: Stress, mental disorders, and health* (pp. 1–25). Washington, DC: American Psychiatric Press.

Klein, D. N., Schwartz, J. E., Rose, S., & Leader, J. B. (2000). Five-year course and outcome of dysthymic disorder. *American Journal of Psychiatry, 157*(6), 931–939.

Kupfer, D. J. (1999). Research in affective disorders comes of age. *American Journal of Psychiatry, 156*(2), 165–167.

Lawson, W. B. (2000). Issues in pharmacotherapy for African Americans. In P. Ruiz (Ed.), *Ethnicity and psychopharmacology* (pp. 37–53). Washington, DC: American Psychiatric Press.

Lenze, E. J., Mulsant, B. H., Shear, M. K., Schulberg, H. C., Dew, M. A., et al. (2000). Comorbid anxiety disorders in depressed elderly patients. *American Journal of Psychiatry, 157*(5), 722–728.

Levy, M. L., & Cummings, J. L. (2000). Parkinson's disease. In E. C. Lauterbach (Ed.), *Psychiatric management in neurological disease* (pp. 41–70). Washington, DC: American Psychiatric Press.

Linde, K., Ramirez, G., Mulrow, C. D., Pauls, A., Weidenhammer, W., & Melchart, D. (1996). St. John's Wort for depression—an overview and meta-analysis of randomized clinical trials. *British Medical Journal, 313,* 1065–1066.

Lisanby, S. H., & Sackeim, H. A. (2000). TMS in major depression. In M. S. George & R. H. Belmaker (Eds.), *Transcranial magnetic stimulation in neuropsychiatry* (pp. 185–200). Washington, DC: American Psychiatric Press.

Lopez, A. D., & Murray, D. J. L. (1998). Global burden of disease 1990–2020. *Nature Medicine, 4,* 1241–1243.

Lynch, A., Glod, C. A., & Fitzgerald, F. (2001). Psychopharmacologic treatment of adolescent depression. *Archives of Psychiatric Nursing, 15*(1), 41–47.

Maj, M., Pirozzi, R., Formicola, A. M. R., & Tortorella, A. (1999). Reliability and validity of four alternative definitions of rapid-cycling bipolar disorder. *American Journal of Psychiatry, 156*(9), 1421–1424.

Martin, A., & Cohen, D. J. (2000). Adolescent depression. *American Journal of Psychiatry, 157*(10), 1549–1551.

McCloskey, J., & Bulechek, G. M. (1996). *Nursing interventions classification (NIC)* (2nd ed.). St. Louis, MO: Mosby.

McElroy, S. L., Altshuler, L. L., Suppes, T., Keck, P. E., Frye, M. A., Denicoff, K. D., et al. (2001). Axis I psychiatric comorbidity and its relationship to historical illness variables in 288 patients with bipolar disorder. *American Journal of Psychiatry, 158*(3), 420–426.

Meltzer, C. C., Price, J. C., Mathis, C. A., Greer, P. J., Cantwell, M. N., Houck, P. R., et al. (1999). PET imaging of serotonin type 2A receptors in late-life neuropsychiatric disorders. *American Journal of Psychiatry, 156*(12), 1871–1879.

Mohr, W. K. (2001). Bipolar disorder in children. *Journal of Psychosocial Nursing, 39*(3), 12–23.

Papolos, D. F., & Papolos, J. (1999). *The bipolar child.* New York: Broadway Books.

Paris, J. (1999). *Nature and nurture in psychiatry.* Washington, DC: American Psychiatric Press.

Parker, G., Gladstone, G., & Chee, K. T. (2001). Depression in the planet's largest ethnic group: The Chinese. *American Journal of Psychiatry, 158*(6), 857–864.

Peden, A. R., Hall, L. A., Rayens, M. K., & Beebe, L. (2000). Negative thinking mediates the effect of self-esteem on depressive symptoms in college women. *Nursing Research, 49*(4), 201–207.

Perraud, S. (2000a). Development of the depression coping self-efficacy scale (DCSES). *Archives of Psychiatric Nursing, 14*(6), 276–284.

Perraud, S. (2000b). Efforts intensify to treat chronic depression. *Nursing Spectrum, 13*(23IL), 16–17.

Preisig, M., Bellivier, F., Fenton, B. T., Baud, P., Berney, A., Courtet, P., et al. (2000). Association between bipolar disorder and monoamine oxidase A gene polymorphisms. *American Journal of Psychiatry, 157*(6), 948–955.

Ratey, J. J. (2001). *A user's guide to the brain.* New York: Pantheon Books.

Robinson, R. G. (2000). Stroke. In E. C. Lauterbach (Ed.), *Psychiatric management in neurological disease* (pp. 219–247). Washington, DC: American Psychiatric Press.

Schreiber, R., Stern, P. N., & Wilson, C. (2000). Being strong: How Black West-Indian Canadian women manage depression and its stigma. *Journal of Nursing Scholarship, 32*(1), 39–45.

Schweiger, U., Weber, B., Deuschle, M., & Heuser, I. (2000). Lumbar bond mineral density in patients with major depression. *American Journal of Psychiatry, 157*(1), 118–120.

Silverstein, B., & Perlick, D. (1995). *The cost of competence.* Oxford, England: Oxford University Press.

Solomon, D. A., Keller, M. B., Leon, A. C., Mueller, T. I., Lavori, P. W., Shea, M. J., et al. (2000). Multiple recurrences of major depressive disorder. *American Journal of Psychiatry, 157*(2), 229–233.

Straub, H., Cross, J., Curtis, S., Iverson, S., Jacobsmeyer, M., Anderson, C., et al. (1998). Proactive nursing: The evolution of a task force to help women with postpartum depression. *Maternal Child Nursing, 23*(5), 262–266.

Sullivan, G. M., Hatterer, J. A., Herbert, J., Chen, X., Roose, S. P., Attia, E., et al. (1999). Low levels of transthyretin in the CSF of depressed patients. *American Journal of Psychiatry, 156*(5), 710–714.

Sullivan, P. R., Neale, M. C., & Kendler, K. S. (2000). Genetic epidemiology of major depression: Review and meta-analysis. *American Journal of Psychiatry, 157*(10), 1552–1562.

Szigethy, E. M., & Ruiz, P. (2001). Depression among pregnant adolescents. *American Journal of Psychiatry, 158*(1), 22–27.

Takeuchi, D. T., Chung, R. C., Lin, K., Shen, H., Kurasaki, K., Chun, C., & Sue, S. (1998). Lifetime and twelve-month prevalence rates of major depressive episodes and dysthymia among Chinese Americans in Los Angeles. *American Journal of Psychiatry, 155*(10), 1407–1414.

Tohen, M., Hennen, J., Zarate, C. M., Baldessarini, R. J., Strakowski, S. M., Stoll, A. L., et al. (2000). Two-year syndromal and functional recovery in 219 cases of first-episode major affective disorder with psychotic features. *American Journal of Psychiatry, 157*(2), 220–228.

Tohen, M., Sanger, T. M., McElroy, S. L., Tollefson, G. D., Chengappa, R., Daniel, D. G., et al. (1999). Olanzapine versus placebo in the treatment of acute mania. *American Journal of Psychiatry, 156*(5), 702–709.

Viguera, A. C., Nonacs, R., Cohen, L. S., Tondo, L., Murray, A., & Baldessarini, R. J. (2000). Risk of recurrence of bipolar disorder in pregnant and nonpregnant women after discontinuing lithium maintenance. *American Journal of Psychiatry, 157*(2), 179–184.

Weinberg, M. K., Posener, J. A., DeBattista, C., Kalehzan, B. M., Rothschild, A. J., & Shear, P. K. (2001). Subsyndromal depression symptoms and major depression in postpar-tum women. *American Journal of Orthopsychiatry, 71*(1), 87–97.

Weiss, E. L., Longhurst, J. G., & Mazure, C. M. (1999). Childhood sexual abuse as a risk factor for depression in women: Psychosocial and neurobiological correlates. *American Journal of Psychiatry, 156*(6), 816–828.

Wolkowitz, O. M., Reus, V. I., Keebler, A., Nelson, N., Friedland, M., Brizendine, L., et al. (1999). Double-blind treatment of major depression with dehydroepiandrosterone. *American Journal of Psychiatry, 156*(4), 646–649.

Wu, J., Buchsbaum, M. S., Gillin, J. C., Tang, C., Cadwell, S., Wiegand, M., et al. (1999). Prediction of antidepressant effects of sleep deprivation by metabolic rates in the ventral anterior cingulate and medial prefrontal cortex. *American Journal of Psychiatry, 156*(8), 1149–1158.

Zimmerman, M., McDermut, W., & Mattia, J. K. (2000). Frequency of anxiety disorders in psychiatric outpatients with major depressive disorder. *American Journal of Psychiatry, 157*(8), 1337–1340.

Zubenko, G. S., Mulsant, B. H., Sweet, R. A., Pasternak, R. E., & Tu, X. M. (1997). Mortality of elderly patients with psychiatric disorders. *American Journal of Psychiatry, 154*(10), 1360–1368.

Zust, B. L. (2000). Effect of cognitive therapy on depression in rural, battered women. *Archives of Psychiatric Nursing, 14*(2), 51–63.

CHAPTER 14

Schizophrenic Disorders

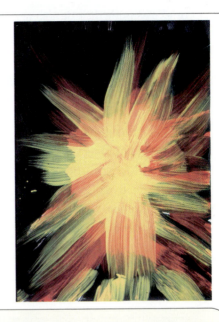

OBJECTIVES

After reading this chapter, you will be able to:

- ASSESS the positive and negative symptoms of schizophrenic disorders.

- DESCRIBE the multiple etiologies of the schizophrenic syndrome.

- IDENTIFY the principles of psychiatric rehabilitation.

- APPLY the nursing process to clients who have schizophrenic disorders.

- PLAN overall goals in the care of clients with schizophrenia.

- INDIVIDUALIZE nursing interventions for clients with schizophrenia.

- EVALUATE care on basis of outcome criteria.

*T*he gold star (religious imagery) is bursting through the blackness of my life.

—*Carlos, Age 49*

MediaLink

CD-ROM
- *Audio Glossary*
- *NCLEX Review*

Animations
- *PET & SPECT Scans*

Companion Web site www.prenhall.com/fontaine
- *Critical Thinking*
- *More NCLEX Review*
- *Case Study*
- *Care Map Activity*
- *Links to Resources*

S chizophrenia is a disorder of the brain like epilepsy or multiple sclerosis. It is diagnosed in about 1 percent of the U.S. population and is a devastating disorder that affects not only the individual but family, friends, and the community as a whole. Although it is referred to as a single disease, it is more accurately a syndrome, characterized by a broad range of symptoms, physiological malfunctions, etiologies, and prognoses. Included in the syndrome of schizophrenia are schizotypal personality disorder, paranoid personality disorder, schizoaffective disorder, schizophreniform disorder, delusional disorder, brief psychotic disorder, shared psychotic disorder, and schizophrenia. Personality disorders are discussed in Chapter 16. Relatives of people who have schizophrenia are often included in the spectrum since they are thought to have a genetic predisposition to schizophrenia but do not necessarily demonstrate full or any clinical manifestations of schizophrenia (Anders, 2000; Cadenhead, Swerdlow, Shafer, Diaz, & Braff, 2000).

Schizophrenia is a combination of disordered thinking, perceptual disturbances, behavioral abnormalities, affective disruptions, and impaired social competency. This means the person has difficulty thinking clearly, knowing what is real, managing feelings, making decisions, and relating to others. Typically, the person is fairly normal early in life, experiences subtle changes after puberty, and undergoes severe symptoms in the late teens to early adulthood. The early age of onset often shatters the lives of its victims and robs them of the opportunity for a productive adult life.

The onset and progression of schizophrenia is quite variable. It is believed that people with an abrupt onset of the illness suffer from a different form of schizophrenia than those whose onset is more insidious. The vast majority develop the disorder in adolescence or young adulthood, with only 10 to 15 percent of cases first diagnosed in people over the age of 45. In some cases, the disorder progresses through relapses and remissions; in other cases, it takes a chronic, stable course; while in still others, a chronic, progressively deteriorating course evolves. Much too often, the illness results in lifelong problems in coping with everyday living that reflect irreversible neurobiological deficits. Early diagnosis and treatment may reduce the chronicity and improve the prognosis of people suffering from schizophrenia. Women tend to have a later onset of illness, better treatment response, shorter and less frequent relapses, and an overall higher quality of life than do their male counterparts (Crespo-Facorro, Piven, & Schultz, 1999; Seeman, 2001).

In **schizoaffective disorder**, clients suffer from symptoms that appear to be a mixture of schizophrenia and the mood disorders. The person experiences one or more of the following psychotic symptoms: delusions, hallucinations, disorganized speech, disorganized behavior, or negative symptoms. In addition, the person experiences symptoms of the mood disorders, which may be major depressive symptoms, manic symptoms, or mixed symptoms. Schizoaffective disorder is most likely a distinct syndrome resulting from a high genetic liability to both mood disorders and schizophrenia. The age of onset, like schizophrenia, is typically late adolescence or early adulthood. Like mood disorders, however, it is much more common in women than in men. Women are also much more likely than men to have their diagnosis switched from schizophrenia to schizoaffective disorder. Clients with schizoaffective disorder often have difficulty maintaining job or school functioning, experience problems with self-care, are socially isolated, and often suffer from suicidal ideation. The prognosis is somewhat better than for schizophrenia but significantly worse than the prognosis for mood disorders (American Psychiatric Association [APA], 2000; Siris, 2000; Tsuang, Stone, & Faraone, 2000).

In **brief psychotic disorder**, there is a rapid onset of at least one of the following psychotic symptoms: delusions, hallucinations, disorganized speech, or disorganized behavior. The episode lasts at least one day but less than one month, after which the person returns to the premorbid level of functioning. The symptoms of **schizophreniform disorder** are the same but last at least one month and less than six months. One third return to their premorbid level of functioning while two thirds progress to the diagnosis of schizophrenia or schizoaffective disorder. In a **shared psychotic disorder**, a person who is in a close relationship with another person who is delusional comes to share the delusional beliefs. This most commonly occurs between two people but may involve more individuals such as when children adopt the parent's delusional beliefs (APA, 2000).

KNOWLEDGE BASE

The classic subtypes described in the *Diagnostic and Statistical Manual of Mental Disorders* (4th ed., Text Revision) (DSM-IV-TR) (undifferentiated, catatonic, paranoid, disorganized, and residual) are difficult to apply and have many symptoms in common. Individuals often get diagnoses changed from one category to another as symptoms fluctuate and thus the classification is unstable (Liddle, 1999). (See DSM-IV-TR feature.) The classic subtypes have given way to new systems of classification. The most widely used system is one of positive symptoms, negative symptoms, and thought disorganization. This arrangement represents symptom types that are probably semi-independent of each other. To make sense of these groups, you must understand that positive does not mean good, and neg-

---

DSM-IV-TR CLASSIFICATIONS

Schizophrenia

Paranoid Type
Disorganized Type
Catatonic Type
Undifferentiated Type
Residual Type

Schizophreniform Disorder

Schizoaffective Disorder
Delusional Disorder
Brief Psychotic Disorder
Shared Psychotic Disorder
Psychotic Disorder due to general medical condition
Substance-induced psychotic disorder
Psychotic Disorder Not Otherwise Specified (NOS)

SOURCE: Reprinted with permission from the *Diagnostic and Statistical Manual of Mental Disorders, Fourth Edition, Text Revision.* Copyright 2000 American Psychiatric Association.

---

ative does not mean bad. Rather, **positive symptoms** are excessive or added behaviors that are not normally seen in mentally healthy adults. For example, healthy adults do not experience delusions; therefore, delusions are a positive symptom (see Table 14.1 ■). Women are more likely to exhibit more positive than negative symptoms. Positive symptoms are most likely the result of physiological changes, including increased dopamine (DA) function in the subcortical areas of the brain and decreased glucose utilization in the brain. Medication is often successful in diminishing positive symptoms (Bryant, Buchanan, Vlader, Breier, & Rothman, 1999).

Negative symptoms are the loss of normal function that is normally seen in mentally healthy adults. For example, healthy adults are able to complete their ADLs; therefore, an inability to care for oneself is a negative symptom of schizophrenia (refer back to Table 14.1). Men are more likely to exhibit prominent negative symptoms. Negative symptoms are most likely related to anatomic changes as well as decreased DA function in the prefrontal cortex. These symptoms have been more treatment resistant.

TABLE 14.1

Symptoms of Schizophrenia

Positive Symptoms	Negative Symptoms
Behavioral	
Hyperactivity	Decreased activity level
Bizarre behavior	Limited speech; conversation difficult
	Minimal self-care
Affective	
Inappropriate affect	Blunted or flat affect
Overreactive affect	Anhedonia
Hostility	
Perceptual	
Hallucinations	Inability to understand sensory information
Sensory overload	
Cognitive	
Delusions	Concrete thinking
Disorganized thinking	Attention impairment
Loose associations	Memory deficits
Suspiciousness	Impaired problem solving
	Lack of motivation
Social	
Aloof and stilted interactions	Social withdrawal, isolation
	Poor rapport with others
	Inadequate social and occupational skills

A *deficit syndrome* has been proposed as a distinct subtype of schizophrenia characterized by significant and persistent negative symptoms. These individuals often experience an insidious onset of schizophrenia, a chronic deteriorating course, and a poor response to treatment. Evidence suggests that the deficit syndrome has important genetic and/or family environmental components (Ross et al., 2000).

BEHAVIORAL CHARACTERISTICS

Positive behavioral characteristics include hyperactivity and bizarre behavior. *Hyperactive behavior* most typically occurs during a period of relapse. The excitement may become so great that it threatens the person's safety or that of others. The behavior may also be very unpredictable. Schizophrenia can cause people to engage in *bizarre behavior* such as repeating rhythmic gestures, doing ritualistic postures, or demonstrating freakish facial or body movements. Some people will imitate other people's movements (*echopraxia*) or words (*echolalia*) or may senselessly repeat the same word or phrase for hours or days. Another positive characteristic is a *decreased awareness of one's own behavior*. It is not unusual to hear clients describe their behavior as being under the influence of alien forces or of other people (Franck et al., 2001).

Negative behavioral characteristics are decreased activity level, limited speech, and minimal self-care.

The *decreased activity level* includes a reduction of energy, initiative, and spontaneity. There is a loss of natural gracefulness in body movements that results in poor coordination; activities may be carried out in a robot-like fashion. People with schizophrenia often have *limited speech*, referred to as *alogia*, which makes it difficult for them to carry on a continuous conversation or say anything new. They may say very little on their own initiative or in response to questions from others; some may be mute for several hours to several days.

Another difficulty for individuals and their significant others is a deterioration in appearance and manners. *Self-care* may become *minimal*; they may need to be reminded to bathe, shave, brush their teeth, and change their clothes. Because of confusion and distraction, they may not conform to social norms of dress and behavior.

AFFECTIVE CHARACTERISTICS

Positive affective characteristics include inappropriate affect, overreactive affect, and hostility. *Inappropriate affect* occurs when the person's emotional tone is not related to the immediate circumstances. An *overreactive affect* is appropriate to the situation but out of proportion to it.

Negative affective characteristics include blunted or flat affect and anhedonia. A *blunted affect* describes a dulled emotional response to a situation, and a *flat affect* describes the absence of visible cues to the person's feelings. Schizophrenia can make it difficult for people to clearly express their emotions. They show less emotion, laugh less, and cry less (see Table 14.2 ■).

Anhedonia, the inability to experience pleasure, causes many people with schizophrenia to feel emotionally barren. They also have an inability to express emotion. These two difficulties may lead to eccentric social interactions and social withdrawal. Consumers may not take much interest in the things around them, even things they used to find enjoyable. If the world feels "flat as cardboard," they may not feel that it is worth the effort to get out and do things.

People with schizophrenia have a normal ability to experience unpleasant emotions and often experience worries and fears. With little warning, some people with schizophrenia become *hostile* as anger turns into aggression with the intent to do harm.

PERCEPTUAL CHARACTERISTICS

Positive perceptual characteristics include hallucinations and sensory overload. A **hallucination** is the occurrence of a sound, sight, touch, smell, or taste without an external stimulus to the corresponding sensory organ. Hallucinations are very real to the person and may be triggered by anxiety and by functional changes in the central nervous system. Researchers, observing brain function through magnetic resonance imaging (MRI), found that the same brain area was activated when clients listened to audible speech as when they were experiencing auditory hallucinations. In other words, the brain reacts as if unable to distinguish between its own internally generated speech and actual, audible speech (Murray, 1999).

TABLE 14.2

Descriptors of Affect

Affect	Example
Inappropriate	When told it's time to turn off the TV and go to bed, Joe begins to laugh uproariously.
Overreactive	When Kathy wins at cards, she jumps up and down and does a cheer for herself.
Blunted	Tom has been looking forward to his wife's visit. When she arrives on the unit, he is only able to give her a small smile.
Flat	When Juanita's mother tells her that her favorite dog has died, Juanita simply says "Oh" and does not give any indication of an emotional response.

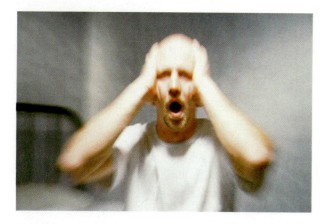

PHOTO 14.1 ■ Many of the symptoms of schizophrenia, including hallucinations and delusions, can be extremely distressing.

SOURCE: Carlton, Chuck/Index Stock Imagery, Inc.

The most common type is *auditory hallucination*, or the hearing of voices or unusual noises. The voice is often that of God, the devil, a neighbor, or a relative; the voice may say either bad or good things; and the voice seems to be coming from an external source. Auditory hallucinations occur in 50 to 80 percent of people with schizophrenia. The next most common type is *visual hallucination*, which is usually nearby, clearly defined, and moving. Visual hallucinations are often accompanied by auditory hallucinations. *Tactile*, *olfactory*, and *gustatory hallucinations* are uncommon and are more likely to occur in people who are undergoing substance withdrawal or abuse.

Hallucinations may considerably control the person's behavior. It is not unusual for people having auditory hallucinations to carry on a conversation with one of the voices. After a period of time, many people realize that if they admit they hear voices, they will be labeled "sick" or "crazy." To avoid being labeled, they may be very evasive about their hallucinations.

Kari, a nurse, is on a home visit with Lisa, a 44-year-old client who lives in supervised housing. Lisa is filling out a piece of paper that Kari gave her yesterday.

Kari: *How are you doing with the self-image exercise?*

Lisa: *He tells me what to say. [laughing softly]*

Kari: *Who tells you what to say?*

Lisa: *He does. I never tell anyone about him. I've only told a couple of people. [makes brief eye contact]*

Kari: *Is he here right now?*

Lisa: *Yes, he just walked around the corner. [looks across the room]*

Kari: *How do you feel when this voice talks to you?*

Lisa: *I'm used to it. I've known him since I was little. Let's see. What do I value the most? Myself. No, he said I can't put that. He says I have to put my loved ones. [looking down at piece of paper]*

Kari: *You value yourself the most, but the voice won't let you write that down?*

Lisa: *Yes.*

Our sensory systems receive information from the environment and from our bodies through stimuli transmitted to the brain. We do not, however, consciously perceive much of this sensory information. Sensory information is processed in a series of relay stations within the brain where irrelevant stimuli are inhibited. This allows us to filter out unnecessary and distracting information—a process called **selective perception**—and focus on what is important at the given moment. Schizophrenia often disrupts the filtering process, causing *sensory overload*. When there are too many messages arriving at the cortex at the same time, thinking becomes disorganized and fragmented (see Figure 14.1 ■).

The negative perceptual characteristic in schizophrenia is the inability to understand sensory information. People with schizophrenia sometimes have a hard time making sense of everyday sights, sounds, and feelings. Their *perception* of what is going on around them may be *distorted* so that ordinary things appear distracting or frightening. They may be overly sensitive to background noises and colors and shapes.

COGNITIVE CHARACTERISTICS

Schizophrenia impairs many cognitive functions, such as thought formation, memory, language, attention,

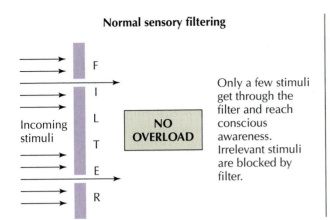

FIGURE 14.1 ■ Impaired sensory filtering in schizophrenia.

and executive functions. Positive cognitive characteristics of schizophrenia are delusions, disorganized thinking, and loose associations.

Delusions are false beliefs that cannot be changed by logical reasoning or evidence. When there is an extensively developed central delusional theme from which conclusions are deducted, the delusions are termed *systematized*. There are a number of delusional types: grandiosity (delusions of grandeur), persecution, control, somatic, religious, erotomanic, ideas of reference, thought broadcasting, thought withdrawal, and thought insertion (see Table 14.3 ■). It is thought that delusions represent dysfunctions in the information-processing circuits within and between the hemisphere. The severity of delusions can be a valuable indicator in monitoring the course of the illness.

Grandiosity, also known as *delusions of grandeur*, is an exaggerated sense of importance or self-worth. It is often accompanied by beliefs of magical thinking.

Shane lives in a group home and is introducing himself to the nursing student who will be there every Wednesday for the next six weeks. "I am Jeremiah the prophet, and this is just the body I reside in. My doctor is the descendent from hell. He has trouble relating to me because I am the Angel of Death. I think you are my girl-friend, but I can't marry you because I am marrying Elaine this afternoon."

People with schizophrenia may experience *delusions of persecution*. They may believe someone is trying to harm them and, therefore, any personal failures in life are the fault of these harmful others.

Vanessa believes she is a victim of a plot. She states that people live in her attic and that they followed her on a recent trip to Florida. She believes these people are spraying her with a toxic chemical that creates somatic symptoms. "They have somehow chosen me to be a victim in an attempt to disrupt the water waves."

Delusions of control occur when the person believes that feelings, impulses, thoughts, or actions are not one's own but are being imposed by some external force.

Samuel believes that a group of doctors are doing long-distance laser surgery on his back. He says his back twitches when they do the surgery, and he can hear the voices of the doctors talking. "I have computer chips in my brain, and the computer sends out electrical impulses and tells me what to do. I really shouldn't be telling you this because now the security people are going to follow you."

Religious delusions involve false beliefs with religious or spiritual themes.

TABLE 14.3

Examples of Delusions

Delusion	Example
Grandiosity	"Within one month I am going to be a billionaire and own 14 houses and 20 cars. I will be so rich and successful that Bill Gates and Allen Greenspan are going to call me for financial advice."
Persecution	"My neighborhood wants me dead or alive. They think I hold all of their secrets. They have tapped my phone and peek through my windows 24 hours a day."
Control	"My mother put a voodoo curse on me. She can control all of my thoughts and emotions through a remote control car. I am completely under her spell."
Religious	"God told me that I am his Chosen One. I can perform miracles. I know this is real because my rosary beads revealed this to me."
Erotomanic	"I can have any guy I want. Matt Damon called me last night but I couldn't go out because I already had a date with Tom Cruise."
Sin and guilt	"I can't do anything right. I always mess everything up. I had so many friends from school but now no one will come and see me because I am a failure."
Somatic	"I have a hammer in my heart. It pounds daggers in it all day long. Don't you hear it? Someday soon it is going to pound so hard that my heart will come flying out of my chest onto the floor."
Ideas of reference	"The headline of the *New York Times* told me that I have been assigned to stop crime. I am issuing a nationwide bulletin telling people to turn in their guns and knives. I take my assignments very seriously."
Thought broadcasting	"I don't have to tell you that. You already know because you can read my mind."
Thought withdrawal	"I'm trying to tell you somehting but I keep losing it because someone keeps stealing my thoughts."
Thought insertion	"You think this is me talking, but it really isn't. My husband keeps putting these thoughts in my head."

The case manager has been called by Miguel's family to make a home visit. He has been sitting in front of a homemade altar and prays with a rosary to God all day long. He has been fasting intermittently for seven weeks and has lost 30 pounds. He tells the case manager that he is being controlled by the devil, needs to be freed by God, and is fasting to atone for his sins. He states, "I don't eat because God is nourishing me."

Erotomanic delusions are beliefs that a person, usually someone famous and of higher status, is in love with her or him. Preoccupation with the "fantasy" lover may lead to stalking. Occasionally, the stalker turns violent, not because of hatred of the person, but because the person cannot fulfill the romantic delusions.

Mandi believes that she is engaged to Brad Pitt and that they will be getting married next month. She is busy planning for the wedding and discussing who, among the rich and famous, will be at the wedding.

Somatic delusions occur when people believe something abnormal and dangerous is happening to their bodies.

Rachel, looking at an orange she is holding, says: "I had a bowel movement yesterday. It looked like this. It was one of my ovaries or it might have been a tumor."

Ideas of reference are remarks or actions by someone else that in no way refer to the person but that are interpreted as related to her or him. *Thought broadcasting* occurs when people believe that their thoughts can be heard by others. *Thought withdrawal* is the belief that others are able to remove thoughts from one's mind. *Thought insertion* is the belief that others are able to put thoughts into one's mind.

Sumidra believes that other people can smell a "bad odor coming from her private parts." She says when she sees two people walking down the street together, they stare at her and she knows they are talking to each other about her terrible smell.

Further information about delusions is found in Chapter 9.

Disorganized thinking is another effect of schizophrenia. Adaptation to the environment and effective coping depend not only on learned responses but also on the flexibility of the brain in organizing this incoming information. Thought disorder is abnormalities in the form of thought and is experienced by the listener as disorganized speech. Because speech is a reflection of cognitive functioning, **loose association** is an indication of disorganized thinking. The person is described as having loose association when verbal ideas shift from one topic to another, there is no apparent relationship between thoughts, and the person is unaware that the topics are unconnected. At times, the person may change topic and direction so frequently that she or he is incoherent or impossible to understand (Goldberg et al., 1998).

Ming Lee states: "The thing in the ozone level is going away and people aren't told about it. Do

you know why my bed is so soft? It doesn't matter. Everybody's got to die and the babies are going away. God bless America."

The negative cognitive characteristics of schizophrenia are concrete thinking, attention impairment, memory deficits, impaired problem solving, lack of motivation, and lack of insight. These symptoms are most likely related to dysfunctions in the cerebral cortex.

Concrete thinking is characterized by a focus on facts and details and an inability to generalize or think abstractly. If you ask a client what brought him to the hospital, he is likely to say "a car." *Attention impairment* interferes with the processing of information and the response to such information. The person has poor concentration and is easily distracted. Disturbances include responding to irrelevant external stimuli and difficulty completing tasks.

You will recall from Chapter 7 that there are two types of long-term memory: declarative and procedural. *Declarative memory* is memory for people and facts, is consciously accessible, and can be verbally expressed. *Procedural memory* does not require conscious awareness and involves the memory of motor skills and procedures. *Memory deficits* in schizophrenia are one of the most severely impaired functions, which explains the day-to-day difficulties encountered by people with schizophrenia. The deficit is primarily in the area of declarative memory. The processes of responding emotionally, forming impressions about people, drawing inferences, and many other high-level cognitive functions are supported by declarative memory. Thus, a person may display inappropriate behavior or make poor judgments when memory is impaired by the disorder (Danion et al., 2001).

Impaired problem solving may occur for a number of reasons. The person may be unaware that a problem exists, have impaired judgment, be unable to think logically, be unable to make a decision, or be unable to plan or follow through on a decision. Since one of the problems with this disorder is faulty information processing, a person with schizophrenia needs more time to think and problem-solve.

Lack of motivation, referred to as *avolition*, is the inability to persist in goal-directed activities. People may have trouble starting projects or following through with things once begun. Their inability to persist at work or school activities gets them into significant employment or academic difficulties. At the extreme, they may have to be reminded to do simple things like taking a bath or changing clothes.

Poor insight, or lack of awareness of one's own mental illness, is more common in people with schizophrenia than in those with schizoaffective disorder or with major depressive disorder. Poor insight means that individuals have difficulty identifying their symptoms, which has implications for agreeing with treatment plans and for recognizing early signs of relapse (Kennedy, Schepp, & O'Connor, 2000).

SOCIAL CHARACTERISTICS

The primary positive social characteristic of schizophrenia is one of aloof and *stilted interactions* with others. People with schizophrenia may use outdated or very formal language and may have difficulty carrying on a conversation.

Nurse: *Hi, my name is Tonya. I am your nurse today.*

Client: *I must say, Miss Tonya, I am very pleased to make your acquaintance. Your profession is certainly to be admired.*

The negative social characteristics of schizophrenia are social withdrawal/isolation, a poor rapport with others, and inadequate social and occupational skills.

Social withdrawal/isolation may result from paranoid delusions, from severe difficulty participating in conversations, or an inability to experience feelings of friendship or intimacy. *Inadequate social skills* can interfere with the ability to develop rapport with others. These ineffective skills may drive away friends and family members who do not understand the behavior, further increasing the sense of isolation. People with schizophrenia may be socially incompetent in part because they are unable to perceive the subtle cues that are critical to interpersonal interactions. In order to understand body cues during an interaction, one must be able to think abstractly. People with schizophrenia understand concrete cues better than abstract cues. For example, while they can identify and recall what someone said and did, they are less able to identify the emotional tone behind the words or comprehend the motivation for the interaction. Occupational skills may be

inadequate because of cognitive disruptions, behavioral abnormalities, inability to manage feelings, or inadequate social skills.

Most people with schizophrenia experience *cycles of relapse and remission*. Families who have a loved one suffering from a chronic medical illness, such as debilitating heart disease, usually receive social support and sympathy. But members of families with a loved one suffering from schizophrenia are often avoided. Many families are drained financially from the expense of long-term therapy, medications, and intermittent hospital stays. Mental health services are poorly covered in most medical insurance policies.

People suffering from schizophrenia are not indifferent to their emotional and social environments. The *emotional climate of the family* has been shown to play a role in the relapse of the disorder. Clients who live in families that are highly critical, hostile, and overinvolved (referred to as *high expressed emotion*) have a significantly higher relapse rate than those who live in a supportive and caring family system. Families who are highly negative or excessively intrusive to the client can accelerate the time to relapse by causing physiological arousal and increased symptoms. On average, the relapse rate among clients who are in family therapy is 24 percent as compared to 64 percent among those not in family therapy (Bustillo, Lauriello, Horan, & Keith, 2001; Paris, 1999).

Approximately one third of the **homeless population** suffers from psychiatric disability, many of these with schizophrenia. The figures rise to 66 percent when chemical dependence is included in the estimate. In addition, all people, if left homeless for a sufficient period, will develop less effective coping skills and demonstrate some type of mental disorder or disability (Mueser, Bond, & Drake, 2001). Perhaps nothing is more upsetting than the sight of an individual who is homeless and clearly experiencing severe psychiatric problems. The image of a disheveled man angrily responding to voices only he can hear is an example of society's failure to address the problem of both homelessness and psychiatric disability. Homeless mentally ill women represent one of the most vulnerable segments of our society. They frequently face a choice between the dangers of life on the street and the hazards of overcrowded, unsafe, and poorly supervised shelters. Rape and physical battery are a daily risk for these women.

Homeless psychiatrically disabled people are often fearful and distrustful of the mental health system. In community health nursing, you must be prepared to work with homeless people in nonclinical settings, including streets, shelters, subways, bus terminals, and other public areas. You will need a combination of patience, persistence, and understanding. Depending on the needs and wants of a particular person, providing food, clothing, or simply company can be essential in developing a therapeutic relationship.

CULTURE-SPECIFIC CHARACTERISTICS

A person's cultural and religious background must be considered when assessing individuals from cultures that are different than your own. In some cultures, experiences that we label as delusional or hallucinatory are expected, normal experiences. In addition, differences in styles of expression of feelings may be misunderstood and labeled as pathologic when in fact they are completely normal for that cultural group (APA, 2000).

Schizophrenia is recognized worldwide and affects about 1 percent of the population in different cultures. For unknown reasons, there are small areas of population with increased incidence, such as second-generation African Caribbeans living in the United Kingdom. The symptoms tend to be universal, with minimal influence by the specific culture (APA, 2000; Harvey, 2001).

AGE-SPECIFIC CHARACTERISTICS

Childhood schizophrenia is diagnosed when the onset of psychotic symptoms occurs before 12 years of age and before the completion of brain maturation. This form of schizophrenia is very severe and may have a stronger genetic predisposition (Sowell et al., 2000).

Most children who develop schizophrenia appear normal at birth and during the first years of life. Subtle behavioral and cognitive characteristics often precede the first psychotic episode. These signs include higher than expected rates of abnormal speech and motor abnormalities such as clumsiness and abnormal movements. In addition, they experience social withdrawal and isolation, decline in IQ over several years, and diminishing school performance. Prior to developing psychotic symptoms there is a high rate of special education placement and failed grades (Nicolson et al., 2000; Nicolson & Rapoport, 2000).

Symptomatology is similar to that seen in adults, although the content of children's hallucinations and delusions comes from their experiences. For example, rather than believing that the FBI is following them, children may believe that a cartoon villain is out to get them.

The majority of *older adults* who have schizophrenia have had the disorder since they were young. A number of these people show substantial improvement in symptoms, especially the positive symptoms, over the course of their lifetimes.

Between 15 and 32 percent of people with schizophrenia have a late onset type, which occurs after age 45 and affects more women than men. The clinical picture is somewhat different than in earlier onset schizophrenia. People with late-onset have more delusions, which are often persecutory and bizarre. They are more likely to exhibit vivid hallucinations but have fewer cognitive disruptions and negative symptoms. It is thought that late-onset schizophrenia may be a less severe form of the disorder (Crespo-Facorro et al., 1999; Zorrilla & Zeste, 2000).

Sensory impairment, such as hearing loss or cataracts, may increase the severity of the symptoms since environmental stimuli are often misinterpreted. In addition, people with hearing and vision loss tend to decrease social contacts and become socially isolated, which may increase suspicious thoughts.

PHYSIOLOGICAL CHARACTERISTICS

Velocardiofacial syndrome is a congenital defect related to chromosome 22. The predominant clinical signs include cleft palate, cardiac abnormalities, minor facial anomalies, and learning disabilities. Among adults with this syndrome, there is an increased incidence of schizophrenia and schizoaffective disorder. These anomalies are considered to develop during the first 16 weeks of gestation and coincide with early brain development. People with velocardiofacial syndrome demonstrate neuroanatomical abnormalities in the temporal lobe as well as decreased total cerebral volume, both of which occur in people with schizophrenia (Eliez et al., 2001; Ismail, Cantor-Graae, & McNeil, 1998).

In comparison to men, women develop schizophrenia several years later and experience less severe symptoms. Research shows that *estrogens* protect against nerve cell loss and preserves connections between neurons. Estrogens also enhance the efficacy of antipsychotic medications. As estrogens decrease in the menopausal years, we find more women than men developing late-onset schizophrenia (Seeman, 2001).

People with schizophrenia have much higher rates of *cigarette smoking* (58 to 88 percent) compared with the general population (25 percent) and twice as high as those with other psychiatric diagnoses. There are three possible reasons for this heavy dependence on nicotine. First, clients may self-medicate with nicotine to improve cognition, lessen auditory hallucinations, and moderate the side effects of medications. Nicotine, like other drugs of addiction such as cocaine and amphetamine, appears to stimulate the reward center of the brain. It does this through stimulation of nicotinic receptors, which increases DA synthesis and decreases DA metabolism. Thus, smoking may be a way to self-medicate a disturbance in the reward center. Second, smoking may be a risk factor for a person who has the genetic vulnerability to schizophrenia. This is supported by the data that those who start smoking at a young age have an earlier onset of their schizophrenia. Third, genetic or environmental factors might work together, contributing to the co-occurrence of nicotine use and schizophrenia (George et al., 2000; Kelly & McCreadie, 1999).

Smoking places clients at greater psychiatric risk because components in cigarette smoke stimulate hepatic enzymes, increasing the rate of metabolism of psychotropic medications. Smoking also places them at increased risk for cardiovascular and respiratory diseases (Weiner et al., 2001).

Abnormalities in the ability to *identify smells* may be a marker of cerebral dysfunction in schizophrenia. Research shows that people with schizophrenia are unable to identify when smells have a pleasing scent, just as they are unable to experience pleasure. The prefrontal brain regions used to assess emotional pleasure and olfactory pleasure appear to have a dysfunction in their circuitry. Just as clients can experience unpleasant emotions, they can identify unpleasant odors. Normally, the limbic system is activated in response to unpleasant odors. Significantly different, people with schizophrenia use their prefrontal regions to recognize unpleasant stimuli, leading to overactivation of these areas. The awareness of unpleasant and potentially dangerous external stimuli may cause individuals to feel threatened and may give rise to paranoid thinking (Crespo-Facorro et al., 2001).

CONCOMITANT DISORDERS

Many people who suffer from schizophrenia use *alcohol* or *drugs* in an effort to self-medicate and feel better. More than 50 percent of people with schizophrenia have problems with alcohol or drugs at some point during their illness. Prompt recognition and treatment of this *dual diagnosis* problem is essential for effective treatment. Substance-related disorders are discussed in Chapter 15.

Suicide accounts for the majority of premature deaths among people with schizophrenia. It is estimated that as many as half of this population experience suicidal ideation, make suicide attempts, or both. Ten percent are successful suicides. Risk factors include more severe illness, frequent relapses, and significant depressive symptoms, especially hopelessness (Radomsky et al., 1999).

Twenty-five percent of people with schizophrenia also experience obsessions and compulsions and of this group, 8 percent can be diagnosed with *obsessive–compulsive disorder*. Most typically, people are preoccupied with the content of their delusions and may ruminate for hours over their upsetting thoughts. Twenty-five percent of people with schizophrenia also experience *depressive episodes*. These depressive symptoms are more likely to occur early in the course of the schizophrenic disorder (Nahas, Molloy, Risch, & George, 2000).

CAUSATIVE THEORIES

Schizophrenia is not a single disorder but rather a syndrome with multiple variations and multiple etiologies, both of which are complex and inadequately understood. In some, a genetic defect may contribute to abnormal development of the brain or a neurochemical malfunction, while in other cases factors such as nutrition, toxins, or trauma might interact in a genetically vulnerable person, resulting in schizophrenia. In other cases the cause may be completely environmental, such as viral infections or birth complications.

Genetic Factors

It is well recognized that there is a genetic component in schizophrenia and it is thought that 85 percent of the susceptibility to schizophrenia may be genetic in origin. However, the exact genetic vulnerability is not known, as no single gene has been identified as a risk factor for schizophrenia. It is likely that a number of genes are involved and that different families may have different genes involved. There may also be a different pattern of inheritance in early-onset versus late-onset type. It is likely that the early-onset type has a higher genetic load for schizophrenia (Paris, 1999).

A person has an 8 percent risk of schizophrenia if a sibling has the disorder, a 13 percent risk if one parent is affected, a 10 to 15 percent risk of sharing the disorder with a dizygotic twin, a 40 to 50 percent risk if both parents are affected, and a 50 percent risk if a monozygotic twin has schizophrenia. In addition, 21 percent of first-degree relatives have schizotypal personality disorder or other traits in the schizophrenic syndrome (Cadenhead et al., 2000; Harvey, 2001) (see Figure 14.2 ■).

In monozygotic twins, prenatal factors do not always affect each twin to the same extent. Because the hands are formed at the same time cells are migrating to the cerebral cortex during the second trimester of pregnancy, they have been a site for indirectly studying brain development. In studying sets of twins in which one has schizophrenia and the other does not, it was found that affected twins had a number of small deformities in their hands and greater differences in their fingerprints compared to their siblings. There was also a significant prenatal size difference between the twins during the second trimester. Conditions that could result in brain injury at this stage of development include anemia, anoxia, ischemia, maternal alcohol or drug abuse, toxin exposure, or viral infection (Tarrant & Jones, 2000).

Neurobiologic Factors

Neurodevelopment studies demonstrate evidence of abnormal brain development. The basic flaw seems to be that certain nerve cells migrate to the wrong areas when the brain is first taking shape, leaving small regions of the brain permanently out of place or miswired. In some cases, the neurons of the cortex may be deficient. From a developmental perspective we do not know whether these cells form normally and then fail to thrive or whether they are malformed from the beginning.

Studies also show higher than expected occurrences of prenatal disruptions and obstetrical complications with increased risk of psychiatric disorders in childhood and adult life. One hypothesis is that exposure to nutritional deficiency during fetal life may be a risk factor for schizophrenia. Other risk factors include fetal hypoxia, exposure to infections during gestation, and fetal growth retardation. It is believed that these risk factors may be related to brain damage (Flashman, McAllister, Andreasen, & Saykin, 2000; Harvey, 2001; Rosso et al., 2000).

You may be wondering why, if schizophrenia begins in utero, does it not manifest for 20 years. Recent studies show that some people with schizophrenia may have early signs that are overlooked or misunderstood. For example, a child might sit up a month later than other children or speak three months later. These signs may indicate a slight maturational lag in brain function that is later associated with schizophrenia. Later in childhood, there may be evidence of lagging development and cognitive perceptual abnormalities.

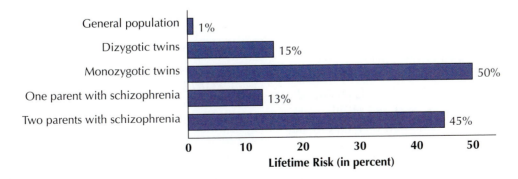

FIGURE 14.2 ■ Average risk of developing schizophrenia.

SOURCES: Cadenhead, K. S., Swerdlow, N. R., Shafer, K. M., Diaz, M., & Braff, D. L. (2000). Sensory gating deficits assessed by the P50 event-related potential in subjects with schizotypal personality disorder. *American Journal of Psychiatry, 157*(1), 55–59; and Harvey, P. D. (2001). Vulnerability to schizophrenia in adulthood. In R. E. Ingram & J. M. Price (Eds.), *Vulnerability to psychopathology* (pp. 355–381). New York: Guilford Press.

One factor related to the delay in the appearance of significant symptoms may be the myelin sheath, which does not form on the outside of many brain cells until late adolescence. Between the ages of 16 and 22, there are also progressive changes in cortical interactions, especially between the left prefrontal and temporal regions. This failure of the cortex to reorganize during adolescence may be the final neurodevelopmental failure of schizophrenia (Sowell et al., 2000).

Neurochemical factors likely involve dopamine (DA), serotonin (5-HT), norepinephrine (NE), glutamate (glu), and gamma-aminobutyric acid (GABA) neurotransmission. At times, neurotransmitters work together (synergistically) to trigger the same biochemical reaction, while at other times they act as antagonists, with one inhibiting the action of another. Glu, involved in learning and memory, may be responsible for some of the cognitive symptoms. In addition, glu is necessary for the breakdown of DA and other transmitters, which affects the efficiency of prefrontal information processing. Glu receptors have a role in regulating the migration and pruning of neurons during brain development and thus may play a role in structural abnormalities that have been seen in schizophrenia. Excessively high levels of NE are associated with positive symptoms, while paranoid symptoms have been related to increased DA activity. No single neurotransmitter is clearly responsible for schizophrenia. The important concept may be homeostasis: the absolute level of any neurotransmitter being much less important than its relative level with respect to all other transmitters. There may also be an undiscovered neurochemical factor yet to be found. It will be a long time before this is understood clearly (Goff & Coyle, 2001; Volk, Austin, Pierri, Sampson, & Lewis, 2001).

A new area of research involves the *fat composition* of cell membranes. The neuronal membrane consists of two layers of fatty molecules, which determines the flexibility of the membrane. Soft and pliable membranes communicate more smoothly than do stiff and rigid membranes. People with schizophrenia are depleted of both DHA (docosahexaenoic acid found in omega-3-type fish oil) and AA (arachidonic acid). These deficiencies may be related to the negative symptoms of schizophrenia (Carper, 2000).

On a larger scale, new brain imaging studies have revealed abnormalities of *brain structure* in schizophre-

nia. Although no single brain region has been found to be involved in the pathology of schizophrenia, the areas most noted for abnormalities include the prefrontal cortex, the temporal lobes, the hippocampus, the limbic system, the thalamus, and the ventricles. The reason people with schizophrenia may not "look the same" clinically may be a function of individual deviations in brain structure. In some cases, there is decreased tissue volume in specific areas, in others there is disrupted cerebral blood flow, in some cases there is decreased utilization of glucose and oxygen, and in others there is increased ventricular size (Gilbert et al., 2001; Perlstein, Carter, Noll, & Cohen, 2001). See Box 14.1 for a list of brain abnormalities.

An example of one deviation is that decreased blood flow to the thalamus may affect the ability of the brain to filter sensory signals, causing the person to be flooded with sensory information (refer back to Figure 14.1). Changes in cerebral blood flow suggest abnormalities in the density, size, or configuration of blood

---

BOX 14.1

CNS Abnormalities in Schizophrenia

Decreased Volume
- Temporal lobes
- Hippocampus
- Prefrontal cortex
- Limbic system
- Thalamus

Decreased Cerebral Blood Flow
- Temporal lobes
- Basal ganglia
- Thalamus

Decreased Blood Glucose and Oxygen Utilization
- Frontal lobes
- Basal ganglia

Decreased Activity
- Prefrontal cortex

Decreased Nicotinic Receptors
- Hippocampus

Increased Ventricular Size

vessels in the person with schizophrenia. Structural abnormalities are really only the end result of some abnormal process and do not tell us much about what that process may be (Sigmundsson et al., 2001).

For some people with schizophrenia, there is a deficiency of **nicotinic receptors** in the hippocampus, an area of the brain important in attention to new sensory stimuli and memory formation. Clients who smoke may be self-medicating with nicotine, which improves their attentiveness and ability to lay down memories.

The *diathesis-stress model* shows the psychosis of schizophrenia as a final common path of neurodevelopmental, neurochemical, and structural decompensation. This is a multiple hit model. In other words, there must be a genetic vulnerability and environmental risk factors, which are then combined with maturational changes or life events that trigger the onset of schizophrenia. The more protective factors a person has, the less the chance he or she has of developing the disorder. Only a few people have such a strong genetic vulnerability that schizophrenia is virtually inevitable. The majority of the population have little or no risk for schizophrenia. In between, are the people who may develop the disorder if stressed enough but who could also survive without schizophrenia if not sufficiently stressed (Siris, 2000; Zorrilla & Zeste, 2000).

PSYCHOPHARMACOLOGICAL INTERVENTIONS

Negative symptoms impose great suffering on people by interfering with their psychosocial functioning. Newer or atypical antipsychotic medications are characterized by:

- Effectiveness in decreasing the negative as well as eliminating the positive symptoms of schizophrenia
- Effectiveness for many people who are not responsive to conventional antipsychotic agents
- Effectiveness for people who also experience depressive symptoms
- A significantly lower incidence of extrapyramidal side effects, which increases clients' ability to continue on the medication.

When added to antipsychotic medications, mood-stabilizing agents such as lithium carbonate, Tegretol (carbamazepine), and Depakote (valproate) enhance

CRITICAL THINKING

Ricardo is a 24-year-old client who is being treated for schizoaffective disorder. He is depressed, withdrawn, and disheveled. He often looks upward and listens intently. He does not offer conversation and reacts in a hostile manner when spoken to, while retreating to the corner of his room.

Mohammed is a 19-year-old client on the same psychiatric unit who is being treated for schizophrenia. Mohammed has a flat affect, paces his room for hours, stomps on spiders that are not present, seldom socializes, and often accuses others of trying to steal his clothing.

1. In what ways does Ricardo's illness differ from Mohammed's?

2. What are the positive and the negative symptoms of schizophrenia?

3. What data support the positive symptoms of schizophrenia for Ricardo? For Mohammed?

4. What data support the negative symptoms of schizophrenia for Ricardo? For Mohammed?

5. Both Ricardo and Mohammed are being treated with antipsychotic drugs that can produce tardive dyskinesia. How will you know if either of these clients is developing this drug side effect?

6. If you were Ricardo's or Mohammed's nurse, how would you intervene during their chronic hallucinatory episodes?

For an additional Case Study, please refer to the Companion Web site for this book.

the effectiveness of the response and improve negative symptoms specifically. They are also effective for people experiencing affective symptoms. Benzodiazepines may also be used as adjuncts to antipsychotic medications. Studies have demonstrated reductions in anxiety, agitation, and psychotic symptoms with the use of these agents. See Chapter 8 for a more detailed explanation of these ancillary medications.

The addition of estrogen in women with acute psychotic episodes often provides a more rapid decrease in positive symptoms as well as a decrease in overall symptoms.

The use of medications in older clients is problematic at times. These individuals are likely to have other

BOX 14.2

Beliefs and Values in Psychiatric Rehabilitation

Beliefs

- The most severely disabled psychiatric client has a potential for productivity.
- The opportunity to be gainfully employed is a generative force in human beings.
- Work can enhance self-esteem and reduce symptoms of mental illness.
- People require opportunities to be together socially.

Values

- Hope, optimism
- Wellness
- Choices
- Self-determination
- Individual responsibility
- Compassion

medical illnesses and to be taking multiple medications. Because of their age, they are at increased risk for drug interactions and side effects. Low doses of the atypical antipsychotics are the drugs of choice.

MULTIDISCIPLINARY INTERVENTIONS

Psychiatric Rehabilitation

The field of **psychiatric** or **psychosocial rehabilitation** grew out of a need to create opportunities for people suffering from psychiatric disabilities. The rehabilitation approach emphasizes the development of skills and supports necessary for successful living, learning, and working in the community. This approach creates *collaborative partnerships* with all interested people—consumers, families, friends, and mental health providers. It is assumed that the consumer will be "in charge" with regard to setting goals for where and how to live, work, learn, socialize, and recreate (see Box 14.2). Rehabilitation is a process, not a quick fix. It is also different than the traditional approach to long-term clients, which assumed that people with schizophrenia could not make decisions and would continue to deteriorate in spite of interventions. We now know that a substantial number of

people with schizophrenia make good adjustments and lead satisfactory lives.

People with mental illness differ little from the general population. They want work that is meaningful and self-enhancing and the opportunity to socialize with others. Psychiatric rehabilitation is anchored in the values of hope and optimism that people can grow, learn, and make changes in their lives. Other values include the promotion of choices, self-determination, and individual responsibility. The essential element of self-help is *power*. People who are psychiatrically disabled need power and control in their relationships with professionals, in their own lives, and in the way resources are allocated. This allows them to take personal responsibility for where they are in their lives and where they are going.

As a nurse who functions as a resource for clients, you must not only be competent but also compassionate and caring. This includes searching for talents and skills until you find them, even when they are obscured by multiple relapses and low self-esteem. Your role is to teach skills, to coach skills as needed in a variety of social and work situations, and to identify supports in the community of choice. In this way you will promote independent living and successful coping for people with psychiatric disabilities (Carling, 1995; Farrell & Deeds, 1997; Palmer-Erbs, 1996).

Group Therapy

Group therapy is an effective psychosocial treatment modality for persons with schizophrenia. It helps prevent the withdrawal and social isolation that may occur for people who are psychiatrically disabled. For people who live alone, the group may be their primary opportunity to relate to others. The group setting also provides an opportunity to discuss and help each other solve problems in everyday living, employment difficulties, or interpersonal conflicts. There are several types of group therapy. Some groups are highly structured, while others may be more spontaneous. Some may have a very narrow topic range such as assertiveness training, while others may have a broader range such as general problems in living in the community. Groups focus on peer support, with an emphasis on development skills and changing behavior. Groups are also used for teaching and social support. See Chapter 10 for more information on group therapy.

Assertive Community Treatment (ACT)

People who are psychiatrically disabled are often ill-prepared to find and maintain the multiple services they need in order to function in the community. A new approach to help clients is the assertive community treatment (ACT) program. Clients are assigned to a specific multidisciplinary team that delivers all services when and where the client needs them. The main goal of the program is to prevent rehospitalization through provision of comprehensive integrated community services. The ACT program provides 24-hour coverage, including emergencies. Studies show that ACT reduces time spent in the hospital, improves housing stability, decreases symptoms, and improves quality of life (Mueser et al., 2001). Various other treatment settings within the community are discussed in Chapter 4.

ALTERNATIVE THERAPIES

Transcranial Magnetic Stimulation

Transcranial magnetic stimulation (TMS) is the use of a magnetic field that passes through the skull, which causes cells in the cerebral cortex to fire. More studies have been conducted in the use of TMS for depression than for schizophrenia. Initial studies indicate that TMS of the left temporoparietal area may decrease the frequency and duration of auditory hallucinations and may modulate other symptoms of schizophrenia (Nahas et al., 2000).

Omega-3 Fatty Acids

Those individuals who may have a deficiency of omega-3 fatty acids will find the addition of fish oil helpful. It may not be that people with schizophrenia have a low intake but rather that they need more to overcome a metabolic disorder that uses up essential fatty acids at a faster rate. The recommended dose is 5 grams per day, which is usually seven or eight capsules. The maximum dose is 15 grams daily. Taking the capsules at night and with orange juice cuts down on the fishy aftertaste (Carper, 2000).

Aromatherapy

Olfactory receptors are the only sensory pathways that open directly to the brain. Nerve cells relay this information directly to the limbic system, influencing emotions and behavior. Inhaling essential oils through the use of a diffuser or using essential oils in massage may be beneficial in inducing a sense of calmness. The following oils are the most helpful: basil, bergamot, chamomile, frankincense, juniper, lavender, lemon balm, and sandalwood. Coriander increases memory and mental function.

Acupuncture

The Chinese claim to have successfully treated schizophrenia with acupuncture. Research in Western medical practice is just beginning in this area. A six-month study in Texas showed a drop in the length of hospital stays for acupuncture-treated individuals (Gerber, 2000).

Complementary/Alternative Therapies

How to Help Clients Improve Body Boundaries and Safe Touch

Massage is an effective method of reducing stress and tension that usually leads to a feeling of relaxation. Touch is a basic need, as necessary for growth and development as food, clothing, and shelter. Sometimes people are "touch starved" because they have few intimate relationships in their lives. This exercise is designed to help you nurture yourself through the sense of touch. It is also designed to help you improve your sense of the boundaries of your body.

1. Use olive oil or sesame oil for this exercise. If possible, warm a quarter cup of oil in the microwave for 10 to 15 seconds being careful not to overheat it.

2. Use one tablespoon of warm oil and rub it into your scalp. Use small, circular motions with the flat of your hand. Massage the forehead from side to side and gently massage your temples using circular motions. Gently rub the outside of the ears and the front and back of the neck.

3. Using more oil, massage your arms and hands.

4. Using more oil, massage your legs. Massage each toe with your fingertips. Vigorously massage the soles of your feet.

5. Sit quietly for a few seconds to relax and then shower or bathe as usual.

SOURCE: Adapted from Chopra, D. (1991). Perfect health. New York: Harmony Books.

NURSING PROCESS

Assessment

The assessment of clients' responses to their illness and their functional status includes assessment of clients' reports, family or caregiver reports, and direct observation of performance. Clients who are not acutely ill are usually able to provide accurate information about their past history with mental illness and their current experiences. It is helpful to ask consumers under what conditions the symptoms improve or worsen. Ask clients how they cope with their symptoms so you can help them maintain and strengthen their effective solutions. Identification of functional abilities and disabilities leads to the formulation of nursing diagnoses (Hagen & Mitchell, 2001).

If clients are acutely ill, it may be difficult to obtain information directly from them. This is especially true for those who are experiencing delusions and hallucinations. Family members, roommates, friends, group home supervisors, or case managers may be the initial data source when there is an admission to the acute care setting. The Focused Nursing Assessment feature provides questions that can be used in the home, the residential or group home setting, or in the acute care setting.

Diagnosis

There are many potential nursing diagnoses for clients suffering from schizophrenia. In synthesizing the assessment data, consider how well clients are functioning in daily life, what their skills and talents are, how stable their affect is, how well they are able to communicate, how well they are getting along with others, and how well they function at work. See the Nursing Diagnoses with NOC & NIC feature for some of the more common nursing diagnoses you may be applying to your clients.

Outcome Identification and Goals

Based on the assessment data, you select outcomes appropriate to the nursing diagnoses. See the Nursing Diagnoses with NOC & NIC feature for outcomes associated with the nursing diagnoses.

Client goals are specific behavioral measures by which you, clients, and significant others identify as realistic and attainable. The following are examples of some of the goals appropriate to people with schizophrenia:

- Communicates clearly
- Completes activities of daily living (ADLs) appropriately
- Exhibits increased attention span
- Makes appropriate decisions
- Affect is appropriate to the situation
- Denies hallucinations
- Verbalizes logical thought processes
- Interacts well with others
- Develops occupational skills

Nursing Interventions

Nurses have many opportunities to assist people with schizophrenia in a variety of settings as previously described. These contacts may be long-term relationships or may be during crisis periods of time. It is important that clients identify their priority concerns if the plan of care is to be effective. Change is more likely to happen when clients are invested in the treatment process.

Families, significant others, or caregivers should be actively involved in the plan of care and be taught to implement many of these interventions. See the Nursing Diagnoses with NOC & NIC feature for interventions associated with the diagnoses and outcomes.

Behavioral: Communication Enhancement

Complex Relationship Building

The nature of the nurse–client relationship is one of the most effective nursing interventions. With rapport, communication, and trust, we are able to help our clients meet the outcome criteria they have identified. Review the material on communicating with clients in Chapter 2. When we listen to clients, accept them for who they are, and understand their perspective, we are more likely to help empower them and thereby help them achieve their highest level of functioning.

Behavior Assessment

What are your responsibilities:
    At home?
    At work?
    At school?

*Signs of hyperactivity

*Evidence of decreased activity level

*Self-care activities

*Behaviors suggestive of hallucinations

Affective Assessment

What kinds of activities/situations give you:
    Pleasure?
    Anxiety?
    Anger?
    Guilt?

*Evidence of problems with affect:
    Inappropriate
    Overreactive
    Blunted
    Flat

*Signs of anhedonia

*Expressions of hostility

Cognitive Assessment

Have you ever heard voices? Are you hearing voices now? What do the voices say to you? What feelings are associated with the voices?

Have you ever seen things other people don't see? What things do you see? What feelings are associated with seeing things?

Do you believe that you are someone very important?

Do you feel anyone is trying to harm you?

Do you feel anyone is controlling you?

Do you think about religion a lot?

Do you believe that you are very guilty for something you have done?

Do you think anything abnormal is happening to your body?

Do you think people are talking about you often?

Do you believe others can hear your thoughts?

Do you believe others can take away your thoughts?

Do you believe others can put thoughts into your head?

Do you have thoughts of harming yourself? Harming others?

Have you ever thought you have special powers that other people do not have?

Sociocultural Assessment

Are you employed?

What are your living arrangements?

*Observations by the nurse

NURSING DIAGNOSES with NOC & NIC

Clients with Schizophrenia

DIAGNOSIS	OUTCOMES	INTERVENTIONS
Altered thought process related to disruptions in cognitive processes such as delusions, loose association, concrete thinking	**Distorted Thought Process:** Self-restraint of disruption in perception, thought processes, and thought control	Complex Relationship Building Active Listening Delusion Management
Social isolation related to withdrawal, preoccupation with symptoms, lack of a supportive network, negative reaction by others to client's social behavior	**Social Interaction Skills:** An individual's use of effective interaction behaviors	Socialization Enhancement
Self-esteem disturbance related to feeling different from others, chronic nature of the disorder	**Self-Esteem:** Personal judgment of self-worth	Self-Esteem Enhancement
Anxiety related to environmental stimuli, reduced contact with reality	**Anxiety Control:** Personal actions to eliminate or reduce feelings of apprehension and tension from an unidentifiable source	Anxiety Reduction
Knowledge deficit related to not understanding disease process; inability to stay on medications	**Knowledge:** Disease Process: Extent of understanding conveyed about a specific disease process **Knowledge:** Medication: Extent of understanding conveyed about the safe use of medication	Teaching: Disease Process Teaching: Prescribed Medications
Fatigue related to hyperactivity	**Knowledge:** Energy Conservation: Extent of understanding conveyed about energy conservation techniques	Energy Management

Active Listening

Sometimes clients are not able to hold thoughts together enough for you to comprehend what is being said. They may not remember how they started a sentence or where their thoughts were taking them (loose association). They are often more able to understand others than to make themselves understood. When this occurs, *interrupt politely* but firmly and ask a question that will help them communicate in a more direct manner. Say something like, "I'm not understanding what you are saying. Could we try that again?" *Listening for themes* in the conversation may help you understand

DIAGNOSIS	OUTCOMES	INTERVENTIONS
Bathing/hygiene self-care deficit related to an inability to remember steps in self-care; low motivation	*Self-Care*: Activities of daily living (ADLs): Ability to perform the most basic physical tasks and personal care activities	Self-Care Assistance
High risk for violence, self-directed, related to command hallucinations	*Suicide Self-Restraint*: Ability to refrain from gestures and attempts at killing self	Suicide Prevention
Sensory-perceptual alterations related to disruptions in temporal lobe causing command hallucinations	*Distorted Thought Control*: Self-restraint of disruption in perception, thought processes, and thought content	Hallucination Management
High risk for violence, directed at others related to suspiciousness, fear	*Aggression Control*: Self-restraint of assaultive, combative, or destructive behavior toward others	Violence Prevention
Caregiver role strain related to fear of unknown, lack of social support, need to care for family member, inappropriate behavior on part of client	*Caregiver Well-Being*: Primary care provider's satisfaction with health and life circumstances	Family Integrity Promotion Family Involvement

SOURCES: Johnson, M., Maas, M., & Moorhead, S. (2000). *Nursing outcomes classification* (NOC) (2nd ed.). St. Louis, MO: Mosby; and McCloskey, J. C., & Bulechek, G. M. (1996). *Nursing interventions classification* (NIC) (2nd ed.). St. Louis, MO: Mosby. North American Nursing Diagnosis Association (1999). *Nursing diagnoses, definitions, and classification 1999–2000*. Philadelphia: Author

the current concerns of the person. When you try to understand the world the client is experiencing, the person is more likely to feel you are being helpful.

Sensory overload or the inability to screen out unimportant stimuli is frustrating and disorienting to clients and interferes with their abilities to listen and communicate. You can teach clients to decrease environmental stimuli by avoiding noise and confusion, including large crowds or large family gatherings.

Socialization Enhancement

Social difficulties frequently accompany schizophrenia, and social skills training is an appropriate nursing intervention. Because of the stigma attached to mental disorders and especially schizophrenia, consumers have had fewer opportunities to develop and practice social skills. This inexperience contributes to inappropriate responses when interacting with others. Poor social functioning has been found to be an important predictor of relapse and rehospitalization (Mueser et al., 2001).

After specific skill deficits are identified, *training strategies* are designed to reduce these deficits and improve the level of functioning. Social skills training is a series of highly structured and organized sessions of practice in basic skills usually conducted in a group format. Specific skills include nonverbal behaviors (facial expression, eye contact), paralanguage (voice loudness, sounds that are not words), verbal content (appropriateness of what is said), and interactive balance (amount of time each person spends talking).

Group leaders *model the appropriate skills*. Through role-play and social reinforcement, members learn the same behaviors, step by step. Social skills training includes such areas as how to initiate a conversation, how to express ideas and feelings appropriately, how to avoid topics that are not appropriate for a casual conversation, how to ask about job openings, and how to interview for a job. The goal of social skills training is to improve social functioning by decreasing problems of daily living, employment, leisure, and relationships. The ability to enjoy interpersonal relationships is a dimension of quality of life that is very important to address with people suffering from schizophrenia. Repeat practice can result in improvements in important areas of social adjustment, leading to less withdrawal and isolation. See Chapter 10 for more information on social skills training.

Behavioral: Coping Assistance

Self-Esteem Enhancement

Many people with schizophrenia desperately desire to be "normal" and thus suffer from low self-esteem. *Self-esteem exercises* can be implemented one to one and in group settings. In a one-to-one exercise, you might ask clients to write out or verbalize their positive qualities. Keeping a self-esteem journal is appropriate for some clients. Look for opportunities to give positive reinforcement. In a group setting, clients may be asked to share their own positive qualities as well as to recognize those of their peers. Group experience is an opportunity to learn how to give and receive positive feedback.

A number of group exercises promote self-esteem. One is having clients make a collage. Materials include magazines, scissors, glue, and blank paper. Have clients look for pictures that tell something about themselves and their interests, cut them out, and glue them on the paper. Have each person take a turn in describing the significance of the collage to the other group members. You can emphasize the positive qualities each collage reveals.

Another self-esteem exercise focuses on the image we present to others and who we really are. Give group members two sheets of paper and crayons or markers. On one sheet of paper, have them draw the "real me," and on the other sheet, the "me others see." Each group member then presents the "me others see" and receives feedback from their peers as to the accuracy of this perception. Then the "real me" is presented and feedback is once again given. This exercise is most successful with clients who have some ability to think abstractly.

Behavioral: Psychological: Comfort Promotion

Anxiety Reduction

Some persons with schizophrenia experience periodic symptoms of anxiety. Since anxiety can be contagious, remain calm and reassuring as you interact with clients. Your presence may help the anxious person feel more secure. Using relaxation techniques or meditation, reducing or eliminating caffeine intake, and moderating environmental stimuli, often lower levels of anxiety. You may encourage clients to go for a walk, work at a simple concrete task, or play a noncompetitive game such as catch. Further interventions are found in Chapter 11.

Behavioral: Patient Education

Teaching: Disease Process

Nursing believes that clients should be actively involved in the management of their illness. Thus, a *psychoeducation program* is an extremely important nursing intervention. The goal is to teach consumers about their illness and to cover the important behavioral, affective, cognitive, perceptual, and social problems they commonly experience. Another facet of psychoeducation is teaching clients to identify early signs of relapse. What exactly those early warning signs are vary from person to person but are repetitive for any one individual. Since early intervention may prevent a relapse, this self-surveillance strategy allows people to influence the course of the disease (McCann, 2001).

Teaching: Prescribed Medication

Some consumers will be unhappy or frustrated with their medication. Discontinuation of medication is a significant factor in relapse. Helping clients understand the need for medication is an important nursing intervention. You may have clients explore the pros and cons of continuing or discontinuing medication. Help them review how medication may be useful in helping them make progress toward personal goals.

The most common reasons for stopping medications include denial of the disorder and the desire to be "normal," an unwillingness to take the amount prescribed when they feel better, self-medicating with drugs or alcohol, and the distress associated with side effects. A recent study indicates that clients' attitudes toward medication may be more positive than health care professionals have previously thought. The majority of consumers recognize that medications are important for their mental health and are necessary for functioning within the community (Mueser et al., 2001).

Assist clients in developing a routine for taking their medication that fits into their daily habits. It may be using a weekly medication box with places for morning, noon, and evening medications. It may be using meal times as natural prompts to remind them of medication. It may be a chart on the wall. Whatever system the client believes will help can usually be adapted for self-management.

Physiological: Basic: Activity and Exercise Management
Energy Management

Some clients pace much of the day and are in danger of exhaustion and must be monitored for evidence of excess physical fatigue. Set limits on hyperactivity by providing firm direction in taking short, frequent rest breaks. They often will manage this better if you stay with them for the designated rest time. Limit environmental stimuli to facilitate relaxation. Design diversional activities that are calming and restful. Clients should monitor their nutritional intake to ensure they have adequate energy resources (McCloskey & Bulechek, 1996).

Physiological: Basic: Self-Care Facilitation
Self-Care Assistance

Some clients will need assistance with self-care because of a change in activity level, confusion, or a perceptual impairment. They may need reminding or assistance with bathing, grooming, personal hygiene, and dressing. This assistance may be in the form of a list of step-by-step directions in the bathroom or bedroom, or gentle reminders such as "It's time for you to brush your teeth," "I think the dress you have chosen is not appropriate for work," or "Did you shower this morning?" Other self-care activities might involve household tasks such as cleaning, cooking, shopping, or money management. As clients progress toward their goals, they are rewarded with greater responsibility and more privileges. Although some clients may never live independently, they often can improve the quality of their lives through increased autonomy.

Safety: Crisis Management
Suicide Prevention

An important priority of care is client *safety*. Command hallucinations may order clients to harm, mutilate, or kill themselves or others. Others have suffered from delusions so intensely for so long that suicide seems like the only way to escape the pain of being persecuted or controlled by others. You must carefully assess for evidence of self-harm and direct care toward protecting clients until they can protect themselves. See Chapter 20 for care of a client who is suicidal.

Safety: Risk Management
Hallucination Management

The experience of hallucinations can be especially troublesome for the person who does not have anyone to talk to about them. Discussion of hallucinations is important to the development of reality-testing skills. Look and listen for clues that the person may be hallucinating, such as grinning or laughing inappropriately, talking to someone whom you cannot see, or slowed verbal responses. Ask the person to describe what is happening. If the person asks if you hear or see what they do, point out simply that you are not experiencing the same stimuli. The goal is to guide the person through the experience and let them know what is actually happening in the environment. Help the individual describe needs that may be reflected in the content of the hallucination. These needs may include having power and control of decisions that affect daily life, the ability to express anger, and self-esteem. For chronic hallucinations, the person might keep a calendar of when hallucinations occur and how long they last in an effort to identify the triggers.

The person experiencing acute hallucinations has no voluntary control over the brain malfunction that is causing this symptom and needs immediate nursing interventions. Do not leave the client alone since the inability to sort out reality may overwhelm her or his ability to cope. You may need to talk slightly louder than usual, but use very short, simple phrases using the person's first name. The person may not be able to hear you but will see that your mouth is moving and know that you are trying to communicate. See Chapter 9 for further information on reduction of hallucinations.

Ask clients what coping methods they have developed for hallucination management so that you can support their efforts. Some people talk with family members, friends, or professionals, some get busy with other activities to take their mind off the hallucinations, and some exercise as a form of distraction. Ineffective coping behaviors include eating or smoking more than usual, using drugs or alcohol, or acting out against other people. Help clients identify effective coping strategies to replace the ineffective strategies. More important than the presence of hallucinations is the ability or inability to effectively cope with the experience.

Clients may wish to become involved in an international self-help movement called "*voice hearer groups*." The goal of the group is to provide support and share practical ways to cope with problems related to experiencing hallucinations. For example, members in one group suggested using a cell phone (real or fake) to respond to the voices when out in public. Rather than being ridiculed for hallucinating, they blend in with others who are using cell phones. See Community Resources for more information on this group (Hagen & Mitchell, 2001).

Delusion Management

Persons experiencing delusions have difficulty processing language; therefore, nonverbal communication is critically important. Approach the person with calmness and empathy. It is very normal to feel confused by a delusion. You must carefully assess the content of the delusion without appearing to probe or patronize the client. Do not attempt to logically explain the delusion nor underestimate the power of a delusion and the person's inability to distinguish the delusion from reality. Assess the duration, frequency, and intensity of the delusion. Since delusions are often triggered by stress, correlate the onset of the delusion with the onset of stress. See Chapter 9 for further information on management of delusions.

Fleeting delusions often will disappear in a short time frame. Fixed delusions may have to be temporarily avoided. Respond to the underlying feelings rather than the illogical nature of the delusion. This will encourage discussion of fears, anxieties, or anger without judging the person. Quietly listen and then give guidance for the immediate task at hand. The client may find it helpful to engage in distracting activities as a way to stop focusing on the delusion.

Environmental Management: Violence Prevention

Some clients may be at high risk for violence directed at others when they misperceive communication from others or when they perceive that they themselves are being threatened. Encouraging clients to *talk out* rather than act out feelings will assist in maintaining control over behavior. Clients often can identify triggering factors such as a noisy environment, unfamiliar people, or other anxiety-provoking situations. If clients begin to escalate and become more agitated, it helps to *remain calm*, use a low tone of voice, give them personal space, and avoid physical contact with them. Set limits on aggressive behavior. Depending on the clinical setting, seclusion may become necessary. See Chapter 9 for further interventions with clients who are at high risk for violence.

The suspicious client is always on the lookout for danger and functions at a steady level of hyperalertness. Avoid frightening these individuals, who may strike out to protect themselves from perceived danger. Always give them plenty of *personal space* and never touch them without specific permission. Because they are hyperalert to everything in the environment, be careful not to behave in ways that could be misinterpreted. A suspicious client could misperceive two people talking together in a soft tone of voice as "They're talking about me." A group of nurses sharing a laugh could be misperceived as "They're all laughing at me."

Among the client population, African Americans are more likely to be perceived as being violent or dangerous than clients from other ethnic groups. This is true even when independent assessment of violent behavior showed they were significantly less likely to be violent. As a result of this racist misperception, African American clients receive more doses, more injections, and higher 24-hour doses of psychotropic drugs than do Euro-Americans (Lawson, 2000).

Family: Life Span Care
Family Integrity

Schizophrenia often strikes adolescents or young adults, leaving their parents confused and frightened. Whether the child is living at home or away, employed or unemployed, parents report feeling a never-ending sense of responsibility for their child, which is at times overwhelming. Parents are likely to experience sorrow and grief as they begin to deal with the impact of their child's illness. Knowing that this is likely to occur, nurses can offer anticipatory guidance and interventions. Parents desire information and some level of involvement in their child's treatment plan. They often seek advice on how to cope with the day-to-day challenges they face, what they might expect in the future, and sources of community support. The question that health care professionals have to answer is how to include the family within the context of client confidentiality.

Family Involvement

Because so many people are afraid of and uninformed about schizophrenia, many families try to hide it from friends and deal with it on their own. We must reach out to these families and offer them support and education. *Family education* often is conducted in a group setting, which enables families to begin to build a support network. You must help them understand that they are not responsible for causing their loved one to develop schizophrenia and have no reason to feel guilty. They need to learn about the nature of schizophrenia and the variety of available treatment programs. They need practical solutions on how to manage on a day-to-day basis. You can assist families in achieving a balance between being protective and encouraging independence. For example, families should try to do things with them rather than for them, so that clients are able to regain their sense of self-confidence. Increased family education often decreases caregiver burden and improves the quality of life for all family members (Czuchta & McCay, 2001). See Box 14.3 for family education.

Families can encourage their loved ones to stick with the treatment program, take their medications, and

---

BOX 14.3

Family Education

- Information about the disorder
- Managing symptoms
- Expectations during recovery
- Role of medications
- Handling crises
- Warning signs of suicide
- Early signs of relapse
- Housing and social resources
- Self-help groups

---

avoid alcohol and drugs. It is important to recognize *early signs of relapse* to prevent acute episodes and rehospitalizations. Family members can ask the person with schizophrenia to agree that, if they notice warning signs of a relapse, it is okay for them to contact the physician so that the medication can be adjusted in an effort to stabilize the condition. All threats of suicide should be taken very seriously. Families should have an identified contact person they can call for help. If the situation becomes desperate, the family should call 911.

The family may need help in *setting expectations* and limits on inappropriate behavior. The positive symptoms of schizophrenia can cause a great deal of family stress. That is also true of the negative symptoms, which are often misinterpreted as laziness or uncooperativeness.

To prevent or delay relapse, it is critical to intervene with families who have high expressed emotion (EE), that is, those who are highly critical, hostile, and overinvolved. Consumers who live in high EE situations have much higher relapse rates than those living in low EE environments. Teach family members to *moderate displays of all emotion* in an effort to provide a neutral emotional climate. They may need assistance in defining and reshaping appropriate boundaries (McCann, 2001).

It is totally within the rights of a family to decide that a member who has an illness must get treatment for it. The family should also establish appropriate rules that must be followed. If the client is unwilling to comply, the family may choose to look for alternative living arrangements. For more information, see Box 14.3 and the Community Resources and Books for Clients and Families features at the end of this chapter.

CLINICAL INTERACTIONS   A Client with Schizophrenia

Sara is 41 years old and has suffered with schizophrenia for the past 15 years. She has a history of childhood sexual abuse. She has been able to live at home with her husband except for a few brief periods of hospitalization. Lately, her thinking has become more disorganized, and her therapist has recommended that she come to the day treatment program. The themes of the interaction below include raping and hurting little children and a desire to return to infancy, a period of time when she felt safe and cared for. In the interaction, you will see evidence of:

■ Labile affect
■ Loose associations
■ Symbolism (attached at waist)
■ Somatic delusions
■ Grandiosity with magical powers

SARA: I killed a man when I was 6 years old, and he was raping and killing little babies. I killed him. Then my friends told me to run, so I ran. I got away with my underpants on. My twin brother died—he committed suicide. [crying]

NURSE: Would you like to talk about this?

SARA: Not right now. I loved my brother. [sobbing] I really miss him. You know I build houses.

NURSE: You do?

SARA: Yes, I start out 14 feet tall and when I'm done I've shrunk to 14 inches. [smiles and laughs]

NURSE: You shrink?

SARA: Yes. The aliens come and get me at night and tell me they'll make me safe and they make me into a baby and take care of me.

NURSE: Do you feel safe as a baby?

SARA: Yes; no one can hurt me then. They protect me. [smiling]

NURSE: [Silence]

SARA: My husband exhibits me, you know. [laughs]

NURSE: Can you explain "exhibits"? I don't understand.

SARA: He took movies of us having sex and set me down and showed them to me. He told me I had grown into a beautiful woman. He still loves me, you know, and I still love him even though I slapped him 3,600 times in the head.

NURSE: How did you feel about his exhibiting you?

SARA: It was okay because I really do love him. I was attached to my husband at the waist in the bedroom. [laughs] [Puts finger to ear and pauses]

NURSE: Are you hearing voices?

SARA: No. I have synthetic eardrums and I hear a buzz sometimes. Do you know I saved little boys from Alcatraz? I saved them to keep them safe. [laughs]

NURSE: I didn't know that. What did you save them from?

SARA: I saved them from the men raping them. They were raping and killing all those little boys. The president gave me permission to save as many as I could.

NURSE: Is it a good feeling when you are able to help others?

SARA: I build spaceships at night and escape to bars for smokes and men buy me whiskey.

NURSE: Could we talk about one thing at a time? You are skipping to other subjects too quickly for me.

SARA: Okay.

Consumers who are discharged from an acute hospitalization with medication as the primary intervention have a 50 percent rehospitalization rate within six to nine months. In contrast, consumers discharged with medication and continuing family therapy only have a 2 to 10 percent rehospitalization rate. Family therapy moves beyond family education and helps people cope with the disorder of schizophrenia. Families learn how to manage conflict, avoid criticizing one another, decrease overprotective behaviors, and develop appropriate expectations of one another. Often, this is best accomplished with the help of a family therapist.

Evaluation

To complete the nursing process, you evaluate clients' responses to nursing interventions based on the outcomes you selected. You determine the appropriate intervals for measurement and document the condition of clients according to each individual's status. Johnson, Maas, and Moorhead (2000) is the resource for identifying measurement scales and specific indicators for each outcome.

Distorted Thought Control

Individuals are able to identify triggers to delusions. They verbalize a decrease in the duration, frequency, and intensity of delusions. They utilize distraction techniques to limit their focus on delusions.

Social Interaction Skills

Social skill deficits are identified and new skills are practiced within a group format. They are able to initiate conversations, express ideas and feelings appropriately, and avoid inappropriate topics.

Self-Esteem

Clients with schizophrenic disorders choose leisure activities that are consistent with their physical, emotional, and social capabilities. They develop a list of pleasurable activities to which they can refer when necessary. Individuals verbalize previous achievements of success and identify their own strengths and abilities. They discuss situations in which they are more autonomous using vocational, social, and community resources. Individuals function as self-advocates and, with persistence, get what they need for themselves.

Anxiety Control

Clients demonstrating improved anxiety control plan and implement effective coping strategies. They rehearse and use techniques such as slow, deep breathing, muscle relaxation, guided imagery, distraction techniques, and a quiet environment to manage their feelings of anxiety.

Knowledge: Disease Process

Client and families acknowledge the reality of schizophrenic disorders. They seek and act on information obtained from reliable sources. Clients are able to manage their disorder by identifying barriers to self-management and problem-solving solutions to these barriers. They develop their own mental health file with information about their diagnoses, medications, self-help strategies, and resources.

Knowledge: Medications

Clients identify their medications by name and describe usual side effects they experience. They verbalize an understanding of the need for continued medication. Clients cite examples of how the medications make their life more functional. They avoid self-

medication with alcohol or drugs. Client implements a routine for taking their medications.

Knowledge: Energy Conservation

Clients limit the extent of episodes of hyperactivity and monitor themselves for signs of excessive physical fatigue.

Self-Care: Activities of Daily Living (ADLs)

Clients respond to environmental cues for ADLs. They live in the least restrictive setting possible.

Suicide Self-Restraint

Clients who are suicidal develop a list of reasons to live or die and goals they hope to achieve with suicide. They develop a list of alternative solutions to their problems. Clients discuss their beliefs regarding death and the impact of suicide on family members. They participate in developing and maintaining a no-suicide contract. Clients formulate a written list of support systems and community resources and remain safe.

Aggression Control

Clients refrain from violating others' personal space and refrain from harming others or destroying property. They identify feelings of anger, frustration, hostility, and aggression. Clients identify alternatives to aggression and maintain self-control without supervision. They communicate their needs appropriately and verbalize control of impulses.[*]

Caregiver Well-Being

Family members acknowledge clients' dependency issues for those who are psychiatrically disabled. They provide appropriate supervision in the least restrictive environment. Clients seek suggestions on how to cope with the day-to-day challenges they face. If relevant, they utilize respite services to maintain their own sense of well-being. They participate in self-help groups within the community and interact with extended family and friends on a regular basis.

To build a care plan for a client with schizophrenia, go to the Companion Web site for this book.

---

[*]These selected outcome indicators are from Johnson, M., Maas, M., & Moorhead, S. (2000). *Nursing outcomes classification (NOC)* (2nd ed.). St. Louis, MO: Mosby.

CHAPTER REVIEW

COMMUNITY RESOURCES

Links to these Web sites can be accessed on the Companion Web site for this book.

American Schizophrenic Association Hotline
800-847-3802
www.schizophrenia.org

ENOSH
P.O. Box 1593
Ramat Hasharon, 47-113
Israel
www.hrisrael.co.il

National Alliance for Research on Schizophrenia and Depression (NARSAD)
60 Cutter Mill Road, Suite 404
Great Neck, NY 11021
516-829-0091
www.mhsource.com

Schizophrenia Association of Ireland
4 Fitzwilliam Place
Dublin 2
Ireland
www.schizophreniaireland.ie/lucia/si/index.htm

Schizophrenia Australia Foundation
223 McKean St.
North Fitzroy
3068 Victoria
Australia
www.sane.org

Schizophrenia Fellowship of New Zealand
P.O. Box 593
Christchurch
New Zealand
www.sfnat.org.nz

Schizophrenia Society of Canada
75 The Donway West, Suite 814
Don Mills, Ontario M3C 3E9
Canada
1-800-809-HOPE
www.schizophrenia.ca

Voice Hearers Group
http://members.aol.com/wmacdo401/voices/group.htm.

BOOKS FOR CLIENTS AND FAMILIES

Amador, X. (2000). *I am not sick, I don't need help! Helping the seriously mentally ill accept treatment: A practical guide for families and therapists.* Peconic, NY: Vida Press.

Hatfield, A. B., & Lefleg, H. P. (1993). *Surviving mental illness: Stress, coping, and adaptation.* New York: Guilford Press.

Holley, T. E., & Holley, J. (1997). *My mother's keeper: A daughter's memoir of growing up in the shadow of schizophrenia.* New York: William Morrow & Co.

Secunda, V. (1997). *When madness comes home: Help and hope for the children, siblings, and partners of the mentally ill.* New York: Hyperion.

Wyden, P. (1998). *Conquering schizophrenia: A father, his son, and a medical breakthrough.* New York: Knopf.

KEY CONCEPTS

Introduction

- Schizophrenia is a syndrome characterized by disordered thinking, perceptual disturbances, behavioral abnormalities, affective disruptions, and impaired social competency.

- Schizoaffective disorder is characterized by symptoms common to both schizophrenia and the mood disorders.

Knowledge Base

- The positive symptoms of schizophrenia are added behaviors not normally seen, such as delusions, hallucinations, loose associations, disorganized thinking, suspiciousness, overreactive affect, hyperactivity, and bizarre behavior.

- The negative symptoms of schizophrenia are the absence of normal behaviors, for example, flat affect, minimal self-care, social withdrawal, low energy level, concrete thinking, lack of insight, attention impairment, lack of motivation, and limited problem-solving ability.

- The most common type of hallucination is auditory followed by visual. Tactile, olfactory, and gustatory hallucinations occur in people undergoing withdrawal from or abuse of alcohol and drugs.

- Delusions are false beliefs that cannot be changed by logical reasoning or evidence. It is thought that they represent dysfunctions in the information-processing circuits between the hemispheres.

- Having no apparent relationship between thoughts is referred to as loose association.

- Concrete thinking is a focus on facts and details and an inability to generalize or think abstractly.

- People with schizophrenia frequently have ineffective social skills, which increases their sense of isolation.

- Childhood schizophrenia is a very severe form with a poor prognosis.

- People with late-onset schizophrenia have more delusions and hallucinations but have fewer cognitive disruptions and negative symptoms.

- Individuals who have velocardiofacial syndrome are at higher risk for schizophrenia.

- Clients who smoke may be self-medicating, or smoking may be a risk factor for schizophrenia, or genetic and environmental factors work together to cause both nicotine use and schizophrenia.

- Concomitant disorders include substance abuse, suicide, and depression.

- Neurobiological factors of schizophrenia include genetic defects, abnormal brain development, neurodegeneration, disordered neurotransmission, and abnormal brain structures.

- It is believed that biological vulnerabilities interact with developmental, environmental, and social processes to produce the schizophrenic syndrome.

- Psychiatric rehabilitation emphasizes the development of skills and supports, considers the consumer to be in control, and promotes choices, self-determination, and individual responsibility.

- Group therapy helps prevent the withdrawal and social isolation that may occur for people who are psychiatrically disabled.

- Assertive community treatment (ACT) programs deliver all services when and where the client needs them.

- Alternative therapies include transcranial magnetic stimulation (TMS), omega-3 fatty acids, and aromatherapy.

The Nursing Process

Assessment

- Nursing assessment is based on interviews with clients, family members, friends, group home supervisors, or case managers.

Diagnosis

- Nursing diagnoses are based on assessment data focusing on how well clients are functioning in daily life, how stable their affect is, how effective their communication is, and how well they are getting along with others.

Outcome Identification and Goals

- Client goals include client safety, improved communication skills, improved social skills, improved self-esteem, compliance with prescribed medication, effective family functioning, and adaptation to living in the least restrictive setting.

Nursing Interventions

- Opportunities to assist people with schizophrenia occur in a variety of settings, in long-term relationships, or in crisis periods.

- A priority of care is client safety, which includes measures to prevent self-harm, suicide, physical exhaustion, and striking out to protect themselves from perceived danger.

- Consumers may need assistance with self-care, ranging from gentle reminders to more step-by-step directions.

- Helping clients understand the need for medication is an important nursing intervention.

- Reduction of anxiety may be accomplished with relaxation techniques, eliminating caffeine, moderating environmental stimuli, walking, or talking out feelings with another person.

- Look and listen for clues that the person might be hallucinating; identify the needs that may be reflected in the hallucination, stay with the person, and speak in short, simple phrases. If asked, simply point out that you are not experiencing the same stimuli.

- Interventions for people who are experiencing delusions include assessing the content, duration, and frequency of the delusion; correlating it with stressful situations; responding to underlying feelings; and providing distracting activities.

- It is necessary to clarify communication when clients' thinking is disorganized. You should listen for themes in clients' conversations.

- Exercises to promote self-esteem include listing positive qualities, keeping a self-esteem journal, making a collage, and focusing on the image we present to others and who we really are.

KEY CONCEPTS *(continued)*

- The goal of psychoeducation is to teach consumers about their illness, the problems they commonly experience, early signs of relapse, and the need for medication.

- Social skills training is a series of highly structured and organized sessions of practice in basic skills, which can result in improvements in important areas of social adjustment.

- Parents of young adult children stricken with schizophrenia often feel a sense of responsibility that, at times, can be overwhelming.

- Family education includes knowledge about the disease, available treatment programs, how to manage on a day-

to-day basis, early signs of relapse, and suicide precautions.

- The family may need help in setting expectations and limits, coping with conflict, and developing appropriate expectations of one another.

Evaluation

- In evaluating clients' responses to nursing interventions, you should determine the appropriate intervals for measurement and documentation of the outcomes according to each individual's status.

EXPLORE *MediaLink*

- Interactive resources, including animations, for this chapter can be found on the Companion Web site at *http://www.prenhall.com/fontaine*. Click on Chapter 14 and select the activities for this chapter.

- For NCLEX review questions and an audio glossary, access the accompanying CD-ROM in this book.

REFERENCES

American Psychiatric Association. (2000). *Diagnostic and statistical manual of mental disorders* (4th ed., Text Revision). Washington, DC: Author.

Anders, R. L. (2000). Assessment of inpatient treatment of persons with schizophrenia: Implications for practice. *Archives of Psychiatric Nursing, 14*(5), 213–221.

Bryant, N. L., Buchanan, R. W., Vlader, K., Breier, A., & Rothman, M. (1999). Gender differences in temporal lobe structures of patients with schizophrenia. *American Journal of Psychiatry, 156*(4), 603–616.

Bustillo, J. R., Lauriello, J., Horan, W. P., & Keith, S. J. (2001). The psychosocial treatment of schizophrenia. *American Journal of Psychiatry, 158*(2), 163–174.

Cadenhead, K. S., Swerdlow, N. R., Shafer, K. M., Diaz, M., & Braff, D. L. (2000). Sensory gating deficits assessed by the P50 event-related potential in subjects with schizotypal personality disorder. *American Journal of Psychiatry, 157*(1), 55–59.

Carling, P. J. (1995). *Return to community.* New York: Guilford Press.

Carper, J. (2000). *Your miracle brain.* New York: HarperCollins.

Crespo-Facorro, B., Piven, M. L. S., & Schultz, S. K. (1999). Psychosis in late life: How does it fit into current diagnostic criteria? *American Journal of Psychiatry, 156*(4), 624–629.

Crespo-Facorro, B., Paradiso, S., Andreasen, N. C., O'Leary, D. S., Watkins, G. L., Ponto, L. L. B., et al. (2001). Neural mechanisms of anhedonia in schizophrenia. *Journal of the American Medical Association, 286*(4), 427–435.

Czuchta, D. M., & McCay, E. (2001). Help-seeking for parents of individuals experiencing a first episode of schizophrenia. *Archives of Psychiatric Nursing, 15*(4), 159–170.

Danion, J. M., Meulemans, T., Kauffmann-Muller, F., & Vermaat, H. (2001). Intact implicit learning in schizophrenia. *American Journal of Psychiatry, 158*(6), 944–948.

Eliez, S., Blasey, C. M., Schmitt, E. J., White, C. D., Hu, D., & Reiss, A. L. (2001). Velocardiofacial syndrome. *American Journal of Psychiatry, 158*(3), 447–453.

Farrell, S. P., & Deeds, E. S. (1997). The clubhouse model as exemplar. *Journal of Psychosocial Nursing, 35*(1), 27–34.

Flashman, L. A., McAllister, T. W., Andreasen, N. C., & Saykin, A. J. (2000). Smaller brain size associated with unawareness of illness in patients with schizophrenia. *American Journal of Psychiatry, 157*(7), 1167–1175.

Franck, N., Farrer, C., Georgieff, N., Marie-Cardine, M., Dalery, J., d'Amato, T., et al. (2001). Defective recognition of one's own actions in patients with schizophrenia. *American Journal of Psychiatry, 158*(3), 454–459.

George, T. P., Ziedonis, D. M., Feingold, A., Pepper, W. T., Satterburg, C. A., Winkel, J., et al. (2000). Nicotine transdermal patch and atypical antipsychotic medications for smoking cessation in schizophrenia. *American Journal of Psychiatry, 157*(11), 1835–1843.

Gerber, R. (2000). *Vibrational medicine for the 21st century.* New York: Eagle Brook.

Gilbert, A. R., Rosenberg, D. R., Harenski, K., Spencer, S., Sweeney, J. A., & Keshavan, M. S. (2001). Thalamic volumes in patients with first-episode schizophrenia. *American Journal of Psychiatry, 158*(4), 618–625.

Goff, D. C., & Coyle, J. T. (2001). The emerging role of glutamate in the pathophysiology and treatment of schizophrenia. *American Journal of Psychiatry, 158*(9), 1367–1376.

Goldberg, T. E., Aloia, M. S., Gourovitch, M. L., Missar, D., Pickar, D., & Weinberger, D. R. (1998). Cognitive substrates of thought disorder. *American Journal of Psychiatry, 155*(12), 1671–1676.

Hagen, B. F., & Mitchell, D. L. (2001). Might within the madness: Solution-focused therapy and thought-disordered clients. *Archives of Psychiatric Nursing, 15*(2), 86–93.

Harvey, P. D. (2001). Vulnerability to schizophrenia in adulthood. In R. E. Ingram & J. M. Price (Eds.), *Vulnerability to psychopathology* (pp. 355–381). New York: Guilford Press.

Ismail, B., Cantor-Graae, E., & McNeil, T. F. (1998). Minor physical anomalies in schizophrenic patients and their siblings. *American Journal of Psychiatry, 155*(12), 1695–1702.

Johnson, M., Maas, M., & Moorhead, S. (2000). *Nursing outcomes classification (NOC)* (2nd ed.). St. Louis, MO: Mosby.

Kelly, C., & McCreadie, R. G. (1999). Smoking habits, current symptoms, and premorbid characteristics of schizophrenia patients in Nithsdale, Scotland. *American Journal of Psychiatry, 156*(11), 1751–1757.

Kennedy, M. G., Schepp, K. G., & O'Connor, F. W. (2000). Symptom self-management and relapse in schizophrenia. *Archives of Psychiatric Nursing, 14*(6), 266–275.

Lawson, W. B. (2000). Issues in pharmacotherapy for African Americans. In P. Ruiz (Ed.), *Ethnicity and psychopharmacology* (pp. 37–53). Washington, DC: American Psychiatric Press.

Liddle, P. F. (1999). The multidimensional phenotype of schizophrenia. In C. A. Tamminga (Ed.), *Schizophrenia in a molecular age* (pp. 1–28). Washington, DC: American Psychiatric Press.

McCann, E. (2001). Recent developments in psychosocial interventions for people with psychosis. *Issues in Mental Health Nursing, 22*, 99–107.

Mueser, K. T., Bond, G. R., & Drake, R. E. (2001). Community-based treatment of schizophrenia and other severe mental disorders: Treatment outcomes. *Medscape mental health 6*(1). *www.medscape.com/Medscape/psychiatry/journal/2001/v06.n01/.*

Murray, R. (1999). Schizophrenia has origins in childhood. *NARSAD Research Newletter, 11*(2), 11–12.

Nahas, Z., Molloy, M., Risch, S. C., & George, M. S. (2000). TMS in schizophrenia. In M. S. George & R. H. Belmaker (Eds.), *Transcranial magnetic stimulation in neuropsychiatry* (pp. 237–251). Washington, DC: American Psychiatric Press.

Nicolson, R., Lenane, M., Singaracharlu, S., Malaspina, D., Giedd, J. N., Hamburger, S. D., et al. (2000). Premorbid speech and language impairments in childhood-onset schizophrenia. *American Journal of Psychiatry, 157*(5), 794–800.

Nicolson, R., & Rapoport, J. L. (2000). Childhood-onset schizophrenia. In J. L. Rapoport (Ed.), *Childhood onset of "adult" psychopathology* (pp. 167–192). Washington, DC: American Psychiatric Press.

Palmer-Erbs, V. (1996). A breath of fresh air in a turbulent health-care environment. *Journal of Psychosocial Nursing, 34*(9),16–21.

Paris, J. (1999). *Nature and nurture in psychiatry.* Washington, DC: American Psychiatric Press.

Perlstein, W. M., Carter, C. S., Noll, D. C., & Cohen, J. D. (2001). Relation of prefrontal cortex dysfunction to working memory and symptoms in schizophrenia. *American Journal of Psychiatry, 158*(7), 1105–1112.

Radomsky, E. D., Haas, G. L., Mann, J. J., & Sweeney, J. A. (1999). Suicidal behavior in patients with schizophrenia and other psychotic disorders. *American Journal of Psychiatry, 156*(10), 1590–1595.

Ross, D. E., Kirkpatrick, B., Karkowski, L. M., Straub, R. E., MacLean, C. J., O'Neill, F. A., et al. (2000). Sibling correlation of deficit syndrome in the Irish study of high-density schizophrenia families. *American Journal of Psychiatry, 157*(7), 1071–1076.

Rosso, I. M., Cannon, T. D., Huttunen, T., Huttunen, M. O., Lonnquist, J., & Gasperoni,

T. L. (2000). Obstetric risk factors for early-onset schizophrenia in a Finnish birth cohort. *American Journal of Psychiatry, 157*(5), 801–807.

Seeman, M. V. (2001). Schizophrenia in women. Presented at the 1st World Congress on Women's Mental Health; March 27–31, 2001. Berlin, Germany. *www.medscape.com/Medscape/CNO/2001/WCWMH/WCWMH-0.5html.*

Sigmundsson, T., Suckling, J., Maier, M., Williams, S. C. R., Bullmore, E. T., Greenwood, K. E., et al. (2001). Structural abnormalities in frontal, temporal, and limbic regions and interconnecting white matter tracts in schizophrenic patients with prominent negative symptoms. *American Journal of Psychiatry, 158*(2), 234–243.

Siris, S. G. (2000). Depression in schizophrenia. *American Journal of Psychiatry, 157*(9), 1379–1388.

Sowell, E. R., Levitt, J., Thompson, P. M., Holmes, C. J., Blanton, R. E., Kornsand, D. S., et al. (2000). Brain abnormalities in early-onset schizophrenia spectrum disorder observed with statistical parametric mapping of structural magnetic resonance images. *American Journal of Psychiatry, 157*(9), 1475–1484.

Tarrant, C. J., & Jones, P. B. (2000). Biological markers as precursors to schizophrenia. In J. L. Rapoport (Ed.), *Childhood onset of "adult" psychopathology* (pp. 65–102). Washington, DC: American Psychiatric Press.

Tsuang, M. T., Stone, W. S., & Faraone, S. V. (2000). Toward reformulating the diagnosis of schizophrenia. *American Journal of Psychiatry, 157*(7), 1041–1050.

Volk, D. W., Austin, M. C., Pierri, J. N., Sampson, A. R., & Lewis, D. A. (2001). GABA transporter-1 mRNA in the prefrontal cortex in schizophrenia. *American Journal of Psychiatry, 158*(2), 256–265.

Weiner, E., Ball, M. P., Summerfelt, A., Gold, J., & Buchanan, R. W. (2001). Effects of sustained-release bupropion and supportive group therapy on cigarette consumption in patients with schizophrenia. *American Journal of Psychiatry, 158*(4), 535–637.

Zorrilla, L. T. E., & Zeste, D. V. (2000). Late-onset schizophrenia. In J. L. Rapoport (Ed.), *Childhood onset of "adult" psychopathology* (pp. 149–165). Washington, DC: American Psychiatric Press.

Substance-Related Disorders

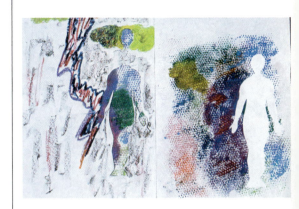

OBJECTIVES

After reading this chapter, you will be able to:

- LIST the commonly abused substances, the actions of these substances, and the signs and symptoms of chemical dependence.

- EXPLAIN the effects of substance abuse on the fetus and the newborn.

- IDENTIFY the effects of substance abuse on the family.

- COMPARE and contrast causative theories of substance abuse.

- USE the substance abuse history and focused nursing assessment when interviewing clients who abuse substances.

- INTERVENE with clients who are chemically dependent.

U nderstand Me

—Brian, Age 19

MediaLink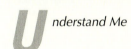

CD-ROM
- *Audio Glossary*
- *NCLEX Review*

Animation
- *Cocaine as Drug of Abuse*

Companion Web site www.prenhall.com/fontaine
- *Critical Thinking*
- *More NCLEX Review*
- *Case Study*
- *Care Map Activity*
- *Links to Resources*

KEY TERMS

*I*n our society, many people use substances recreationally to modify mood or behavior. However, there are wide sociocultural variations in the acceptability of chemical use. Alcohol, caffeine, and tobacco are legal drugs, but the social acceptability of using them varies. Narcotics, sedatives, stimulants, and hallucinogens are illegal drugs, and the general population considers recreational use to be socially unacceptable.

There are other forms of addiction, often referred to as *process addictions*, which are beyond the scope of this chapter. These process addictions include workaholism, gambling, shopping, spending and indebtedness, eating disorders, and sexual addiction. Process addictions involve compulsive behaviors that serve to reduce anxiety.

The *Diagnostic and Statistical Manual of Mental Disorders* (4th ed., Text Revision) (DSM-IV-TR) classifies the pathological use of chemicals as psychoactive substance-related disorders. The words *substance* and *chemical* are used interchangeably. **Substance abuse** is defined as recurrent use that results in a failure to manage work, school, or home roles, or in hazardous situations such as driving a car, or resulting in substance-related legal problems or related interpersonal problems. This diagnosis can be used only for someone who has never been diagnosed as dependent. **Substance dependence** occurs when the use of the drug is no longer under control and continues despite adverse effects. Substance-dependent individuals experience tolerance with a need for increasing amounts of the drug, withdrawal symptoms, and increasingly higher doses. People who are dependent on drugs may spend a great deal of time in obtaining drugs and limit their usual social, occupational, or recreational activities because of the substance use (American Psychiatric Association [APA], 2000). This chapter focuses on substance dependence, which is the more severe form of the substance-related disorders.

Substance **withdrawal** is physiological, behavioral, cognitive, and affective symptoms that occur after reduction or discontinuance of a drug that has been used heavily over a long period of time. When experiencing withdrawal, most individuals find themselves craving the drug, which they know would reduce the withdrawal symptoms. Withdrawal symptoms are specific for each drug (APA, 2000).

Chemical dependence is a complex, chronic, progressive *disease* that can be fatal if left untreated. While it is true that a disease is not defined as a deficiency of willpower, this disease is comprised of several biochemical processes that are subject to voluntary control. In addition, there are psychological, sociological, and spiritual aspects to chemical dependence.

A number of types of psychoactive substances are associated with chemical dependence. The days of the so-called "pure" drug addict or alcoholic are gone. Most people who are chemically dependent are polydrug abusers. They may use amphetamines or cocaine to get high, and alcohol, Valium, or marijuana to come down off the high. Some use sedatives to sleep and amphetamines to wake up. Whatever the pattern, clients must be treated for all secondary as well as primary addictions. See the DSM-IV-TR Classifications of substance use disorders.

DSM-IV-TR CLASSIFICATIONS

Alcohol-Related Disorders

Amphetamine-Related Disorders

Caffeine-Related Disorders

Cannabis-Related Disorders

Cocaine-Related Disorders

Hallucinogen-Related Disorders

Inhalant-Related Disorders

Nicotine-Related Disorders

Opioid-Related Disorders

Phencyclidine-Related Disorders

Sedative-, Hypnotic-, or Anxiolytic-Related Disorders

Polysubstance-Related Disorders

Other Substance-Related Disorders

SOURCE: Reprinted with permission from the *Diagnostic and Statistical Manual of Mental Disorders,* Fourth Edition, Text Revision. Copyright 2000 American Psychiatric Association.

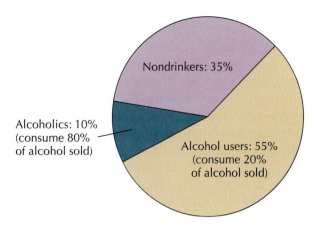

FIGURE 15.1 ■ Alcohol use in the United States.

Substance use disorders in the United States cost over $500 billion a year, including the costs of treatment, related health problems, absenteeism, lost productivity, drug-related crime and incarceration, and efforts in education and prevention. Alcoholism (alcohol dependence) is a major health problem, one that is responsible for 100,000 deaths annually in the United States. More than 6 million persons in the United States are in severe need of substance abuse treatment but only 37 percent of them will receive needed treatment. Approximately 35 percent of the population does not drink, and 55 percent consume only 20 percent of the alcohol. The remaining 10 percent consumes 80 percent of the alcohol. The number of inmates in American prisons more than tripled over the last 20 years to nearly 2 million, with 60 to 70 percent testing positive for substance abuse on arrest (Kalb, 2001; Washington, 2001) (see Figure 15.1 ■).

Studies indicate that alcohol is a factor in 30 to 55 percent of motor vehicle fatalities, 50 percent of domestic violence cases, 53 percent of all deaths from accidental falls, 64 percent of all fatal fires, and 80 percent of suicides. Alcoholism is the most expensive addiction for business and industry; 40 percent of

industrial deaths and 47 percent of industrial injuries are caused by the use of alcohol (APA, 2000; Yi, Stinson, Williams, & Bertolucci, 1999) (see Figure 15.2 ■).

In general, women drink less heavily than men do. However, the level of drinking for women age 35 to 64 has increased. Drinking typically begins during adolescence, with 92 percent of high school students and 90 percent of college students reporting the use of alcohol; 30 percent report drinking regularly. This rate has remained fairly stable for the past 20 years (Pfefferbaum, Rosenbloom, Deshmukh, & Sullivan, 2001).

Statistics on the number of drug abusers are difficult to provide. The illicit nature of drug use makes it nearly impossible to retrieve accurate information. As many as 33 percent of all Americans age 12 and older have used an illegal drug during their lives.

In the 1960s, hallucinogens and amphetamines were the illegal drugs most commonly used. In the 1970s, heroin, marijuana, and sedatives were the most popular drugs. The 1980s was the decade of cocaine. Judging by the increase in cocaine-related visits to hospital emergency departments, we continue to have hard-core cocaine abuse problems in the United States. Eight million Americans use cocaine regularly, with 2.2 million considered to be dependent. Heroin has become a more popular drug with adolescents and young adults with the change from injecting it to smoking it. Unfortunately, users mistakenly believe that smoking heroin is not addicting. The rapidly escalating abuse of amphetamines, especially Ecstasy, is a significant problem at

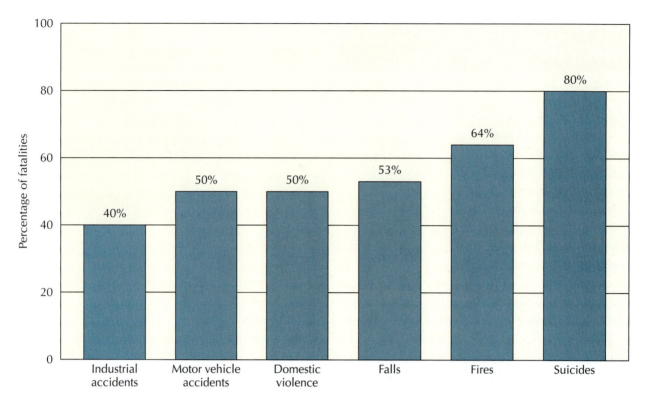

FIGURE 15.2 ■ Fatal events in which alcohol is a factor.

dance clubs and dance parties known as "raves." Young people take these "love drugs" for increased energy and sexual desire (Klitzman, Pope, & Hudson, 2000).

Adolescents are quicker than adults to initiate and extend poly-drug abuse. Most adolescents abuse a wide number of substances, whereas adults tend to focus on one or two "drugs of choice." (For a list of the risk factors in teenagers, see Box 15.1.) Men are more likely to abuse cocaine, marijuana, and opioids; women are more likely to abuse sedatives, antianxiety agents, and amphetamines (Naegle & D'Avanzo, 2001).

Recent attention has been given to *impaired health professionals*, including nurses and physicians. For the most part, substance abuse among nurses is not much higher or lower than that of the general population. Nurses and other health professionals have the same risk factors as others in developing addiction. Workplace stress, work-related injuries, and easy access to prescription drugs may place nurses at greater risk of substance abuse.

When nurses have an addiction, the shame and guilt is magnified. After all, nurses are healers and nurturers. They are not expected to have their own prob-

lems, certainly not an addiction that could lead them to take drugs from clients or be less than 100 percent in control when they are at work. Prior to 1982, nurses identified as addicted or abusing alcohol or drugs were either fired or reported to state boards of nursing and

---

BOX 15.1

Substance Dependence Risk Factors in Teenagers

- Peer pressure, group norms: Prosubstance use
- A greater here-and-now orientation than adults; drugs provide immediate gratification
- Rebellion against authority
- Alienation from traditional social and religious values; drugs viewed as a way to individuate and disconnect
- Stressful situations, such as a dysfunctional family
- Insecurity and low self-esteem: Powerful triggers for compensatory substance abuse

Signs of Substance Abuse Among Nurses

- Frequent or unexplained disappearances from the unit
- Increasing difficulty meeting schedules or deadlines
- Sloppy or illogical charting
- Excessive number of mistakes
- Smell of alcohol on breath
- Labile emotions
- Diminished alertness
- Isolation from co-workers
- Frequent reports of medication spills or other waste
- Discrepancies in end-of-shift medication counts
- Increase in patients' complaints of unrelieved pain

disciplined by censure, suspension, or having their professional license revoked. Nurses now have access to peer assistance and statewide programs to seek treatment and save their licenses. Nurses with substance abuse problems are required to stop practicing and enter a 12-step treatment program for monitoring. Those who abuse alcohol are not allowed to perform patient care or handle controlled substances for 6 months. For those who abuse substances other than alcohol, the ban is for one year (Naegle & D'Avanzo, 2001; Trinkoff, Zhou, Storr, & Soeken, 2000). See Box 15.2 for signs of substance abuse among nurses.

KNOWLEDGE BASE

This section begins with an overview of the commonly abused substances and provides specific information for each of the categories (see Table 15.1 ■). The discussion then moves to the general characteristics of substance-abusing individuals and their families.

ALCOHOL

Types of alcohol include liquor, beer, and wine. Common street names for alcohol and mode of administration include:

- *Street names:* Booze, hooch, moonshine, sauce
- *Mode of administration:* Oral

Site of Action

Alcohol acts as a central nervous system depressant in two ways. Alcohol potentiates gamma-aminobutyric acid (GABA) activity, a major inhibitory neurotransmitter. Alcohol decreases glutamate activity, a major excitatory neurotransmitter. In both cases, the outcome is depression of the central nervous system (CNS) (Tabakoff & Hoffman, 1999).

Effects

The *pattern of dependence* on alcohol varies from person to person. Some have a regular daily intake of large amounts of alcohol. Others restrict their use to drinking heavily on the weekends or days off from work. Some may abstain for long periods of time and then go on a drinking binge. The behavior may be inconsistent at the beginning of dependence. At times, people with alcohol dependence can drink with control, and at other times, they cannot control the drinking behavior. As the course of alcoholism continues, there may be behaviors such as starting the day off with a drink, sneaking drinks through the day, gulping alcoholic drinks, shifting from one alcoholic beverage to another, and hiding bottles at work and at home. They may give up hobbies and other interests in order to have more time to drink. It is not unusual for alcoholics to engage in what is known as telephonitis, making telephone calls to family and friends at inappropriate times, such as the middle of the night.

Mayfield, McCleod, and Hall (1974) developed the *CAGE Questionnaire*, which is simple and can be incorporated into any nursing assessment. One positive answer raises concern, and more than one positive answer is a strong indication of alcohol problems:

C Have you ever felt that you should **c**ut down on your drinking?

A Have people **a**nnoyed you by criticizing your drinking?

G Have you ever felt bad or **g**uilty about your drinking?

E Have you ever taken a drink in the morning, as an "**e**ye-opener"?

Complications

Alcohol is a chemical irritant and has a direct toxic effect on many organ systems (see Table 15.2 ■).

Blackouts, a fairly early sign of alcoholism, are a form of amnesia for events that occurred during the drinking period. The alcoholic may carry out conversa-

TABLE 15.1

Frequently Abused Substances

Substance	Psychological Effects	Physiological Effects	Overdose	Withdrawal
Alcohol	Hostility, crying, shame, despair, blackouts, talkativeness	Slurred speech, lack of coordination, flushed face	Confusion, stupor, coma, possible death	6–8 hours after last drink: Irritability, tremors, elevated pulse and blood pressure 6–96 hours: Seizures, hallucinations 3–14 days: Alcohol withdrawal delirium
Sedatives	Sedation, euphoria, talkativeness, irritability, impaired attention and memory	Drowsiness, sleep, lowered pulse and blood pressure	CNS depression, respiratory arrest	Similar to alcohol withdrawal, seizures, anxiety, tremors, psychosis
Narcotics	Euphoria, sedation, attention and memory, motivation, apathy	Drowsiness, pinpoint pupils, pain motor retardation	Lowered respirations, pulse, and blood pressure; coma, death	Few hours to few days lasting 1–2 days; craving, flulike symptoms, fearfulness
Cannabis	Pleasure, euphoria, slowed sense of time, altered perceptions	Dry mouth, fast pulse, appetite, fatigue, reddened eyes	Hallucinations	Craving, anxiety
Amphetamine	Elation, energy, anxiety, grandiosity, rapid speech, confusion	Elevated pulse and blood pressure, arrhythmias, visual disturbances, insomnia	Agitation, hallucinations, cardiovascular collapse, suicide	Sleep, fatigue, anhedonia, depression
Cocaine	Euphoria, energy, talkativeness, grandiosity, impaired judgment, paranoia, violence	Insomnia, anorexia, elevated pulse and blood pressure, runny nose, irritated nasal membrane	Delirium, hyperthermia, seizures, respiratory or cardiac arrest, cerebral hemorrhage	Severe craving, irritability
Hallucinogens	Euphoria, hallucinations, impulsiveness, paranoia, impaired judgment, body image changes	Intensified perceptions, sense of slowed time, elevated pulse and blood pressure, tremors, lack of coordination	Confusion, delirium, psychosis, accidents, suicide	No symptoms
Inhalants	Euphoria, uninhibited behavior, floating sensation, illusions, drowsiness, amnesia	Perceptual changes, hallucinations, eye irritation, sensitivity to light, nose/mouth irritation	Cardiac and respiratory arrest	No symptoms

TABLE 15.2

Physiological Complications from Alcohol Dependence

Body Systems	Toxic Effects
Gastrointestinal	Esophageal reflux, esophagitis, esophageal varices, gastritis, decreased appetite, malabsorption, recurrent diarrhea, acute or chronic pancreatitis (75% of cases related to alcohol abuse)
Liver	Hepatomegaly, fatty liver, alcoholic hepatitis, cirrhosis, cancer. Elevated gamma-glutamyl transpeptidase (GGT) results
Cardiovascular	Hypertension, cardiomyopathy, arrhythmias, increased risk for stroke, coronary artery disease, sudden cardiac death
Respiratory	Pneumonia, bronchitis, tuberculosis
Hematologic	Bone marrow depression, anemia, leukopenia, blood clotting abnormalities
Neurologic	Seizures, peripheral neuropathy, optic neuropathy, Wernicke's encephalopathy, Korsakoff's syndrome, alcoholic dementia, impaired cognitive function, labile moods, sleep disturbances
Endocrine	Hyperglycemia, decreased thyroid function
Reproductive	Erectile problems, decreased testosterone, decreased sex drive, menstrual irregularities
Nutritional	Thiamine deficiency, folic acid deficiency, vitamin A deficiency, magnesium deficiency, zinc deficiency

SOURCES: American Psychological Association. (2000). *Diagnostic and statistical manual of mental disorders* (4th ed., Text Revision). Washington, DC: Author; Dunphy, L. M., & Winland-Brown, J. E. (2001). *The art and science of advanced practice nursing*. Philadelphia: Davis; and Naegle, M. A., & D'Avanzo, C. E. (2001). *Addictions and substance abuse: Strategies for advanced practice nursing*. Upper Saddle River, NJ: Prentice Hall.

tions and elaborate activities with no loss of consciousness, but have total amnesia for those activities the next day. This may be explained by the toxic effects of alcohol on glutamate transmission necessary for memory storage. A more advanced CNS problem is *Wernicke's encephalopathy*, which is characterized by ataxia (lack of coordination), abnormal eye movements, and confusion. These symptoms result from chronic thiamine deficiency. About 80 percent of people with Wernicke's encephalopathy also develop *Korsakoff's syndrome*, characterized by intact intellectual functioning but an inability to retrieve long-term memory events or retain new information. **Confabulation**, making up information to fill memory blanks, develops in the person's attempt to protect self-esteem when confronted with memory loss. *Alcoholic dementia* is characterized by impaired abstract thinking and judgment, personality changes, and impaired memory. This is often seen in chronically heavy drinkers (APA, 2000).

Withdrawal

Alcohol withdrawal syndrome (AWS) typically begins about six to eight hours after the last drink. Early symptoms include irritability, anxiety, insomnia, tremors, sweating, and a mild tachycardia. In rare cases, the person may experience grand mal seizures or intermittent visual, tactile, or auditory hallucinations. Symptoms of withdrawal usually peak during the second day of abstinence and are likely to show significant improvement by the fourth or fifth day. For individuals who repeatedly withdraw from alcohol, symptoms become worse each time (Reoux, 2001).

Alcohol withdrawal delirium, formerly referred to as delirium tremens (DTs), usually occurs on days 2 and 3 but may appear as late as 14 days after the last drink. The person experiences confusion, disorientation, hallucinations, tachycardia, hypertension or hypotension, extreme tremors, agitation, diaphoresis, and fever. Death may result from cardiovascular collapse or hyperthermia. With improved diagnosis and medical treatment, the mortality rate has dropped from 20 percent to 1 percent (APA, 2000).

Overdose

Signs of alcohol intoxication include nausea, vomiting, lack of coordination, slurred speech, staggering, disorientation, irritability, short attention span, loud and frequent talking, poor judgment, lack of inhibition, labile emotions, and, for some, violent behavior. Alcohol intoxication may result in accidents or falls that may cause contusions, sprains, fractures, and facial or head trauma. High blood alcohol levels may result in unconsciousness, coma, respiratory depression, and death (see Table 15.3 ■). This becomes a critical situation in the emergency department and necessitates careful triage. Treatment of alcohol intoxication is dependent on the presenting physical complications.

SEDATIVES/HYPNOTICS/ ANTIANXIETY AGENTS

Types of sedatives/hypnotics/antianxiety agents include barbiturates (Seconal, Nembutal, Amytal, Tuinal, Phenobarbital, Quaaludes) and benzodiazepines (Valium, Librium, Xanax, Halcion, Ativan). Common street names for sedatives/hypnotics/ antianxiety agents and mode of administration include:

- ■ *Street names*: Downers, ludes, red devils, reds, blue angels, blues, yellow jackets, trenks, barbs
- ■ *Mode of administration*: Taken orally but can be used intravenously (IV)

Site of Action

They act by enhancing the action of GABA in the limbic system of the brain. They may cause significant CNS depression.

Effects

People using these drugs may experience drowsiness, sedated appearance, lack of coordination, euphoria, labile emotions, irritability, anxiety, impaired attention, and working memory loss.

Complications

Two new designer drugs, Rohypnol (roofies, forget pills, R2) and GHB (G-riffic, Grievous Bodily Harm, Liquid G), have been called "date rape" drugs since they have been used to render rape victims unconscious. They also cause short-term memory loss, leading to horrifying stories of women whose only memory is of waking up naked with a stranger. Initially, they give a feeling of euphoria but combined with alcohol can lead to unconsciousness, coma, or, in some cases, death.

TABLE 15.3

Blood Alcohol Levels and Symptoms

Blood Alcohol Level (Percentage of Alcohol in Blood)	Behavior
0.05	Changes in mood and normal behavior; loosening of judgment and restraint; person feels carefree
0.08–0.10	Voluntary motor action clumsy; legal level of intoxication
0.20	Brain motor area depression causes staggering; easily angered; shouting; weeping
0.30	Confusion; stupor
0.40	Coma
0.50	Death (usually due to medullar respiratory blocking effects)

Withdrawal

Symptoms of withdrawal are similar to alcohol withdrawal: altered perceptions, hallucinations, depression, diaphoresis, marked agitation, tachycardia, anxiety, tremors, seizures, and delirium. If the individual has been taking high doses or has been taking these drugs for a long period of time, the withdrawal process should be medically supervised. Abrupt cessation can lead to serious problems, such as seizures and psychosis, and may even end in death. The medication is carefully titrated downward until the withdrawal process is completed.

Overdose

An overdose of sedative–hypnotics is very dangerous. Symptoms include weak and rapid pulse, shallow respirations, cold and clammy skin, and possible coma and death. When combined with alcohol, serious overdose can occur rapidly, with death from respiratory depression.

OPIOIDS

Types of opioids include morphine, heroin, codeine, Dilaudid, Percodan, Demerol, methadone, Nubain, Darvon, Oxyfast, Percocet, Vicodin, Ultram, and Talwin. Common street names of opioids and mode of administration include:

- **Street names**: Smack, dope, H, horse (heroin); shit, Miss Emma, lords, D, dollies, china white
- **Mode of administration**: Oral, smoking, inhalation, injection, IV

Site of Action

Endorphins, enkephalins, and dynorphins are the naturally occurring substances that stimulate the opiate receptors in the brain, providing pain relief, pleasure, and motivation and in regulating temperature, respiration, endocrine, and gastrointestinal activity. External opioids attach to those same opiate receptors (Jaffe & Jaffe, 1999).

Effects

When opioids are injected IV or inhaled, brain levels rise rapidly giving a brief, intense sensation called a rush or thrill. This is followed by a longer-lasting period called a high, which includes a sense of calmness. The effects of opioids are a sedated appearance, motor retardation, slurred speech, impaired attention and memory, decreased awareness, and reduction of instinctual drives. Euphoria, pleasure, and relaxation also occur. Physically, opioids depress respiration, suppress coughs, and inhibit gastrointestinal motility. Cocaine and heroin may be used together as heroin maintains the euphoria after cocaine loses its effect. Continued use decreases the body's production of endorphin and enkephalin, resulting in a very low tolerance of pain and discomfort during withdrawal.

Complications

Poisoning may be a problem because heroin is often "cut" with substances that may contain impurities to increase the quantity for sale. Because the potency of street heroin is unknown and because today's heroin is considerably more potent than it was 30 years ago, a number of overdose deaths occur every year. Since most users "shoot up" and share needles, they are at high risk for hepatitis, HIV infection, and AIDS. Other complications from heroin use include liver problems, malignant hypertension, strokes, and kidney failure largely as the result of infections and impurities (Naegle & D'Avanzo, 2001).

Withdrawal

Withdrawal symptoms usually begin within a few hours to a few days after the last dose. Symptoms are subjectively distressful include craving, muscle aches, backaches, severe abdominal cramps and diarrhea, watery eyes, running nose, yawning, tremors, chills, sweating, and a crawling skin sensation. Symptoms peak in two to three days, and the discomfort may last as long as two weeks (McCabe, 2000).

Overdose

Signs of overdose include clammy skin, shallow respirations, pinpoint pupils (may be dilated with severe hypoxia), coma, and death from respiratory depression or sudden irreversible pulmonary edema. Narcan (naloxone), a narcotic antagonist, 0.4 to 2 mg may be given IV to reverse respiratory depression and coma. The reversal is rapid but short-lived; thus, repeated treatments are needed every two to three minutes. Lasix may be helpful for pulmonary edema.

CANNABIS

Types of cannabis include marijuana and hashish. The most common street names and mode of administration are:

- *Street names*: Grass, joint, pot, ganja, blang, reefer, weed, Mary Jane, Acapulco gold, Colombian, roach
- *Mode of administration*: Smoking in cigarettes or pipes. Inhaling the smoke through a water-cooled apparatus called a "bong" lessens irritation and aids deeper inhalation. Occasionally taken orally when mixed with food.

Site of Action

Delta-9-tetrahydrocannabinol (THC) is the psychoactive ingredient in cannabis. The content of THC ranges from 2 to 5 percent in marijuana, while hashish can contain up to 15 percent THC. THC acts on the cardiovascular and central nervous system. Recently, scientists have discovered a cannabis receptor in the brain. It is believed that we make our own endogenous cannabis in the form of anandamide, a derivative from arachidonic acid (Martin, 1999).

Effects

Cannabis is the most widely used illegal drug in the United States. Sixty million people have tried cannabis, and some 20 million use it regularly. Effects of cannabis include pleasure that may progress to euphoria, anxiety, apathy, detachment, passivity, enhanced appetite, slowed sense of time, altered perceptions, and sexual arousal.

The debate regarding medical marijuana continues at the federal level, although several states have approved the use of marijuana for medical purposes. Marijuana as a medical herb has been known for centuries, much longer than its use as a recreational drug. Marijuana appears to be a more potent antiemetic than prescription antiemetics. It is also useful in treating glaucoma, epilepsy, multiple sclerosis, hypertension, anorexia, and pain. A number of state nursing associations are considering the endorsement of medical use of marijuana (Martin, 1999).

Complications

Since cannabis results in slowed response time and inattention, users should not drive motor vehicles for 12 hours after using the drug. Untoward effects include acute panic reactions, hostility, or vomiting. Cannabis is often used with other drugs, for example, to extend a heroin high or to lessen anxiety when snorting cocaine (Naegle & D'Avanzo, 2001).

Embalming fluid is becoming an increasingly popular drug for users looking for a new and different high—one that often comes with violent and psychotic side effects. Users are buying marijuana cigarettes that have been soaked in the fluid and then dried. They are called by any number of names including "wet," "fry," and "illy."

Withdrawal

Withdrawal produces few symptoms.

Overdose

Overdose may result in a psychotic episode characterized by bizarre behavior, paranoia, and hallucinations. Cannabis is not lethal even at very high doses.

COCAINE

The most common street names for cocaine and mode of administration include:

- *Street names*: Coke, crack, blow, snow, C, powder, dust, flake, nose candy
- *Mode of administration*: Smoking, inhalation, injection, IV. When smoked, brain delivery rate is similar to IV.

Cocaine can be used in several ways. Snorting powdered cocaine into the nose, where it is absorbed through the mucous membrane, is a common method. There remains a persistent but erroneous belief that snorting cocaine is not addictive. It is addictive; it just takes longer. Snorting on a regular basis causes ulcerations of the nasal mucous membrane and may lead to perforation of the septum. The high is achieved about two to three minutes after use and may last as long as 20 to 30 minutes.

Smoking purified chips of cocaine, known as crack, has a higher potential for addiction and leads to more compulsive use than snorting. It is the most efficient way to deliver cocaine, taking only six to seven seconds for the drug to reach the brain. The high lasts only two to five minutes, and the crash is more severe than with snorting.

Site of Action

The primary reason people use cocaine is to stimulate the CNS. It is believed that cocaine binds to the dopamine (DA) transporters, preventing them from picking up DA, resulting in an accumulation of DA and an out-of-control reward system. The cumulative effect is an intense feeling of euphoria. Persistence blockage of DA transporters may eventually lead to depletion of DA levels. Research animals permitted to self-administer cocaine with no limitations will often overdose and die (Smock, 1999).

Effects

Because of its action on the CNS, cocaine is a uniquely addicting drug. With its powerful rewarding properties, cocaine is even capable of making obsessive users of well adjusted and mature individuals. **Positive reinforcement** occurs through the mood-altering effects of generalized euphoria, increased energy and mental alertness, a feeling of self-confidence, and increased sexual arousal. Tension, fatigue, and shyness disappear, and the person becomes more talkative and playful. Judgment may be impaired, and the person may become paranoid or even violent. The initial rush of euphoria lasts only 10 to 20 seconds followed by a less intense feeling of euphoria lasting 15 to 20 minutes.

Following cocaine use, the intense pleasure is replaced by equally unpleasant feelings. This is referred to as a rebound dysphoria, or "crash." **Negative reinforcement** occurs when the person experiences the crash and takes more cocaine to overcome the dysphoria. Both positive and negative reinforcement sustain the use of cocaine. With increased use, there is a progressive tolerance of the positive effects while the negative effects steadily intensify. In other words, the highs are not as high and the lows are much lower.

Complications

Cocaine induces constriction of coronary and cerebral vessels, leading to cardiac and cerebral infarcts with the risk being higher for those who smoke crack. Positron emission tomography (PET) studies in chronic cocaine users demonstrate decreased glucose utilization and a generalized decreased blood flow in the frontal cortex (Gottschalk, Beauvais, Hart, & Kosten, 2001).

Complications from snorting cocaine may be loss of the sense of smell and necrosis leading to perforation of the nasal septum. Smoking cocaine can cause pulmonary damage and IV use may contribute to hepatitis. Since 27 to 75 percent of cocaine abusers also meet the criteria for alcohol abuse or dependence, there are added complications (Brown et al., 1998).

Crack cocaine can lead to marathon binge use, known as a "run," lasting many hours or even days. A run can cost hundreds or thousands of dollars and leave the person in a state of total dysfunction.

Some people try speedballing, in which cocaine is mixed with heroin and injected intravenously. The high is reached in about 30 to 60 seconds. The appeal of a speedball is that the heroin decreases the unpleasant jitteriness and crash from cocaine. Speedballs are extremely dangerous. Heroin decreases the respiratory rate, as does cocaine in high enough doses. Heroin decreases the threshold for seizures, and cocaine is capable of inducing seizures. Mistakenly believing that the effects cancel each other out, some users overdose.

Space-basing is smoking crack cocaine that has been sprinkled with phencyclidine (PCP). This method may lead to intense panic and terror. People who have space-based sometimes become violent, and their behavior is uncontrollable.

Withdrawal

Symptoms of cocaine withdrawal include severe craving for cocaine and depression, which may be important triggers for relapse. Other symptoms include fatigue, irritability, vivid and unpleasant dreams, and insomnia or hypersomnia.

Overdose

Signs of cocaine intoxication include the feelings of euphoria, grandiosity, anger, combativeness, and impaired judgment. In addition, the person may experience tachycardia, elevated blood pressure, perspiration or chills, nausea and vomiting, seizures, respiratory depression, cardiac arrhythmias, hyperpyrexia, and death. Death can occur in as little as two to three minutes or up to 30 minutes after smoking crack (APA, 2000).

Treatment of cocaine overdose may require ventilation of the client. Medications include lidocaine or propranolol IV for ventricular dysrhythmias, acetaminophen or Dantrium for hyperthermia; propranolol or calcium channel blockers for tachycardia; hydralazine or nitroprusside for hypertension, and diazepam or phenobarbital for seizures.

AMPHETAMINES

Types of amphetamines include benzedrine, methedrine, dexedrine, methamphetamine, and MDMA (methylenedioxymethamphetamine—a synthetic designed drug). Common street names of amphetamines and mode of administration include:

- *Street names*: Bennies, speed, dexies, hearts, uppers, pep pills (amphetamine); crystal, crank, meth, speed, ice (methamphetamine); Ecstasy, Adam (MDMA)
- *Mode of administration*: Oral, smoking, and IV

Site of Action

The stimulant effect on the neurotransmitters is similar to cocaine. It both blocks reuptake of DA and increases release of DA. The long-lasting effects on the brain are much greater than the changes found in people who abuse heroin, alcohol, or cocaine. One or two doses can cause permanent brain damage from vasoconstriction and neurotoxicity (Volkow et al., 2001).

Effects

In small amounts, amphetamines create a sense of mental alertness, euphoria, self-confidence, and increased sex drive. As use increases, people become hypervigilant, grandiose, agitated, and irritable. Some individuals alternate between using amphetamines to "get going" and sedatives to "calm down."

Methamphetamine and MDMA are the most potent amphetamines and can cause addiction after only one try. Ice, the smokable form of methamphetamine, is sometimes used as a substitute for cocaine because it is more easily available and less expensive. The effects of ice are similar to those of crack cocaine except that the euphoric state comes on a little slower and may last as long as 12 to 30 hours. People who use ice are more likely to become violent and unpredictable in their behavior.

Instead of euphoria, MDMA users experience a warm state of empathy and good feelings for all those around them. This state of positive feelings has been described as a decrease in fear and aggression and an increase in connectedness.

Complications

Amphetamines greatly increase cardiac and respiratory rates and blood pressure. Chronic abuse frequently leads to paranoid, often violent psychotic states accompanied by auditory and tactile hallucinations. Other complications include motor disturbances similar to Parkinson's disease and poor memory performance, as well as tachycardia, arrhythmias, hypertension, altered respiration, headache, visual disturbances, and insomnia. Death may occur from cerebrovascular accident,

cardiovascular collapse, or suicide (Volkow et al., 2001).

Withdrawal

Withdrawal symptoms include exhaustion, fatigue, excessive need to sleep, unpleasant dreams, enhanced appetite, and depression. Drug craving may occur in some individuals. Depression may last for weeks and be accompanied by suicidal ideation.

Overdose

Amphetamine intoxication is often associated with impaired social or occupational functioning. Other symptoms include euphoria, hyperactivity, hypervigilance, interpersonal sensitivity, talkativeness, anxiety, anger, fighting, and impaired judgment. The person may experience tachycardia, arrthymias, coronary artery spasms, myocardial infarction, hypertension, hyperthermia, and seizures. Medications include propranolol or calcium channel blockers for tachycardia; hydralazine or nitroprusside for hypertension, and Valium or phenobarbital for seizures. A protective environment may be necessary to prevent injury or suicide.

MDMA can cause death when combined with high levels of physical activity, such as at a rave dance. Death is usually the result of greatly increased body temperature, hypertension, muscle breakdown, and kidney failure.

HALLUCINOGENS

Types of hallucinogens include lysergic acid diethylamide (LSD), mescaline, PCP, psilocybin, ketamine, and gamma-hydroxybutyrate (GHB). Common street names of hallucinogens and mode of administration include:

- *Street names*: Acid, cid, microdots, windowpane, barrel, blotter, sugar cubes, trips (LSD); mesque (mescaline); angel dust, crystal, hog, tranks, tea (PCP); magic mushrooms, shrooms (psilocybin); green mauve, L.A., special coke, Special K, bumps (ketamine); G, Liquid G (GHB)
- *Mode of administration*: Oral, smoking, inhalation, IV

Site of Action

These substances affect DA, serotonin (5-HT), norepinephrine (NE), and opioid receptors in the brain. The

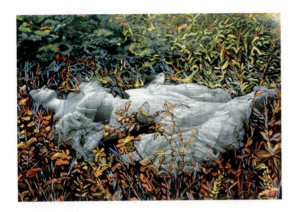

PHOTO 15.1 ■ Hallucinogenic drugs distort and intensify visual perceptions.

SOURCE: A. Rousseau/The Image Works.

effects on the brain are somewhat unpredictable and may be influenced by the environment, the experience, and the expectations of the user (Glennon, 1999).

Effects

People who take hallucinogens described vivid visual images, altered perceptions, and a sensation of slowed time. They may also experience euphoria, anxiety, labile emotions, hostility, and depression. They may be impulsive or unable to perform simple tasks.

Hallucinogens are the only drugs that animals will not self-administer, indicating that they do not like the effects. The underlying reason is that the sensory, visual, and auditory misinterpretations have no beneficial effect for survival.

Complications

One of the dangers is a "bad trip," during which the person is in a psychotic state and terrified by perceptual changes. Flashbacks occur when the person is drug free but relives the experience of being on the drug. Hallucinogens can lead to violent and out-of-control behavior.

Herbal ecstasy, also known as Cloud 9, X, and Ultimate Xphoria, is a legal (in many states) combination of herbs and other ingredients available cheaply at health food stores and truck stops as pills or tea. The main active ingredients are caffeine and ephedrine. Both of these drugs give a sense of euphoria and energy that lasts several hours. High doses can cause increased heart rate and blood pressure, heat stroke, stroke, and

death. The Food and Drug Administration (FDA) has issued warnings against the use of these drugs (Duke, 2000).

Withdrawal

Withdrawal is generally believed not to occur.

Overdose

Hallucinogen intoxication is evidenced by marked anxiety, ideas of reference, inattention, fear of losing one's mind, paranoia, and impaired judgment. Other changes include intensification of perceptions, depersonalization, illusions, hallucinations, dilated pupils, tachycardia, sweating, tremors, and incoordination. In most cases the person knows that the effects are substance induced. Cause of death may be due to accidents or suicide.

INHALANTS

Types of inhalants include volatile solvents (gasoline, lighter fluid, paint thinner, spray paint, wax removers, hair spray, odorants, air fresheners, dry cleaning fluid, spot remover, analgesic sprays), propellant gases used in aerosols such a whipped cream dispensers, nitrates (amyl nitrite, butyl nitrite), and anesthetics (nitrous oxide). Common street names of inhalants and mode of administration include:

- *Street names*: Poppers, rush (nitrates); laughing gas (nitrous oxide)
- *Mode of administration*: Fumes are inhaled directly from an open container or from a surface upon which the substance has been applied (sniffing), from a plastic bag (snorting, bagging), or from inhalant-soaked rag next to or over the mouth or nose (huffing).

Site of Action

Substances displace oxygen and cause tachycardia.

Effects

Volatile substances produce a quick form of intoxication with effects such as lightheadedness, tingling, euphoria, giddiness, impaired judgment, sense of well-being, sense of power, slurred speech, salivation, and loss of contact with reality. Other effects are sensations of floating and perceptual changes including hallucinations.

Nitrates have been used by individuals to enhance sexual experience and pleasure. Nitrates may cause euphoria and alter perceptions. Nitrous oxide, often sold in large balloons from which the gas is released, induces a state of giggling and laughter.

Complications

Chronic use of inhalants can cause multiple organ damage. In the cardiovascular system, they can lead to myocarditis and fibrosis. Some cause direct pulmonary irritation with chemical pneumonitis. Toluene, the active substance in airplane glue, may cause chronic renal failure, peripheral neuropathy, and dementia. Contact dermatitis may be seen on the hands, nose, or around the mouth. Problems associated with nitrites include panic reactions, nausea, dizziness, and hypotension. Nitrous oxide can cause a paranoid psychosis with confusion.

Withdrawal

There are no known withdrawal symptoms related to the use of inhalants.

Overdose

Anytime someone uses inhalants, she or he can die, even from the first experience. "Sudden sniffing death" is associated with arrhythmias, ventricular fibrillation, decreased cardiac output, respiratory depression, and accidents while intoxicated.

ANABOLIC STEROIDS

Types of anabolic steroids include Anadrol, Anavar, Dianobol, Durabolin, Equipose, Finajet, Halotestin, Maxibolin, Winstrol, Durabolin, and Depo-testosterone. Common street names of anabolic steriods and mode of administration include:

- *Street names*: Roids, Andro
- *Mode of administration*: Oral or IM injection. Users may "stack" steroids—mixing oral and injectable forms. Users often "pyramid"—set up a 6- or 12-week cycle beginning with low doses, slowly increase the doses, midway start decreasing the doses, ending with zero use. This may be a continuous cycle, or the user may take a break from steroid use between cycles.

Site of Action

Anabolic steroids act on testosterone receptors concentrated in certain muscle groups, genitalia, hair follicles, and a few brain regions. Steroids increase calcium

uptake in bones, increase protein synthesis, and alter the distribution of body fat (Naegle & D'Avanzo, 2001).

Effects

Athletes and body builders use anabolic steroids to build body muscle mass and strength and improve physical appearance. There is little evidence that athletic skill is enhanced by steroids, although the ability to train longer and harder is enhanced. Some people report an increase in energy and may even experience a "high."

Complications

There is a potential for liver tumors, jaundice, kidney problems, fluid retention, hypertension, and cardiovascular problems. Women using anabolic steroids may increase muscle mass, develop a deeper voice, develop a larger clitoral size, have absent menses, and be infertile. Steroids may cause a decreased sex drive, shrinking of the testicles, and infertility in males. A less well-known side effect is referred to as *roid rage*, with dramatic mood swings, manic-like episodes and a tendency toward aggressive behavior and violence (Anabolic Steroid Abuse, 2001).

Withdrawal

There are no known withdrawal effects related to the use of anabolic steroids.

Overdose

Toxicity may be evidenced by abnormal liver function tests.

CAFFEINE

Caffeine is ingested orally. Common street names for caffeine and mode of administration include:

- *Street names*: Java, Jo
- *Mode of administration*: Ingestion of liquids and food. Average amounts: brewed coffee, 125 mg/cup; instant coffee, 90 mg/cup; tea, 60 mg/cup; caffeinated soft drinks, 40 mg/cup. Chocolate and over-the-counter medications account for less than 10 percent of caffeine consumption by U.S. adults. Heavy use is daily or near-daily consumption of 625 mg or more of caffeine.

Site of Action

Absorption of caffeine occurs within minutes, and brain levels remain stable for at least one hour.

Caffeine is an adenosine receptor antagonist. Blockage of this receptor results in mental alertness, reduction in cerebral blood flow, and bronchodilation.

Effects

People use caffeine to decrease fatigue, increase alertness, and enhance a sense of well-being. People with asthma say that caffeine makes breathing easier. Caffeine is probably the most widely used drug in the world. Eighty percent of adults drink at least three cups of coffee a day (Kendler & Prescott, 1999).

Complications

The most well known side effect is nervousness. For individuals who are susceptible to hypertension, caffeine may increase blood pressure. For those who are prone to anxiety, caffeine may increase levels of anxiety. Some people who consume large doses of caffeine experience gastroesophogeal reflux.

Withdrawal

Caffeine withdrawal, occurring within 24 to 48 hours, is marked by headaches, marked fatigue or drowsiness, anxiety or depression, irritability, muscle tension, and nausea or vomiting.

Overdose

Caffeine toxicity results in feeling ill, shaky or jittery.

NICOTINE

Types of nicotine include tobacco products: cigarettes, cigars, pipes, and chewing tobacco. Common street names of nicotine and mode of administration include:

- *Street names*: smokes, fags, chaw
- *Mode of administration*: Inhalation, chewing, prescription gum or patch

Site of Action

Nicotine acts as an agonist at the nicotinic receptor, a subtype of acetylcholine receptor. It acts as a stimulant to the CNS by releasing DA in the nucleus accumbens, the reward center of the brain (Salokangas et al., 2000).

Effects

Nicotine produces feelings of alertness, increases blood pressure and heart rate, increases irritability, and decreases appetite.

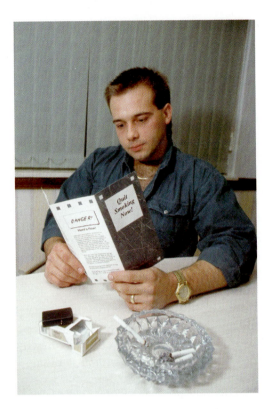

PHOTO 15.2 ■ Smoking is one of the greatest preventable hazards to health.

SOURCE: Dennis MacDonald/PhotoEdit.

Complications

Nicotine is still the leading cause of preventable, premature death in the world. The long-term health problems are related to the tars and other compounds released when burned. The most common complications are lung disease, cancer of the lung, and cardiovascular disease. People who chew tobacco are at higher risk for cancer of the mouth. Use of nicotine is more common among people with other mental disorders (APA, 2000).

Withdrawal

Symptoms of withdrawal include craving, anxiety, restlessness, decreased concentration, overeating, irritability, frustration, constipation, and headaches. Nicotine gum and nicotine patches relieve withdrawal symptoms.

Overdose

Symptoms of nicotine overdose include heart palpitation, anxiety, and sleep disturbance.

BEHAVIORAL CHARACTERISTICS

Lack of control in using chemicals is the central behavioral characteristic. Because alcohol and drugs decrease inhibitions, many substance abusers become hostile, argumentative, loud, boisterous, and even violent when they are under the influence of the chemical. Compulsive and long-term substance abusers are at higher risk for violence than are recreational or intermittent users. Other users become withdrawn, tearful, and socially isolated when they are under the influence.

Behavioral characteristics are exhibited in the workplace as frequent absences. If workers are abusing substances at noon, their productivity decreases in the afternoon. They often have interpersonal problems at work that are related to their chemically dependent behavior. They may fail to get promoted or may lose a job, and frequent job changes are common.

Users who obtain their drugs through prescriptions may be able to live normally without arousing suspicion, but those who use illegal drugs may have to alter their lifestyle. The latter group often becomes involved in a drug subculture in which self-protection, prostitution, theft, and burglary prevail. As a result of this kind of lifestyle, they often find themselves in legal difficulties.

AFFECTIVE CHARACTERISTICS

Psychoactive substances are used by some people as stimulants to overcome feelings of boredom and depression. Others use these substances to manage their anxiety and stress. The overall intention is to decrease negative feelings and increase positive feelings.

People who abuse substances are often *emotionally labile*. They may be grandiose or irritable at one moment and morose and guilty the next. When they try to control their use of drugs and fail in this attempt, they experience feelings of guilt and shame. When the problem becomes public knowledge, they are likely to feel embarrassed and humiliated.

Ellen is a 29-year-old woman who was recently released from an outpatient detoxification facility. Ellen's older daughter came home from school and found her mother drinking. When the daughter tried to take the bottle from Ellen,

Ellen slapped her across the face. Realizing what she had done, Ellen tried to grab her daughter to comfort her, but the girl ran away screaming, "I hate you!"

COGNITIVE CHARACTERISTICS

Some people have *low self-esteem* prior to their chemical dependence. They may have turned to drugs as a way to feel better about themselves. Others develop low self-esteem as a result of their problems with substance abuse. Grandiose thoughts may be an attempt for both groups to compensate for low self-esteem (Boyd, 2000).

Denial is the major defense mechanism that helps maintain a chemical dependence. Denial, which is self-deception and an unconscious attempt to maintain self-esteem in the face of out-of-control behavior, enables a person to underestimate the amount of drugs used and to avoid recognizing the impact of abusing behavior on others. Denial results from cultural standards of what is or is not appropriate behavior. Supporting the denial is the use of projection, minimization, and rationalization. *Projection*, seeing others as being responsible for one's substance abuse, is heard in: "My three teenagers are driving me crazy. It's their fault I drink." *Minimization*, not acknowledging the significance of one's behavior, is heard in: "Don't believe everything my wife tells you. I wasn't so high that I couldn't drive." *Rationalization*, giving reasons for the behavior, is heard in: "I only use Valium because I'm so unhappy in my marriage." These defense mechanisms are considered consequences, not causes, of chemical dependence. They serve to protect self-esteem by giving an explanation that helps the person conform to cultural standards (Wing, 1996).

Alcoholic denial has many aspects, including denial of facts, denial of implications, denial of change, and denial of feelings. *Denial of facts* is the outermost layer of protection and the most frequently used form of denial. It functions to avoid negative consequences. It is heard in: "I have not been drinking," and "I only had one or two beers." *Denial of implications* is used when some threatening fact gets established and that fact is made public, as in a DUI (driving under the influence). It functions to avoid the image of failure and is heard in: "Okay, I had a few, but I wasn't drunk," "I only smoke pot," and "Your sister drinks more than I do." *Denial of change* helps people resist making any real change. It functions to protect them from assuming responsibility for their own behavior. It is heard in: "So, I'm an alcoholic, so what," "I'll try to stop," and "I wanted to stay sober, but I couldn't." *Denial of feelings* is aimed at shutting off feelings and protects people from being overwhelmed by strong emotions. It is heard in: "It doesn't bother me" and "I'm not angry!" Denial can be a major obstacle to treatment, for no treatment will be effective until the individual acknowledges that the substance abuse is out of control.

Blackouts are a form of amnesia for events that occurred during the drinking period. The person may carry out conversations and activities with no loss of consciousness, but have total amnesia for those activities the next day.

Marian, a 53-year-old woman has been a "closet drinker" for more than 15 years. She has tried to keep her drinking a secret from her husband and friends by using a strong mouthwash to cover up the alcohol odor of her breath, which was not very effective. Her husband has become more concerned as she seems to have frequent falls and bruising. His concern was heightened one day when Marian misplaced the mail, and he finally found it in the refrigerator.

SOCIAL CHARACTERISTICS

Social values contribute to the problem of substance abuse in the United States. The mass media promote the desire for immediate gratification and self-indulgence. Complex family problems are solved in 30 minutes on television. All forms of media push over-the-counter medications for minor ailments, contributing to the expectation of a pain-free existence. Values such as these indirectly support the use and abuse of chemical substances.

Effects on the Family

Substance abuse is a family problem, and the most devastating impact occurs when the abuser is a parent. Power struggles between abusing and nonabusing partners destroy couples and contribute to a *dysfunctional*

family system. Family relationships begin to deteriorate, and family members become trapped in a cycle of shame, anger, confusion, and guilt. In some families, substance abuse is a contributing factor to emotional neglect and physical or sexual abuse. Often, family members and old friends will be abandoned for new relationships within the drug subculture. In other cases, chemically dependent people simply become more isolated as alcohol or drugs become the main focus of their lives. Some are successful in keeping their substance abuse hidden from their colleagues and most of their significant relationships.

Financial problems may arise from underemployment or unemployment as the compulsion to use chemicals takes precedence over work. However, many substance abusers continue to be employed. For those using illegal substances, the cost can be incredibly expensive. Illegal substance abusers may be criminally involved with the legal system. Some use prostitution or drug dealing as a way to pay for their drugs. Some become involved in minor crimes such as pickpocketing or shoplifting to obtain money for the drugs. Yet others turn to robberies and burglaries to support the high cost of their habit.

Kendal, age 36, has a 20-year history of poly-drug abuse. At 16, he smoked pot every day, drank beer and wine, and used downers, Valium, and phenobarbital. He dropped out of school in the middle of his sophomore year. His sporadic employment history includes being a laborer and a short-order cook. The longest Kendal has ever been employed is 8 months. His wife has filed for divorce because of his financial problems, drinking, and verbal abuse. He has been living with his mother, but she recently told him to leave because he continues to abuse alcohol and other drugs. He has been charged with public intoxication five times and has been picked up on assault charges for disturbing the peace and resisting arrest while being intoxicated. Kendal appears to be dependent on others to take care of him or make decisions for him.

Ineffective communication patterns contribute to anxiety and anger. In an attempt to create the illusion of normality, substance abuse is never discussed within or outside of the family system. This refusal to acknowledge there is a problem contributes to family denial. To avoid embarrassment, family members make excuses to outsiders for the user's behavior. A nonabusing partner may remain in a relationship because of emotional dependency, money, family cohesion, religious compliance, or outward respectability. Other nonabusing partners may threaten to or actually leave the abuser. At this point, the abuser promises never to drink or use again, the family is reunited, the promise is usually broken, and the family becomes locked into a dysfunctional pattern.

Co-dependency

Co-dependency is a relationship in which a non–substance-abusing partner remains with a substance-abusing partner. The relationship is dysfunctional—the nonabusing partner is overresponsible and the abusing partner is underresponsible. Co-dependents operate out of fear, resentment, helplessness, and hopelessness. They are obsessively driven to control the user's behavior and to solve the problems created by the user. When this is not effective, co-dependents become exhausted and depressed but are unable to stop the "helping" behaviors. They often suffer from low self-esteem and fear of abandonment. Co-dependents are *caretakers*, and this caretaking activity may be a compensation for feelings of inadequacy. Women may be more vulnerable to co-dependent behavior because they have been socialized to be responsible for the family and often feel they are expected to be loyal to their partner at all costs. As professionals, we must be careful not to pathologize women by blaming them for the user's behavior (Martsolf, Sedlak, & Doheny, 2000; Stafford, 2001).

Co-dependents often engage in **enabling behavior**, which is any action by a person that consciously or unconsciously facilitates substance dependence. Enabling behaviors, such as making excuses for the partner with the employer and lying to others about the abuse, protect the substance abuser from the natural consequences of the problem. Enabling is a response to addiction, not a cause of addiction. The purpose of enabling is the family's instinctual desire to stay together. It is a process of compensating for the dysfunction in one family member and avoiding the issues that threaten the breakup of the family.

Children of Alcoholics

It is estimated that one out of every eight Americans is a child of an alcoholic parent. Children who grow up in homes where one or both parents are alcoholics often suffer the effects their entire lives. Dysfunctional family roles develop around the impact of alcoholism. Despite mysterious events, nonsense language, and threats of impending doom, everyone in the family acts as if the situation were perfectly normal. It is extremely frightening to have a parent who switches from being a joking, pleasant person to a raging tyrant in the blink of an eye. It is terrifying to live with a drunken father who not only screams that he is going to kill the child but then attempts to do just that. At the same time, the parent convinces the child that if it weren't for what the child did, the parent would not be acting that way.

Very early in life, children of alcoholics learn to *keep the secret* and not talk about the alcohol problem, even within the family. They are taught not to talk about their own feelings, needs, and wants; they learn not to feel at all. Eventually, they repress all feelings and become numb to both pain and joy. The children become objects whose reason for existence is to please the alcoholic parent and serve his or her needs. Children of alcoholics are expected always to be in control of their behavior and their feelings. They are expected to be perfect and never make mistakes. However, within the family system, no child can ever be perfect "enough." Consistency is necessary for building trust, and alcoholic parents are very unpredictable. Children learn not to expect reliability in relationships. They learn very early that if you don't trust another person, you won't be disappointed.

Children of alcoholics tend to develop one of four patterns of behavior. The *hero*, often the oldest child, becomes the competent caretaker and works on making the family function. The *scapegoat* acts out at home, in school, and in the community. This child takes the focus off the alcoholic parent by getting into trouble and becoming the focus of conflict in the family. The behavior may also be a way to draw attention to the family in an unconscious attempt to seek help. The *lost child* tries to avoid conflict and pain by withdrawing physically and emotionally. The *mascot*, often the youngest child, tries to ease family tension with comic relief used to mask his or her own sadness (Williams, 1996).

In dysfunctional families, designated roles keep the family balanced. Each role is a way to handle the distress and shame of having an alcoholic parent. Every family member has a sense of some control, even though the roles do not change the family system's dysfunction.

Leticia, a 14-year-old high school student, had been an excellent student when suddenly her grades dropped dramatically. She tearfully confessed to her school counselor that personal problems were affecting her grades. Leticia explained that her father had a "drinking problem" but had been going to AA for several years. Three months ago, Leticia's father lost his job and was unable to get another. A month ago, he started a pattern of binge drinking. Leticia was reluctant to talk because she knew her mother would be furious if she knew Leticia had revealed the family secret. Leticia's mother was working overtime to keep the family going. When Leticia's mother was home, she fought constantly with her husband about his drinking. Her father tried to get Leticia to buy alcohol for him after her mother poured his supply down the drain. When Leticia tried to explain that she was too young to purchase alcohol, her father screamed at her, "Get out of my sight! You're useless!" When her father was sober, he tried to be Leticia's best friend. Leticia stopped bringing friends home because she didn't know what to expect. She was too nervous to do homework, always worrying about what her father might do. Leticia told the counselor, "I don't want him to be my friend. I don't even want him for a father anymore!"

Adult children of alcoholics grow up denying the stresses of their dysfunctional families. Denial becomes a frequent defense mechanism that only makes things worse as they proceed through life. The sense of total obligation to the alcoholic parent makes it extremely difficult for adult children to criticize the addicted parent.

Adult children of alcoholics have grown up without mature adult role models and without experiencing healthy family dynamics. They expect all relationships to be based on power, violence, deceit, and misinformation. They often have difficulty expressing emotion and receiving expressions of feelings. Some grow up to repeat the family pattern by either becoming addicted themselves or marrying an addicted person.

Adult children of alcoholics often feel a need to change others or to control the environment for the good of others. They typically deny powerlessness and try to solve all problems alone. They blame themselves for not being able to achieve what no one can achieve. Obsessions are common forms of defense, such as constant worrying, preoccupations with work or other activities that bring about good feelings, and compulsive achievement. The obsessive pattern covers the feelings of helplessness and blocks the feelings of anxiety, inadequacy, and fear of abandonment.

Social Morality

Most Americans have a moralistic attitude about substance dependence. It is viewed as a sin or as the result of a weak will. Addicts are seen as totally responsible for their situation and are expected to use willpower to control themselves and become respectable members of society once again. Social class may also influence one's perspective of substance abuse. For example, nurses who have moralistic views may have difficulty accepting the disorder in a clergyperson yet have no reservations acknowledging alcoholism among gang members or the homeless population (Wing, 1996).

This moralistic perspective especially *stigmatizes women*. Men's drinking tends to be more public and more socially acceptable than women's, which often drives women's alcohol problems underground. Women are expected to be "ladylike" at all times, and when they drink too much or get high, they are quickly labeled "loose women," "sleaze-bags," or "drunks." Most treatment programs are developed for and serve men. Often unacknowledged is the fact that women have different clinical courses and treatment needs than do men. Mothers may avoid treatment for fear of triggering investigations by child welfare services and losing custody of their children. Another difficulty is that there may be no safe place for their children while they are in treatment (Ehrmin, 2001).

Even more stigmatized by American society are *lesbian alcoholics*. They suffer as women in a male-dominated culture and also carry the double stigma of being lesbian and being alcoholic. Lesbian women have a higher rate of alcohol consumption than heterosexual women do. They also attempt suicide seven times more often and have higher rates of completed suicide than do heterosexual, nonalcoholic women. In a homophobic culture, coming to terms with one's homosexuality and accepting a gay identity are very painful. It is thought that depression, alcohol use, and suicide among lesbians may be related to the effects of stigmatization (Alexander, 1996).

Women who have been abused physically and sexually are at greater risk for becoming alcoholics than nonabused women. It is believed that using alcohol may be an attempt to self-medicate while coping with the physical and emotional consequences of abuse. (Domestic violence is covered fully in Chapter 21, and sexual abuse is covered in Chapter 22.)

Several states have enacted legislation to decriminalize nonviolent drug use. The goal is to order drug treatment rather than incarceration. First- and second-time nonviolent offenders are treated as medical patients instead of criminals. This is a major philosophical shift whose evolution will be interesting to follow.

High-Technology Lifestyle

The digital revolution has transformed some young adults' lives into a combination of excessive wealth, driving ambition, long work hours, and a pressure to perform. Illicit drug activity is booming among high-tech workers, and drugs are the latest "secret" of the industry—speed to work on, coke to play on, and smoking heroin to come down on. It is too early for formal research studies that quantify the problem, but there are obvious signs of its growth within the computer industry.

CULTURE-SPECIFIC CHARACTERISTICS

The social consequences of abuse of substances are increasing in more and more countries as well as in the United States. The problem has increased and become more complex with the arrival of hard drugs in third world countries. Many countries cannot cope with basic health needs, much less substance-use disorders (Olatawura, 2000).

There are many different ethnic groups in the United States, each having its own unique values regarding the definition of substance abuse and how it should be regarded and treated. Sociocultural factors often determine the choice of the substance and the extent to which it is abused. The use of naturally produced drugs is deeply rooted in many cultures. In some contexts, such as in communion in Christian churches or in ceremonies of the Native American church, substances are considered sacred. The use of mind-altering drugs for treatment of medical conditions is legally permitted but controlled. In other circumstances, the use of these same drugs is considered criminal. In some cultures, alcohol is consumed as part of normal mealtime activities and used to celebrate social events, and does not contribute to the development of substance use problems (Paris, 1999).

Euro-Americans have the highest overall rates of alcohol consumption. Euro-American men are much more likely to be heavy drinkers, while only 8 percent of the women are classified as heavy drinkers. Heavy drinking among males is highest is the 18 to 29 age group. One third of the women abstain completely (Naegle & D'Avanzo, 2001).

African Americans abstain more and drink less than Euro-Americans. Only 4 percent of the women are classified as heavy drinkers, and more than 50 percent abstain completely. However, the leading cause of death among African American males between the ages of 15 and 34 is homicide, and alcohol and/or drugs are implicated in at least 70 percent of these incidents. African Americans are more likely to be arrested than to be treated for substance-related disorders (Wright, 2001).

Hispanic Americans are the largest minority population in the United States. Mexican Americans are the largest subgroup followed by Puerto Ricans and Cuban Americans. There are significant differences in the patterns of alcohol and drug use among the various subgroups. Puerto Ricans have the highest use of marijuana and cocaine, while among Mexican Americans, alcohol is the most abused substance. Hispanic American men typically increase their drinking from their 20s to their 30s, then decrease it after age 40. The ability to consume large amounts of alcohol without appearing intoxicated is associated with "machismo." Hispanic American women are similar to African American women in that nearly half abstain from any use of alcohol (Arboleda-Florez & Weisstub, 2000; Naegle & D'Avanzo, 2001).

Asian Americans have the lowest consumption levels and rates of alcohol-related problems of all the major racial and cultural groups. Fifty percent of Asian Americans lack the active form of the enzyme aldehyde dehydrogenase. This genetic deficiency leads to the accumulation of acetaldehyde when drinking, resulting in the "flushing" response—facial flushing and cardiac palpitations. This genetic predisposition may, in actuality, be a protective factor (Pi & Gray, 2000).

Chinese culture, for example, discourages solitary drinking and emphasizes social drinking associated with eating. Sharing a meal with others includes ritualistic toasting, which increases social interactions and increases the bonds of friendship. Japanese Americans have the highest rate of alcohol, tranquilizer, marijuana, and cocaine use (Liu, 2000).

Alcohol use among Arab Americans is rare. One of the protective factors may be the influence of Islam, which condemns the use of alcohol. Little is known about substance abuse problems among this ethnic group. There is also not much data on Asian Indian Americans. It appears that they are more prone to use alcohol or drugs after migration to a foreign country (Abudabbeh & Hamid, 2001; Sandhu & Malik, 2001).

The Europeans introduced alcohol to the Native People population. Because Native Peoples are not a homogeneous group, there is considerable tribal variation in drinking patterns. In general, the magnitude of alcohol problems is greater among Native Peoples than among other groups in the United States. The percentage of Native Peoples who abstain is about the same as in the general population. Among those who do drink, however, there are significantly fewer light or moderate drinkers (23 percent) and over twice as many heavy drinkers. As with other cultural groups, the men drink more than the women do. Alcohol is associated with social situations, and there is little solitary drinking. Men tend to drink in groups and pass the bottle. It is considered rude or insulting to refuse the offer of a drink. Alcohol is the drug of choice for Native youth, although marijuana and inhalants are also used more than in the general population. Hawk Littlejohn, the medicine man of the Cherokee Nation, Eastern Band, attributes this problem to the fact that Native Peoples have lost the opportunity to make choices. They can no longer choose how they live or how they practice their religion. He believes that once people return to a sense of identification, they will begin to rid themselves of alcoholism (Spector, 2000; Weaver, 2001).

AGE-SPECIFIC CHARACTERISTICS

Children and Adolescents

In American society, the use of alcohol and cannabis during the teen and young adult years is a common practice. For many, it is a stage of experimentation, with use decreasing with age. For others, alcohol use continues and expands until the stage of addiction is reached.

Adolescent substance use is related to many factors. If parents are users, there may be a genetic influence as well as a modeling influence. Research shows that all types of parental substance use are associated with children's substance use. Alcohol and drug use is often accepted in the teen peer group. Developmentally, adolescents may abuse substances as a means of rebelling against parents, in a search for identity, and in an effort to separate from the family. Other risk factors include sensation-seeking tendencies, risk-taking tendencies, and the availability of drugs. Some teens experiencing family dysfunction, problems in school, problems with peers, and/or emotional or physical trauma may feel overwhelmed and attempt to escape through the use of substances. Some adolescents suffering from mental disorders try to self-medicate with alcohol or drugs (Johnson, 1999; Richter & Richter, 2001).

Peak initiation for alcohol and cigarette use is between the 6th and 9th grades. Initiation of marijuana peaks between the 9th and 11th grades while other illegal drug initiation peaks between the 10th and 12th grades (Chassin & Ritter, 2001).

Substance-related disorders progress more rapidly in adolescents than in adults. Adults may take from two to seven years from the first use to full dependency. Teens may make this progression in 6 to 18 months. Research shows that the earlier the age at which young people take their first drink of alcohol, the greater the risk of developing serious problems. Over 40 percent of all people who drink alcohol between the ages of 11 and 14 become alcohol dependent. That is four times the rate (10 percent) for those who have their first drink at ages 20 and older (Chassin & Ritter, 2001; DeWit, Adlaf, Offord, & Ogborne, 2000).

The use of denial is often stronger since teens do not have years of negative consequences. They often experience developmental delays: Growth and development slows down, they fall behind in academics, their social skills stagnate, they experience poor impulse control, and they are intolerant of delayed gratification. They typically shift to a peer group composed solely of other drug-using adolescents. In a two-parent home, the roles may be polarized, with one parent being the enabler and the other parent the enforcer. This creates much family conflict and distress.

The National Institute on Drug Abuse (1999) tracks prevalence of alcohol use among adolescents. Alcohol consumption among high school seniors has shown a steady decrease since 1979. In 1979, 88 percent of seniors used alcohol in the past year, 72 percent used alcohol in the past month, and 7 percent drank on a daily basis. In 1999, 74 percent of seniors used alcohol in the past year, 51 percent used alcohol in the past month, and 3.4 percent drank on a daily basis. Data has also been collected regarding adolescents who drink and drive. In 1997, 21 percent of males and 12 percent of females drove a car one or more times when they had been drinking. In the same year, 38 percent of males and 34.5 percent of females rode one or more times in a car driven by someone who had been drinking.

For teens under the age of 18, inhalants are the fourth most abused drug, after alcohol, tobacco, and marijuana. About 17 percent of adolescents in the United States say that they have sniffed inhalants at least once in their lives. Inhalant abuse is more common among early teens, with usage dropping off as they grow older. In addition, there is an extraordinary amount of online information on how to obtain, synthesize, extract, and ingest a wide range of hallucinogens. This Web-based information is proving to be of significant danger to vulnerable individuals (Halpern & Pope, 2001).

Older Adults

Illicit drug use, such as cocaine or opiates, is more unusual in older adults compared to young adults. Alcohol abuse, however, is a problem for 10 to 15 percent of older adults. Often, they go undiagnosed because in old age the symptoms can be subtle or atypical, or mimic symptoms of other geriatric illnesses. Clients may present with erratic changes in mood or behavior; malnutrition; bladder and bowel incontinence; gait disorders; and recurring falls, burns, or head trauma.

Older adults have less social, legal, occupational, and interpersonal consequences of their alcohol abuse because they are often not working and often live alone. Two thirds of this group have had long-standing problems with alcohol and have multiple medical complications. One third develop the drinking problem late in life, often in response to bereavement, retirement, loneliness, relationship stress, and physical illnesses. Denial of substance abuse is common at all ages but may be more intense in older adults because of memory problems and the shame-based belief of this generation that substance abuse is immoral (Eliopoulos, 2001).

Abuse of prescription drugs among the elderly is two to three times higher than the general population. Benzodiazepine dependence is most common and may have been prescribed for long periods of time. Of individuals who have a history of long-term use (more than one year), 70 percent are over the age of 50 and often have physical health problems. Among older people who are institutionalized, the abuse is even more widespread. Benzodiazepine abuse in the elderly results in excessive daytime sedation; ataxia, which increases the risk of falls and accidents; and cognitive impairments such as attention and memory problems (Coogle, Osgood, & Parham, 2000).

PHYSIOLOGICAL CHARACTERISTICS
Central Nervous System Effects

An addicted brain is different, both physically and chemically, from a normal brain. Substances of abuse alter the brain's reward system by artificially boosting DA effects. Cocaine blocks the DA transporter, leaving excess DA in the synapse, which keeps the pleasure circuit firing. Heroin and nicotine stimulate the release of DA. Amphetamines block DA transporters and stimulate the release of DA. Alcohol alters DA, 5-HT, glutamate, and GABA neurotransmission. Low levels of 5-HT are related to increased aggression. Chronic use of mind-altering drugs decreases the number of DA receptors. With fewer receptors, the drugs do not have the effect they originally did and higher doses are needed to get the same effect (Krakowski, 2000).

Withdrawal is also a result of the altered DA system. Withdrawal and abstinence deprive the brain of the only source of DA that produces a sense of pleasure. Without the drug, life seems not worth living. Continued abstinence, however, allows DA receptors and the DA system to return to normal.

Professionals are concerned not just with the direct effects of alcohol and drugs on the brain but also with residual effects that cause *craving* and a return to compulsive substance abuse. It is believed that each time a drug is used, specific brain structures are activated, leaving a memory trace that remains long after the drug has disappeared from the body. There is growing evidence that the cerebellum is involved in this learned memory association. Each incidence of drug use is paired with environmental cues of persons, places, and things, which then have the ability to trigger the same brain circuits even in the absence of the drug. Addicts begin to crave their drugs when they see, hear, or smell a reminder of past use. Brain imaging techniques have been able to measure changes in the amygdala, the anterior cingulate, and the prefrontal cortex in response to environmental triggers (Schneider et al., 2001).

Sexual Effects

A rapid increase in *sexually transmitted infections (STIs)* has been associated with substance abuse, especially crack cocaine. Users of illegal substances may trade sex for the drug. Cocaine abusers often get involved in multiple-partner sex and are unable to consider safer sex practices when high. Since alcohol decreases inhibitions and judgment, there has been a rise in STIs among adolescents and young adults. Contaminated needles are a leading cause of the spread of hepatitis, HIV infection, and AIDS. As this problem grows, the premature death rate from drug abuse may approach that of alcohol abuse (Anderson & Mathieu, 1998; Harsch et al., 2000).

Substance-related disorders have a number of *sexual consequences*. Chronic *alcohol* abuse leads to erection problems for 40 percent of men as well as ejaculation difficulties in 10 to 25 percent of men. Among women entering treatment for alcoholism, 70 to 80 percent have difficulty achieving orgasm, 30 to 40 percent have problems with sexual arousal, and 30 percent have lost their desire for sex. People who use *marijuana* report enhanced sexual enjoyment with an intensification of touch and perception. They have increased attentiveness to their partner, although sexual behavior remains the same. The initial use of *amphetamines* increases sex drive and sensations; long-term use leads to problems with arousal, function, and the sense of pleasure. Use of *hallucinogens* can create both extremely positive and negative sexual effects. The heightened sensory-perceptual stimuli may enhance or intensify sex or create a terrifying experience. Sexual performance may be impossible because of intoxication. People using *opioids* find their desire for sex has been replaced with their desire for the drug. They also experience decreased sexual arousal and difficulties with orgasm/ejaculation.

Cocaine is associated with hypersexuality. Seventy percent of males and 30 percent of females report a strong link between cocaine use and a variety of sexual acting-out behaviors. Cocaine is a CNS stimulant that relaxes inhibitions, increases sexual fantasies, and increases sexual desire. High doses of cocaine can produce compulsive masturbation, multipartner marathons, group sex, and even sexual abuse of children. It is not uncommon for cocaine abusers to go on marathon binges of cocaine and sex (Crenshaw & Goldberg, 1996).

Intrauterine Substance Exposure

It is known that many of these chemicals cross the placental barrier and have harmful effects on unborn children. Prenatal substance use screening by primary care professionals has become an established public health priority, and women are advised to abstain completely during pregnancy.

Tobacco, the most abused substance by pregnant women, increases the flow of carbon monoxide to the fetus and decreases placental blood flow. Smoking is a risk factor for miscarriage, ectopic pregnancy, preeclampsia, abruptio placenta, placenta previa, and premature rupture of membranes. Effects on the infant include low birth weight, prematurity, higher risk for sudden infant death syndrome (SIDS), and an increase in respiratory illness and ear infections (Naegle & D'Avanzo, 2001; Richter & Richter, 2001).

Alcohol is the second most abused substance by pregnant women (19 percent) and causes abnormalities ranging from the subtle cognitive-behavioral impairments of **alcohol-related birth defects (ARBDs)** to the symptoms of **fetal alcohol syndrome (FAS)**. Individuals with ARBDs or FAS often develop significant mental illness as they mature. It is believed that alcohol causes faulty central nervous system cell migration during fetal development. FAS is the third leading cause of birth defects in the United States including heart defects, malformed facial features, and low IQ or mental retardation. Other effects are low

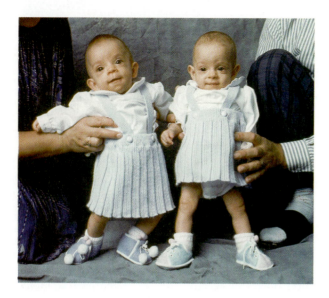

PHOTO 15.3 ■ Fetal alcohol syndrome. Fetal alcohol syndrome is the result of women consuming alcohol during pregnancy, and it can have many severe effects on the child; among them are physical malformations such as those shown here.

SOURCE: George Steinmetz/San Francisco AIDS Foundation.

birth weight, slow growth rate, hyperactivity, maladaptive behavior, and severe reading and math disabilities. Some children with FAS show improvement over time, but academic problems and behavioral disorders seem to persist for most of them (Richter & Richter, 2001).

Recent studies suggest that poverty and the use of cigarettes and alcohol while pregnant may be more responsible for fetal damage than cocaine. Cocaine is especially dangerous to the fetus if it is used during the first trimester of pregnancy when the brain is developing. Cocaine is such a potent vasoconstrictor that reduced blood supply to the fetus causes neurological abnormalities that may result in learning and behavioral problems. After birth, these infants tend to experience abnormal sleep patterns, tremors, poor feeding, irritability, and sometimes seizures. Many of the effects disappear as the infant develops (Ratey, 2001).

Children who have been exposed to opioids prior to birth are very sensitive to noise and are irritable and tremulous. They may have uncoordinated sucking and swallowing reflexes, which cause feeding problems (Naegle & D'Avanzo, 2001).

CONCOMITANT DISORDERS/ DUAL DIAGNOSIS OF MENTALLY ILL CHEMICAL ABUSER

Clients must be assessed for **dual diagnosis**, the presence of substance abuse with a concurrent psychiatric disorder. A dual diagnosis indicates one of three things: Two independent disorders occur together, substance abuse caused the other mental disorder, or the person with the mental disorder uses substances in an effort to self-medicate and feel better. Whatever the original cause of substance abuse, it usually complicates all other problems so much that it must be dealt with immediately. Substance abuse can precipitate prolonged psychotic relapses and contribute to medication noncompliance, as well as unstable relationships, financial mismanagement, disruptive behavior, and unstable housing. One study found that untreated dually diagnosed persons are 12 times more likely to have a history of violence (Dixon & DeVeau, 1999).

Individuals with a psychiatric disorder are at higher risk for having a substance abuse disorder. Of the general population, 13 percent abuse alcohol and 6 percent abuse drugs. The risk is twice as high for those suffering from depression, bipolar disorder, or an anxiety disorder. For those who are young and psychiatrically disabled, the substance abuse rate is around 50 percent. Antisocial behavior is predictive of both adolescent and adult involvement in substance abuse, and about 70 percent of those diagnosed with antisocial personality disorder are chemically dependent. One study found that more men become depressed as a result of alcohol abuse while more women experience depression first and then self-medicate with alcohol. People who seek treatment for either posttraumatic stress disorder (PTSD) or substance use disorder have relatively high rates of co-morbidity for the other disorder. The rates of co-morbidity from substance abuse (excluding tobacco) and pathological gambling, range from 34 to 80 percent, among those in treatment. The substance most abused by pathological gamblers is alcohol (Boyd & Mackey, 2000; Hall et al., 2000; Wu, Kouzis, & Leaf, 1999).

People with mental illnesses report that their reasons for using substances include attempting to improve unpleasant moods such as anxiety and depression, increasing social interactions, and increasing pleasure by feeling high. It is clear, however, that drugs and alcohol often increase psychotic symptoms and are a factor in relapse of mental illness. Violence against others and violence against oneself also occur more frequently in substance-abusing persons with mental illness (Miller, 1997).

CAUSATIVE THEORIES

Extensive research on the causes of substance dependence has yielded theories that combine biological and sociocultural components. It is obvious that there are multiple pathways for substance use disorders. The high risk factors are a genetic predisposition, an exposure to substances, and social reinforcement. Those individuals with the strongest predisposition may develop substance use disorders in any cultural setting where substances are available. Although the theories are presented separately, remember that they interact in ways that are not yet clearly understood.

Genetics

Substance-related disorders are heterogeneous. Many studies have focused on families in an attempt to determine whether a predisposition to alcoholism or substance abuse is inherited. Twins and adoptees have been studied to determine the role of genetics, and it has been found that alcoholism clearly runs in families, with inheritability estimates of 40 to 60 percent. This means that approximately half the risk for alcohol abuse disorders in the population can be explained by genetic factors. Early-onset alcoholism is a marker for a stronger genetic predisposition. Though we know there is an inheritable component, we do not know exactly what is inherited. It may be poor self-regulation, sensation seeking, or negative affect with a need to self-medicate (Chassin & Ritter, 2001).

The genetic susceptibility is complicated and involves multiple genes. Each gene alone may not have power to cause alcoholism, but a group of genes acting together has a stronger influence. If the individual inherits a set of predisposing genes and encounters the necessary environmental influences, then there will be a high probability that substance abuse disorder will result (Paris, 1999; Prescott & Kendler, 1999).

Genetic defects lead to deficiencies and imbalances in neurotransmitters, neuropeptides, and receptors. These chemical changes may give rise to a wide range of behavioral disturbances and a variety of compulsive disorders.

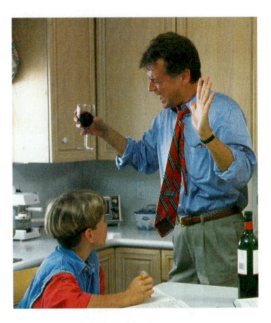

PHOTO 15.4 ■ Alcoholism runs in families because of a combination of genetic and environmental factors.

SOURCE: Tom & Dee Ann McCarthy/Corbis/Stock Market.

Neurobiological Theory

Craving for a drug is a cardinal feature of addictive disorders and is significant because of its potential to trigger drug use and relapse. Both stress and internal and external cues prompt craving in people who abuse substances. Internal cues might be the feeling of anxiety, anger, depression, or frustration. External or environmental cues include drug-using friends, drug-using places, or seeing drug paraphernalia.

Cravings for alcohol, drugs, and food share a mechanism involving the reward system in the brain. Dopamine (DA) is not just the neurotransmitter that transmits pleasure signals, but it may, in fact, be the master molecule of craving and addiction. Genetic defects may alter DA neurotransmission by (Wexler et al., 2001):

- Interfering with the normal release of DA at critical receptor sites in the reward centers of the brain
- Changing the structure of DA receptors, resulting in decreased DA binding
- Decreasing the number of DA receptors, leading to decreased DA binding

Addictive substances such as alcohol, cocaine, heroin, coffee, nicotine, and chocolate temporarily offset or overcome these defects by artificially inducing the release of abnormal amounts of DA. Moderate levels of stimulation or excitement have a similar effect. Increased DA transmission in the basal ganglia, particularly the nucleus accumbens, is directly responsible for the exhilarating rush that reinforces the desire to get more of the substance (Kalivas, 2001). Thus, these substances move normal brain processes into an exaggerated state. Glucose probably has the same effect, thus causing a compulsive craving for food in some eating disorders.

Some individuals may begin with low levels of neurotransmitters. The first use of a substance corrects for this deficiency, which explains why people often enjoy their first experience with the alcohol or drug. The problem is that the psychoactive substance then creates an even greater deficiency of neurotransmitters, which contributes to craving for more of the substance.

We still have a lot to learn about addiction. Researchers are looking at different roles that DA receptor subtypes play in creating and maintaining addiction. Other researchers have vaccines for substance abuse in clinical trials. It is important to remember that all genetic and neurobiological theories leave room for the substantial impact of environmental, social, and individual factors.

Intrapersonal Theory

For many years, intrapersonal theories were the only causative explanations for substance dependence, and they contributed to the moral perspective that still exists in the general population today. These theories describe substance dependence as being determined by personality traits and developmental failures. More recent research has made these theories much less popular.

One hypothesis is that the person's basic nature is to search for altered states of consciousness. The result of this unconscious search is chemical dependence. Another hypothesis is related to the person's desire to seek out and discover new experiences. Impulsive personality traits are another consideration. Rebellion has also been proposed as an explanation for initiating the use of substances. Unlawful or undesirable behavior is one of the most effective means of expressing contempt or defiance of authority.

Behavioral Theory

Behavioral theory looks at the antecedents of substance use behavior, prior experiences with use, and the beliefs and expectations surrounding the behavior. This perspective considers which reinforcement principles operate in substance dependence. Consequences for continuing to use or deciding not to use, such as increasing pleasure or decreasing discomfort, are studied. Behavioral theorists also look at the activities associated with substance dependence, social pressures, rewards, and punishments.

Learning Theory

Learning theory states that chemically dependent people have learned maladaptive ways of coping. It is thought that substance dependence is a learned, maladaptive means of decreasing anxiety. Abusive behavior is viewed on a continuum from no use to moderate use, through excessive to dependent use. All these behaviors are learned responses. Learning theorists look at childhood exposure to role models, customs surrounding the use of chemicals, and the symbolic meaning of the drug. Risk factors include the degree of effort required to search out and obtain substances; the frequency and intensity of negative events while obtaining and using the substance; the availability of nondrug, pleasurable resources; and family context in terms of modeling, conflict, and degree of parental supervision (Higgins, 1999).

Sociocultural Theory

Sociocultural theory considers how cultural values and attitudes influence substance abuse behavior. Cultures whose religious or moral values prohibit or extremely limit the use of alcohol or drugs have lower rates of chemical dependence.

Sociocultural theory is based on the idea that values, perceptions, norms, and beliefs are passed on from one generation to another. Alcohol is part of everyday life in some families, while in other families; there is infrequent use or abstinence. The United States is a *drug-oriented society*. Advertisements offer medicinal cures not only for minor aches and pains but also for major health problems. Adolescents and young adults see their parents use various substances such as alcohol, caffeine, nicotine, antianxiety agents, and sedatives. With sanction from television advertising and parental examples, these young people see nothing wrong with trying various drugs.

It is unclear if the physical environment of poverty is a cause or a consequence of substance use. It is known that people in poor neighborhoods have more access to substances, with a high density of liquor stores and sellers of illegal drugs (Chassin & Ritter, 2001).

Peer group pressure can cause drug use. Being in a peer group is important for adolescents and young adults. If some members are experimenting with drugs, other members are likely to follow suit.

One of the primary causes of substance abuse and dependence among African Americans and Hispanic Americans is sociocultural. Substance abuse is symptomatic of larger social problems. *Racism* creates a disparity in the socioeconomic systems of minority groups, who must manage the oppression that accompanies this inequality. Racism results in unemployment, and it is very painful to live in poverty in a culture with a materialistic ethic. Racism also results in dense clustering in substandard housing, environmental pollution, inadequate health care, and lack of power. When all this is combined with the relatively excessive availability of alcohol and other drugs, it is not surprising that there is a high rate of substance dependence among young people from minority populations.

One example of sociocultural theory is seen in substance-related disorders among Native People who have suffered the loss of their historical traditions. The federal government made them relocate to reservations, forcing subservience on them. The *stress of acculturation* has been very high. Economically, most residents of the reservations are chronically depressed. Native Peoples suffer from extreme poverty, poor health, inadequate health care, housing problems, and transportation problems. Short-term relief through drinking or using drugs may appear to outweigh the long-term damage that results from substance dependence.

Feminist Theory

Feminist theory looks at the high cost of conforming to gender roles. Rigid gender socialization may keep people from experiencing life to the fullest. Women are denied access to their powerful selves, and men are denied access to their nurturant and expressive selves. Feminist theory believes that addiction may be a response to suppressed identity and self-concept. Women frequently have childhood histories of physical, sexual, or emotional abuse and often state that addiction occurred as a response to severe stressors. Victimization results in feelings of low self-esteem, and women use alcohol and drugs to cope with these negative feelings. When women's relationships fail or are dysfunctional, the use of substances often increases. Their feelings of alienation from others contributes to feeling lonely, unloved, unwanted, and depressed (Boyd & Mackey, 2000; Mynatt, 1998).

PSYCHOPHARMACOLOGICAL INTERVENTIONS

Alcohol withdrawal is a serious medical problem, and the primary treatment goal is the prevention of delirium. Benzodiazepines are the medications of choice as they decrease withdrawal symptoms by preventing CNS hyperexcitability and prevent seizures. Dosage is determined by withdrawal symptoms. One of the following medications will be used: Librium (chlordiazepoxide), 25 to 50 mg, orally or IV, every four to six hours; Valium (diazepam), 5 to 10 mg, orally or IV, every four to six hours; Tranzene (clorazepate), 15 mg, orally, every four to six hours; or Ativan (lorazepam), 2 mg, PRN. These medications are titrated downward over a period of five days. High doses of thiamine are given during alcohol withdrawal to decrease the rebound effect of the nervous system as it adapts to the absence of alcohol. For clients with delirium, delusions, or hallucinations, antipsychotic medications may be used.

Some people suffering from alcoholism take Antabuse (disulfiram) as part of their rehabilitation treatment program. Antabuse inhibits aldehyde dehydrogenase and leads to an accumulation of acetaldehyde if alcohol is ingested. The reaction occurs within 5 to 10 minutes and may last from 30 minutes to several hours. Symptoms include flushing, nausea and copious vomiting, thirst, diaphoresis, dyspnea, hyperventilation, throbbing headache, palpitations, hypotension, weakness, and confusion. In severe reactions, coma, seizures, cardiovascular collapse, respiratory depression, and death can occur. Antabuse should be used only under careful medical and nursing supervision, and clients must understand the consequences of the therapy. Antabuse is contraindicated for people with cardiovascular disease, depression, or schizophrenia. See Box 15.3 for client teaching regarding Antabuse.

Antabuse

- Avoid all exposure to alcohol and substances containing alcohol, including food, liquids, and substances applied to the skin.
- Read all product labels to ensure that they do not contain alcohol.
- Common products that contain alcohol include mouthwash, cough syrups, shaving lotion, and cologne.
- If you are exposed to alcohol while taking Antabuse, you will experience a reaction within 5 to 10 minutes, and it may last from 30 minutes to several hours.
- Symptoms of an Antabuse reaction include flushing, nausea and severe vomiting, thirst, sweating, shortness of breath, hyperventilation, throbbing headache, heart palpitations, low blood pressure, weakness, and confusion. In a severe reaction, you may experience seizures, coma, and cardiac or respiratory arrest.
- Antabuse takes 14 days to be removed from your body following discontinuation of the medication. Do not drink or become exposed to alcohol during this time.

The opiate antagonists naltrexone (ReVia, Trexan) and acamprosate (Campral) have been shown to significantly decrease craving for alcohol and narcotics and lower the relapse rate. There are three possible dosage schedules: (1) 50 mg daily and 100 mg on Saturdays; (2) 100 mg every other day; (3) 150 mg every third day. A similar drug, nalmefene, is currently under study. These medications interfere with the intoxicating effects in the brain by blocking the opiate receptors. People who take naltrexone or acamprosate and drink or use narcotics report that they feel less "high," less uncoordinated, and less intoxicated than usual. Side effects can include difficulty sleeping, nervousness, and gastrointestinal distress. Since these drugs can interfere with the use of narcotic analgesics in emergencies, the person must carry a medical alert card at all times. Some AA groups disagree with the use of naltrexone or acamprosate since the person is not "drug free," while other AA groups support the use of this medication (Farren & O'Malley, 1999).

Ondansetron (Zofran), an antinausea drug, helps modulate alcohol craving, especially for those who began drinking at a young age. It may be used alone or in combination with naltrexone. Studies also suggest that baclofen (Lioresal), an antispastic analgesic, may reduce obsessional thinking about alcohol (King, Licata, & Podell, 2001).

Opiate withdrawal symptoms may be alleviated with clonidine (Catapres) and should be used under supervision in an inpatient detoxification center. Since clonidine lowers blood pressure, vital signs should be carefully monitored. Other medications include acetaminophen for headaches, ibuprofen for muscle aches, hydroxyzine for anxiety or insomnia, dicyclomine for abdominal cramps, and an antacid for indigestion.

Ultra-rapid detoxification of opiates is a new treatment approach designed to almost completely eliminate the distressful symptoms of withdrawal. Rather than the 5 to 15 days with traditional detox procedures, ultra-rapid detox can be accomplished within four to six hours. This approach, done in a hospital or surgical setting, uses general anethesia to ensure comfort during this procedure. The individual is then given Revia or Trexan (naltrexone), which blocks the opiate receptors and assists the receptors to begin to reestablish normal sensitivity. When the anesthesia is discontinued, the individual awakens being physically detoxed. The greatest advantage of this approach is humanistic, that is, it lessens the very distressing withdrawal symptoms of opiate addiction. The only risk is that of a reaction to the general anesthesia. This approach does not relieve the psychological withdrawal symptoms, and clients must agree to intensive follow-up programs to maintain their drug-free state (McCabe, 2000).

Methadone maintenance programs are used for some people who are addicted to heroin. The daily dose is titrated upward over a period of two weeks, with a daily maintenance dose of 60 to 80 mg. Unlike heroin, methadone can be taken orally, and its effects last 24 hours instead of four. Levomethadyl (Orlaam, LAAM) is a longer-acting preparation that can be administered three times a week. Since it cannot be sent home with clients, they must ingest it at the clinic. Extreme care must be taken to protect children from accidentally ingesting methadone, as it may result in death to the child. A new form of buprenorphine

(Puprenex, Suboxone, an under-the-tongue lozenge) acts like extra-mild methadone at low doses. Unlike methadone, this form of buprenorphine is neither intoxicating nor dangerous at high doses. Both methadone and buprenorphine may be used with pregnant and nursing women (Barnett, Rodgers, & Bloch, 2001).

The purpose of methadone is to reduce the craving to ward off withdrawal symptoms. The typical course of this narcotic substitution therapy program is two to four years, but some researchers believe lifelong maintenance may be necessary.

There is some anecdotal evidence that gabapentin (Neurontin) may reduce craving in those who have a long history of cocaine addiction. Repeated cocaine use inhibits GABA release, and gabapentin increases brain GABA levels (Raby, 2000).

Sustained-release bupropion (Zyban), an antidepressant, is helpful for some individuals who wish to quit smoking. The dosage is 150 mg one time a day for three days, and twice a day thereafter. The client is instructed to pick a day to quit smoking somewhere in the neighborhood of three weeks after beginning the medication.

MULTIDISCIPLINARY INTERVENTIONS

No single treatment is appropriate for all individuals, and overcoming addiction is never an easy process. Effective treatment attends to the multiple needs of individuals, not just their drug use. Treatment approaches must address medical, psychological, social, vocational, and legal problems. Unfortunately, the relapse rate is 25 to 50 percent of those who are admitted for treatment. But with medications and intensive, long-term support, many people can recover (Ehrmin, 2001).

Treatment options include brief therapy, intensive outpatient or inpatient treatment, and residential treatment. Trained professionals at a community drug treatment center usually provide brief therapy. Clients learn specific behavioral methods for stopping or reducing their substance use, such as goal setting, self-monitoring, and identifying high-risk situations. Outpatient-intensive programs allow clients to remain in their work and home settings while participating in treatment for four or five hours every day. It is appropriate for those who require intensive care but have a reasonable chance for abstinence

outside a restricted setting. Inpatient treatment occurs in the emergency department and on acute care inpatient units. Hospitalization is appropriate for those at risk for severe withdrawal syndromes, those who are psychiatrically disabled, those who are a danger to themselves or others, and those who have not responded to less intensive treatment efforts. Residential treatment usually lasts 7 to 21 days and offers a safe and structured environment for those who lack social and vocational skills and drug-free social supports to be abstinent in a less restricted setting. Inpatient programs are downsizing and closing as third-party reimbursement is rapidly decreasing.

Most older adults still resist referral to chemical dependency programs and are more comfortable in senior-oriented programs. In addition, a significant number are unable or unwilling to leave their homes. Thus, programs must be specifically designed for older adults, including community outreach, home visitation, and social services. Alcohol problems should be presented to them in the context of problems of adjusting to aging. They may need special approaches such as slow-paced therapy and emotionally supportive therapy rather than the confrontive style used with younger adult males. Social bonding with age peers often improves outcomes.

Drug rehabilitation is the recovery of optimal health through medical, psychological, social, and peer group support for chemically dependent people and their significant others. **Abstinence** is merely stopping the intake of the drug; it does not imply that any other behaviors have changed. People who abstain are often referred to as "dry drunks" because they continue all their other unhealthy behaviors. In contrast, **sobriety** implies that not only have these individuals stopped using the drug, but they have also achieved a centered or balanced state. Emotional growth is achieved through the development of positive values, attitudes, beliefs, and behaviors. Sobriety is the overall goal of drug rehabilitation.

The **recovery model** is a vital part of rehabilitation that views chemical dependence as a chronic, progressive, and often fatal disease. The responsibility for recovery is on the client, and any attempt to shift responsibility to others, such as family or friends, is confronted directly. Recovery is considered a lifelong, day-to-day process and is accomplished with the support from peers with the same addiction. Recovery programs typically are *12-step programs*, first introduced by Alcoholics Anonymous (AA), in which honesty is a very high value. These programs are deeply spiritual, and recovery is thought to depend, in part, on faith in a higher power. See Chapter 10 for more detailed information on 12-step programs. Clients are referred to AA, Cocaine Anonymous, or Narcotics Anonymous. Partners are encouraged to join Al-Anon, children to join Alateen or Alatots, and adult children to join Adult Children of Alcoholics (ACOA). (The 12 steps of AA are found in Chapter 10, Box 10.2.)

Treatment programs have traditionally been designed for men, and many people believe that women require different, gender-specific approaches. Believing that causes of substance abuse are poor self-esteem, relationship problems, and histories of abuse and depression, treatment focuses on competence, strengths, and confidence. Confrontational models are less effective for women than are treatment approaches framed in terms of relationships. *Women for Sobriety (WFS)* is the first self-help support group founded specifically for women who are alcoholics. It is an emotional and spiritual growth program in which members use positive affirmation and share experiences to aid in the recovery process. The group process helps decrease the isolation and loneliness many substance-abusing women experience. Box 15.4 shows the 13 affirmations of WFS.

Family therapy helps family members identify situations in which they acted as enablers. They then suggest alternative actions or statements they could have used in those situations. These new behaviors are practiced in a variety of settings. The family then moves on to making a contract with the client to use new, nonenabling strategies in the future.

Preventive education is another multidisciplinary intervention. Adolescents and preteens who have not used either alcohol or other drugs need some anticipatory guidance to help them cope with the inevitable choices they will have to make. Many community alcohol and drug projects and school-based prevention programs are helpful for parents and children and offer support groups and literature. The goal is to protect children from the many adverse consequences of smoking, drinking, and illicit drug use.

The need for *community education* continues. The medical community recognizes addictive disorders as brain diseases, but the concept of moral failure is still evident in the thinking of U.S. citizens. Our country has a higher investment in criminal justice rather than

---

BOX 15.4

Levels of the New Life Program and Thirteen Affirmations: Women for Sobriety

Level I: Accepting Alcoholism as a Physical Disease

I have a drinking (life-threatening) problem that once had me.

Level II: Discarding Negative Thoughts, Putting Guilt Behind, and Practicing New Ways of Viewing and Solving Problems

Negative thoughts destroy only myself.
Problems bother me only to the degree I permit them to.
The past is gone forever.

Level III: Creating and Practicing a New Self-Image

I am what I think.
I am a competent woman and have much to give life.

Level IV: Using New Attitudes to Enforce New Behavior Patterns

Happiness is a habit I will develop.
Life can be ordinary or it can be great.
Enthusiasm is my daily exercise.

Level V: Improving Relationships as a Result of Our New Feelings About Self

Love can change the course of my world.
All love given returns.

Level VI: Recognizing Life's Priorities: Emotional and Spiritual Growth, Self-Responsibility

The fundamental object of life is emotional and spiritual growth.
I am responsible for myself and my actions.

SOURCE: Reprinted with permission from Women for Sobriety Inc., PO Box 618, Quakertown, PA 18951.

---

treatment, including the denial of health insurance payment for addictive disorders. There is a beginning movement in some states to offer treatment options in place of jail for nonviolent offenders. As nurses, we

CRITICAL THINKING

You are doing your clinical rotation in a clinic for the homeless. You expect to find many clients with substance use problems, and you do. You have never worked with clients who have these problems, and you are a little concerned about the rotation. Your first day you attend the team meeting, hoping that this will provide you with important information about the clients and the treatment services that are offered in the clinic. You realize that these clients have complex problems—from medical and psychiatric to social and economic problems. From the discussion, you learn that the two commonly abused substances by the clinic's clients are alcohol and opiates.

During the morning, you see a client enter the clinic. She is staggering and talking to everyone. Her speech is slurred. You sit in on an interview with this client, Ms. Johnston. She cannot seem to keep up with the conversation and says she cannot remember what she did yesterday when asked to describe her day. The clinic nurse tells you Ms. Johnston has a long history of excessive drinking. The nurse asks Ms. Johnston when she had her last drink. She tells the nurse sometime during the morning, and she has no money. From the client's appearance, the nurse wonders if the client is pregnant. When asked, Ms. Johnston says she is maybe three months pregnant. The physician orders a pregnancy test and a blood alcohol level (BAL).

Later, another client, Mr. Cahill, comes to the desk and demands to see the doctor. "I am having awful pain and need help." His eyes are watery, his nose is running, and he is sweating. The nurse asks you to go into the examining room with the physician. The nurse tells you that Mr. Cahill has never been to the clinic. His clothes are dirty, and he has not combed his hair. He is smoking and is told that he cannot smoke in the clinic. Mr. Cahill yells back, "I am in severe pain. Get me some help, and I will leave." During the exam, you and the physician notice that Mr. Cahill has needle marks on both arms. The client denies drug use and says he has severe abdominal pain.

1. The night before your clinical, you read about drug dependence and tolerance. What are they and how are they related?

2. Alcohol is a stimulant. Why is this a false statement?

3. What data support the concern that Ms. Johnston might be abusing alcohol? If she is, what are other signs and symptoms that you might expect?

4. When the pregnancy test returns, it indicates that Ms. Johnston is pregnant. What impact will her alcohol usage have on intrauterine development and her child?

5. From the data provided, what might Mr. Cahill be experiencing?

6. When you attend a meeting for family members of alcoholics, you hear them discussing co-dependency. How does co-dependency affect the client's treatment?

7. The recovery model is an important component of substance abuse treatment. Why is the model so challenging for the client?

8. Clients with substance abuse problems are often treated with psychopharmacologic interventions. What are some of these interventions that might be used for alcohol abuse and opiate abuse? What aspects of their use are important to consider when these interventions are implemented?

For an additional Case Study, please refer to the Companion Web site for this book.

---

must continue to fight for innovative treatment programs for those with substance use disorders. Effective drug treatment reduces crime, reduces the spread of infectious disease, and restores the ability of addicted people to be functional, contributing members of society rather than a drain on public resources.

ALTERNATIVE THERAPIES
Herbs and Nutrients

A nutritional supplement called SAMe (pronounced "sammy") may be effective in substance use disorders. SAMe (S-adenosylmethionine), a compound made by every cell in the body, helps produce DA, 5-HT, and NE. SAMe may be used for depression that accompanies withdrawal from psychoactive substances. It may also reverse some of the effects of alcoholic hepatitis and cirrhosis. The dose is 800 to 1,600 mg/day and is best taken 30 minutes before meals. SAMe should be used with caution in people who have a history of cardiac arrhythmias. Infants normally have a three to four times naturally higher level of SAMe than do adults. Given this knowledge, the amount of SAMe passing to infants through breast milk may be inconsequential (Brown & Gerbarg, 2000).

Herbs may also be useful in easing withdrawal symptoms. Chamomile is helpful during withdrawal from a number of substances. Evening primrose oil is used for alcohol withdrawal. Ginseng eases cocaine withdrawal, while valerian decreases the effects of benzodiazepine withdrawal. Milk thistle is thought to speed the production of new liver cells and bind to the outside of liver cells, slowing the entry of liver-damaging toxins. This appears to be effective in people with hepatitis and cirrhosis. Kudzu kudzu is in clinical trials for decreasing the craving for alcohol. Heantos, a mixture of 13 herbs, is in clinical testing for the treatment of heroin and cocaine addiction (Fontaine, 2000).

Omega-3 fatty acid is made up of DHA (docosahexaenoic acid) and EPA (eicosapentaenoic acid). DHA makes up one half of all fat in brain cell membranes especially in the cortex and the photoreceptors of the retina. Excessive alcohol depletes the brain of omega-3 fatty acids, especially DHA, which contributes to cortical damage and visual impairment. The recommended dose is 5 g/day of fish oil, which is usually seven or eight capsules. The maximum dose is 15 g/day. Taking the capsules at night and with orange juice cuts down on the fishy aftertaste (Carper, 2000).

Individuals who are malnourished from the effect of drugs as well as inadequate nutritional intake, need to supplement all the known vitamins and minerals. These nutrients include free-form amino acid complex (1,500 mg/day) and L-cysteine or N-acetylcysteine (1,000 mg/day) for withdrawal and improvement in brain and liver function; glutathione 3,000 mg/day for decreasing the craving for alcohol; and B-complex vitamins for absorption of nutrients and formation of red blood cells. In addition to depleting the body of B-complex vitamins, alcohol also depletes magnesium, and vitamins C, D, E, and K. Caffeine depletes the body of biotin, inositol, potassium, thiamine, and zinc. Heavy caffeine users should replace these substances. Tobacco use depletes vitamins A, C, and E (Balch & Balch, 2000).

Health care professionals now advocate precursor amino acid loading in the diet to facilitate the restoration of neurotransmitters. Tryptophan is the precursor for serotonin, and tyrosine is the precursor for epinephrine. Two vitamins, ascorbic acid and folic acid, are necessary for the metabolism of tyrosine. Tropamine includes precursors for most of the neurotransmitters as well as substances that inhibit the destruction of neuropeptides. Tropamine may also decrease drug and alcohol craving.

Acupuncture

Acupuncture is an effective treatment for substance use disorders. It eases the symptoms of withdrawal and decreases the intensity of cravings. Researchers in one study (Avants, Ragan, Jones, & Hommer, 2000) found that participants assigned to acupuncture were significantly more likely to abstain from cocaine than were the participants in the two control groups. Acupuncture shows promise not only for cocaine addiction but also for addiction to narcotics, amphetamine, cortisone, antianxiety agents, nicotine, alcohol, and even food addictions. In alcoholism, acupuncture both relieves the symptoms of withdrawal as well as decreasing the number of relapses. Acupuncture is a safe and relatively low-cost form of treatment (Bernstein, 2000; Gerber, 2000).

NURSING PROCESS

Assessment

People who abuse substances rarely seek treatment because they believe they are drinking too much alcohol or using too many drugs. Typically, what brings them into the health care system are problems with their jobs, relationships, money, and/or the legal system. All who enter treatment are ambivalent about giving up the chemicals they have become dependent on. If clients are coerced into treatment, expect them to feel angry, controlled, humiliated, fearful, defensive, and mistrustful.

The nursing assessment should be conducted in a nonjudgmental and matter-of-fact way. Give positive recognition that it was a personal choice to come into treatment. State that your goal is not to force them into doing anything but rather to help achieve an assessment and understanding of the nature of their use of substances. Following the assessment, you will be able to provide them with realistic feedback about their substance use behavior. Begin with less intrusive questions, such as "How many cigarettes do you smoke a day?" before asking questions about other substances. Follow with questions related to the use of prescription drugs. Then proceed to ask questions about the past and present use of alcohol and illegal drugs. Box 15.5 is an overview of a substance abuse assessment.

The Focused Nursing Assessment feature provides questions for assessing clients who are substance dependent. The assessment has a twofold purpose: to identify problems and to increase clients' awareness of the toll that substance use may be taking on their lives.

Clients being detoxified from alcohol abuse should be assessed on an ongoing basis using the *Clinical Institute Withdrawal Assessment (CIWA-Ar)* tool. The tool measures the severity of alcohol withdrawal based on 10 common signs and symptoms: nausea and vomiting; tremor; paroxysmal sweats; anxiety; agitation; tactile, auditory, and visual disturbances; headache; and orientation. The maximum score is 67, and clients who score higher than 20 should be admitted to a hospital (see Table 15.4 ■).

BOX 15.5

Substance Abuse History

- Assess for each substance
- Age begun
- Method of use (oral, smoking, inhaling, injecting)
- Amount and frequency of use
- Most recent use
- Withdrawal symptoms in the past
- Setting and circumstances of use (people, places, things, moods, and emotional states associated with use; how and where drugs are procured
- Benefits of use
- Proportion of income or savings spent on drugs
- Financial consequences of drug use (overdue bills, credit card debts, does person sell drugs to offset cost)
- Relationship, vocational, social problems associated with use

---

Physical Assessment

Forty-five percent of all cases of cirrhosis in the United States are alcoholic cirrhosis, also called Laennec's cirrhosis. Liver disease is the cause of 75 percent of medically related deaths among those who abuse alcohol, with the peak age between 40 and 50 years. Women tend to develop cirrhosis more quickly and with less alcohol intake than men do (Dunphy & Winland-Brown, 2001).

Physical assessment is a critical task, especially for clients who have a history of abusing alcohol. A complete physical assessment is necessary because alcohol affects so many body systems. Look first at the client's general appearance, take vital signs, and then examine the person in head-to-toe order.

Depending on the stage of alcoholism, the type of trauma the person may have been exposed to, poor hygiene, and malnutrition, you need to examine for changes in the integrity of the *skin and scalp*. Ecchymosis, lacerations, color, evidence of healed injuries, bumps, scars, and diaphoresis may be present. Bruises, lacerations, and numerous scars may be evidence of frequent trauma from bumps, falls, or fights. Decreased prothrombin production in advanced liver disease causes easy bruising. Dermatitis, seborrhea, and skin sensitivity to light results from vitamin B deficiencies. Spider angiomas are found on the face and sometimes on the chest of people with advanced liver disease. Diaphoresis may be a sign of impending withdrawal. Dependent edema may indicate liver problems. Statis dermatitis indicates the edema has been present for some time.

You observe the client's *head* for shape and symmetry of facial structures. Orbital ridges and bony areas around the eyes should be palpated for evidence of fractures. Advanced disease frequently causes facial edema or a "puffy face" with flushed cheeks and nose.

The *eyes* need to be inspected thoroughly. Icterus may be present in the sclera from hepatitis or cirrhosis. Extraocular movements are assessed to look for nystagmus and palsies of the lateral and conjugate gaze. When these signs are positive, Wernicke's encephalopathy is suspected. Pupil shape, equality, and reactivity to light evaluate normal nerve function.

The *ear* canals need to be examined. Increased redness is an indication of infection. Since trauma is often seen in alcoholics, the ear canal is inspected for exudate, blood, and lesions.

Behavior Assessment	Affective Assessment	Cognitive Assessment	Social Assessment
When did you begin to have problems with substances?	In what way does your drug use decrease your: Anxiety? Boredom? Depression?	What kinds of things do you have difficulty remembering?	Who do you consider to be the most significant people in your life?
Have you ever missed work/school because of drug use?	What kinds of comments have others made to you about rapid mood swings?	Have you ever had blackouts?	Can you confide in these people?
What kinds of employment/school problems have you experienced?	What drug-abusing behavior has led you to feel: Guilty? Embarrassed? Ashamed? Humiliated?	Have you invented information or stories to make up for forgetting?	Which of these individuals abuse substances with you?
Have you missed family/social events because of drug use?		What reasons do you give others for your use of drugs?	Who knows about your substance abuse?
How hostile and argumentative do you become when using substances?		Have you experienced hallucinations?	Describe family arguments relating to your substance abuse.
Have you ever attempted to harm yourself or others while under the influence these drugs?		Do you believe you have a chemical dependence that is out of your control?	Who protects you from the consequences of your abuse?
Have you had periods in your life when you were drug free? How long did these last?			How has your sexual behavior changed with your substance use?
Have you ever received treatment for using drugs?			
If so, what kind?			

The *mouth* is observed for signs of trauma and infection. Lip peeling and corner fissures are early signs related to vitamin B deficiencies. People who are homeless may have difficulty maintaining oral hygiene. Teeth need to be inspected for caries, cracks, tenderness, and missing teeth. Observe the gums for color, inflammation, consistency, bleeding, or retraction.

The *neck* is observed for color, skin texture, masses, symmetry, range of motion, and visible pulsations. Chronic alcoholism may lead to cardiomyopathy, with congestive heart failure causing increased venous pressure, which results in distended jugular veins.

Inspect the *chest* since debilitated substance abusers are at risk for pneumonia and tuberculosis. Note the rate and character of respirations. Auscultation can reveal breath sounds with lung consolidation. Gynecomastia is common with cirrhosis or chronic liver disease since the liver can no longer inactivate estrogen.

Observation of the *abdomen* may reveal bulging flanks indicative of abdominal fluid retention and tense glistening skin resulting from ascites. The abdomen is percussed to identify enlarged organs, fluid retention, gaseous distention, and masses. An enlarged liver, percussed as greater than 12 centimeters at the midclavicular line, can indicate alcoholic hepatitis or

TABLE 15.4

Clinical Institute Assessment (CIWA-Ar)

Patient: _____ Date: /_____/_____/_____ Time: _____
                                          Y   M   D   (24-hour clock, midnight = 00:00)

Pulse or heart rate, taken for one minute: _____ Blood pressure: _____

NAUSEA AND VOMITING—Ask, "Do you feel sick to your stomach? Have you vomited?" Observation.

0 no nausea and no vomiting

1 mild nausea with no vomiting

2

3

4 intermittent nausea with dry heaves

5

6

7 constant nausea, frequent dry heaves and vomiting

TREMOR—Arms extended and fingers spread apart. Observation.

0 no tremor

1 not visible, but can be felt fingertip to fingertip

2

3

4 moderate, with patient's arms extended

5

6

7 severe, even with arms not extended

PAROXYSMAL SWEATS—Observation.

0 no sweat visible

1 barely perceptible sweating, palms moist

2

3

4 beads of sweat obvious on forehead

5

6

7 drenching sweats

TACTILE DISTURBANCES—Ask, "Have you any itching, pins and needles sensations, any burning, or any numbness, or do you feel bugs crawling on or under your skin?" Observation.

0 none

1 mild itching, pins and needles, burning, or numbness

2 mild itching, pins and needles, burning, or numbness

3 moderate itching, pins and needles, burning, or numbness

4 moderately severe hallucinations

5 severe hallucinations

6 extremely severe hallucinations

7 continuous hallucinations

AUDITORY DISTURBANCES—Ask, "Are you more aware of sounds around you? Are they harsh? Do they frighten you? Are you hearing anything that is disturbing to you? Are you hearing things that you know are not there?" Observation.

0 not present

1 very mild harshness or ability to frighten

2 mild harshness or ability to frighten

3 moderate harshness or ability to frighten

4 moderately severe hallucinations

5 severe hallucinations

6 extremely severe hallucinations

7 continuous hallucinations

VISUAL DISTURBANCES—Ask, "Does the light appear to be too bright? Is its color different? Does it hurt your eyes? Are you seeing anything that is disturbing to you? Are you seeing things that you know are not there?" Observation.

0 not present

1 very mild sensitivity

2 mild sensitivity

3 moderate sensitivity

4 moderately severe hallucinations

5 severe hallucinations

6 extremely severe hallucinations

7 continuous hallucinations

(*continued*)

TABLE 15.4

Clinical Institute Assessment (CIWA-Ar) *(continued)*

ANXIETY—Ask, "Do you feel nervous?" Observation.

0 no anxiety, at ease

1 mildly anxious

2

3

4 moderately anxious or guarded so anxiety is inferred

5

6

7 equivalent to acute panic states as seen in severe delirium or acute schizophrenic reactions

HEADACHE, FULLNESS IN HEAD—Ask, "Does you head feel different? Does it feel like there is a band around your head?" Do not rate for dizziness or lightheadedness. Otherwise, rate severity.

0 not present

1 very mild

2 mild

3 moderate

4 moderately severe

5 severe

6 very severe

7 extremely severe

AGITATION—Observation.

0 normal activity

1 somewhat more than normal activity

2

3

4 moderately fidgety and restless

5

6

7 paces back and forth during most of the interview or constnatly thrashes about

ORIENTATION AND CLOUDING OF SENSORIUM—Ask, "What day is this? Where are you? Who am I?" Observation.

0 oriented and can do serial additions

1 cannot do serial additions or is uncertain about date

2 disoriented for date by no more than 2 calendar days

3 disoriented for date by more than 2 calendar days

4 disoriented for place and/or person

Total CIWA-Ar Score:

Rater's Initials:

Maximum Possible Score: 67

---

cirrhosis. Complaints of anorexia, nausea, vomiting, fever, and presence of liver tenderness are all early signs of hepatitis. Later signs of hepatitis are pale stools, dark urine, and jaundice. Jaundice may be more readily identified on the abdomen because of less exposure to the sun.

Portal hypertension may be indicated if you find dilated veins at the umbilicus, gastrointestinal bleeding, and hemorrhoids. Check for black or tarry stools or frank rectal bleeding. Esophageal varices, secondary to portal hypertension, are usually discovered when the person vomits bright red blood, passes red blood through the rectum, or has dark, tarry stools from the upper gastrointestinal tract. Esophageal varices are especially susceptible to life-threatening hemorrhage. Other signs of portal hypertension are dilated or varicose veins at the umbilicus and hemorrhoids.

The major areas observed in assessing the *neurologic status* are consciousness, cognitive function, and motor function. Consciousness is assessed as you converse with clients. Deviations may be observed in relation to arousability, responses to commands, and response to painful stimuli. Note the orientation to time, place, and person. Individuals suffering from Korsakoff's syndrome may have intact intellectual functioning but an inability to retrieve long-term memory events or retain new information. Alcoholic dementia is characterized by impaired abstract thinking and judgment, personality changes, and impaired memory. Wernicke's encephalopahy is characterized by ataxia, abnormal eye movements, and confusion.

Diagnosis

After completing the assessment and appraising the knowledge base, you are ready to analyze and synthesize the information. Answer the following questions:

1. How does the client view substance abuse?
2. How does the client view alcoholics or addicts?
3. What is the client's concept of disease?
4. What does the client claim to want out of treatment?
5. Is the client being forced to seek treatment by family, employer, or the legal system?

See the Nursing Diagnoses with NOC and NIC feature for clients with substance-related disorders. Nursing diagnoses relating to acute overdose and chronic physical complications of substance dependence are beyond the scope of this text. Refer to your medical–surgical text to review these diagnoses and the appropriate nursing responses.

Outcome Identification and Goals

Based on the assessment data, you select outcomes appropriate to the nursing diagnoses. See the Nursing Diagnoses with NOC and NIC feature for outcomes associated with the nursing diagnoses.

Client goals are specific behavioral measures by which you, clients, and significant others identify as realistic and attainable. The following are examples of some of the outcomes appropriate to people who have substance-related disorders:

■ Remains safe during the withdrawal process
■ Acknowledges the reality of the disorder
■ Acknowledges the negative consequences of substance-abusing behavior
■ Identifies triggers to relapse

■ Utilizes spiritual support resources
■ Demonstrates improved problem-solving skills
■ Improves levels of physical health and fitness
■ Participates in self-help groups
■ Family members participate in relapse prevention education
■ Parents abstain from substance use/abuse

Nursing Interventions

Substance dependence is not hard to see, but it is hard to treat. Clients must become invested in treatment and require intensive support from others.

Behavioral: Behavior Therapy

Substance Use Treatment: Alcohol Withdrawal

Review Table 15.1 for signs of overdose and withdrawal. Emergency management of acute alcohol intoxication is necessary to save lives. Clients must be quickly assessed for life-threatening situations requiring immediate response. Blood alcohol levels (BALs) are generally obtained to determine the level of intoxication, and you should be alert for the problem of mixed addiction. Monitor vital signs frequently. Place the client in a quiet environment to avoid excessive stimulation that could increase agitation. Lighting in the room should be maintained, especially at night, to decrease the possibility of misinterpretation of stimuli and shadows. Provide verbal reassurance and reality orientation as necessary. If there is no one to stay in constant attendance, it may be necessary to restrain the client for protection from injury. Restraints, however, often increase confusion and agitation.

Complete recovery from withdrawal may take as long as two or three weeks. An important component to successful treatment is consistent contact and development of a relationship with another person such as a nurse or nurse-therapist.

Substance Use Treatment: Drug Withdrawal

Review Table 15.1 for signs of overdose and withdrawal. Some clients are at high risk for violence related to the psychotic effects of chemicals (hallucinations and delusions), impulsive behavior when intoxicated, and the process of withdrawal from chemicals (agitation, paranoia). Try to determine if there is a his-

NURSING DIAGNOSES with NOC & NIC

Clients with Substance-Related Disorders

DIAGNOSIS	OUTCOMES	INTERVENTIONS
Ineffective individual coping related to using chemicals as a way to cope with life	**Risk Control:** Alcohol Use: Actions to eliminate or reduce alcohol use that poses a threat to health **Risk Control:** Drug Use: Actions to eliminate or reduce drug use that poses a threat to health	Substance Use Treatment: Alcohol Withdrawal Substance Use Treatment: Drug Withdrawal
Ineffective denial related to believing that there is no problem with use of substances	**Risk Control:** Alcohol Use: Actions to eliminate or reduce alcohol use that poses a threat to health **Risk Control:** Drug Use: Actions to eliminate or reduce drug use that poses a threat to health	Substance Use Treatment
Powerlessness related to an inability to control the use of drugs	**Knowledge:** Substance Use Control: Extent of understanding conveyed about managing substance use safely	Substance Use Treatment
Self-esteem disturbance, altered role performance related to lifestyle disrupted by substance abuse	**Substance Addiction Consequences:** Compromise in health status and social functioning due to substance addiction	Substance Use Treatment
Social isolation related to a lifestyle of substance abuse	**Social Involvement:** Frequency of an individual's social interactions with persons, groups, or organizations	Support Group
Ineffective family coping related to co-dependent and enabling behavior; neglect or abuse of family members	**Family Coping:** Family actions to manage stressors that tax family resources	Family Support Family Therapy
High risk for violence, self-directed, related to psychotic symptoms; hyperactivity; panic anxiety; hopelessness; suicidal ideation	**Knowledge:** Substance Use Control: Extent of understanding conveyed about managing substance use safely	Impulse Control Training
Spiritual distress related to alienation from others; loss of faith in a higher being	**Psychosocial Adjustment:** Life Change: Psychosocial adaptation of an individual to a life change	Spiritual Support Hope Instillation
Knowledge deficit related to parents' use of alcohol, nicotine, or other drugs; need for early drug prevention education	**Knowledge:** Health Behaviors	Learning Facilitation

SOURCES: Johnson, M., Maas, M., & Moorhead, S. (2000). *Nursing outcomes classification (NOC)* (2nd ed.). St. Louis, MO: Mosby; McCloskey, J. C., & Bulechek, G. M. (1996). *Nursing interventions classification (NIC)* (2nd ed.). St. Louis, MO: Mosby; and North American Nursing Diagnosis Association (1999). *Nursing diagnoses, definitions, and classification 1999–2000.* Philadelphia: Author.

tory of violence, since that is one of the best predictors of present or future violence. Early intervention with diversional activities can prevent some outbursts by channeling energy into other activities. The type of diversional activity, whether it is a passive or a vigorous activity, depends on the level of the client's agitation. Decrease environmental stimuli or remove the person to a quieter area, as this may decrease the risk. If the client is experiencing hyperthermia, a cooling blanket may be helpful. Explain what is happening to the client to increase contact with reality. Reassure that the effect of the drug will wear off. Clients must be closely observed to prevent injury or suicide. If the client has overdosed on an oral drug activated charcoal or gastric lavage may be necessary.

Substance Use Treatment

An important nursing intervention is helping clients *overcome denial* and recognize the significance of the substance dependence. Keep in mind that it is very painful for clients to stop denying that alcohol and drugs are causing problems for themselves and others. Together, you begin to identify the situations in which substance abuse occurs, the type and amount of substances used, and the frequency of the abuse. You can then help the client identify what the negative consequences of this behavior have been and connect problems in life directly to the drug dependence. Using the one-day-at-a-time philosophy will minimize their feelings of being overwhelmed. Clients must identify a personal motivation for abstinence and then make a commitment to it. You can help them through this process by listening and through active support. Finally, it is very important to help clients identify their strengths and abilities, to decrease their feelings of helplessness and hopelessness.

Teach clients *problem-solving skills.* Many clients who abuse substances have avoided problems in life through the use of drugs. In order to abstain, they will need to develop alternative solutions to a broad range of life situations. (For a detailed discussion on teaching clients how to problem-solve, see Chapter 2.)

In working with clients who have abused alcohol or drugs, you often provide *vocational guidance.* If there are educational deficiencies, they must be addressed. Clients must determine how to keep the jobs they currently have or how to obtain new jobs. Attaining financial stability is one of the goals of recovery. You can

help clients plan short-term and long-range goals related to education and employment. It is often helpful to role-play employment situations such as on-the-job pressures and getting along with peers and supervisors.

You can encourage clients to improve their physical health and *fitness.* Many will benefit from a regular exercise program, which will in itself reduce anxiety and depression. For some, exercise becomes a leisure activity to replace the activity of substance abuse. Exercise is also helpful in avoiding relapse. Physiologically, the brain is stimulated by endogenous endorphins instead of alcohol or other drugs. Those who get involved in running often describe the natural "high" of running as a replacement for the old "high" of drugs. Exercising with other people aids in socialization as new "drug-free" friendships are developed. Exercise also provided a focus and outlet for emotions and a sense of mastery over one's physical body (Hays, 1999).

Impulse Control Training

Impulse control training is an important part of *relapse prevention.* The first step is to help clients identify and verbalize feelings and explore the origins of these feelings. Through discussion, you can help them recognize how they used alcohol and drugs to avoid the pain of their emotions. Another step in relapse prevention is having clients identify high-risk situations, such as specific people (friends who also use), places (bars), or specific activities ("coke" parties). Clients must also identify internal as well as external cues that trigger the urge to use chemicals. If possible, help them identify techniques from the past that led to success in avoiding substance abuse. The next step is to help clients anticipate and plan for problem situations by developing strategies for avoiding or actively coping with them when faced with such situations. Active strategies include self-statements to remind oneself of the commitment, assertiveness skills, and relaxation techniques. Provide opportunities to role-play these strategies.

Having a great deal of unstructured time is not helpful to people in early recovery. In the past, they spent a great deal of time and energy thinking about and using chemicals. Having to change daily activities can pose a problem for newly sober people who have no substitutes. Give them the task of planning a daily schedule, especially for the days off work. This promotes the creation of a healthy balance of activities and aids in preventing relapse. Finally, clients must learn to identify early warning signals of impending relapse in order to seek support and help as early as possible.

While attempting to help clients prevent recurrences of substance use, acknowledge the possibility that slips will occur, and develop strategies to limit the duration and intensity of any relapse episodes. It is believed that it takes 9 to 15 months to adjust to a lifestyle free of chemical use. Most treatment failures and relapses occur in the first 15 months after abstinence begins. There is also a lifelong vulnerability to relapse. Close to half of recovering people fail to maintain abstinence after a year—about the same proportion of people with diabetes and hypertension who fail to comply with their diet, exercise, and medications. With the limitations on the length of intensive treatment programs, clients are often discharged well before the plan of care has been fully evaluated.

Recovery is total abstinence from all drugs, not just the drug of choice. Once people have crossed the line from chemical use to chemical dependence, they can never return to controlled use without rekindling the addiction. A reasonably motivated client involved in an effective treatment program can have a better prognosis than previously thought. A variety of factors, such as social support, level of functioning before the addiction, and willingness to accept the need for lifestyle changes, influence the treatment outcome.

Behavioral: Coping Assistance

Support Group

Refer clients and their families to *self-help groups*. Mutual support makes people feel useful and valuable. At the beginning of rehabilitation, you may need to monitor client attendance at group meetings. Within each category there are special interest groups, including AA meetings for nurses, AA meetings for gays and lesbians, and women's groups such as Women Reaching Women or Women for Sobriety. Refer to the Community Resources feature at the end of this chapter.

Many people have developed a lifestyle revolving around substance abuse. Their social interactions have been largely restricted to drinking or using "buddies." Facilitate clients in developing an appropriate social support system and discuss the importance of regular social contacts. Help clients identify alcohol- and drug-free social activities. *Group therapy* is a treatment of choice in most programs. Clients learn to accept themselves as recovering individuals and help themselves while helping others. The group provides a sense of belonging and a source of friendships. Realizing that they are not alone, people feel less ashamed and despairing. Group members can also monitor one another for signs of relapse.

Spiritual Support

Most chemical dependency treatment approaches have a strong spiritual basis and stress that people need to feel connected to a greater power. Review the 12 Steps of Alcoholics Anonymous in Box 10.2 in terms of the spiritual focus. Facilitate clients' use of meditation, prayer, and other religious traditions and rituals. Refer clients to spiritual advisors of their choice. Some clergy are trained and skilled in substance abuse counseling and serve as a resource for people trying to find meaning in life.

Hope Instillation

Demonstrate hope by responding to clients' worth and dignity and viewing their substance use disorder as only one facet of each person. Encourage clients to realistically view themselves in the present after sorting through past experiences and to "let go" and move on. Promote anticipated positive experiences and the hope that life will be better without alcohol or drugs. Attitudes to be encouraged are hoping, having faith, trusting, anticipating the positive, looking forward to the future, and believing.

Behavioral: Patient Education

Learning Facilitation

When working with parents and/or families, we need to ask parents about their use of alcohol, nicotine, and other substances. We need to help the adults of the family understand the influence of their behavior in terms of their children's attitudes and future behavior. Parents who smoke may be more motivated to quit when they recognize the relationship between secondhand smoke and respiratory infections, asthma, and otitis media.

It is also important to assess family members for alcohol or drug problems, which may be stressing the entire family system. Children may be abused or neglected or exhibit behavioral problems as a symptom of family dysfunction. During routine interactions with

Complementary/Alternative Therapies

How to Help Clients Meditate

Research has demonstrated that people using meditation experience a significant decrease in tobacco,
alcohol, and illicit drug use. All sitting meditative
practices begin with finding a comfortable but erect
position. The posture itself is a meditation. Slumping
reflects low energy and passivity, while a ramrod-
straight posture reflects tension and effort. It is easiest
to meditate if the spine is straight and the body posture is symmetrical. Some people sit on the floor
cross-legged using a firm cushion under their backside to support the spine. Others sit in a chair with a
straight back with both feet on the ground. Many people use focus words or phrases such as love, peace,
let it be, relax, Our Father who art in heaven, Shalom,
or Om.

1. Pick a focus word or short phrase that is firmly
   rooted in your belief system.
2. Sit quietly in a comfortable position.
3. Close your eyes.
4. Relax your muscles.
5. Breathe slowly and naturally, and as you do,
   repeat your focus word, phrase, or prayer silently
   to yourself as you exhale.
6. Assume a passive attitude. Don't worry about how
   well you're doing. When other thoughts come to
   mind, simply say to yourself, "Oh, well," and gently return to the repetition.
7. Continue for 10 to 20 minutes.
8. Do not stand immediately. Continue sitting quietly
   for a minute or so, allowing other thoughts to
   return. Then open your eyes and sit for another
   minute before rising.
9. Practice this technique once or twice daily.

SOURCE: Benson, H. (1997). Timeless healing. New York:
Fireside Books.

children, such as back-to-school physicals or immuniza-
tions, ask about concerns children may have about what
is or is not happening within the family (Tweed, 1998).

By preadolescence, you should be screening children for evidence of risk factors as well as evidence of
substance use. If the child is to be open with you, you
must be nonjudgmental and matter-of-fact. Physical

signs that may alert you include frequent "cold" or
"allergies or other respiratory problems, unexplained
frequent injuries, altered sleep pattern, and loss of
appetite. Suspicious emotional signs include social isolation, sexual acting out, aggression, mood swings, and
depression. Behavioral cues include changing friends
to ones who have multiple problems, decline in school
performance, problems with teachers, poor judgment,
and loss of interest in hobbies or sports (Tweed, 1998).

Family: Life Span Care
Family Support, Family Therapy

Because of enabling behaviors and co-dependent family
members, many families have ineffective coping skills.
Encourage the recognition that chemical dependency is
a family disease and abstinence is impacted by the family process. All family members need relapse prevention
education to help identify triggers to relapse and coping
strategies for dealing with trigger events.

Help co-dependent members *talk about feelings* of
pain and anger since they have most likely been prevented from expressing their feelings directly. Help
them learn how to respect and take care of themselves,
decrease their need for perfectionism, and "own" their
full range of feelings. They must become empowered
in order to give up co-dependent behavior. Identify
enabling behaviors by nonabusing family members
since they are often unaware of their own problematic
behaviors. Help family members acknowledge and
change overresponsible behaviors such as covering up
for and protecting the client. To equalize power in
adult relationships, help the family develop a list of
responsibilities. Encourage role playing of these new
behaviors to reinforce the change in behavior.

Other groups affiliated with AA serve as *support
groups* for families of those who abuse substances. Al-
Anon is designed to help family members share common experiences and to gain an understanding of substance-related disorders. Alateen is another group
designed to help the family and the person come to
terms with the problem of substance abuse. Adult
Children of Alcoholics (ACOA) helps people deal with
past family issues and the impact of these issues on present life. If the family is to remain intact, expectations,
role behaviors, and communication patterns must be
assessed and modified, often with the support of
appropriate 12-step groups.

CLINICAL INTERACTIONS   A Substance-Abusing Client

Jim, age 34, has two daughters who live with his ex-wife. His parents are still living, and he has a twin sister and two older brothers. He has been living with his parents and has maintained a close relationship with all family members until recently, when his cocaine abuse problems worsened. He has recently entered a drug rehabilitation program. In the interaction, you will see evidence of:

■ Grandiose thinking
■ Use of cocaine to decrease anxiety about the family's response
■ Denial
■ Deterioration of family relationships
■ Lack of control in the use of cocaine

NURSE: Would you tell me a little about what led up to your coming into the program?

JIM: Well, I was on my way to work and I had to stop and get more coke before I went in. I was on my bike going about 110 mph. I always push it like that—going real fast. I don't worry about it because I know I'll always get away with it. They all know who I am.

NURSE: Who is "they"?

JIM: The police. All I have to do is show them a picture of my dad and they know right away who it is—he was a fireman and battalion chief for years. I was always getting pulled over when I was a kid, and they would just take the booze and tell me to go home because they knew who I was because of my dad. So, anyway, I'm driving along and my bike runs out of gas, so I'm trying to push it to get some gas and I get too tired and just push it to the side of the road, lay down on it, and go to sleep. It must have been about 2 hours later when one of these roadside helper vans came by and woke me up. They filled my tank and by then it was too late to go to work and I knew I couldn't go home because I think my family had decided they were going to get me to go for some help. So I went into the city, met these guys I deal with all the time, and traded them my bike for an 8-ball [an eighth of an ounce of cocaine] and a little money so I could get something to eat.

NURSE: Are you saying that your family was aware of your drug use and that's why you came in for treatment?

JIM: I don't really have a problem. I could quit any time, but they know there was something wrong. I had gotten to the point I would light up and smoke it in front of my sister.

NURSE: How did she react to that?

JIM: She asked me not to do it in front of her. She didn't like the way it made me act. My mom even told me she didn't like the way I had been acting. She told me the other day that she had gotten to the point she didn't even know who I was anymore. She wanted her Jimmy back. [Hands the nurse a sheet of paper.] I wrote this the other day. I don't know . . . maybe you'd like to read it and maybe not.

NURSE: Do you want me to read it?

JIM: Well . . . yeah.

[This was a poem about cocaine where cocaine is an entity calling out to the victim, promising euphoria, and taking away all his troubles.]

NURSE: You write here about this taking away all your troubles and cares. Is that how you feel about using cocaine?

JIM: When you're high you don't care about anything.

NURSE: How do you feel when you don't have the high?

JIM: Like going and getting more. Not now, though. I'm through. I've given it up and I'm not going to do it anymore.

NURSE: You sound pretty determined.

JIM: I am. I've got to get back to how I was before. My oldest daughter called me and told me she didn't like me the way I had become. She said I wasn't like her dad anymore. But she realizes now it was the drugs. She wants me to get better so I'll be more fun than I have been lately. I used to be a pretty friendly guy, smiled a lot, liked to have a good time. Before I came here, I usually just stayed at home and got high or was out trying to get more.

Evaluation

The future of drug and alcohol treatment is uncertain; the problems are great and the needs are many. There is increasing reluctance to expend resources on people who may show little gratitude and who seem to have brought their troubles on themselves. Programs often suffer from the burdens of inadequate staff and unreliable funding. Waiting lists are long and the average length of treatment—days to several months—is generally thought to be insufficient.

To complete the nursing process, you evaluate clients' responses to nursing interventions based on the outcomes you selected. You determine the appropriate intervals for measurement and document the condition of clients according to each individual's status. Johnson, Maas, and Moorhead (2000) is the resource for identifying measurement scales and specific indicators for each outcome.

Risk Control: Alcohol/Drug Use

Clients identify situations in which substance abuse occurs. They verbalize a personal motivation for and a commitment to abstinence. They utilize problem-solving skills to find alternatives to the abuse of substances. They obtain and maintain job and financial security.

Knowledge: Substance Use Control

Individuals acknowledge the extent of their substance abuse problems. They verbalize the connection between substance use and the avoidance of painful feelings. They identify personal high-risk situations that are triggers to relapse. They formulate a list of strategies to cope with triggers. They verbalize a need for significant lifestyle changes.

Substance Addiction Consequences

Clients who abuse alcohol and/or drugs have minimal long-term physical complications from their abuse of substances. They participate in a regular exercise pro-gram. They identify the negative consequences and connect problems in life directly to the substance addiction.

Social Involvement

Clients and families participate in self-help groups and verbalize a sense of belonging. They develop a new social support system to replace their substance-using friends.

Family Coping

Dependent children of substance-abusing parents remain free from harm and exhibit normal growth and development. All family members verbalize that chemical dependency is a family disease and participate in family therapy and support groups. There is no evidence of co-dependent behavior within the family system.

Psychosocial Adjustment: Life Change

Clients acknowledge to themselves and others their "new" identity as a recovering person. They use meditation, prayer, and other religious traditions and rituals if desired. They verbalize a hope for the future and an anticipation of long-term abstinence.

To build a Care Plan for a client with a substance-related disorder, go to the Companion Web site for this book.

CHAPTER REVIEW

COMMUNITY RESOURCES

Links to these Web sites can be accessed on the Companion Web site for this book.

Adult Children of Alcoholics (ACOA)
310-534-1815
www.recovery.org

Al-Anon/Alateen
800-344-2666
www.Al-Anon-Alateen.org

Alcoholics Anonymous
World Services Office
P.O. Box 459, Grand Central Station
New York, NY 10163
212-870-3400
www.alcoholics-anonymous.org

Asian American Drug Abuse Program
5318 S. Crenshaw
Los Angeles, CA 90043
323-293-6284
www.aadapinc.ws

800 Cocaine Information
800-262-2463
www.drughelp.org

Co-Dependents Anonymous
602-277-7991
www.ourcoda.org

Indian Health Service
Alcoholism and Substance Abuse Program
301-443-4297
www.his.gov

International Nurses Anonymous
1020 Sunset Drive

Lawrence, KS 66044
913-842-3893
www.suresite.com

Mothers Against Drunk Driving
800-438-MADD
www.madd.org

Narcotics Anonymous
800-992-0401
www.wsoinc.com

National Association for the Dually Diagnosed
132 Fair Street
Kingston, NY 12401
800-331-5362
www.thenadd.org

National Black Alcoholism and Addiction Council (NBAC)
1101 14th Street NW
Suite 630
Washington, DC 20005
202-296-2696
www.borg.com/~nbac/

National Council of La Raza
202-785-1670
www.nclr.org

Nurses and Recovery
800-872-9998
www.tktucker.net/nir/

Women for Sobriety, Inc.
P.O. Box 618
Quakertown, PA 18951
215-536-8026
www.womenforsobriety.org
www.NewLife@nni.com

BOOKS FOR CLIENTS AND FAMILIES

Brown, S., & Lewis, V. M. (2000). *The family recovery guide.* Oakland, CA: New Harbinger.

Horvath, A. T. (1998). *Sex, drugs, gambling, and chocolate: A workbook for overcoming addictions.* Atascadero, CA: Impact.

How to get sober and stay sober. (2000). Center City, MN: Hazelden.

Nakken, C. (2000). *Reclaim your family from addiction.* Center City, MN: Hazelden.

Twelve steps and twelve traditions. (1995). New York: Alcoholics Anonymous World Services.

KEY CONCEPTS

Introduction

- Chemical dependence is a chronic and progressive disease that can be fatal if untreated.

- Most people who are chemically dependent are poly-drug abusers.

- Substance abuse contributes to other illnesses, fetal syndromes, accidents, suicides, and homicides.

- Substance abuse among nurses is not much higher or lower than that of the general population. There are statewide programs that help nurses seek treatment and save their licenses.

Knowledge Base

- The pattern of alcohol abuse varies from person to person. Some abuse daily, some abuse on weekends, and others abuse on periodic binges.

- Blackouts are a form of amnesia for events that occur during the drinking period.

- Wernicke's encephalopathy results from thiamine deficiency and is characterized by ataxia, abnormal eye movements, and confusion.

- Korsakoff's syndrome is an inability to retain new information and a disruption in long-term memory. People may use confabulation when confronted with memory loss.

- Alcoholic dementia is characterized by impaired thinking, judgment, and memory as well as personality changes.

- Alcohol withdrawal syndrome usually begins about six to eight hours after the last drink and is characterized by irritability, anxiety, insomnia, and tremors.

- In alcohol withdrawal, the person may experience seizures, hallucinations, disorientation, confusion, tachycardia, hypertension or hypotension, diaphoresis, and fever.

- Overdose of alcohol may result in unconsciousness, coma, respiratory depression, and death.

- Sedatives, hypnotics, and anxiolytics provide a sense of well-being and relaxation. There is a great risk for addiction and overdose.

- Rohypnol and GHB, the "date rape" drugs, are used to render rape victims unconscious.

- Overdose of sedative-hypnotics and/or when combined with alcohol can lead to respiratory depression and death.

- Opioids create a feeling of euphoria, pleasure and relaxation. Withdrawal symptoms may last as long as a week.

- Overdose on opioids can lead to death from respiratory depression. Narcan (naloxone) may be given IV to reverse respiratory depress and coma. The client is likely to need repeated doses.

- Cannabis, the drug category that includes marijuana and hashish, is the most widely used illegal drug in the United States.

- Overdose of cannabis may result in a psychotic episode but is not lethal.

- The primary reason people use cocaine is to stimulate the CNS reward center. Positive reinforcement includes euphoria, increased energy, and increased sexual arousal. Negative reinforcement occurs when the person takes more cocaine to overcome the rebound dysphoria.

- Use of cocaine can result in cardiac and cerebral infarct and perforation of the nasal septum.

- Signs of cocaine withdrawal include severe craving, depression, fatigue, and irritability.

- Cocaine intoxication can result in rapid death.

- Amphetamines stimulate the CNS by increasing DA in the reward system. Ice, the smokable form of methamphetamine, may substitute for cocaine as a stimulant because it is more easily available, is less expensive, and produces a much longer high.

- Chronic abuse of amphetamine may lead to paranoid and often violent psychotic states.

- MDMA can cause death when combined with high levels of physical activity, such as at a rave dance.

- Hallucinogens can lead to accidents, out-of-control behavior, and a psychotic state. Cause of death may be due to accidents of suicide.

- Inhalants produce euphoria, perceptual changes, impaired judgment, sense of well-being, sense of power, and a loss of contact with reality.

- Chronic use of inhalants can cause significant damage to the cardiovascular, pulmonary, and renal systems.

- Sudden death with inhalants is associated with arrhythmias, ventricular fibrillation, or respiratory depression.

- Some athletes and bodybuilders use anabolic steroids to build body mass and strength. A side effect may be "roid rage" with dramatic mood swings, manic-like episodes, and a tendency toward violence.

- Caffeine is the most widely used drug in the world. Side effects include nervousness, anxiety, and gastroesophageal reflux.

- Nicotine acts as a CNS stimulant by releasing DA in the reward center. It is still the leading cause of preventable, premature death in the world.

- Lack of control in using chemicals is the central behavioral characteristic of people who are chemically dependent. They may become loud, hostile, argumentative, and even violent. They may experience work or school problems and may become involved in a drug subculture.

- The overall intention of substance dependence is to decrease negative feelings and increase positive feelings. People who are chemically dependent are emotionally labile and experience guilt and shame.

- Alcoholic denial includes denial of facts, denial of implications, denial of change, and denial of feelings. Other defense mechanisms include projection, minimization, and rationalization.

- Substance abuse is a family problem, and the most devastating impact occurs when the abuser is a parent. To avoid embarrassment, family members often deny the severity of the problem.

- Co-dependency may occur in non–substance-abusing partners when they become overresponsible and the substance-abusing partner becomes underresponsible.

- Co-dependents engage in enabling behavior, which is any action that facilitates substance dependence.

- Children growing up in a substance-abusing home learn not to talk about the problem, not to talk about their own needs and wants, and not to feel. They become objects whose reason for existence is to please the abusing parent. They are expected to be perfect and always in control. They learn very early not to trust other people.

- Children of alcoholics suffer the consequences of a dysfunctional family. They expect all relationships to be based on power, violence, deceit, and misinformation. Some grow up to repeat the family patterns by either becoming addicted themselves or marrying an addicted person.

- Most Americans view substance dependence as a sin or the result of a weak will. Women are more stigmatized than men are, and lesbians suffer the double stigma of being lesbian and being alcoholic.

- Illicit drug activity is a growing problem among high-tech workers.

- Men abuse substances at a higher rate than women do. Among women, twice as many European American women drink heavily compared to African American, Hispanic American, Asian American, and Native American women.

- Substance-related disorders progress more rapidly in adolescents than in adults. They often experience developmental delays and shift to a peer group of other drug users.

- Alcohol abuse often goes undiagnosed in old age since the symptoms can be subtle or mimic symptoms of other geriatric illnesses.

- Abuse of prescription drugs among the elderly is two to three times higher than the general population.

- Sexually transmitted infections and AIDS are on the rise among people who abuse substances.

- Sexual consequences of substance-related disorders include decreased desire, erection problems, and orgasmic difficulties. Cocaine is linked to sexual acting-out behaviors.

- Tobacco is the most abused substance by pregnant women and is a risk factor for miscarriage, ectopic pregnancy, preeclampsia, and placental problems.

- Fetal alcohol syndrome (FAS) is the third leading cause of birth defects in the United States. Effects include heart defects, malformed facial features, mental retardation, a slow growth rate, hyperactivity, and learning disabilities.

- Cocaine use during pregnancy may result in learning and behavioral problems.

- Children who have been exposed to opioids prior to birth are very sensitive to noise, are irritable and tremulous, and may have feeding problems.

- Dual diagnosis indicates that there is a substance abuse problem as well as another coexisting mental disorder. The risk for a substance use disorder is twice as high for those suffering from major psychiatric disorders as compared to the general population.

- Neurobiological theorists believe that an underlying predisposition to substance abuse is the result of genetic defects. Genetic defects lead to deficiencies and imbalance in neurotransmitters, neuropeptides, and receptors. An abnormal mechanism involving the reward center of the brain creates compulsive behaviors involving alcohol and drugs. The primary neurotransmitter involved is DA.

- Behavioral theory considers reinforcement principles that maintain substance dependence. Learning theory states that it is a result of learned maladaptive ways of coping.

- Sociocultural theory considers cultural and family values regarding the use of chemicals, peer group pressure, the impact of racism, and the stress of acculturation in the development of chemical dependence.

- Feminist theory believes that addiction may be a response to an inadequate self-concept. There is often a history of abuse, dysfunctional relationships, or both.

- Antabuse, naltrexone, acamprosate, ondansetron, and baclofen may be used by some individuals to help avoid craving.

- Clonidine may ease opiate withdrawal symptoms and methadone, levomethadyl, and buprenorphine are used for heroin withdrawal.

- Drug rehabilitation is the recovery of optimal health through medical, psychological, social, and peer group support. The recovery model is a lifelong, day-to-day process, typically includes 12-step programs, and places the responsibility for recovery on the client.

- Nutritional supplements and herbs useful for substance abusing clients are SAMe, chamomile, evening primrose oil, ginseng, milk thistle, kudzu kudzu, heantos, and fish oil.

- Acupuncture eases the symptoms of withdrawal and decreases the intensity of craving.

The Nursing Process

Assessment

- The nursing assessment begins with a substance abuse followed by a focused nursing assessment designed to elicit understanding of the impact of substance abuse on the client and family.

- Abnormal physical findings in individuals who have chronic use of alcohol include liver disease; effects of trauma; easy bruising; spider angiomas on the face; facial edema; teeth and gum problems; congestive heart failure; ascites; esophageal varices; gastrointestinal bleeding; and impaired consciousness, cognitive function, and motor function.

Diagnosis

- Nursing diagnoses include Ineffective individual coping, Social isolation, Ineffective family coping, Powerlessness, Disturbance in self-esteem, Ineffective denial, High risk for violence, and Spiritual distress.

Outcome Identification and Goals

- Client goals include acknowledging the disorder and its negative consequences, sobriety, rehabilitation, and improved family coping.

Nursing Interventions

- Emergency management of acute alcohol intoxication or drug overdose is vitally important to save the client's life. Common problems include respiratory depression, seizures, and cardiovascular disorders. Clients may need ventilatory support, cardiac monitoring, seizure precautions, medications to support blood pressure, and treatment for hyperthermia.

- Nursing interventions include helping clients overcome denial and recognize the significance of their problem. This must occur before clients can make a commitment to abstinence and recovery.

- Most substance-abusing clients need to learn how to solve problems rather than avoid problems through the use of drugs.

- Clients may need vocational guidance such as educational programs and job training.

- A regular exercise program is an important component of rehabilitation.

- Relapse prevention includes self-control training. Clients are taught to identify and manage feelings, high-risk situations, and active coping strategies.

- Self-help groups for clients and families are an important part of the recovery process.

- A client's history of violent behavior is one of the best predictors of current potential for violence. Clients must be assessed frequently and provided with outlets for anxiety and energy. Other interventions include a quiet environment, PRN medication, and, if absolutely necessary, seclusion or restraints.

- Spiritual support and hope installation promote recovery from substance abuse.

- Family members need help in identifying and changing co-dependent and enabling behaviors. They must learn new ways to respond to the client and how to respect and care for themselves.

Evaluation

- Recovery is total abstinence from all drugs. The recovering person can never return to controlled use without rekindling the addiction.

EXPLORE *MediaLink*

- Interactive resources, including animations, for this chapter can be found on the Companion Web site at *http://www.prenhall.com/fontaine.* Click on Chapter 15 and select the activities for this chapter.

- For NCLEX review questions and an audio glossary, access the accompanying CD-ROM in this book.

REFERENCES

Abudabbeh, N., & Hamid, A. (2001). Substance use among Arabs and Arab Americans. In S. L. Ashenberg (Ed.), *Ethnocultural factors in substance abuse treatment* (pp. 275–290). New York: Guilford Press.

Alexander, C. J. (1996). *Gay and lesbian mental health: A sourcebook for practitioners.* New York: Harrington Park Press.

American Psychiatric Association. (2000). *Diagnostic and statistical manual of mental disorders* (4th ed., Text Revision). Washington, DC: Author.

Anabolic Steroid Abuse (2001). *National Institute on Drug Abuse: Research Report Series. www.nida.nih.gov/ResearchReports/steroids/AnabolicSteroids.html.*

Anderson, P. B., & Mathieu, D. (1998). Drinking and safer sex: Are college students at risk? *Journal of Sex Education and Therapy, 23*(4), 297–301.

Arboleda-Florez, J., & Weisstub, D. N. (2000). Conflicts and crises in Latin America. In A. Okasha, J. Arboleda-Florez, & N. Sartorius (Eds.), *Ethics, culture, and psychiatry: International perspectives* (pp. 29–45). Washington, DC: American Psychiatric Press.

Avants, S. K., Ragan, P., Jones, D. W., & Hommer, D. (2000). A randomized controlled trial of auricular acupuncture for cocaine dependence. *Archives of Internal Medicine, 160*(15), 2305–2312.

Balch, J. F., & Balch, P. A. (2000). *Prescription for nutritional healing* (2nd ed.). Garden City, NY: Avery.

Barnett, P. G., Rodgers, J. H., & Bloch, D. A. (2001). A meta-analysis comparing buprenorphine to methadone for treatment of opiate dependence. *Addiction, 96,* 683–690.

Bernstein, K. S. (2000). The experience of acupuncture for treatment of substance

dependence. *Journal of Nursing Scholarship, 32*(3), 267–272.

Boyd, M. R. (2000). Predicting substance abuse and comorbidity in rural women. *Archives of Psychiatric Nursing, 14*(2), 64–72.

Boyd, M. R., & Mackey, M. C. (2000). Alienation from self and others: The psychosocial problem of rural alcoholic women. *Archives of Psychiatric Nursing, 14*(3), 134–141.

Brown, R. A., Monti, P. M., Myers, M. G., Martin, R. A., Rivinus, T., Dubreuil, M. E., et al. (1998). Depression among cocaine abusers in treatment. *American Journal of Psychiatry, 155*(2), 220–225.

Brown, R. P., & Gerbarg, P. L. (2000). Integrative psychopharmacology. In P. R. Muskin (Ed.), *Complementary and alternative medicine and psychiatry* (pp. 1–66). Washington, DC: American Psychiatric Press.

Carper, J. (2000). *Your miracle brain.* New York: HarperCollins.

Chassin, L., & Ritter, J. (2001). Vulnerability to substance use disorders in childhood and adolescence. In R. E. Ingram & J. M. Price (Eds.), *Vulnerability to psychopathology* (pp. 107–134). New York: Guilford Press.

Coogle, C. L., Osgood, N. J., & Parham, I. A. (2000). Addictions services. *Community Mental Health Journal, 36*(2), 137–148.

Crenshaw, T. L., & Goldberg, J. P. (1996). *Sexual pharmacology.* New York: Norton.

DeWit, D. J., Adlaf, E. M., Offord, D. R., & Ogborne, A. C. (2000). Age at first alcohol use: A risk factor for the development of alcohol disorders. *American Journal of Psychiatry, 157*(5), 745–750.

Dixon, L. B., & DeVeau, J. M. (1999). Dual diagnosis: The double challenge. *NAMI Advocate, 20*(5), 16–17.

Duke, J. A. (2000). *The green pharmacy herbal handbook.* Emmaus, PA: Rodale Reach.

Dunphy, L. M., & Winland-Brown, J. E. (2001). *The art and science of advanced practice nursing.* Philadelphia: Davis.

Ehrmin, J. T. (2001). Unresolved feelings of guilt and shame in the maternal role with substance-dependent African American women. *Journal of Nursing Scholarship, 33*(1), 47–52.

Eliopoulos, C. (2001). *Gerontological nursing* (5th ed.). Philadelphia: Lippincott.

Farren, C. K., & O'Malley, S. S. (1999). Occurrence and management of depression in the context of naltrexone treatment of alcoholism. *American Journal of Psychiatry, 156*(8), 1258–1262.

Fontaine, K. L. (2000). *Healing practices: Alternative therapies for nursing.* Upper Saddle River, NJ: Prentice Hall.

Gerber, R. (2000). *Vibrational medicine for the 21st century.* New York: Eagle Brook.

Glennon, R. A. (1999). Neurobiology of hallucinogens. In M. Galanter & H. D. Kleber (Eds.), *Textbook of substance abuse treatment* (2nd ed.) (pp. 33–37). Washington, DC: American Psychiatric Press.

Gottschalk, C., Beauvais, J., Hart, R., & Kosten, T. (2001). Cognitive function and cerebral perfusion during cocaine abstinence. *American Journal of Psychiatry, 158*(4), 540–545.

Hall, G. W., Carriero, N. J., Takushi, R. Y., Montoya, I. D., Preston, K. L., & Gorelick, D. A. (2000). Pathological gambling among cocaine-dependent outpatients. *American Journal of Psychiatry, 157*(7), 1127–1133.

Halpern, J. H., & Pope, H. G. (2001). Hallucinogens on the Internet: A vast new source of underground drug information. *American Journal of Psychiatry, 158*(3), 481–483.

Harsch, H. H., Pankiewicz, J., Bloom, A. S., Rainey, C., Cho, J., Sperry, L., et al. (2000). Hepatitis C virus infection in cocaine users—a silent epidemic. *Community Mental Health Journal, 36*(3), 225–233.

Hays, K. F. (1999). *Working it out: Using exercise in psychotherapy.* Washington, DC: American Psychological Association.

Higgins, S. T. (1999). Principles of learning in the study and treatment of substance abuse. In M. Galanter & H. D. Kleber (Eds.), *Textbook of substance abuse treatment* (2nd ed.) (pp. 67–73). Washington, DC: American Psychiatric Press.

Jaffe, J. H., & Jaffe, A. B. (1999). Neurobiology of opiates/opioids. In M. Galanter & H. D. Kleber (Eds.), *Textbook of substance abuse treatment* (2nd ed.) (pp. 11–19). Washington, DC: American Psychiatric Press.

Johnson, C. A. (1999). Determinants of effective school and community programs for tobacco, alcohol, and drug abuse prevention. In S. B. Kar (Ed.), *Substance abuse prevention: A multicultural perspective* (pp. 219–230). Amityville, NY: Baywood.

Johnson, M., Maas, M., & Moorhead, S. (2000). *Nursing outcomes classification (NOC)* (2nd ed.). St. Louis, MO: Mosby.

Kalb, C. (2001, February 12). *Newsweek,* 48–50.

Kalivas, P. W. (2001). Drug addiction: To the cortex . . . and beyond! *American Journal of Psychiatry, 158*(3), 349–350.

Kendler, K. S., & Prescott, C. A. (1999). Caffeine intake, tolerance, and withdrawal in women. *American Journal of Psychiatry, 156*(2), 223–228.

King, W., Licata, B., & Podell, R. N. (2001). New hope for alcohol treatment. *Nursing Spectrum, 14*(7IL), 36.

Klitzman, R. L., Pope, H. G., & Hudson, J. I. (2000). MDMA ("ecstasy") abuse and high-risk sexual behaviors among 169 gay and bisexual men. *American Journal of Psychiatry, 157*(7), 1162–1164.

Krakowski, M. (2000). Impulse control: Integrative aspects. In M. L. Crowner (Ed.), *Understanding and treating violent psychiatric patients* (pp. 147–165). Washington, DC: American Psychiatric Press.

Liu, X. (2000). Ethics and psychiatry in China. In A. Okasha, J. Arboleda-Florez, & N. Sartorius (Eds.), *Ethics, culture, and psychiatry: International perspectives* (pp. 119–132). Washington, DC: American Psychiatric Press.

Martin, B. R. (1999). Neurobiology of marijuana. In M. Galanter & H. D. Kleber (Eds.), *Textbook of substance abuse treatment* (2nd ed.) (pp. 39–45). Washington, DC: American Psychiatric Press.

Martsolf, D. S., Sedlak, C. A., & Doheny, M. O. (2000). Codependency and related health variables. *Archives of Psychiatric Nursing, 14*(3), 150–158.

Mayfield, D. G., McCleod, G., & Hall, P. (1974). The CAGE Questionnaire. *American Journal of Psychiatry, 131,* 1121–1123.

McCabe, S. (2000). Rapid detox: Understanding new treatment approaches for the addicted patient. *Perspectives Psych Care, 36*(4), 113–120.

Miller, D. T. (1997). Dual diagnosis: A clinical challenge. *Nursing Spectrum,* 14–15.

Mynatt, S. (1998). Increasing resiliency to substance abuse in recovering women with comorbid depression. *Journal of Psychosocial Nursing, 36*(1), 28–36.

Naegle, M. A., & D'Avanzo, C. E. (2001). *Addictions and substance abuse: Strategies for advanced practice nursing.* Upper Saddle River, NJ: Prentice Hall.

National Institute on Drug Abuse. (1999). National survey results on drug use from the monitoring the future study. NIH Publication Nos. 98–4345, 99–4661. Rockville, MD: National Institutes of Health.

Olatawura, M. O. (2000). Ethics in sub-saharan Africa. In A. Okasha, J. Arboleda-Florez, & N. Sartorius (Eds.), *Ethics, culture, and psychiatry: International perspective* (pp. 103–108). Washington, DC: American Psychiatric Press.

Paris, J. (1999). *Nature and nurture in psychiatry.* Washington, DC: American Psychiatric Press.

Pfefferbaum, A., Rosenbloom, M., Deshmukh, A., & Sullivan, E. V. (2001). Sex differences in the effects of alcohol on brain structure. *American Journal of Psychiatry, 158*(2), 188–197.

Pi, E. H., & Gray, G. E. (2000). Ethnopsychopharmacology for Asians. In P. Ruiz (Ed.), *Ethnicity and psychopharmacology* (pp. 91–113). Washington, DC: American Psychiatric Press.

Prescott, C. A., & Kendler, K. S. (1999). Genetic and environmental contributions to alcohol abuse and dependence in a population-based sample of male twins. *American Journal of Psychiatry, 156*(1), 34–40.

Raby, W. N. (2000). Gabapentin therapy for cocaine craving. *American Journal of Psychiatry, 157*(12), 2058–2059.

Ratey, J. J. (2001). *A user's guide to the brain.* New York: Pantheon Books.

Reoux, J. P. (2001). Searching for new detoxification strategies. *www.eurekalert.org/pub_releases/2001-09/ace-sfn091001.php.*

Richter, L., & Richter, D. M. (2001). Exposure to parental tobacco and alcohol use: Effects on children's health and development. *American Journal of Orthopsychiatry, 71*(2), 182–198.

Salokangas, R. K. R., Vilkman, H., Ilonen, T., Taiminen, T., Bergman, J., Haaparanta, M., et al. (2000). High levels of dopamine activity in the basal ganglia of cigarette smokers. *American Journal of Psychiatry, 157*(4), 632–634.

Sandhu, D. S., & Malik, R. (2001). Ethnocultural background and substance abuse treatment of Asian Indian Americans. In S. L. Ashenberg (Ed.), *Ethnocultural factors in substance abuse treatment* (pp. 368–392). New York: Guilford Press.

Schneider, F., Habel, U., Wagner, M., Franke, P., Salloum, J. B., Shah, N. J., et al. (2001). Subcortical correlates of craving in recently abstinent alcoholic patients. *American Journal of Psychiatry, 158*(7), 1075–1083.

Smock, T. K. (1999). *Physiological psychology: A neuroscience approach.* Upper Saddle River, NJ: Prentice Hall.

Spector, R. E. (2000). *Cultural diversity in health & illness* (5th ed.). Upper Saddle River, NJ: Prentice Hall.

Stafford, L. L. (2001). Is codependency a meaningful concept? *Issues in Mental Health Nursing, 22,* 273–286.

Tabakoff, B., & Hoffman, P. L. (1999). Neurobiology of alcohol. In M. Galanter & H. D. Kleber (Eds.), *Textbook of substance abuse treatment* (2nd ed.) (pp. 3–10). Washington, DC: American Psychiatric Press.

Trinkoff, A. M., Zhou, Q., Storr, C. L., & Soeken, K. L. (2000). Workplace access, negative proscriptions, job strain, and substance use in registered nurses. *Nursing Research, 49*(2), 83–90.

Tweed, S. H. (1998). Intervening in adolescent substance abuse. *Nursing Clinics of North America, 33*(1), 29–45.

Volkow, N. D., Chang, L., Wang, G., Fowler, J. S., Franceschi, D., Sedler, M. J., et al. (2001). Higher cortical and lower subcortical metabolism in detoxified methamphetamine abusers. *American Journal of Psychiatry, 158*(3), 383–388.

Washington, O. G. M. (2001). Using brief therapeutic interventions to create change in self-efficacy and personal control of chemically dependent women. *Archives of Psychiatric Nursing, 15*(1), 32–40.

Weaver, H. N. (2001). Native Americans and substance abuse. In S. L. Ashenberg (Ed.), *Ethnocultural factors in substance abuse treatment* (pp. 77–96). New York: Guilford Press.

REFERENCES *(continued)*

Wexler, B. E., Gottschalk, C. H., Fulbright, R. K., Prohounik, I., Lacadie, C. M., et al. (2001). Functional magnetic resonance imaging of cocaine craving. *American Journal of Psychiatry, 158*(1), 86–95.

Williams, T. G. (1996). Substance abuse and addictive personality disorder. In F. W. Kaslow (Ed.), *Handbook of relational diagnosis and dysfunctional family patterns.* New York: Wiley & Sons.

Wing, D. M. (1996). A concept analysis of alcoholic denial and cultural accounts. *Advanced Nursing Science, 19*(2), 54–63.

Wright, E. M. (2001). Substance abuse in African American communities. In S. L. Ashenberg (Ed.), *Ethnocultural factors in substance abuse treatment* (pp. 31–51). New York: Guilford Press.

Wu, L. T., Kouzis, A. C., & Leaf, P. J. (1999). Influence of comorbid alcohol and psychiatric disorders on utilization of mental health services in the national comorbidity survey. *American Journal of Psychiatry, 156*(8), 1230–1236.

Yi, H., Stinson, F. S., Williams, G. D., & Bertolucci, D. (1999). Alcohol epidemiologic data system. *Surveillance Report #49.* Rockville, MD: National Institute on Alcohol Abuse and Alcoholism, Division of Biometry and Epidemiology.

Personality Disorders

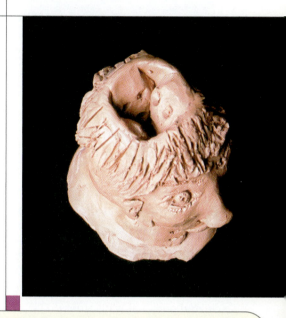

OBJECTIVES

After reading this chapter, you will be able to:

- DESCRIBE the concepts of personality and personality disorders.

- IDENTIFY the characteristics of the three clusters of personality disorders.

- DISCUSS the causative theories of personality disorders.

- SPECIFY assessment criteria for clients with personality disorders.

- IDENTIFY your own feelings when caring for clients with personality disorders.

- IDENTIFY basic approaches when working with clients in the three clusters of personality disorders.

- PLAN, implement, and evaluate care based on identified priorities.

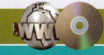

MediaLink

CD-ROM
- *Audio Glossary*
- *NCLEX Review*

Companion Web site www.prenhall.com/fontaine
- *Critical Thinking*
- *More NCLEX Review*
- *Case Study*
- *Care Map Activity*
- *Links to Resources*

I f I let you help me you'll want something in return. There's always a price. I give a little and you squeeze harder wanting more and more of me. You hold me so tight there's no way to get away. You're always there, never letting go. I don't want to talk or feel or look at what's making me sick. I just want to learn how to not feel and not think so I can get back to my old life.

—Kay, Age 40

To understand the nature of personality disorders, it is helpful to review the concept of personality. Personalities develop as people adapt to their physical, emotional, social, and spiritual environments. *Personality* refers to stable patterns of thoughts, feelings, behaviors, and motivation. Personality determines how people cope with feelings and impulses, how they see themselves and others, how they respond to their surroundings, and how they find meaning in relationships and cultural values. Personality can also be thought of as a style of adaptive functioning. These patterns are noticeable in a wide variety of situations.

The psychobiological model of personality considers both temperament and character. *Temperament*, heavily influenced by genetic variables, refers to the features of personality that are present in infancy. A person's temperament is highly stable over time. *Character*, heavily influenced by environmental variables, refers to enduring traits and behavior patterns. It is those aspects of personality that are the product of learning and interaction with the environment. Although these distinctions appear clear-cut in theory, the reality is that the separation of genetic and environmental influences is not possible (Jang & Vernon, 2001; Livesley, 2001).

A personality becomes *disordered* when the patterns are exaggerated, inflexible and maladaptive. Personality disorders represent the extremes of normal variation of personality. The dysfunction may be a failure to establish personal identity, an inability to initiate or maintain intimate relationships, and/or a lack of social skills interfering with cooperative relationships. Some people with personality disorders suffer intense emotional pain, while others seem invulnerable to painful feelings. Some are able to maintain relationships and careers, while others become functionally impaired.

Clients with personality disorders are among the most difficult to treat. Most will never enter a psychiatric hospital, seek or receive outpatient treatment, or even undergo a diagnostic evaluation. Some will enter the mental health system through family pressure or because of a court order. With those who do come into the system, mental health professionals find their expertise tested. In the majority of cases, the personality problems are **ego-syntonic**. They perceive their difficulties in dealing with other people to be external to them. Incapable of considering that their problems have anything to do with them personally, they will describe being victimized by specific others or by "the system." Some may develop an awareness of their self-defeating behavior but remain at a loss as to how they got that way or how to begin to change.

Personality disorders are diagnosed or coded on Axis II of the *Diagnostic and Statistical Manual of Mental Disorders* (4th ed., Text Revision) (DSM-IV-TR) (American Psychiatric Association [APA], 2000). See the DSM-IV-TR Classifications feature. There is a high degree of overlap among the personality disorders, and many individuals exhibit traits of several disorders. Typically, personality disorders become apparent before or during adolescence and persist throughout life. In some cases, the symptoms become less obvious by middle or old age.

It is extremely difficult to estimate the incidence of personality disorders. Many people with personality

DSM-IV-TR CLASSIFICATIONS

Paranoid Personality Disorder
Schizoid Personality Disorder
Schizotypal Personality Disorder
Antisocial Personality Disorder
Borderline Personality Disorder
Histrionic Personality Disorder
Narcissistic Personality Disorder
Avoidant Personality Disorder
Dependent Personality Disorder
Obsessive–Compulsive Personality Disorder
Personality Disorder Not Otherwise Specified (NOS)

SOURCE: Reprinted with permission from the *Diagnostic and Statistical Manual of Mental Disorders,* Fourth Edition, Text Revision. Copyright 2000 American Psychiatric Association.

disorders never come to the attention of the mental health system. The best estimate is that 6 to 18 percent of the general population suffers from some disruption serious enough to be diagnosed as a personality disorder. Currently, the most commonly diagnosed is borderline personality disorder, which appears to occur three times more often in women than in men. This group accounts for 50 percent of the diagnoses, and all the other disorders together make up the remaining 50 percent. Of all psychiatric clients, 15 to 25 percent are diagnosed with borderline personality disorder (Brown & Dodson, 1999; Gunderson & Gabbard, 2000; Nehls, 1999).

KNOWLEDGE BASE

There are 10 personality disorders, grouped into three clusters. The disorders within each cluster are considered to have similar characteristics (see Table 16.1 ■). The clusters are traditional but likely to be challenged as new information in behavioral genetics and developmental psychology alter our understanding of the nature, origins, and treatment of personality disorders. The DSM-IV-TR clusters and corresponding disorders are:

Cluster A
1. Paranoid (PPD)
2. Schizoid (SZPD)
3. Schizotypal (STPD)

Cluster B
4. Antisocial (APD)
5. Borderline (BPD)
6. Histrionic (HPD)
7. Narcissistic (NPD)

Cluster C
8. Avoidant (AVPD)
9. Dependent (DPD)
10. Obsessive–Compulsive (OCPD)

People with diagnoses from **Cluster A personality disorders** usually appear eccentric, and they exhibit many withdrawal behaviors. People with diagnoses from **Cluster B personality disorders** appear dramatic, emotional, or erratic. They tend to be very exploitive in their behavior. People with diagnoses from **Cluster C personality disorders** are those who appear anxious or fearful. Their behavior pattern is one of compliance. People with diagnoses from the anxious Cluster C improve more than those from the erratic Cluster B who in turn improve more than those with the eccentric and withdrawn Cluster A (Perry, Banon, & Ianni, 1999).

An additional category, *Personality Disorder Not Otherwise Specified* refers to those that do not meet criteria for any specific personality disorder. This category also includes disorders currently being researched, in this case passive–aggressive personality disorder and depressive personality disorder.

CLUSTER A PERSONALITY DISORDERS
Paranoid Personality Disorder

Behaviorally, people with **paranoid personality disorder (PPD)** are very *secretive* about their entire existence. Confiding in other people is perceived as dangerous and is not likely to occur, even within family relationships. Paranoid people are hyperalert to danger, search for evidence of attack, and become argumentative as a way of creating a safe distance between themselves and others. They rarely seek help for their personality problems, and they seldom require hospitalization.

TABLE 16.1

Characteristics of Personality Disorders

Cluster	Behavioral	Affective	Cognitive	Sociocultural
A	Eccentric, craves solitude, argumentative, odd speech	Quick anger, social anxiety, blunted affect	Unable to trust, indecisive, poverty of thoughts	Impaired or nonexistent relationships; occupational difficulties
B	Dramatic, craves excitement, wants immediate gratification, self-mutilates	Intense, labile affect; no sense of guilt; anxious; depressed	Considers self special and unique, egocentric, identity disturbances, no long-range plans	Manipulates and exploits others; stormy relationships
C	Tense, rigid routines, submissive, inflexible	Anxious, fearful, depressed	Moralistic, low self-confidence	Dependent on others, avoids overt conflict, seeks constant unconditional love

Affectively, paranoid people typically *avoid sharing their feelings* except for a very quick expression of anger. They may never forgive perceived slights and may bear grudges for long periods of time. There is a prevalent fear of losing power or control to others. These individuals experience a chronic state of tension and are rarely able to relax.

Cognitively, paranoid people are very *guarded* about themselves and secretive about their decisions. They expect to be used or harassed by others. When confronted with new situations, they look for hidden, demeaning, or threatening meanings to benign remarks or events, and they respond by criticizing others. For example, if there is an error in a bank statement, the paranoid person may say the bank did it to ruin his or her credit rating.

Socially, paranoid people have great difficulty with intimate relationships. They interact in a cold and *aloof manner*, thus avoiding the perceived dangers of intimacy. Because they expect to be harmed by others, they question the loyalty or trustworthiness of family and friends. *Pathological jealousy* of the spouse or sex partner frequently occurs.

Devin's boss has been critical of Devin's inability to get his work done in a timely fashion. Although Devin is constantly trying to hear what others are talking about and is easily distracted, he is unable to relate this behavior to his job difficulties. Instead he states, "People at work keep bothering me and talking to each other just to slow me down. They are trying to turn my boss against me. Every little thing I do or say is used against me."

Schizoid Personality Disorder

Behaviorally, people with **schizoid personality disorder (SZPD)** are *loners* who prefer solitary activities because social situations and interactions increase their level of anxiety. They may be occupationally impaired if the job requires interpersonal skills. However, if work may be performed under conditions of social isolation, such as being a night guard in a closed facility, they may be capable of satisfactory occupational achievement.

Affectively, people with schizoid personality disorder are stable but have a limited range of feelings. Their *affect* is *blunted* or flat. Because they do not express their feelings either verbally or nonverbally, they give the impression that they have no strong positive or negative emotions. However, if they are forced into a close interaction, they may become very anxious.

Cognitively, they could be described as having

poverty of thoughts. The thoughts they do express are often vague. Some of their beliefs are these: "It doesn't matter what other people think of me" and "Close relationships are undesirable."

Socially, they interact with others in a cold and aloof manner, have *no close friends*, and prefer not to be in any relationships. They are indifferent to the attitudes and feelings of others, and thus are not influenced by praise or criticism.

Charlie, age 34, lives alone in a residential hotel. He is employed as a night guard in a warehouse. He interacts minimally with the other night guards and always eats his meals by himself. He has no friends and no social contacts outside of work. He describes people as "replaceable." He visits his parents, who live a mile away, once a year.

Schizotypal Personality Disorder

Behaviorally, people with **schizotypal personality disorder (STPD)** have a considerable disability. With peculiarities of thinking, appearance, and behavior that are not severe enough to meet the criteria for schizophrenic disorder, this disorder appears to be related to schizophrenia. It is assumed that some people with schizotypal personality disorder will progress to schizophrenia. Some studies have shown a greater prevalence of this personality disorder among biological relatives of people suffering from schizophrenia. Under periods of extreme stress and anxiety, they may experience transient psychotic symptoms that are not of sufficient duration to make an additional diagnosis (Cadenhead, Swerdlow, Shafer, Diaz, & Braff, 2000; Voglmaier et al., 2000).

People with this disorder exhibit *odd speech*. It is coherent but often tangential and vague or, at times, overelaborate. They prefer solitary activities and often experience occupational difficulties.

Affectively, they are typically constricted, and their affect may be *inappropriate* to the situation at times. Social situations create anxiety for those with schizotypal personality disorder.

Cognitively, these individuals experience the most severe distortions of any of the personality disorders. The disturbances include *paranoid ideation*, suspi-

ciousness, ideas of reference, odd beliefs, and magical thinking. They may experience illusions such as seeing people in the movement of shadows. They usually experience *difficulty in making decisions*.

Socially, they fear intimacy and desire no relationships with family or friends. Thus, they are very isolative and are usually *avoided by others*.

Carol, a 24-year-old unemployed single woman, lives in a rooming house. She keeps to herself, and most of the other boarders in the rooming house find her to be eccentric. Carol is preoccupied with the idea that her dead father was a movie star who left her a fortune with which her guardian absconded. Carol has a habit of saying odd things like, "So go the days of our lives." Most of the rooming house boarders avoid Carol because of her strange behaviors.

CLUSTER B DISORDERS

The three unstable disorders in this category—borderline, histrionic, and narcissistic—can barely be distinguished from one another. More so than with other disorders, the diagnosis may be influenced by personal bias, gender stereotypes, and cultural prejudices on the part of the professional.

Antisocial Personality Disorder

A diagnosis of **antisocial personality disorder (ASPD)** requires that the characteristics appear before the age of 15, and the client is usually given the diagnosis of conduct disorder. The diagnosis of antisocial personality disorder is not applied until after the age of 18. In boys, the behavior typically emerges during childhood, while for girls it is more likely to occur around puberty. There are at least twice as many males as females diagnosed with ASPD. They are at risk for substance abuse, criminal behavior, and becoming a victim of violence (Kaylor, 1999).

Behaviorally, actions may range from fairly mild to moderate severity, to very severe. Predominant childhood manifestations are lying, stealing, truancy, vandalism, fighting, and running away from home. In adulthood, the pattern changes to failure to honor financial obligations, an inability to function as a responsible parent, a tendency to lie pathologically, and an inability to sustain consistent appropriate work behavior. They may engage in nonviolent sexual offenses such as voyeurism or exhibitionism. A few commit violent crimes such as sadistic acts and murder. People with ASPD conform to rules only when they are useful to them. Their behavior is often *impulsive* and they have difficulty delaying gratification (Stone, 2000).

Affectively, people with ASPD express themselves quickly and easily but with very little personal involvement. Thus, they can profess undying love one minute and terminate the relationship the next. In addition, they are very *irritable* and *aggressive*. They have no concern for others and experience no guilt when they violate society's rules.

Cognitively, people with ASPD are *egocentric* and *grandiose*. They make no long-range plans and they are extremely confident that everything will always work out in their favor because they believe they are more clever than everyone else is. The disorder is ego-syntonic, they assume no responsibility for their actions, and they have no desire to change in any way.

Socially, these individuals are generally unable to sustain lasting, close, warm, and responsible relationships. Their sexual behavior is impersonal and impulsive. They *exploit others* in a cold and calculating way, while disregarding others' feelings and rights. With their quick anger, poor tolerance of frustration, and lack of guilt, they are often emotionally, physically, and sexually abusive to others (Kaylor, 1999).

Stephen, a divorced 20-year-old, works as a busperson at a pizza parlor, but he has a new job every other month. Stephen has an arrest record going back to high school. There, he was often truant and was picked up many times by the police for using marijuana and receiving stolen goods. Stephen often took money from his mother's purse, and he once fenced the family silver for drug money. Stephen married when he was 18, but the marriage lasted only six months. Stephen liked having women on the side, and his wife wasn't very understanding. When she nagged him about going out, Stephen beat her up. Stephen is working as a busperson to get enough money together to start a marijuana crop. As soon as he has enough money to buy some starter plants, he plans to go into business for himself.

Borderline Personality Disorder

Individuals with **borderline personality disorder (BPD)** exhibit a heterogeneous mixture of symptoms. In many ways, borderline personality would be more appropriately called cyclical personality because of the erratic moods or an impulse control disorder because of unpredictable behavior.

Behaviorally, people with BPD are generally impulsive, unpredictable, and manipulative. They engage in such *self-destructive behaviors* as reckless driving, substance abuse, binge eating, risky sexual practices, financial mismanagement, and violence. Self-mutilation, suicide threats, and attempted suicide are maladaptive responses to intense pain or attempts to relieve the sense of emptiness and gain reassurance that they are alive and can feel pain. Physically self-damaging actions, such as cutting or burning, may be precipitated by threats of separation from others, by rejection, or by demands of parenting or intimacy. Self-mutilation is a "severity" marker for the disorder, and those who self-mutilate are at higher risk for suicide (Brown & Dodson, 1999). See Chapter 9 for a full discussion of self-mutilation.

They may *manipulate others* to act against them in a negative or aggressive way. They alternate between

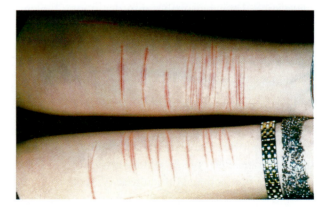

PHOTO 16.1 ■ Some people with borderline personality disorders engage in recurrent suicidal gestures or self-mutilating behaviors.

SOURCE: Dr. P. Marozzi/Science Photo Library; Photo Researchers, Inc.

periods of competence and incompetence. Although they do not deliberately avoid responsibility, they cannot explain how such avoidance occurs. They may be arrogant and challenging one minute and eager to please and submissive the next (Brown & Dodson, 1999).

Affectively, people with BPD are intense and unstable. They often have difficulty managing anxiety. Some are *anxious* most of the time, some have recurrent bouts of anxiety, and others experience intermittent panic attacks. People with BPD have difficulty tolerating and moderating strong feelings, which rapidly escalate to intense states of emotion. Irritation jumps to rage, sadness to despair, and disappointment to hopelessness. Their emotions are *labile* without any apparent reason or stimulus. Anger is often the predominant feeling. Some are incapable of caring for or loving others because of their feelings of inferiority. They might say they don't deserve to exist. In contrast, most have an inability to experience empathy in interactions with others or guilt for personal wrongdoings (Krakowski, 2000).

Cognitively, people with BPD are characterized by *identity disturbance*. Their self-descriptions tend to be vague and confusing. These individuals often suffer from changing identity and body image and changing sexual orientation, all of which may be indications of transient dissociative states. Some take on the identity of the people with whom they are interacting. Self-evaluation of abilities and talents alternates between grandiosity and depreciation. At times, they feel entitled to special treatment and, at other times, unworthy of anyone's attention. Believing that the world is dangerous and hostile, they feel powerless and vulnerable. Another cognitive characteristic is *dichotomous thinking*—things are either all good or all bad. For example, people with BPD are unable to see both positive and negative qualities in the same person or in themselves at the same time. The result is a shifting view of the self with rapidly shifting roles such as victim and victimizer, dominant and submissive. Psychotic episodes are common for some clients with BPD. These episodes may be brief or lengthy and are likely to result in repeated hospitalizations (Wilkinson-Ryan & Westen, 2000).

Socially, people with BPD have a history of intense, unstable, and *manipulative relationships*. Inside is a deprived, fragile child who may have grown up in a dysfunctional family. As adults, they desperately seek the love and nurturing they never received as a child. At the same time, they fear they will be abused and abandoned by others. This fear leads to rapid shifts from extremes of dependency to extremes of autonomy. Desperate clinging alternates with accusations and fights, in a frantic effort to avoid abandonment (Sanislow, Grilo, & McGlashan, 2000).

There is a great overlap between BPD and all the other personality disorders. Because symptoms vary in any given client at any given time, the disorder is both difficult to diagnose and difficult to treat. These clients use a large amount of mental health resources, often present themselves in acute crisis, and frequently drop out of treatment programs. Two thirds of people diagnosed with BPD are female. Some professionals believe that the borderline diagnosis has become the negative catch-all of psychiatric diagnoses. There is also a prejudice associated with this label and clients are seen as manipulative and noncompliant rather than sick (Nehls, 2000). There is concern that any female client who is resistant to an authoritarian therapist is labeled BPD.

Other explanations for the high rate of occurrence among females include the stresses of being female in a sexist culture, gender differences for "normal" behavior, and differences in the socialization of boys and girls. Many people with BPD have been sexually abused as children. For these individuals, a better diagnosis might be atypical posttraumatic stress disorder or severe survivor syndrome, neither of which are standard diagnoses in the DSM-IV-TR (Wilkinson-Ryan & Westen, 2000).

Julie, a 25-year-old part-time college student, frequently tells her friends how inconsiderate her parents are because they don't take care of her the way they "should" and, conversely, how awful it is because she can't become independent and live on her own. At times, she tries to manipulate her friends into doing things for her, and at other times she barely acknowledges that they exist. After dating Greg for only two weeks, she has told everyone he is absolutely perfect and they are "madly in love." One afternoon, Greg tells Julie he can't see her that evening because he must study for an exam. Julie flies into a rage, jumps into her car, and (continued) goes to a local bar, where she impulsively picks up a stranger and has sex with him in the parking lot. Returning home, she scratches her wrists with a broken bottle and calls Greg to tell him it's all his fault that she slashed her wrists and is going to die.

Histrionic Personality Disorder

Behaviorally, people with **histrionic personality disorder (HPD)** are most prominently characterized by *seeking stimulation* and excitement in life. Their behavior and appearance focus attention on themselves in an attempt to evoke and maintain the interest of others. They are seen as colorful, extroverted, and seductive individuals who seem always to be the center of attention. When they don't get their own way, however, they believe they are being treated unfairly and may even have a temper tantrum. They may resort to assaultive behavior or suicidal gestures to punish others.

Affectively, people with HPD are overly *dramatic*. Even minor stimuli cause emotional excitability and an exaggerated expression of feelings. They often seem to be on a roller coaster of joy and despair.

Cognitively, they are very *self-centered*. They become overly concerned with how others perceive them because of a high need for approval. Thoughts are, for example: "I need other people to admire me in order to be happy," "People are there to admire me and do my bidding," and "I cannot tolerate boredom." Histrionic people are guided more by their feelings than by their thinking, which tends to be vague and impressionistic. The basic belief is: "I don't have to bother to think things through—I can go by my gut feeling."

Socially, they constantly seek assurance, approval, or praise from family and friends. There is often exaggeration in their interpersonal relationships, with an emphasis on acting out the *role of victim or princess*. People with HPD commonly have flights of romantic fantasy, though the actual quality of their sexual relationships is variable. They may be overly trusting and respond very positively to strong authority figures, whom they think will magically solve their problems.

Leticia, a 25-year-old hairdresser, is popular with her clients. Leticia is very attractive, with long black hair and elegantly sculptured nails.

She always wears the latest fashions and lots of jewelry. Leticia enjoys entertaining her customers with tales of exploits with the many men in her life. Recently, she told of meeting a handsome cowboy in a bar and deciding to go to Las Vegas with him for the weekend. She claimed he treated her like a queen, hiring a chauffeured limo, dining by candlelight, and dancing until dawn. However, Leticia doesn't plan to see the young man again because she lives by the motto, "So many men, so little time!"

NARCISSISTIC PERSONALITY DISORDER

Behaviorally, those with **narcissistic personality disorder (NPD)** strive for power and success. Failure is intolerable because of their own *perfectionistic standards*. They do what they can to maintain and expand their superior position. Thus, they may seek wealth, power, and importance as a way to support their "superior" image. They tend to be highly competitive with others they view as also being superior.

Affectively, people with NPD are often labile. If criticized, they may fly into a *rage*. At other times, they may experience anxiety and panic and short periods of depression. They try to avoid feelings of blame and guilt because of intense fear of humiliation. When their needs are not met, they may react with rage or shame but mask these feelings with an aura of cool indifference.

Cognitively, those with narcissistic personality disorder are *arrogant* and *egotistical*. They are even more grandiose than people with HPD are. They have a tendency to exaggerate their accomplishments and talents. They expect to be noticed and treated as special whether or not they have achieved anything. Their feelings of specialness may alternate with feelings of special unworthiness. They are preoccupied with fantasies of unlimited success, power, brilliance, beauty, and ideal love. Underneath this confident manner is very low self-esteem.

Socially, people with NPD have *disturbed relationships*. They have unreasonable expectations of favorable treatment and exploit others to achieve personal goals. Friendships are made on the basis of how they can profit from the other person. Romantic partners are used as objects to bolster self-esteem. They are unable to develop a relationship based on mutuality.

Santo, a 43-year-old attorney, lives in an expensive house and drives a foreign sports car. He thrives on letting others know how successful his law practice is and about all the luxuries it affords him. He pays meticulous attention to his appearance. He has had multiple affairs during his marriage and justifies these by saying that his wife isn't living up to his expectations. He doesn't believe others have a right to criticize him and becomes irate if his wife makes requests of him.

classes, especially those that require him to speak in front of the group. He frets for hours over being embarrassed by something he might say that will make him look foolish. In class, Eric never sits next to the same person twice because this helps him avoid having to socialize. He has been admiring a girl named Jennie in his philosophy class, but he has never attempted to speak to her. Eric has been trying to find a way to ask Jennie out. However, everything he plans to say seems foolish. He is afraid Jennie will say no.

CLUSTER C DISORDERS
Avoidant Personality Disorder

Behaviorally, social discomfort is the primary characteristic of people with **avoidant personality disorder (AVPD)**. Any social or occupational activities that involve significant interpersonal contact are avoided. The belief underlying this behavior is: "If people get close to me, they will discover the 'real' me and reject me."

Affectively, these individuals are fearful and *shy.* They are easily hurt by criticism and devastated by the slightest hint of disapproval. They are distressed by their lack of ability to relate to others and often experience depression, anxiety, and anger for failing to develop social relationships.

Cognitively, people with AVPD are overly sensitive to the opinions of others. They suffer from an *exaggerated need for acceptance.* The thought is: "If others criticize me, they must be right."

Socially, they are reluctant to enter into relationships without a guarantee of uncritical acceptance. Since unconditional approval is not guaranteed, they have few close friends. In social situations, people with AVPD are afraid of saying something inappropriate or foolish or of being unable to answer a question. They are *terrified of being embarrassed* by blushing, crying, or showing signs of anxiety to other people.

Eric, a 22-year-old college senior, is considered to be shy by other students. Eric stays in his room studying and generally avoids parties. He has no real friends at college and spends his time watching television when he has no homework. Eric has a hard time in some of his

Dependent Personality Disorder

Behaviorally, dependence and submissiveness are the major features of **dependent personality disorder (DPD)**. People with DPD have difficulty doing things by themselves and getting things done on their own. They go to great lengths not to be alone and always

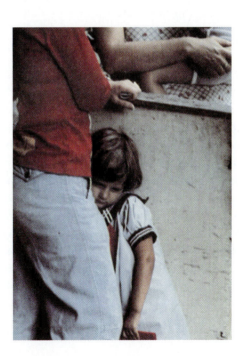

PHOTO 16.2 ■ Parental overprotectiveness may encourage dependence and interfere with the child's opportunities to learn skills that are necessary for more independent behavior.

SOURCE: Lester Sloan/Woodfin Camp & Associates.

agree with others to avoid rejection. With a strong need to be liked, dependent people volunteer to do unpleasant or demeaning things to increase their chances of acceptance. They avoid occupations in which they must perform independent functions.

Affectively, they *fear rejection* and abandonment. They feel totally helpless when they are alone. They are easily hurt by criticism and disapproval and are devastated when close relationships end. These fears contribute to a chronic sense of anxiety, and they may develop depression.

Cognitively, people with DPD have a severe *lack of self-confidence* and belittle their abilities and assets. Unable to make everyday decisions without an excessive amount of advice and reassurance from others, they often allow others to make choices for them. They exercise dichotomous thinking, such as: "One is either totally dependent and helpless or one is totally independent and isolated."

Socially, those with DPD desire *constant companionship* because they feel helpless when they are alone. Passively resisting making decisions, they often force their spouses or partners into making important choices for them, such as where to live, where to work, with whom to socialize, and in what activities to participate.

Min, a 32-year-old homemaker, married at 18 and moved directly from relying on her parents to relying on her husband. She was unable to go to any stores alone and unable to drive. She relied on her husband to pick out her clothing because she felt she had no taste. She stayed in the marriage for 10 years, even though her husband was verbally abusive and had multiple affairs. When she separated from her husband, she felt devastated, even though it was a terrible relationship. Within a few months, Min remarried and felt very relieved to be taken care of again.

Obsessive–Compulsive Personality Disorder

Behaviorally, people with **obsessive–compulsive personality disorder (OCPD)** exhibit *perfectionism* and *inflexibility*. The need to check and recheck objects and situations demands much of their time and energy.

They are industrious workers, but because of their need for routine, they are usually not creative. They may fail to complete projects because of the unattainable standards they set for themselves. No accomplishment ever seems good enough.

People with OCPD are polite and formal in social situations, where they can maintain emotional distance from others. They are very protective of their status and material possessions, so they have difficulty freely sharing with other people.

Affectively, they are *unable to express emotions*. To alleviate the anxiety of helplessness and powerlessness, they need to feel in control. Total control means that emotions, both tender and hostile, must be held in check or denied. Life and interpersonal relationships are intellectualized. The blocking of feelings and emotional distance are attempts to avoid losing control over themselves and their environment.

Because defenses are rarely adequate to manage anxiety, they develop a number of *fears*. They fear disapproval and condemnation from others and therefore avoid taking risks. They dread making mistakes. When mistakes occur, they experience a high level of guilt and self-recrimination, thus becoming their own tormentors. They also fear losing control. Rules and regulations are an attempt to remain in control at all times. Still fearful that things could go wrong, people with OCPD invent rituals in an attempt to ensure constancy and increase their feelings of security. As they try to control fear with a narrow focus on details and routines, the need for order and routine escalates.

People with OCPD have three types of *cognitive* distortions: perfectionism, a need for certainty, and a belief in an absolutely correct solution for every problem. *Procrastination* and *indecision* are common because they would rather avoid commitments than experience failure. Before making a decision, they accumulate many facts and try to figure out all the potential outcomes of any particular decision. When a decision is finally made, they are plagued by *doubts* and fears that an alternative decision would have been better. Since there is a constant striving to be perfect in all things, doing nothing is often considered better than doing something imperfectly. The underlying belief is: "I must avoid mistakes to be worthwhile."

Questioned as to how they view themselves, they say they are conscientious, loyal, dependable, and responsible—descriptions that conflict with an underlying low self-esteem and belief of inadequacy.

Socially, their need for control extends to interpersonal relationships. Regarding themselves as *omnipotent* (all-powerful) and *omniscient* (all-knowing), they expect their opinions and plans to be acceptable to everyone else; compromise is hardly considered. Frequent demands on their families to cooperate with their rigid rules and detailed routines undermine feelings of intimacy within the family system. Because they view dependency as being out of control and under the domination of the partner, they may abuse or oppress their partners so that an illusion of power and control can be maintained.

When interacting, people with OCPD have an overintellectual, meticulous, detailed manner of speaking designed to increase feelings of security. They unconsciously use language to confuse the listener. By bringing in side issues and focusing on nonessentials, they distort the content of the subject, which is a source of great frustration to the listener.

Jim, a 42-year-old midlevel executive for a food-processing plant, is always in trouble with the plant manager because he fails to get reports in on time. Jim blames his secretary for the problem, saying, "I can't get anything done right unless I do it myself." However, Jim's secretary promptly types exactly what he gives her. Jim then adds new details and reorganizes the report, and she has to type a new version. Jim keeps all the drafts of the report and documents the time it takes for the secretary to type them. He stores these in a file that only he is allowed to use. Jim lost his "to do" list one morning and had his secretary help him try to find it for over half an hour. Jim yelled at the secretary when she suggested that he try to remember what was on the list.

Obsessive–compulsive personality disorder (OCPD) must be distinguished from obsessive–compulsive disorder (OCD). In the past, it was thought that OCD was a more severe form of OCPD. Research indicates distinct differences between the disorders, with only 20 percent of people with OCD exhibiting characteristics of the personality disorder. People with OCD do not experience rigid patterns of many behaviors, the restricted affect, nor the excessive passion for productivity. OCD is ego-dystonic, while OCPD is *ego-syntonic* (Paris, 1999).

PERSONALITY DISORDERS NOT OTHERWISE SPECIFIED

The label personality disorder not otherwise specified is used when a person does not meet the full criteria for any one personality disorder, yet there is significant impairment in social or occupational functioning or in subjective distress.

Depressive Personality Disorder

People with **depressive personality disorder** are persistently gloomy and unhappy and are unable to experience the feelings of pleasure, joy or humor. They tend to worry and obsess on negative subjects. Their view of the future is *pessimistic* and they are unable to believe that their lives will ever improve. They have a low self-esteem as evidenced by their focus on their inadequacies and failures. This disorder occurs equally among women and men (APA, 2000).

Passive–Aggressive Personality Disorder

Individuals with **passive–aggressive personality disorder** oppose and resist others' expectations and demands. This persistent behavior occurs in work and social situations. Forms of passive–aggressive behavior include: procrastination, forgetfulness, intentional inefficiency, chronic lateness, and no carryover of learning. Overtly, the behavior is passive and submissive, but beneath this façade is a great deal of hostility and resentment.

Passive–aggressive people are often seen as "nice" people, and it is only when their "victims" are completely frustrated, that their hidden defiance becomes apparent. They say they did not do it "on purpose" and present themselves as innocent and well intentioned. The victim feels guilty and avoids confrontation for fear of being called a nag.

Chronic forgetters, for example, are unable to say they don't want to do something. Instead, they passively agree to everything and then proceed to "forget" to do it. Eventually, others learn not to count on them to do anything important and thus they avoid tasks and responsibilities. *Procrastinators* passively aggress with their annoying delays and refusal to be held to a fixed date or time. They also trigger guilt feelings in others by saying such things as, "Relax, you'll live longer!" Their hostility is passively expressed by keeping others waiting. People who are *chronically late* for appointments, dates, or social events are indirectly expressing their hostility for the person or persons kept waiting. They are also usually creative apologizers who have amazing excuses for their lateness. Those who have *no carryover of learning* express their aggression by never anticipating the needs of significant others or never learning from previous experience. Instead, they force the victim to make repeated requests each and every time. They may further manipulate victims by saying such things as, "Relax. If you want me to do something, just tell me!" Table 16.2 summarizes the characteristics related to types of disorders.

CULTURE-SPECIFIC CHARACTERISTICS

When assessing for the presence of personality disorders, practitioners must consider the cultural context and life circumstances influencing ways of thinking, feeling, and behaving. For example, immigrants or refugees might be perceived as being suspicious or paranoid when, in reality, they are simply unfamiliar with American culture. They may also be perceived as cold, hostile, or indifferent as they struggle to blend in to the dominant society. Some ethnic and cultural norms emphasize politeness and passivity, which might be misinterpreted as traits of dependent personality disorder. Since personality is somewhat a reflection of one's culture, nurses must be careful not to inadvertently label normal behavior as pathological.

Personality disorders can be diagnosed in clinical populations all over the world. Social expectations of any given culture encourage some kinds of behavior and suppress others. Thus, if culture has some influence in shaping personality, these disorders should have different prevalence rates. For example, antisocial personality disorder is rapidly increasing in North America and has very low rates in certain East Asian societies such as Taiwan. It is thought that North American families increase risk factors by failing to discipline their children effectively. In contrast, the Taiwanese have a strong belief in discipline and suppress most of the impulsive behaviors in children and adolescents (Paris, 1999; Paris 2001).

AGE-SPECIFIC CHARACTERISTICS

Personality disorders may become apparent in childhood and adolescence. Those prone to Cluster A disorders may have poor peer relationships; social anxiety and withdrawal; underachievement in school; and peculiar thoughts, language, and fantasies. They may become victims of teasing because they appear "odd" or "eccentric" (APA, 2000).

Childhood behavioral disorders such as conduct disorder and attention deficit/hyperactivity disorder, contribute to the development of adult antisocial personality disorder. The validity of borderline personality disorder in children and adolescents is a controversial topic. Some researchers believe that BPD in young people can be reliably diagnosed. Others believe that the symptoms are relatively unstable over time and therefore a personality disorder is not an accurate diagnosis (Becker, Grilo, Edell, & McGlashan, 2000; Kaylor, 1999). See Chapter 17 for more information on the spectrum disorders.

Extreme shyness beginning in infancy may be associated with Cluster C disorders. Overanxious children are more likely to be overprotected and vulnerable to developing dependent traits. It is critical, however, that labels not be attached to behavior that is developmentally appropriate (APA, 2000).

Since personality, and therefore personality disorders, is relatively stable over time, the disorders persist into late life. There may be some modification of symptoms since impulsiveness decreases with age (Kennedy, 2000).

CONCOMITANT DISORDERS

There is a high correlation between *substance abuse* and antisocial personality disorder. At times, it is difficult to separate these disorders, as substance abuse is itself an antisocial behavior that causes problems similar to those of the personality disorder. Thus, substance abusers are divided into two groups: *primary antisocial addicts*, whose antisocial behavior is independent of the need to obtain drugs, and *secondary antisocial addicts*, whose antisocial behavior is directly related to drug use (Skodol, Oldham, & Gallaher, 1999).

Substance abuse is also a common symptom of borderline personality disorder. The addiction may be associated with poor impulse control and erratic mood changes. Substance use may be an attempt to self-medicate.

TABLE 16.2

Characteristics Related to Types of Disorders

Behavioral Characteristics

Impulsive

ASPD—difficulty delaying gratification; criminal behavior

BPD—behavior unpredictable; self-destructive

Rigid

OCPD—perfectionism interferes with task completion

AVPD—doesn't want to be embarrassed by trying new activities

Affective Characteristics

Intense, unstable, inappropriate affect

BPD—affect instability; difficulty moderating strong feelings

HPD—rapidly shifting and shallow expression of emotions; overly dramatic

ASPD—irritable, aggressive

PPD—quick expression of anger; bears grudges; pathological jealousy

Restricted, flat affect

SZPD—cold and detached

STPD—inappropriate or constricted

OCPD—unable to express emotions; fearful

AVPD—fearful; shy

Cognitive Characteristics

Hostile, paranoid world view

STPD, BPD—transient paranoid ideation

PPD—hyperalert to danger; secretive

Negative sense of self

NPD—envious of others or believes others are envious of them

AVD—views self as socially inept or inferior

DPD—can't do things on own; lack of self-confidence in judgment or abilities

Lack of sense of self

BPD—unstable self-image or sense of self

Exaggerated sense of self

HPD—needs to be the center of attention

NPD—grandiose sense of self-importance

ASPD—egocentric and grandiose

Peculiar thought processes

- Odd beliefs, magical thinking

- Poverty of thoughts (schizoid)

Social Characteristics

Overly close relationships

BPD—unstable and intense; alternate between idealization and devaluation

HPD—considers relationships to be more intimate than they actually are

DPD—goes to excessive lengths to obtain nurturance and support from others

Distant/avoidant relationships

OCPD—excessively devoted to work to exclusion of friendships; unable to compromise

PPD—argumentative; fear information and relationships will be used against them

(*continued*)

TABLE 16.2

Characteristics Related to Types of Disorders *(continued)*

Social Characteristics (continued)	
Distant/avoidant relationships *(continued)*	SZPD—doesn't want relationships
	STPD—only maintains contact with family
	AVPD—fears criticism, disapproval, or rejection from others
Lack of concern for other's needs	ASPD—indifferent to others' feelings; no remorse for hurting others
	NPD—unreasonable expectations of others; exploits others

PPD, paranoid; SZPD, schizoid; STPD, schizotypal; ASPD, antisocial; BPD, borderline; HPD, histrionic; NPD, narcissistic; AVPD, avoidant; DPD, dependent; OCPD, obsessive–compulsive

SOURCES: Geiger, T. C., & Crick, N. R. (2001). A developmental psychopathology perspective on vulnerability to personality disorders. In R. E. Ingram & J. M. Price (Eds.), *Vulnerability to psychopathology* (pp. 57–102). New York: Guilford Press; Livesley, W. J. (2001). Conceptual and taxonomic issues. In W. J. Livesley (Ed.), *Handbook of personality disorders* (pp. 3–38). New York: Guilford Press; and Paris, J. (1999). *Nature and nurture in psychiatry*. Washington, DC: American Psychiatric Press.

Psychotic episodes or disorders often co-occur with schizotypal, borderline, and dependent personality disorders. Mood disorders co-occur more often with avoidant and borderline personality disorders, and anxiety, eating, and somatoform disorders co-occur with avoidant, dependent, and borderline personality disorders (Dolan-Sewell, Krueger, & Shea, 2001).

Recurrent *suicidal behavior* is characteristic of borderline personality disorder. Suicides are often associated with anger and often the result of impulsive behavior in the context of interpersonal relationship problems. Other factors contributing to suicide in persons with personality disorders include depression and substance abuse. A history of prior attempts is the strongest predictors of future attempts and suicide completion (Soloff, Lynch, Kelly, Malone, & Mann, 2000).

CAUSATIVE THEORIES

As with other psychiatric disorders, a number of theories have been offered to identify the causes of personality disorders. With continuing refinement of diagnostic criteria for each cluster of disorders, it will become possible to conduct useful research on specific populations that have been accurately diagnosed. In the past, wide differences in the application of specific diagnostic labels precluded the gathering of reliable data. Since there was so little agreement about whether a person should be included in the category at the outset, it is easy to understand why the search for any common factors—in genetics, early experiences, family patterns, or any other variable—failed to yield results from which general conclusions could be drawn.

Remaining obstacles are the refusal to seek treatment on the part of the client and the relatively infrequent need for psychiatric hospitalization. These obstacles have limited research to those seeking therapy (most often with borderline personality disorder) or those being referred through the criminal system (most often with antisocial personality disorder).

There is no single cause of the personality disorders. Most likely, they arise from an interaction between biological factors and the environment. Just as one's biology or constitution can alter experiences in life, so, too, many experiences alter one's basic biology. The brain constantly changes to absorb new experiences.

Genetic Theory

Studies suggest a common genetic factor in schizotypal personality disorder and schizophrenia. Individuals in both groups have an equal probability of having a sibling with schizophrenia. This shared genetic vulnerability has led many people to consider schizotypal per-

Neurobiological Theory

Some of the personality disorders are primarily disorders of impulse control. There may be problems with limbic system regulation. Brain imaging studies report reduced glucose utilization in the limbic system and the prefrontal cortex of people who exhibit impulsive aggression when compared to normal controls. People diagnosed with BPD and ASPD appear to have lower serotonin (5-HT) activity than control groups. The lower the 5-HT levels, the more likely the client is to self-mutilate, experience intense rage, and behave aggressively toward others. A concurrent high level of norepinephrine (NE) creates hypersensitivity to the environment and is related to aggressive behavior. Abnormalities in levels of dopamine (DA) may explain the psychotic episodes experienced by some clients with BPD and schizotypal personality disorder (Coccaro, 2001; Krakowski, 2000; Leyton et al., 2001).

Recent research has found that there may be a relationship between criminal behavior and physiological underarousal to stimulation. Heart rate, skin conductance, and electroencephalogram (EEG) readings are lower in people with ASPD than in those without the disorder. This underarousal can be interpreted in two ways: Either the person seeks inappropriate stimulation to counteract the underaroused state or it can be seen as a marker of low fear levels, which would interfere with the anticipation of danger (Ratey, 2001).

Intrapersonal Theory

The idea that most children are *resilient* to adversity is critical for understanding the impact of negative events in childhood. Some aspects of resilience are biological. Children with positive personality traits and higher levels of intelligence are more adept at finding ways to cope with adversity. In contrast, children with negative personality traits and lower levels of intelligence experience more stress as they attempt to cope with adversity. Psychosocial aspects of resiliency are positive relationships, which buffer negative experiences. Thus, growing up in a dysfunctional family can be offset by attachments to competent extended family members (Paris, 2001).

People with Cluster A personality disorders have been studied minimally because they seldom request or are forced into treatment. Intrapersonal theory suggests that the primary defense mechanism is one of projection; that is, they project their own hostility on others and respond to them in a fearful and distrustful

sonality disorder as one of the schizophrenia spectrum disorders (Voglmaier et al., 2000).

A strong predictor of the development of antisocial behavior is antisocial personality disorder in one or both parents. This seems to be due to both genetic and environmental factors. There also appears to be a genetic link between antisocial and borderline personality disorders. It is believed that people with both disorders are born with an innate biological tendency to react intensely to low levels of stress (Herpertz, Kunert, Schwenger, Eng, & Sass, 1999; Paris, 2001).

manner. It is also thought that they defensively with-draw from others for fear they will be hurt.

Intrapersonal theory explains ASPD as a develop-mental delay or failure. It is believed that people with ASPD have an underdeveloped superego, in that authority and cultural mores have not been internal-ized. Conformity to cultural expectations is situational and superficial, and there is an inability to experience guilt when rules are violated.

Individuals with BPD often think, feel, and behave more like toddlers than adults. When young children experience inadequate parenting, their basic needs and desires remain unsatisfied. Unmet needs lead to hostil-ity toward those on whom their lives depend. At the same time, these children are terrified by the destruc-tiveness of their anger. They begin to believe that they have been, or will be, abandoned, and the parents are unable to provide good experiences to balance the intense feelings of neglect. All of this contributes to making adults who feel so utterly empty inside that they can never get enough attention and nurturing. At the same time, they are terrified of intimacy because of their fears of abandonment. This constant tension between need and fear leads to acting out feelings of rage and self-destructive behavior to manage the guilt.

Social Theory

Negative childhood experiences do not necessarily lead to mental disorders in adulthood. Risk factors may, however, increase the likelihood of negative outcomes. In community populations, psychosocial stressors con-tribute to pathology in only a minority of those who are exposed. In clinical populations, people with a vari-ety of mental disorders report more psychosocial stres-sors during childhood than do those without mental disorders. In other words, most people are resilient to adversity but those who develop mental disorders have an underlying vulnerability to stress (Paris, 2001).

A variety of social conditions lead to low self-esteem, negative self-concept, and even self-hatred. When one is on the receiving end of social oppression, it is more difficult to develop self-esteem and a healthy identity.

Social expectations encourage some kinds of behav-ior and suppress others. Traditional societies are more tolerant of dependence, and people are expected to conform to family and group norms. Some believe that industrialization has contributed to a changing value

system and that Cluster B personality disorders may be a response to society's increasing complexity. We have come to recognize current values such as these: Personal needs are more important than group needs, expediency is more important than morality, and appearance is more important than inner worth. Believing that survival depends solely on themselves, those with Cluster B personality disorders develop a value system of "Every person for herself or himself" and "Take care of number one first."

Family Theory

Many individuals diagnosed with personality disorders report dysfunctional families of origin. This may reflect some reality but may also reflect how distressed adults account for their present difficulties by blaming their parents. Multiple negative experiences in child-hood are more likely to cause problems than one or two negative experiences. Abnormal parenting (abuse, neglect, overcontrol) may also be a risk factor for per-sonality disorder (Paris, 1999).

The diathesis-stress model states that biology and social environment of the family interact in such a way as to produce personality disorders. For example, chil-dren who are born with a temperament of impulsivity and mood instability may be badly treated, in response, by family members. Other children who are born with an anxious temperament and who have problems with peer relationships may be overprotected or rejected by parental caregivers. Children with diffi-cult temperaments come into conflict with peers and parents, increasing the likelihood of either social rejec-tion or physical abuse (Paris, 1999).

People with ASPD are thought to come from fami-lies with inconsistent parenting that resulted in emo-tional deprivation in the children. Because of their own personality or substance abuse problems, parents may be unable to supervise and discipline their children, or they may even model antisocial behavior for the chil-dren. Others seem to come from healthy families and had good childhood experiences (Nehls, 1999).

Family theorists view BPD as a dysfunction of the entire family system across several generations, with sim-ilar dynamics of blurred generational boundaries of the incestuous family (see Chapter 22). BPD usually occurs in an enmeshed family system. With a high family value on children's loyalty to parents, adult children cling to their parents even after marriage. As a result, the marital couple is unable to bond with each other. When children are born, they are encouraged to cling, and normal separation behavior is discouraged. Often, the children end up in a caretaking role with parents and must assume a high level of family responsibility. During late adolescence, they are unable to separate from their parents because of an incorporated family theme that separation and loss are intolerable. It is within the third or fourth generation of enmeshed families that borderline traits develop into the personality disorder. Male children with BPD tend not to marry and remain connected with their families of origin. Female children with BPD often marry but tend to pick passive and distant partners who are enmeshed with their own families (Bartholomew, Kwong, & Hart, 2001).

It is believed that a chaotic, depriving, abusive, or brutalizing environment is a major factor in the development of BPD. Research shows that 50 to 70 percent of clients diagnosed with BPD have a history of abuse. Tentative findings at this point indicate that the abuse began at an early age, that the child was neglected as well as abused, that sexual abuse was often combined with physical abuse, and that there was usually more than one perpetrator. It must be noted that abuse within the family is not a single incident but rather part of a dysfunctional family behavior pattern that is either chaotic or coercively controlling. Dysfunctional families distort all interactions and relationships (Krakowski, 2000).

Feminist Theory

Girls and boys are socialized very differently in America. Boys are encouraged to be independent, self-sufficient, active, and thinking rather than feeling individuals. Girls are taught to be dependent, submissive, passive, and feeling individuals who are more concerned with the needs of others than with their own needs. Such rigid role expectations can lead to identity difficulties. The same behaviors that may be considered acceptable in men (impulsiveness, expressing anger, argumentativeness, making demands) are labeled pathological in women. It is more likely that men are diagnosed as having antisocial personality disorder and women are diagnosed as having BPD when exhibiting similar behaviors. These differences in diagnoses reflect the real and unfortunate consequences of gender-role stereotyping in American culture (Brown & Dodson, 1999).

PSYCHOPHARMACOLOGICAL INTERVENTIONS

Studies are being conducted on the effectiveness of medications in treating personality disorders. Medications may be used to modify temperament, address specific symptoms, or to treat co-morbid Axis I disorders. Psychotic symptoms appear to respond to low doses of the antipsychotic agents. These medications are best used for relief of acute symptoms and are typically discontinued when the psychotic features disappear. A number of medications are being tried to decrease the impulsive, aggressive, and self-destructive behavior patterns of BPD. Selective serotonin reuptake inhibitors (SSRIs), Catapres (clonidine) and Tenex (guanfacine) diminish rage and rapid mood swings as well as decrease aggression and impulsive and self-destructive behavior. SSRIs are also used to treat obsessive ruminations in people with personality disorders. SSRIs include Prozac (fluox-

Complementary/Alternative Therapies

How to Help Clients Relax

Throughout the day you may find hundreds of opportunities to integrate some deep breathing, relaxation, self-massage, and gentle movement techniques into usual activities. Try this:

- You are sitting at a stoplight. Take a deep breath.
- You are just about to fall asleep or have just awakened. Breathe deeply and allow your whole body to become completely relaxed.
- You are in the shower washing your hair. As you apply shampoo, massage your scalp vigorously; rub your ears, relax, take several deep breaths.
- As you apply lotion or oil to your body following your bath, do so with the intent of relaxing each muscle group as you gently massage your entire body.
- You are watching television. During each commercial break, massage your hands, feet, and ears. Breathe deeply and relax.
- You are vacuuming the house. Relax your shoulders, breathe deeply, and coordinate your movements with your breathing.

SOURCE: Adapted from Jahnke, R. (1997). *The healer within.* San Francisco: Harper San Francisco.

etine), Paxil (paroxetine), and Zoloft (sertraline). Medications should be viewed as a means of controlling symptoms that are disabling. The overall treatment plan includes individual, group, family, and behavioral therapy. As more is learned about these disorders, improved techniques can be designed to better meet individual client needs (Bender et al., 2001).

ALTERNATIVE THERAPIES

There are no specific alternative therapies for individuals with personality disorders. Those who experience anxiety may find chamomile tea or the herb kava to be helpful. Yoga and meditation may also decrease levels of anxiety. People who have a concomitant mild or moderate depression may find St. John's Wort or SAMe helpful. Vitamin B_{12} is necessary for the production of dopamine and serotonin, which may be lowered in depressive states.

NURSING PROCESS

Assessment

As with other psychiatric disorders, data collection serves as the starting point for the nursing process for clients with personality disorders. The main obstacle to assessment is the probability that the client will not perceive that a problem exists. If possible, interview family members for their perceptions of the problem. Exercise professional judgment in seeking information from others about their relationships with the client. Although the objective is to obtain a description of the client's functioning within various family and social contexts, you must be certain that the client's rights are protected. By remaining alert to the potential for a breach of confidentiality, you can ensure that neither the legal nor the ethical limits of the professional domain are exceeded. The Focused Nursing Assessment feature lists assessment questions for clients with personality disorders.

Diagnosis

Probable nursing diagnoses can be identified for each cluster of personality disorders. Remember that no client fits neatly into any theoretically determined diagnostic category and that no standardized list or table can provide a comprehensive description of the problems specific to individual clients. The Nursing Diagnoses with NOC and NIC feature serves as a framework for nursing care, but they cannot replace a comprehensive, individualized plan for the client.

Outcome Identification and Goals

Based on the assessment data, you select outcomes appropriate to the nursing diagnoses. The most common outcomes are found in the Nursing Diagnoses with NOC and NIC feature.

Client goals are specific behavioral prescriptions which you, the client, and significant others identify as realistic and attainable. The following are examples of some of the outcomes appropriate to people with personality disorders:

- Implements behavioral contract to reduce self-destructive activities
- Incidents of self-mutilation decrease
- Decreases suicidal behavior
- Utilizes the problem-solving process
- Verbalizes an internal locus of control
- Interacts socially with others
- Verbalizes decreased anxiety
- Decreases perfectionistic behavior

Nursing Interventions

Approach clients with *Cluster A* personality disorders in a gentle, interested, and nonintrusive manner that is respectful of the client's need for distance, privacy, and respites from interpersonal interactions. Demands for trust or self-disclosure may heighten anxiety and even precipitate a transient psychotic state. The staff needs to understand that clients' social withdrawal and lack of feeling or responses are self-protective rather than unappreciative.

Clients with *Cluster B* personality disorders require much more patience and structure from nurses. The approach must be one of consistency and limit setting.

Behavior Assessment	Affective Assessment	Cognitive Assessment	Social Assessment
What is your usual pattern of daily activities?	Describe your usual mood.	Would you describe yourself as independent or dependent?	How do you usually relate to others?
What is your work history?	What happens when you feel frustrated? Angry? Fearful? Happy? Peaceful?	What do you like about yourself?	When do you prefer to be alone? To be with others?
Describe your functioning at work/school.	What causes you to be upset with others?	What would you like to change about yourself?	Describe the differences between your business and social relationships.
Has anyone ever told you your behavior was a problem? If so, what did they tell you?	How do you react to criticism?	What are your expectations for the future?	How many close relationships with others do you have? Describe the relationships.
Describe any problematic behavior you displayed as a teenager.	Do others ever describe you as detached, cool, or aloof? If so, what do they say?		Are other people out to discredit or hurt you?
Describe both successful and unsuccessful attempts you have had in trying to modify your behavior patterns.	How do you feel when you are with groups of people?		Are you able to say "no" to other people?
How do you resolve conflicts with others?	How often are you rejected or do you feel others reject you?		
When did you have your last drink? When did you last use drugs?	Would you consider yourself to be affectionate and empathetic toward others?		

It is critically important that staff members keep open and clear lines of communication with one another.

Clients with *Cluster C* diagnoses will find it helpful when you point out their avoidance behavior and secondary gains. Assertiveness training helps these clients manage their dependency and anger. Anxiety may lessen when they learn to modify their perfectionistic standards.

Three fundamental beliefs guide your approach in working with persons experiencing personality disorders. The first is *self-determination*. Clients are partners in treatment and have the right to choose their own course in life. Second, the focus is on *role functioning* while recognizing that not all symptoms will disappear. Third is *maintaining hope*. These clients are particularly susceptible to loss of hope for change and giving up on treatment. See the Nursing Diagnoses with NOC and NIC feature for people with personality disorders.

Behavioral: Behavior Therapy
Impulse Control Training

The first priority of care is client *safety*. These clients, especially those with BPD, are often suicidal or they self-mutilate. Take all suicidal thinking seriously. It is an indication they are not feeling safe. The immediate goal of crisis management is to ensure safety and manage emotions and impulses. (Nursing interventions for clients who are suicidal are covered in Chapter 20, and for those who self-mutilate in Chapter 9). Intense emotional pain and poor impulse control contribute to self-destructive behavior. The most helpful initial

NURSING DIAGNOSES with NOC & NIC

Clients with Personality Disorders

DIAGNOSIS	OUTCOMES	INTERVENTIONS
Cluster A Fear related to perceived threats from others or the environment	**Fear Control:** Personal actions to eliminate or reduce disabling feelings of alarm aroused by an identifiable source	Presence
Social isolation related to inadequate social skills, craving of solitude	**Social Support:** Perceived availability and actual provision of reliable assistance from other persons	Social Skills
Spiritual distress related to lack of connectedness to others	**Spiritual Well-Being:** Personal expressions of connectedness with self, others, higher power, all life, nature, and the universe that transcent and empower the self	Presence
Cluster B Impaired social interaction related to manipulation of others, unstable mood, poor impulse control, extreme emotional reactions, extreme self-centeredness, seductive behavior	**Impulse Control:** Self-restraint of compulsive or impulsive behavior **Social Interaction Skills:** An individual's use of effective interaction behaviors	Impulse Control Training Limit Setting Social Skills
High risk for violence, self-directed (suicide or self-mutilation), related to intense emotional pain, poor impulse control	**Impulse Control:** Self-restraint of compulsive or impulsive behavior	Impulse Control Training

response is to talk in a calm, monotone voice, repeating a phrase such as: "You are with me. I will help you remain safe."

Often, clients regress to an earlier age and thus your interventions should match the presenting age. For example, if they are acting like 3- or 4-year-olds in a rage, use a kind, soothing approach with simple, firm directions to contain the behavior. Once clients are able to control behavior, there are a number of nursing interventions directed toward the goal of remaining safe and increasing impulse control. Establish an hour-by-hour or day-by-day *anti-harm contract* with clients. This may be either a verbal or a written agreement. Help them identify and label feelings (self-monitoring) in order to learn to recognize that self-destructive behaviors are responses to feelings and that these responses can be changed over time. This is the beginning of the problem-solving process.

DIAGNOSIS	OUTCOMES	INTERVENTIONS
Cluster B *(continued)* High risk for violence directed at others or objects related to intense rage, poor impulse control	***Impulse Control:*** Self-restraint of compulsive or impulsive behavior	Impulse Control Training
Anxiety related to feelings of abandonment	***Anxiety Control:*** Personal actions to eliminate or reduce feelings of apprehension and tension from an unidentifiable source	Anxiety Reduction
Cluster C Ineffective individual coping related to high dependency needs, rigid behavior/thoughts, inadequate role performance, high need for approval from others, inability to make independent decisions	***Social Support:*** Perceived availability and actual provision of reliable assistance from other persons	Social Skills
Anxiety related to feelings of abandonment, disapproval, losing control, conflict	***Anxiety Control:*** Personal actions to eliminate or reduce feelings of apprehension and tension from an unidentifiable source	Anxiety Reduction

SOURCES: Johnson, M., Maas, M., & Moorhead, S. (2000). *Nursing outcomes classification (NOC)* (2nd ed.). St. Louis, MO: Mosby; McCloskey, J. C., & Bulechek, G. M. (1996). *Nursing interventions classification (NIC)* (2nd ed.). St. Louis, MO: Mosby; and North American Nursing Diagnoses Association (1999). *Nursing diagnoses definitions and classification 1999–2000*. Philadelphia: Author.

Next, ask clients to identify *triggers* to and *patterns* in their self-destructive behavior. Diaries can be used to track the changes in feelings and to identify the specific stimuli that caused the change. Self-monitoring via diary cards provides more accurate recall and detail about the relationship between mood, triggers, self-harm behavior, and effective coping strategies. Brainstorm ideas on what other behaviors might be substituted for the harmful ones. Clients need to learn how to tolerate dysphoric emotions and how to solve problems rather than acting impulsively. They then decide which response they will implement the next time they feel like hurting themselves. When that has been done, evaluate the effectiveness of the new behavior with the client. Clients need a great deal of support, reminding, and guidance from nurses before they are able to develop any consistency in new behaviors. They need to be encouraged to identify and use sources of support during this time. Remember that competency is often achieved by the gradual substitution of progressively more adaptive behaviors. For example, clients may be encouraged to seek help from a crisis center before engaging in self-harming behaviors. The next step would be to develop alternative behaviors until the next scheduled therapy appointment. And finally, clients learn how to manage and tolerate distress without engaging in harmful behavior. With a gradual approach, change is not so overwhelming.

Personality disorders often have a negative impact on the family and friends surrounding the individual. It is important to *include families* in the treatment process. See Chapter 3 for more information on family intervention. Families need information about the nature of the condition, its course, and the available treatments. Teach them practical strategies to cope with everyday interactions and behaviors that are disruptive to family life. They need to learn how to respond with understanding and compassion rather than anger and defensiveness. See Box 16.1 for topics to include in family education.

Limit Setting

Many of these clients tend to test nurses and behave in a manipulative manner. To help you identify when this is occurring, consider how the following behaviors might be manipulative. The client:

- Appears helpless
- Lies
- Uses rationalization or minimization of responsibility for own behavior
- Engages in seductive behavior
- Compliments or flatters staff
- Asks for special privileges
- Makes demands of or threatens staff
- Gets other clients to confront staff
- Works on other clients' problems and not on own issues
- Uses role reversal with staff

Clients who are manipulative respond best to a high level of structure and *clear ground rules*. Explain the reasons for the rules as well as the consequences when expectations are not met. You must maintain a careful balance between being an authority figure while not

---

BOX 16.1

Family Education

- Personality disorders are long-standing and inflexible patterns of relating to the world and other people.
- Affected people usually have little insight into their behavior.
- Their loved one is handicapped but not disabled.
- There are frequent co-morbid conditions such as depression, anxiety disorders, psychotic episodes, and substance abuse.
- Life stresses make clients more vulnerable to relapse.
- Go slowly. Recovery takes time.
- Maintain family routines as much as possible.
- Don't ignore threats of self-harm.

---

being harsh or judgmental. If you try to be their "friend," you will be open to manipulation. If you take a strong authority stance, you will create frequent power struggles. The best approach is straightforward and businesslike. Together, develop the goals of treatment and behavioral contracts to reduce inappropriate activities. The focus is always on the client's behavior, as they tend to blame others for their problems. Do not be dissuaded by their excuses and rationalizations. Convey expectations in a clear, direct manner and request clarification from clients of their understanding. This decreases the use of manipulation through misunderstanding.

Pay attention to your own emotional responses to these clients. It is very easy to internalize the client's sense of chaos, anger, and frustration. In a residential home or inpatient unit, power struggles often develop, and the milieu becomes chaotic for everyone. Remaining therapeutic may require supervision or consultation from an unbiased colleague. One staff member may see a client as vulnerable and needy, while another might perceive the same client to be aggressive, provocative, and in need of clear limits. The client is an expert at playing one person off another in a manipulative attempt. Without outside supervision, debates among staff members can become highly personalized and polarize the staff into several factions.

Teach friends and family members how to set limits with individuals who are passive–aggressive. To avoid the "misunderstandings," have the person repeat back the instructions you have given before they set out to perform the task. Family members and friends should never take it for granted that the person has understood. To deal with a person who procrastinates, they should set a precise, never vague deadline and establish a penalty for delays. The same is true for latecomers—a clearly set consequence is established for late behavior. Family and friends must consistently enforce all consequences if the passive–aggressive behavior is to lessen.

Behavior Modification: Social Skills

The goal of nursing interventions with clients who are helpless and dependent is to increase their coping skills and encourage *independent functioning*. The first step is to communicate to clients that you recognize their feelings of helplessness and fears of becoming more independent. This expression of empathy will help them be more collaborative in the problem-solving process. Explore examples of dichotomous thinking, such as "One is either totally dependent and helpless or one is totally independent and isolated." Often clients view nurses as all-powerful rescuers who will make everything better. But carefully avoid rescuing behavior because it would reinforce the client's feeling of helplessness and the external locus of control. The next step is to help clients identify what would be different, what they would gain, and what they would lose if they were less helpless. Focus on one issue at a time. Begin with a fairly insignificant situation, and help them identify what they would like out of this situation. They can then problem-solve ways to achieve their goals. With each subsequent use of the problem-solving process, their skills will increase, and they will become more confident in their ability to handle problems as they arise.

Interventions designed to decrease socially isolative behaviors and reward socially outgoing behaviors are often accomplished through *social skills training* and *assertiveness training*. Be sure to respect a client's need to be distant or isolative, while encouraging and supporting interactions with others. Help clients identify interpersonal problems resulting from social skill deficits. Encourage them to verbalize their feelings associated with these problems, and assist them in identifying alternative ways to relate without seduction or intimidation. Role play and provide feedback about the appropriateness of their responses. Encourage them to evaluate their behavior in social situations.

Group therapy is often an adjunct to individual therapy. The process of group therapy helps clients focus on interpersonal issues as well as individual issues. Clients not only get feedback from more than one person, they also have the opportunity to be therapeutic with other group members. Since clients with personality disorders have inadequate social skills, group therapy is one way to develop and foster better relationships with others, decrease real isolation, and increase the sense of feeling understood.

Behavioral: Psychological Comfort Promotion

Anxiety Reduction

Some clients avoid making decisions to avoid the anxiety of failure. Whenever possible, encourage them to *make their own decisions* to reinforce a sense of competence and an internal locus of control. Point out the destructive effects of indecision to further their understanding that an imperfect decision may be less harmful than no decision. Explain that there are no absolute guarantees of the future for any of us. Explore how many decisions in life can be remade, as these clients often believe that decisions are always final. Anxiety is increased when they fear failure if the "perfect" decision is not made. Teach clients the *problem-solving process*. This increases their skills in decision making and helps them see that there are a variety of choices that can be made, tested, and evaluated. Give feedback for decisions they make to reinforce positive changes in behavior. The problem solving process is covered in more detail in Chapter 2.

Some clients become perfectionistic to guard against the anxiety of feeling inferior. To help clients gain insight into the need for perfectionistic behavior, comment on the link between this behavior and feelings of anxiety and helplessness. Explore their fear of being judged inferior by others and help them evaluate whether this is a realistic appraisal of others' responses. *Promote realistic self-appraisal* through discussion of abilities and limitations. Some clients benefit from being assigned three purposeful, nonharmful mistakes per day, such as setting the table incorrectly, giving wrong directions, putting postage stamps on upside down, or wearing two different socks. They are to use a journal to record their feelings in response to the mistakes. This exercise serves to increase clients' sense of control over errors and helps them recognize that many mistakes are not serious. Provide feedback for positive changes to reinforce behavior and increase their ability to accurately appraise themselves. Help clients acknowledge that an anxiety-free life is impossible, which may help them give up striving for perfection.

Some clients keep others at a distance and reduce anxiety by the need to always "be right." Do not get caught up in a struggle for control in being right, as this will reinforce maladaptive behavior. Facilitate clients' *acceptance of responsibility for their own behavior* and explore how this affects other people. When they see themselves more realistically, they may be able to behave in more socially effective ways. Use relevant humor and laughter regarding perfectionism as a relief from tension and anxiety. Humor allows clients to risk speaking about the need to be right without fear of ridicule. Teach clients that humor used appropriately is a highly valued attribute in this culture. Humor allows people to experience pleasure and decreases emotional distance from others.

Anxiety prevents some clients from *asking for help* when it is needed. Have clients identify expectations that will occur should help be sought. They need to recognize that fear of rejection precludes seeking help. Use appropriate self-disclosure regarding situations in which you have sought help, to enable clients to recognize that asking for assistance need not result in rejection. Role play with clients as to how to ask for help in a particular situation to increase the use of unfamiliar skills. After seeking help, have clients evaluate the situation in terms of feelings and how others responded. This helps them assess the reality of their anticipated fears.

Clients can also choose environments that are less stressful and have a better fit with their personality traits. For example, people who are highly introverted will manage better in a very predictable environment and often do better when they can work alone. Clients who are highly extroverted respond best in an environment that presents challenges and a high level of interaction with others.

Behavioral: Coping Assistance

Presence

Priority is given to establishing and maintaining a *therapeutic relationship* because individuals with personality disorders have great difficulty with relationships. It is critical that clients feel secure enough to discuss problems. The style of interaction must be one of respect and collaboration. It is helpful to use words such as "we" and "together" to promote a collaborative working relationship. Listen to clients' concerns and communicate your empathetic understanding of their situations. If verbal interactions are too intense, remain physically present without expecting verbal responses. Let clients know that you are there to help them but do not reinforce dependent behaviors. Recognize and support strengths and areas of competence without minimizing their pain and distress. Change is difficult and painful, and consumers need to be supported and motivated to stay in treatment.

Evaluation

Personality traits are almost always too ingrained for radical change through therapy. Because the problems associated with personality disorders have been with most clients for their entire lives, clients respond to intervention strategies very slowly. You must define small steps toward the achievement of therapeutic goals. You can assist them most by helping them see how their behavior affects their lives so that they can learn to modify patterns enough to develop a more adaptive lifestyle. Some clients are in enough pain that they wish to grow and change. Others do not see that they have any problems and choose not to be involved in the therapeutic process.

To complete the nursing process, you evaluate clients' responses to nursing interventions based on the outcomes you selected. You determine the appropriate intervals for measurement and document the condition of clients according to each individual's status. Johnson, Maas, and Moorhead (2000) is the resource for identifying measurement scales and specific indicators for each outcome.

Impulse Control

Clients identify situations that require thoughtful action and stop and think before acting impulsively. They plan alternative behaviors before particular situations arise. Clients exhibit no self-mutilative or suicidal behavior. They respond appropriately to clear rules and limit setting. Clients acknowledge responsibility for their own behavior.

Social Interaction Skills

Social skill deficits are identified and new skills are practiced within a group format. Clients are able to initiate

CLINICAL INTERACTIONS   A Client with Borderline Personality Disorder

Enid, age 34, is an inpatient with a diagnosis of borderline personality disorder. She has been in and out of relationships with many different men and does not stay in a job for more than a year. She has a history of self-mutilation and numerous suicide attempts. During the past year, she has been writing love letters to her psychiatrist. She has just demanded one-to-one contact with her nurse. In the interaction, you will see evidence of:

■ Attempted manipulation of the nurse
■ Self-mutilation as a way to decrease anxiety
■ Labile affect

ENID: First, my doctor doesn't see me until after he sees all his other patients. Then you're too busy doing group. I just don't have anyone to talk to.

NURSE: Enid, I do one group per day, and I'm available most of the other hours of my shift. You need to deal directly with me, but if necessary, there are other staff members available.

ENID: But you are the only nurse who understands me.

You are the only one I feel I can really open up to. I can't talk about my issues with anyone but you!

NURSE: Enid, what is making you so upset?

ENID: Do you promise not to tell anyone else if I tell you? You must promise me this! My doctor made me talk about the letters I've written him. They were beautiful. He sat there and read them to me . . . like he was reading the newspaper . . . totally devoid of the emotion they were written with. So I did this [pulls up sleeves to reveal multiple new longitudinal superficial lacerations]. Now you have to promise me not to tell anyone else!

NURSE: I can't promise that. I will need to inform the other members of your treatment team. Any time there is a significant event or change in a client's status, that information needs to be shared. But why don't we talk about it first.

ENID: You are just like all the others. You are going to betray me! How dare you!

NURSE: If I failed to share this information, that would be unfair to you.

conversations, express ideas and feelings appropriately, and avoid inappropriate topics.

Social Support

Clients and families utilize group therapy and self-help support groups in managing the impact of their personality disorder on others. They verbalize increased trust of others, a feeling of empathy for group members, and a heightened sense of connectedness. Clients behave more assertively and communicate more directly. They are able to effectively negotiate stressful interpersonal situations.

Fear Control

Clients verbalize lessening of physical tension. They experience a relatively stable mood state. Clients verbalize fears appropriately.

Anxiety Control

Clients demonstrating improved anxiety control, plan and implement effective coping strategies. They rehearse and use techniques such as slow, deep breathing, muscle relaxation, guided imagery, distraction techniques, and a quiet environment to manage their feelings of anxiety. Clients utilize journal writing as a self-monitoring technique.

Spiritual Well-Being

Clients with adequate spiritual well-being express a sense of hope and of meaning and purpose in life. They participate in spiritual experiences such as meditation, prayer, worship, song, and/or spiritual reading. Clients express feelings of serenity, and a connectedness with others.[*]

To build a care plan for a client with a personality disorder, go to the Companion Web site for this book.

[*]These selected outcome indicators are from Johnson, M., Maas, M., & Moorhead, S. (2000). *Nursing Outcomes Classification* (*NOC*) (2nd ed.). St. Louis, MO: Mosby.

CHAPTER REVIEW

COMMUNITY RESOURCES

Links to these Web sites can be accessed on the Companion Web site for this book.

The Center: Post-Traumatic Disorders
800-369-2273
www.psychinstitute.com

Emotional Intelligence
www.eqi.org

BOOKS FOR CLIENTS AND FAMILIES

Alberti, R., & Emmons, M. (1995). *Your perfect right: A guide to assertive living* (7th ed.). San Luis Obispo, CA: Impact.

McKay, M., Davis, M., & Fanning, P. (1997). *How to communicate: The ultimate guide to improving your personal and professional relationships.* New York: Fine.

Santoro, J., & Cohen, R. (1997). *The angry heart: Overcoming borderline and addictive disorders.* Oakland, CA: New Harbinger.

Sorensen, M. J. (1998). *Breaking the chain of low self-esteem.* Sherwood, OR: Wolf.

KEY CONCEPTS

Introduction

- Personality disorders are inflexible and maladaptive behavior patterns by which certain people cope with their feelings, the way they see themselves and others, how they respond to their surroundings, and how they find meaning in relationships.

- Usually, the personality problems are ego-syntonic and clients perceive their difficulties in dealing with other people to be external to them.

- There is a high degree of overlap among the personality disorders, and many people exhibit traits of several disorders. The most commonly diagnosed is borderline personality disorder.

Knowledge Base

- The common characteristics of Cluster A disorders are odd, eccentric behavior and social isolation.

- Paranoid personality disorder refers to clients who are suspicious, secretive, and pathologically jealous.

- Schizoid personality disorder refers to clients who have a restricted range of emotions, are loners, and are not influenced by praise or criticism.

- Schizotypal personality disorder may be related to chronic schizophrenia. People with this disorder have an odd style of speech and their affect is often inappropriate. They may be suspicious and experience ideas of reference and magical thinking.

- The common characteristics of Cluster B disorders are dramatic, emotional, or erratic behavior, and behavior that exploits others.

- Antisocial personality disorder (ASPD) refers to clients who consistently violate the rights of others as well as the values of society. They are unable to experience guilt for their inappropriate behavior. They are more often found in prisons than in hospitals.

- Borderline personality disorder (BPD) sufferers often have other mental disorders such as mood disorders, eating disorders, and substance abuse. Symptoms vary in any given person at any given time. Their behavior is impulsive and manipulative, and they are at high risk for suicide and self-mutilation. Their moods are intense and unstable.

- Histrionic personality disorder (HPD) refers to clients who are overly dramatic and self-centered, and who need people to admire them constantly.

- Narcissistic personality disorder (NPD) refers to clients

who strive for power and success, mask their feelings with aloofness, and are extremely grandiose. They exploit others to achieve personal goals.

■ The common characteristics of Cluster C personality disorders are anxiety, fear, and overtly compliant behavior.

■ Avoidant personality disorder (APD) refers to clients who are shy, introverted, lacking in self-confidence, and extremely sensitive to rejection.

■ Dependent personality disorder (DPD) refers to clients who are unable to do things by themselves, fear abandonment, and force others into making their decisions.

■ Obsessive–compulsive personality disorder (OCPD) refers to clients who have a high need for routines, are unable to express feelings, fear making mistakes and therefore have difficulty making decisions, and attempt to control all interpersonal relationships.

■ Depressive personality disorder and passive–aggressive personality disorder are coded under personality disorder not otherwise specified.

■ Forms of passive–aggressive behavior include procrastination, forgetfulness, intentional inefficiency, chronic lateness, and no carryover of learning.

■ Since personality, and therefore personality disorder, is relatively stable over time, they begin at a young age and continue on throughout life.

■ Concomitant disorders include substance abuse, chronic anxiety, panic attacks, depression, and suicide.

■ There is no single cause of personality disorders. They likely arise from an interaction between biological factors and the environment. Neurobiological factors include limbic system dysregulation, low levels of 5-HT, high levels of NE, and abnormal levels of DA.

■ Intrapersonal factors include projection of hostility, perfectionistic standards, underdeveloped superego, and fear of abandonment.

■ Social oppression and changing value systems may contribute to the development of personality disorders.

■ Family factors include an inability to manage conflict, lack of individuation from the parents, and a chaotic and abusive environment.

■ Feminist theorists consider rigid sex-role stereotyping to be a factor in personality disorders.

■ Medications used for clients with personality disorders include SSRIs and antipsychotic agents.

The Nursing Process

Assessment

■ Clients typically do not see that a problem exists within themselves. It is often helpful to interview family and friends, if possible.

■ You must maintain a sensitivity in the interview process so that the client does not become guarded or defensive.

Diagnosis

■ Based on the typical characteristics, nursing diagnoses can be made for each cluster and individualized for each client.

Outcome Identification and Goals

■ Outcomes include fear control, social support, spiritual well-being, impulse control, social interaction skills, and anxiety control.

■ Goals include a decrease in self-destructive behavior, verbalization of less anxiety, utilization of the problem-solving process, and the development of healthy peer relationships.

Nursing Interventions

■ You should approach people with Cluster A disorders in a gentle, interested, and nonintrusive manner that is respectful of the client's need for distance and privacy.

■ Clients with Cluster B disorders require much more patience and structure on your part. The milieu must be consistent to avoid manipulation and power struggles.

■ In clients with Cluster C disorders, it is helpful to point out their avoidance behaviors and secondary gains. Problem solving and assertiveness training help them become more independent.

■ The three fundamental beliefs guiding nursing practice are self-determination, role functioning, and maintaining hope.

■ The first priority of care is safety from suicide and self-mutilation. Clients must be protected until they can protect themselves. Antiharm contracts may help maintain safety.

■ The problem-solving process is used to determine positive coping alternatives in response to thoughts of self-harm.

■ Manipulative clients need a highly structured approach. Nurses may need frequent staff reports and supervision to counteract the client's ability to play one staff member against the other.

■ Helpless and dependent clients need interventions to increase their coping skills and develop a more independent style of functioning. Problem solving, social skills training, and assertiveness training are effective interventions.

■ Group therapy helps clients focus on interpersonal issues as they get feedback from more than one person and have the opportunity to be therapeutic with other group members.

- Clients need to learn how to make their own decisions to reinforce an internal locus of control. Using the problem-solving process helps them see the variety of choices that can be made, tested, and evaluated.

- Promote clients' realistic self-appraisal through discussion of abilities and limitations.

- Help clients acknowledge that an anxiety-free life is impossible, which may help them give up striving for perfection.

- Avoid power struggles and help clients' accept responsibility for their own behavior.

- Discuss how fear of rejection may interfere with seeking help from others when appropriate.

- Provide enough distance and privacy to prevent escalation of anxiety.

Evaluation

- In evaluating the care of clients with personality disorders, it is important to remember that these disorders are often lifelong and are not likely to yield readily to intervention strategies.

EXPLORE *MediaLink*

- Interactive resources, including animations, for this chapter can be found on the Companion Web site at *http://www.prenhall.com/fontaine*. Click on Chapter 16 and select the activities for this chapter.

- For NCLEX review questions and an audio glossary, access the accompanying CD-ROM in this book.

REFERENCES

American Psychiatric Association (2000). *Diagnostic and Statistical Manual of Mental Disorders* (4th ed., Text Revision). Washington, DC: Author.

Bartholomew, K., Kwong, M. J., & Hart, S. D. (2001). Attachment. In W. J. Livesley (Ed.), *Handbook of personality disorders* (pp. 196–230). New York: Guilford Press.

Becker, D. F., Grilo, C. M., Edell, W. S., & McGlashan, T. H. (2000). Comorbidity of borderline personality disorder with other personality disorders in hospitalized adolescents and adults. *American Journal of Psychiatry, 157*(12), 2011–2016.

Bender, D. S., Dolan, R. T., Skodol, A. E., Sanislow, C. A., Dyck, I. R., McGlashan, T. H., et al. (2001). Treatment utilization by patients with personality disorders. *American Journal of Psychiatry, 158*(2), 295–302.

Brown, A., & Dodson, K. (1999). Borderline personality disorder. *NARSAD Research Newsletter, 11*(3), 18–21.

Cadenhead, K. S., Swerdlow, N. R., Shafer, K. M., Diaz, M., & Braff, D. L. (2000). Modulation of the startle response and startle

laterality in relatives of schizophrenic patients and in subjects with schizotypal personality disorder. *American Journal of Psychiatry, 157*(10), 1660–1668.

Coccaro, E. F. (2001). Biological and treatment correlates. In W. J. Livesley (Ed.), *Handbook of personality disorders* (pp. 124–135). New York: Guilford Press.

Dolan-Sewell, R. T., Krueger, R. F., & Shea, M. T. (2001). Co-occurrence with syndrome disorders. In W. J. Livesley (Ed.), *Handbook of personality disorders* (pp. 84–104). New York: Guilford Press.

Gunderson, J. G., & Gabbard, G. O. (2000). Foreword. In J. G. Gunderson & G. O. Gabbard (Eds.), *Psychotherapy for personality disorders* (pp. xv–xvii). Washington, DC: American Psychiatric Press.

Herpertz, S. C., Kunert, H. J., Schwenger, U. B., Eng, M., & Sass, H. (1999). Affective responsiveness in borderline personality disorder. *American Journal of Psychiatry, 156*(10), 1550–1556.

Jang, K. L., & Vernon, P. A. (2001). Genetics. In W. J. Livesley (Ed.), *Handbook of personal-*

ity disorders (pp. 177–195). New York: Guilford Press.

Johnson, M., Maas, M., & Moorhead, S. (2000). *Nursing outcomes classification (NOC)* (2nd ed.). St. Louis, MO: Mosby.

Kaylor, L. (1999). Antisocial personality disorder: Diagnostic, ethical and treatment issues. *Issues in Mental Health Nursing, 20,* 247–258.

Kennedy, G. J. (2000). *Geriatric mental health care.* New York: Guilford Press.

Krakowski, M. (2000). Impulse control: Integrative aspects. In M. L. Crowner (Ed.), *Understanding and treating violent psychiatric patients* (pp. 147–165). Washington, DC: American Psychiatric Press.

Livesley, W. J. (2001). Conceptual and taxonomic issues. In W. J. Livesley (Ed.), *Handbook of personality disorders* (pp. 3–38). New York: Guilford Press.

Leyton, M., Okazawa, H., Diksic, M., Paris, J., Rosa, P., Mzengeza, S., et al. (2001). Brain regional methyl-l-tryptophan trapping in impulsive subjects with borderline personality disorder. *American Journal of Psychiatry, 158*(5), 775–782.

Nehls, N. (2000). Recovering: A process of empowerment. *Advanced Nursing Science, 22*(4), 62–70.

Nehls, N. (1999). Borderline personality disorder: The voice of patients. *Research in Nursing & Health, 22*(4), 285–293.

Paris, J. (2001). Psychosocial adversity. In W. J. Livesley (Ed.), *Handbook of personality disorders* (pp. 231–241). New York: Guilford Press.

Paris, J. (1999). *Nature and nurture in psychiatry.* Washington, DC: American Psychiatric Press.

Perry, J. C., Banon, E., & Ianni, F. (1999). Effectiveness of psychotherapy for personality disorders. *American Journal of Psychiatry, 156*(9), 1312–1321.

Ratey, J. J. (2001). *A user's guide to the brain.* New York: Pantheon Books.

Sanislow, C. A., Grilo, C. M., & McGlashan, T. H. (2000). Factor analysis of the DSM-III-R borderline personality disorder criteria in psychiatric inpatients. *American Journal of Psychiatry, 157*(10), 1629–1633.

Skodol, A. E., Oldham, J. M., & Gallaher, P. E. (1999). Axis II comorbidity of substance use disorders among patients referred for treatment of personality disorders. *American Journal of Psychiatry, 156*(5), 733–738.

Soloff, P. H., Lynch, K. G., Kelly, T. M., Malone, K. M., & Mann, J. J. (2000). Characteristics of suicide attempts of patients with major depressive episode and borderline personality disorder. *American Journal of Psychiatry, 157*(4), 601–608.

Stone, M. H. (2000). Gradations of antisociality and responsivity to psychosocial therapies. In J. G. Gunderson & G. O. Gabbard (Eds.), *Psychotherapy for personality disorders* (pp. 95–130). Washington, DC: American Psychiatric Press.

Voglmaier, M. M., Seidman, L. J., Niznikiewicz, M. A., Dickey, C. C., Shenton, M. E., & McCarley, R. W. (2000). Verbal and nonverbal neuropsychological test performance in subjects with schizotypal personality disorder. *American Journal of Psychiatry, 157*(5), 787–793.

Wilkinson-Ryan, T., & Westen, D. (2000). Identity disturbance in borderline personality disorder. *American Journal of Psychiatry, 157*(4), 528–541.

CHAPTER 17

Spectrum Disorders

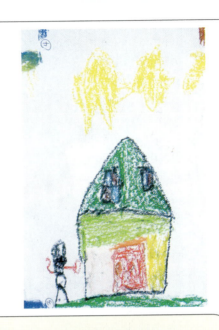

OBJECTIVES

After reading this chapter, you will be able to:

- EXPLAIN genetic loading in relation to the spectrum disorders.

- COMPARE and contrast individuals with one or more of the spectrum disorders.

- EXPLAIN the neurobiologic alterations in the spectrum disorders.

- ANALYZE the sociocultural factors that contribute to or result from the spectrum disorders.

- APPLY the nursing process to clients who have spectrum disorders.

*A*way From My Family

—George, Age 8

Removed from home due to disruptive and assaultive behaviors toward family

MediaLink

CD-ROM
- *Audio Glossary*
- *NCLEX Review*

Companion Web site www.prenhall.com/fontaine
- *Critical Thinking*
- *More NCLEX Review*
- *Case Study*
- *Care Map Activity*
- *Links to Resources*

Spectrum disorders are mental disorders linked by overlapping signs and symptoms and genetic similarities. Although the *Diagnostic and Statistical Manual of Mental Disorders* (4th ed., Text Revision) (DSM-IV-TR) encourages health care professionals to limit their diagnoses to one, most clinicians recognize that people with spectrum disorders often have two or three of these problems concurrently. This chapter looks beyond the limitations of categories to the commonalities of the disorders presented here.

Spectrum disorders include attention deficit/hyperactivity disorder, oppositional defiant disorder, conduct disorder, Tourette's disorder, bipolar disorder, Asperger's disorder, pervasive developmental disorder not otherwise specified, and autistic disorder (see the

DSM-IV-TR Classifications feature). Children who develop these disorders experience severe disruption in their social and emotional lives. Inattention, hyperactivity, and impulsivity characterize **attention deficit/ hyperactivity disorder (ADHD)**. **Oppositional defiant disorder (ODD)** is a recurrent pattern of disobedient and hostile behavior toward authority figures. More severe in symptoms is **conduct disorder (CD)**, which is characterized by a persistent pattern of aggres-

DSM-IV-TR CLASSIFICATIONS

Attention Deficit and Disruptive Behavior Disorders

Attention Deficit/Hyperactivity Disorder
Combined Type
Predominantly Inattentive Type
Predominantly Hyperactive–Impulsive Type

Conduct Disorder
Childhood-Onset Type
Adolescent-Onset Type
Unspecified Onset

Oppositional Defiant Disorder

Disruptive Behavior Disorder NOS

Tic Disorders

Tourette's Disorder
Chronic Motor or Vocal Tic Disorder
Transient Tic Disorder
Tic Disorder NOS

Mood Disorders

Bipolar Disorders

Pervasive Developmental Disorders

Autistic Disorder
Asperger's Disorder
Pervasive Developmental Disorder NOS

SOURCE: Reprinted with permission from the *Diagnostic and Statistical Manual of Mental Disorders*, Fourth Edition, Text Revision. Copyright 2000 American Psychiatric Association.

sive and destructive behavior with disregard for the rights of others and the norms of society. **Tourette's disorder (TD)** appears to be ADHD with chronic motor and vocal tics. **Bipolar disorder** is characterized by the occurrence of one or more manic episodes and one or more depressive episodes. **Asperger's disorder** involves severe impairment in social interactions as well as repetitive patterns of behavior and activities. Children with **pervasive developmental disorder (PDD) not otherwise specified (NOS)** have severe impairment in social interaction and very limited verbal communication. This is considered by many to be a milder form of autism. Social isolation, communication impairment, and strange repetitive behaviors characterize **autistic disorder**.

Spectrum disorders are polygenetic caused by the coming together from both parents of a number of genes affecting dopamine (DA), serotonin (5-HT), and norepinephrine (NE) transmission (see Figure 17.1 ■). As the genetic load increases, the symptoms increase from the milder one of ADHD through the most severe one seen in autism. In addition, the more genetic load-ing, the more co-morbid the disorders. For example, although ADHD is a distinct clinical condition, it is common for it to co-occur with one or more of the other disorders, creating a distinctive set of problems. In addition, the same child may experience different disorders over time. For example, at age 4, Sam is diagnosed with ADHD. At age 6, he develops tics and the diagnosis of Tourette's disorder is made. By 8 years of age, he is defiant of authorities (ODD), and by 10, he has become extremely destructive and disruptive (CD).

In the general population, 90 percent of people do not experience spectrum disorders. Of the remaining 10 percent, 7 to 9 percent have ADHD, 4 percent have oppositional defiant disorder, 3 percent have conduct disorder, 1 percent have Tourette's disorder, 1 percent have bipolar disorder, 0.5 percent have Asperger's disorder, 0.5 percent have pervasive developmental disorder, and 0.1 percent have autistic disorder (Paris, 1999). Nearly half of the children with ADHD also have many of the other spectrum disorders. In addition, ADHD-like symptoms are sometimes actually manifestations of childhood-onset bipolar disorder. As you can see, these disorders are so intertwined that it is often difficult to sort them out. Until more is known about these disorders, no diagnosis should be discounted because another disorder is present. Spectrum disorders are clear examples that health care providers need to treat the symptoms the individual is experiencing, not the diagnosis (Mannuzza, Klein, Bessler, Malloy, LaPadula, 1998; Oie & Rund, 1999; Spencer et al., 2001).

□ Genes common to two or more disorders

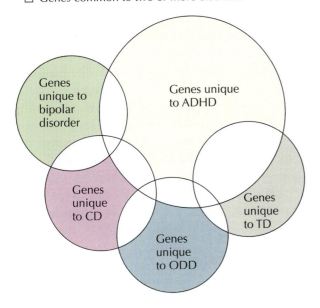

FIGURE 17.1 ■ Diagram illustrating the concept of spectrum disorders as polygenetic disorders sharing some, but not all, genes in common with co-morbid disorders.

SOURCE: Original concept by David E. Cummings, MD, 1998.

KNOWLEDGE BASE

No two children or adults present with spectrum disorders in the same way. Different individuals experience different family and cultural environments, different complications, and have different personalities and characteristics. The first section of the knowledge base considers behavioral, affective, cognitive, and social characteristics that are common to all the spectrum disorders. Following that, you will find those characteristics that are specific to each disorder.

BEHAVIORAL CHARACTERISTICS

Common to the spectrum disorders is **hyperactive behavior**. As early as the first few weeks of life, a child may demonstrate signs of hyperactivity. Infants sleep little, are active in the crib, and cry frequently. Sometimes, an infant manages to escape the confines of the crib to begin a journey of rapid, impulsive activity. Toddlers cannot sit still, and they leave a trail of destruction. The degree of activity may be comparable to that of peers, but the child with hyperactive behavior is unable to stop being active even when appropriate, as in not being able to sit down to eat. Older children frequently leave their classroom seats or constantly fidget in their chairs. They appear to be in constant motion with fingers or feet tapping, legs swinging, or wiggling in the chair. Adults may experience hyperactivity as a difficulty in relaxing or sitting still. They may often feel a restlessness and have a powerful urge to move around. Not all adults are hyperactive and this is the symptom that is least likely to persist in adulthood. There is a small group of individuals who experience **hypoactive behavior** in which they move much less than other children and may even seem lethargic. These children may be misdiagnosed with chronic fatigue syndrome.

People with spectrum disorders are often characterized by *impulsivity*. They do not stop to think before they speak or act. Most of us process our thoughts before we speak them. We may meet someone and think, "She's ugly," or "He's fat," but do not say those words out loud. Someone with a spectrum disorder will say their words even as they are thinking them and are sorry before they finish. They do not learn from these experiences because they cannot pause long enough to reflect before they act. Impulsive children have difficulty waiting their turn and often interrupt or intrude on others. In adults with spectrum disorders, impulsivity may lead to serious problems such as impulse buying, foolish business investments, or hasty marriages.

Obsessions (recurrent persistent ideas, thoughts, images, impulses) and **compulsions** (repetitive behavior performed in a stereotyped fashion) may be clinical manifestations of spectrum disorders. They may engage in compulsive checking, touching, counting, or lining up. Rituals may develop related to "evening things up" such as running around a circle three times in one direction and then three times in the opposite direction to "unwind." Routines must be followed exactly; objects must be returned to their "rightful" place or the child will become agitated. Some children may spend hours in *repetitive behavior* such as stacking blocks or examining and fondling objects. In the more severe disorders the child may have repetitive physical movements such as clapping, hand flapping, finger snapping, rocking, dipping, and swaying.

People with spectrum disorders tend to be *inflexible*. They have difficulty with transitions or changes and prefer sameness. They may even panic at the slightest change of a daily routine. Any request to change or to transition from one activity to another is perceived as a stressor and a threat. For example, if the parent asks the child to turn off the television and come to dinner, the response may be one of anger and the child quickly becomes oppositional and defiant. This oppositional behavior is defensive in nature and arises out of an attempt to maintain control when experiencing stress. Adults with spectrum disorders often become frustrated with changes in social plans. If the plan is to go to a specific movie that is then sold out, the response may be one of extreme frustration and anger.

AFFECTIVE CHARACTERISTICS

Affective symptoms of spectrum disorders include *labile mood*, that is, variations in mood characterized by rapid, wide swings of emotion and levels of arousal. Having multiple difficulties in school as well as family and friendship problems, these children feel inadequate and frustrated. Some may internalize their feelings, becoming withdrawn and depressed. Others may act out these feelings, becoming aggressive, getting into fights, or impulsively striking out. They may seem like Jekyll and Hyde moving from being pleasant and compliant to angry, argumentative, and controlling in a split second.

Individuals with spectrum disorders tend to be extraordinarily irritable and almost all experience periods of explosive *rage* over which they have no control. They have tantrums for hours at a time, often for no obvious reason. They may be aware or unaware of the effects of their temper on other family members.

COGNITIVE CHARACTERISTICS

Inattention is a hallmark of spectrum disorders. Inattention or distractibility is defined as the inability to regulate attention or concentration during the performance of a task. People with spectrum disorders may be easily distracted by sights (movements of people around them, clouds moving in the sky), sounds (conversations, traffic noises), or internal thoughts that intrude on the task at hand. Although most people have occasional problems with inattention, for these individuals the problem is so pervasive that it interferes with their day-to-day life and they often miss important information.

Maria issues an invitation to Jose by saying, "Come to dinner on Friday. It's a potluck and the party starts at 7." Jose shows up at 5 on Friday without a dish to share since all he heard Maria say is "dinner on Friday."

An extremely short attention span and distractibility are sometimes accompanied by *learning disabilities*. The ability to think abstractly, conceptualize, and generalize are disturbed, as is the ability to assimilate, retain, and recall. Even without learning disabilities, there can be no learning if the child is unable to pay attention. Compared to those without spectrum disorders, these children have more academic problems, underachieve at school, and a higher rate of being placed in special education (Valente, 2001).

A common frontal lobe problem is evidenced by difficulties with **executive function** in which affected individuals are unable to set goals or plan ahead. They are unable to anticipate what may happen and are unable to change plans when necessitated by the situation.

Before long, children with spectrum disorders begin to recognize that they cannot conform to the expectations of parents and teachers. Some children accept that these expectations are "correct," and their inability to achieve them results in loss of self-esteem, helplessness, and depression. This is more typical of girls and is less disruptive to society. Others, more frequently boys, decide that parents and teachers are "wrong" and develop a defiant attitude and may act out their frustrations in a hostile manner.

SOCIAL CHARACTERISTICS

Spectrum disorders cause *impaired social interactions*. The primary cause of this difficulty is impulse control problems. For example, when children cannot wait their turn, interrupt and intrude on others, say whatever comes into their minds, or explode in rage, their

social inappropriateness leads to peer rejection and social exclusion. The combination of intensity and inflexibility that these children bring to social interactions cannot help but produce conflict with parents, siblings, friends, and teachers. The rejection may lead to low self-esteem, which in turn leads to further acting out behavior. The lack of social experiences limits the possibilities for healthy interactions that might provide a sense of self-esteem (Cooper, 1999; Papolos & Papolos, 1999).

Social interactions are severely impaired in those individuals suffering with Asperger's disorder or autism. There is an inability to share activities or interest with other people as well as a lack of social or emotional reciprocity that is the basis of interpersonal relationships. Nonverbal behaviors, such as eye contact, and body postures and gestures that regulate interactions are impossible for these individuals. For those who are autistic, it is unlikely that they will be capable of adult intimate relationships (American Psychiatric Association [APA], 2000).

As the symptoms become more severe and obvious to people outside the family, others start *blaming the parents* for having no control over the child. Since parents never know when a violent rage will occur, they describe themselves as walking on eggshells. When a rage attack occurs in public, strangers often feel free to give "advice" on parenting skills. Parents end up feeling criticized, humiliated, incompetent, and extremely angry. Over time, the family may withdraw socially to avoid exposing themselves and their children to public attention and possible ridicule (Papolos & Papolos, 1999).

Spectrum disorders in childhood predict multiple problems in adulthood. These problems include occupational problems, lowered educational level, higher rate of divorce/separation, and less contact with supportive others (Faraone et al., 2000).

At age 38, Brian has been diagnosed with ADHD and is being treated with Ritalin. He recalls being given some medication for about a year sometime in his early years of elementary school. He describes himself as a very lonely child who was constantly being teased by other children. He couldn't concentrate at school or home and his father repeatedly told him how inadequate he was. He says the teachers just passed him along so they wouldn't have to teach him for a second year. Before being diagnosed and treated for ADHD, his fellow workers would make fun of him when he couldn't follow directions from the supervisor. They used to tell him he had a hamster for a brain and would try to provoke him into a physical fight.

PHYSIOLOGICAL CHARACTERISTICS

For those with bipolar disorder, there are increased manic or depressed episodes in response to seasonal variation as well as during periods of hormonal change that occur during the menstrual cycle in females. There is also difficulty in the thermoregulatory system as evidenced by persistently low body temperature and asynchronization of circadian rhythms of appetite, energy production, and activity (Papolos & Papolos, 1999).

Children with spectrum disorders have difficulties with the integration of sensory information. They may overreact to normal social cues such as misinterpreting a casual touch as a threatening gesture. In response, they can become hypervigilant and develop paranoid tendencies. The limbic system, or "emotional brain"—particularly the amygdala—dictates the response to the perceived threats in 100ths of a second, even before the stimulus reaches the cognitive centers of the brain. Dysfunction in the amygdala, in individuals with spectrum disorders, contributes to inappropriate fear, rage, and anxiety (Ratey, 2001).

The brain of people with autism seems to register sensory experiences too intensely sometimes and barely at all at other times. When overaroused by sensations (internal or external), the person reacts as if the stimulus is irritating or even threatening. Children with autism may shut down or try to get away from the stimuli by screaming, covering their ears, or running away. Often overly sensitive to sounds, tastes, smells, and sights, they may prefer soft clothing and certain foods, and may be bothered by sounds or sights no one else seems to hear or see. At other times, they may be completely oblivious to what is occurring in the environment (Papolos & Papolos, 1999; Ratey, 2001).

Sleep problems are very common for individuals with spectrum disorders. Those who have difficulty falling asleep describe the problem as not being able to "slow down and stop thinking." Others are restless sleepers who waken at the slightest noise and who are then unable to return to sleep. About one third of children with ADHD have nocturnal enuresis, or bedwetting, which is usually outgrown by the age of 10.

CULTURE-SPECIFIC CHARACTERISTICS

The prevalence of the spectrum disorders appears to be similar in countries where the population has been studied. The exception to this is the low prevalence of ADHD in Asian populations. The speculation is that there may be an association between ADHD and the 7-repeat allele of the dopamine 4-gene. This particular allele is low in Asian populations (Faraone et al., 1999).

It is estimated that approximately 9 to 19 percent of children in the United States have serious emotional and behavioral disturbances. Many of these children receive no treatment or receive treatment that is inappropriate or inadequate, especially minority youth. As with adults, children and adolescents should receive services in the least restrictive setting that is appropriate for their needs. In a study comparing placements for African American versus Euro-American youth, several differences were found. First, there were a disproportionate number of African American youth in the mental health system. Secondly, the Euro-American youth had more presenting substance abuse and emotional problems compared to the African American youth. Thirdly, African American youth were more likely to be placed in correctional facilities and foster care while Euro-American youth would more likely be hospitalized. It appears that race and ethnicity may be determinants of the type of placements provided to American youth. More information is needed about inequity in health care in order that uniform levels of care are achieved (Sheppard & Benjamin-Coleman, 2001).

CHARACTERISTICS SPECIFIC TO THE DISORDERS

Attention Deficit/Hyperactivity Disorder

Attention deficit/hyperactivity disorder is characterized by inattention, hyperactivity, and impulsivity. In spite of much publicity, there is no increase in the incidence of ADHD in the United States compared to 20 years ago. The 7 to 9 percent prevalence rate in the general population makes ADHD more common than cancer and many other disorders. In general, boys with ADHD out number girls with the disorder by a rate of about three to one. The earlier the onset the more likely ADHD will continue into adulthood.

There are actually three different types of ADHD, each with different symptoms: (a) predominantly inattentive, (b) predominantly hyperactive/impulsive, and (c) combined. The combined type is the most common type of ADHD. A diagnosis of ADHD is made when a person displays at least six symptoms from either list (see Table 17.1 ■), with some of the symptoms having started before age seven. For a valid diagnosis, symptoms of ADHD should be present in two or more settings (e.g., home and school/work) and the

---

TABLE 17.1

Symptoms of ADHD

Those with predominantly inattentive type often:

- Fail to pay close attention to details or make careless mistakes in schoolwork, work, or other activities
- Have difficulty sustaining attention to tasks or leisure activities
- Do not seem to listen when spoken to directly
- Do not follow through on instructions and fail to finish schoolwork, chores, or duties in the workplace
- Have difficulty organizing tasks and activities
- Avoid, dislike, or are reluctant to engage in tasks that require sustained mental effort
- Lose things necessary for tasks or activities
- Are easily distracted by extraneous stimuli
- Are forgetful in daily activities

Those with predominantly hyperactive–impulsive type often:

- Fidget with their hands or feet or squirm in their seat
- Leave their seat in situations in which remaining seated is expected
- Move excessively or feel restless during situations in which such behavior is inappropriate
- Have difficulty engaging in leisure activities quietly
- Are "on the go" or act as if "driven by a motor"
- Have accidental injuries
- Talk excessively
- Blurt out answers before questions have been completed
- Have difficulty awaiting their turn
- Interrupt or intrude on others
- Experience peer rejection

Those with the combined type:

- Have a combination of the inattentive and hyperactive–impulsive symptoms

SOURCE: American Psychiatric Association. (2000). *Diagnostic and statistical manual of mental disorders* (4th ed., Text Revision). Washington, DC: Author.

person's behavior must adversely affect social, academic, or occupational functioning (APA, 2000).

ADHD can be thought of as an addiction to the present. It appears that individuals with ADHD are unable to complete tasks that will provide a later reward. Immediate pleasure and gratification are their driving force. An interesting perspective on ADHD, which may be applied to some of the other spectrum disorders, suggests that persons with ADHD are hunters among farmers. This analogy serves to explain the "roaming" characteristics. The hunter thinks visually, is excited by the hunt, but becomes easily bored with mundane tasks. The hunter constantly monitors the environment and readily changes strategies at a moment's notice. Hunters are often very creative and people with higher levels of activity may have functioned better in hunter–gatherer societies. While spectrum disordered children appear disruptive in school, it must be noted that there is no biological advantage to sitting quietly in a classroom. While parents may be frustrated, it is helpful for them to remember the many "hunters" who have made positive changes in the world (Paris, 1999).

At one time, ADHD was considered strictly a childhood condition, outgrown in adolescence and of little consequence for adults. Research indicates, however, that the disorder persists into adulthood in 30 to 70 percent of affected individuals, often with serious consequences. ADHD is a known risk factor among adults for antisocial behavior, substance abuse, academic underachievement, and low occupational success. In adults, inattention is more persistent than hyperactivity or impulsivity. Physical hyperactivity often changes to verbal hyperactivity in adults (Biederman, Mick, & Faraone, 2000; Murphy & Schachar, 2000; Wilens et al., 2001).

Oppositional Defiant Disorder

Oppositional defiant disorder (ODD) is a recurrent pattern of disobedient and hostile behavior toward authority figures. Children with ODD are frequently disruptive, argumentative, hostile, irritable, and commonly annoy people. They often deliberately defy adult rules but tend to blame others for their own mistakes and difficulties. Such disruptive behavior occurs at a more frequent rate, at greater intensity, and for longer periods of time than the usual behavioral problems of peers. Disturbances in behavior lead to social

problems with peers and adults, and impaired academic functioning. For the majority of these individuals, the problem behaviors end in adolescence.

Christopher's mother describes him as a very tenacious child who seems like a "pit bull who gets hold of my neck and doesn't let go until I give in to him." One day when they were visiting his grandmother, Christopher persistently begged for an ice cream cone. In an effort to make the visit more pleasant, his mother gave in to his demands and made him an ice cream cone. After about two licks, Christopher threw the cone in the garbage and walked away with a sense of having "won a battle."

Conduct Disorder

Conduct disorder (CD) is one of the more common diagnoses given to adolescents and is characterized by a persistent pattern of aggressive and destructive behavior with disregard for the rights of others and the norms of society. One third of these teens go on to develop antisocial personality disorder especially those with early onset and severe and wide-ranging symptoms. (See Chapter 16 for a complete discussion of personality disorders.)

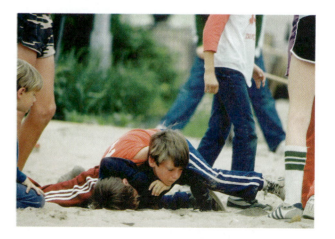

PHOTO 17.1 ■ Many fights among children are caused by their attributing hostile intent to others and then retaliating.

SOURCE: Pearson Education/PH College

There are two subtypes of conduct disorder: (a) childhood-onset type and (b) adolescent-onset type. Both subtypes can be further described as mild, moderate, or severe. Individuals with childhood-onset type are usually male, are frequently physically aggressive to others, and have disturbed peer relationships. Those with the adolescent-onset type are less likely to be physically aggressive and have better peer relationships (APA, 2000).

Children and adolescents with moderate and severe conduct disorder engage in significant and persistent antisocial behavior that violates the rights of others at home, in school, and in the community. Antisocial behavior may be solitary in nature, or it may occur in a peer group such as a gang. Physical aggression is common, and cruelty to other people and animals may occur. Youths with conduct disorder may destroy other people's property, set fires, steal, and rob.

Fifteen-year-old Ruben has been admitted to a residential setting for aggressive behavior. His mother was raped when she was 15, and Ruben is the result of the rape. His mother has been married and divorced twice. He has three younger siblings ages 11, 9, and 5 years. For the past several months, Ruben has been cutting school and getting into gang fights. He has been expelled for truancy and fighting. His mother was disciplining him by making Ruben go to work with her. He recently told his mother that if she continued to make him go to work, he would kill her. His younger siblings are afraid of him and his friends. He becomes very angry with anyone who doesn't agree with his views. He states that he is in the residential placement only because his mother is "crazy and a bitch." When asked about future expectations, he states, "to hang with friends and not go back to school."

Anger resulting from self-hatred, depression, and helplessness is directed outward. These youths lack guilt or remorse over their deviant behavior. Maladjustment to school, truancy, and dropping out of school are common. The unacceptable behavior and lack of social controls bring about social alienation, unless they are part of a similar group of teens. Rela-

tionships with peers and adults are manipulative and used for personal advantage (Pajer, 1998).

Tourette's Disorder

Tourette's disorder appears to be ADHD with chronic motor and vocal tics. Tourette's disorder usually starts between 5 and 9 years of age. It can, however, begin as early as 1 and as late as the teens. This is a disorder of the brain characterized by sudden, rapid, recurrent **motor tics** (involuntary movements) and **vocal tics** (involuntary vocalizations). These tics are further subdivided into simple and complex (see Table 17.2 ■). Motor tics include eye blinking, facial grimacing, head jerking, neck movements, shoulder shrugging, and hand movements. Common vocal tics include throat clearing, grunting, coughing, sniffing, yelling, or screaming. A much smaller group of children exhibit *coprolalia*—the involuntary use of obscene words. Many people consider Tourette's disorder to be ADHD with tics (Kiessling, 2001; Papolos & Papolos, 1999).

When Jaycee was 6 years old he developed a motor tic of rapid and recurrent eye blinking. At age 9, he developed a vocal tic of sniffing and was also diagnosed with moderate ADHD. By age 12, Jaycee had frequent periods of eye blinking, side-to-side head turning, foot stamping, and repeatedly inserting his fingers into his mouth. He was able to voluntarily suppress these tics only for short periods of time. His tics increased in severity during periods of stress, anxiety, and fatigue.

An estimated 100,000 people in the United States have Tourette's disorder and as many as one in 200 have partial symptoms of the disorder. Tourette's disorder is more frequent among males. It is thought that the dysfunction occurs in the caudate nucleus, part of the basal ganglia, an area of the brain that helps control movement (Ward, 2001).

Bipolar Disorder

Almost half of children first diagnosed with depression go on to develop the bipolar form of a mood disorder. Bipolar disorder is characterized by both manic episodes and depressed episodes with intervals of normal mood. In contrast to the typical adult characteristics, children with bipolar disorder have more irritable

TABLE 17.2
Types of Tics

	Vocal Tics	Motor Tics
Simple	Throat clearing	Eye blinking
	Sniffing	Shoulder shrugs
	Grunting	Facial grimacing
	Coughing	Head jerking
Complex	Animal sounds	Smelling objects
	Repeating words	Hopping
	Coprolalia	Touching people
	Stuttering	Pulling on clothes

moods with explosive outbursts, and their cycles of mania and depression are far more rapid. The rapidity of the mood swings, occurring multiple times a day, is referred to as ultra-ultra rapid cycles. The vast majority also experience recurrent rageful and often violent temper tantrums, which may last as long as an hour (Papolos, 2001). (See Chapter 13 for information about bipolar disorders in adulthood.) Psychotic symptoms such as delusions and hallucinations can occur in both the manic and depressive phases of bipolar disorder. The content of these may reflect the current mood state.

When Rachel experiences a manic state she often talks about playing golf with Tiger Woods, winning over him, and being invited to play on the Olympic golf team. When she is clinically depressed, Rachel's believes that her parent's want to kill her to prevent her from becoming famous.

Bipolar disorder in children is an under-identified problem. It is estimated that one third of all the children in the United States who are being diagnosed with ADHD also meet the criteria for bipolar disorder. Hyperactivity and distractibility are symptoms for both mania and ADHD. The distinguishing feature is

elation and grandiosity, characteristic of the manic state (Geller et al., 2001).

Asperger's Disorder

Asperger's disorder involves severe impairment in social interactions as well as repetitive patterns of behavior and activities. People with Asperger's disorder exhibit a variety of characteristics and the disorder can range from mild to severe. By definition, those with Asperger's disorder have a normal IQ and many exhibit exceptional skill or talent in a specific area. They often become obsessively preoccupied with a particular subject, which may lead to a career at which they may be successful as adults. Some experience obsessions that are bizarre in nature. They are often viewed as eccentric or odd and easily become victims of teasing and bullying.

On the surface, language development seems normal and children with Asperger's disorder have extraordinarily rich vocabularies. They often, however, sound like "little professors" and have difficulty using language in a social context. Their attempts at conversation result in one-sided, long-winded lecturing (Volkmar, Klin, Schultz, Rubin, & Bronen, 2000).

By age 4, Westin was very interested in, and quite knowledgeable about, astronomy. He would pursue this interest at any opportunity.

In conversations with peers, he inevitably brought the conversation or play around to stars and planets. He was quickly seen as a rather eccentric child. By age 10, he had significant social problems. He did not always respond to other people's facial expressions or gestures. He actively avoided eye contact and seemed to look through people. When interacting with others he engaged in long monologues describing the history of the universe, in spite of repeated attempts by others to change the subject.

Asperger's disorder sufferers are not solitary or withdrawn but they put people off by abrupt and awkward approaches. They may have difficulty making eye contact and may actually turn away at the same moment as greeting another person. They have a great deal of difficulty reading nonverbal cues and body language and very often have difficulty determining proper body space. As a result they have significant impairment in social and occupational functioning.

Autistic Disorder

Autistic disorder, or autism, is the most severe form of pervasive developmental disorders, although it varies in severity from victim to victim. It is characterized by social isolation, communication impairment, and strange repetitive behaviors. In infancy, the symptoms of autism may be subtle and almost unnoticeable, but it is unusually clear by age 2 or 3 that something is wrong. The most striking feature of autistic disorder is profound social isolation. Children with autism dislike being touched or looking people in the eye, and they seem to take no pleasure in sharing experiences with others. They have little sense of human relations, or even their parents being their parents, and have difficulty experiencing affection and cannot anticipate the thoughts and actions of others.

Disturbances in motor behavior such as whirling, lunging, daring, rocking, and toe walking present a bizarre picture. Some behavior may be self-mutilative, such as head banging or hand biting. They may throw tantrums for no apparent reason. They often *perseverate*, that is, show an obsessive interest in a single toy, activity, or person. They insist on sameness and resist changes in routine.

Language development is almost always slow. What

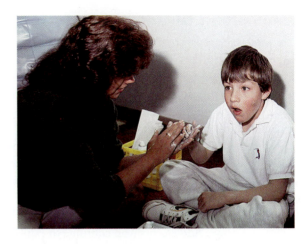

PHOTO 17.2 ■ Children with autistic disorder, like the child in this picture, are normal in physical appearance. The communication problems, autistic aloneness, and need to preserve sameness are readily apparent among children with autism, however.

SOURCE: George Goodwin.

first seems a "creative" choice of words turns out to be the beginning of abnormal language patterning. Communication with others is seriously impaired. Children with autism may be mute, may make unintelligible sounds, or may say words repeatedly. They may be unable to name objects and cannot use or understand abstract language.

About half of children with autism will be mentally disabled. Ten percent have unusual talents and are known as "savants." Savants possess unusual talents that appear at an early age—an exceptional rote memory, a capacity for lightening calculation, precocious musical gifts or drawing ability, or the ability to name the day of the week corresponding to any calendar date. Although they possess rare talents, they may or may not be mentally disabled in other respects. The movie *Rainman* is a dramatic example of autism, with Dustin Hoffman portraying a savant with unusual counting abilities (Brown & Weaver, 1998).

Follow-up studies of children with autism have found that only 5 to 10 percent become independent as adults, 25 percent progress but still require supervision, and the remainder continue to be severely impaired and in need of a high level of care (Brown & Weaver, 1998).

Concomitant Disorders

Depression is the most common concomitant condition of spectrum disorders. It is particularly frequent in adolescents and young adults, although it is sometimes overlooked. Depression is thought to arise from not feeling good enough, not feeling loved, and not feeling connected to others (Volkmar et al., 2000).

Studies show a high risk for *substance use disorders* for people with ADHD, oppositional deviant disorder, conduct disorder, and bipolar disorders. The potential for substance use disorders is high during adolescence, a time when individuals may begin to experiment with alcohol and drugs. Adolescents who continue to exhibit antisocial or delinquent behavior after age 15 are much more likely to develop substance problems. Researchers are currently asking the following questions: Is the association due to an attempt to self-medicate? Is the tendency to use substances something in the genes common to spectrum disorders and substance use disorders? Does substance abuse trigger the genes for spectrum disorders? Are substance use disorders another variation of spectrum disorders (Disney, Elkins, McGue, & Iacono, 1999; Papolos & Papolos, 1999)? See Chapter 15 for further information on substance use disorders.

There is co-morbidity associated with mental disorders and delinquent behavior in the adolescent population. Similar antecedents include family dysfunction, parental mental health problems, low academic achievement, relationships with other troubled peers, and chaotic neighborhoods. It is estimated that as many as 60 percent of youth incarcerated in juvenile correctional facilities suffer from emotional illnesses. The juvenile justice system is beginning to respond to this problem and make efforts to provide mental health care. It is not easy to provide services for adolescents whose behaviors involve both the mental health system and the juvenile justice system (Shelton, 2001).

CAUSATIVE THEORIES

The exact cause of the spectrum disorders remains unknown, but it is likely that they involve genetic factors, anatomical abnormalities, neurotransmission problems, and environmental factors.

Genetics

Spectrum disorders are polygenic disorders. The candidates for further study include dopamine D1, D2, and D4 receptor genes, dopamine transporter gene, monoamine oxidase gene, 5-HT genes, NE genes, gamma-aminobutyric acid (GABA) genes, and androgen receptor genes. Because spectrum disorders are the result of many genes acting together, each of these genes individually exerts only a small effect on the disorders.

Biological relatives of children with ADHD are at higher risk for the disorder. Twin studies demonstrate that there is a genetic factor in some cases of ADHD. In 50 to 80 percent of monozygotic twins, both twins have ADHD. Among dizygotic twins, both twins have the disorder 30 percent of the time. Adoption studies suggest that the transmission is biological (Faraone, Doyle, Mick, & Biederman, 2001).

In one study of monozygotic twins that were discordant (only one twin affected) for Tourette's disorder, the twin with the disorder consistently had a lower birth weight than the unaffected twin. In the monozygotic twins who both had Tourette's disorder, the twin with the lower birth weight had a more severe tic disorder than the other (Volkmar et al., 2000).

Monozygotic twin studies of people with bipolar disorder found a concordance rate of 76 percent. For those twins raised apart from each other, the concordance rate was 67 percent. Studies of Asperger's disorder show that there appears to be a significantly greater incidence of the disorder in first-degree relatives. Twin and family studies show that autism is strongly genetically determined (Constantino & Todd, 2000; Papolos & Papolos, 1999).

Making genetic associations to human behavior and temperament is the most complex area of study in molecular genetics. The attempt to solve this puzzle will require massive testing of the entire human genome.

Neurobiologic Factors

Abnormalities in people with spectrum disorders have been observed in different brain regions. Structural brain imaging studies have shown size abnormalities of the frontal lobes, basal ganglia, corpus callosum, and parietal lobes. Small frontal lobes have been found to correlate with inability to change or transition from one activity to another. Researchers have also discovered that in adults with autism, the brain as a whole is larger and they are trying to find out where the extra tissue is concentrated (Brown & Weaver, 1998; Rubia et al., 1999).

The results of functional imaging studies have demonstrated low brain activity in prefrontal cortex, the caudate nucleus, and parietal brain regions. It appears that in hyperactive adolescents there is a delayed development of the frontal lobes. This may explain why much of the physical hyperactivity lessens or disappears in adulthood. The response inhibition system of the brain is located in the right prefrontal lobe and its underactivation seems to be related to a lack of control. This means that people with spectrum disorders have greater problems than most in inhibiting or delaying a behavioral response. Prefrontal lobe dysfunction has been suggested as a potential biological deficit in antisocial behavior. The prefrontal area of the brain is responsible for motivation, mood regulation, and executive function. Abnormalities in this area contribute to impulsivity, short attention span, mood instability, difficulty planning or delaying gratification, and poor motivation; problems very common to the spectrum disorders (Pajer, 1998; Rubia et al., 1999).

Hyperactivity, impulsivity, and inattention suggest neurotransmission dysfunction. NE is related to a person's ability to sustain attention and mental effort. DA is responsible for physical movement, reward-motivated behaviors, and body temperature regulation. It is thought that people with ADHD actually have an increase in the DA transporter molecule, which reduces DA levels by taking the neurotransmitter back up into the transmitting cell. Abnormal variations may contribute to highs and lows in mood and physical and verbal hyperactivity. In some cases, it is thought that there are DA abnormalities in the frontal lobe and NE abnormalities in the parietal lobe—two sites for the process of attention. Others believe that the basic difficulty is related to the balance between DA and NE. Disturbances in 5-HT may contribute to problems in social relatedness and communication, ritualistic characteristics, and aggressive and impulsive behavior (Bragdon & Gamon, 2000; Ernst, 1999).

Acetylcholine (ACh) and its nicotinic receptors influence learning and memory and are involved in emotional regulation. Recent studies suggest that **nicotinic dysregulation** may play a role in spectrum disorders. People with many of the spectrum disorders have a greater risk and earlier age at onset, of cigarette smoking than other individuals. In addition, maternal smoking during pregnancy appears to increase the risk for ADHD in children. In one study, adults with ADHD treated with commercially available transdermal nicotine experienced a significant improvement in their symptoms and neuropsychological functioning. Nicotine appears to specifically improve attention and executive function problems and decrease aggression (Wilens et al., 1999).

Recent studies of autism suggest that some individuals may have an autoimmune basis for the disorder. Immune abnormalities include problems in the numbers of T cells, abnormal B- and T-cell function, and poor antibody production. Autoimmune findings have also been demonstrated in Tourette's disorder (Hollander, 1999).

Psychosocial Factors

The genetic and neurobiological factors do not exist in isolation but rather interact with psychosocial factors in people's social, cultural, and physical environments. For example, abnormal brain structure and function lead to cognitive deficits, which then lead to behavioral manifestations. The extent, and to some degree the nature, of the behaviors are influenced by social and psychological factors. These factors include people's experiences, which may or may not enable them to compensate for cognitive deficits or provide them with a low or high degree of motivation, which in turn affects their ability to cope. Even where biological factors are clearly implicated, it is the social and cultural environment that determines whether or not the observed behaviors are determined to be desirable or undesirable. If the judgment is one of deviancy, the judgment itself has an effect on the self-image and behavior of the individual. Because the biological and psychosocial factors are so intertwined, it is impossible to determine the extent of the impact of each (Cooper, 1999).

PSYCHOPHARMACOLOGICAL INTERVENTIONS

Spectrum disorders are neurobiologic, disabling conditions for which a number of medications may be used to normalize the neurobiology. Medication must not be seen as a magic cure and must always be used in conjunction with multidisciplinary interventions. However, the change induced by medication is frequently striking. The purpose of the treatment plan is to help people become productive members of the community. Attempting this without trying to correct

TABLE 17.3

Therapeutic Effects of CNS Stimulant Medications

Increase	*Decrease*
■ Attention	■ Aggression
■ Accuracy	■ Daydreaming
■ Concentration	■ Defiance
■ Learning	■ Distractability
■ Memory	■ Destructiveness
■ Coordination	■ Hyperactivity
■ On-task behavior	■ Mood swings

the problem with medications is like trying to teach reading to people with very poor vision and no glasses. A person with poor vision would not be told that if they just tried harder they could read the blackboard. Yet, that is often what is said to children with spectrum disorders, "Just try harder to sit still and pay attention."

Medication should be seen as providing a "window of opportunity" to allow other strategies to be more effective. There is clearly little point in attempting complex teaching strategies, behavioral management, or psychotherapy if children are excessively impulsive and unable to pay attention.

Stimulants are the most widely used drugs for treating ADHD (see Table 17.3 ■). The most commonly used stimulants are Ritalin, Methylin, Concerta (methylphenidate); Dexedrine (dextroamphetamine); Adderall (amphetamine and dextroamphetamine); and Cylert (pemoline). These drugs increase activity in parts of the brain that are underactive, improving attention and reducing impulsiveness, hyperactivity, and/or aggressive behavior. Provigil

TABLE 17.4

Medication Dosage for ADHD

Generic Name	Trade Name	Recommended Dosage
Methylphenidate	Ritalin, Methylin	5–30 mg every 4–6 hours; adults need higher doses
Dextroamphetamine, destroamphetamine, and amphetamine	Dexedrine Adderall	5–15 mg every 4–6 hours 5–30 mg every 4–6 hours
Pemoline	Cylert	Up to 112 mg once a day
Modafinil	Provigil	200–400 mg once a day
Atomoxetine*		1.2 mg/kg/day

*Not yet approved by the FDA.

BOX 17.1

Side Effects of Stimulant Medications

- Appetite suppression—most frequent side effect; often decreases over first few weeks.
- Abdominal pain/headaches—occasionally occur in first few days; rarely persist.
- Transient change in personality—some children become irritable, weepy, and agitated; more common with Dexedrine.
- Sleep problems—too high a dosage too late in day may make it difficult for child to fall asleep.
- Rebound effect—some children become worse as drug wears off; more frequent doses may be necessary.
- Itchy skin, rashes, mood change, or nausea can occasionally occur.
- Tolerance and dependence can occur with Dexedrine and Adderal.

SOURCE: Cooper, P. (1999). ADHD and effective learning: Principles and practical approaches. In P. Cooper & K. Bilton (Eds.), *ADHD: Research, practice, and opinion* (pp. 138–157). London: Whurr.

Side effects of the stimulant medications are short term and last only for the duration of each dose, about four hours. Adverse reactions are usually dose related, and there is no evidence at this time of harmful long-term effects of therapeutic use (Zwi, 2000). The most common side effects are found in Box 17.1, and client and family teaching information is found in Box 17.2.

Since people with spectrum disorders suffer from a variety of symptoms, a number of other medications may be used. The symptoms that are most bothersome in terms of social and academic functioning are treated first. Antidepressants are used for depressed or manic mood states; mood stabilizers are used for mood swings, tantrums, and rage; antipsychotic agents are used for rage episodes, oppositional defiant disorder, conduct disorder, and Tourette's disorder. The antihypertensive medication Catapres (clonidine) has been found to reduce motor tics in many of the people with Tourette's disorder, and may also be a treatment option for ADHD. Other drugs under study for Tourette's disorder include two antihypertensives—Inversine (mecamylamine) and Tenex (guanfacine)—and Botox (botulinum toxin). Initial studies have shown that the use of a nicotine patch may have a beneficial effect in relieving some of the symptoms of Tourette's disorder. Studies are just beginning on Provigil (modafinil) for ADHD (Cowdry, 2001; Ward, 2001).

(modafinil) is used for the hypoactive form of ADHD and for nacrolepsy.

Ritalin increases the synaptic concentration of dopamine by blocking more than 50 percent of the dopamine transporters. The time to reach peak action in the brain is 60 minutes. It is rapidly metabolized and out of the body in four hours. Thus, dosage may be as frequent as five times a day. The typical dose is 0.3 to 0.8 mg/kg/dose given two to three times a day. Dexedrine and Adderall increase the release of dopamine, thus increasing the concentration in the synapse. Dexedrine and Adderall may be too stimulating for the hyperactive person, but appropriate for the hypoactive form of ADHD. Provigil blocks dopamine reuptake in the basal ganglia and reticular activating system (RAS) (Volkow, 1998).

Dosage and timing adjustments are critical to effective management. This can often make the difference between successful and unsuccessful management (see Table 17.4 ■). Dosages should be titrated slowly in order to achieve the lowest satisfactory dose. The goal is to achieve a tolerable suppression of the symptoms. Spectrum disorders have ever-changing symptoms so medications must be adjusted, increased or decreased in a rational fashion.

BOX 17.2

Medication Teaching

Stimulant Medications
- No caffeine; increases feeling jittery
- No cough medicine with ephedrine; increases feeling jittery
- Do not take on a empty stomach
- No drug "holidays"; this is a life problem, not an academic problem

Dexedrine/Adderall
- Do not eat or drink citrus foods within 1 hour of taking; interferes with absorption

Ritalin
- Antihistamines nullify effect

MULTIDISCIPLINARY INTERVENTIONS

Effective management of spectrum disorders is collaborative, involving a combination of education, nursing, medical, and psychological strategies, where appropriate. Day-to-day interaction is very much in the hands of the educator. Spectrum disorders often go undiagnosed until the child is enrolled in a school setting. As children begin school, issues of emotional and behavioral health and learning disorders become much more important.

School nurses are responsible for meeting the health needs of emotionally and mentally disabled students. The single most frequently used medication in schools is Ritalin (methylphenidate). As part of the zero-tolerance policy, students are not allowed to carry prescribed medication. The school nurse, typically, is responsible for medication administration during school hours (Kronenfeld, 2000).

Because of the impaired abilities in communication and social relatedness in children with Asperger's disorder and Autistic disorder, more positive outcomes are shown in children who receive early intervention services. The *LEAP* (Learning Experiences . . . An Alternative Program for Preschoolers and Parents) intervention model focuses on children's social development. The theoretic basis of LEAP is social learning theory. Proponents believe that learning can take place through observation of others' behavior and its consequences. They recognize that children with developmental disorders need support and assistance in order to learn vicariously, through others. Typically developing peers serve as models in integrated preschool classrooms. The goal is to provide children with autism the opportunity to observe and imitate peer behavior in natural settings (Erba, 2000).

Floor time is a developmental approach to intervention with children who have severe difficulties in relating and communicating. This model is a child-directed play period with the parents functioning as the first and primary play partners. Parents are challenged to follow their children's lead while creating situations that address emotional needs. For example, if a child's problem-solving abilities are limited, the parent may set up several problems during the course of a session (e.g., a toy gets stuck in a hole or a part of a puzzle is missing). Through this playful process, it is hoped that children will be able to master developmental milestones (Erba, 2000).

TEACCH (Treatment and Education of Autistic and Related Communication Handicapped Children) provides a lifelong continuum of services for individuals and families. Services include assessment, diagnosis, treatment, utilization of community resources, and supported employment and living situations. The goal of TEACCH is for the adult with the disorder to fit as well as possible into the community (Erba, 2000).

ALTERNATIVE THERAPIES

Hyperactive children and children who avoid touch often benefit from positive physical contact with their parents. Touch is a primal need, as necessary for growth and development as food, clothing, and shelter. Touch can be thought of as a nutrient transmitted through the skin in many different ways: holding, cuddling, caressing, and massage. *Massage* is combined with *aromatherapy* when essential oils are used in the massage oil. Molecules of essential oils are so tiny they are quickly absorbed through the skin and enter the intercellular fluid and the circulatory system, bringing healing nutrients to the cells. Benefits are gained not only from the penetration of the oil through the skin but also from inhalation of the vapor and from direct massage of the skin and muscles. Soothing oils are chamomile, lavender, clary sage, and marjoram. They have significant calming effects and are also useful for children who are angry and aggressive. A whole body massage, a back massage, or a simple massage of the hands and feet may decrease anxiety and tension and

Complementary/Alternative Therapies

How to Help Clients Decrease Anger and Frustration

Massage provides a valuable tactile approach, which, when combined with verbal approaches, communicates nurses' care and compassion. Children and adolescents with poor impulse control, short attention, and low tolerance for frustration may accept and benefit from hand massage (see Figure 17.2 ■).

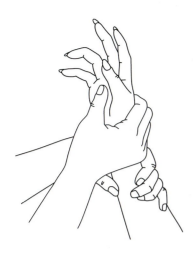

A

While holding the client's hand, place massage oil or lotion on the hand. Gently bend the hand backward and forward to limber the wrist. Grasp each finger and do range of motion exercises.

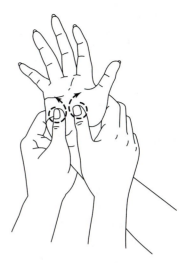

B

With the client's elbow resting on the table, hold the hand upright and massage the palm of the hand with the cushions of your thumbs, using circular movements in opposite directions.

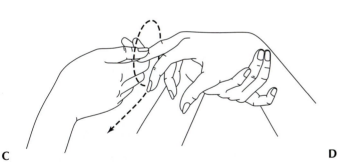

C

Massage each finger from the base to the tip, along all surfaces of the finger.

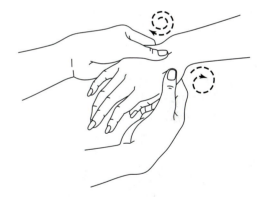

D

Use your thumbs to massage the wrist and top of the hand, using circular movements. Repeat three times. Repeat the entire procedure on the other hand.

FIGURE 17.2 ■ Procedure for hand massage.

SOURCE: Fontaine, K. L. (2000). *Healing practices: Alternative therapies for nursing.* Upper Saddle River, NJ: Prentice Hall.

increase the sense of well being. The two most suitable essential oils for babies and small children are chamomile and lavender (Fontaine, 2000).

Reflexology is able to stimulate the natural healing processes of the body. Some people find this very useful for hyperactive children. After a few sessions, children will often treat their own hands when upset. Too much work on the tip of the thumb or the great toe will overstimulate rather than calm down the child (Cooper, 1999).

Electroencephalographic *biofeedback* records information about brain wave activity from sensors placed on the scalp. The electrodes feed the information to a computer that registers the results on a visual monitor that produce a kind of video game of brain waves. When the person produces waves associated with concentration, the game speeds up. The game slows down when brainwaves associated with daydreaming are produced. This type of computer system is used for mind quieting and attention control in people with spectrum disorders; it also makes learning control of attention and concentration more interactive and fun, especially for children (Fontaine, 2000).

Melatonin has been used to treat insomnia in people with autism. It appears that the melatonin not only improved sleep but also decreased irritability and improved alertness and sociability. *SAMe* has had some success with mood changes secondary to the spectrum disorders. The amino acid *tyrosine* may help increase levels of dopamine (Amen, 2001; Brown & Gerberg, 2000).

Omega-3 fatty acids are critical for neural development and are important cognitive enhancers. In individuals with ADHD there may be a genetic dysfunction that interferes with people's ability to metabolize needed fats. Research shows abnormally low levels of omega-3 fatty acids in aggression and impulsivity. Omega-3 fatty acids can be found in salmon, tuna, trout, sardines, and anchovies. Flax is the best plant source of these acids. For people who dislike fish, fish oil capsules may be helpful (Brown & Gerberg, 2000).

NURSING PROCESS

Assessment

The type of nursing assessment you conduct will depend on the child or adolescent's growth and developmental level. Observations of behavior and interactions with others may be the most important tool you will use. Play and art therapy techniques are often used in the assessment process. Family members must also be assessed if your data are to be accurate. Teachers often provide valuable data for a total assessment picture. See the Focused Nursing Assessment feature for general guidelines. As a nurse, you always learn from your clients. Listen very carefully to what it is like to have one or several of the spectrum disorders.

Diagnosis

Based on the assessment data, you develop any number of nursing diagnoses for the individual child or adolescent as well as for the family. Some of the more common diagnoses are listed in the Nursing Diagnoses with NOC and NIC feature.

Outcome Identification and Goals

Based on the assessment data, you select outcomes appropriate to the nursing diagnoses. The most common outcomes are found in the Nursing Diagnoses with NOC and NIC feature.

Client goals are specific behavioral prescriptions which you, the client, and significant others have identified as realistic and attainable. The following are examples of goals that may be pertinent to clients with spectrum disorders:

- Acknowledge the effect of own behavior on social interactions.
- Improve social interaction skills such as cooperation, assertiveness, trustworthiness, and responsibility.
- Acknowledge personal strengths.
- Identify factors that precipitate violent behaviors.
- Practice behaviors that generate self-confidence.
- Identify alternative ways to cope with problems.
- Stay on task.

Nursing Interventions

Goals and outcome criteria help focus your nursing care. Children experiencing such a range of difficulties need help in many aspects of their lives. The overall goal is to help clients function more effectively in their social and emotional lives and achieve balance in their behavior. That means you provide nurturing, compassionate care balanced with a strong emphasis on self-discipline, personal accountability, and social responsibility. As a nurse, you are verbally and physically assertive and provide consistent, confident messages without demeaning the client (Greene, 1998). See the

Behavior Assessment	Affective Assessment	Cognitive Assessment	Social Assessment	Physiological Assessment
Do your friends comment that your behavior is in any way unusual?	Do your moods or feelings seem to change frequently?	How well do you think you are able to concentrate?	Has there been increasing conflict with your parents or siblings?	Do others comment that you seem clumsy?
Do you see your behavior as being different from that of others your age?	Are there certain seasons of the year when you feel better or worse?	How difficult is it to get your attention?	Who do you get into physical fights with?	Do you dislike other people touching you?
Are there exact routines that you follow on a daily basis?		Do others say they have trouble understanding you?	Are you having any problems with school? Attendance? Academic performance? Interactions with your friends?	Do you seem to be more sensitive to sights and smells than others?
Can you give me an example of ways you have gotten into trouble with your parents? Teachers? Other adults?		Who is responsible for the mistakes you make?		(Observe use of eye contact, bizarre movements, use of personal space)
Have you been in trouble with the police?				

Nursing Diagnoses with NOC and NIC feature for a list of nursing interventions.

Behavioral: Behavioral Therapy

Assertiveness Training

Individuals with spectrum disorders are often so aggressive and belligerent that they offend and alienate others. It is important to teach them the difference between passive, aggressive, and assertive behavior. *Passive behavior* is behavior in which people fail to express their needs and feelings and allow their rights to be violated by others. *Aggressive behavior* is inconsiderate of other's rights and feelings and destructive to interpersonal relationships. Aggressive behavior results in arguments and power struggles. *Assertive behavior* is asking for what one wants (respect for self) or acting to get it in a way that respects other people. Assertiveness is often associated with positive self-esteem. It is also an attitude that says, "Here I am, a person with unique gifts to give the world. Who are you? What do you bring?"

Assertiveness training is a program that teaches individuals ways to change negative self-concepts, reduce anxiety, identify strengths, and increase self-awareness. Assertiveness training typically includes discussion of ideas concerning assertiveness, practice of communication skills, making requests, refusing request, giving and receiving positive comments, and handling criticism. Assertiveness training programs teach people how to *manage their anger*. See Box 17.3 for teaching examples of assertive self-statements in dealing with anger.

Along with assertiveness training exercises, clients need to learn how to *resolve interpersonal conflict*. As a

NURSING DIAGNOSES with NOC & NIC

Clients with Spectrum Disorders

DIAGNOSIS	OUTCOMES	INTERVENTIONS
Impaired social interactions related to motor and vocal tics; difficulty using language in a social context; difficulty reading body language; impulsive behavior; inability to share pleasurable experiences with others; bizarre motor behaviors	*Social Interaction Skills:* An individual's use of effective interaction behaviors *Social Involvement:* Frequency of an individual's social interactions with persons, groups, or organizations *Loneliness:* The extent of emotional, social, or existential isolation response	Socialization Enhancement
Self-esteem disturbance related to low achievement in school; beliefs that others do not understand them; frequent criticism from others; inability to conform to the expectations of parents and teachers; rejection from peers and adults	*Self-Esteem:* Personal judgment of self-worth	Self-Esteem Enhancement
Altered thought processes related to poor concentration; inability to focus attention; difficulties with executive functions	*Concentration:* Ability to focus on a specific stimulus *Decision Making:* Ability to choose between two or more alternatives *Information Processing:* Ability to acquire, organize, and use information	Behavior Modification: Social Skills

nurse you discuss and model the processes of compromising, negotiating, and dealing with frustration. Teaching the *problem-solving* process will help clients generate alternative solutions to problems and teaches children how to resolve their own problems. See Chapter 2 for more detail in problem solving.

Behavioral Management/Overactivity

Clients who are hyperactive or in a manic episode may become exhausted when excessive levels of activity are combined with decreased awareness of fatigue. When intervening, you must first get the person's attention by calling his or her name or lightly touching the arm. If the environment (a person or situation) is overstimulating, you may need to redirect or remove the client to a *quieter area* to facilitate self-control. Clients experiencing hypomanic or manic episodes should avoid stimulating places such as school sporting events, dances, or shopping malls. Limiting intake of caffeinated food and fluids may also facilitate self-control. Clients should

DIAGNOSIS	OUTCOMES	INTERVENTIONS
High risk for violence, directed at others related to impulsivity, aggression; antisocial behavior; lack of guilt or remorse over deviant behavior	***Aggression Control:*** Self-restraint of assaultive, combative, or destructive behavior toward others ***Impulse Control:*** Self-restraint of compulsive or impulsive behaviors	Assertiveness Training Limit Setting Patient Contracting Anger Control Assistance
Altered family processes related to intensified parent–child conflict; parents feeling criticized, humiliated, and incompetent	***Caregiver–Patient Relationship:*** Positive interactions and connections between the caregiver and care recipient ***Caregiver Emotional Health:*** Feelings, attitudes, and emotions of a family care provider while caring for a family member or significant other over an extended period of time	Family Involvement
Impaired memory related to inattention, difficulties with executive function	***Memory:*** Ability to cognitively retrieve and report previously stored information	Memory Training

SOURCES: Johnson, M., Maas, M., & Moorhead, S. (2000). *Nursing outcomes classification (NOC)* (2nd ed.). St. Louis, MO: Mosby; McCloskey, J. C., & Bulechek, G. M. (1996). *Nursing interventions classification (NIC)* (2nd ed.). St. Louis, MO: Mosby; and North American Nursing Diagnoses Association (1999). *Nursing diagnoses definitions and classification 1999–2000.* Philadelphia: Author.

establish a routine that includes a balance of structured time (activities at school, homework, and physical exercises) and quiet times and post this in a visible place.

If you are helping clients who are hyperactive to follow a procedure, give instructions or *explanations in simple, concrete language* and ask them to repeat what they heard before beginning the task. Allow clients to carry out one instruction before being given another and provide positive feedback for the completion of each step (McCloskey & Bulechek, 1996).

Behavioral Modification: Social Skills

It is important to help children and adolescents with spectrum disorders to become socially integrated and not a disruptive influence in the family, in school, or with peers. These individuals have found, in the past, that any attention is better than no attention at all. Children sometimes learn that it is easier to get noticed by behaving in negative or foolish ways, than by being "good." The best thing you can do in these circumstances is to minimize the amount of attention given

Teaching: Self-Statements for Dealing with Anger

Preparing for Instigation

- This is going to upset me, but I know how to deal with it.
- I can work out a plan to handle this.
- I can manage the situation. I know how to regulate my anger.
- There won't be any need for an argument.
- Easy does it. Remember to keep your sense of perspective.

Impact and Confrontation

- Stay calm. Just continue to relax.
- As long as I keep my cool, I'm in control.
- I don't need to prove myself.
- I'm not going to let him get to me.
- There is no need to doubt myself. What he says doesn't matter.

Coping with Arousal

- My muscles are starting to feel tight. Time to relax and slow things down.
- I have a right to be annoyed, but let's keep the lid on.
- Time to take a deep breath.
- He would probably like me to get really angry. Well, I'm going to disappoint him.
- Let's try a cooperative approach. Maybe we are both right.

Reflecting on the Provocation: Conflict Unresolved

- Forget about the aggravation. Thinking about it only makes me upset.
- There are difficult situations, and they take time to straighten out.
- I'll get better at this with practice.
- Don't take it personally.
- Take a deep breath and think positive thoughts.

Reflecting on the Provocation: Conflict Resolved

- I handled that one pretty well. It worked!
- That wasn't as hard as I thought.
- It could have been a lot worse.
- I guess I've been getting upset for too long when it wasn't even necessary.
- I'm doing better at this all the time.

for negative behavior and to *maximize the amount of attention given for positive behavior*. Obviously, it is not always possible to ignore negative behavior. When necessary, deal with the behavior immediately, decisively, and as quietly as possible.

People who are impulsive may not stop to consider consequences before acting. They tend to become intrusive and interruptive and are totally unaware that their behavior is irritating to others. You will need to *teach* them *social skills*, that is, all the things we say and do when we interact with others. *Discuss likability factors* such as trustworthiness, responsibility, and a sense of humor. People who are trustworthy do what they say they will do. Responsible people acknowledge their contributions to situations in which they are involved. Healthful humor must be distinguished from harmful humor. Harmful humor ridicules other people by laughing *at* them. Healthful humor occurs when you laugh *with* others. An appropriate sense of humor can help people adapt in difficult situations.

You will need to teach clients social skills through discussion, modeling, and practice. They need to learn what the social rules of the group are. Most people will not tell others when a rule is violated because it is considered rude. Some people with spectrum disorders get lost in their own world. They need to learn how to socially connect with others. It is *social competence*, not academic success that determines our success as an adult. See Chapter 10 for detail on social skills training.

Limit Setting

All children, and particularly those with spectrum disorders, benefit from clear, predictable routine and structure. *Rules and expectations must be clearly stated*. Children and adolescents need frequent, immediate, and *consistent feedback* on behaviors. Establish reasonable and meaningful consequences for both compliant and noncompliant behavior.

During *time-outs*, clients can be sent for a short, specified period (3 to 10 minutes depending on the developmental level of the child) when they are behaving inappropriately. It should be a place where they will not receive stimulation or attention. You must clearly explain to the client why it is being done (the offense) and what it is intended to do (cool off). If the client remains out of control when the time period is up, the time-out is extended with a careful explanation.

Client Contracting

Behavioral contracts are another way of establishing expectations, discussing them with clients, and reinforcing them. An agreement is made between the client and nurse/parent/teacher that establishes clear behavioral expectations, states how these are to be achieved, and relates achievement to rewards. *Token economies* involve the giving of tokens, in the form of points, stickers, or other "currency," as rewards for positive, rule-compliant behavior. These tokens are then exchanged for a more concrete reward such as a privilege or a favorite activity.

Behavioral: Cognitive Therapy

Anger Control Assistance

Children and adolescents with spectrum disorders do not start the day planning on screaming obscenities at or threatening parents, teachers, or nurses. Instead, they get caught up in situations that seem beyond their control. It is helpful to *identify* in advance specific *situations* that may routinely lead to explosive episodes. That way, you may be able to deescalate clients before things reach the point of no return. Ask yourself: What is the source of frustration? What is the client capable of right now? What issues are essential to address right now? What situations should be avoided now? What situations can be adapted now? If the behavior escalates, try backing off and giving some emotional and physical space (Greene, 1998). See Chapter 9 for managing clients who are aggressive.

When the situation is calm, provide comfort and assurance. Show confidence in clients' abilities to adapt to change as it occurs. Explain that everyone experiences anger and discuss "real life" situations and how anger can be managed in a positive way.

Memory Training

There are a number of *coping techniques* that can be taught to people who are experiencing short-term memory problems. Post-it notes are great visual reminders and can be put on bathroom mirrors, staircases, notebooks, dashboards, or any other place that may catch people's attention. Some people keep tape recorders nearby to record assignments, appointments, due dates, and so on. A home answering machine can be used in a similar way. People can call home with a reminder of something and have their memory "tweaked" when they listen to their messages.

Behavioral: Communication Enhancement

Socialization Enhancement

People with spectrum disorders are often unable to read nonverbal communication. Because two thirds of communication is considered to be nonverbal, it is critical that they learn to observe, understand, and respond to nonverbal cues. They must also learn how to be a "self-observer," paying attention to what messages they are communicating nonverbally. (Review nonverbal communication in Chapter 2.) If their listening skills are inappropriate, they must be *taught the body language of active listening*. Use the mnemonic device, **OFFER**, as a way to help them remember:

O = open posture
F = face person
F = lean forward
E = make eye contact
R = relax

Teaching clients to *repeat what they have heard* can prevent many problems. If the teacher gives an assignment verbally, these individuals need to tell the teacher what was heard. Chances are, important information will be missed the first time around. It is also important to teach them not to blurt out whatever comes to mind. Unfiltered thoughts can indeed cause harm, even when harm is unintended. It is critical to relationships that clients learn to *stop and process silently* before speaking. Another social difficulty is that of speaking too much and conducting a one-sided conversation. Since they have little perception of how they monopolize conversations, they should ask friends and family members to let them know when they are talking too much. It may be helpful to buy a vibrating watch and set it for three minutes at the beginning of interactions. This is a silent reminder to stop talking and give the other person a chance.

Behavioral: Coping Assistance

Self-Esteem Enhancement

Self-esteem enhancement means that you support people's persistence, competence, and their overall ability to deal effectively with life's problems. Children with spectrum disorders need assistance to maintain a healthy self-esteem in the face of their difficulties. You further this assistance by giving them a sense of acceptance, belonging, and security. Acknowledge their talents and skills and *celebrate their achievements*, however small. Encourage hobbies and interests. *Teach clients positive self-talk*—"I can do this, I am a worthwhile person." Encourage self-reliance. Having responsibilities at home helps them feel needed and gives them a sense of purpose and achievement. Let them know that mistakes are okay. Mistakes are a minor set back and an opportunity for learning. At the end of the day have them ask the following questions:

■ What have I tried that was new today?

■ What have I done today better than before?

■ Who are the people I have helped today?

■ Who has helped me today?

■ What gave me the most pleasure today?

Be sure to praise any areas where clients make progress. As these children and teens develop better self-control, their self-esteem rises.

Family: Life Span Care
Family Involvement

The experience of having a spectrum disorder profoundly changes the life of the person with the disorder as well as those who care for her or him. Symptoms are often disruptive and social impairments can stress the family system. Parents of children with autism report more family problems, more marital problems, more depression, and more social isolation than do parents of typically developing children or parents of children who are mentally disabled. The more severe the child's symptoms, the greater the degree of parental stress.

Family members are an important resource to clients and professionals. You need to understand and empathize with the distress relatives experience when trying to cope with the disruption created by spectrum disorders (Dunn, Burbine, Bowers, & Tantleff-Dunn, 2001).

In order for family members to become active participants in clients' treatment, they must be taught about the disorder and be able to solve common problems. They need to be educated about psychotropic medications, helping them to recognize possible side effects and facilitate compliance with medication. Families also benefit from learning how to *communicate better* with one another. Good communication is necessary for supportive relationships. Helping families utilize the *problem-solving process* enables them to deal more effectively with the stress associated with having a family member with a spectrum disorder.

Parents who use a style of escape–avoidance to manage their children's problems are at higher risk for depression, isolation, and relationship problems. Examples of this style of coping include hoping for miracles, fantasy solutions, distancing or avoiding others, and food or drugs. Discourage the use of escape–avoidance patterns. Encourage them to spend time with supportive peers. Help them face reality through the problem-solving process. It may be appropriate to refer parents to couple or *family therapy* (Dunn, Burbine, Bowers, & Tantleff-Dunn, 2001).

Physiological: Basic: Activity and Exercise Management
Exercise Promotion

All children and adolescents behave and pay attention better under circumstances in which their needs for physical activity are met. Encourage them to plan a daily schedule for *physical activities*. They may find that keeping an exercise diary or log will help them maintain an exercise program. Finding a friend with whom to exercise is another way to stay on task with the program.

If you are in a group setting, you may schedule stretching exercises as well as competitive games such as volleyball, basketball, or soccer. Not only do clients get the benefit of exercise, they also learn how to function as team members and how to play by the rules.

Physiological: Basic: Immobility Management
Physical Restraint

Some children in a rage can do great damage to a home or hospital unit. A therapeutic hold can help them gain control and calm down. To prevent injury to the child or yourself, you should not attempt a therapeutic hold without additional specific training. In a therapeutic hold, you get behind the child and slide your back down the wall, taking the child with you. You then put your legs over the child's, wrap the child's hands around the child's middle, and hold your arms over the child's hands. All the time you should be saying in a calm, soft voice: "I will not let you hurt yourself or me or destroy things. I will hold you until your rage is over. I will hold you until we are all safe."

Evaluation

To complete the nursing process, you evaluate clients' responses to nursing interventions based on the out-

CRITICAL THINKING

The community mental health center conducts a clinic once a month for evaluation of children and adolescents who might be having problems at home or in school. You are observing an assessment of an adolescent. The adolescent, Steve, is 12 years old and was referred to the clinic by his school counselor. Steve has a long history of problems in school, such as hyperactivity with increasing inability to sit still in class and difficulty concentrating on content. Steve also interrupts during the class, which has become a more serious problem. His grades have been below average. Steve says he has been having problems sleeping, and his mother says that he has lost weight. His mother comments that he has always been very active, and it was difficult to care for him in the early years. Most recently, he was caught stealing some CDs from a local music store. Steve's explanation is he wanted to try to take the CDs so he did. His mother commented that it was surprising since he owned two of the CDs already. During the interview, Steve responds but does not seem to understand that he might be having serious problems.

After the assessment, you attend the team meeting in which Steve is discussed as well as other issues related to clients who have recently been evaluated by the clinic staff. The team consists of two nurses, a psychiatrist, a psychologist, an educational specialist, and a social worker.

1. One of the first things that you hear in the team meeting is the importance of treating the symptoms and not the diagnosis. Why would you support this statement?
2. Considering the data that are supplied, what other data might be disclosed in further assessment of Steve?
3. What interventions are most important for Steve at this time?
4. The clinic recommends that Steve be placed on Ritalin (methylphenidate). How would you know that this medication is effective?
5. Families are very important in the evaluation and treatment of children and adolescents with problems; however, family blame is a major concern and must be carefully considered. How would you best intervene with Steve's family and consider the issue of family blame?
6. How would you compare and contrast ADHD and conduct disorder?

For an additional Case Study, please refer to the Companion Web site for this book.

comes you selected. You determine the appropriate intervals for measurement and document the condition of clients according to each individual's status. Johnson, Maas, and Moorhead (2000) is the resource for identifying measurement scales and specific indicators for each outcome.

Social Interaction Skills

Clients with spectrum disorders develop social and emotional reciprocity that is the basis of interpersonal relationships. Their interactions with others are warm, genuine, and considerate. Clients interact in an assertive manner and utilize appropriate confrontation skills.

Social Involvement

Clients socialize with peers in nonaggressive ways. They identify the benefits of interpersonal relationships. Clients participate in support groups and verbalize a sense of belonging.

Loneliness

Clients express feelings of being understood by and included in activities with others. They establish contact with other people and express decreasing feelings of isolation.

Impulse Control

Clients identify situations that require thoughtful action and stop and think before acting impulsively. They plan alternative behaviors before particular situations arise. Clients respond appropriately to clear rules and limit setting. They acknowledge responsibility for their own behavior.

Communication Ability

Clients pay attention to what is being communicated to them. They acknowledge what they hear and understand and respond back appropriately. Clients do not interrupt and intrude on others. They repeat what they have heard others say and demonstrate the body language of active listening.

Self-Esteem

Clients verbalize previous achievements of success and identify their own strengths and abilities. They describe improved thoughts about their worth and abilities, utilizing positive self-talk. Clients refrain from acting out.

A Client with Bipolar Disorder and Oppositional Defiant Disorder

Seventeen-year-old Ben was brought to the hospital after his mom called the police and told them Ben was attacking her. Ben states that he often lives with his dad, which he much prefers. He verbalizes a lot of anger toward his mother. He says she didn't treat him well growing up. She was always yelling at him and punishing him instead of giving him the love he needed and wanted. In the interaction you see evidence of:

- Concrete thinking
- Dichotomous thinking
- Hyperactive behavior
- Hostility
- Flight of ideas
- Grandiose thinking

NURSE: Earlier in group it was suggested that everyone write two goals they want to achieve when they go home. Would you like to work on that for a while? [offers pencil and paper]

BEN: Yeah sure, that would be great. [tapping fingers, running fingers through hair] Well, I already know what my short-term goals are. You see, when I go home I want to be close to my father. Like tell him stuff and talk with him. [His writing is scratchy and unclear] I definitely want to be close to my dad. And I want to clean up the house. That helps me calm down. Oh yeah, I want to recycle. [laughs]

NURSE: Are you close to your dad now?

BEN: Oh yeah. I live with him. I'm 17 years old. I'm not close to my mother though. I hate her right now, like I hate her actual being. I mean I love her unconditionally, but I hate her right now. [Starts a very fast rap song about all of the negative things his mom did to him as a child. Ends with him singing angrily how he wished she could have taught him and shown him love instead of anger.]

NURSE: You seem angry about how your mom treated you when you were growing up.

BEN: Yeah, well that's the way it was. Heck, she cares more about the kids she babysits than me. And I do have another short-term goal. I want to get into the music business. You know get into the studio. [tapping fingers, running fingers through hair, looking around]

NURSE: What are some ways you could get information about getting into the studio?

BEN: Oh, I could look in the phone book. [writes that down] Hmm . . . my friend Andy has connections. I could call him up and hook up with him. [writes that down]

NURSE: Those seem like good ways of starting.

BEN: Man, you help me so much. [smiling]

NURSE: Make sure you keep that paper so you can refer back to it. That way, if you forget what your plan is, you will have everything written down.

BEN: [is distracted by other clients and starts laughing]

NURSE: In group, you mentioned you also wanted to go into the Navy eventually.

BEN: Yeah, maybe. I want to be a seaman. Or maybe go into the reserves. That's long term though, because you have to stay a while. And I don't want to stay in for two years.

NURSE: You would have to make that commitment if that is what you decide.

BEN: Yeah, I guess. [nonchalant]

NURSE: You said earlier that you also wanted to go to college.

BEN: You know what else I am going to do after that? A preacher. [nodding] I was told at a young age that I would be a preacher. You know that flea market near here? Well, there was a psychic there once when I was a little shorty who said that is what I would do and I believe her. I do. [starts a rap about putting fear of the holy ghost into people] Cuz I only have one life to live and I've got to keep going. Keep it going smooth. I used to drive an '84 Riviera. Then I sold it for $800. Then I bought an '86 Camaro yellow and black just like your name badge. Those are the colors of the gang I used to be in that I told you about.

NURSE: You have looked at your goals now. How do you feel about that?

BEN: I feel great. I can't wait to get out of here. [Starts another rap. This time it makes no sense and is not understandable.] Okay. I gotta go now. Thanks for talking to me.

Concentration

Clients are able to regulate their attention and concentration during the performance of tasks.

Decision Making

Clients set goals and plan ahead. They are able to change plans if the situation demands it. Clients verbalize an internal locus of control and a sense of empowerment.

Information Processing

Clients communicate logical thought processes to others. They think before speaking or acting impulsively. Their attention span increases.

Aggression Control

Clients refrain from violating others' personal space and refrain from harming others or destroying property. They identify feelings of anger, frustration, hostility, and aggression. They identify alternatives to aggression and maintain self-control without supervision. Clients communicate their needs appropriately and verbalize control of impulses.[*]

Caregiver–Patient Relationship

Clients and their families report less confrontation and oppositional behavior. They verbalize a mutual sense of attachment. Clients communicate effectively and solve problems to the best of their abilities.

Caregiver Emotional Health

Parents report decreased feelings of disappointment, guilt, and irritation. They participate in social activities with others and report a sense of connectedness with friends and family. They utilize community resources.

The Serenity Prayer, an important piece of 12-step self-help groups can also be utilized by people with spectrum disorders. It would look like this:

God, grant me the serenity to accept the things I cannot change *(do not deny the disorder, meet it head on)*

Courage to change the things I can *(social and communication skills, medications)*

And the wisdom to know the difference.

To build a Care Plan for a client with a spectrum disorder, go to the Companion Web site for this book.

---

[*]These selected outcome indicators are from Johnson, M., Maas, M., & Moorhead, S. (2000). *Nursing outcomes classification (NOC)* (2nd ed.). St. Louis, MO: Mosby.

CHAPTER REVIEW

Links to these Web sites can be accessed on the Companion Web site for this book.

ARCH National Resource Center for Crisis Nurseries and Respite Care Services
800-773-5433

Child and Adolescent Bipolar Foundation
1187 Willmette Ave., #Pmb 331
Willmette, IL 60091
847-256-8525
www.cabf.org

Children and Adolescent Service System Programs (CASSP)
202-687-5000

Children and Adults with Attention Deficit/Hyperactivity Disorder (CHADD)
8181 Professional Pl, Suite 201
Landover, MD 20785
800-233-4050
www.chadd.org

Family Voices
P.O. Box 769
Algodones, NM 87001
505-867-2368
www.familyvoices.org

National Alliance for Autism Research
414 Wall St.
Research Park
Princeton, NJ 08540
888-777-NAAR
www.naar.org

National Clearinghouse on Family Support and Children's Mental Health
800-628-1696

Tourette Syndrome Association
42-40 Bell Blvd.
Bayside, NY 11361-2820
800-237-0717
www.tsa.mgh.harvard.edu

United Kingdom
www.tourettesyndrome.co.uk

BOOKS FOR CLIENTS AND FAMILIES

Friends in Recovery. (1996). *The twelve steps—A key to living with attention deficit disorder.* San Diego: RPI.

Frith, U. (1991). *Autism and Asperger's syndrome.* Cambridge, MA: Cambridge University Press.

Jamison, K. R. (1995). *An unquiet mind: A memoir of moods and madness.* New York: Random House.

Richardson, W. (1997). *The link between ADD & addiction: Getting the help you deserve.* Colorado Springs, CO: Pinon Press.

Shimberg, E. F. (1995). *Living with Tourette syndrome.* New York: Fireside Books.

Waltz, M. (2000). *Bipolar disorders: A guide for helping children and adolescents.* Sebastopol, CA: O'Reilly and Associates, Inc.

KEY CONCEPTS

Introduction

- Spectrum disorders are neurobehavioral disorders linked by overlapping signs and symptoms, dual diagnoses, and that are genetically interrelated.

- Attention deficit/hyperactivity disorder is characterized by inattention, hyperactivity, and impulsivity.

- Oppositional defiant disorder is a recurrent pattern of disobedient and hostile behavior toward authority figures.

- Conduct disorder is characterized by a persistent pattern of aggressive and destructive behavior with disregard for the rights of others and the norms of society.

- Tourette's disorder appears to be ADHD with chronic motor and vocal tics.

- Bipolar disorder is characterized by the occurrence of one or more manic episodes and one or more depressive episodes.

- Asperger's disorder involves severe impairment in social interactions as well as repetitive patterns of behavior and activities.

- Children with pervasive developmental disorder not otherwise specified (NOS) have severe impairment in social interaction and very limited verbal communication.

- Social isolation, communication impairment, and strange repetitive behaviors characterize autistic disorder.

Knowledge Base

- People with spectrum disorders exhibit hyperactive and impulsive behavior.

- They tend to be inflexible and have difficult with transitions or changes.

- People with spectrum disorders experience marked variations in mood leading to multiple difficulties in school as well as family and friendship problems. They may have tantrums for hours at a time, often for no obvious reason.

- Inattention or distractibility is a hallmark of spectrum disorders.

- Difficulties with executive functions contribute to the inability to set goals, plan ahead, anticipate what may happen, and change plans when necessary.

- The brains of people with spectrum disorders seem to register sensory experiences too intensely sometimes and barely at all at other times.

- Concomitant disorders include depression and substance use disorders.

Causative Theories

- Structural and functional brain imaging studies have shown size abnormalities and abnormal brain activity of the frontal lobes, basal ganglia, corpus callosum, and parietal lobes.

- Abnormalities in the prefrontal areas responsible for motivation, mood regulation, and executive functions result in impulsivity, short attention span, mood instability, difficulty planning or delaying gratification, and poor motivation.

- Neurotransmission dysfunction includes NE, DA, 5-HT, and nicotine.

Psychopharmacological Interventions

- Medications provide a window of opportunity to allow other strategies to be more effective.

- The most commonly used medications are Ritalin, Methylin, Concerta, Dexedrine, Adderall, and Cylert.

Multidisciplinary Interventions

- Day-to-day interaction is very much in the hands of the educator who must collaborate with health care providers to determine appropriate strategies.

Alternative Therapies

- Soothing oils used in massage therapy include chamomile, lavender, clary sage, and marjoram. A whole body massage or a simple massage of the hands and feet may decrease anxiety and tension.

- Reflexology is helpful for some children who experience hyperactivity.

- Biofeedback has been successfully used to attention control.

The Nursing Process

Assessment

- The type of nursing assessment you conduct depends on the child or adolescent's growth and developmental level.

Diagnosis

- Nursing diagnoses include impaired social interactions, self-esteem disturbance, impaired physical mobility, altered thought processes, high risk for violence, impaired verbal communication, and altered family processes.

Outcome Identification and Goals

- The most common outcomes include social interaction skills, social involvement, loneliness, impulse control, communication ability, self-esteem, concentration, decision making, information processing, aggression control, caregiver–patient relationship, and caregiver emotional health.

Nursing Interventions

- Behavioral interventions include assertiveness training, social skills training, limit setting, and patient contracting.

- Cognitive interventions include anger control assistance, memory training, socialization enhancement, and self-esteem enhancement.

- Life span care encourages family involvement.

- Physiologic interventions include exercise promotion and physical restraint.

KEY CONCEPTS *(continued)*

Evaluation

■ To complete the nursing process, you evaluate clients' responses to nursing interventions based on the outcomes you selected.

EXPLORE *MediaLink*

■ Interactive resources, including animations, for this chapter can be found on the Companion Web site at *http://www.prenhall.com/fontaine.* Click on Chapter 17 and select the activities for this chapter.

■ For NCLEX review questions and an audio glossary, access the accompanying CD-ROM in this book.

REFERENCES

Amen, D. G. (2001). *Healing ADD.* New York: Putnam's Sons.

American Psychiatric Association. (2000). *Diagnostic and statistical manual of mental disorders* (4th ed., Text Revision). Washington, DC: Author.

Biederman, J., Mick, E., & Faraone S. V. (2000). Age-dependent decline of symptoms of attention deficit hyperactivity disorder. *American Journal of Psychiatry, 157*(5), 816–820.

Bragdon, A. D., & Gamon, D. (2000). *Brains that work a little bit differently.* Cape Cod, MA: The Brainwaves Center.

Brown, A., & Weaver R. (1998). How related are autism and childhood schizophrenia? *NARSAD Research Letter, 10*(3), 13–20.

Brown, R. P., & Gerbarg, P. L. (2000). Integrative psychopharmacology. In P. R. Muskin (Ed.), *Complementary and alternative medicine and psychiatry* (pp. 1–66). Washington, DC: American Psychiatric Press.

Constantino, J. N., & Todd, R. D. (2000). Genetic structure of reciprocal social behavior. *American Journal of Psychiatry, 157*(12), 2043–2045.

Cooper, P. (1999). ADHD and effective learning: Principles and practical approaches. In P. Cooper & K. Bilton (Eds.), *ADHD: Research, practice and opinion* (pp. 138–157). London: Whurr.

Cowdry, R. (2001). Preliminary studies offer promising results for alternative treatments for ADHD. *NAMI Advocate,* Spring, 19–20.

Disney E. R., Elkins, J. J., McGue, M., & Iacono, W. G. (1999). Effects of ADHD, conduct disorder and gender on substance use and abuse in adolescence. *American Journal of Psychiatry, 156*(10), 1515–1521.

Dunn, M. E., Burbine, R., Bowers, C. A., & Tantleff-Dunn, S. (2001). Moderators of stress in parents of children with autism. *Community Mental Health Journal, 37*(1), 39–52.

Erba, H. W. (2000). Early intervention programs for children with autism: Conceptual frameworks for implementation. *American Journal of Orthopsychiatry, 70*(1), 82–93.

Ernst, M., Zametkin, A. J., Matochik, J. A., Pascualvaca, D., & Jons, P. H. (1999). High midbrain DOPA accumulation in children with attention deficit hyperactivity disorder. *American Journal of Psychiatry, 156*(8), 1209–1215.

Faraone S. V., Biederman, J., Weiffenbach, B., Keith, T., Chu, M. P., Weaver, A., et al. (1999). Dopamine D4 gene 7-repeat allele and attention deficit hyperactivity disorder. *American Journal of Psychiatry, 156*(5), 768–770.

Faraone S. V., Biederman, J., Mick, E., Williamson, S., Wilens, T., Spencer, T., et al. (2000). Family study of girls with attention deficit hyperactivity disorder. *American Journal of Psychiatry, 157*(7), 1077–1082.

Faraone, S. V., Doyle, A. E., Mick, E., & Biederman, J. (2001). Meta-analysis of the association between the 7-repeat allele of

the dopamine D4 receptor gene and attention deficit hyperactivity disorder. *American Journal of Psychiatry, 158*(7), 1052–1057.

Fontaine, K. L. (2000). *Healing practices: Alternative therapies for nursing.* Upper Saddle River, NJ: Prentice Hall.

Geller, B., Craney, J. L., Bolhofner, K., DelBello, M. P., Williams, M., & Zimerman, B. (2001). One-year recovery and relapse rates of children with a prepubertal and early adolescent bipolar disorder phenotype. *American Journal of Psychiatry, 158*(2), 303–305.

Greene, R. W. (1998). *The explosive child.* New York: HarperCollins.

Hollander, E., DelGiudice-Asch, G., Simon, L., Schmeidler, J., Cartwright, C., DeCaria, C., et al. (1999). B lymphocyte antigen D8/17 and repetitive behaviors in autism. *American Journal of Psychiatry, 156*(2), 317–320.

Johnson, M., Maas, M., Moorhead, S. (Eds.), (2000). *Nursing outcomes classification (NOC)* (2nd ed.). St. Louis, MO: Mosby.

Kiessling, L. S. (2001). Tourette's syndrome: It's more common than you think. *Brown University Child and Adolescent Behavior Letter, 17*(7), 1, 6–7.

Kronenfeld, J. J., (2000). *Schools and the health of children.* Thousand Oaks, CA: Sage Publications.

Mannuzza, S., Klein, R. G., Bessler, A., Malloy, P., & LaPadula, M. (1998). Adult psychiatric status of hyperactive boys grown up. *American Journal of Psychiatry, 155*(4), 493–498.

McCloskey, J., & Bulechek, G. M. (1996). *Nursing interventions classification (NIC)* (2nd ed.). St. Louis, MO: Mosby.

Murphy, P., & Schachar, R. (2000). Use of self-ratings in the assessment of symptoms of attention deficit hyperactivity disorder in adults. *American Journal of Psychiatry, 157*(7), 1156–1159.

Oie, M., & Rund, B. R. (1999). Neuropsychological deficits in adolescent-onset schizophrenia compared with attention deficit hyperactivity disorder. *American Journal of Psychiatry, 156*(8), 1216–1222.

Pajer, K. A. (1998). What happens to "bad" girls? A review of the adult outcomes of antisocial adolescent girls. *American Journal of Psychiatry, 155*(7), 862–870.

Papolos, D. (2001). Childhood-onset bipolar disorder: Under-diagnosed, under-treated and under discussion. *NARSAD Research Newsletter, 12*(4), 11–13.

Papolos, D., & Papolos, J. (1999). *The bipolar child.* New York: Broadway Books.

Paris, J. (1999). *Nature and nurture in psychiatry.* Washington, DC: American Psychiatric Press.

Ratey, J. J. (2001). *A user's guide to the brain.* New York: Pantheon Books.

Rubia, K., Overmeyer, S., Taylor, E., Brammer, M., Williams, S. C. R., Simmons, A., et al. (1999). Hypofrontality in attention deficit hyperactivity disorder during higher-order motor control. *American Journal of Psychiatry, 156*(6), 891–896.

Shelton, D. (2001). Emotional disorders in young offenders. *Journal of Nursing Scholarship, 33*(3), 259–263.

Sheppard, V. B., & Benjamin-Coleman, R. (2001). Determinants of service placements for youth with serious emotional and behavioral disturbances. *Community Mental Health Journal, 37*(1), 53–64.

Spencer, T. J., Biederman, J., Faraone, S., Mick, E., Coffey, B., Geller, D., et al. (2001). Impact of tic disorders on ADHD outcome

across the life cycle. *American Journal of Psychiatry, 158*(4), 611–617.

Valente, S. M. (2001). Treating attention deficit hyperactivity disorder. *Nurse Practitioner, 26*(9), 14–26.

Volkmar, F. R., Klin, A., Schultz, R. T., Rubin, E., & Bronen, R., (2000). Asperger's disorder. *American Journal of Psychiatry, 157*(2), 262–267.

Volkow, N. D. (1998). Dopamine transporter occupancies in the human brain induced by therapeutic doses of oral methylphenidate. *American Journal of Psychiatry, 155*(10), 1325–1331.

Ward, R. G. (2001). Tourette's syndrome. *Nursing Spectrum, 14*(6IL), 22–24.

Wilens T. E., Spencer, T. J., Biederman, J., Girard, K., Doyle, R., Prince, J., et al. (2001). A controlled clinical trial of bupropion for attention-deficit hyperactivity disorder in adults. *American Journal of Psychiatry, 158*(2), 282–288.

Zwi, M. (2000). Evidence and belief in ADHD. *British Medical Journal, 321,* 975–976.

PART FIVE

Neurobehavioral Brain Disorders

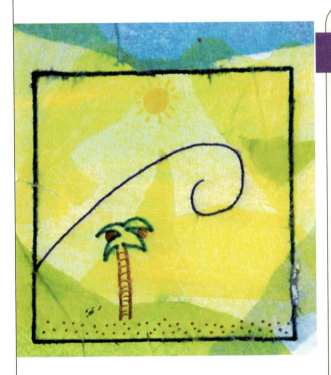

*T*his is where I would like to be 5 years from now when I'm 20: In California.

—Rachel, Age 15

CHAPTER 18

Cognitive Impairment Disorders

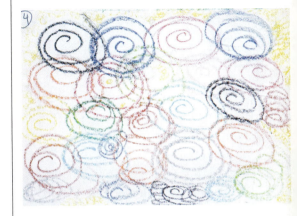

OBJECTIVES

After reading this chapter, you will be able to:

- DIFFERENTIATE between dementia and delirium.

- ASSESS clients with dementia and delirium and differentiate these disorders from pseudodementias.

- INTERVENE with clients suffering from cognitive impairment disorders.

- ASSIST families in planning care for clients with dementia.

- EVALUATE the plan of care based on the outcome criteria.

Lost in an unending maze
Circling round and round
Never stopping to ask questions
Never slowing down

The walls just seem to grow and grow
With no end in sight
Overlapping,
Overflowing
Drowning me in fright

Alone am I
In this crazy maze
Alone
Each night and day

My biggest fear is
To be alone,
Alone
With nowhere to go

—Anna, Age 19

The process of mental deterioration related to cognitive impairment disorders has a profound effect on clients, their families, and society as a whole. This chapter presents dementia and delirium, the two most common forms, in which there are diffuse disturbances in cognitive performance. In general, they differ in both symptoms and outcomes.

Dementias are chronic, irreversible brain disorders characterized by impairments in memory, abstract thinking, and judgment, as well as changes in personality. Loss of autonomy, loss of dignity, and loss of the self result in despair of victims and families. Stroke-related dementia, also known as *vascular dementia*, accounts for about 7 percent of all the dementias. Another type of dementia, typically affecting younger people, is *AIDS dementia complex (ADC)*, caused by HIV infection of the brain. It is estimated that ADC occurs in 15 to 25 percent of people with AIDS, with a widely varied but progressively deteriorating course. Symptoms include psychomotor slowing, decreased speed in processing information, impaired memory, and impaired executive functioning. *Frontal lobe dementias (FLDs)*, caused by a variety of brain diseases, are often misdiagnosed as mental disorders because personality, sociability, and executive function are prominently impaired (Chun, 1998; Yeaworth & Burke, 2000). Frontal lobe dementias are discussed in more detail in Chapter 19.

Alzheimer's disease (AD) accounts for about 80 percent of dementing illness and currently affects about 4.8 million Americans. It strikes 1 out of 12 people over the age of 65, 1 out of 3 over age 80, and almost 1 out of 2 over the age of 85. Onset generally

DSM-IV-TR CLASSIFICATIONS

Delirium

Delirium due to . . . (general medical condition)
Substance intoxication delirium
Substance withdrawal delirium
Delirium due to multiple etiologies
Delirium NOS

Dementia

Dementia of the Alzheimer's type, with early onset
Dementia of the Alzheimer's type, with late onset
Vascular dementia
Dementia due to HIV disease
Dementia due to head trauma
Dementia due to Parkinson's disease
Dementia due to Huntington's disease
Dementia due to Pick's disease
Dementia due to Creutzfeldt–Jakob disease
Substance-induced persisting dementia
Dementia due to multiple etiologies
Dementia NO

Cognitive Disorder NOS

SOURCE: Reprinted with permission from the *Diagnostic and Statistical Manual of Mental Disorders*, Fourth Edition, Text Revision. Copyright 2000 American Psychiatric Association.

occurs in late life but in rare cases the disorder appears in the 40s and 50s. More women than men are affected, in part because women live longer. The impact of AD will be felt more severely in the twenty-first century, when the baby boom generation reaches old age. By the middle of the twenty-first century, it is estimated that 14 million Americans will experience the destruction of AD (Haight, 2001; Kennedy, 2000).

Approximately 15 to 20 percent of Alzheimer's cases are believed to be inherited; this form is known as *familial Alzheimer's disease (FAD)*. Because FAD often begins at a much younger age, it is also referred to as early-onset AD.

Delirium is an acute, usually reversible brain disorder characterized by clouding of the consciousness (a decreased awareness of the environment), a reduced ability to focus and maintain attention, and altered perception. Delirium is the most common cognitive disorder. See the DSM-IV-TR Classifications feature. Ten to 30 percent of individuals hospitalized for a medical condition, 25 percent of inpatients with cancer, 51 percent of postoperative clients, and 30 to 40 percent of hospitalized AIDS clients develop delirium as a complication of their primary illness. The presence of delirium indicates that a medical illness is affecting the brain, and rapid medical intervention is needed to prevent irreversible deterioration or death. People with dementia are more susceptible to delirium ("Practice Guidelines," 1999). (For a comparison of dementia and delirium, see Table 18.1 ■).

KNOWLEDGE BASE: DEMENTIA

Because multi-infarct dementia and AD demonstrate many of the same characteristics and the latter is believed to be more prevalent, AD is used as the model for dementia. The average course of AD is 5 to 10 years, but the range may be 2 to 20 years. People who have early onset often deteriorate more rapidly. The progression is roughly divided into three stages: Stage 1 (mild) typically lasts two to four years, stage 2 (moderate) may continue for several years, and stage 3 (severe) usually lasts only one to two years before death occurs (see Table 18.2 ■).

BEHAVIORAL CHARACTERISTICS

The most notable changes in behavior during stage 1 are difficulties performing complex tasks, related to a *decline in recent memory*. People suffering from AD are unable to balance their checkbooks or plan a well-balanced meal. They may have difficulty remembering to buy supplies for the home or responding to different schedules within the home. At work, the ability to plan a goal-directed set of behaviors is seriously limited, resulting in missed appointments and incomplete verbal or written reports.

Personal appearance begins to decline, and they need help selecting clothes appropriate for the season or particular event. They remain capable of independent living. During stage 1, these people recognize their confusion and are frightened by what is happening. Fearing the diagnosis, they attempt to cover up and rationalize their symptoms.

In stage 2, behavior deteriorates markedly and client *safety* becomes an issue. The most common accidents are falls, followed by injuries resulting from difficulty using sharp objects. *Wandering behavior* poses a potential danger because AD sufferers get lost easily and are unable to retrace their steps back home. Lost and confused, they may become victims of street crime.

During stage 2, they need assistance with the sequence of skills for *activities of daily living (ADLs)*. They also need help in dressing, toileting, and bathing. The inability to carry out skilled and purposeful movement or the inability to use objects properly is called **apraxia**. Also evident is **hyperorality**, the need to taste, chew, and examine any object small enough to be placed in the mouth. People in this stage need to be protected from accidentally eating harmful substances such as soaps or poisons.

Although there may be a sharp increase in appetite and food intake, there is seldom a corresponding weight gain. In contrast, some individuals have limited or no recognition of mealtimes or even food. Behavior in this stage is characterized by continuous, repetitive acts that have no meaning or direction. These repetitive behaviors—which may include lip licking, tapping of fingers, pacing, or echoing others' words—are referred to as **perseveration phenomena**.

Many long-lived adults, including those suffering from Alzheimer's disease, become disoriented at the end of the day; this is usually referred to as **sundown syndrome**. Orientation seems to decrease as daylight recedes. It becomes more difficult to distinguish shapes from shadows and to pinpoint the source of sounds in

TABLE 18.1

Dementia and Delirium Compared

Dementia	Delirium
Onset	
Onset of impairment generally slow and insidious	Onset usually sudden. Acute development of impairment of orientation, memory, cognitive function, judgment, and affect
Essential Feature	
Not based on disordered consciousness; however, delirium, stupor, and coma may occur	Clouded state of consciousness
Etiology	
Generally caused by irreversible alteration of brain function	Caused by temporary, reversible, diffuse disturbances of brain function
Course	
No diurnal fluctuations. The clinical course usually progresses over months or years, ending in death	Short, diurnal fluctuations in symptoms. The clinical course is usually brief, although it may last for months. Untreated, prolonged delirium may cause permanent brain destruction and lead to dementia
History	
Onset: Insidious	Onset: Sudden
Duration: Months to years	Duration: Hours to days
Course: Consistent deterioration with occasional lucid moments	Course: Fluctuating arousal
Motor Signs	
None (until late)	Postural tremor, restless, hyperactive, or sluggish
Speech is usually normal in early stages, but word-finding difficulties progress	Slurred speech, reflecting disorganized thinking
Mental Status	
Attention generally normal in early stages; inattention progresses	Attention fluctuates
Memory	
Memory impairment; recent memory affected before remote	Impaired by poor attention
Language	
Aphasia in later stages	Normal or mild misnaming of objects
Perception	
Hallucinations not prominent, although cognitive impairment may lead to paranoid delusions	Visual, auditory, and/or tactile hallucinations

TABLE 18.1

Dementia and Delirium Compared *(continued)*

Mental Status (continued)	
Pronounced Mood/Affect	
Disinterested and/or disinhibited	Fear and suspiciousness may be prominent; anxiety, depression, anger, irritability, or euphoria may occur
Review of Systems	
Extraneural organ systems usually uninvolved	History of systemic illness or toxic exposure
EEG	
Normal or mildly slow	Pronounced diffuse slowing of fast cycles related to state of arousal

the environment. Sundown syndrome is more pronounced when clients are fatigued. Various behaviors relating to sundown syndrome include wandering, confusion, hyperactivity, restlessness, and aggression.

In the middle and later stages of AD, psychotic symptoms are common and are a leading cause of institutionalization (Garand & Hall, 2000). Disruptive, *agitated behavior* occurs in 13 percent of clients with mild dementia, 24 percent in moderate dementia, and 29 percent in severe dementia. Exhibiting poor impulse control, they may have outbursts and tantrums, and their behavior is often socially unacceptable. Verbally agitated behavior includes negative comments, repetitive questions, inappropriate laughing, verbal outbursts or screaming, and verbal resistance of daily routines. As it escalates, verbal agitation becomes aggressive when clients call names, curse, yell, and make threats. Physically agitated behavior includes pacing, perseveration phenomena, hoarding, wandering, and being uncooperative with personal care activities. As it escalates, physical agitation becomes aggressive when clients hit, bite, spit, grab, or throw things. Verbal and physical aggression also affects caregivers leading to frustration, depression, injury, and a higher risk for elder abuse. Risk factors for aggression include male gender, more severe dementia, delusions or hallucinations, earlier age of onset, wandering, sleep disorder, and underlying medical illnesses. Agitation and aggression often results from physical discomfort, sensory deprivation, or social isolation. Frequently, the person is unable to explain an

unmet need such as pain, fecal or urinary urgency, constipation, anxiety, or depression (Lyketsos, et al., 1999; Rowe, Straneva, Colling, & Grabo, 2000).

Almost half of clients with AD become withdrawn and *apathetic* as the disease advances. This is evidenced in passive behaviors such as decreased interaction with others, withdrawal from activities, less interest in a variety of experiences, and less willingness to try new activities (Colling, 2000; Lyketsos et al., 2000).

Wandering is another problem at this time. Wandering may be a substitute for social interaction and thus is a way to alleviate loneliness and separation from others. Wandering may also be an expression of agitation, boredom, pain, or discomfort. Within a safe environment, wandering can be beneficial since it stimulates circulation and oxygenation and promotes exercise.

In stage 3 of AD, a syndrome like Klüver–Bucy syndrome develops, which includes the continuation of hyperorality and the development of periodic binge eating. Behavior is also characterized by **hyperetamorphosis**, the need to compulsively touch and examine every object in the environment. There is a sharp deterioration in motor ability that progresses from an inability to walk to an inability to sit up, and finally to an inability even to smile.

AFFECTIVE CHARACTERISTICS

In stage 1 of AD, anxiety and depression may occur as affected people become aware of and try to cope with noticeable deficits. They frequently experience feelings

TABLE 18.2

Changes in Normal Aging and Changes in Alzheimer's Disease Compared

Normal Aging	Alzheimer's Disease
Recent memory more impaired than remote memory	Recent and remote memory profoundly affected
Difficulty in recalling names of people and places	Inability to recall names of people and places
Decreased concentration	Inability to concentrate
Writing things down is helpful in stimulating memory	Inability to write; nothing stimulates memory
Changes do not interfere with daily functioning	Changes cause an inability to function at work, in a social relationship, and at home
Insight into forgetful behavior is preserved	With progression, the person has no insight into changes that have occurred

of helplessness, frustration, and shame in relation to their deficits. Diagnosis of a concomitant depression is important because depression can worsen the symptoms of dementia and for that reason must not be ignored.

In the beginning of AD, clients may lack spontaneity in verbal and nonverbal communication. They are less enthusiastic, less cheerful, and less affectionate. As the disease progresses, there is an increased *lability* of emotions from flat affect to periods of marked irritability. Delusions of persecution may precipitate feelings of intense fear. *Catastrophic reactions*, resulting from underlying brain dysfunction, are common. In response to everyday situations, the person may overreact by exploding in rage or suddenly crying. In the severe stage, response to environmental stimuli continues to decrease until the person is wholly nonresponsive (Colling, 2000).

COGNITIVE CHARACTERISTICS

The primary cognitive deficit in stage 1 is memory impairment with a *decrease in concentration*, an increase in distractibility, and an appearance of absent-mindedness. The ability to make accurate judgments also declines. People suffering from early AD may have difficulty managing their finances or may give away large amounts of money in response to radio and television

solicitations. It is difficult to decide when to prevent them from driving. Because they are easily distracted, they may forget the meaning of road signs, may confuse the meaning of red and green lights, and may not look to see that no other cars are coming; they are also extremely accident prone.

They may be disoriented about time but remember people and places. Transitory *delusions* of persecution may develop in response to the memory impairment. The person may make such statements as "You hid my keys. I know you don't want me to be able to get out of the house and drive"; "Where are my shoes? Everybody keeps hiding things to make me crazy"; "Why didn't you tell me there was a party tonight? You just don't want me to go and have any fun." It is difficult for sufferers of AD and their families to balance the need for independence with situations in which they need help. Caregivers may be accused of treating them like children on the one hand, and not giving them enough attention on the other.

Language skills begin to deteriorate in stage 1 as individuals have problems in thinking of what to say and *language processing* takes longer. They may have word-finding and object-naming difficulties. They have problems with complex conversations, rapid speech, and speech in noisy and distracting environments. At this stage, they may self-correct or apologize for communication problems.

In stage 2 of AD, there is a *progressive memory loss*, which includes both recent and remote memory. New information cannot be retained, and there is no recollection of what occurred 10 minutes or an hour ago. Loss of remote memory becomes obvious when there is no recognition of family members or recall of significant past events. This loss may be the most painful aspect of AD, erasing a whole lifetime of memories for that person.

Confabulation, the filling in of memory gaps with imaginary information, is an attempt to distract others from observing the deficit. Comprehension of language, interactions, and significance of objects is greatly diminished. During this stage, the person becomes completely disoriented in all three spheres of person, time, and place.

Many people with AD develop *psychotic symptoms* of delusions and hallucinations. Delusions often involve themes of persecution such as believing that misplaced items have been stolen. Paranoia can also take the form of delusional jealousy with accusations of infidelity, which can be heartbreaking for the partner. Hallucinations can occur in all of the senses, but visual hallucinations are the most common and occur in more than 20 percent of clients with AD. The hallucinations are distressing and are associated with more rapid cognitive decline. **Misidentification syndrome** frequently occurs, in which familiar people are seen as unfamiliar and vice versa. They may even believe that people on television are really present (Chapman, Dickinson, McKeith, & Ballard, 1999).

As the disease progresses, communication breakdowns become more frequent and more severe. Stressful and confusing situations compound the difficulty in understanding others or expressing thoughts. An increase of **aphasia**—the loss of the ability to understand or use language—occurs, which begins with the inability to find words and eventually limits the person to as few as six words. Concurrently, **agraphia**, the inability to read or write, develops. Finally, the inability to recognize familiar situations, people, or stimuli evolves; this is known as **agnosia**. *Auditory agnosia* is the inability to recognize familiar sounds such as a doorbell, the ring of a telephone, or a barking dog. *Tactile agnosia*, **astereognosia**, occurs when the person is unable to identify familiar objects placed in the hand, such as a comb, pencil, or paintbrush. *Visual agnosia*, or **alexia**, occurs when the person can look at a frying pan, a telephone, or a toothbrush and have no idea what to do with these objects.

The following interchange illustrates the aphasic characteristics of AD. Pat is able to give a variety of descriptors but cannot think of the one necessary word.

Sue called her mother, Pat, to see how she was doing.

Sue: *It sounds like you are eating, Mom. What are you eating?*

Pat: *I can't tell you.*

Sue: *Is it hot or cold?*

Pat: *It's cold.*

Sue: *Did you get it out of the refrigerator?*

Pat: *No, it's like bread.*

Sue: *Is it a sandwich?*

Pat: *Sort of. I put butter on it.*

Sue: *Is it crackers?*

Pat: *No. I used to buy a lot of it and put it in the freezer.*

Sue: *Is it cookies?*

Pat: *No. Usually I have it for breakfast. I took the last slice.*

Sue: *Is it coffee cake?*

Pat: *Yes, that's what it is.*

In stage 3 of AD, there is a severe decline in cognitive functioning. Clients may be oblivious to others in the home and may be unable to recognize themselves in the mirror. They may scream or yell spontaneously or be able to say only one word or unable to say anything. In addition, there is no longer any nonverbal response to internal and external stimuli; the person degenerates to a *vegetative state*.

Mr. Goldstein, a 67-year-old engineer, began to forget where he placed familiar objects around the house and, as his wife noted, had difficulty balancing the checkbook. His co-workers began
(continued)

to notice impaired judgments in the workplace. Mr. Goldstein tended to project on others his increasing inability to handle usual tasks efficiently. Within two years, he was in stage 2, and Mrs. Goldstein had to label objects in the home so that he could identify them by name. He responded with fear to sounds he could no longer identify. He needed assistance with eating, bathing, and dressing and constant supervision because of his wandering behavior. Mrs. Goldstein found that a regular routine was helpful and continually repeated, "My husband is still in there, I just have to go in and draw him out."

SOCIAL CHARACTERISTICS

There are at least two victims of AD: the person with the disease and the caregiver(s). Remember that for every client, there is a family in distress. Spouses or partners may experience the loss of growing older together as planned, fear for one's own future, and the anguish of watching a life partner deteriorate. Children and siblings may wonder if they will inherit this disease. AD has been called by some "death by a thousand subtractions" and by former First Lady Nancy Reagan as "the long goodbye."

Families are the primary providers of long-term care for people who suffer from dementia. Most often, the sufferer is elderly. Elderly spouses, who are most likely to provide care, have limited strength and energy to meet the demands of the situation. Middle-aged children, most typically daughters, must manage their own problems as well as the role reversal that occurs with a dependent parent. Caring for a person with dementia is among the most difficult of family responsibilities and the one for which caregivers receive minimal support and training.

Concerns about intimacy and *sexuality* are important for most couples, regardless of sexual orientation. Most of us have been socially conditioned to think that old people are—or should be—nonsexual, and especially old, demented people. The reality is that sexuality ranges along a continuum of no interest to active, ongoing interest. Severity of the disease is not always the standard by which to judge the appropriateness of sexual behavior. Some healthy partners have no interest in continuing a sexual relationship with an ill partner. This may be in response to feeling more like a parent to the partner

or feeling insignificant when not recognized by the ill person. Some healthy partners are interested in maintaining sexual intimacy but may be physically exhausted or feel guilty about being sexual with a partner who is unable to clearly consent. Other healthy partners express no interest in genital sex but remain interested in emotional intimacy (loving words) and physical intimacy (holding, kissing, stroking). Others are able to maintain all types of intimacy, including genital sex, and feel satisfied and joyful with the interaction. A satisfactory sex life is a comfort to these couples as their bodies remember and celebrate this pleasure.

Communication problems cause more caregiver stress, as clients are unable to take part in family conversations and fail to start or sustain conversations, all of which leads to caregivers feeling frustrated, lonely, and isolated.

The changes that occur in AD are frightening to family members, and witnessing the steady deterioration of their loved ones is extremely painful. Many families eventually become exhausted and suffer from emotional, physical, and financial problems. Outside relationships may have to be forfeited. Custodial care in an appropriate facility may be necessary. Many couples, however, cannot afford day care early and full-time nursing care late in the disease process. Finding the money to hire sitters or housekeepers can be stressful for the well partner.

The necessity of drastically altering lifestyles may lead to overwhelming feelings of anger, resentment, depression, and hopelessness. These feelings may be displaced onto the ill person, who then may become more vulnerable to elder abuse. (Elder abuse is discussed in Chapter 21.) Research indicates that caregivers who are at high risk for abusing are those who have been in the caregiving role for many years, who have been providing care for many hours every day, and whose loved one is severely impaired (Kennedy, 2000).

While clients are still able to participate and make their wishes known, family members can seek their guidance regarding long-term plans. A *living will* or an *advance directive* may be formulated. A durable power of *attorney for health* care should be named as well as a *durable power of attorney* for financial matters.

PHYSIOLOGICAL CHARACTERISTICS

Deterioration of the central nervous system (CNS) results in physical changes throughout the body (see

Table 18.3 ■). People with dementia may suffer from **hypertonia**, an increase in muscle tone that results in muscular twitching. While hyperactivity may occur, eventually there is a loss of energy and increasing fatigue with physical activity. The sleep cycle is impaired; there is a decrease in total sleep time and more frequent awakenings. This disruption leads to *sleep deprivation*, which magnifies the already disturbed cognitive functions (Kovach, 2000).

People suffering from AD are susceptible to injuries from *falls*. About half the falls are secondary to medical problems such as orthostatic hypotension, arrhythmias, and impaired vision. Other falls are related to such factors as poor lighting or loose rugs. Some people will fall because of poor judgment, as in putting a chair on top of a table and climbing up to reach something. Because of changes in the CNS, people suffering from AD people have a decreased reaction time. Thus, it is more difficult to regain balance when beginning to fall.

As the disease progresses, incontinence of both urine and stool occurs. In the final stage, anorexia leads to an emaciated physical condition. *Death* usually occurs from pneumonia, urinary tract infection leading to sepsis, malnutrition, or dehydration.

Pathophysiological changes associated with Alzheimer's disease are degenerative and result in gross atrophy of the cerebral cortex. As the disease destroys brain cells, two types of abnormalities occur. *Neurofibrillary tangles* are thick, insoluble clots of protein inside the damaged brain cells or neurons. *Amyloid plaques*, found on the outside of dead and damaged neurons, consist of bits of dying cells mixed with beta-amyloid protein. The enzyme, beta-secretase, appears to play a key role in the buildup of plaques. At present, it is unclear which pathology is most responsible for the disease process.

Galanin is a neuropeptide that is thought to play a role in the pathophysiology of AD. One of the many functions of galanin is to rescue neurons that are in distress by slowing the cells down and eventually immobilizing them so that repairs can be made. The destruction of cells in AD leads to twice the normal level of galanin as the condition worsens. Excess galanin

TABLE 18.3

CNS Pathways of Destruction

Area	Function	Symptoms
Limbic system	Memory, interpretation of emotion	Problems with recent and later remote memory; depression; apathy; unstable affect
Hippocampus	Memory storage	Decreased ability to learn; memory loss
Frontal lobe	Cognition, planning; motor aspects of speech; control of movement; control of outbursts; insight into own behavior	Problems with planning activities; inability to carry out skilled, purposeful movement; catastrophic reactions and emotional outbursts; delusions; inability to walk, talk, swallow
Parietal lobe	Sensory speech and ability to recognize written words; proprioception; ability to recognize objects and their function	Inability to recognize familiar places, people, and purpose of common household objects; expressive aphasia; agraphia; agnosia; hallucinations; seizures; falls
Temporal lobe	Memory, judgment, learning; ability to understand spoken words	Receptive aphasia; problems with memory and learning new concepts or activities
Occipital lobe	Ability to understand written words	Inability to read with comprehension; hallucinations

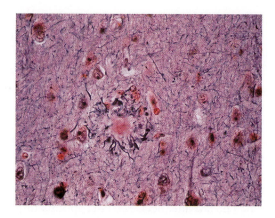

PHOTO 18.1 ■ This microscopic photograph illustrates senile plaques, which are found throughout the cortex and hippocampus of patients with Alzheimer's disease.

SOURCE: Martin M. Rotker/Science Source/Photo Researchers, Inc.

inhibits memory, especially visual memory, which may explain why people with AD get easily lost in their own neighborhood because they cannot remember landmarks. Drug antagonists to galanin do not cross the blood–brain barrier and have to be directly injected into the brain. Researchers are trying to develop oral antagonists because of their potential to slow the progression of this disease (Miller, 2001).

There is a specific pattern in the death of neurons in AD. The first nerves to die are in the *limbic system*, the center for emotion and memory. The limbic system interprets emotional responses coming from the cerebral cortex, and the hippocampus, a part of the limbic system, is involved in memory storage. Destruction of the hippocampus results in recent memory loss. Remote memory loss is slower to occur, possibly because the memories are stored in more than one location in the brain. AD often brings on depression related to limbic system damage, as well as damage to the locus ceruleus, which modulates mood and stress response (Garand & Hall, 2000).

AD causes a progressive loss of most neurotransmitters and a reduction of synaptic binding sites. Decreased serotonin (5-HT) in the brain is associated with increased aggressive behavior, anxiety, agitation, and psychosis. Decreased levels of dopamine (DA) lead to movement difficulties, blunted affect, and apathy. Lowered levels of acetylcholine (ACh) lead to memory difficulties,

agitation, and psychotic symptoms. The balance between DA and ACh may also influence aggression in persons with Alzheimer's disease. High levels of norepinephrine (NE) lead to anxiety, agitation, anorexia, and insomnia (Garand & Hall, 2000; Porter et al., 2000).

The destruction of neurons spreads toward the surface of the brain, killing off nerve cells in the *cerebral cortex*. A wide variety of symptoms appear as the destruction spreads throughout the four lobes (see Table 18.4 ■). Computed axial tomography (CAT) scans may demonstrate brain atrophy, widened cortical sulci, and enlarged cerebral ventricles. Positron-emission tomography (PET) scans can detect Alzheimer's-related abnormalities by the way certain sugars are processed in the brain, especially in the temporal and parietal lobes. Early Alzheimer's is suspected if there is a decreased use of glucose in the areas where language processing and memory storage takes place.

CONCOMITANT DISORDERS

There are several reversible disorders that simulate or mimic dementia. Referred to as **pseudodementias**, these include drug toxicity, metabolic disorders, infections, and nutritional deficiencies. Chronic lung disease and heart disease can lead to cerebral hypoxia and symptoms of dementia. The most common cause of pseudodementia is depression, which is often overlooked by health care professionals. Up to 50 percent of people with AD experience a concomitant depression. It is imperative that such disorders be recognized and differentiated from irreversible dementia (see Table 18.4). Only through recognition can appropriate treatment measures be initiated (Chemerinski, Petracca, Sabe, Kremer, & Starkstein, 2001).

CAUSATIVE THEORIES
Genetic Theory

The cause of AD is unknown but is likely to be a combination of aging and genetic and environmental factors. Research continues in an effort to understand the biochemical events responsible for the destruction of brain cells and is currently focusing on the role of chromosomes 1, 14, 19, and 21 and the *amyloid precursor protein (APP)* gene. APP is the precursor of beta-amyloid protein that accumulates into plaques in AD.

People with Down syndrome, who have an extra copy of *chromosome 21*, which includes the amyloid precursor protein (APP) gene, are at high risk for

TABLE 18.4

Depression and Dementia Compared

Depression	Dementia
Relatively rapid onset	Insidious onset
Symptoms progress rapidly	Symptoms progress slowly
Able to recall recent events	Has difficulty recalling recent events
Has long-term memory	As disease progresses, loses long-term memory
"Don't know" answers are common	Uses confabulation rather than admitting "don't know"
Attention span normal	Impaired attention span
Affect is depressed	Affect is shallow and labile
Oriented to person, time, and place	Unable to recognize familiar people and places; becomes lost in familiar environments; disoriented as to time
Apathetic in relationship to ADLs	Struggles to perform ADLs and is frustrated as a result

developing lesions in the brain similar to those seen in AD. Seventy-five percent of persons with Down syndrome over the age of 60 have dementia, with neurobiological changes postmortem that are indistinguishable from those of AD (Huang et al., 1999).

It is not yet known how the genes and their various mutations cause AD. In familial Alzheimer's disease (FAD), the mutations of the APP gene that occur on *chromosomes 14* and *1* are the likely genes. The defective gene on chromosome 14 is called presenilin 1, while the defective gene on chromosome 1 is referred to as presenilin 2. If a person inherits one of the presenilin-producing genes, they are likely to develop AD at an early age. These two defects account for approximately 50 percent of the cases of FAD (Garand & Hall, 2000).

Chromosome 19 is the linkage with late-onset FAD and sporadic AD. Scientists are looking for the link between genes and the production of *apolipoprotein E (APOE)*. APOE is associated with the transport of cholesterol and the formation of plaques in the brain. APOE comes in three varieties: E2, E3, and E4. The E2 version of the gene protects people from getting AD, while E4 increases risk and causes AD to start at a younger age. Those with two copies of E4 are at a very

high risk of AD. The risk from E3, the most common APOE gene, falls in between, which gives individuals an intermediate risk of AD. APOE plays a role in cholesterol transport, cerebral amyloid deposition, neuronal plasticity, and cholinergic activity.

Currently, the consensus is against *genetic testing* for AD. Tests are promising but lack the sensitivity and specificity for routine use. At this time, we also do not know all of the possible genetic mutations, which limit the predictability of genetic testing. If testing is available in the future, it will be necessary to protect against genetic discrimination by employers and insurers (Roberts, 2000).

Cholinergic Hypothesis

Memory and learning are, to a certain extent, dependent on acetylcholine (ACh). The enzyme choline-acetyl transferase (ChAT) synthesizes ACh from choline and acetyl coenzyme A. The enzyme cholinesterase (ChE) inactivates ACh. It is believed that individuals with AD have low levels of ChAT and ACh and high levels of ChE when compared to control groups. Researchers are seeking ways to raise and maintain ACh levels in those suffering from AD (Adams & Page, 2000; Keltner, Zielinski, & Hardin, 2001).

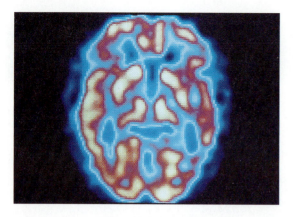 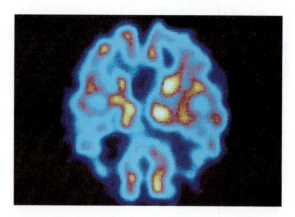

PHOTO 18.2 ■ PET scan of the brain (basal ganglia level) of a normal person and a patient with Alzheimer's disease. The scans show brain activity from low (blue) to high (yellow). Normal brain metabolic activity produces a roughly symmetrical pattern in the yellow areas of the left and right hemispheres (left). The patchy appearance of the patient's scan indicates degeneration of brain tissue.

SOURCE: Tim Beddow/Science Photo Library/Photo Researchers, Inc.

Inflammation

Low-level inflammation may be a factor in the development of AD. *Prostaglandin*, an inflammatory fatty acid, is neutralized by nonsteroidal anti-inflammatory drugs (NSAIDs). Researchers have been able to detect high levels of prostaglandin in the brains of people with AD as compared to control groups. These prostaglandins are neurotoxic and cause degeneration of the brain (Prasad, 1998).

Environmental Risk Factors

One environmental risk factor for AD is *traumatic head injury.* People who have experienced severe head injuries have a significant increase in the deposition of amyloid protein in their brains. The injury may decrease the brain's functional reserves. It is also possible that damage to the blood–brain barrier allows entry of toxic products or somehow makes the brain more susceptible to the effects of aging (Heyman, 1998).

Protective Factors

Estrogen, through its sustaining action on axons and dendrites, may be a protective factor for AD. Estrogens are also antioxidants, which protect neurons against beta-amyloid, and they also modulate the secretion of ACh in the brain. Menopausal women who take estrogen replacement are at lower risk for and slower pro-

gression of AD. *NSAIDs* may also be a protective factor. Researchers have long observed that people with arthritis are less likely to get AD than the general population and think their drugs may be the reason. *Cigarette smoking* may be a protective factor in both early- and late-onset AD. Smoking facilitates nicotinic receptor function and appears to delay signs and symptoms of AD. The better-educated people are, the less likely they are to experience dementia. It is believed that *mental stimulation* actually builds many more synapses between neurons, which allows individuals to better withstand the damages of disease (Chun, 1998; Folstein & Folstein, 1998; Seeman, 1997).

PSYCHOPHARMACOLOGICAL INTERVENTIONS

No known treatment can stop or reverse the mental deterioration of AD. Researchers are looking for ways to increase the amount of ACh in the brain. Because it is digested in the gastrointestinal tract, ACh cannot be taken orally. Three medications currently approved by the Food and Drug Administration (FDA) increase the availability of ACh in the synapses by inhibiting the enzyme cholinesterase responsible for the breakdown of ACh. These medications are Aricept (donepezil), Exelon (rivastigmine), and Reminyl (galantamine). Reminyl is a cholinesterase inhibitor that also includes nicotinic receptor modulating activity. A previous drug, Cognex (tacrine), has been withdrawn from the market because of liver toxicity.

Cholinesterase inhibitors do not cure AD but may slow the progression of the disorder. In some cases, this is almost as good as a cure: Because the AD usually strikes late in life, delaying its onset by a year would decrease the incidence and delay nursing home placement. Cholinesterase inhibitors are not effective for those with advanced AD. The side effects are usually transient, occurring at the onset of treatment, and include nausea, diarrhea, sweating, bradycardia, and insomnia. Taking the medication after breakfast may decrease side effects. Additional cholinesterase inhibitors, physostigmine, metrifonate, and eptastigmine, are in development at the present time (Cummings, 2000; Kennedy, 2000).

NSAIDs may reduce the inflammatory response to amyloid protein deposits. At this time, researchers are not recommending the use of NSAIDs to prevent AD since they have side effects such as dizziness, fluid retention, gastrointestinal problems, and nervousness. *Hormone replacement therapy* may lower the risk of AD and prevent normal age-related decline in cognition. Estrogen promotes neuronal sprouting and enhances cholinergic activity in the brain. Estrogen also appears to increase blood flow and glucose metabolism in the brain along with its anti-inflammatory and antioxidative properties (Garand & Hall, 2000; Shepherd, 2001).

Because a concomitant depression may increase functional disability, *antidepressant medications* are prescribed for people with depressive symptoms. Antipsychotic medications may decrease agitation, aggression, paranoid thinking, and poor impulse control. Eldepryl (selegiline), a selective monoamine oxidase B inhibitor that is approved for motor dysfunction of Parkinson's disease, may delay functional decline but does not improve cognitive performance.

Medication should not be overused to sedate and calm clients. For those clients experiencing sleep problems, the use of hypnotics is contraindicated because the medication does not improve sleep patterns and often increases confusion and sedation during awake periods. The newer antipsychotic medication, *Risperdal (risperidone)* may be helpful in promoting sleep as well as in regulating agitated and aggressive behavior. Other medications used for agitation and aggression include Desyrel (trazodone), BuSpar (buspirone), Tegretol (carbamazepine), and Depakote (valproate).

Memantine, a drug under FDA investigation, is being tested for the treatment of moderate to severe AD. This new drug targets the excitatory amino acids such as glutamate (glu). Excess glu is associated with neuronal nerve cell death found in the neurodegenerative disorders. The drug appears to correct the glu imbalance by acting as a receptor antagonist (Brown University Geriatric Psychopharmacology Update, 2001).

MULTIDISCIPLINARY INTERVENTIONS

The most effective approach to AD occurs with the coordinated efforts of the multidisciplinary team. *Speech therapists* may be able to slow down the aphasic process as well as restore partial swallowing function. *Physical therapists* can maintain or increase range of motion, improve muscle tone, improve coordination, and increase endurance for exercise. *Occupational therapists* can provide additional sensory stimulation and self-care training programs. *Social workers* can provide individual or group therapy for families of people with AD; moreover, they can help with community resources or institutional placement. *Pastoral counselors* can help clients and families meet religious and spiritual needs.

ALTERNATIVE THERAPIES
Antioxidants

Antioxidants are a group of vitamins, minerals, enzymes, and herbs that help protect the body from naturally occurring free radicals. As the body goes through its normal processes, and oxygen is used to provide cellular fuel, some of the oxygen molecules lose one of their pair of electrons. When they do, the formerly stable oxygen molecules become dangerous free radicals that try to stabilize themselves by stealing another electron from stable molecules, thus damaging them and creating more free radicals. An excess of free radicals is, in part, responsible for the effects of aging and is implicated in degenerative conditions such as AD (Fontaine, 2000).

As people age, they produce fewer antioxidants and may benefit from dietary antioxidants such as vitamin C, vitamin E, carotenoids, the mineral selenium, and the hormone melatonin. Herbs with antioxidant properties include bilberry, ginkgo, grape seed extract, green tea, and flavonoids. Fruits and vegetables are the primary sources for antioxidants, though they are also available in the form of supplements. At the top of the list in providing antioxidants are fruits and vegetables with the deepest colors such as prunes, raisins, blueberries, blackberries, raspberries, garlic, kale, cranberries, strawberries, spinach, broccoli, and beets (Carper, 2000).

Coenzyme Q10 is a substance whose actions resemble those of vitamin E. It is the only one of the coenzyme Qs found in human tissue. It may be one of the most powerful antioxidants. It has been found to be helpful for people with Alzheimer's disease (Balch & Balch, 2000).

Omega-3 Fish Oil

Omega-3 fish oil, an essential fat, especially the component DHA (ducosahexaenoic acid), is essential for optimal functioning of neuronal synapses in the brain. Good sources of omega-3 fish oil include salmon, mackerel, herring, sardines, and cod liver oil. Eating too many omega-6 vegetable fats such as corn oil and other processed oils, makes the neuronal membranes rigid and can also destroy DHA. Low levels of DHA are a risk factor for low mental performance and the development of AD (Brown & Gerbarg, 2000).

Phosphatidyl Serine

Phosphatidyl serine (Ptd Ser) is a component of the nerve cell membrane that helps keep nerve cell membranes flexible. A dose of 300 mg/day for one month followed by 100 mg/day thereafter often improves memory. Ptd Ser from cow brains is rich in DHA and increases levels of DA and NE. As a supplement, it may be combined with ginkgo (Brown & Gerbarg, 2000).

Melatonin

Insomnia is a frequent problem among persons suffering from AD. Melatonin, a hormone secreted by the pineal gland, plays a critical role in the regulation of the day–night cycle. As we age, we produce less melatonin, and for those with AD the disturbance is even more pronounced. Studies have shown that melatonin is effective in inducing sleep and has no notable side effects. Slow-release melatonin often improves the sleep pattern in people with AD.

Dehydroepiandrosterone

Dehydroepiandrosterone (DHEA) is a corticosteriod produced primarily in the adrenal glands. In addition to serving as a precursor to testosterone and estrogen, DHEA may be involved in regulating mood and one's sense of well-being. The method of action is unclear but it may stimulate gamma-aminobutyric acid (GABA) receptors or increase 5-HT levels. Since there is little known about long-term risks, it is probably best used under medical supervision. The usual dose is up to 90 mg per day (Wolkowitz, Petracca, Chemerinski, & Kremer, 1999).

SAMe

SAMe (S-adenosylmethionine), a compound made by every cell in the body, helps produce DA, 5-HT, and NE. In addition, SAMe improves cell membrane flexibility. Low levels of SAMe have been found in persons with AD. SAMe should be used with caution in people who have a history of cardiac arrhythmia.

Lecithin

Lecithin is a major component of cell membranes. Nerve cells and the protective membranes surrounding the brain are largely composed of lecithin. High doses of lecithin may be helpful for people with AD. Most lecithin is derived from soybeans but recently egg lecithin has become popular (Balch & Balch, 2000).

Music Therapy

Neurohormone and neurotransmitter levels may change as a result of music therapy. One study of people with AD found that 30 to 40 minutes of music therapy in the morning, five days a week for four weeks, resulted in significant increases in serum melatonin concentration. Levels continued to rise even after the music therapy had been discontinued for six weeks. Some of the clinical effects were clients' ability to sign and learn new songs, an increased ability to follow rhythmic patterns, an ability to anticipate endings of phrases and songs, an improved ability to follow changes in tempo, and increased social interaction with peers and therapists (Kumar, Tims, & Gruess, 1999).

KNOWLEDGE BASE: DELIRIUM

Delirium, an acute disorder of cognition and attention, has become increasingly recognized as a common and serious problem for hospitalized individuals. Delirium occurs in 10 to 40 percent of hospitalized

Complementary/Alternative Therapies

Interacting with a Pet

Individuals suffering from Alzheimer's disease often have fewer episodes of anxiety, depression, and outbursts of verbal aggression when they are also able to interact with a companion pet or therapy animal. Caregivers can encourage interaction with the animal, such as a dog or a cat, when the individual seems to be more upset.

■ Note the physical and emotional signs of tension: Are the hands clenched? Body trembling? Restlessness? Unable to relax? Breathing more rapidly?

■ Encourage interaction with the animal for at least 20 minutes. You may have to join in to model appropriate interaction with the pet such as gentle play, stroking, petting, and talking to the animal.

■ Note any changes that would indicate less anxiety and less aggression.

elderly clients, 30 to 40 percent of hospitalized people with AIDS, and up to 60 percent of nursing home residents over the age of 75. In the general hospital population, the rate is 10 to 30 percent. Nearly 80 percent of terminally ill people develop delirium near death (American Psychiatric Association [APA], 2000).

Delirium develops quickly and usually lasts about one week unless the underlying disorder is not corrected. Prompt medical attention is vital in order to prevent permanent brain damage or death. If the cause is not found and treated, death may occur in a matter of days or weeks. The course of the disorder is one of fluctuation; that is, periods of coherence alternate with periods of confusion ("Practice Guidelines," 1999).

BEHAVIORAL CHARACTERISTICS

People suffering from delirium generally display an alteration in *psychomotor activity* and *poor impulse control*. Some are apathetic and withdrawn, others are agitated and tremulous, and still others shift rapidly between apathy and agitation. Hyperactivity is typical of a drug withdrawal state, whereas hypoactivity is typ-

ical of a metabolic imbalance. Speech patterns may be limited and dull, or they may be fast, pressured, and loud. There may be a constant picking at clothes and bed linen as the result of an underlying restlessness. This combination of restlessness and cognitive changes interferes with the person's ability to complete tasks. Bizarre and destructive behavior, which worsens at night, may occur as they attempt to protect themselves or escape from frightening delusions or hallucinations. This behavior may take the form of calling for help, striking out at others, or even attempting to leap out of windows ("Practice Guidelines," 1999).

Over the course of the past two days, Mary has exhibited abrupt behavioral changes. Sometimes, she seems apathetic and withdrawn, barely responding to questions or environmental stimuli. Most of the time, however, particularly at night, she becomes agitated and calls out loudly. She vacillates between being verbally aggressive and abusive and being very vulnerable and frightened, asking for help and whimpering like a small child. Much of the verbal content of her messages has to do with snakes that are in bed with her. She desperately keeps trying to remove these snakes from her bed linens.

AFFECTIVE CHARACTERISTICS

In the state of delirium, a person's affect may range from apathy to extreme irritability to euphoria. Emotions are *labile*; they can change abruptly and fluctuate in intensity. A person may be laughing and suddenly become extremely sad and tearful, reflective of the CNS insult. The predominant emotion in delirium is *fear*. Illusions, delusions, and hallucinations are vivid and extremely frightening.

Mary is terrified by the visual hallucinations of snakes on her bed. She perceives her safety to be threatened and cries for help in removing the snakes. During a family interview, the nurse in charge learns that Mary has always been extremely frightened of snakes, which increases the impact of her hallucinations.

COGNITIVE CHARACTERISTICS

The primary cognitive characteristics of delirium are disorganized thinking and a diminished ability to maintain and shift attention. *Disorganized thinking* is evidenced by rambling, bizarre, or incoherent speech. Lack of judgment and reason severely impairs the decision-making process. Delirious people have difficulty focusing their attention and are *easily distracted* by environmental stimuli; therefore, interactions are difficult, if not impossible. Attention problems result in an impairment in recent memory. Remote memory problems may result from changes in the neurotransmitters, making the retrieval of information difficult.

Another cognitive disruption is *disorientation*, which often results from attention deficits. Disorientation as to time and place is common, whereas identity confusion is rare. Almost all people suffering from delirium misperceive sensory stimuli in the environment. The result is usually visual or auditory *illusions*. For example, the person may believe that spots on the floor are insects. Visual *hallucinations* are also common and may involve people, animals, objects, or bright flashes of light or color. *Delusional beliefs* exist, supporting the illusions and hallucinations. These changes often extend into sleep, which may be accompanied by vivid and terrifying dreams ("Practice Guidelines," 1999).

Marie is an 18-year-old, extremely thin, anorexic client. Laboratory analysis reveals her blood glucose level to be 40 mg/dL. She is agitated and incoherent. Owing to her inability to think logically and also to the fact that she is trying to communicate to others not actually present, she is unable to give a history. She is completely disoriented as to time and place. In terms of orientation to people, she is able to state her own name but does not recognize the boyfriend who brought her to the hospital. In fact, she is convinced that Ron, a nurse, is her boyfriend.

SOCIAL CHARACTERISTICS

Because of the sudden and often unexplained onset of delirium, *families* are usually anxious and frightened.

They may not know how to respond to the agitation, pressured speech, destructive behavior, and labile moods. Equally confusing to families are the disorientation, illusions, hallucinations, and delusions. Because delirious individuals are unable to make decisions, family members must temporarily assume that responsibility.

PHYSIOLOGICAL CHARACTERISTICS

People with delirium experience a disturbance in the *sleep cycle*. Some have hypersomnia and sleep fitfully throughout the day and night. Others have insomnia and sleep very little, day or night. There are obvious signs of *autonomic activity*, including increased cardiac rate, elevated blood pressure, flushed face, dilated pupils, and sweating. Respiratory depth or rhythm may be altered as a result of brain stem depression, or in an attempt to correct an acid–base imbalance that results from the underlying disorder.

Delirious individuals may experience irregular *tremors* throughout the body. Those in a resting position may have myoclonus, a sudden, large muscle spasm. Although they occur most frequently in the face and shoulders, these spasms, which are a result of irritation of the cerebral cortex, can happen anywhere in the body. If the hand is hyperextended, there will be an involuntary palmar flexion called *asterixis*. Generalized seizures may also occur ("Practice Guidelines," 1999).

CONCOMITANT DISORDERS

Delirium occurs in people of all ages. However, the incidence increases with age because of the accompanying illnesses and medication use. Physiological changes of aging such as decreased blood flow to the liver and kidneys predispose long-lived adults to delirium. People with AD are also predisposed to delirium because their CNS function is already compromised. Other groups at high risk include people with terminal cancer and those with HIV/AIDS.

The term **pseudodelirium** is used to describe symptoms of delirium that occur without any identifiable organic cause. The symptoms may occur from sensory deprivation or from the effects of psychosocial stress. Those most vulnerable to pseudodelirium have some preexisting cerebral disease such as a mood disorder, anxiety, schizophrenia, and dementia ("Practice Guidelines," 1999).

CRITICAL THINKING

Theresa is a nurse who works part time in a senior citizens' center. It is a unique position that allows her to apply her nursing experience in a community setting. Teaching the seniors about their health, helping them when they are ill by advocating for their needs, and giving them the information that they need to advocate for themselves are important aspects of her position. She also spends time helping the seniors deal with Medicare and Medicaid issues. Sometimes, she thinks that too much of her time is spent on reimbursement, but Theresa understands how important this assistance is to the seniors. Since she has been at the center, she has begun a class on nutrition, arranged for exercise classes, and conducted screenings on blood pressure, depression, and other relevant health care concerns. She works with some seniors individually on their particular health care needs, such as diabetes, recovery from a myocardial infarction, and hypertension.

Theresa also conducts a caregiver group. This group met today, and Theresa is concerned about one of the members, Mrs. Wiley. Her husband has Alzheimer's disease dementia, and for several years, Mrs. Wiley has cared for her husband at home. Mr. Wiley has attended the Alzheimer's disease group that Theresa leads at the center. Mr. Wiley is 70 and has experienced a gradual reduction in recent memory. Early on in his illness, he was very frightened about what was happening to him. He developed apraxia. He stopped driving when he became distracted and could not remember what the lights or road signs meant. Mr. Wiley did not attend his group meeting last week. Mrs. Wiley was very upset in the caregiver meeting. She said that this week her husband seemed so much worse at the end of the day, very disoriented. Then three days ago, he left the house without her knowledge. She was so frightened she called her neighbors. They all went out looking for him and found him in the nearby park, sitting on a bench. Mr. Wiley could not remember how he got to the park or how to get home.

1. What is the relationship between Mr. Wiley's new symptoms and the progress of his AD?

2. What would concern you about Mr. Wiley's recent symptoms? What interventions might be taken to assist Mr. Wiley and Mrs. Wiley with these recent symptoms?

3. What are some of the likely symptoms that Mr. Wiley will experience as he moves from stage 2 to stage 3? Considering these symptoms, describe several interventions that may be required.

4. Theresa is getting ready to begin her class on diabetes when she overhears two of the seniors talking about Mrs. Collins, a member of the group. Mrs. Collins has been hospitalized with pneumonia and complications from her diabetes. The two seniors discuss how Mrs. Collins has developed Alzheimer's, and it is so sad. Theresa interrupts their conversation and asks them why they thought Mrs. Collins had Alzheimer's disease. They said that when they visited Mrs. Collins she was totally disoriented, picking at the bed linens, and was crying and laughing almost at the same time. Her daughter said that Mrs. Collins had almost hit the nurse the night before. Is it possible that Mrs. Collins has developed Alzheimer's disease while in the hospital? What other cause might you infer from this data about Mrs. Collins?

5. Formulate an education plan that would include critical information about Alzheimer's disease that Theresa might provide for the senior citizens' center.

For an additional Case Study, please refer to the Companion Web site for this book.

CAUSATIVE THEORIES

By affecting the CNS, many conditions may lead to delirium. Cerebral metabolism is dependent on sufficient amounts of oxygen, glucose, and metabolic cofactors. Brain hypoxia may result from pulmonary disease, anemia, or carbon monoxide poisoning. A decreased cerebral blood flow leads to ischemia of the CNS. *Ischemia* may result from cardiac arrhythmias or arrest, congestive heart failure, pulmonary embolus, decreased blood volume, systemic lupus erythematosus, or subacute bacterial endocarditis. A lack of adequate glucose for cerebral metabolism occurs during a state of *hypoglycemia*. Certain metabolic cofactors are essential for cerebral enzyme actions. *Co-factor deficiencies* involve thiamine, niacin, pyridoxine, folate, and vitamin B_{12} ("Practice Guidelines," 1999).

Endocrine disorders of the thyroid, parathyroid, and adrenal glands are associated with delirium. Hepatic and renal failure may be contributing disorders. Fluid and electrolyte imbalance—particularly acidosis, alkalosis, potassium, sodium, magnesium, and calcium imbalances—are additional causes of delirium.

Toxicity from substances such as alcohol, sedatives, antihistamines, parasympatholytics, opioids, cerebral stimulants, digitalis, antidepressants, and heavy metals may also lead to a delirious state. (See Chapter 15 for a thorough discussion of alcohol and drug abuse.) Other likely offenders include anticholinergics and analgesics, which induce CNS depression.

Any direct or primary CNS disturbance—trauma, infection, hemorrhage, neoplasm, or a seizure disorder—is likely to trigger delirium. In addition, drugs used for the treatment of hypertension and Parkinson's disease has been implicated in causing delirium.

The use of physical restraints may be a contributing factor to delirium. The use of restraints with older adults is often said to be for their personal safety and avoidance of harm. Yet restraint use has many negative affects, such as decreased mobility, skin breakdown, cardiac stress, agitation, confusion, and lowered self-esteem. Physical restraints can precede the onset of delirium, thus precipitating this acute disorder (Sullivan-Marx, 1994).

PSYCHOPHARMACOLOGICAL INTERVENTIONS

The medical treatment of *delirium* involves the swift identification of the organic cause. Appropriate treatment requires removal of an offending substance, stabilization in the presence of trauma, administration of antibiotics for infection, or reestablishing of nutrition and metabolic balance. Medications used in managing substance withdrawal delirium are discussed in Chapter 15.

Controlling the symptoms of delirium may be accomplished through the administration of Haldol (haloperidol) intravenously over a period of one to three minutes. When combined with Ativan (lorazepam), there is often a rapid reduction of delirium and severe agitation. IM administration of Haldol has an unpredictable rate of absorption and is more likely to produce extrapyramidal side effects. The usual dose is 1 to 2 mg. Doses may be repeated every 20 to 30 minutes but should not total more than 5 mg every 15 minutes, with a maximum of 240 mg in a 24-hour period. The desired clinical effect is a person who is drowsy but arousable. Once the person is calm, 0.5 to 3 mg of Haldol may be administered orally. If a client develops extrapyramidal symptoms, 25 to 50 mg of Benadryl (diphenhydramine) may be given intravenously ("Practice Guidelines," 1999).

NURSING PROCESS

Assessment

Assessing clients with cognitive impairment disorders—and, specifically, AD—can be a challenge to a nurse's ingenuity and patience. Some clients can respond appropriately when questions are asked simply and enough time is given. Others are so disoriented and confused that they are unable to answer questions; in these situations, you must rely on family members to provide the necessary assessment data. Functional impairment, such as the ability to manage finances and household chores, is more accurately assessed with family members. See the Focused Nursing Assessment feature for clients with cognitive impairment disorders and their family members.

Investigators at McGill University in Montreal have developed a Safety Assessment Scale (SAS) to assess the risk of accidents for people with AD living at home. The categories of questions cover living arrangements; fire and burn risk; nutrition and poisoning; health and medication problems; wandering and getting lost; safety of the home environment; and driving safety. See the Web sites at the end of this chapter for accessing the Safety Assessment Scale.

Hamdy and colleagues (1994) developed a *differential diagnosis tool* based on the word "dementia." It is critical that all other disease processes be identified and treated before a person is diagnosed with AD.

D **Drugs and alcohol.** Long-lived people often purchase many over-the-counter medications, have many medications prescribed, and sometimes borrow medication from friends.

E **Eyes and ears.** People who cannot hear or see well often appear confused.

M **Metabolic and endocrine diseases.** Disruptions such as electrolyte imbalance, hypothyroidism, and uncontrolled diabetes may mimic dementia.

E **Emotional disorders.** Mood and schizophrenic disorders may be mistaken for AD.

N **Nutritional deficiencies.** These may mimic dementia.

T **Tumors and trauma.** Disorders of the CNS may be confused with AD.

I **Infection.** Infections of the urinary tract and pneumonia in long-lived people may lead to confusion. Clients may not have an elevated temperature.

A **Arteriosclerosis.** A decreased blood flow to the brain, brain attacks, and multi-infarct dementia often mimic AD.

Caregivers must also be assessed for *caregiver burden*. Multiple stressors need to be considered when you assess caregivers. Questions to consider are:

- How is care giving interfering with employment or other family roles?
- Can stress be decreased through anticipation and prioritization?
- Is respite care an option?
- What are the quality and extent of supportive relationships for the caregiver?
- Is there evidence of anxiety or depression?

Support for caregivers is essential at all times while caring for clients with AD.

Diagnosis

There are many potential nursing diagnoses for clients experiencing cognitive disorders. In synthesizing the assessment data, consider how well clients are functioning in daily life, what skills they still retain, how well they are able to communicate, and how the caregivers are coping. See the Nursing Diagnoses with NOC and NIC feature for some of the more common nursing diagnoses you may be applying to your clients.

Outcome Identification and Goals

Once you have established diagnoses, you select outcomes appropriate to the nursing diagnoses. The more common outcomes are listed in the Nursing Diagnoses with NOC and NIC feature.

Client goals are specific behavioral measures by which you and significant others determine progress toward goals. The following are examples of some of the outcomes appropriate to people (and their caregivers) with cognitive impairment disorders:

- Improves orientation as delirium clears
- Participates in appropriate social activities
- Participates in a gentle exercise routine
- Establishes routines to decrease confusion
- Remains safe from harm
- Utilizes support groups and respite care

Nursing Interventions

Most clients with *delirium* will be in the acute care setting. In caring for these clients, all measures must be taken to ensure that permanent brain damage or death does not occur. Because delirium is acute and short term, plans of care are directed toward short-term goals, with the long-term medical and nursing goal of correcting the underlying disorder.

Over 50 percent of people with *AD* live in the community. The goal of nursing intervention is to facilitate optimal quality of life for both clients and caregivers and to manage problems as they arise. *Home care* can be a great challenge to families and health care professionals. The role of the nurse is to build therapeutic alliances with significant others and teach specific skills for caregiving. All of the following nursing interventions are *skills to be taught to caregivers*. In caring for clients with AD, patience and compassion are the guiding principles, with innovation and flexibility as the key elements. What works today may not work tomorrow. Because cognition underlies and directs behavior, clients' cognitive abilities guide the selection of appropriate nursing interventions. Even though the disorder is progressive and eventually terminal, it is

Behavior Assessment	Affective Assessment	Cognitive Assessment	Social Assessment
How much assistance is needed in: • Bathing? • Toileting? • Dressing? • Eating? Describe any difficulties in performing complex tasks at home and at work. Give me an example of something that has confused you recently. Have you ever become lost when you went out for a walk?	What kinds of things make you feel anxious? When do you feel sad? How often do you feel irritable? What are your major frustrations in life? How do you feel about growing older?	What month is it? What year is it? Who is the President of the United States? What is your telephone number (or address)? Where are you right now? Tell me your complete name. What did you do for activity this morning? What is the purpose of (show the objects to the client) a comb? Toothbrush? Pencil? Telephone book? Shoe? What is the meaning of the proverb "People in glass houses shouldn't throw stones"? What would you do if someone shouted "Fire!" right now?	How close do you feel to your family members? How do you handle disagreements?

important to support and encourage clients to remain at the highest possible level of functioning.

Safety: Risk Management

Delirium Management

Management of clients who are experiencing delirium includes initiating therapies to reduce or eliminate the factors that are causing the delirium. The neurological status of clients must be monitored on an ongoing basis. Clients benefit from nursing interventions designed to prevent or manage agitation, anxiety, and perceptual or cognitive disturbances. Whenever possible, interventions other than restraints, such as sitters, a foot or back massage, good lighting, and frequent observation, should be used to prevent delirious clients from harming themselves or others. Restraints often increase agitation and carry risks for injuries and are used only when other interventions fail. (For nursing care of clients who have hallucinations and/or delusions, see Chapter 9.)

Frequent contact, repeating of information, and reassurance will increase the client's orientation. Brief, simple statements are better understood than lengthy explanations. Give the client and family information about what is happening and what can be expected to occur in the future. Orient the client as necessary and avoid frustra-

Families of Clients with Cognitive Impairment Disorders

Behavior Assessment	Affective Assessment	Cognitive Assessment	Social Assessment
How much assistance is needed in activities of daily living?	Describe the degree of spontaneity to verbal and non-verbal stimuli.	Have there been changes in her or his ability to concentrate?	Is there a family history of organic brain disorder?
Tell me about her or his wandering away from home.	How anxious does she or he seem to you?	Describe any confusion about person, time, or place.	What are previous hobbies/interests? Family activities?
Is there difficulty in carrying out psychomotor activities?	How depressed does she or he seem to you?	Describe any suspicious thinking.	Who has been the primary caregiver?
Is she or he picking up and putting things in the mouth?	In what way is irritability increasing?	Describe any recent memory loss.	Describe the stresses in care-giving (emotional, physical, financial).
Does she or he touch everything in sight?	Does she or he have wide mood swings? Describe.	Describe any remote memory loss.	Describe the positive aspects of caregiving.
What kinds of repetitive movements does she or he make?		Does she or he make up answers when facts cannot be remembered?	What kinds of support systems are you able to use? Family? Friends? Religious? Self-help groups?
Describe her or his interactions with other people.		Is there difficulty in finding the right word for objects?	What kinds of discussions have taken place regarding placement?
Is she or he withdrawn? Agitated? Aggressive?		Has she or he lost the ability to read and write?	What other kinds of living arrangements are possible?
Are the behavior problems worse at night?		Is there an inability to identify familiar sounds?	Who is involved in making these decisions?
		Give me examples of irrational decision making.	How united is the family in providing care?
		Has she or he thought that strangers were family members? Please give examples.	

tion through quizzing with questions that cannot be answered. Delirium is aggravated by visual and auditory impairment, and it is important that clients be given their glasses and hearing aids if appropriate. Make certain there is a visible clock and calendar in the room. All who come in contact with clients should provide reorientation by reminding them of where they are, the date and time, and what is happening to them.

Since both sensory deprivation and sensory overstimulation can worsen symptoms, you will need to adjust the environment according to the client's response. This is often a process of trial and error. Intensive care units are noisy environments with beeps, alarms, pumps, and respirators. This ongoing noise level may overstimulate the confused person with delirium. On the other hand, too quiet an environment may contribute to clients' intense focus on their altered perceptions and thoughts. In general, you will want enough light at all times to minimize shadows that may contribute to illusions (McCloskey & Bulechek, 1996).

Following recovery, clients and their families should be educated about the apparent cause of the delirium. It is important that they and future health care providers are aware of risk factors that may lead to delirium in the future.

NURSING DIAGNOSES with NOC & NIC

Clients with Cognitive Impairment Disorders

DIAGNOSIS	OUTCOMES	INTERVENTIONS
Impaired home maintenance management related to disorientation, wandering behavior, poor impulse control	*Safety Behavior:* Home Physical Environment: Individual or caregiver actions to minimize environmental factors that might cause physical harm or injury in the home	Dementia Management Environmental Management: Safety
Bathing/hygiene/dressing/grooming/feeding/self-care deficit related to an inability to sequence these skills	*Self-Care:* Activities of Daily Living: Ability to perform the most basic physical tasks and personal care activities	Dementia Management
Altered thought processes related to distractibility, decreasing judgment, memory loss, confabulation	*Cognitive Orientation:* Ability to identify person, place, and time	Reality Orientation
Impaired verbal communication related to aphasia, agraphia, agnosia	*Communication Ability:* Ability to receive, interpret, and express spoken, written, and nonverbal messages	Dementia Management
Caregiver role strain related to changing roles, physical exhaustion, financial problems	*Caregiver Lifestyle Disruption:* Disturbances in the lifestyle of a family member due to caregiving *Caregiver Well-Being:* Primary care provider's satisfaction with health and life circumstances	Family Involvement
Risk for violence directed at others related to labile emotions, aggressive behavior	*Aggression Control:* Self-restraint of assaultive, combative, or destructive behavior toward others	Environmental Management: Safety

SOURCES: Johnson, M., Maas, M., & Moorhead, S. (2000). *Nursing outcomes classification (NOC)* (2nd ed.). St. Louis, MO: Mosby; McCloskey, J. C., & Bulechek, G. M. (1996). *Nursing interventions classification (NIC)* (2nd ed.). St. Louis, MO: Mosby; and North American Nursing Diagnoses Association (1999). *Nursing diagnoses definitions and classification 1999–2000.* Philadelphia: Author.

Dementia Management

Focusing on the strengths and abilities of people with dementia, as opposed to problems and disabilities, may counteract negative views held by some health care providers. This positive focus may also prevent excess disability. Caregivers should identify small, achievable goals on which they can build success as opportunities arise. Flexible consistency is the most effective approach when caring for people with dementia (Wells & Dawson, 2000).

Communication with clients is an extremely important nursing intervention. See Box 18.1 for ways to improve communication with clients. Attempts to communicate are more likely to be successful when

---

BOX 18.1

Improving Communications

- Reduce background noise.
- Speak only when you can be seen so your facial expression can provide visual cues to the meaning of your words.
- Address by name.
- Speak slowly to compensate for decreased ability to process information.
- Ask only one question at a time and wait for the response.
- Give instructions one step at a time.
- When possible, demonstrate actions you want the person to take—miming and gestures can increase understanding.
- Pictures may increase understanding.
- Learn the limits of the person's attention span.
- Be quick with praise and encouragement.

---

environmental distractions and noise are kept to a minimum. Begin each conversation by identifying yourself and addressing clients by name to orient them and get their attention. Speak slowly and distinctly, in a low tone or voice, conveying a sense of calm. Because these clients may not be able to comprehend complex language, use clear, simple sentences. Do not demean the person or use baby talk; clients can often comprehend the emotional tone of speech even when they can no longer understand the words. Closed-ended questions are easier to respond to than open-ended questions; ask only one question at a time. Pronouns are often misunderstood, and clients may respond more appropriately to direct address, as in "Mary, it is time to eat now." Using nonverbal communication such as smiles, hugs, gestures, and handholding will reinforce verbal communication. Above all, remember that these clients are adults and should be treated with respect and dignity.

Life review or *reminiscence therapy* is a guided recollection in which clients are encouraged to remember the past and share their memories with family, peers, or staff. Reminiscence therapy focuses on strengths and does not encourage people to dwell on losses. It can raise self-esteem and increase social intimacy. When doing a life review, choose a comfortable setting and set aside adequate time. Use pictures and memorabilia as cues. Encourage verbal expression of feeling of past

events. Comment on the feelings that accompany the memories in an empathic manner. Use direct questions to refocus back to life events if clients digress. By encouraging older adults to tell you about their lives, you can learn about hope, grief, achievement, and loss. It is a way you can communicate caring while helping them maintain their sense of identity (Haight, 2001).

Involvement with their environment is important for clients with AD. Caregivers should plan regular *social activities.* Clients are often more capable than either they or their families realize, and there may be any number of simple tasks they could do by themselves. Performing simple tasks around the home keeps them busy and helps them feel good about themselves.

Studies have shown that *exercise* decreases disruptive behaviors and increases appropriate interactions with others. It is important that they be provided with regular exercise such as walking, group exercise, or dancing. The rhythmic motions of exercise may be a way to meet the need for the repetitive behavior that occurs in Alzheimer's clients. They may participate in exercise more willingly if others exercise with them. Having a regular routine (same time, same exercises) will minimize confusion. If the client is unsteady, a supportive person should be nearby to prevent falls and injuries. Consistent, low-impact exercise will increase the oxygenation of the brain, slow the loss of motor function, and increase energy and feelings of well-being and accomplishment.

Music therapy is used to reduce the effects of stress and improve the quality of life for clients with AD. Singing, drumming, or moving to music may decrease aggressive outbursts, reduce agitation, lessen anxiety, improve affect, and increase perceptual, motor, and verbal skills.

Because many clients suffering from Alzheimer's disease experience sleep problems, actions to *improve sleep* will benefit both clients and families. Encourage clients and family members to keep a sleep journal to establish baseline data. The journal should answer such questions as: How many daytime naps are being taken? How many times a night does the client awaken? What medications are being taken? Several factors may exacerbate sleep problems. Pain, as from arthritis, can make sleep more difficult. Caffeine intake, eating rich foods near bedtime, fluid intake in the evening, and exercising too close to bedtime can be detrimental. Interventions include minimizing napping during the

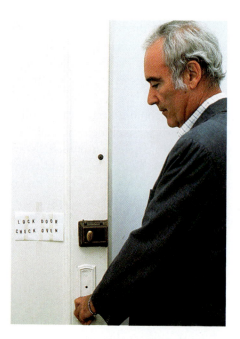

PHOTO 18.3 ■ People with dementia can remain active longer by using signs to prompt their behavior. This man is reminded to lock the door when he leaves his apartment.

SOURCE: Ira Wyman/Corbis/Sygma.

daytime, regular exercise but not too close to bedtime, modifying the environment by decreasing noise, and providing comfort measures such as back rubs.

Instruct caregivers to maintain a *regular schedule* of mealtimes to prevent confusion that is caused by change. Limit the number of foods in front of clients since they may have difficulty deciding which food to eat. Provide utensils with large built-up handles or use finger foods when lack of coordination interferes with eating. Try using bowls rather than plates, and offer soup in a mug. This is easier because food is not pushed off a plate and liquid is not spilled from a spoon. Remove other distractions from the eating area to maintain the focus on eating. Do not rush eating, since people with AD often eat slowly.

Encourage *ADL skills* that are still present to maintain independence and provide opportunities for clients to feel a sense of competence. Try to follow old routines as much as possible, such as time of day for a bath or preference for a bath or a shower. If there is a severe short-term memory problem, frequent reminders about the activity may be necessary. Clients should be encour-

aged to make as many decisions as possible in ADLs. This increases their sense of control and prevents the disengagement that occurs when all responsibility is taken away. Lay out clean clothes in the order to be put on. Velcro tape instead of buttons and zippers is often helpful (Kolanowski & Whall, 2000).

Environmental Management: Safety

Even first-stage AD can impair driving to some extent, and the risk of accidents increases with increasing severity of the dementia. Discuss the *risks of driving* with clients and caregivers. Explore clients' current driving patterns, transportation needs, and possible alternatives. These issues should be reassessed frequently. At some point, caregivers will need to prevent clients' driving. Encourage them to lock the car keys in a cabinet, hide the garage door controller, and learn easily reversible ways to disable the car.

Caregivers must *minimize hazards* in the home because people with Alzheimer's disease suffer from poor judgment. Objects that may be potentially dangerous must be locked up or removed, including irons, power tools, paints, solvents, stove knobs, and cleaning agents. The water heater should be turned to a lower temperature to prevent accidental burning. Paint hot water faucets and knobs red. Remove footstools, extension cords, and throw rugs that can lead to tripping, as well as table lamps, vases, and other breakables that are easily knocked over.

The client should be prohibited from smoking or be provided with supervision in order to prevent burns or fires. Prescribed medications can become a hazard when clients take the wrong medication, too much medication, or the right medication at the wrong time. Since memory loss interferes with correct self-administration, it is often appropriate for caregivers to administer the medications. Rid the home of firearms and poisonous plants and put safety locks on cabinets containing harmful substances.

Family members and/or institutional staff members need to be taught measures to *reduce potential injury from wandering* or becoming lost. Provide clients with an ID bracelet and ID card. Have the family register with the Safe Return program through the Alzheimer's Association (1-800-621-0379). If the client can still read and comprehend, a family member can write out simple directions home, along with the home phone number. Family members should assess the neighborhood for potentially dangerous areas such as busy streets, swimming pools, rivers, and bridges. Other people living in the neighborhood can be alerted to the situation, which will increase protection for the client. If the client is wandering away from the home, the yard can be fenced in with locked gates. The doors to the house should be kept locked, and an alarm system can be connected to the doors. This will prevent the person from slipping out unnoticed. Wandering is often decreased in clients who are provided regular outlets for exercise.

Many clients will require *safety measures* regarding impaired physical mobility, which might be evidenced by stiffness, awkwardness, and unsteadiness. Keep furniture in the same places and provide good lighting. Pad sharp corners, and discard throw rugs to minimize the likelihood of falls. If the client is unsteady, a supportive person should be nearby to help maintain balance. Handrails on staircases and in bathrooms provide additional support. If the client is unable to sit unassisted, a posey chair may be helpful.

As many as 33 percent of clients with AD become physically abusive to their caregivers. Steps should be taken to ensure the safety of client, family, and staff. *Catastrophic reactions* may occur when clients feel overwhelmed and overstimulated. Rapid questions, excessive commands, and too much noise and activity can provoke the response. Criticism and conflict may also contribute. Clients may respond with anger, stubbornness, agitation, and combativeness. The first step is to respond calmly and not retaliate with anger. Remember that the client's anger is often exaggerated and displaced. Remove objects in the environment that may be used to harm self or others. Try to understand what precipitated the aggressive behavior. Some clients may perceive that they are being threatened, and the aggressive behavior may be an attempt to defend themselves. Determine whether the client behaves this way toward everyone in the environment or only to specific people. Some clients become aggressive when they have pain and believe nothing is being done to help them. Accurately identifying precipitating events increases one's ability to prevent or minimize recurrence. Finally, clients should be removed from the upsetting situation or environment. Distractions are often effective because impaired memory makes them forget what caused the immediate anger. Catastrophic reactions can be avoided by:

- Keeping requests relatively simple to avoid frustration
- Avoiding confrontation and deferring requests if client becomes angry
- Being consistent and avoiding unnecessary change
- Providing frequent reminders, explanations, and orientation cues
- Ignoring inappropriate behavior that is not harmful
- Avoiding crowds, strangers, confusion, and noise

Behavioral: Cognitive Therapy
Reality Orientation

Use the name clients prefer to reinforce their identity. *Provide aids* that assist with orientation, such as large-print calendars, clocks, and labels on objects in the environment. Be selective regarding media and avoid programs with intricate plots or frightening content. If clients are using confabulation to reduce their shame or embarrassment about memory losses, give cues to help them remember reality and gently remind them of what actually occurred by filling in information gaps. Routinely and frequently orient clients to who, where, and what is happening, which allows them to become oriented without shame. Do not argue or persist in trying to convince clients of actual reality. When confusion is irreversible, this will only increase confusion and frustration. Discuss topics meaningful to clients, such as work, hobbies, children, or significant life events, as these topics promote their identity.

Caregivers can establish measures to decrease agitation and disorientation. The *physical environment* should be kept stable to increase comfort and decrease frustration and agitation. ADLs should be scheduled at a regular time. As much as possible, encourage clients to participate in decisions regarding their care. If appropriate, you should make certain that clients are wearing their glasses and hearing aids. Poor vision and hearing deficits will increase the potential for confusion.

Family: Life Span Care
Family Involvement

As a nurse, you must be an *advocate* for family caregivers. Families are often in need of teaching and counseling, support groups, and respite care. Help them locate local resources and develop support networks (see Community Resources feature at the end of this chapter). Peer support through dementia caregiver groups

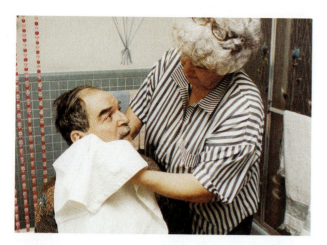

PHOTO 18.4 ■ Individuals who care for people with dementia assume an enormous burden. Respite programs attempt to provide assistance to these individuals.

SOURCE: Richard Falco/Black Star.

lessens the alienation and the sense of inadequacy that caregivers often experience. Other benefits of support groups include caregiving tips, suggestions on negotiating with community agencies, and overcoming practical and emotional barriers. By decreasing caregiver burden, these groups may improve the quality of life for clients and their families. Other resources that might help include social service agencies, home health agencies, cleaning services, Meals on Wheels, transportation programs, geriatric law specialists, and financial planners.

There are three typical conflicts that family member's experience in caring for their loved one with dementia. There are disagreements over the diagnosis and treatment plan, conflict over the quantity and quality of care, and different ideas about who should provide care and to what extent various family members share in the care. *Family meetings* are often necessary to help individuals express their views and for the family to gain consensus when possible.

In the early stage of the disease, clients and families should discuss *end-of-life care* issues. Advanced directives regarding feeding tubes, respirators, hemodialysis, and cardiac resuscitation should be carefully discussed. The appointment of a durable power of attorney for health care decisions and for financial decisions should be made while the client is still able to participate in the decision-making process.

Caregivers need breaks from a very stressful job. They may need assistance in developing coping strategies that deal directly with specific problems, as well as the multitude of emotions they are experiencing. *Respite care* provided by other family members or through adult day care programs may limit the sense of being overwhelmed by the combination of hard work and personal loss associated with caring for a person with AD. Discuss the need for periods of rest and recreation to prevent total emotional and physical fatigue of caregivers. Since clients are unable to provide positive feedback to caregivers, discuss how they might seek rewards and recognition apart from clients. Families need to keep their expectations realistic. Their loved ones with AD will not get better, but with good caregiving, clients can maintain independence and dignity for a long time.

Evaluation

To complete the nursing process, you evaluate clients' responses to nursing interventions based on the outcomes you selected. You determine the appropriate intervals for measurement and document the condition of clients according to each individual's status. Johnson, Maas, and Moorhead (2000) is the resource for identifying measurement scales and specific indicators for each outcome.

Safety Behavior: Home Physical Environment

Clients stop driving and smoking when safety becomes a concern. Clients self-administer medications correctly. Clients do not wander and get lost in the neighborhood. They do not fall accidentally.

Self-Care: Activities of Daily Living

Caregivers support clients' abilities in bathing, toileting, and dressing themselves. When independence is no longer possible, appropriate assistance is provided.

Cognitive Orientation

Clients remain oriented in all spheres when cues are provided. Family members use pictures to label objects and rooms in the home.

Communication Ability

Clients acknowledge that someone is speaking to them. They respond to nonverbal communication. Clients discuss topics meaningful to them personally.

CLINICAL INTERACTIONS — A Client with Dementia of the Alzheimer's Type

Ray, 72 years old, has been experiencing symptoms of Alzheimer's disease for the past several years. For the past year he has been attending a day program for persons with Alzheimer's disease. His daughter drops him off on her way to work and picks him up on her way home. If outside appointments need to be scheduled during that time, the staff of the day program provides transportation. Ray's daughter has forgotten to inform the staff about Ray's appointment to have his hair cut. In the interaction, you will see evidence of:

- Confusion with pronouns: Ray uses "we" to mean "I."
- Difficulty comprehending even small changes in schedule
- Loss of short-term memory
- An inability to remember the word *barber*

NURSE: Ray, we are going to have lunch 30 minutes earlier today because it is the day for the music therapist to be here with us.

RAY: We go to lunch at 12.

NURSE: It is necessary to have lunch now.

RAY: We don't want to go now.

NURSE: Please come with me. It is time to go to lunch.

RAY: We won't go now.

NURSE: It's time to go to lunch.

RAY: We go at 12!

NURSE: It's time for lunch.

RAY: [throwing up his hands] Okay, okay. [Ray eats and returns to the day room.]

RAY: We have an appointment at 2 P.M.

NURSE: Can you tell me what that appointment is for?

RAY: It's at 2 P.M.

NURSE: Do you know where you are supposed to go for the appointment?

RAY: Main Street.

NURSE: Do you know where you are supposed to go on Main Street?

RAY: Main Street. That's where we have to go.

NURSE: Can you give me any other hints as to where you are supposed to go?

RAY: We need the wallet.

NURSE: You need your wallet. Is it a store?

RAY: We need the wallet.

NURSE: Do you need to buy something?

RAY: Hair.

NURSE: Hair. Did you make an appointment at the barbershop?

RAY: Yes.

NURSE: I need to take you to your barbershop on Main Street at 2 P.M.

RAY: We have an appointment at 2 P.M.

NURSE: I will make certain that you get to your hair appointment by 2 P.M.

Aggression Control

Clients exhibit less agitation and combativeness. They verbalize a feeling of safety. Family members identify precipitating events and minimize their occurrence.

Caregiver Lifestyle Disruption

Families utilize support groups and respite care. They report an increased sense of competency and decreased sense of caregiver burden. Clients and families discuss end-of-life care issues while the client is still able to do this.

To build a Care Plan for a client with a cognitive impairment disorder, go to the Companion Web site for this book.

CHAPTER REVIEW

COMMUNITY RESOURCES

Links to these Web sites can be accessed on the Companion Web site for this book.

Alzheimer's Association
919 North Michigan Ave.
Chicago, IL 60611-1676
800-272-3900
www.alz.org

Alzheimer's Outreach
www.zarcrom.com/users/alzheimers

ALZwell Alzheimer's Caregivers' Page
www.alzwell.com

Eldercare Locator
800-677-1116

National Family Caregivers Association
10605 Concord St., Suite 501
Kensington, MD 20895-2504
800-896-3650

BOOKS FOR CLIENTS AND FAMILIES

Hendershott, A. (2000). *The reluctant caregivers.* Westport, CT: Bergin & Garvey.

Hodgson, H. (1998). *The Alzheimer's caregiver: Dealing with the realities of dementia.* Minneapolis, MN: Chronimed.

Hoffman, S., & Platt, C. (2000). *Comforting the confused: Strategies for managing dementia.* New York: Spinger.

Mace, N., & Rabins, P. (1999). *The 36-hour day: A family guide to caring for persons with Alzheimer's disease* (3rd ed.). Baltimore, MD: Johns Hopkins University Press.

Marcell, J. (2001). *Elder rage or take my father . . . please: How to survive caring for aging parents.* Irvine, CA: Impressive Press.

KEY CONCEPTS

Introduction

- Dementias are chronic, irreversible brain disorders characterized by impairments in memory, abstract thinking, and judgment, as well as changes in personality. Dementia of the Alzheimer's type (AD) accounts for 80 percent of dementing illnesses. Familial Alzheimer's disease (FAD) begins at a much younger age, and first-degree relatives have a 50 percent risk of developing the disorder.

- Other forms of dementia result from multiple infarctions in the CNS and from degenerative nervous system disorders, and are secondary to other disorders such as AIDS, drug intoxication, Korsakoff's syndrome, CNS neoplasms, and head injuries.

- Delirium is an acute, usually reversible brain disorder characterized by clouding of the consciousness, a reduced ability to focus and maintain attention, and altered perception. It may be the result of a wide variety of pathophysiological conditions.

Knowledge Base: Dementia

- Behavioral characteristics of dementia include a decline in personal appearance, socially unacceptable behavior, wandering, apraxia, hyperorality, perseveration phenomena, hyperetamorphosis, sundown syndrome, and a deterioration in motor ability. Psychotic symptoms may occur with hallucinations, delusions, and aggressive behavior.

- Affective characteristics of dementia include anxiety, depression, helplessness, frustration, shame, lack of spontaneity, and irritability. Moods are often labile, and catastrophic reactions are common.

- Cognitive characteristics of dementia include memory loss, poor judgment, disorientation, language problems, delusions of persecution, confabulation, aphasia, agraphia, and agnosia.

- Families are typically the primary caregivers for people with dementia. As such, they risk emotional and physical fatigue and financial hardship. They need to be encouraged to use supportive resources.

■ Deterioration of the CNS results in physical changes such as hypertonia, impaired sleep cycles, injuries from falls, slowed reaction time, and eventually, death.

■ As the disease progresses, tangles and plaques develop in the brain. The first cells to die are in the limbic system. The destruction of neurons then spreads throughout the four lobes of the cerebral cortex. Symptoms correlate with destruction of various parts of the brain.

■ There are several reversible disorders that can masquerade as dementia. Referred to as pseudodementias, these include depression, drug toxicity, metabolic disorders, infections, and nutritional deficiencies.

■ FAD has a stronger genetic link. It appears that chromosomes 1, 14, 19, and 21 may play a role in the development of this disease. APOE, produced in the brain, changes the form of amyloid, the principal component of the plaques associated with AD.

■ Individuals with AD have low levels of ChAT and ACh.

■ An environmental risk for AD is traumatic head injury.

■ Protective factors for AD include estrogen, NSAIDs, and cigarette smoking.

■ The drugs Aricept (donepezil), Exelon (rivastigmine), and Reminyl (galantamine) slow the breakdown of ACh, thereby increasing the amount available for neurotransmission. Vitamin E and Eldepryl (selegiline) may slow the rate of functional decline. Haldol (haloperidol), an antipsychotic, may help regulate sleep.

■ Alternative therapies include antioxidants, omega-3 fish oil, Ptd Ser, melatonin, DHEA, SAMe, lecithin, and music therapy.

Knowledge Base: Delirium

■ Behavioral characteristics of delirium include an alteration in psychomotor activity, poor impulse control, apathy and withdrawal, agitation, and bizarre and destructive behavior.

■ Affective characteristics of delirium may range from apathy to irritability to euphoria, and they may change abruptly.

■ The main cognitive characteristics are disorganized thinking, difficulty focusing attention, and easy distractibility. Additional characteristics include recent memory difficulties, disorientation, illusions, hallucinations, and delusions.

■ Because of the sudden and often unexplained onset of delirium, families are usually anxious, frightened, and confused.

■ Physiological characteristics of delirium include disturbance in sleep cycles, increased autonomic activity, and irregular tremors throughout the body.

■ Delirium occurs in people of all ages, but the incidence increases with age. Any physical illness has the potential to cause delirium.

■ Concomitant disorders that increase the risk of delirium include decreased blood flow to the liver and kidneys, AD, terminal cancer, and AIDS. The use of physical restraints can contribute to the onset of delirium.

■ Pseudodelirium describes symptoms of delirium that occur without any identifiable organic cause.

■ Intravenous Haldol is the most effective method of controlling the symptoms of delirium.

The Nursing Process

Assessment

■ Client assessment must include the family's perception of changes because the client is not considered a reliable source of accurate information.

■ Nurses must assess for other disorders that may mimic dementia. These include drug and alcohol abuse, visual or hearing problems, metabolic and endocrine diseases, emotional disorders, nutritional deficiencies, CNS tumors or trauma, infections, and arteriosclerosis.

Diagnosis

■ Nursing diagnoses relevant to caring for clients with cognitive impairment disorders range from impaired home maintenance, to altered thought processes, impaired verbal communication, risk for violence, and caregiver role strain.

Outcome Identification and Goals

■ Since dementia is a progressive disorder, outcomes are developed to maintain the highest level of functioning that is possible at any given time.

Nursing Interventions

■ In caring for clients with delirium, all measures must be taken to ensure that permanent brain damage or death does not occur.

■ Keeping the client safe is a priority. Interventions include measures to reduce potential injury from wandering or becoming lost, measures to decrease agitation and disorientation, measures to manage aggressive behavior, safety measures regarding impaired physical mobility, and steps to minimize specific hazards in the environment.

KEY CONCEPTS *(continued)*

■ Finding ways to communicate with clients is an extremely important nursing intervention. You will be most successful when you decrease environmental distractions, identify yourself and clients by name, speak slowly and distinctly, use simple sentences, give instructions one step at a time reinforced with demonstrations, and use touching and smiling to reinforce verbal communications.

■ Develop plans to include clients in regular social activities and exercise routines. Many clients can be responsible for simple daily tasks.

■ Interventions to improve sleep patterns will benefit both clients and families.

■ Encourage clients and families to seek legal guidance early in the disease process, when clients are still able to make their wishes known.

■ The overall goal of nursing intervention is to help maintain the quality of life in spite of impairments. Nurses must also function as advocates for family caregivers.

■ For the client who is experiencing delirium, the environment must be adapted according to the client's response.

Evaluation

■ Evaluation of nursing care is based on progress toward the outcome criteria by the client and family.

EXPLORE *MediaLink*

■ Interactive resources, including animations, for this chapter can be found on the Companion Web site at *http://www.prenhall.com/fontaine.* Click on Chapter 18 and select the activities for this chapter.

■ For NCLEX review questions and an audio glossary, access the accompanying CD-ROM in this book.

REFERENCES

Adams, T., & Page, S. (2000). New pharmacological treatments for Alzheimer's disease: Implications for dementia care nursing. *Journal of Advanced Nursing, 31*(5), 1183–1188.

American Psychiatric Association. (2000). *Diagnostic and statistical manual of mental disorders* (4th ed., Text Revision). Washington, DC: Author.

Balch, J. F., & Balch, P. A. (2000). *Prescription for nutritional healing* (3rd ed.). Garden City Park, NY: Avery.

Brown, R. P., & Gerbarg, P. L. (2000). Integrative psychopharmacology. In P. R. Muskin (Ed.), *Complementary and alternative medicine and psychiatry* (pp. 1–66). Washington, DC: American Psychiatric Press.

Brown University Geriatric Psychopharmacology Update. (2001). Memantine looks promising for moderate to severe AD. 5(8), 1–3, *www.medscape.com/ Manisses/GPU/2001/v05.n08.*

Chapman, F. M., Dickinson, J., McKeith, I., & Ballard, C. (1999). Association among visual hallucinations, visual acuity, and specific eye pathologies in Alzheimer's disease. *American Journal of Psychiatry, 156*(12), 1983–1985.

Carper, J. (2000). *Your miracle brain.* New York: HarperCollins.

Chemerinski, E., Petracca, G., Sabe, L., Kremer, J., & Starkstein, S. E. (2001). The specificity of depressive symptoms in patients with Alzheimer's disease. *American Journal of Psychiatry, 158*(1), 68–72.

Chun, M. R. (1998). The epidemiology of dementia among the elderly. In M. F. Folstein (Ed.), *Neurobiology of primary dementia* (pp. 1–26). Washington, DC: American Psychiatric Press.

Colling, K. B. (2000). A taxonomy of passive behaviors in people with Alzheimer's disease. *Journal of Nursing Scholarship, 32*(3), 239–244.

Cummings, J. L. (2000). Cholinesterase inhibitors: A new class of psychotropic compounds. *American Journal of Psychiatry, 157*(1), 4–15.

Folstein, S. E., & Folstein, M. F. (1998). Genetic counseling in Alzheimer's disease and Huntington's disease. In M. F. Folstein (Ed.), *Neurobiology of primary dementia* (pp. 329–364). Washington, DC: American Psychiatric Press.

Fontaine, K. L. (2000). *Healing practices: Alternative therapies for nursing.* Upper Saddle River, NJ: Prentice Hall.

Garand, L., & Hall, G. R. (2000). The biological basis of behavioral symptoms in dementia. *Issues in Mental Health Nursing, 21*(1), 91–107.

Haight, B. K. (2001). Life reviews: Helping Alzheimer's patients reclaim a fading past. *Leadership, 27*(1), 20–25.

Hamdy, R. C., Turnball, J. M., & Edwards, J. (1994). *Alzheimer's disease: A handbook for caregivers.* (2nd ed.). St. Louis, MO: Mosby.

Heyman, A. (1998). Head trauma as a risk factor for Alzheimer's disease. In M. F. Folstein (Ed.), *Neurobiology of primary dementia* (pp. 205–212). Washington, DC: American Psychiatric Press.

Huang, W., Alexander, G. E., Daly, E. M., Shetty, H. U., Krasuski, J. S., Rapoport, S. J., et al. (1999). High brain myo-inositol levels in the predementia phase of Alzheimer's disease in adults with Down's syndrome. *American Journal of Psychiatry, 156*(12), 1879–1886.

Johnson, M., Maas, M., & Moorhead, S. (2000). *Nursing outcomes classification (NOC)* (2nd ed.). St. Louis, MO: Mosby.

Keltner, N. L., Zielinski, A. L., & Hardin, M. S. (2001). Drugs used for cognitive symptoms of Alzheimer's disease. *Perspectives in Psychiatric Care, 37*(1), 31–34.

Kennedy, G. J. (2000). *Geriatric mental health care.* New York: Guilford Press.

Kolanowski, A. M., & Whall, A. L. (2000). Toward holistic theory-based intervention for dementia behavior. *Holistic Nursing Practice, 14*(2), 67–76.

Kovach, C. R. (2000). Sensoristasis and imbalance in persons with dementia. *Journal of Nursing Scholarship, 32*(4), 379–384.

Kumar, A. M., Tims, F., & Gruess, D. G. (1999). Music therapy increases serum melatonin levels in patients with Alzheimer's disease. *Alternative Therapies, 5*(6), 49–57.

Lyketsos, C. G., Steinberg, M., Tschanz, J. T., Norton, M. C., Steffens, D. C., & Breitner, J. C. S. (2000). Mental and behavioral disturbances in dementia. *American Journal of Psychiatry, 157*(5), 708–714.

Lyketsos, C. G., Steele, C., Galik, E., Rosenblatt, A., Steinberg, M., Warren, A., et al. (1999). Physical aggression in dementia patients and its relationship to depression. *American Journal of Psychiatry, 156*(1), 66–71.

McCloskey, J. C., & Bulechek, G. M. (1996). *Nursing interventions classification* (2nd ed.). St. Louis, MO: Mosby.

Miller, M. A. (2001). Regulation of galanin in memory pathways. In J. T. Hokfelt, T. Bartfal, & J. Crawley (Eds.), *Galanin: Basic research discoveries and therapeutic implications* (pp. 652–679). New York: Annals of New York Academy of Science.

Porter, R. J., Lunn, B. S., Walker, L. L. M., Gray, J. M., Ballard, C. G., & O'Brien, J. T. (2000). Cognitive deficit induced by acute tryptophan depletion in patients with Alzheimer's disease. *American Journal of Psychiatry, 157*(4), 638–640.

Practice guidelines for the treatment of patients with delirium. (1999). *American Journal of Psychiatry: Supplement, 156*(5), 1–20.

Prasad, K. N. (1998). Prostaglandins as putative neurotoxins in Alzheimer's disease. *Proceedings Society of Experimental Biology and Medicine, 219,* 120–125.

Roberts, J. S. (2000). Anticipating response to predictive genetic testing for Alzheimer's disease: A survey of first-degree relatives. *Gerontologist, 40*(1), 43–52.

Rowe, M. A., Straneva, J. A., Colling, K. B., & Grabo, T. (2000). Behavioral problems in community-dwelling people with dementia. *Journal of Nursing Scholarship, 32*(1), 55–56.

Seeman, M. V. (1997). Psychopathology in women and men: Focus on female hormones. *American Journal of Psychiatry, 154*(12), 1641–1646.

Shepherd, J. E. (2001). Effects of estrogen on cognition, mood, and degenerative brain disease. *Journal of American Pharmacology Association, 41*(2), 221–228.

Sullivan-Marx, E. M. (1994). Delirium and physical restraint in hospitalized elderly. *IMAGE, 26*(4), 295–300.

Wells, D. L., & Dawson, P. (2000). Description of retained abilities in older persons with dementia. *Research Nursing & Health, 23,* 158–166.

Wolkowitz, O. M., Petracca, G., Chemerinski, E., & Kremer, J. (1999). Double-blind treatment of major depression with dehydroepiandrosterone. *American Journal of Psychiatry, 156*(4), 646–649.

Yeaworth, R. C., & Burke, W. J. (2000). Frontotemporal dementia: A different kind of dementia. *Archives of Psychiatric Nursing, 14*(5), 249–253.

CHAPTER 19

Neuropsychiatric Problems

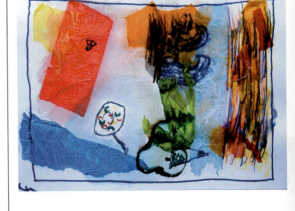

OBJECTIVES

After reading this chapter, you will be able to:

- IDENTIFY psychiatric problems associated with selected neurological disorders.

- ASSESS clients with selected neurological disorders for psychiatric symptoms.

- TEACH caregivers intervention strategies for managing psychiatric symptoms.

- EVALUATE the plan of care.

MediaLink

CD-ROM
- *Audio Glossary*
- *NCLEX Review*

Animation
- *T-cell Destruction by HIV*

Videos
Extrapyramidal Side Effects
- *Tremor—hands and arms*
- *Grasping tremor*
- *Lateral tremor*
- *Akinesia and pill rolling*
- *Bradykinesia—shuffling gait*

Companion Web site
www.prenhall.com/fontaine
- *Critical Thinking*
- *More NCLEX Review*
- *Case Study*
- *Care Map Activity*
- *Links to Resources*

C louds cover my face
I can only feel my fear
My eyes won't see, my lips won't breathe
I'm lost in a lonely breeze

I can only feel my fear
It wraps its wretched claws too tight
Knowing more than I
And as fear laughs with delight
Time passes slowly by

Knowing more than I
And not stopping to see if I care
Time passes slowly by
While I live in despair

—Anthony, Age 17 (painting)
—Anna, Age 19 (poetry)

T he focus of this chapter is on psychiatric problems associated with specific neurological disorders. The disorders presented in this chapter have variable causes, but all impose psychiatric disability to a greater or lesser extent. Helping you see the connection between central nervous system disruption and the psychiatric sequelae illustrates how the principles and skills of mental health nursing are basic to all nursing specialties. Anxiety, depression, delirium, dementia, psychosis, and aggression complicate the progression and treatment of these disorders. Psychiatric disorders must be considered on an ongoing basis since they can appear or resolve during the course of the illness (see Table 19.1 ■).

Other than a brief definition of each disorder, the concentration of this chapter is on the psychiatric components. You are referred to a medical–surgical or neurology text for detailed information on other aspects of these disorders. Likewise, you will find more detail about these mental health problems in the anxiety, mood, schizophrenia, and suicide disorders chapters. The disorders used to illustrate concepts of mental health nursing include degenerative disorders, dementias, seizure disorders, multifocal disruptions, infections, and traumatic brain injury.

KNOWLEDGE BASE

DEGENERATIVE DISORDERS
Parkinson's Disease

Parkinson's disease (PD) is a degenerative disease of the central nervous system caused by a deficit of dopamine (DA) secreted by cells of the basal ganglia. Muscle rigidity, difficulty initiating movement, resting tremor, weakness, gait disturbances, and a masklike face characterize the disorder. Parkinson's disease and the drugs used to treat it can also cause a wide range of psychiatric symptoms.

Dopamine not only plays an important role in motor ability, but is also involved in the motivation to act. *Apathy*, or reduced motivation, results from low levels of dopamine. People lose interest in activities previously enjoyable. Apathy interferes with the ability to be productive and the interest to try new activities. As a result, persons with Parkinson's disease may become increasingly withdrawn.

Thirty to fifty percent of sufferers develop *depression* at some time during their illness. Symptoms include feelings of hopelessness, helplessness, decreased self-esteem, and disruptions in eating and sleeping. Risk factors for depression include female gender, early age at onset, greater right-sided symptoms, and gait instability. In some instances, depression appears before motor symptoms. Protective factors for depression include low level of disability, positive social support, effective coping strategies, and an internal locus of control (Levy & Cummings, 2000).

About 40 percent of individuals with Parkinson's disease develop *anxiety disorders*, the most common being phobias, panic disorder, generalized anxiety disorder, and obsessive–compulsive disorder. The anxiety may occur with or without a concurrent depression. As Parkinson's disease progresses, individuals may become anxious in situations that earlier would not have

TABLE 19.1

Psychiatric Symptoms of Neuropsychiatric Problems

	Emotional Lability	Aggression	Anxiety	Depression	Cognitive Problems	Psychosis	Delirium	Dementia
Parkinson's disease			X	X				X
Huntington's disease	X	X	X	X	X	X		X
Pick's disease		X			X			
Creutzfeldt–Jakob disease					X		X	X
Epilepsy	X			X	X	X		
Multiple sclerosis	X			X	X			
Brain attack	X			X	X			
HIV/AIDS	X		X	X	X		X	X
PANDAS	X		X					
Lyme disease				X	X			
Traumatic brain injury			X	X				X

caused anxiety. In some instances, the anxiety is severe enough to cause people serious disruptions in their lives (Weiner, Shulman, & Lang, 2001).

Cognitive disruptions generally are not apparent until late in the disorder. Between 25 and 40 percent of individuals develop *dementia* with profound memory loss, confusion, and disruption in day-to-day functioning.

The medications used to treat Parkinson's disease may, in themselves, cause behavior changes and psychiatric symptoms. This is related to the length of time taking medications, higher doses over time, and the prescription of multiple medications. Many people experience vivid dreams and nightmares, so realistic as to be frightening. During the nightmare they may talk, scream, or make violent threatening movements referred to as *REM behavioral disorder*. Some develop *hallucinations,* which are usually visual and which may be threatening or nonthreatening in nature. Others develop *delusions,* which are often paranoid in nature. If the individual becomes extremely agitated and diffi-

cult to control, it is considered a medical emergency and admission to a safe environment is necessary until the medications are readjusted. These problems may be reduced or eliminated with a decreased dosage of antiparkinson medications (Barnes, David, Holroyd, Currie, & Wooten, 2001; Weiner et al., 2001).

Huntington's Disease

Huntington's disease (HD) is a hereditary neurodegenerative disorder characterized by an excess of undesired movement and lack of muscle tone. As the disorder progresses, movements become uncontrolled, resulting in purposeless, rapid motions such as flexing and extending the fingers, raising and lowering the shoulders, or grimacing. The duration of this disorder is typically 15 years.

Psychiatric symptoms are among the most common features of Huntington's disease and include affective and cognitive changes. About 30 percent of affected individuals develop severe *irritability* and episodic *aggressive* behavior. Some are unable to tolerate frustration, while others cannot delay gratification. Some obsess about a single request and become irritable when they are not accommodated. Irritability may alternate with *apathy* during which there is little desire to do anything. Families may label this behavior as "laziness," not understanding this as a symptom of the disease. Sadly, those with the disease may have little insight into this dramatic change in their personality (Kennedy, 2000).

Mood swings and bouts of *depression* are common experiences for about 30 percent of those with Huntington's disease. *Bipolar disorder* is a complication for 10 percent of sufferers. *Anxiety* over minor issues occurs early on in the illness. Obsessive–compulsive symptoms occur in about 25 percent of clients. Other complications include generalized anxiety disorder and panic disorder (Anderson, Louis, Stern, & Marder, 2001; Ranen, 2000).

People with Huntington's disease suffer from a global decrease in cognitive functioning. The changes begin with slowed thinking, decreased concentration and problem solving, and deterioration in quality of work. Visual *memory impairment* occurs early, while verbal memory remains intact until fairly late in the disease. For example, they may not be able to reproduce a design they saw, such as a square or a circle, but may remember words and stories. Orientation is usually intact until the late stages. Paranoid *delusions* are common but hallucinations are much less common. *Dementia* appears in all people with Huntington's disease, although the rate of progression and the extent of symptoms vary from individual to individual (Hayden, 2000; Williams, Schutte, Evers, & Forcucci, 1999).

FRONTAL LOBE DEMENTIAS

Frontal lobe dementias, caused by a variety of brain diseases, are often misdiagnosed as mental disorders because personality, sociability, and executive function are prominently impaired (Chun, 1998; Yeaworth & Burke, 2000). Frontal lobe dementias include Pick's disease and Creutzfeldt–Jakob disease.

Pick's Disease

Pick's disease is a rare form of a progressive dementia involving abnormal ballooning of neurons accompanied by atrophy of the frontal and temporal lobes. The disorder usually begins in middle age with a life span of 2 to 10 years following diagnosis. At the present time there is no known cause, treatment, or cure.

Pick's disease often begins with *socially uninhibited behaviors* and sudden *changes in personality*. Poor judgment, socially inappropriate interactions, and impulsive sexual behavior cause embarrassment to family and friends. Early in the disorder behaviors may include illegal acts such as stealing, sex crimes, or aggression toward others. These behaviors may contribute to a misdiagnosis of a primary mental disorder (e.g., schizophrenic or mood disorders) rather than a dementia.

Other psychiatric symptoms include euphoria, jealous delusions, poor insight, a lack of concern for loved ones, and inattentiveness to surroundings. In interactions with others, individuals with Pick's disease either lose attention to the conversation or simply repeat the words of the other person. As the disease progresses they may no longer recognize family and friends. Some experience *hyperorality*, the need to taste, chew, and examine any object small enough to be placed in the mouth. It is thought that a deficit of serotonin (5-HT) contributes to carbohydrate craving, overeating, and weight gain (Garand, Buckwalter, & Hall, 2000; Yeaworth & Burke, 2000).

Creutzfeldt–Jakob Disease

Creutzfeldt–Jakob disease (CJD) is rare fatal brain disorder that causes inevitable death within 2 to 12 months. CJD is the human equivalent of bovine spongiform encephalopathy or mad cow disease (CDJ Info, 2001; Windl & Kretzschmar, 2000). There are two different forms of CJD: (1) *classic*, which can arise spontaneously, be genetically transmitted, or be contracted via infection, and (2) *variant*, which is caused by eating diseased meat or cattle products. An infectious agent unlike any previously known pathogen causes CJD. This newly discovered pathogen is called a prion, short for proteinaceous infectious particle. **Prions** are small particles that resist inactivation and are thought to transform normal protein molecules into infectious ones, eventually eating spongy holes in the brain, that destroy the person's ability to function.

CJD has signs and symptoms similar to Alzheimer's disease, except that the mental deterioration occurs very rapidly. Affected persons suffer a bizarre range of symptoms such as *hallucinations*, seeing things upside down, ataxia, and hyperreflexia. *Memory* problems lead to confusion and disorientation. Speech becomes difficult for others to understand. Personality changes are obvious and there is a rapid decline into *delirium* and *dementia*. In the final stages, people lose all mental and physical function.

EPILEPSY

Epilepsy is unprovoked, recurring seizures caused by sporadic electrical discharge of neurons in the cerebral cortex leading to a wide spectrum of problems. It is one of the most common neurological disorders in the United States. The association between epilepsy and *schizophrenia-like psychosis* has long been noted. Psychotic symptoms are classified according to the phase of clinical seizures: *ictal* (the onset of an epileptic seizure) or *postictal* (after an epileptic seizure).

Ictal psychosis is usually brief, lasting hours to days. There may be a wide range of perceptual, behavioral, cognitive, and affective symptoms. Clients may experience *hyperorality* or *stereotypic behaviors* such as constant picking at clothing. They may become mute during the psychotic episode. *Hallucinations* and *thought distortions* are not uncommon. There is no change in the level of consciousness, and insight is usually maintained. Individuals with ictal psychosis often have amnesia for the episode (Sachdev, 1998).

Postictal psychosis usually follows seizure clusters or a recent increase in seizure frequency and occurs in as many as 7 to 10 percent of clients. The psychotic episode occurs within a few hours to a few days following the last seizure. Cognitive symptoms include grandiose, somatic, or religious *delusions* and ideas of reference. There may be some clouding of consciousness. Perceptual symptoms involve auditory *hallucinations*. Affective symptoms may be either *manic* or *depressive* in nature. Postictal psychosis disappears within a few days (Sachdev, 1998).

Sam, age 19, has a history of temporal lobe seizures. He has experienced a recent increase in the frequency of his seizures. For the last several days he has been bothering the neighbors at all times of the day and night wanting to discuss religion and asking if they have been saved. He explained his actions by telling everyone he was God. Even though the neighbors threatened to call the police, Sam wasn't worried because "who would call the police on God?"

MULTIFOCAL DISRUPTIONS
Multiple Sclerosis

Multiple sclerosis (MS) is a chronic disorder of the central nervous system (CNS) caused by destruction of the myelin sheath. The resulting scar tissue slows or blocks transmission of nerve impulses. Symptoms of MS range from relatively benign to somewhat disabling to devastating.

Psychiatric symptoms, which may appear even before the typical neurological symptoms, include cognitive dysfunction and mood disorders. Cognitive impairment is present in 55 to 65 percent of persons with MS. Basic language skills and verbal intelligence are not affected. Decreased *attention span* and *slowed information processing* are common problems. Clients are able to encode and store memories but may not be able to spontaneously recall those memories. Given cues, people with MS are able to retrieve memories. Repeated presentations of new material results in improved learning. *Executive functions* may be interrupted, resulting in decreased judgment, loss of the ability to think abstractly, and loss of the ability to generalize (Schwid, Weinstein, Wishart, & Schiffer, 2000).

When people cannot control their laughing and crying, they are said to have *labile affect*. This occurs for about 22 to 29 percent of people with MS. Laughing or crying may be exaggerated or completely inappropriate to the situation or the person's overall mood. As many as 10 percent of people with MS develop *bipolar disorder*, compared to less than 1 percent of the general population. Sixty percent of clients develop a *major depression* sometime during their illness and disability. The *suicide* rate is almost eight times higher than the general population. Affective symptoms are not necessarily correlated with the degree of disability, suggesting that they are independent of physical and mental deficits (Daly, Komaroff, Bloomingdale, Wilson, & Albert, 2001; Feinstein, 1999).

Linnea was diagnosed with MS three years ago and bipolar disorder 18 months ago. She has only very mild neurological symptoms with occasional tingling and numbness, mostly of the upper extremities. Her mother states that she is more confused lately, is getting messages from the television (ideas of reference), and
(continued)

disappears for days at a time. Linnea says that she has periods of severe fear during which she stays in her car in parking lots, afraid to go home, to the police, or to the hospital. During one of these episodes, she stayed in a stranger's home and during another one, she gave a stranger a ride home. Her family is very concerned because Linnea acts as if nothing is wrong and refuses to take responsibility for her behavior.

Brain Attack

Brain attack, also called a *stroke*, is a major cause of cerebrovascular dementia. The vast majority of brain attack (77 percent) is thrombic or embolic, leading to ischemia of brain tissue. The remaining 23 percent are hemorrhagic in origin. Brain attack is second only to Alzheimer's disease as a leading cause of dementia. Psychiatric symptoms include cognitive impairment, apathy, pathological emotions, and mood disorders (Chun et al., 1998).

Cognitive impairment is the most frequent psychiatric symptom following a brain attck. Individuals with left hemisphere destruction have difficulty with *orientation*, language, *executive functions* such as decreased judgment, and abstract thinking. *Apathy* is a frequent cognitive impairment that interferes with pleasure and activities of daily living and contributes to increased social withdrawal.

Affective problems include *emotional lability* as demonstrated by pathological laughing and crying. These episodes may be excessive to the situation, may appear spontaneously, or may be in response to non-emotional events. *Depression* is the most common mood disorder, affecting 20 to 50 percent of people who have experienced a brain attack. Half will suffer a major depression, and half will have a less severe form of depression (Robinson, 2000).

Interestingly, people who suffer from a primary depression may be at higher risk for a brain attack. Depressed people have a greater platelet activation and responsiveness than nondepressed individuals. 5-HT secretion by platelets produces aggregation or clumping of blood cells, which makes people with depression more susceptible to atherosclerosis, thrombosis, and vasoconstriction (Lenze, Cross, McKeel, Neuman, & Sheline, 1999).

George, who is 73 years old, has been admitted for major depression. He is upset that most of his children do not take care of him except his youngest son, who "respects" him. He recently went to his granddaughter's birthday party and thought family members ignored him. He claims his wife is abusing him physically and mentally. On admission he states, "People think I'm nuts. I'm not nuts. I'm just angry that my gun and car were taken away. I've been robbed of my independence." Three days after admission, the staff noticed that George was having difficulty following verbal directions and alternating between lethargy and agitation. He was noted to have difficulty swallowing food and liquids. His speech was slurred and he was drooling. Further assessment determined that George had suffered a brain attack.

INFECTIONS
HIV/AIDS

Direct involvement of the brain by HIV is known as HIV/AIDS encephalopathy. CNS involvement in HIV infection can result either from the direct effect of the virus on the brain or from secondary opportunistic infections and malignancies. HIV enters the brain by infecting monocytes that are able to cross the blood–brain barrier. This typically occurs early in the course of the infection and initially it is usually asymptomatic. Later psychiatric manifestations include delirium, dementia, mood disorders, and anxiety disorders (Maldonado, Fernandez, & Levy, 2000; Ungvarski & Trzcianowska, 2000).

Delirium is the most frequent psychiatric complication of AIDS, affecting as many as 40 to 65 percent of HIV-infected persons. Rapid recognition and treatment is necessary to prevent permanent brain damage (American Psychiatric Association Practice Guidelines, 2000).

Seventy percent of individuals with AIDS will develop HIV-associated minor cognitive disorder. Abnormalities of minor cognitive disorder include impaired attention or concentration, mental slowing, impaired memory, personality change, irritability, or emotional lability. Since orientation and insight are preserved, clients become very concerned and depressed over their loss of functioning. As neurotoxicity continues, problems become more pronounced and as many as 20 to 30 percent of infected individuals will develop HIV-associated *dementia* often referred to as AIDS dementia complex. At this point, individuals have difficulty processing information, impaired executive function, memory and learning problems, apathy, labile emotions, and inappropriate social behavior (American Psychiatric Association Practice Guidelines, 2000; Ungvarski & Trzcianowska, 2000).

Depression may be related to chronic stress such as social stigma, long-term physical discomfort and illness, and the prospect of eventual death. Only 10 percent of people with AIDS experience a major depression, leading researchers to believe that depression is not a direct result of HIV infection of the brain (Ciesla & Roberts, 2001).

Anxiety is a frequent problem among AIDS victims. It is estimated that 17 to 36 percent of clients will have an anxiety disorder sometime during their disability. The most common disorders are panic disorder, generalized anxiety disorder, and posttraumatic stress disorder (Maldonado, Fernandez, & Levy, 2000).

Although AIDS affects all people regardless of their age, gender, ethnicity, or sexual orientation, some populations may be at higher risk. One such group is persons who are psychiatrically disabled. The prevalence of HIV infection in the general population is 0.3 percent compared to 4 to 23 percent of psychiatrically disabled individuals. One of the risk factors is the high rate of alcohol and substance use among this population. Infection occurs directly through the sharing of contaminated needles. Substance use is also associated with unsafe sexual activities such as multiple partners, exchanging sex for money or drugs, and not using condoms. Psychiatrically disabled people are also at higher risk because of poor judgment, ineffective problem-solving skills, sexual impulsivity, a tendency toward taking chances, low motivation to alter sexual behaviors, and transient social relationships (Stoff, 1998).

Pediatric Autoimmune Neuropsychiatric Disorders

Pediatric autoimmune neuropsychiatric disorders (PANDAS) are a neurological complication associated with streptococcal infections in some children. The antibodies produced to fight the streptococci bacteria can trigger an autoimmune reaction. This reaction is most frequently directed against cells in the heart and joints (rheumatic fever) but in 20 to 30 percent of the cases it reacts with the basal ganglia, causing an antibody-mediated inflammation leading to CNS dysfunction (Swedo & Pekar, 2000).

There is some correlation between PANDAS and obsessive–compulsive disorder (OCD), Tourette's disorder, and attention deficit/hyperactivity disorder (ADHD). (See Chapter 17 for more information on these disorders.) Some children develop these disorders simultaneously with or subsequent to the autoimmune reaction. A number of children, however, have ADHD, tic disorders, and OCD before the occurrence of streptococcal infection. It is thought that these mental disorders may reflect a vulnerability to PANDAS (Hoekstra et al., 2001; Mercadante et al., 2000).

The symptoms of PANDAS are a sudden and dramatic onset of *obsessive–compulsive disorder (OCD), ADHD,* and/or *Tourette's disorder.* Affected children are described as having changed overnight. They exhibit classic OCD symptoms such as excessive handwashing, nighttime rituals, checking behavior, and obsessions about death. They may develop tics and sudden uncontrollable movement, grunts, and facial grimaces. They demonstrate a peculiar "squirminess" in which they try very hard to sit still but constantly wiggle and fidget in their chairs. Other symptoms include separation anxiety, age-inappropriate behavior, and nighttime difficulties including severe nightmares and new bedtime fears or rituals. Over 90 percent experience emotional lability with unprecipitated bouts of crying or hysterical laughter and increased irritability. In some children, PANDAS resolve completely; in others, the symptoms continue with less severity, and a few will have periods of acute symptom relapse (Giedd, Rapoport, Garvey, Perlmutter, & Swedo, 2000; Hoekstra et al., 2001; Swedo et al., 1998).

Lyme Disease

A small percentage of people with Lyme disease develop CNS symptoms months to years after diagnosis and treatment. **Lyme disease** is a tick-borne infection that may affect the skin, joints, heart, eyes, and CNS. Lyme meningitis may occur within the first few months after infection. Symptoms include irritability, headache, lethargy, and cognitive dysfunctions (Estanislao & Pachner, 1999).

Late-stage Lyme disease CNS involvement leads to

symptoms such as memory loss, naming problems, difficulty concentrating, fatigue, and depression. It is thought that these changes are the result of a diffuse inflammatory process in the basal ganglia and cerebral cortex. This is an extremely rare complication and usually responds to antibiotic therapy (Kaplan et al., 1999).

TRAUMATIC BRAIN INJURY

Traumatic brain injury is defined as a head injury caused by car accidents, falls, assaults, or sport injuries. In comparison with the general population, a higher percentage of people who have had a traumatic brain injury develop psychiatric illnesses within a year. The period of greatest risk for traumatic brain injuries is from the mid-teens through the mid-20s, before the onset of many major psychiatric disorders, contributing to the belief that the injury itself is associated with the onset of the psychiatric disorder. Behavioral, affective, and cognitive symptoms are more likely to prevent the return to work and social activities than are the physical deficits related to the injury (Deb, Lyons, Koutzoukis, Ali, & McCarthy, 1999).

Depression is the most common complication, occurring in 39 percent of people with a mild injury and in 77 percent of those with a severe injury. Depressive symptoms usually begin within the first six months after injury. *Anxiety* symptoms occur in 24 to 28 percent of people with traumatic head injury. Anxiety disorders include panic disorder and obsessive–compulsive disorder. There is also a high rate of sleep disorders, especially *nightmares*.

Psychosis following traumatic brain injury resembles schizophrenia. Reported rates range from 0.07 to 10 percent, with an increasing risk over time, compared to a rate of 0.8 percent of schizophrenia in the general population. The exact relationship between schizophrenia and traumatic brain injury is unclear. It may be a result of a gene–environment interaction. The traumatic brain injury (environment) may lower the threshold for the development of schizophrenia in those with genetic vulnerability to the disorder. Another possibility is that early symptoms of schizophrenia such as agitation or psychosis might increase vulnerability to traumatic brain injury. This vulnerability might be related to impaired attention and/or cerebellar dysfunction (Malaspina et al., 2001).

People with traumatic brain injury may be more susceptible to *Alzheimer's disease*. Traumatic brain injury may not cause Alzheimer's disease but may reduce the time to disease onset for those with a predisposition. People who have experienced severe head injuries have a significant increase in the deposition of amyloid protein in their brains. The injury may decrease the brain's functional reserves. It is also possible that damage to the blood–brain barrier allows entry of toxic products or somehow makes the brain more susceptible to the effects of aging (Malaspina et al., 2001).

CULTURE-SPECIFIC CHARACTERISTICS

In most of these neuropsychiatric disorders, we do not know why one person develops the disorder and another does not. Some have a genetic component, such as Parkinson's disease, Huntington's disease, CJD, and brain attack. Others such as seizure disorders, MS, HIV/AIDS, PANDAS, traumatic brain injury, and Lyme disease have a much stronger environmental risk. Most likely, most these neuropsychiatric disorders are caused by a combination of environmental and genetic factors.

Parkinson's disease is one of the most common neurodegenerative disorders in the United States and Canada. The racial distribution remains unclear. Some studies indicate similar frequency of Parkinson's disease for Euro-Americans and African Americans. Other studies suggest that the frequency is higher among Euro-Americans. Among the Japanese and some Europeans, there is a higher rate of young-onset Parkinson's disease (Gasser & Oertel, 2000; Weiner et al., 2001).

Little is known about the impact of race and culture on Huntington's disease. It appears to be less frequent in Japan, China, Finland, and Africa. The variant form of CJD appears to be related to the presence of infected cattle, which is then consumed by humans living in that geographical area. All but one case have been in the United Kingdom. Multiple sclerosis is more common in Euro-Americans of northern and central European ancestry. Groups that appear to be resistant to MS include Native People, Chinese, Japanese, and Lapps (Hayden, 2000; Sadovnick & Dyment, 2000).

The adult ticks that cause Lyme disease depend on the presence of deer for their survival. The population of ticks is determined by the number of deer in any given area. As many as 92 percent of the cases are found in 10 states: Connecticut, Rhode Island, New Jersey, New York, Pennsylvania, Delaware, Massachusetts, Wisconsin, Minnesota, and Maryland (Estanislao & Pachner, 1999).

AGE-SPECIFIC CHARACTERISTICS

The average age of onset of Parkinson's disease is 60 years, with 80 percent of all affected persons developing the disorder between 40 and 70 years. About 5 percent of sufferers are diagnosed between the ages of 30 and 40, which is referred to as young-onset Parkinson's disease. It is highly unusual for someone below the age of 30 to be diagnosed with this disorder, but there are a few cases of juvenile onset before the age of 20 (Weiner et al., 2001).

The average age of onset of Huntington's disease is 40 years. Ten percent develop the disorder before the age of 20 and 25 percent develop it after the age of 50. CJD affects most people in their 60s. The average age of onset for the variant type of CJD is younger with an average age of 29 years. Variant CJD has a longer duration, the average being 16 months before death. Pediatric autoimmune neuropsychiatric disorder is by definition a childhood disorder. The average age of onset is between 10 and 11 years (Mercadante et al., 2000; Windl & Kretzschmar, 2000).

Epilepsy has the highest occurrence in individuals under the age of 20. The next highest age group is over the age of 70 years. It is possible to determine the cause of epilepsy only in less than half of the cases. Common causes include congenital brain malformations, high fevers, head trauma, brain tumors, and brain attacks (Schachter, 2001).

PSYCHOPHARMACOLOGICAL INTERVENTIONS

Medications are prescribed to manage the specific *psychiatric symptoms* people are experiencing. The preferred drug for depression in Parkinson's disease is Paxil (paroxetine), which eases the depression without increasing motor fluctuations. Two antipsychotic medications, Clozaril (clozapine) and Seroquel (quetiapine) appear to improve memory and concentration while decreasing psychiatric symptoms. Risperdal (risperidone) and Zyprexa (olanzapine) are not prescribed, as they worsen the symptoms of Parkinson's disease (*Well-Connected*, 2001).

When people with post–brain attack depression are given antidepressants, their depression eases, as does the cognitive and social impairment that complicates the recovery from brain attack. Aventyl or Pamelor (nortriptyline) is a better choice than Prozac (fluoxetine) for individuals who have concurrent depression and medical illness. The side effects such as nausea, anorexia, and weight loss occur more frequently with Prozac (fluoxetine) in the elderly population (Robinson et al., 2000).

NURSING PROCESS

Assessment

In addition to a complete physical assessment, a careful history is needed from the client and family members. To maintain clients' sense of self-determination, the mental status assessment should begin with family members present and progress to an individual interview. If possible, you need to gain clients' permission to share information with the family. Emphasis is on openness and full disclosure, which is essential in the management of future deterioration, if that is the likely outcome.

Client assessment includes activities of daily living (ADLs). Obtaining information from family members may more accurately assess functional impairment, since the client may be unaware of impairments. Assessment of ADLs covers hygiene and grooming, household chores and responsibilities, quality of schoolwork or outside employment, and management of finances. Clients may appear in immaculate condition as a result of attentive caregivers, yet not be able to shop, cook, bathe, dress, or pay bills without total assistance.

Psychiatric symptoms or mental disorders may occur or remit during the course of the neurological illness and must be assessed on an ongoing basis. See the Focused Nursing Assessment feature for some general questions. More specific questions can be found in the chapters on anxiety, mood, schizophrenic, and spectrum disorders.

Behavior Assessment	Affective Assessment	Cognitive Assessment	Social Assessment
Describe any difficulties in performing complex tasks at home, school, or work.	What kinds of things make you feel anxious?	What year is it? Month?	How close do you feel to your family members?
Give me an example of something that has confused you recently.	When do you feel sad?	What is your telephone number? Address?	How do you handle disagreements?
Do you find yourself repeatedly checking or counting things?	How often do you feel irritable?	What would you do if you found a stamped, addressed envelope on the sidewalk?	
How much help do you need in ADLs?	What are your major frustrations?	Which one of the following objects does not belong in this group: car, dog, wagon, truck?	
		Do you hear voices that others say they do not hear?	

Diagnosis

Based on the assessment data, you develop any number of nursing diagnoses for the child or adult client. In synthesizing the assessment data, consider how well clients are functioning in daily life. See the Nursing Diagnoses with NOC and NIC feature for some of the more common nursing diagnoses you may be applying to your clients.

Outcome Identification and Goals

Once you have established diagnoses, you select outcomes appropriate to the nursing diagnoses. The more common outcomes are listed in the Nursing Diagnoses with NOC and NIC feature.

Client goals are specific behavioral measures by which you and significant others determine progress toward outcomes. The following are examples of some of the goals appropriate to people with neuropsychiatric disorders:

- Improved orientation as delirium clears
- Establishes routines to decrease confusion
- Remains oriented to person, time, and place
- Completes ADLs appropriate to functional level
- Improved levels of anxiety and depression
- Interacts appropriately with others

Nursing Interventions

Goals and outcome criteria help focus your nursing care. The overall goal is to help clients function more effectively in their social and emotional lives. The majority of nursing interventions appropriate to these clients are found in the chapters on anxiety, mood, cognitive, and spectrum disorders. You are encouraged to review and integrate that knowledge when working with people who are experiencing neuropsychiatric disorders. Physical nursing care is found in your medical–surgical and neurological nursing texts.

Safety: Risk Management
Delirium Management

The neurological status of clients experiencing delirium must be monitored on an ongoing basis. Clients benefit from nursing interventions designed to prevent or manage agitation, anxiety, and perceptual or cognitive disturbances. Whenever possible, interventions

Families of Clients with Neuropsychiatric Problems

Behavior Assessment	Affective Assessment	Cognitive Assessment	Social Assessment
Has there been a sudden change in behavior?	How anxious does she or he seem to you?	Have there been changes in her or his ability to concentrate?	Describe interactions with other people.
Is it difficult to get her or him involved in activities?	How depressed does she or he seem to you?	Describe any confusion about person, time, or place.	Does she or he embarrass you in social situations?
How much assistance is needed in ADLs?	In what way is irritability increasing?	Describe any recent or remote memory loss.	What are previous hobbies/interests? Family activities?
Is she or he withdrawn? Agitated? Aggressive?	Does she or he laugh and/or cry inappropriately?	Give me examples of irrational decision making.	What kinds of discussions have taken place regarding the future?
Does she or he have bizarre, uncontrolled physical motions?		Is there any evidence of delusions?	Who is involved in making these decisions?

other than restraints, such as sitters, should be used to prevent delirious clients from harming themselves or others. Restraints often increase agitation and carry risks for injuries and are used only when other interventions fail.

Frequent contact, repeating of information, and reassurance will increase the client's orientation. Brief, simple statements are better understood than lengthy explanations. Give the client and family information about what is happening and what can be expected to occur in the future. Orient the client as necessary and avoid frustration through quizzing with questions that cannot be answered. Provide a written schedule of ADLs and daily activities. Delirium is aggravated by visual and auditory impairment, and it is important that clients be given their glasses and hearing aids if appropriate. Make certain there is a visible clock and calendar in the room. All who come in contract with clients should provide reorientation by reminding them of where they are, the date and time, and what is happening to them.

Since both sensory deprivation and sensory overstimulation can worsen symptoms, you will need to adjust the environment according to the client's response. This is often a process of trial and error.

Behavioral: Psychological Comfort Promotion
Calming Technique

Calming techniques such as muscle relaxation and deep breathing are useful for managing the physiological dimensions of anxiety. Deep breathing replaces the shallow breathing that highly anxious people adopt unconsciously and prevents hyperventilation. The goal is to provide clients with a skill response so that they can experience anxiety without feeling overwhelmed. In addition to focusing on and relaxing specific muscle groups, teach clients to take a deep breath though the nose, inhaling to the count of five, and then exhaling to the count of five. Progressive relaxation should be practiced twice a day for 20 minutes. It will be several weeks before clients experience significant benefit. Even fairly young children can be taught this technique. Children often enjoy this exercise, and it helps them recognize when their bodies are tightening up. Eventually, they learn how to cope with stress by breathing deep and then shaking it off.

Other calming techniques you can teach clients involve changing their sensory experiences or getting involved in activities. Some people like to take a walk or read a book, others like to hold on to a pillow or rub a worry stone, and others find that talking to a friend

NURSING DIAGNOSES with NOC & NIC

Clients with Neuropsychiatric Problems

DIAGNOSIS	OUTCOMES	INTERVENTIONS
Acute confusion related to clouding of consciousness, disorientation, sensitivity to environmental stimulation	**Cognitive Ability:** Ability to execute complex mental processes	Delirium Management
Anxiety related to chronic or terminal prognosis, emotional lability, impaired cognitive abilities	**Anxiety Control:** Personal action to eliminate or reduce feelings of apprehension and tension from an unidentifiable source	Calming Technique
Family Coping: Potential for growth related to care-taking responsibilities, support of all family members, development of effective coping strategies.	**Family Normalization:** Ability of the family to develop and maintain routines and management strategies that contribute to optimal functioning when a member has a chronic illness or disability	Family Support

SOURCES: Johnson, M., Maas, M., & Moorhead, S. (2000). *Nursing outcomes classification (NOC)* (2nd ed.). St. Louis, MO: Mosby; McCloskey, J. C., & Bulechek, G. M. (1996). *Nursing interventions classification (NIC)* (2nd ed.). St. Louis, MO: Mosby; and North American Nursing Diagnoses Association (1999). *Nursing diagnoses definitions and classification 1999–2000*. Philadelphia: Author.

or singing a song calms them down. They can say positive affirmations aloud such as: "I am calm and happy," "My breathing is slow and even," or "I am very relaxed."

Family: Life Span Care

Family Support

Effective family nursing interventions depend on your understanding of the effects of neurological disorders on family caregivers. The goal is to identify and reduce any negative perceptions, improve coping skills, and increase social supports.

It is important that you listen to each family member's perspective of the disease process and prognosis. Point out discrepancies in expectations and provide education regarding realistic prognosis. Normalizing the family's experience involves addressing family fears and helping the family adjust to the life changes that occur. It may be appropriate to introduce the family to other families undergoing similar experiences. Peer groups help families in problem solving and decreasing caregiver distress and social isolation. Equalizing caregiving tasks involves reducing disproportionate care taking burdens on individual family members. Provide necessary knowledge of options to family that will assist them to make decisions about care of their loved ones. If appropriate and desired, help families arrange for respite care.

Evaluation

To complete the nursing process, you evaluate clients' responses to nursing interventions based on the outcomes you selected. You determine the appropriate intervals for measurement and document the condition of clients according to each individual's status. Johnson, Maas, and Moorhead (2000) is the resource for identifying measurement scales and specific indicators for each outcome.

CRITICAL THINKING

Your clinical group is meeting for a conference in your clinical site, which is a medical unit. Your instructor announces that he thinks a good topic to discuss is neuropsychiatric disorders. All of the students are confused and comment that they are not taking psychiatric nursing. The instructor asks all of the students to list the types of problems that their clients have at this time. The diagnoses listed are HIV/AIDS, stroke, and Parkinson's disease, and one client is hospitalized with diabetes complications but also has epilepsy. The instructor continues the discussion by asking you to list some of the symptoms you have identified in your assessments of these clients.

You finally arrive at the conclusion that your clients may have psychiatric problems associated with specific neurological disorders, such as the ones that your clients exhibit. You discuss how the disruption of the central nervous system affects clients' behavior, affect, cognition, and social interactions. You begin to realize the psychiatric content has relevance wherever you are practicing.

1. How would you compare and contrast the cognitive and affect characteristics related to HIV/AIDS, stroke, epilepsy, and Parkinson's disease?

2. Based on the data about the illnesses/disorders noted in question 1 and this case, what key outcomes would you identify that would relate to all of them?

3. You are working with the family of the patient who has Parkinson's disease. How might you explain the patient's emotional responses?

4. How might you intervene to assist the families of these clients?

5. One of your students states that he would expect to see depression in all HIV/AIDS clients as the virus affects the brain in ways that causes depression to develop. How would you dispute this suggestion?

For an additional Case Study, please refer to the Companion Web site for this book. 🌐

Cognitive Ability

Clients remain safe from harm. They verbalize an understanding of what is being communicated to them. Clients remain oriented.

Anxiety Control

Individuals demonstrating improved anxiety control plan and implement effective coping strategies. They rehearse and use techniques such as slow, deep breathing, muscle relaxation, guided imagery, distraction techniques, and a quiet environment to manage their feelings of anxiety.

Family Normalization

Family members verbalize their perspective of the disease process and prognosis. They are able to express fears and describe home management problems. Clients seek out peer and group support. They utilize respite care when necessary.

To build a care plan for a client with a neuropsychiatric problem, go to the Companion Web site for this text. 🌐

CHAPTER REVIEW

COMMUNITY RESOURCES

Links to these Web sites can be accessed on the Companion Web site for this book.

Creutzfeldt–Jakob Disease Foundation
P.O. Box 611625
North Miami, FL 33261-1625
954-436-7591 (Fax)
www.cjdfoundation.org

Huntington's Disease Society of America
158 West 29th St., 7th Floor
New York, NY 10001-5300
800-345-hdsa
www.hdsa.org

National Institute of Neurological Disorders and Stroke
National Institutes of Health
31 Center Dr., MSC 2540
Bethesda, MD 20892
301-496-4000
www.nih.gov

National Multiple Sclerosis Society
733 Third Ave.
New York, NY 10017
800-344-4867
www.nmss.org

National Parkinson Foundation
1501 Northwest 9th Ave.
Miami, FL 33136
800-327-4545
www.parkinson.org

National Stroke Association
8480 East Orchard Road
Suite 1000
Englewood, CO 80111
800-STROKES
www.stroke.org

BOOKS FOR CLIENTS AND FAMILIES

Dumont, R. (1996). *The sky is falling.* New York: Norton.

Mace, M., & Rabins, P. (1999). *The 36-hour day: A family guide to caring for persons with Alzheimer's disease,* *related dementing illness and memory loss in later life* (3rd ed.). Baltimore, MD: Johns Hopkins University Press.

KEY CONCEPTS

Knowledge Base

- People with Parkinson's disease have difficulty with problem solving and abstract thinking, memory problems, and slowed thinking. Many go on to develop dementia.

- Affective symptoms of Parkinson's disease include apathy, depression, and anxiety.

- Psychiatric symptoms are among the most common features of Huntington's disease and include dementia, irritability and aggressiveness. Mood and anxiety disorders may also occur.

- Individuals with Pick's disease experience sudden changes in personality and socially uninhibited behavior that is embarrassing to family and friends.

- Creutzfeldt–Jakob disease leads to confusion, disorientation, personality changes, delirium, and dementia.

- People with epilepsy may experience a temporary psychosis in the ictal or postictal phase.

- Psychiatric symptoms of multiple sclerosis include decreased attention span, slowed information processing, disordered executive function, pathological laughing/crying, bipolar disorder, and major depression.

- Brain attacks may result in people having difficulty with orientation, language, executive functions, abstract thinking, emotional lability, and depression.

- Delirium is the most frequent psychiatric complication of AIDS, followed by dementia, depression, and anxiety.

- Psychiatrically disabled individuals are at higher risk for HIV/AIDS because of higher rates of substance abuse, poor judgment, sexual impulsivity, and multiple sex partners.

- PANDAS, resulting from streptococcal infections, present with a sudden and dramatic onset of obsessive-compulsive disorder and/or Tourette's disorder.

- Depression is the most common complication following a traumatic brain injury. Up to 10 percent of victims experience a psychosis that resembles schizophrenia.

- People with traumatic brain injury may be more susceptible to Alzheimer's disease.

The Nursing Process

Assessment

- Assessment involves both clients and their families.

- Functional assessment includes ADLs such as hygiene and grooming, household responsibilities, school or employment responsibilities, and financial management.

Diagnosis

- Nursing diagnoses are developed from assessment data and are related to clients' responses to psychiatric dysfunctions such as mood, anxiety, schizophrenic, and spectrum disorders.

Outcome Identification and Goals

- Examples of outcomes include established routines, completion of ADLs appropriate to the functional level, anxiety control, and cognitive ability.

Nursing Interventions

- Nursing interventions are designed to prevent or manage agitation, anxiety, and perceptual or cognitive disturbances in clients who are experiencing delirium.

- Interventions designed to improve orientation include frequent contact, repeating of information, reassurance, written schedules, clocks and calendars, and an environmental balance to prevent sensory deprivation or sensory overstimulation.

- Calming techniques such as muscle relaxation and deep breathing are useful in managing anxiety.

- Other calming techniques include distracting activities and positive affirmations.

- Therapeutic family interventions include listening to the family, normalizing their experience, and facilitating equalization of caregiving tasks.

Evaluation

- Clients will be able to communicate clearly and maintain their attention and concentration.

- They will manage their anxiety through effective coping strategies.

EXPLORE *MediaLink*

- Interactive resources, including animations and videos, for this chapter can be found on the Companion Web site at *http://www.prenhall.com/fontaine*. Click on Chapter 19 and select the activities for this chapter.

- For NCLEX review questions and an audio glossary, access the accompanying CD-ROM in this book.

REFERENCES

American Psychiatric Association Practice Guidelines. (2000). *Practice guidelines for the treatment of patients with HIV/AIDS.* Washington, DC: American Psychiatric Press.

Anderson, K. E., Louis, E. D., Stern, Y., & Marder, K. S. (2001). Cognitive correlates of obsessive and compulsive symptoms in Huntington's disease. *American Journal of Psychiatry, 158*(5), 799–801.

Barnes, J., David, A. S., Holroyd, L., Currie, L., & Wooten, G. F. (2001). Visual hallucinations in Parkinson's disease. *American Journal of Ophthalmology, 123*(5), 807–808.

CDJ Info. (2001). Creutzfeldt–Jakob Disease Foundation, Inc. *www.cdjfoundation.org/CJDInfo.html.*

Chun, M. R. (1998). The epidemiology of dementia among the elderly. In M. F. Folstein (Ed.), *Neurobiology of primary dementia* (pp. 1–26). Washington, DC: American Psychiatric Press.

Ciesla, J. A., & Roberts, J. E. (2001). Meta-analysis of the relationship between HIV infection and risk for depressive disorders. *American Journal of Psychiatry, 158*(5), 725–731.

Daley, E., Komaroff, A. L., Bloomingdale, K., Wilson, S., & Albert, M. S. (2001). Neuropsychological function in patients with chronic fatigue syndrome, multiple sclerosis, and depression. *Applied Neuropsychology, 8*(1), 12–22.

Deb, S., Lyons, I., Koutzoukis, C., Ali, I., & McCarthy, G. (1999). Rate of psychiatric illness 1 year after traumatic brain injury. *American Journal of Psychiatry, 156*(3), 374–379.

Estanislao, L. B., & Pachner, A. R. (1999). Spirochetal infection of the nervous system. *Neurologic Clinics, 17*(4), 783–800.

REFERENCES *(continued)*

Feinstein, A. (1999). *The clinical neuropsychiatry of multiple sclerosis.* Cambridge, MA: Cambridge University Press.

Garand, L., Buckwalter, K. C., & Hall, G. R. (2000). The biological basis of behavioral symptoms in dementia. *Issues in Mental Health Nursing, 21*(3), 91–107.

Gasser, T., & Oertel, W. H. (2000). Genetics of Parkinson's disease and other movement disorders. In S. M. Pulst (Ed.), *Neurogenetics* (pp. 351–372). New York: Oxford Press.

Giedd, J. N., Rapoport, J. L., Garvey, M. A., Perlmutter, S., & Swedo, J. E. (2000). MRI assessment of children with obsessive-compulsive disorder or tics associated with streptococcal infection. *American Journal of Psychiatry, 157*(2), 281–283.

Hayden, M. R. (2000). Huntington's disease. In S. M. Pulst (Ed.), *Neurogenetics* (pp. 265–280). New York: Oxford University Press.

Hoekstra, P. J., Bijzet, J., Limburg, P. C., Steenhuis, M. P., et al. (2001). Elevated D8/17 expression on B lymphocytes, a marker of rheumatic fever, measured with flow cytometry in tic disorder patients. *American Journal of Psychiatry, 158*(4), 605–610.

Johnson, M., Maas, M., & Moorhead, S. (2000). *Nursing outcomes classification (NOC)* (2nd ed.). St. Louis, MO: Mosby.

Kaplan, R. F., Jones-Woodward, L., Workman, K., Steere, A. C., et al. (1999). Neuropsychological deficits in Lyme disease patients with and without other evidence of central nervous system pathology. *Applied Neuropsychology, 6*(1), 3–11.

Kennedy, G. J. (2000). *Geriatric mental health care.* New York: Guilford Press.

Lenze, E., Cross, D., McKeel, D., Neuman, R. J., & Sheline, Y. I. (1999). White matter hyperintensities and gray matter lesions in physically healthy depressed subjects. *American Journal of Psychiatry, 156*(10), 1602–1607.

Levy, M. L., & Cummings, J. L. (2000). Parkinson's disease. In E. C. Lauterbach (Ed.), *Psychiatric management in neurological disease* (pp. 41–70). Washington, DC: American Psychiatric Press.

Malaspina, D., Goetz, R. R., Friedman, J. H., Kaufmann, C. A., et al. (2001). Traumatic brain injury and schizophrenia in members of schizophrenia and bipolar disorder pedigrees. *American Journal of Psychiatry, 158*(3), 440–446.

Maldonado, J. L., Fernandez, F., & Levy, J. K. (2000). Acquired immunodeficiency syndrome. In E. C. Lauterbach (Ed.), *Psychiatric management in neurological disease* (pp. 271–295). Washington, DC: American Psychiatric Press.

Mercadante, M. T., Busatto, G. F., Lombroso, P. J., Prado, L., et al. (2000). The psychiatric symptoms of rheumatic fever. *American Journal of Psychiatry, 157*(12), 2036–2038.

Ranen, N. G. (2000). Huntington's disease. In E. C. Lauterbach (Ed.), *Psychiatric management in neurological disease* (pp. 71–92). Washington, DC: American Psychiatric Press.

Robinson, R. G. (2000). Stroke. In E. C. Lauterbach (Ed.), *Psychiatric management in neurological disease* (pp. 219–247). Washington, DC: American Psychiatric Press.

Robinson, R. G., Schultz, S. K., Castillo, C., Kopel, R., Kosier, B. S., et al. (2000). Nortriptyline versus fluoxetine in the treatment of depression and in short-term recovery after stroke. *American Journal of Psychiatry, 157*(3), 351–359.

Sachdev, P. (1998). Schizophrenia-like psychosis and epilepsy: The status of the association. *American Journal of Psychiatry, 155*(3), 325–336.

Sadovnick, A. D., & Dyment, D. (2000). Multiple sclerosis and other demyelinating diseases. In S. M. Pulst (Ed.), *Neurogenetics* (pp. 373–388). New York: Oxford Press.

Schachter, S. C. (2001). Epilepsy. *Neurologic Clinics, 19*(1), 57–78.

Schwid, S. R., Weinstein, A., Wishart, H. A., & Schiffer, R. B. (2000). Multiple sclerosis. In E. C. Lauterbach (Ed.), *Psychiatric management in neurological disease* (pp. 249–270). Washington, DC: American Psychiatric Press.

Stoff, D. M. (1998). HIV infection in people with severe mental illnesses. *NAMI Advocate, 20*(2), 25–26.

Swedo, S. E., Leonard, H. L., Garvey, M., Mittleman, B., et al. (1998). Pediatric autoimmune neuropsychiatric disorders associated with streptococcal infections. *American Journal of Psychiatry, 155*(2), 264–271.

Swedo, S. E., & Pekar, M. (2000). PANDAS: A new "species" of childhood-onset obsessive–compulsive disorder? In J. L. Rapoport (Ed.), *Childhood onset of "adult" psychopathology* (pp. 103–119). Washington, DC: American Psychiatric Press.

Ungvarski, P. J., & Trzcianowska, H. (2000). Neurocognitive disorders seen in HIV disease. *Issues in Mental Health Nursing, 21*(1), 51–70.

Weiner, W. J., Shulman, L. M., & Lang, A. E. (2001). *Parkinson's disease.* Baltimore, MD: Johns Hopkins University Press.

Well-Connected. (2001). What drugs other than L-dopa are used for Parkinson's disease? *Health.medscape.com/cx/viewarticle/402930.*

Williams, J. K., Schutte, D. L., Evers, C. A., & Forcucci, C. (1999). Adults seeking presymptomatic gene testing for Huntington disease. *Image, 31*(2), 109–114.

Windl, O., & Kretzschmar, H. A. (2000). Prion diseases. In S. M. Pulst (Ed.), *Neurogenetics* (pp. 191–218). New York: Oxford University Press.

Yeaworth, R. C., & Burke, W. J. (2000). Frontotemporal dementia: A different kind of dementia. *Archives of Psychiatric Nursing, 14*(5), 249–253.

PART SIX

Dysinhibition Syndromes

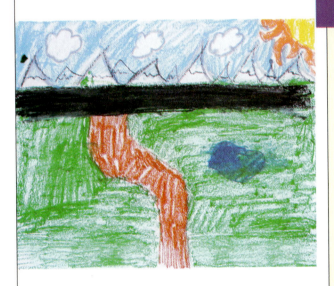

As I walk through obstacles, my problems lie behind.

I am hoping to cross the mountains to see what future I can find.

I must pass through the fog because my life is unclear.

So I can pass through the dangers I always have feared.

—Kenny, Age 12

Suicide

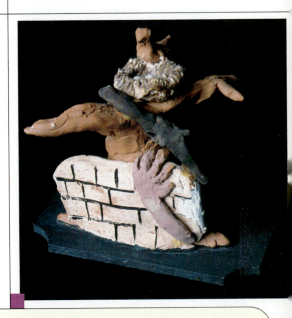

OBJECTIVES

After reading this chapter, you will be able to:

- IDENTIFY people who are at high risk for suicide.
- DISCUSS some of the reasons people have for committing suicide.
- ASSESS individuals who are at risk for suicide.
- IMPLEMENT a plan of care for clients who are suicidal.

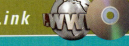

MediaLink

CD-ROM
- *Audio Glossary*
- *NCLEX Review*

Companion Web site www.prenhall.com/fontaine
- *Critical Thinking*
- *More NCLEX Review*
- *Case Study*
- *Care Map Activity*
- *Links to Resources*

A lifetime of fear and hiding behind a wall that no one could get through. The wall kept me alive. It blocked everything so I could survive. Now people want the wall to come down. Without the wall my only choice is the gun. The tree of life with 3 eggs in the nest: My children. How do I fit them into a life where my only choices are the wall or the gun?

—*Kay, Age 40*

Suicide is a worldwide, national, local, and familial problem. While the definitions of suicidal behavior and suicide overlap, there are slight differences. **Suicidal behavior** can be defined in two ways:

1. The behavior and thoughts leading up to the act of suicide
2. The act of taking one's own life

The word **suicide** is defined in the following three ways:

1. The act of taking one's own life
2. A person who takes his or her own life
3. The end result—survival or death—described as either attempted or completed

Worldwide, there are almost 2 million suicides every year. Every 15 minutes, another American commits suicide, for a total of 30,600 people a year. The reported numbers in the United States are actually low because many suicides are reported as accidental deaths. The real rate may be three to five times higher. Even with this underreporting, suicide remains the eighth leading cause of death in the general population. The impact of these statistics becomes even greater when we recognize that for every completed suicide, there are 10 to 20 unsuccessful attempts. There are more than four male suicides for every female suicide. However, at least twice as many females as males attempt suicide (Centers for Disease Control and Prevention [CDC], 2001; Grunebaum et al., 2001; Mann, 1998). Such data can also be viewed on the CDC resource link provided on the Companion Web site for this book.

Over 90 percent of suicide victims have a psychiatric disorder at the time of death. Most psychiatric clients, however, do not commit suicide. People who are psychiatrically disabled often commit suicide from years of pain, frustration, and low self-esteem, which contribute to demoralization and depression. Spiritually, they may perceive themselves as hopelessly damaged and lose all sense of purpose and meaning in life.

Nurses have higher rates of completed suicide than the general population. The most common method chosen by nurses is drug overdose, and nurses have easier access to drugs than most people do in the general population. Knowing how drugs work and how much to take may increase the lethality of the behavior. The daily stress of caring for people suffering from violence and trauma, serious illness, and impending death may be a risk factor for suicide of nurses (Goetz, 1998).

Suicide is a public health crisis. In 1999, U.S. Surgeon General David Satcher (U.S. Department of Health and Human Services [USDHHS], 1999) announced a national strategy for suicide prevention using the acronym **AIM:**

Access: to services and programs
- Improve recognition, referral, and treatment for mental disorders.
- Increase accessibility of mental health services.
- Reduce access to lethal means.
- Develop community crisis management plans.

Illumination: broaden the public's awareness
- Reduce the stigma of mental illness.
- Increase awareness of suicide as a preventable problem.
- Build multidisciplinary partnerships for prevention.

Methodology: advance the science of suicide prevention
- Intensify research into causal factors.
- Expand culturally appropriate prevention programs.
- Identify and expand successful programs and strategies.

Such data can also be viewed on the USDHHS Web site, which can be accessed through a resource link on the Companion Web site for this book. 🌐

KNOWLEDGE BASE

There are various *philosophies* about suicide, ranging from believing it is wrong to believing it has a positive value. See Box 20.1 for details of these philosophies.

People commit suicide for hundreds of *reasons*. Here are a few of the reasons:

- Some are driven by delusions or command hallucinations.
- Because of depressed feelings related to a chronic or terminal illness, some see no hope for the future.
- For some, suicide is a relief from intolerable and inescapable physical or emotional pain.
- Some individuals have experienced so many losses that life is no longer valuable.
- Some have been beset with multiple crises, which have drained their internal and external resources.
- For some, suicide is the ultimate expression of anger toward significant others.

Suicide can be precipitated by many factors. It carries a great variety of meanings to the victims as well as the survivors. Despite this variety, potential suicide victims have a number of characteristics in common that can alert you to the danger. *Previous suicide attempts* and a sense of *hopelessness* are the most powerful clinical predictors of future completed suicide (Malone et al., 2000).

BEHAVIORAL CHARACTERISTICS

Suicide is not a random act. It is a way out of a problem, dilemma, or unbearable situation. Suicidal individuals suffer intensely, and people contemplating suicide often make subtle or even overt comments that indicate as much. They may mention all the pressure and stress they are experiencing and how helpless they feel. Some may discuss beliefs concerning life after death. *Verbal cues* are such statements as:

- "It won't matter much longer."
- "Will you miss me when I'm gone?"
- "I can't take this much longer."

BOX 20.1 ■

Philosophies About Suicide

Suicide Is Wrong

- Suicide does violence to the dignity of human life.
- Suicide is an irrevocable act that denies future learning or growth.
- It is only for God to give and to take away human life.
- Suicide does violence to the natural order of things.
- Suicide adversely affects the survivors.

Suicide Is Sometimes Permissible

- Suicide is permissible when the person's life is unbearable.

Suicide Is Not a Moral or Ethical Issue

- Suicide is a fact of life that can be studied like other life events.
- Suicide is a morally neutral act in that every person has a free will and the right to act according to that will.

Suicide Is a Positive Response to Certain Conditions

- When life ceases to be enjoyable, people have the right to end their lives.
- There are certain times in life when death is less an evil than dishonor.
- Some suicides are demanded by society as a way of dispensing justice.

Suicide Has Intrinsic Positive Value

- Suicide has a positive value when it is the way people can enter a meaningful afterlife that they desire.
- Suicide has a positive value because it is a way in which people can be immediately reunited with valued ancestors and loved ones.

- "The pain will be over soon."
- "I won't be here when you come back on Monday."
- "You won't have to worry about the money problems much longer."
- "The voices are telling me to hurt myself."

Certain *behaviors* may indicate suicidal intentions. Obtaining a weapon such as a gun, a strong rope, or a collection of pills is a high indicator of impending suicide. Often, people contemplating suicide begin to withdraw from relationships and become more isolative. There may be a change in school or work performance. An increased tendency toward accidents might indicate initial suicidal behavior. Some may show a sudden interest in their life insurance policy, whereas others may make or change their will and give personal belongings away. Signs of substance abuse may also be present.

Willis, 16, was the youngest of four children and had enjoyed a stable family life. Two years earlier, he cut himself just enough to draw a little blood following a breakup with a girlfriend. There was no follow-up to this incident. His friends described Willis as very tense on some days and his relationship with his current girlfriend as "rocky." The day before he killed himself, Willis gave his music collection to his older brother, saying that where he was going, he would no longer need it. He told his girlfriend that if she would not see him anymore, he would be watching her from above. At the time, she didn't understand what he meant. The next day, Willis took the gun his family kept for protection, put it to his head, and pulled the trigger.

Behavioral characteristics also include choosing a method for suicide. **Lethality** is measured by four factors:

1. The degree of effort it takes to plan the suicide
2. The specificity of the plan
3. The accessibility of the weapon or method
4. The ease by which one may or may not be rescued

More people kill themselves with *guns* than by all other methods combined, and death by firearms is the fastest-growing method of suicide. More than half of the teenagers who commit suicide shoot themselves with a gun kept at home. An important social issue is the alarming increase in the number of guns purchased in the United States. Two hundred million guns are now in the hands of individual Americans, which is more than double the number held in 1969. Those who are most vulnerable to impulsive suicide are

clearly the most affected by availability of guns. The dramatic increase in suicide in children and adolescents is almost solely due to guns (American Foundation for Suicide Prevention [AFSP], 2001; Pearson, 1998).

Studies show that people who live in homes where there is a gun are five times more likely to experience a suicide than are people where guns are not present. Most gun owners state that they keep a gun in their home for "protection" or "self-defense." The reality is, however, that only 2 percent of gun-related deaths in the home are the result of a homeowner shooting an intruder. Three percent are accidental child shootings, 12 percent are the result of adult partners shooting one another, and 83 percent are the result of a suicide, often by a young person (AFSP, 2001).

The next most commonly used methods for committing suicide are cutting/piercing; hanging; and poisoning by liquids, solids, and gases such as carbon monoxide. The suicide methods most often chosen by younger children are hanging and jumping from a window or in front of a car (CDC, 2000).

AFFECTIVE CHARACTERISTICS

All the affective characteristics indicative of depression may be associated with people who are suicidal. These include feelings of desolation, guilt, failure, shame, and loss of emotional attachments. A pervading sense of *hopelessness* has the highest association with suicide. Life is seen as intolerable, with no hope for change or improvement.

People have a high degree of *ambivalence* before making the final decision to commit suicide. An internal conflict exists between the wish to die and the wish to live. If the part that wants to live can be adequately supported during this struggle, the balance may shift in favor of life. Once the decision has been made to commit suicide, conflict and anxiety cease, and the person may appear calm and untroubled. Others may interpret this change in the affective state as an improvement. What appears to be a change for the better may in fact be an indication of the decision to die.

COGNITIVE CHARACTERISTICS

Suicidal behavior has a variety of cognitive components. Suicidal people tend to think dichotomously, that is, all-or-none reasoning such as good or bad, right or wrong. This *rigid cognitive style* makes it difficult for people who are suicidal to problem-solve. Recurring thoughts of self-blame, negative self-evaluation, and dire expectations of the future contribute to a hopeless outlook. When people choose to die, they are so distorted by pain—physical, mental, or emotional—that the world is reduced to a solitary alternative. There seems to be only one answer: to die.

Another cognitive component involves *fantasies*. Unable to see the finality of death, suicidal people sometimes have fantasies about continuing on after their own death. They may talk about being able to see how people will react to their death or how their children will grow up. Others have expectations about meeting up with departed loved ones after death. Many people eagerly look forward to this reunion with family and friends.

A smaller percentage of people hopes or believes a suicide attempt will force a solution to interpersonal problems. For some, it is a cry for help. In either case, the suicidal behavior is a form of *manipulation*. They are so desperate that they can see no other method to resolve problems or get the necessary help.

People with sensory or thought disorders may be potentially suicidal. *Command hallucinations* are common and may often direct the person to commit suicide. At first, the person may be frightened by the voices, but later the person may be compliant and carry out the command. People with *delusions* of control or persecution may also be at risk for suicide. If these delusions cannot be managed with treatment, they may believe the only way to escape those who are controlling or persecuting them is to die. It is the ultimate method of getting relief from their extremely painful thoughts.

Kendall had a 15-year history of delusions of control. His delusional system was fixed, and he had responded poorly to a variety of interventions. His system centered on the belief that there was an electrode in his ear by which his family controlled him. They woke him up, they put him to sleep, they thought for him, and they talked for him through this electrode. Three weeks before his suicide, he expressed feelings of desperation. He said the doctors had done everything, but they either couldn't or wouldn't

remove the electrode from his ear. He said he couldn't go on this way, not being himself and being controlled by hateful family members. His final solution was to kill himself to escape the total control that had plagued him for 15 years.

For those rescued from their suicidal behavior, there is often a change of mind. Either they return to the ambivalent state of thought or they decide they do want to live. Throughout their lives, however, they remain at *higher risk* for suicide than the general population. It seems that once the decision to die was made in the past, that decision may be easier to make again.

SOCIAL CHARACTERISTICS

People who attempt or commit suicide are often in periods of *high stress* in their lives. Stressors include under- or unemployment, family disruption, rejection by a significant other, abrupt changes in career responsibilities, and recent catastrophic events. They often have a limited social network, and when their attempts to get support fail, their level of distress increases. When people either have not developed their own coping skills or have exhausted their ability to cope, suicide may be a last, desperate attempt to cope with stress and resolve problems.

Social pressures and a lack of resources often result in depression in adolescents who are *gay, lesbian, bisexual, or transgendered (GLBT)*. They are vulnerable to all the stressors of adolescence as well as the many stressors related to a stigmatized sexual orientation. GLBT youth feel ostracized from the dominant culture because of an absence of role models and distorted media presentations. They may suffer intimidation ranging from ridicule to threats and physical violence from beatings to rape. For reasons of acceptance and personal safety, GLBT youth remain hidden from their families and the community in which they live. Given this type of social climate, it is no surprise that lesbian and gay youths are six times more likely to commit suicide than heterosexual youths (Saulnier, 1998).

When teenage suicides are publicized by the news media or when there are television dramas about suicide, the rate of adolescent suicide increases several weeks following the event. Suicides that are inspired by suicides in this way are called **copycat suicides**. Copycat suicide seems to be an adolescent phenomenon, with girls more susceptible than boys are. The potential copycat appears to be a troubled adolescent who empathizes with the pain of the suicidal person and is easily influenced by the media.

Some people who are suspicious, or who are prone to violence as a method of coping with feelings, may combine *homicide–suicide*. The perpetrator, usually a male, commits one or more homicides and shortly thereafter commits a violent suicide. Homicide–suicide often occurs within a family. Most cases are adults who are spouses or partners but children may also be victims (Cohen, Llorente, & Eisdorfer, 1998).

On December 13, 2001, Jeffrey Wein, age 30, shot and killed his wife, Kristin Lynn Wein, age 31, as well as his 5-month-old daughter Emma. Jeffrey then drove several miles to his parent's home, where he killed both his parents and himself in their home. Jeffrey purchased the gun the day before the murders and suicide. Their northern Indiana community was stunned as the family was very active in the community and had no known marital or family problems. (Gary Post-Tribune, December 14–19, 2001).

Whatever way the act of suicide is committed, it has a *traumatic effect* on the family and friends of the victim. In addition to the grief, these people must cope with the stigma and cultural taboos associated with suicide. Family and friends are frequently unaware of the danger signs and respond to the suddenness of the death with shock and bewilderment. Some people respond with anger toward the victim and the event. Others feel betrayed and abandoned. Because society assumes that all survivors must feel guilty and responsible for the suicidal behavior, those who do not experience guilt may wonder why and may feel guilty about not feeling guilty. Some survivors experience a sense of relief when a suicide ends the physical or mental suffering of a loved one. Other survivors blame themselves with such thoughts as "If only I had done [had not done] . . . this would not have happened." Shame and guilt cast family members in the role of murderers, when in truth they, too, are victims. The death of a child, in particular, puts extreme strain on the parents. Because they were unable to protect their child, they may be overwhelmed with feelings of guilt and powerlessness (Hendin, Lipschitz, Maltsberger, Haas, & Wynecoop, 2000).

Many survivors are plagued with real or imagined images of the death scene. Families must also cope with other people seeking details about the death, with others' inability to acknowledge the death, or others even blaming them for the death. Some people develop obsessions about their own suicide. Family survivors enter a higher risk category for suicide; about 20 percent of them will exhibit suicidal behavior themselves. Having a loved one die is traumatic at any time, but having a loved one die as a result of suicide can be overwhelming.

CULTURE-SPECIFIC CHARACTERISTICS

Suicide continues to be an urgent problem in all countries of the world, especially among the youth, where suicide may be the second or third leading cause of death. Acts of suicide relate to a range of social, political, and psychological factors. Philosophies about suicide are deeply rooted in cultural traditions. Because it is highly stigmatized and illegal in many places, suicide is thought to be grossly underreported.

Euro-Americans have the highest rates of suicide in the United States, accounting for over 90 percent of all suicides. The peak for females is around age 50. For males, the suicide rate continues to increase throughout life, with those over 65 having the highest suicide rate of all groups (CDC, 2001; CDC, 2000; Shea, 1998).

Native People are not a culturally homogeneous population. There are wide variations in the suicide rates of different Native tribes. For example, the Chippewa have the lowest rate, with 6 suicides out of 100,000 people, and the Black Feet have the highest rate, at 130 out of 100,000. The suicide rate for Alaskan natives is twice that of the general population of the United States. Suicide rates in the Canadian Native population are more than three times the rate of the same age group of non-Native Canadians. Tribes that have maintained traditions have the lowest rates. High rates of suicide are related to multiple factors such as the breakdown of traditional values, enforced residence on reservations, geographic isolation, isolation of children from their families of origin, inadequate housing, high unemployment, extreme poverty, and a high incidence of alcoholism (CDC, 2001; Robinson, 2001).

Hispanic Americans are at highest risk for suicide during young adulthood. This is thought to be related to the stress of acculturation because the rates are higher in the United States than in their countries of origin. Stressors include the language barrier, discrimination, poverty, and educational disadvantages (Malone et al., 2000).

Asian Americans are one of the fastest-growing ethnic groups in the United States. Having never been treated with the same courtesy given to immigrants from Europe, they have suffered a long history of discrimination. Typically, the suicide rate increases with age among Asian Americans (Malone et al., 2000).

The rate of suicide for African Americans remains well below the rate for Euro-Americans. African Americans experience the highest rate of suicide between the ages of 25 and 34, after which there is a general decline to low levels in old age. Among African Americans, older adults have more purposeful roles, higher status, and much lower rates of suicide than Euro-Americans of the same age group do. The very low rate of suicide among African American women is attributed to their participation in community activities, including church, and to the strong psychosocial support they share, which contributes to positive self-esteem and minimal need for approval from the dominant culture (Malone et al., 2000).

Judaism has a general prohibition against taking one's own life, based on two religious reasons. The first is that people belong to God and therefore have no right to destroy that which is not theirs. The second reason is that people are created in God's image, and suicide is the destruction of the divine image. In Christianity, the commandment against murder has been interpreted to apply to taking one's life. Suicide offends God, who offers life as a gift, and suicide also offends the human community (Cohen, 1998; Zohar, 1998). (See Table 20.1 ■.)

AGE-SPECIFIC CHARACTERISTICS

In the United States, suicide rates vary dramatically by age groups. Although suicide occurs at all stages throughout life, people continue to be surprised when they learn about suicide in a child younger than 12. The fact is, children as young as age 3 to 5 have been known to commit suicide. Suicide is the fourth leading cause of death for children ages 10 to 14 (an increase of 100 percent since 1950) and the third leading cause of

death for young people 15 to 24 years old (tripled since 1950). The risk for suicide among young people is greatest among Euro-American males. The suicide rate for African Americans aged 10 to 14 has increased the most (233 percent), while increasing 126 percent for those aged 15 to 19. The Centers for Disease Control and Prevention (CDC, 1998) reported that 20.5 percent of students in grades 9 through 12 had seriously thought about attempting suicide, 16 percent had made a specific suicide plan, and 8 percent had actually attempted suicide in the past year (Lyon et al., 2000; Prigerson et al., 1999).

People who are 65 and older have the highest suicide rate of all age groups. They make up only 13 percent of the population, but they account for 25 percent of all suicides. In the United States, someone 65 years or older completes suicide every 90 minutes, most frequently with firearms. Suicide rates for men are relatively constant from ages 25 to 64, but increase significantly after age 65, and men account for 83 percent of suicides among persons age 65 and older. With the increasing number of older adults in the United States, this fact has serious implications for future health care planning (CDC, 2001; CDC, 2000).

ASSISTED SUICIDE

Physician-**assisted suicide** has received increased attention over the past decade. Among the general public, support for the "right to die" has grown steadily, with 64 percent of the population supporting assisted dying for people with terminal illness. At issue is whether the dying should have the right to request and receive aid in dying from physicians. Legal safeguards include multiple requests from the person over a two-week period, witnessed and documented discussion of treatment options and hospice care, a confirmation of the terminal condition by another physician, and psychiatric assessment that the person is not impaired by a mental illness.

Those who are against the issue believe that the greater good for the society demands keeping the prohibitions in place. It is seen as a form of medical killing in violation of social, ethical, and medical traditions, which would turn physicians from healers into killers. There is concern that it will be applied in an involuntary way against elderly, poor, handicapped, or otherwise disadvantaged people. A further concern is that some individuals will be pressured to end their lives as

TABLE 20.1

Suicide and Homicide as Leading Causes of Death According to Age, Gender, and Ethnicity

Group	1–4	5–9	10–14	15–24	25–34	35–44	45–54	55 and over
All males	H-4th	H-4th	S-3rd H-4th	H-2nd S-3rd	S-2nd H-3rd	S-5th H-6th	S-5th	S-8th
All females	H-4th	H-4th	H-4th S-5th	H-2nd S-4th	H-4th S-6th	S-4th	S-8th	
African American Males	H-2nd	H-3rd	H-2nd S-4th	H-1st S-3rd	H-1st S-5th	H-5th S-7th	H-8th	
African American Females	H-2nd	H-3rd	H-2nd S-7th	H-2nd S-6th	H-4th S-9th	H-6th		
Euro-American Males	H-4th	H-4th	S-3rd H-4th	S-2nd H-3rd	S-2nd H-3rd	S-4th H-7th	S-4th	S-8th
Euro-American Females	H-4th	H-4th	S-4th H-6th	S-2nd H-4th	S-3rd H-5th	S-4th	S-6th	S-10th
Native People Both genders	H-4th	H-2nd S-9th	S-2nd S-3rd	S-2nd H-3rd	S-5th H-3rd	H-7th H-6th	S-10th	
Asian American Both genders	H-4th	H-4th	H-3rd S-5th	S-2nd H-3rd	S-3rd H-4th	S-4th H-6th	S-5th H-7th	S-9th

H = homicide
S = suicide
If no rank of death listed, it was not among the top 10 leading causes of death.
SOURCE: CDC, 2000.

---

an economic sacrifice for their families. The American Nurses Association opposes nurse participation in assisted suicide, believing that such actions are a breach of the Code for Nurses and the ethical traditions of the nursing profession (Schwarz, 1999). In contrast, the Oregon Nurses Association supports people's rights to self-determination and believes that nurses have a primary role in end-of-life decision (Nurse News, 2000).

There is little research regarding nurses' responses to dying people who request assisted suicide or euthanasia. In one study, 30 percent of terminally ill clients asked their oncology nurse for large amounts of drugs (for intentional self-overdose) and 25 percent asked for injections to end their lives (euthanasia). Nurses in this study indicated that they had a need to discuss these end-of-life situations, but in reality had few, if any, discussions with their peers and supervisors. It is important that further research be conducted on nurses' responses to such requests (Matzo & Schwarz, 2001).

In 2001, the Netherlands became the first country to legalize euthanasia fully, after 30 years of debate. Euthanasia has been tolerated for years, but most Dutch citizens wanted a legal framework to protect participating physicians (Cloud, 2001). In 1994, Oregon passed the Death with Dignity Act, which made it legal for physicians to provide a prescription for lethal drugs for terminally ill clients who request them. In 1997, the United States Supreme Court recognized states' decisions in the matter of physician-assisted suicide. This decision meant that battles must be fought out in each of the states. These are not just legal debates but moral, medical, social, political, and religious debates as well (Battin, Rhodes, & Silvers, 1998). In 2002, Oregon was involved in new litigation with the federal government. The attorney general authorized federal drug-enforcement agents to identify and punish physicians who prescribe federally controlled drugs to help terminally ill patients die. This is viewed as an effort to nullify Oregon's Death with Dignity Act.

Those who support assisted suicide believe a change in the law is necessary based on reasons of compassion and freedom of choice in the face of intolerable suffering. The desire to have medical help in ending one's life is seen as an extension of the right to refuse to be sustained on life support systems or to request not to be resuscitated. It must be remembered that many people with life-threatening illnesses are already taking matters into their own hands and ending their lives, with or without help and regardless of laws. Most people have no one with whom they can discuss these issues and no place to turn for advice. Proponents believe that everyone has the right to open dialogue, counseling, and involvement of family, partners, and friends regarding the wish to die when further living is intolerable.

CONCOMITANT DISORDERS

Although the vast majority of people with mental disorders do not commit suicide, more than 90 percent who do commit suicide have a diagnosable mental illness at the time of their death. Among people with schizophrenia, 10 to 13 percent commit suicide; for those with mood disorders, the rate is 20 percent; for those with personality disorder, the rate is 5 to 10 percent; and 7 percent of people with alcohol dependence die by suicide. People with more than one of these disorders may be at very high risk for suicide (AFSP, 2001).

It is important that you remember people are at risk for suicide throughout the course of treatment for their mental disorder. In some cases, the risk increases as individuals improve. This transient higher risk may be because they have the energy and the capacity to act on

---

BOX 20.2

Factors Contributing to High Suicidal Risk

- Euro-American
- Elderly people, especially men, followed by adolescents and college students
- People who are isolated without support systems
- Individuals who are recently unemployed
- Recent loss of a significant relationship
- Separated, divorced, or widowed people
- Presence of a substance use disorder
- Presence of a mental disorder
- Feelings of failure and hopelessness
- Presence of a gun in the home
- Previous suicide attempts
- Positive family history of completed suicide

---

self-destructive plans made earlier in the course of their illness.

People with chronic medical diseases are more likely to commit suicide than those with acute illnesses or no illness. At highest risk are people suffering from progressive diseases such as cardiovascular disease, multiple sclerosis, and cancer. Moreover, people who take a large number of medications may, as a direct result of the chemical effects on the body, experience a depressive episode leading to suicide. Substance abuse is a contributing factor for some suicidal people, particularly older men who live alone and have few or no support systems. The use of chemicals may be an attempt to self-medicate to control the symptoms of depression, or it may be a way to overcome inhibitions over the actual act of suicide. See Box 20.2 for a list of factors contributing to suicidal behavior.

CAUSATIVE THEORIES

Suicide is a complex act, and a variety of factors contribute to the behavior. The degree of influence of each factor varies from individual to individual. When risk factors are combined, the likelihood of suicidal acts is greater, either because internal restraints decrease or excess stress increases suicidal impulses.

Genetic Theory

Adoption studies in the United States and Denmark indicate that there may be a genetic factor in suicidal

CRITICAL THINKING

Alice is a nurse at a community mental health center in an urban area. She is working in the crisis intervention services, which includes a 10-bed short-term unit and ambulatory care services. Alice has worked at the center for five years but has recently transferred to the crisis service as she wanted a change and saw this as a place she could utilize her assessment skills and work with the community more directly.

Alice has just finished an admission assessment on a 30-year-old woman who was admitted following a suicide attempt with an overdose. She is now medically stable. Alice found that the assessment provided her with some important data that can be used to help the client. The client, Ms. Simmons, is single and has never been married. She did have a baby at the age of 16, but this baby was given up for adoption. Ms. Simmons works as a secretary. When Alice asked the client how she was feeling, the client responded, "I could not take it anymore. It's no use." Ms. Simmons has had one known previous overdose, two years ago. This time she overdosed with medication that was given to her for insomnia that she had been saving for several months so that she would have a large enough dose. She would not talk further about it. Alice knows from the ER report that Alice was found by a neighbor who had been concerned about Ms. Simmons's low mood and had not seen her leave for work, which was unusual. The neighbor had a key from Ms. Simmons. When asked about her family, Ms. Simmons said her parents were living in a different city, and that yesterday she went to a baby shower for a cousin. Alice wondered about this last comment, as it did not seem quite connected to the question about her family. Most people respond with information about their immediate family.

1. How does Ms. Simmons demonstrate the key predictors of suicide?

2. Alice must determine the lethality of Ms. Simmons's intent. How would you do this for this client?

3. What behavioral, affective, cognitive, and social characteristics of suicide does Ms. Simmons exhibit?

4. Alice asks Ms. Simmons the following: "What made you want to hurt yourself?" What is not helpful about this approach? What might be Ms. Simmons's response?

5. Given Ms. Simmons's status at the time of admission, how might you implement crisis management for her?

6. In addition to Alice's responsibility for assessment and working with clients on the short-term unit, she often acts as a community liaison and provides education for various community groups on mental health issues. After she finishes her shift, Alice goes to a community meeting of elderly citizens to discuss depression. One of the attendees asks Alice her opinion of assisted suicide. This is a "hot" topic today for health care professionals. What is your personal opinion of assisted suicide?

For an additional Case Study, please refer to the Companion Web site for this book.

---

behavior. Individuals who were adopted at birth and later committed suicide were found to have significantly more biological relatives who had committed suicide than the control group. It is believed that this genetic factor may be an inability to control impulsive behavior, and that either environmental stress or a mental illness may drive the impulsive behavior toward suicide (Mann et al., 1999).

Neurobiological Theory

Recent research indicates that the primary neurobiological factor in suicide is a disturbance related to serotonin (5-HT) dysfunction. 5-HT is the constraining and anti-impulsive neurotransmitter. Sufficient 5-HT may be related to people's tolerance for adversity, the ability to resist impulsive urges, and the means to find solutions to problems. In both attempted and completed suicides there is a significant *decrease* in 5-HT irrespective of the primary psychiatric diagnosis. As levels of 5-HT decrease, people become more impulsive, more aggressive, and lose control more quickly. Interestingly, 5-HT levels rise during pregnancy and pregnant women are at very low risk for suicide. The fetus produces much of the excess 5-HT, which may be self-protective, by inhibiting self-destructive behaviors by the mother.

Suicide risk is also related to past head injury. Aggressive, impulsive children and adults are more likely to sustain a head injury, and head injuries can cause impulsive and aggressive behaviors. The final decision to commit suicide may be an impulsive act that is the result of powerful biological processes (Krakowski, 2000; Mann et al., 1999).

Sociocultural Theory

Suicide may result when people experience social isolation, and become alienated from society, family, and friends. Another sociocultural factor is rapid social change resulting in the loss of previous patterns of social integration. People who have difficulty adapting to the demand of new roles are more likely to view suicide as a solution to their problems.

Loss is another factor closely related to suicide. Certainly, the impact of any loss depends on the significance the person attributes to that loss. Whenever the most important and significant aspects of a person's life are threatened or destroyed, suicide is likely to be considered. Women's motives tend to be *interpersonal*, that is, related to painful or lost relationships. Men's motives tend to be *intrapersonal*, that is, related to financial problems or the loss of a job.

Behavioral Theory

Behavioral theorists believe that suicide is often a learned problem-solving behavior. They consider the *reinforcements* prior to and following attempted suicidal behavior. The internal reinforcement is that the behavior itself serves to decrease anxiety. Following the suicidal behavior, the external reinforcement is that the person is removed from the stressful environment and freed from daily pressures. Significant others who were critical may now become supportive. These types of reinforcement are essential in the repetition of suicidal behavior.

Developmental Theory

In addition to these general causes of suicide, there are more specific causes for various age groups. Some of the reasons *children* commit suicide are to escape from physical or sexual abuse, a chaotic family situation, feeling unloved or constantly criticized, anticipation of disciplinary action, humiliation in school, and the loss of significant others.

Adolescents may commit suicide for the same reasons children do. Additional age-specific causes include the absence of meaningful relationships, difficulties in maintaining relationships, sexual problems, and acute problems with parents. Additional suicidal factors for college students include competition for success, anxiety over academic work, and academic failure signifying a loss of parental love or esteem.

Suicide among *older adults* may be related to a change in status from autonomy to dependency, accompanied by decreased participation in social activities. Many of the changes experienced by older adults may contribute to a higher incidence of suicide. Those who experience illness that results in a lower level of functioning may become suicidal. Other factors include loneliness and social isolation, loss of partner and friends, loss of work deemed important by the culture, and outliving resources.

NURSING PROCESS

Assessment

You may be apprehensive about assessing people who are at risk of attempting or committing suicide. Your reasons may include fear of giving the person the idea of suicide, fear of being incorrect, fear of the person's reaction, and reluctance to discuss a taboo subject. It is important for you to recognize that *you cannot give the idea of suicide to anyone.* By late childhood or early adolescence, every person knows that suicide is one alternative to solving problems. Most youngsters, without being actively suicidal, have thoughts of suicide in times of stress. An example is the child who is angry with his parents and thinks, "If I went out and got run over by a car, they'd be sorry they were so mean to me!" Many adults have considered what method they would choose if they were to commit suicide. Thus, even though the topic is taboo under most social conditions, the majority of people have thought about and formed an opinion about suicide.

Remember that people who are suicidal are *afraid.* They fear that no one cares. They may not introduce the topic because they fear being judged or considered weak or "crazy." When confronted with your own fears about discussing suicide, remember that no nursing intervention will be effective unless the suicide threat is assessed. If the person is not suicidal, asking the questions will do no damage. But if the person is suicidal and the topic is not discussed, the person has been abandoned while in a dangerously vulnerable position. Remember that the answers you get depend on the questions you ask.

When assessing people for suicidal potential, *use specific words* such as *kill yourself or commit suicide.* If you use a more vague term, such as *want to hurt yourself,* some suicidal people will respond negatively. They may not want to cause themselves pain, but they do want to kill themselves. People need to know what you are talking about, and you cannot risk misunderstandings. You might introduce the topic of suicide by saying something like: "Often, when people are feeling very upset or depressed, they have thoughts of killing themselves. Have you had any thoughts of wanting to kill yourself?" (Shea, 1998).

It is also important that you assess for protective factors against suicidal acts. *Protective factors* include a social support system, problem-solving and coping history, a sense of responsibility to children, hopefulness, fear of suicide, fear of social disapproval, and moral objections to suicide. The more protective factors individuals have, the less likely it is that they will act on suicidal thoughts at vulnerable times.

You may find yourself struggling with ambivalence about suicide. The conflict centers on the issue of people's right to choose their own time and method of dying. Many of us have thought about the conditions under which we would choose not to live, such as with a chronic or terminal illness. Having considered suicide as an option, you may question whether you have the right to prevent another person's suicide, or you may not experience this conflict at all because you believe that all suicides should be prevented.

You and the families of clients should not expect that an accurate assessment will prevent all suicides. This expectation would contribute to unrealistic guilt when a person does successfully commit suicide. Not all victims exhibit cues before their death; many people cannot be correctly identified before they kill themselves. This is not intended to minimize the importance of a suicide assessment; rather, it is to establish realistic professional expectations. If a person is intent on suicide, it is difficult to intervene effectively. However, if a person is still ambivalent, intervention may save that person's life. Therefore, it is always vital that, for those at risk, a suicide assessment be done.

See the Focused Nursing Assessment feature for specific questions to ask when assessing a person's potential for suicide. Box 20.3 describes the levels of suicide severity.

BOX 20.3

Levels of Severity of Suicide

Nonexistent
- No identifiable suicidal ideation

Mild
- Suicidal ideation of limited frequency, intensity, and duration
- No plan for suicide
- Mild dysphoria
- Good self-control
- Few risk factors
- Identifiable protective factors

Moderate
- Frequent suicidal ideation with limited intensity and duration
- Some specific plans
- No intent to die
- Good self-control
- Limited dysphoria
- Some risk factors
- Identifiable protective factors

Severe
- Frequent, intense, and enduring suicidal ideation
- Specific plans
- Some intent to die
- Method is available/accessible
- Impaired self-control
- Severe dysphoria
- Multiple risk factors
- Few protective factors

Extreme
- Frequent, intense, and enduring suicidal ideation
- Specific plans
- Clear intent to die
- Method is available/accessible
- Impaired self-control
- Severe dysphoria
- Multiple risk factors
- No protective factors

SOURCE: Rudd, M. D., Joiner, T., & Rajab, M. H. (2001). *Treating suicidal behavior.* New York: Guilford Press.

Behavior Assessment	Affective Assessment	Cognitive Assessment	Social Assessment
Are you thinking about suicide?	How would you describe your overall mood?	What will your suicide accomplish for you?	What kinds of losses have you sustained during the past year? Relationships? Separations? Divorce? Deaths? Jobs? Roles? Self-esteem?
By what method would you commit suicide?	What kinds of things make you feel guilty?	What will your suicide accomplish for others?	
Do you have the means on hand?	In what areas of life do you feel like a failure?	What would have to change for you to decide to live?	What kinds of stress have you been under during the past six months?
Have you done a practice session of the suicide?	What does the future look like to you?	What are your thoughts about death?	Which people are able to provide support for you?
When do you plan to commit suicide?	To what degree do you feel hopeless or out of control of your life?	Is there a way for you to continue on in life after death?	Have any of your friends or family members committed suicide? What is the anniversary date? What thoughts and feelings do you have about this suicide?
Have you tried to kill yourself before?	To what degree do you feel hopeful about the future?	Do you hope to meet dead loved ones after you die?	
How have things been going at school/work for you?	What part of you wishes to die?	How well do you think you solve problems?	
Are you still interested in visiting with friends?	What part of you wishes to live?	Do you hear voices that others say they do not hear?	Who will benefit from your suicide? How?
Who depends on you to take care of them?	What will other people think of you if you commit suicide?	What do the voices say to you?	
How much have you been drinking lately?		Is suicide a way for you to escape control or persecution by others?	
How often do you use street drugs?			
Have you made or changed your will recently? Have you checked your life insurance policy?			
What kinds of personal belongings have you given away?			
Have you planned your funeral?			

Diagnosis

Based on the assessment data, you develop any number of nursing diagnoses. For a person who is actively suicidal, the most obvious nursing diagnosis is: High risk for violence, self-directed, related to acute suicidal state.

If a person has successfully committed suicide, the family may become your client—in the short term, as in the emergency department, or for a longer period, in a community or home setting. Possible nursing diagnoses may be: Ineffective family coping, compromised, related to the suicide of a family member; and Spiritual distress related to questions regarding the death, anger at the deceased, or a struggle with the sense of life's injustices.

Outcome Identification and Goals

Based on the assessment data, you select outcomes appropriate to the nursing diagnoses. See the Nursing Diagnoses with NOC and NIC feature for outcomes.

Client goals are specific behavioral measures by which you, clients, and significant others determine progress toward goals. The primary goal in a suicidal crisis is simply to keep the person alive. The following are examples of some of the other goals appropriate to people who are suicidal:

- Remains safe from self-injury
- Verbalizes a decrease in suicidal thoughts and related behaviors
- Utilizes the problem-solving process
- Discusses personal philosophy of death
- Develops a no-suicide contract
- Verbalizes a sense of hopefulness regarding the immediate future
- Identifies realistic protective factors

Nursing Interventions

Safety: Crisis Management

Suicide Prevention

In planning nursing care, use the following questions to guide the process:

- Is the client actively suicidal? At what level of severity?
- What is the degree of lethality of the plan?
- Does the client need to be in a protected environment?
- What is the extent of protective factors?

When clients are severely or extremely suicidal, the first priority of care is *client safety*. If clients are not in the hospital, someone must remain with them at all times until they can be moved to a safe environment. Clients should be transported to the hospital by family members, friends, or police to ensure accurate evaluation and possible admission.

Upon admission, all dangerous objects will be removed, such as pocket knives, glass articles, belts, razors, and pills. If the client is on medication, be certain that all medication is swallowed, not stockpiled for a future suicide attempt. *Suicidal precautions* include checking clients' whereabouts and status every 10 to 15 minutes on an irregular schedule of observation. If the client is acutely suicidal, constant observation is necessary. Constant observation can be demoralizing and dehumanizing. Thus, it is important that you gently explain to clients that the protection is necessary until they are able to resist suicidal impulses.

Clients should never be lectured about the negative consequences of suicide. The main goal is to *protect* clients who are suicidal until they are able to protect themselves. Through active intervention, it is hoped that clients will be able to develop alternative solutions to the difficulties fostering their suicidal intentions.

The role of the nurse is one of active participation in *problem solving*. The first step is to have clients write a list of reasons to live and reasons to die, to help them conceptualize the conflict more clearly. The next step is to have them describe the goal they hope to achieve with suicide. At this time, remind them that suicide is only one of several possible alternatives. Together, you and the client develop a list of alternatives for meeting the stated goal. Discussion of the potential outcomes of suicide is the next step in the problem-solving process. The following questions are appropriate: "What is the likelihood that you will injure yourself seriously if your attempt is not successful?" "Will death be the most successful method of meeting your goal?" Clients have often not considered the negative outcomes, such as permanent bodily damage and failure to achieve the goal. Next, focus the discussion on potential outcomes of other alternatives. The rationale for this phase is to support the part of the client that wishes to live.

People who are suicidal may not have thought past the act of self-injury, that is, the reality and finality of death. It is appropriate to *discuss death*: what it means, feelings about death, and what they think it will be like. The next step is reviewing the reasons to continue living and a list of meaningful supportive network systems. This focus on available support systems will decrease feelings of isolation and helplessness. Some clients have not considered the impact of their suicide on family members. It may be helpful to discuss the

NURSING DIAGNOSES *with NOC & NIC*

Clients Who Are Suicidal

DIAGNOSIS	OUTCOMES	INTERVENTIONS
High risk for violence, self-directed related to acute suicidal state, a desire to kill oneself as a solution to problems, an increased risk of suicide in the future	*Suicide Self-Restraint*	Suicide Prevention

SOURCES: Johnson, M., Maas, M., & Moorhead, S. (2000). *Nursing outcomes classification (NOC)* (2nd ed.). St. Louis, MO: Mosby; McCloskey, J. C., & Bulechek, G. M. (1996). *Nursing interventions classification (NIC)* (2nd ed.). St. Louis, MO: Mosby; and North American Nursing Diagnoses Association (1999). *Nursing diagnoses definitions and classification 1999–2000*. Philadelphia: Author.

impact on survivors: grief, anger, shame, guilt, and the increased risk for family members to commit suicide themselves. This external focus and concern may reduce the possibility of impulsive behavior.

Contracts are verbal or written agreements with clients regarding specific goals or outcomes. Clients are often asked to write their own **no-suicide contract** that specifies their intent to remain safe and sign it. Your signature on the contract indicates that you will help them keep their contract. In some settings the contracts may be verbal agreements. The purpose of the contract is to formalize their agreement not to act on suicidal impulses and evoke a commitment to life (Drew, 2001).

Assist clients in developing a *crisis card* to enable them to use existing support systems and community resources. Names and phone numbers of competent and willing family and friends are written on the card as well as numbers of community resources such as hotlines, mental health center emergency services, and local emergency departments.

When clients are successful with suicide, you must quickly intervene to *support the family* through the crisis. Provide opportunities for family members to discuss the death; many of their friends will avoid the topic because of discomfort. Most family members have a desperate need to talk in an environment of acceptance and understanding. The family should be allowed to express anger at the victim for abandonment and anger at themselves for not being able to prevent the suicide. This will normalize anger as an important part of the grieving process. Offer information on literature, community resources, and available support groups. Anticipatory guidance, as in foreseeing the stress of holiday times and the anniversary of the death, will decrease the impact of these situations. If family issues remain unresolved, those involved should be referred for family therapy. The Community Resources and Books for Clients and Families features at the end of this chapter provide resource information for clients with suicide potential and surviving family members.

Evaluation

To complete the nursing process, you evaluate clients' responses to nursing interventions based on the outcomes you selected. You determine the appropriate intervals for measurement and document the condition of clients according to each individual's status. Johnson, Maas, and Moorhead (2000) is the resource for identifying measurement scales and specific indicators for each outcome.

Suicide Self-Restraint

Individuals who are suicidal develop a list of reasons to live or die and goals they hope to achieve with suicide. They develop a list of alternative solutions to their problems. They discuss their beliefs regarding death and the impact of suicide on family members. They participate in developing and maintaining a no-suicide contract and remain safe. They formulate a written list of support system and community resources.

When clients are successful at suicide, ask yourself several questions to resolve any unnecessary self-blame and guilt:

■ Did I take the client's suicidal intentions seriously?

■ Did I provide as safe an environment as possible?

■ Was the client willing to find alternative solutions?

■ Do I have a right to prevent all suicides?

■ Does the client have a right to determine her or his own death?

■ Am I the only one who is blaming myself?

■ What do I need to do to feel less guilty about this death?

It is necessary for staff members to discuss their feelings and responsibilities in regard to a client's suicide. They will find it helpful to explore concepts of life and death, as well as their moral obligations. If feelings of guilt and failure are not thought about and expressed, individual staff members may project anger and blame onto others or even onto the dead client.

CHAPTER REVIEW

COMMUNITY RESOURCES

Links to these Web sites can be accessed on the Companion Web site for this book.

Crisis Line
800-521-4000

American Association of Suicidology
4201 Connecticut Ave., NW, Suite 408
Washington, DC 20008
202-237-2280
www.suicidology.org

American Foundation for Suicide Prevention
120 Wall St., 22nd Floor
New York, NY 10005
888-333-AFSP
www.afsp.org

Light for Life Foundation for the Prevention of Youth Suicide
P.O. Box 644
Westminster, CO 80030-0644
303-429-3530
www.yellowribbon.org

Suicide Hotline
888-SUICIDE
888-784-2433

Suicide Prevention Advocacy Network (SPAN)
www.spanusa.org/home.htm

BOOKS FOR CLIENTS AND FAMILIES

After Suicide: A Unique Grief Process
Ray of Hope, Inc.
1518 Derwen Dr.
Iowa City, IA 52240

The Ultimate Rejection
Suicide Prevention Center, Inc.
184 Salem Ave.
Dayton, OH 45406

BOOKS FOR CLIENTS AND FAMILIES *(continued)*

Afterwords: A Letter for and About Suicide Survivors
A. Wrobleski (Editor)
5124 Grove St.
Minneapolis, MN 55436-2481

Shamoo, T. K., & Patros, P. G. (1997). *Helping your child cope with depression and suicidal thoughts.* San Francisco: Jossey-Bass.

Steel, D. (1998). *His bright light.* New York: Delacorte Press.

KEY CONCEPTS

Introduction

- For every completed suicide, there are 10 to 20 unsuccessful attempts.

- Over 90 percent of suicide victims have a psychiatric disorder at the time of death.

- Nurses have higher rates of completed suicide than the general population, which is partly attributed to access to and knowledge about lethal medications.

Knowledge Base

- Suicide can be precipitated by hopelessness, delusions, hallucinations, intractable pain, multiple crises, and/or unexpressed anger.

- Previous attempts and a sense of hopelessness are the most powerful indicators of future completed suicide.

- Behavioral cues to potential suicide are verbal comments, obtaining a weapon, social isolation, giving away belongings, and substance abuse.

- Lethality is measured by the degree of effort it takes to plan the suicide, the specificity of the plan, the accessibility of the method, and the ease by which one may be rescued.

- In the United States, more people kill themselves with guns than by all other methods combined. Of gun-related deaths in the home, 83 percent are suicides.

- Affective cues to potential suicide are ambivalence, desolation, guilt, failure, shame, hopelessness, and helplessness.

- Cognitive cues to potential suicide are a rigid cognitive style, fantasies about death, interpersonal problems, command hallucinations, and delusions.

- Stressors related to suicide include unemployment, family disruption, rejection by significant others, abrupt changes in career responsibilities, and recent catastrophic events.

- Gay, lesbian, bisexual, or transgendered teens are ostracized from the dominant culture and are six times more likely to commit suicide than heterosexual youth.

- Copycat suicide seems to be an adolescent phenomenon, with girls more susceptible than boys are.

- Homicide–suicide often occurs within a family, and the perpetrator is usually a male.

- In addition to grief, survivors of suicide must cope with the stigma and cultural taboos associated with the death. They may experience shock, bewilderment, guilt, shame, anger, or relief.

- Euro-Americans have the highest rates of suicide in the United States.

- People over 65 have the highest suicide rate of all age groups followed by teens and young adults.

- At issue in assisted suicide is whether the dying should have the right to request and receive aid in dying from physicians.

- Oregon has a Death with Dignity Act, and the Netherlands is the first country to fully legalize euthanasia.

- People with mood disorders, schizophrenia, substance use disorders, and personality disorders are at risk for suicide.

- Suicide may be caused by many factors, including serotonin dysfunction, genetics, rapid social change, interpersonal or intrapersonal losses, a learned method of problem solving, and developmental crises.

The Nursing Process

Assessment

- Health care professionals must initiate suicide assessments. If the topic is not discussed, the person will have been abandoned while in a dangerously vulnerable position.

KEY CONCEPTS *(continued)*

- You cannot give the idea of suicide to anyone.

- Use specific language such as *kill yourself* or *commit suicide* when assessing clients.

- Assess for protective factors against suicidal acts.

- Accurate assessment will not prevent all suicides.

Diagnosis

- The most appropriate nursing diagnosis is high risk for violence, self-directed, related to acute suicidal state.

Outcome Identification and Goals

- The main goal is that the client remains safe from self-harm.

- Other goals include a decrease in suicidal thoughts, ability to problem solve, willingness to sign a no-suicide contract, and the development of a sense of hopefulness.

Nursing Interventions

- The first priority of care is to keep the client safe. Clients may need to be on suicide precautions or under constant observation.

- Encourage clients to implement the problem-solving process for alternative solutions to the difficulties fostering their suicidal intentions.

- It is appropriate to discuss the meaning of death with clients who are thinking about killing themselves.

- Clients may be asked to write and sign a no-suicide contract.

- Help clients develop a crisis card for community resources.

- If the suicide is successful, families will need active and supportive intervention.

Evaluation

- The most successful outcomes of the plan of care are that clients remain safe from self-harm, and that they improve their problem-solving skills.

EXPLORE *MediaLink*

- Interactive resources, including animations, for this chapter can be found on the Companion Web site at *http://www.prenhall.com/fontaine*. Click on Chapter 20 and select the activities for this chapter.

- For NCLEX review questions and an audio glossary, access the accompanying CD-ROM in this book.

REFERENCES

American Foundation for Suicide Prevention. (2001). *Facts about suicide*. www.afsp.org.

Battin, M. P., Rhodes, R., & Silvers, A. (1998). Introduction. In M. P. Battin, R. Rhodes, & A. Silvers (Eds.), *Physician assisted suicide*. (pp. 1–10). New York: Routledge.

Centers for Disease Control and Prevention. (2001). Suicide in the United States. *www.cdc.gov/ncipc/factsheets/suifacts.htm*.

Centers for Disease Control and Prevention. (2000). Leading causes of death reports. *www.cdc.gov*.

Centers for Disease Control and Prevention. (1998). Youth risk behavior surveillance—

United States. *Morbidity and Mortality Weekly Report, 47*, 1–89.

Cloud, J. (2001). A license to kill? *Time*, April 23, p. 66.

Cohen, C. B. (1998). Christian perspectives of assisted suicide and euthanasia. In M. P. Battin, R. Rhodes, & A. Silvers (Eds.), *Physician assisted suicide* (pp. 334–346). New York: Routledge.

Cohen, D., Llorente, M., & Eisdorfer, C. (1998). Homicide–suicide in older persons. *American Journal of Psychiatry, 155*(3), 390–396.

Drew, B. L. (2001). Self-harm behavior and

no-suicide contracting in psychiatric inpatient settings. *Archives of Psychiatric Nursing, 15*(3), 99–106.

Goetz, C. (1998). Are you prepared to S.A.V.E. your nursing student from suicide? *Journal of Nursing Education, 37*(2), 92.

Grunebaum, M. F., Oquendo, M. A., Harkavy-Friedman, J. M., Ellis, S. P., Li, S., Haas, G. L., et al. (2001). Delusions and suicidality. *American Journal of Psychiatry, 158*(5), 742–747.

Hendin, H., Lipschitz, A., Maltsberger, J. T., Haas, A. P., & Wynecoop, S. (2000). Therapists' reactions to patients' suicides.

American Journal of Psychiatry, 157(12), 2022–2026.

Johnson, M., Maas, M., & Moorhead, S. (2000). *Nursing outcomes classification (NOC)* (2nd ed.). St. Louis, MO: Mosby.

Krakowski, M. (2000). Impulse control: Integrative aspects. In M. L. Crowner (Ed.), *Understanding and treating violent psychiatric patients* (pp. 147–165). Washington, DC: American Psychiatric Press.

Lyon, M. E., Benoit, M., O'Donnell, R. M., Getson, P. R., Silber, T., & Walsh, T. (2000). Assessing African American adolescents' risk for suicide attempts. *Adolescence, 35*(137), 121–134.

Malone, K. M., Oquendo, M. A., Haas, G. L., Ellis, S. P., Li, S., & Mann, J. J. (2000). Protective factors against suicidal acts in major depression. *American Journal of Psychiatry, 157*(7), 1084–1088.

Mann, J. J., Waternaux, C., Haas, G. L., & Malone, K. M. (1999). Toward a clinical model of suicidal behavior in psychiatric patients. *American Journal of Psychiatry, 156*(2), 181–189.

Mann, J. J. (1998). Brain biology influences the risk for suicide. *Decade of the Brain, 8*(4), 3–4.

Matzo, M. L., & Schwarz, J. K. (2001). In their own words: Oncology nurses respond to patient requests for assisted suicide and euthanasia. *Applied Nursing Research, 14*(2), 64–71.

Nurse News. (2000). Oregon RNs and assisted suicide. *Nursing Spectrum, 13*(5IL), 9.

Pearson, J. (1998). Suicide in the United States. *Decade of the Brain, 8*(4), 1–2.

Prigerson, H. G., Bridge, J., Maciejewski, P. K., Berry, L. C., Rosenheck, R. A., Jacobs, S. C., et al. (1999). Influence of traumatic grief on suicidal ideation among young adults. *American Journal of Psychiatry, 156*(12), 1994–1995.

Robinson, B. A. (2001). Suicide among Canada's Native people. Ontario Consultants on Religious Tolerance. *www.religioustolerance.org/sui_nati.htm.*

Saulnier, C. F. (1998). Prevalence of suicide attempts and suicidal ideation among lesbian and gay youth. In L. M. Sloan, N. S. Gustavsson (Eds.), *Violence and social injustice against lesbian, gay, and bisexual people* (pp. 81–101). New York: Haworth Press.

Schwarz, J. K. (1999). Assisted dying and nursing practice. *Image, 31*(4), 367–373.

Shea, S. C. (1998). *Psychiatric interviewing: The art of understanding* (2nd ed.). Philadelphia: Saunders.

U.S. Department of Health and Human Services. (1999). *Mental Health: A Report of the Surgeon General—Executive Summary.* Rockville, MD: U.S. Department of Health and Human Services, Substance Abuse and Mental Health Services Administration, Center for Mental Health Services, National Institutes of Health, National Institute of Mental Health.

Zohar, N. J. (1998). Jewish deliberation on suicide. In M. P. Battin, R. Rhodes, & A. Silvers (Eds.), *Physician assisted suicide* (pp. 362–372). New York: Routledge.

CHAPTER 21

Domestic Violence

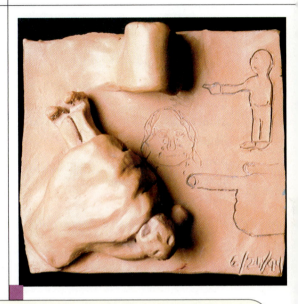

OBJECTIVES

After reading this chapter, you will be able to:

- IDENTIFY people who are at high risk for domestic violence.
- ASSESS all clients for evidence of domestic violence.
- IDENTIFY multidisciplinary treatment interventions.
- EVALUATE the short-term and long-term effectiveness of the plan of care.
- REPORT suspected incidents of child and elder abuse.

A tunnel is nothing but walls. You go into a long tunnel and all you see behind you and in front of you are more walls. You lose track of how long you've been there and you don't know how long it will take you to get out. If you do get out, what will be on the other side?

—Kay, Age 40

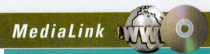

CD-ROM
- *Audio Glossary*
- *NCLEX Review*

Companion Web site www.prenhall.com/fontaine
- *Critical Thinking*
- *More NCLEX Review*
- *Case Study*
- *Care Map Activity*
- *Links to Resources*

KEY TERMS

Healthy People 2010, published by the U.S. Department of Health and Human Services (2000), describes domestic violence as a very significant problem in the United States. Domestic violence—violence within the family—occurs at all levels of society. The myth is that violence occurs only among the poor and undereducated, but the reality is that violence occurs also among the middle and upper classes and professional elite. See Box 21.1 for myths and facts about domestic violence. In the past, these problems among wealthy or prominent people were kept hidden from the general public. With an increase in national concern, however, more publicity is being given to cases of domestic violence at all socioeconomic levels. These objectives can be viewed on the *Healthy People 2010* Web site, which can be accessed through a resource link on the Companion Web site for this book.

In this chapter, the word family refers to any one of these three categories: (a) those who are related by birth, adoption, or marriage; (b) those in an intimate relationship; and (c) those who are in a domestic relationship, that is, sharing the same household.

BOX 21.1

Myths and Facts About Domestic Violence

Myth: Family violence is rare.
Fact: Every year, 10 million Americans are abused by a family member.

Myth: Family violence is confined to mentally disturbed or sick people.
Fact: Fewer than 10 percent of all cases involve an abuser who is mentally ill. The vast majority of abusers seem to be totally normal and are often charming, persuasive, and rational.

Myth: Violence is trivial—a joking matter.
Fact: A woman is beaten every 15 seconds in the United States, and 2,000 to 4,000 women are murdered by their husbands or boyfriends every year. Every year, 2.5 million children are abused, and 1,200 die from the abuse. There are 1 million cases of elder abuse annually.

Myth: Family violence is confined to the lower classes.
Fact: Social factors are not relevant. There are doctors, ministers, psychologists, and nurses who beat their family members. Violence occurs at least once in two thirds of all marriages.

Myth: All members of the family participate in the family dynamics; therefore, all must change in order for the violence to stop.
Fact: Only the perpetrator has the ability to stop the violence. A change in the victim's behavior will not cause the abuser to become nonviolent.

Myth: Family violence is usually a one-time event, an isolated incident.
Fact: Violence is a pattern, a reign of force and terror. It becomes more frequent and severe over time.

Myth: Abused women like being hit; otherwise, they would leave.
Fact: Abused women are forced to stay in the relationship for many reasons. The perpetrator dramatically escalates the violence when a woman tries to leave.

Although the image or fantasy of the American family is one of happiness and harmony, this ideal is often in conflict with the underlying reality of domestic violence. The home is the most frequent place for violence of all types. Women and children are more likely to be assaulted, raped, and killed by people who claim to love them. Perpetrators of violence do to intimates in their homes what they would not dare do any place else. The U.S. culture does not condone violence in schools, at work, or on the streets, but it continues to "allow" it within the privacy of the family. It is time that hitting licenses be canceled for all people.

Abuse, interchangeable with **violence** in this chapter, refers to a pattern of behavior that dominates, controls, lowers self-esteem, or takes away freedom of choice. It is systematic persecution of another individual ranging from subtle words or actions to violent battering—acts of commission. Abuse also includes various types of neglect—acts of omission. See Box 21.2 for definitions of types of abuse.

The incidence of domestic violence can only be estimated. Studies often include only those people who are willing to respond to surveys. Typically underrepresented in such studies are those who do not speak English, the very poor, the homeless, and those who are hospitalized or incarcerated at the time of the survey. The actual rates of domestic violence are probably much higher than reported.

In all 50 states, nurses are required by law to report suspected incidents of child abuse, and in every state, there is a penalty—civil, criminal, or both—for failure to report child abuse. In addition, not reporting child abuse is considered to be nursing malpractice. State laws vary for reporting the abuse of adults and the elderly. Forty-three states have mandatory reporting laws for elder abuse, with the other seven states saying elder abuse "may" be reported. In 1994, the Violence Against Women Act made it a federal crime to cross state lines to assault a spouse or domestic partner. This act was renewed in 2000 and funded with $300 million through 2005. Domestic violence is now considered to be a violent crime against which the victim has the right to be protected and for which the perpetrator can be arrested and prosecuted.

SIBLING ABUSE

The form of domestic violence most unrecognized occurs between siblings. Many people assume it is natural and even appropriate for children to use physical force with one another. Parents say things like "It's a

---

BOX 21.2

Types of Abuse

Emotional Abuse

Frequent belittling or demeaning; words or behaviors that undermine sense of self, competence, safety; psychological intimidation; accusations; demand obedience to every order; destruction of property, pets

Physical Abuse/Battering

Hitting, punching, grabbing, shoving, slapping, kicking, biting, hit with objects, use of weapons

Sexual Abuse

Inappropriate sexual behavior, including peeping, touching, rape, use of objects, forced sex with other people or animals

Social Abuse

Isolation from actual and potential support systems; controlling use of time and space; continual watching/spying

Economic Abuse

Little or no access to assets; minimal input into family expenditures

Neglect

Physical

Failure to provide adequate food, shelter, sleeping arrangements, clothing, and general physical care

Emotional

Failure to nurture, love, support; failure to validate self-worth

Medical

Failure to provide adequate medical care, especially when serious or life threatening

Educational

Failure to enroll child in school or alternative means of education; failure to get child to school; failure to assist child in completing educational tasks. Generally applied to child under age 11

Abandonment

Leaving child alone without adequate supervision; abandoning child, throwing child out of home, not allowing a runaway to return home

good chance for him to learn how to defend himself," "She had a right to hit him; he was teasing her," and "Kids will be kids." With these attitudes, children learn that physical force is an appropriate method of resolving conflict among themselves. Children who are hit by their parents have more than double the rate of violence against siblings than children whose parents did not hit them. Hitting children increases the probability that they will be violent. Parents should not be complacent about sibling aggression; 3 percent of all child homicides in the United States is caused by siblings. Even though violence decreases with age, studies indicate that 63 to 68 percent of adolescent siblings use physical violence to resolve conflict (Bloom & Reichert, 1998).

Charlie, age 13, is the eldest child of four: Jane, age 11, Trevor, age 8, and Taylor, age 6. Both parents work long hours just to make ends meet, so Charlie is left in charge when everyone gets home from school. Charlie constantly yells at Jane to pick up the house, cook dinner, and take care of the younger kids. When Jane says "no" Charlie curses at her and often kicks or punches her, saying "Why should I have to do everything around here?"

One day in gym class, the PE teacher noticed bruises on Jane's arm and a black-and-blue mark around her eye. When questioned about the bruises, Jane said, "Oh my brother and I were just roughhousing." Suspicious, the PE teacher documented what he had seen. When Jane appeared in class a week later with more bruises, the teacher filed a report and Social Services was alerted. A full physical examination revealed contusions, bruises, and lacerations on Jane's face, back, and legs from repeated beatings. When questioned, Charlie was stone-faced and stated that "he was just doing what it took to be in charge."

Closely related to sibling abuse is peer abuse that occurs at the junior high school level. Unlike any older age, at this level there is more female-to-male violence than male to female. Boys of this age still obey what their parents have told them: "Don't hit girls." Junior high school girls, however, feel empowered to hit boys when they tease, and the schools ignore this form of peer violence. Ultimately, young men abandon what they were told and strike back. We must tell young girls very clearly that if a boy teases them, a kick in the groin is *not* appropriate and that there are other ways to defend their honor.

CHILD ABUSE

Each year, approximately 2.8 million American children experience at least one act of physical violence, and 1.4 million are otherwise abused or neglected. Children who live in homes in which a parent is being abused are 1,500 times more likely to be abused than the national average. Younger parents are more likely to *physically abuse* children than older parents and the abuse is often disguised as discipline. For many, hitting begins when they are infants and does not end until they leave home. Younger children are spanked, punched, grabbed, slapped, kicked, bitten, and hit with fists or objects. Boys are at a higher risk for serious and/or fatal injuries. Adolescents are more likely to be beaten up and have a knife or gun used against them. Both men and women are equally likely to abuse young children. During adolescence, however, the abuser is more likely to be male (Hansen, Sedlar, & Warner-Rogers, 1999).

Shaken baby syndrome is one of the most serious yet frequently overlooked forms of child abuse. It involves vigorous shaking of babies who are being held by the extremities or shoulders that causes whiplash-induced intracranial and intraocular bleeding. It is estimated that one third have significant and permanent brain damage and one third of the victims die. Not recognizing the dangers, many parents shake rather than hit the child, mistakenly believing it is less violent (Ewing, 1997).

Clydell, a 19-year-old father, has been found guilty of murdering his 2-month-old son. He sobs uncontrollably at his sentencing, saying that he never meant to hurt his son—he just wanted him to stop crying. He didn't know that picking the baby up and shaking him would kill him.

Neglect is the most frequently reported type of child maltreatment. It differs from abuse in that it is an act of *omission* that results in harm. Neglect includes lack of adequate physical care, nutrition, and shelter. It also includes unsanitary conditions that often contribute to health and developmental problems. Lack of human contact and nurturance is considered to be emotional neglect (Gershater-Molko & Lutzker, 1999).

In the United States, **homicide** is one of the five leading causes of death before the age of 18. Sixty percent of children who are killed by their parents/caretakers are under the age of 4, and 40 percent are less than 1 year old. Most of these deaths are from battering in response to colic in the infant, toilet training difficulties in the toddler, and to special needs children. A small percentage of children are killed because they are unwanted, as the result of mercy killings, at the hands of a mentally ill parent, or in retaliation when one parent kills the child to inflict hurt on the other parent (Bloom & Reichert, 1998; Busby & Smith, 2000).

Shallane, age 12, was beaten to death by her parents. She had lost her jacket and when she was unable to find it she was severely punished. Her parents said they were acting on the Biblical injunction of 39 lashes times 3. Shallane's mother tied her to the bed and watched as her father beat her with an electrical cord. Before the beating was finished, Shallane died of internal injuries. Shallane had in fact been beaten 39 lashes times 3.

Although it is a rare event, each year more than 300 parents are killed by their children in the United States. This accounts for 1.5 to 2.5 percent of all homicides. Both victims and perpetrators tend to be Euro-Americans, with 30 percent of the perpetrators being under age 18. The most frequent situation, 90 percent of cases, is one in which the teen has been severely abused and/or the mother is a victim of abuse. The adolescent's attempts to get help have failed and the family situation becomes increasingly intolerable prior to the murder. A critical factor is the easy availability of guns in the home. The other 10 percent of cases involve either a severely mentally ill child who experiences hallucinations and delusions or the dangerously antisocial child who has extreme conduct problems (Ewing, 1997).

Munchausen syndrome by proxy (MSBP) often goes unrecognized as a form of child abuse. A parent, often the mother, persistently lies about symptoms the child is experiencing or actually induces symptoms in the child with the intent of keeping in contact with health care providers and hospitals. For example, she may add blood to a child's emesis, urine, or feces, purposefully create wounds and infect them, or even inject feces, poisons, or other toxins directly into the bloodstream. In a sense, the child is doubly abused, by both the parent's action and by frequent hospitalizations, extensive medical testing, and even a number of surgeries. Approximately 10 percent of the cases are fatal. The mother often seems to be a very concerned and loving parent, and it may take months or years and multiple "illnesses" before the manipulation is discovered. The victims are often young because older children would be more likely to tell health care professionals the truth about their so-called symptoms. The motivation for this type of child abuse is unknown. It is thought that women with a history of childhood abuse, who feel unloved and insecure, may seek love and support from their children's health care providers. As the mother is consulted and included in the care she receives the secondary gains of attention and support. Other thoughts are that some mothers may be expressing anger through MSBP or may be using the sick child to develop a closer relationship with her adult partner (Dowdell & Foster, 1999).

Milka, age 9 months, has been admitted to the hospital for episodes of breathing difficulties. Her mother seems to be needy of a great deal of staff attention. After several days, the staff noticed that Milka experienced breathing difficulties only when her mother was in the room. Through very careful observation, the staff identified that the mother would periodically put the pillow over Milka's face until she stopped breathing and the alarms went off. The mother would then quickly remove the pillow and hover over her daughter with great concern.

PARTNER ABUSE— HETEROSEXUAL

Although no class, ethnic group, religion, or age group is immune from domestic violence, most victims are *women*. And if the abused are mothers of dependent children, their children are likely to be victims also. Female partner abuse in heterosexual relationships is the most widespread form of family violence in the United States. It is thought that one woman in six is physically abused by her partner, and that 3 to 4 million women are severely assaulted every year. If verbal and emotional assaults were included, the numbers would be much higher. Violence is the single largest cause of injury to women in the United States, with 20 percent of emergency department visits resulting from physical abuse. Three to four battered women are killed every day in the United States (Bloom & Reichert, 1998; Torres & Han, 2000).

Half the women who are abused suffer beatings several times a year. The other half may be beaten as often as once a week. The intensity and frequency of attacks tend to escalate over time. Compared to nonabused women, abused women are five times more likely to attempt suicide, 15 times more likely to abuse alcohol, and nine times more likely to abuse drugs (Torres & Han, 2000).

Overwhelmingly, the first acts of partner violence occur in *dating relationships*. Physical abuse occurs among as many as 30 to 40 percent of college students and in 10 to 20 percent of high school students who are dating. Sadly, more than 25 percent of victims and 30 percent of offenders interpret violence as a sign of love. Common reasons teens and young adults give for the violence is betrayal and jealousy. Boys and girls are just as likely to be perpetrators or victims of physical abuse. Girls, however, are more likely to be victims of sexual violence. Victims of child abuse are more likely to become victims or perpetrators of violence in dating relationships (Centers for Disease Control and Prevention [CDC], 2000; O'Keefe, 1998). For early warning signs of teenage dating violence, see Box 21.3.

It is estimated that there are between 100,000 and 150,000 heterosexual *male partners* who are abused by women who initiate the violence. They are generally not recognized as "real" victims, and when they do tell others they are criticized for not standing up for themselves or for not fighting back.

BOX 21.3

Early Warning Signs of Teenage Dating Violence

The teenage perpetrator:

■ Believes that men should be in control and women should be submissive
■ Is jealous and possessive of his girlfriend, won't let her have friends, and checks up on her
■ Tries to control his girlfriend by giving orders and making all the decisions
■ Threatens his girlfriend with violence
■ Uses or owns weapons
■ Has a history of losing his temper quickly and fighting
■ Brags about mistreating others
■ Blames his girlfriend when he is violent; says she provoked him and made him do it
■ Has a history of abusive relationships

PARTNER ABUSE— HOMOSEXUAL

Until very recently, there has been a public minimization or denial of physical abuse in lesbian and gay relationships. This denial has been supported by the myths that women are not violent people and that men can defend themselves. In reality, violence does occur in some gay and lesbian families, for the same reasons as in heterosexual families: to demonstrate, achieve, and maintain **power** and **control** over one's partner. In addition to physical or emotional abuse, the violent partner may use *homophobic control*—the threat of telling ("outing") family, friends, neighbors, or employers about the victim's sexual orientation.

In the United States, domestic violence is the third largest health problem for gay men, following substance abuse and HIV/AIDS. It is estimated that 20 to 25 percent of coupled gay men and lesbians are victims. Men rarely talk about being victims for fear of being considered feminine if they admit that their partners are hurting them. Looking at violence in same-sex relationships demonstrates clearly that violence is not a gender issue but rather a power issue.

Homophobia and hatred of homosexuals in the

United States contributes to difficulties of battered lesbians and gays. They are cut off from the usual support systems available to heterosexual victims such as specialized counseling services and shelters. Most state laws regarding domestic violence exclude gays and lesbians with the use of terms such as *spouse* and *battered wife*. Gays and lesbians of color and those who live in rural areas are even more isolated than their counterparts. Because same-sex partnerships are not recognized as "legitimate," victims have no access to the legal system. Often, being victimized by one's lover is less frightening than being victimized by the legal system. Fear of being identified as gay or losing custody of children adds to the silence about the violence. Members of lesbian and gay communities are currently making an attempt to intervene with and support victims (Levy & Lobel, 1998; West, 1998a).

ELDER ABUSE

One and a half million elderly people are mistreated each year nationwide. *Elder abuse* is any deliberate action or negligence that harms elderly people. *Physical abuse* is the nonaccidental use of physical force that results in bodily injury, pain, or impairment. Some older adults may have their basic physical needs *neglected* and suffer from dehydration, malnutrition, decubiti, urine burns, and oversedation. Families may deprive them of necessary articles such as glasses, hearing aids, and walkers. *Emotional neglect* can mean leaving a person for long periods of time or failing to provide social contact. Some older people are *psychologically abused* by verbal assaults, threats, intimidation, humiliation, and/or harassment. Remarks such as "One of these days I am going to poison your food and you won't know when" are considered psychological abuse.

Families may *violate* an older person's *rights* by refusing appropriate medical treatment, forcing isolation or unreasonable confinement, denying privacy, providing an unsafe environment, or demanding involuntary servitude. Some elders are *financially exploited* by their relatives through theft or misuse of property or funds. Others are beaten and even *sexually abused* or raped by family members.

Perpetrators of elder abuse may be a spouse, child, grandchild, niece, nephew, or some other relative. The abuse is most likely to be inflicted by a person with whom the victim lives. Those elders with mental or physical disabilities are at greatest risk. A number of factors contribute to abuse of older adults. Perpetrators may have personal problems such as lack of support in caring for the older family member, alcohol or drug addiction, or a family history of violence. Family factors include unresolved previous conflicts and power struggles. The perpetrator may be retaliating for previous abuse suffered at the hands of the elder person. Elderly people are often resistant to intervention because they fear that losing a caregiver will mean they will have to be put in an institution (Adelman, Lachs, & Breckman, 1999; Raphel & Berry, 1998).

EMOTIONAL ABUSE

Although the focus of violence in this chapter is on physical abuse, it must be remembered that emotional abuse is often equally as damaging. Words can hit as hard as a fist, and the damage to self-esteem can last a lifetime. Emotional abuse involves one person shaming, embarrassing, ridiculing, or insulting another either in private or in public. It may include destruction of personal property or the killing of pets in an effort to frighten or control the victim. Such statements as "You can't do anything right," "You're ugly and stupid—no one else would want you," and "I wish you had never been born" are devastating to self-esteem.

ABUSE OF PREGNANT WOMEN

Pregnancy is a time of increased risk for abuse. There are more incidents of violence during pregnancy than of hypertension, gestational diabetes or placenta previa, all of which are screened for regularly. Indeed, 16 to 25 percent of women report abuse during pregnancy. A past history of abuse is one of the strongest predictors of abuse during pregnancy. Nonpregnant women are usually beaten in the face and chest. But pregnant women tend to be beaten in the abdomen, which can lead to miscarriage, placenta abruptio, fetal loss, premature labor, fetal fractures, pelvic fractures, rupture of the uterus, and hemorrhage. Battering during pregnancy is associated with severity of abuse. The man who beats his pregnant partner is an extremely violent and dangerous man. Battering during pregnancy is also a risk factor for eventual homicide of the female partner (Bloom & Reichert, 1998).

The first prenatal visit is often related to abuse status. Abused women are twice as likely to delay prenatal care until the third trimester. Many abused women report that the abuser forced them to avoid prenatal care by denying them access to transportation.

Physical abuse during pregnancy may be related to ambivalent feelings about the pregnancy, competition for attention with the developing fetus, increased vulnerability of the woman, increased economic pressures, and decreased sexual availability. Unfortunately, abuse of pregnant women is often overlooked by health care professionals, even when the victim appears in the emergency department with bruises, cuts, broken bones, and abdominal injuries.

STALKING

The term *stalking* has become not only a part of the American vocabulary but also a new classification of crime and all 50 states have passed stalking laws. **Stalking** is the act of following, viewing, communicating with, or moving threateningly toward another person. Property damage and assault may accompany stalking. Most victims are exposed to a number of different stalking behaviors by the same perpetrator such as (Kamphuis & Emmelkamp, 2001):

- Unwelcome mail, phone calls, and visits
- Harass at work or home
- Follow on the street
- Threaten or use violence
- Make threats against family members
- Damage property
- Order items and charge to victim's account
- Spread rumors and lies

In the United States, 8.2 million women and 2 million men report being stalked at some time in their lives. Women are far more likely to be victims, and men are far more likely to be perpetrators (Reno, 1999).

Domestic stalking occurs when a former partner, spouse, or family member threatens or harasses a per-

son. The stalker often makes it clear that the victim is his "property." The stalker is usually motivated by a desire to continue the relationship, which can evolve into an attitude of "If I can't have her/him, no one can." In some cases, the stalker is angry and retaliating against the victim whom he perceives as rejecting him. Frequently, there is a history of domestic violence, and the stalking often ends in a violent attack on or killing of the victim (Mullen, Pathe, Purcell, & Stuart, 1999).

Victims often feel trapped in an environment filled with anxiety, stress, and fear that often result in their having to make drastic changes in how they live their lives. Most victims seek legal counsel, restraining orders, change their phone numbers and daily travel routes, avoid going out of their home, and increase their home security. In spite of these responses, the stalking may continue for several years (Kamphuis & Emmelkamp, 2001).

After three years of living together, Gwen left Brian because of his moodiness, violent temper, and infidelities. Shortly after Gwen moved out, Brian would leave threatening notes on her car windshield and would call her constantly at work and at her new apartment threatening to kill her if she would not marry him. Gwen would often find that her tires had been flattened and on more than one occasion, Brian attempted to run her off the road. Gwen filed a restraining order but the stalking continued. Gwen was afraid to go out of the house because Brian would just seem to show up wherever she was. It took Brian beating up Gwen for authorities to notice. Brian screamed in court that he would kill Gwen for what she had done to him. The stalking had gone on for over a year.

Cyberstalking refers to the use of the Internet, e-mail, or other electronic communications to stalk another person. It is a serious problem that is likely to become more widespread. Similar to other forms of stalking, cyberstalkers wish to establish control over the victim. In many cases there was a prior relationship between perpetrator and victim, but there are also a number of situations of cyberstalking by strangers. With the anonymity and lack of direct confrontation, some individuals feel empowered to stalk via electronic media. A common form of cyberstalking is repeated sending of threatening or harassing messages. Some perpetrators post "supposed messages" from the victim on bulletin boards or in chat rooms, thus tricking other Internet users into further harassment of the victim. For example, a perpetrator "posted information on the Web claiming her 9-year-old daughter was available for sex. The Web posting included their home phone number with instructions to call 24 hours a day. They received numerous calls" (Reno, 1999, p. 8).

KNOWLEDGE BASE

As a nurse, you must be involved in the prevention, detection, and treatment of domestic violence. Development of the knowledge base and the ability to identify factors that contribute to family violence will help you arrive at early detection and an accurate diagnosis of the problem. Male perpetrator–female victim is used as the model for ease in reading.

BEHAVIORAL CHARACTERISTICS

Domestic violence is the deliberate and systematic pattern of abuse used to establish *power* and *control* over the victim through fear and intimidation. The behavior is always intentional. Perpetrators choose to be violent and give themselves permission to be violent. Perpetrators are not out of control, as is commonly assumed. They may be enraged or cool and calculating, but in either case they have made a choice. The victim cannot "make them do it." Generally, perpetrators of domestic violence are law abiding and are dangerous only to their loved ones

To the victim, domestic violence often happens without warning and without a buildup of tension. A pattern of violence usually develops. Frustration or stress may precipitate the first incident. If the victim immediately refuses to accept the violence and seeks outside help, there are often no further episodes. If the victim submits to the violence, then physical force, without the stimulus of frustration or stress, becomes a way of relating, and the pattern becomes resistant to change. A typical cycle occurs when conflict escalates into a violent episode, after which the perpetrator begs for the victim's forgiveness. The victim stays in the system because of promises to reform. With the next episode of conflict, the **cycle of violence** begins again and becomes part of the family dynamics (see Table 21.1 ■).

Acts of violence against children range from a light slap to severe beating to homicide. Hitting or *spanking children* is condoned and even approved of as being necessary and good for the child. Many parents, how-

---

TABLE 21.1

The Cycle of Violence

Perpetrator	Victim
Tension Building Phase	
Moody, withdraws affection, isolates victim, name-calling, verbally abusive, destroys property	Attempts to calm partner, nurturing, stays away from support systems, passive, feels as if walking on eggshells
Battering Phase	
Pushing, shoving, hitting, other acts of violence	Protects self any way possible; someone else calls police; victim leaves
Contrition Phase	
Says sorry, begs forgiveness, promises never again	Agrees to stay or return; attempts to stop legal proceedings; hopeful

SOURCE: Adapted from Dutton, D. G. (1998). *The abusive personality.* New York: Guilford Press.

ever, do not realize the underlying messages they are giving to the child by hitting (Straus, 1994):

- If you are small and weak, you deserve to be hit.
- People who love you hit you.
- It is appropriate to hit people you love.
- Violence is appropriate if the end result is good.
- Violence is an appropriate method of resolving conflict.

No studies have demonstrated that spanking is an effective method of discipline beyond the initial effect. Only nonphysical interventions, such as time-outs, are effective in the long run in helping children modify their unwanted behavior. When spanking is not effective, some parents increase physical punishment in an effort to maintain control and demand obedience (Bauman & Friedman, 1998). See Box 21.4 for myths that surround the use of spanking.

Parental violence often becomes chronic in that it occurs periodically or regularly. In extreme cases, it ends in the death of the infant or child. Child victims are helpless captives because they are dependent on the adults in the family. Abused children often try to please the abusing parent and may become overly compliant to all adults. They may avoid peers and withdraw from outside contacts. It is not unusual for child victims to act out with aggressive behavior later, during adolescence.

Jerry, age 18, was brought to the psychiatric unit by the police. He had been arrested at home for threatening the lives of his family. Jerry describes his mother as abusive, neglectful, and alcoholic. He states that he has always been blamed for any trouble. When he was younger he was locked in the closet for hours on end. At times, his mother forced his older siblings to hold Jerry down while he was beaten by her and his stepfather. Sometimes, she would place an open coat hanger in his mouth and twirl it around. Jerry remembers being forced to stand all night with his hands in the air until his mother would finally fall asleep. Jerry's brothers both ran away from home at the age of 16. Jerry, unable to distance himself from his mother and her cruelty, has remained at home. He has a history of violence as well as alcohol and drug abuse.

BOX 21.4

Myths That Surround the Use of Spanking

Myth: Spanking is harmless.
Fact: Spanking makes parenting more difficult because it reduces parents' ability to influence their children, especially when the children are teens and are too big to control by physical force. Also, authority figures should be trusted and respected, not feared.

Myth: I was spanked, and I'm okay.
Fact: You made it despite being hit; hitting increases the probability that you are more likely to use aggression to handle conflicts.

Myth: If you don't spank, your children will be spoiled or run wild.
Fact: Nonspanked children are better behaved than are children of parents who spank. Nonspanking parents tend to pay more attention to their children's behavior and tend to do more explaining and reasoning, which helps children develop internal controls.

Myth: Spanking is needed as a last resort.
Fact: If spanking is done at all, "last resort" may be the worst since parents are usually very angry and act impulsively. It teaches children that being extremely angry justifies hitting.

Myth: Parents spank rarely or only for serious problems.
Fact: Parents who spank tend to use this method for almost any misbehavior; many do not even give the child a warning—they spank before trying other things.

Myth: It is unrealistic to expect parents to never spank.
Fact: It is no more unrealistic to expect parents to not hit a child than to expect that husbands not hit their wives or that a supervisor never hit an employee.

SOURCE: Adapted from Straus, M. A. (1994). *Beating the devil out of them: Corporal punishment in American families.* Lexington, MA: Lexington Books.

Among adult family members, women commit fewer violent acts than men do. Women do more hitting, kicking, and throwing of objects, and their violent behavior is often in self-defense. Men are more likely to push, shove, slap, beat up, and even use knives or guns against their partner. The acts that men commit against women are more dangerous and result in more severe injuries. While the victim is being beaten, she is also being verbally abused, often by being called a slut, a bad housekeeper, or a rotten mother. The abuser attacks aspects of life that women use to measure their success: homemaking, child care, attractiveness, sex appeal, and sexual fidelity.

The abuser is the most powerful person in the life of the victim. The abuser's purpose is to *enslave the victim*, while simultaneously demanding respect, gratitude, and love. Control over the victim is established by repetitive emotional abuse that instills terror and helplessness. Threats of serious harm or threats against other family members keep the victim in a constant state of fear. In order to have complete domination, the abuser isolates the victim. She often is forced to give up work, friends, and family. He may stalk her, eavesdrop, and intercept letters and phone calls. Control and scrutiny of the victim's body and bodily functions further destroy her sense of autonomy. She is shamed and demoralized when told what to eat, when to sleep, what to wear, when to go to the bathroom, and so on. For a victim who has been deprived long enough, the hope of a meal, a bath, or a kind word can be a powerful reward. All this abusive behavior alternates with unpredictable outbursts of physical violence. Such domestic captivity of women, along with traumatic bonding to the batterer, often goes unrecognized.

Homicide is the ultimate expression of male control over females. Of women who are murdered, 50 percent are killed by a past or present husband or lover. At least two thirds of these women have been abused by their murderer prior to their death. The vast majority have previously turned to the police and courts for help. The risk of death increases as the victims resist or try to take control over their lives by leaving the abuser. In the case of a joint homicide–suicide, the perpetrator is almost always male and the victim is almost always female.

Women sometimes kill their husbands or lovers, almost invariably in response to years of abuse. Those victims who kill typically have suffered more frequent abuse with serious injuries, have been threatened with death, and have fewer coping resources than battered women in general. They most often murder their partners in self-defense, fearing for their lives and the lives of their children. One third of the murders occur during the course of battering incidents. The remainder occurs while the abuser is asleep or otherwise preoccupied. The battered woman syndrome is a permissible legal defense in all 50 states (Ewing, 1997; O'Leary & Murphy, 1999).

AFFECTIVE CHARACTERISTICS

Violent people are often extremely *jealous* and *possessive*. They view other family members in terms of property and ownership and believe that they are entitled to control others. Abusers use violence in an attempt to prove to themselves and others that they are superior and in control. The use of physical force temporarily obliterates their sense of inadequacy and compensates for a lack of internal resources.

Victims may be immobilized by a variety of affective responses to the abuse such as anxiety, helplessness, and depression. Feelings of self-blame may be expressed in such statements as "If I hadn't talked back to my mother, she wouldn't have hit me," and "If I were a better wife, he wouldn't beat me." Guilt can contribute to depression, which further immobilizes victims and keeps them from leaving or seeking help for the family system.

Fear contributes to women's inability to leave abusive relationships. Often threatened with death at the idea of leaving, they live in fear of physical reprisal. Fearing loneliness, some women may believe that being in a bad relationship is better than being alone. Also, leaving the relationship does not necessarily ensure the end of the abuse. The abuser is often most dangerous when threatened with or faced with separation. Some choose to kill when they believe that death is better than divorce. See Box 21.5 for reasons why people stay in or return to abusive relationships.

Michael, age 45, is a very successful physician. During recent divorce proceedings, he has confessed to periodically beating his wife Maria. At times he would yank her around by the hair or hold her out of a second-story window and threaten to let her fall. During each of Maria's three pregnancies, Michael would beat her, particularly in her abdomen, saying he wished he could kill both her and the unborn child. This periodic abuse has continued throughout the 20-year marriage but was kept a family secret until the divorce proceedings.

BOX 21.5

Why Do They Stay? Why Do They Go Back?

Fear

They fear physical reprisal if they resist, of being found and beaten again, or of their children being hurt. Those who attempt to leave risk suffering worse violence and even death.

Learned Helplessness

They believe they have no choices and no control and they have come to believe that violence is an accepted way of life.

Traumatic Bonding

Traumatic bonding results from alternating good and bad treatment and is worsened by no sense of autonomy.

Emotional Dependency

They are convinced that they are weak and inferior and do not deserve better treatment. The thought of potential autonomy is frightening because of their insecurity.

Financial Dependency

They may not have a source of income. If the abuser is arrested, he may lose his job and the family will have no income. They have been taught that they have to be submissive in exchange for financial support.

Guilt/Shame

They have been convinced that they provoked the abuse and often feel guilt over the failure of the relationship. There may be family/religious/cultural values against divorce or separation. They may feel shame about remaining in the abusive relationship.

Severe depression

Severe depression often accompanies abuse. Victims who are depressed do not have the energy to take action.

Isolation

They have few, if any, friends and little support from extended family. Abuser often allows no phone or mail contact, no use of a car, and may even confine the victim in the home.

Children

Victims may believe two parents are better than one. They may have been threatened with loss of custody or the abuser may threaten to harm or kidnap the children.

Hope

They hope that if they change in the way the abuser wants them to, the abuse will stop. They continue to hope that the abuser will keep promises and stop the assaults.

Fear also contributes to the inability to leave for a partner in an abusive gay or lesbian relationship. Because many couples share close friends within the same community, victims may fear shaming their partners. They may also fear friends will either deny the problem or take the abuser's side. Homophobia contributes to the victim's reluctance to seek help. Calling the police may result in ridicule or hostile responses from the officers. Victims may not seek help from family members to avoid reinforcing negative stereotypes about homosexuality, which might exacerbate the family's homophobia (West, 1998a).

COGNITIVE CHARACTERISTICS

Many abusive people have *perfectionistic standards* for family members. An unrealistically high standard results in rigidity and an obsession with discipline and control. Inflexibility hinders the abuser's ability to find alternative solutions to conflict. Some abusers have a self-righteous belief that they have a prerogative to use physical force to make others comply with their wishes. Many abusers lack an understanding of the effect of their behavior on the victims and may even blame their abusive behavior on the victims, evidence of the use of denial, projection, and an external locus of control. See Box 21.6 for examples of how people "explain" their violent behavior.

Abusers shape reality for and create significant *cognitive distortions* in their victims. Using fear and isolation, abusers construct a reality in which the victim is defective, incompetent, lazy, careless, ugly, undesirable, promiscuous, stupid, and bad. The abuser then justifies the abuse as punishment for these negative traits.

BOX 21.6

How Perpetrators Explain Violent Behavior

Denial

Denial of all or part of their violent behavior—"It never happened."

Forgetting

Blanking out their behavior—"I can't remember."

Minimization

Minimizing the extent, frequency, and effects—"It was just . . ." or "It was only . . ."

Removal of Self

Separation of the sense of self from the abusive behavior—"I'm not a violent person."

Event Without Intention

Abuse has an independent dynamic of its own—"If she hadn't ducked down, she wouldn't have been hit in her face. She would have only been hit in her belly."

Excuses

Accepts the blame but not the responsibility—"I was abused as a kid, that's why I do it" or "I couldn't help it, I had too much to drink."

Justifications

Accepts the responsibility but not the blame—"You're a lousy mother—I'll teach you to keep these kids quiet."

Confessions

These can be with or without remorse. Confessions become normalized as part of a violent way of life—"I didn't mean to hit you so hard."

Many parents who abuse their children suffered emotional deprivation or abuse when they themselves were children. As parents, they may lack information about the normal growth and development of children and therefore have unrealistic expectations. Anger may turn to violence when a child is unable to meet the parent's unreasonable demands.

Victims of abuse often begin with or develop *low self-esteem*. They begin to believe the violence itself is evidence of personal worthlessness. Some victims even absolve the abuser from responsibility by blaming violent behavior on a high level of stress or too much alcohol.

SOCIAL CHARACTERISTICS

The abuser's *family history* is an important factor in understanding domestic violence. Much of adult behavior is determined by childhood experiences within the family system. The experience of violence in the family of origin teaches that the use of physical force is appropriate. Children may cope with exposure to abuse by identifying with either the aggressor or the victim. Often, these children grow up to become another abuser or adult victim. In addition, the media provide ample opportunity for children to see violence and learn to identify with and tolerate violent behavior (Ewing, 1997).

The violent family is often *socially isolated*. In some families, the isolation precedes the violence. In others, the isolation is in response to the violence. Family members, ashamed of what is occurring, withdraw from interactions with others to avoid the humiliation that might occur if the violence became known.

Abused women experience significant *stress* when they leave their abusers. Women who are forced to flee from their abusers to seek safety must give up their homes, their jobs, their system of child care, and perhaps financial security. Women who experience these significant life changes and have few supportive networks are at risk for problems such as depression and posttraumatic stress disorder (Torres & Han, 2000).

CULTURE-SPECIFIC CHARACTERISTICS

Violence is a complex behavior, and, like all behaviors, it occurs in the context of culture. Severe and ongoing domestic violence has been documented in almost every country in the past 25 years. The vast majority of victims are females. In a study of 90 societies throughout the world, wife beating was present in 75 societies. There appear to be four cultural factors that are strong predictors of wife abuse. The strongest factor is (a) gender economic inequality, followed by (b) male authority and decision making in the home, (c) divorce restrictions for women, and (d) a pattern of using physical violence for conflict resolution. The more women are completely dependent on men, the more vulnerable they are to violent action with no options for escape. The following are some examples of violence against women (Desjarlais et al., 1995; McCloskey & Eisler, 1999):

- Afghanistan—All women are victims of extreme violence, including severe mutilation and murder.
- Papua, New Guinea—56 to 67 percent of women are beaten.
- Bangladesh—50 percent of all murders are husbands killing their wives.
- Sri Lanka—60 percent of women are beaten.
- Mexico—60 percent of women are physically abused.
- Kenya—42 percent of wives say they are beaten regularly.
- Chile—80 percent of women have suffered abuse by male partner or relative.
- Japan—59 percent of women report abuse.
- Korea—38 percent of women are abused.
- Thailand—more than 50 percent of married women are beaten regularly.
- Peru—33 percent of women who come to the emergency department are victims of domestic violence.
- Norway—25 percent of women have been physically and/or sexually abused.
- New Zealand—17 percent of women are abused.
- Italy—The highest court has ruled that it is not a crime to beat your wife, as long as you do it only once in a while.

Domestic violence resulting in death is a serious problem in some parts of the world. In India, the illegal "dowry death" or "bride-burning" occurs in some areas. The relatives of married sons demand large sums of material goods from the families of daughters-in-law. If this is not provided, they may kill the young woman. Female infanticide has increased in parts of Asia over the past decade. Not only is this a tragic loss of life, but it also has a tremendous impact on the mental health of mothers and other family members. Women are forced from family pressures and agonizing circumstances to make desperate moral choices. These choices are not easily made nor ever forgotten (Desjarlais et al., 1995).

Since the early 1990s women have been systematically beaten, terrorized, and oppressed in Afghanistan.

The Taliban forced them to wear burkas—heavy head-to-toe coverings that are very hot, restrict airflow, and limit movement. Women were not allowed out of their homes unless accompanied by a male family member. They could not attend school or hold a job. Women could not laugh in public, and had to walk in such a way that no part of their body was exposed. Any male who witnessed an infraction was free to beat, stone, mutilate, or murder the "offending" woman. There is a political advocacy group called the Revolutionary Association of Women of Afghanistan, or *RAWA*, which is agitating to gain basic rights for women in Afghanistan.

The United States has a higher rate of intrafamily homicide than the overall rate of homicide in European countries such as England, Germany, and Denmark. Women of all racial and ethnic backgrounds are exposed to acts of violence by their male partners. Some studies indicate that African American women are twice as likely to experience severe violence as are Euro-American women. Risk factors include young age, low socioeconomic status, and unemployment/underemployment of men. Among the Latino American population, Puerto Rican husbands are twice as likely than Euro-American husbands and 10 times more likely than Cuban American husbands to assault their wives. Domestic violence often arises out of dysfunctional adaptation to extreme economic pressure. Among Hispanic American couples, the rates vary according to immigration status. Mexican Americans born in the United States report rates 2.5 times higher than those born in Mexico do. No studies have been conducted on partner violence among Asian Americans (Taylor, 2000; West, 1998b).

If the immigrant family had negative experiences with authorities in their native country, they may wish to avoid contact with the police or social service agencies. If they are undocumented immigrants, they may fear that their illegal status will be discovered if they report domestic violence.

Domestic violence is not traditional in Native People's life but has evolved in modern times. The sanctions and protections against battering have decreased, and women are increasingly vulnerable to violence. As with other minority groups, family tension is increased by unemployment, undereducation, and financial strain. Elders believe the long-term solution is to return to traditional values that nurture children, give them self-esteem, and teach boys to love and respect women (Spector, 2000).

CONCOMITANT DISORDERS

The effect of living in a climate of fear and uncertainty contributes to an increased risk for several mental disorders. Problems associated with child abuse include depression, substance abuse, self-mutilation, eating disorders, and dissociative disorders. Conduct disorder is nine times as likely to occur in abused adolescents compared to the nonabused population. Sixty to eighty-five percent of abused children and adults are at risk for posttraumatic stress disorder (PTSD). The more severe the battering episodes and injuries, the greater the intensity of PTSD symptoms. Family violence has the worst mental health outcomes of any form of interpersonal violence because there is no safe and supportive place for retreat. Even civilians caught up in a war still experience the family as a place of safety and security (Hall, 2000; Widom, 1999; Woods, 2000).

Research suggests that there is an association between domestic violence and premature infants. This may be a result of direct physical abuse causing the onset of labor or death of the fetus. It is believed that premature delivery may also be related to the psychosocial stress of the abuse (Horan, Hill, & Schulkin, 2000).

CAUSATIVE THEORIES

Domestic violence is easy to describe but difficult to explain. There is no single cause of this type of violence. It results from an interaction of biogenic, personality, situational, and societal factors that have an impact on families.

Neurobiological Theory

Biogenic theorists propose that genes and neurotransmitters may contribute to causing violent behavior. Although a genetic predisposition may make certain behaviors more likely, it does not make them inevitable. Serotonin (5-HT) plays an important role in mood and aggressive behavior. 5-HT calms us through inhibitory control over aggression. Abnormally low levels of 5-HT result in a lack of control, loss of temper, and explosive rage (Ratey, 2001).

Childhood abuse and neglect lead to permanent alternations in the parts of the central nervous system that are known to be stress responsive. Corticotropin-releasing factor (CRF) is a major regulator of the

endocrine, autonomic, immune, and behavioral stress responses. It is thought that stress early in life results in sensitization of the brain to even mild stressors in adulthood, thus contributing to mood and anxiety disorders long after the abuse or neglect has stopped (Heim, Newport, Bonsall, & Miller, 2001).

Intrapersonal Theory

Intrapersonal theory suggests that the cause of violence lies in the personality of the abuser. It is thought that people who are violent *choose not to control their expressions of anger and hostility.* As many as 80 percent of male abusers grew up in homes in which they were abused or observed their mothers being abused. Sometimes these children try unsuccessfully to intervene, and sometimes they just try to get out of the way. Typically, they are afraid to go for help because of the code of family secrecy regarding the abuse and because they recognize that they too will be abused if they tell. Some children "externalize" their responses and become aggressive to siblings and peers, destructive, and noncompliant with adults. Some children "internalize" their responses and become fearful and withdrawn. Both of these responses contribute to a delay in social development by being unpopular and rejected or by being too anxious to participate in activities.

This early emotional deprivation contributes to an adult who is very needy of nurturance and support. He comes to adult relationships with unrealistic demands for time and attention. As the relationship develops, he discourages his partner's relationships with other people because of his low self-esteem and fear of abandonment (Sudermann & Jaffe, 1999).

Parents who abuse their children often have inappropriate expectations of themselves and their children. They may have inadequate parenting skills and a lack of resources. Often, they lack empathy toward children's needs and there may even be role reversal between parent and child.

Social Learning Theory

Social learning theory proposes that violence is a *learned behavior* and people are conditioned to respond aggressively and violently. Young boys are encouraged to demonstrate strength and dominance rather than empathetic and caring attributes. Children learn about violence from observation, from being a victim, and from behaving violently themselves. If the use of violence is rewarded by a gain in power or a reduction in anxiety, the behavior is reinforced. If there is immediate negative reinforcement within the family, a decrease in violent behavior will result. Learning to abuse is the first step in the battering process but it does not necessarily lead vulnerable individuals to abuse. The social environment impacts how the potentially abusive person behaves. In other words, the person must have the *opportunity to abuse* without suffering negative consequences. There is the perception that he can "get away with it." Although learning may have occurred and opportunity is present, the potentially abusive person makes a *conscious choice* to abuse. The batterer is solely responsible for the violence.

In addition to family models, the media provide many models of violence to which children are exposed. Some movies and television shows demonstrate that "good" people use force to achieve "good" ends. Many of the stories make no attempt to justify the use of force for "good" ends; they simply present endless, senseless acts of cruelty by one human being upon another. With these types of family and media examples, children develop values that tolerate, and even accept as normal, everyday violence between people.

Feminist Theory

Feminist theory describes the *sexist structure* of the family and society as an important factor in domestic violence. The cultural value is that men have a right to keep women subordinate through power and privilege. Men abuse because they believe they have a right to do so and because they can get away with it. Domestic violence is a power issue. Victims are sometimes labeled as co-dependent in the abusive relationship, but such labeling is just another way of blaming the victim for the abuse. Women are sexualized as objects, restricted in state and federal participation in decision making, dehumanized with labels, controlled over the rights to their own bodies, and demeaned in value (Gamache, 1998).

The sexist economic system helps entrap women, who often are forced to choose between poverty and abuse. It is difficult for women to find advocates and solutions within the male-dominated legal, religious, mental health, and medical systems. Society sanctions male violence by neglecting female victims. What remains unacknowledged is that women are being murdered on a regular basis, not by strangers but by husbands and lovers.

CRITICAL THINKING

Branko and Drenka, a Serbian/American couple, dated for nine months prior to their marriage, during which time Branko was attentive and adoring of Drenka but often jealous and possessive. Following their marriage, Branko insisted that Drenka quit her job and stay home even though Drenka enjoyed working and feared becoming bored. Drenka became pregnant right away. During her pregnancy, Branko became totally possessive of Drenka, keeping her from family or friends. After the birth of their daughter, Branko began criticizing Drenka for her care of the baby, her care of the house, and the time she devoted to him. Drenka always felt that Branko's criticism was justified because she didn't enjoy being a housewife. Eventually, Branko's criticism gave way to pushing, shoving, hitting, and threatening Drenka's life. He maintained that she forced him to be violent because she didn't perform her duties as well as he expected. After each violent episode, Branko would vow his undying love for Drenka and promise that he would never hit her again. Drenka feels frightened and ashamed but does not report Branko's violence because she believes that if she works harder, Branko's behavior will change.

1. What affective and cognitive characteristics in Branko's behavior may have forewarned of his abusive tendency?

2. Based on data about domestic violence, what social characteristic was likely present in Branko's past that predisposed him to becoming violent?

3. What is the fallacy in Drenka's belief that if she works harder, Branko's behavior will change?

4. What is the prediction based on the interaction between Drenka and Branko if he seriously injured her and she had to be cared for in a health care setting?

5. Based on your understanding of domestic violence and spousal abuse, what are the greatest dangers to Drenka if she does not seek help?

6. As a mental health nurse, if you were Drenka's friend and she confided in you that she was in an abusive relationship, how might you respond?

For an additional Case Study, please refer to the Companion Web site for this book.

NURSING PROCESS

Assessment

Given the incidence of abuse, it is logical to assume that you will encounter victims in a variety of clinical settings. Although one third of all women's visits to emergency departments are caused by domestic violence, fewer than 10 percent are identified. Women are treated for the immediate injury or complaint and dismissed without assessing for the life-threatening condition—abuse—that caused the immediate injury.

There are clues that you need to recognize that would indicate the possibility of domestic violence. One of the behaviors to look for is the man speaking for the woman in response to questions about the injury. She may seek his approval before answering questions. He may criticize or correct her answers. Often, he may not want health care professionals to talk to the woman alone. You need to ask questions related to abuse when the woman is by herself and away from significant others. Make certain that no one can walk into the room or overhear what is said.

Unexplained bruises, lacerations, burns, fractures, multiple injuries on more than one side of the body, or old injuries in various stages of healing should alert you to the possibility of abuse. A body map can be used to document physical injuries. Be aware that some victims use makeup, clothing, or hair to cover injuries. See the Focused Nursing Assessment feature for indicators of physical abuse.

Further assessment is needed if the victim says her partner has problems with alcohol or drug abuse or has a history of violent behavior. If she has concerns about the safety of her children or expresses a fear of returning home, more in-depth assessment must be completed.

During the assessment of every client, in all types of health settings, one or two introductory questions should be asked. In assessing a child, say, for example, "Moms and dads try to help their children learn how to behave well. What happens to you when you do something wrong?" Or ask, "What is the worst punishment you ever received?" In assessing adolescents for dating violence you may ask, "Is hitting okay when your boyfriend/girlfriend flirts with other people or catches you flirting with someone else, or if you get hit first?"

In assessing adults, you may begin with this approach: "One of the sources of stress in our lives is family disagreement. Could you describe how disagreements affect you? What happens when you disagree?" If the responses to these questions are indicative of violence, a focused nursing assessment must be conducted; see the Focused Nursing Assessment feature. Obviously, the assessment questions must be adapted to the client's age, gender, and family situation.

For clients who do not speak English, it is important to use a non–family member who speaks their language to assist in the assessment process. The use of a non–family member helps assure confidentiality and safety of clients. Those who are immigrants may need to be reassured that reporting of abuse will not change their immigrant status (Raphel & Berry, 1998).

Diagnosis

There are a number of nursing diagnoses for victims and perpetrators of domestic violence. Priority must be given to critical and serious physical injuries. The severity and potential fatality of the situation must be considered, as well as the needs of dependent children and legal issues surrounding the case. See the Nursing Diagnoses with NOC and NIC feature for examples of nursing diagnoses appropriate for clients after critical and serious injuries have been managed.

Outcome Identification and Goals

Based on the assessment data, you select outcomes appropriate to the nursing diagnoses. See the Nursing Diagnoses with NOC and NIC feature for outcomes associated with the nursing diagnoses.

Client goals are specific behavioral prescriptions which you, the client, and significant others have identified as realistic and attainable. The following are examples of goals that may be pertinent to clients involved in domestic violence:

- Remains safe and free from harm
- Develops an escape plan
- Manages conflict appropriately
- Verbalizes an internal locus of control

Behavior Assessment	Affective Assessment	Cognitive Assessment
What types of things cause conflict within your family? How is this managed or resolved?	Who do you view as responsible for the use of physical force within the family?	Do you believe or hope the violence will not recur?
Who in your family loses control when angry?	How much guilt are you experiencing at this time?	What are your beliefs about keeping the family together?
Have you been emotionally abused by someone in your family?	Are you afraid of your partner/parent/sibling or anyone else?	Describe your personal strengths and abilities.
Have you been slapped? Hit? Punched? Thrown? Shoved? Kicked?	Tell me about your fears: Financial problems? Child care problems? Loneliness? Further physical injury?	What are the rules about using physical force within your family?
Has anyone forced you to have sexual activities?	Do you feel safe living in your home?	
Have you attempted to leave the relationship in the past? What occurred then?	How hopeless do you feel about your situation?	

- Verbalizes an understanding of normal growth and development of children
- Implements appropriate and safe parenting techniques
- Utilizes community resources

Nursing Interventions

Most victims of domestic violence would like it to end, but they may not know how to seek the help they need. It is extremely important that you be nonjudgmental in your interactions with all family members. Initially, clients may be unwilling to trust you because of family shame and fears of being accused for remaining in the violent situation. It is vital that you not impose your own values by offering quick and easy solutions to the very complicated problem of domestic violence.

Treatment of families experiencing violence requires a multidisciplinary approach, with a broad range of interventions. Nurses, social workers, physi-

cians, family therapists, vocational trainers, police, protective services personnel, and lawyers must coordinate to intervene effectively in a domestic violence situation. See the Community Resources feature at the end of this chapter for referrals for both victims and perpetrators of domestic violence.

Safety: Risk Management
Abuse Protection

In the initial contact with family members, assure their *physical safety* as much as possible. It is critical to assess the level of danger for the victim; homicide may be a real possibility if previous threats have been made. If an adult is being abused, there is a likelihood that children are being abused. Even if the children are not being physically abused, witnessing domestic violence can be devastating. It is also important to assess the level of danger for the abuser. The severity and duration of the violence are the factors that contribute the most directly to victims killing their abusers in self-defense. If the level of danger is high, protective services or the

Social Assessment

How did your parents relate to each other?

What type of discipline was used when you were a child?

Describe your relationships with people outside your basic family unit.

Who can you turn to for support in times of stress?

Are you kept alone for long periods of time?

What types of contact have you had with the legal system: Phoned police? Restraining order? Obtained a lawyer? Court cases? Protective services?

If family members are present, what is the quality of their interactions?

Physiological Assessment

Is there a history of unexplained injuries?

Is there evidence of trauma such as bruises, burns, bites, punctures, irregular areas of hair loss, or old scars?

Are there any fractured bones or dislocated joints?

Does the client have problems with mobility?

Is there any evidence of internal injuries such as abdominal distension, absent bowel sounds, persistent vomiting, injury to organs, or hypovolemic shock?

Does the client complain of abnormal sensations, numbness, or pain?

Assess for signs of neglect—poor hygiene, cleanliness, proper clothing for the weather, over- or undermedication.

Assess for sexual abuse such as sexually transmitted infections, dysmenorrhea, pelvic inflammatory disease, or genital or rectal tearing.

Is growth and development normal for the client's age?

---

police should be contacted for emergency custody placement or removal to a shelter.

You should help women develop a *"safe plan"* or "escape plan" to use when their safety is threatened. They should plan a quick, safe exit from their home as well as a safe place to go and teach it to their children. You may suggest that they have all important documents such as birth certificates and orders of protection, some money, a list of important phone numbers, and a couple days' clothing gathered in one secure location. They should have a second set of car keys so they can leave quickly if they need to.

Families experiencing violence often have poor communication skills. Nursing interventions can be designed to improve the family members' *effective communication*. The skills you can teach include active listening with feedback, clear and direct communication, and communication that does not attack the personhood of others. Identify the normality of conflict within all families by discussing how disagreements are inevitable. From there, discuss the use of the demo-

cratic process in conflict resolution and decision making. It is best to practice with minor, unemotional family problems at first.

Family interventions also include helping identify methods to *manage anger* appropriately. All family members must assume responsibility for their own behavior. They can learn and practice talking out anger as it occurs. Make suggestions for appropriate expression, such as relaxation, physical exercise, and striking safe, inanimate objects (a pillow, a couch, or a punching bag). Guide the family in establishing limits and defining consequences if violence recurs. Emphasize that violence within the family will not be tolerated.

Feminist-sensitive therapy can and should be practiced by all professionals, female and male, who are involved with victims of domestic violence. This might also be called a *survivor-centered approach*—not specific techniques, but rather a perspective or way of seeing and understanding the context in which women and children live, recognizing the cultural values that underlie

NURSING DIAGNOSES with NOC & NIC

Victims of Domestic Violence

DIAGNOSIS	OUTCOMES	INTERVENTIONS
Ineffective family coping, disabling, related to an inability to manage conflict without violence	**Abusive Behavior Self-Control:** Self-restraint of own behavior to avoid abuse and neglect of dependents or significant others	Impulse Control Training
	Abuse Cessation: Evidence that the victim is no longer abused	Abuse Protection
High risk for violence, directed at others, related to a history of the use of physical force within the family	**Aggression Control:** Self-restraint of assaultive, combative, or destructive behavior toward others	Impulse Control Training
	Abuse Recovery: Physical: Healing of physical injuries due to abuse	
Altered parenting related to abuse or neglect of children	**Abuse Protection:** Protection of self or dependent others from abuse	Abuse Protection: Child
	Neglect Recovery: Healing following the cessation of substandard care	Abuse Protection: Elder
Powerlessness related to feelings of being dependent on the abuser	**Abuse Recovery:** Financial: Regaining monetary and legal control or benefits following financial exploitation	Abuse Protection: Elder
Self-esteem disturbance related to feeling guilty and responsible for being a victim	**Abuse Recovery:** Emotional: Healing of psychological injuries due to abuse	Crisis Intervention
Social isolation related to control by perpetrator and shame regarding family violence	**Social Support:** Perceived availability and actual provision of reliable assistance from other persons	Environmental Management Crisis Intervention

SOURCES: Johnson, M., Maas, M., & Moorhead, S. (2000); *Nursing outcomes classification (NOC)* (2nd ed.). St. Louis, MO: Mosby; McCloskey, J. C., & Bulechek, G. M. (1996). *Nursing interventions classification (NIC)* (2nd ed.). St. Louis, MO: Mosby; and North American Nursing Diagnoses Association (1999). *Nursing diagnoses definitions and classification 1999–2000*. Philadelphia: Author.

domestic violence. Using this approach, you speak up and say that violence is wrong and will not be tolerated.

One of the primary goals of feminist-sensitive therapy is the *empowerment* of victims. The process of violence removes all power and control from a person, resulting in low self-esteem, anxiety, depression, and somatic problems. The following principles are basic to the empowerment of victims:

- A commitment to the belief that women and men are inherently equal

- An egalitarian approach to the nurse–client relationship in which the client is viewed as an equal partner rather than a helpless recipient of nursing interventions

- That you cannot keep your partner/parent from being violent by trying to "do better"
- Interventions that focus on the enhancement of the victim's power
- An emphasis on the victim's strengths and abilities
- That everyone deserves relationships that are non-violent
- Respect for the victim's ability to understand her or his own experiences
- Family interventions that change destructive roles and expectations within the family system
- A willingness to state clear value positions about domestic violence

Through this approach, clients can become aware that they have choices in, and control over, their lives. Avoid trying to convince adult victims to leave their abuser. As difficult as it may be, you must be willing to support clients in their pain, rather than telling them what to do about their problems. For the most positive adaptive outcome, adult victims must be their own rescuers and take charge of their own safety and protection plan. If they need help with this process, they must be taught to ask for that help directly. This is not meant to imply in any way that you would abandon clients; rather, you stand by, support, and affirm the positive choices and decisions they make.

Adult clients must begin identifying ways in which they are dependent on their abusers. High levels of dependency make it difficult for victims to leave abusers without intense support. You can help them *identify* intrapersonal and interpersonal *strengths* to decrease their feelings of powerlessness. From there, clients can move on to identifying aspects of life that are under their control. Offer *assertiveness training* to help them develop new skills for relating to others in the future. But caution them, if they are still in the abusive relationship, that assertive behavior may escalate the violence.

Abuse Protection: Child

Parents who are physically abusive need help in developing and improving their *parenting skills*. Begin by recognizing their current positive parenting skills, to increase their self-worth and help them engage in the learning process. Share your understanding that the use of violence is a desperate attempt to cope with their children. Confirming that they care about their children will increase the likelihood of their active participation in the treatment process.

Because domestic violence is often transgenerational, discuss with the parents how they were punished as children. Teach them about the normal growth and development of children. Unrealistic demands for children to comply beyond their developmental ability often result in violence. The first step in the problem-solving process is helping parents identify specific problems they experience with raising children. They can then go on to identify types of discipline, other than physical force, that are age appropriate for their children. Positive discipline includes such parental behaviors as:

- Tell children what is allowed as well as what is not allowed.
- Offer choices rather than threats.
- Requests should be realistic and age appropriate.
- Choose your battles—don't argue over every small transgression.
- Acknowledge and reward appropriate behavior.

Parents need support in implementing, practicing, and evaluating these new skills. They need to help their children develop their own self-control as they manage each developmental stage.

Abuse Protection: Elder

Support the elder person and caretakers in identifying and expanding *social support networks*. These outside individuals may be able to help with activities of daily living (ADLs), transportation, financial advice, and assistance with personal problems. Assist the caretakers in exploring their feelings about the older person in their care. Help them identify factors that are disturbing to them and which may contribute to neglect or abuse. Determine the caretakers' ability to meet their loved one's needs, and provide appropriate teaching. Provide community resource information, including addresses and phone numbers of agencies that offer senior service assistance. See the Community Resource feature at the end of this chapter.

Environmental Management: Community

All nurses should evaluate their professional obligations and practice in counteracting those aspects of society that foster domestic violence. Domestic violence is a mental health problem of national and international importance, and nurses should be leaders in helping prevent it in future generations.

Primary prevention includes educating the general population on the existence of domestic violence and its devastating effects. Nursing interventions include parent education, family life education and conflict resolution programs in schools, referral for appropriate child or elder care, establishment of support groups, and education of fellow nurses about the problem of domestic violence. It is important to challenge the belief that violence is a normal part of loving relationships. As a professional, you can monitor the media and keep the pressure on to decrease the amount of violence that is portrayed. It is tragic that some young people's popular music contains messages that support violence against females. Similar to the seat belt campaign, state and federal campaigns should be developed for zero tolerance against domestic violence.

Secondary prevention includes working with children who are victims or who have seen their mothers beaten, and making referrals for multidisciplinary intervention. Teen victims and perpetrators of dating violence benefit from peer support and feedback in a group format. This allows them to learn from one another as well as provide support to other victims.

Nurses must be *community advocates* in supporting hotlines, crisis centers, and shelters for victims of domestic violence. Battered women's shelters need volunteer nurses to help support their programs. Domestic violence information flyers should be available in health care facilities. Public women's bathrooms should have local domestic violence hot line numbers posted in an easily visible site. On the political level, nurses must make their voices heard in regard to policies and laws affecting children, women, and older people. Questions to guide the evaluation of nursing practice include the following:

■ What action have I taken to decrease violence in the media?

■ Have I been an advocate for gun control?

■ Have I confronted the use of physical punishment within families?

■ Have I volunteered to teach parenting classes at grade schools and high schools?

■ Have I written to legislators to protest funding cuts in programs designed to help children, women, and older people?

■ Have I spoken out on the need to increase the number of bilingual/bicultural counselors, lawyers, nurses, and physicians to attend to the cultural needs of families?

Safety: Crisis Management
Crisis Intervention

Crisis intervention is an intensive, short-term counseling process based on assessment and diffusion of volatile domestic violence situations. It is a time-limited approach to problem identification designed to promote the victim's return to a pre-crisis level of function within four to six weeks. Intervention is directed toward developing rapport with the victim, clarifying the presenting problems, and enhancing the victim's existing problem-solving ability. See Chapter 10 for further information on crisis intervention.

Crisis intervention focuses on the immediate problem and seeks an answer to the question, "Why have you come for help now?" A precipitating event of major consequence usually has occurred within a few days of seeking therapy. Safety of the victim(s) is of primary importance. Once safety is assured, nursing interventions include (McCloskey & Bulechek, 1996):

■ Identification of effective and ineffective coping skills

■ Emphasis on victim's strengths and abilities

■ Development of problem-solving skills and new coping behaviors

■ Identification of available support systems

■ Participation in group therapy with other victims and survivors of domestic violence

■ Evaluation of the effectiveness of new coping strategies

A thorough assessment of supports and previous coping behaviors and their effectiveness precedes and provides direction for crisis intervention strategies.

Behavioral: Behavior Therapy
Impulse Control Training

Most abusers do not seek treatment unless it is court ordered or there are custody issues involved. It is frustrating to intervene with abusers who deny the reality of or the responsibility for the violence. *Group therapy* for abusers is sometimes helpful. The group setting is more effective than individual therapy because interactions with a number of people more successfully address the anger and control problems. The responsibility for aggression is always placed on the aggressor. Issues regarding the patriarchal and power views of relationships are discussed in great depth. Types of abuse are examined as well as the underlying belief systems. Participants are asked to specify their abusive behaviors, identify the intentions behind those behaviors, and examine the effects of the abuse on their victims. The goal is to establish new skills and techniques of coping with life's problems. Abusers learn that anger can be controlled and that violence is always a choice.

The federal *Gun Control Act of 1968* prohibits anyone who has been convicted of a felony from owning or possessing a firearm or ammunition. The 1996 amendment to the act prohibits anyone who has been convicted of a misdemeanor involving domestic violence from owning or possessing a firearm or ammunition. There are no exceptions to this law including police or military personnel. Violation of this act results in 10 years in prison and a fine of $250,000. Victims of domestic violence should be able to turn to the police and have their partner arrested. This law, however, has been difficult to enforce and is being challenged by the National Rifle Association.

Evaluation

Nurses in long-term settings or within the community have an opportunity to evaluate the effectiveness of the multidisciplinary treatment plan over an extended period of time. When violence no long exists within the family system, the plan has succeeded. Sharing in the process of family growth and adaptation can be a tremendous source of professional satisfaction.

To complete the nursing process, you evaluate clients' responses to nursing interventions based on the outcomes you selected. You determine the appropriate intervals for measurement and document the condition of clients according to each individual's status.

Johnson, Maas, and Moorhead (2000) is the resource for identifying measurement scales and specific indicators for each outcome.

Abuse Cessation

The victim reports cessation of emotional, physical, sexual, and/or financial abuse.*

Abuse Protection

The victim develops an adequate escape plan to use when safety is threatened. If the level of danger is high, restraining orders are obtained. If the abuser continues to be violent, the relationship is ended.*

Abuse Recovery: Emotional

Victims identify intrapersonal and interpersonal strengths. They determine what aspects of life are under their control. They utilize assertive skills in interactions with others. Victims report a sense of empowerment.

Abuse Recovery: Financial

Child and elder protective services are notified. Victims identify intrapersonal and interpersonal strengths. They determine what aspects of life are under their control. They utilize assertive skills in interactions with others. Victims report a sense of empowerment.

Abuse Recovery: Physical

Child and elder protective services are notified. Victims develop, and implement when necessary, an escape plan. Victims identify intrapersonal and interpersonal strengths. They determine what aspects of life are under their control. They utilize assertive skills in interactions with others. Victims report a sense of empowerment.

Abusive Behavior Self-Control

Abusive parents identify positive parenting skills appropriate to the developmental stage of their children. They identify and utilize nonviolent methods of discipline. Teen victims and perpetrators of dating violence use peer support and participate in group therapy. Abusers participate in group therapy and utilize

---

*These selected outcome indicators are from Johnson, M., Maas, M., & Moorhead, S. (2000). *Nursing outcomes classification (NOC)* (2nd ed.). St. Louis, MO: Mosby.

relevant community resources. Perpetrators assume responsibility for all aggressive behaviors.

Aggression Control

Perpetrators refrain from emotionally, financially, or physically violating other individuals. They identify feelings of anger, frustration, hostility, and aggression. They identify alternatives to aggression and maintain self-control without supervision. They communicate their needs appropriately and verbalize control of impulses.[*]

Neglect Recovery

Child and elder protective services are notified. Dependent children or elders remain free from harm and exhibit age-appropriate behaviors, feelings, and cognitions.

Social Support

The family regularly interacts with family and friends. Victims and perpetrators effectively negotiate stressful interpersonal situations.

CHAPTER REVIEW

COMMUNITY RESOURCES

Links to these Web sites can be accessed on the Companion Web site for this book.

Nursing Network on Violence Against Women
  International (NNVAWI)
PMB 165
1801 H St., Suite B5
Modesto, CA 95354-1215
888-909-9993
www.nnvawi.org

Victims
Bridgework Ministries, Inc.
1226 Turner St., Suite C
Clearwater, FL 34616
813-530-1499
www.bridgeworkministries.com

Child Abuse Prevention—Kids Peace
800-257-3223
www.kidspeace.org

Domestic Violence Hotline
800-799-SAFE
Hearing impaired
800-787-3224

Gay Men's Domestic Violence Project
P.O. Box 9183
Cambridge, MA 02139
617-497-7317
www.gmdvp.org

KIDS USA
800-543-7025

National Council on Child Abuse and Family Violence
800-222-2000

National Organization for Victim Assistance (NOVA)
717 D St. NW
Washington, DC 20004
202-393-NOVA
www.try-nova.org

National Victim Center
307 West 7th St.
Fort Worth, TX 76102
817-877-3355
www.nvc.org

---

[*]These selected outcome indicators are from Johnson, M., Maas, M., & Moorhead, S. (2000). *Nursing outcomes classification (NOC)* (2nd ed.). St. Louis, MO: Mosby.

Network for Battered Lesbians and Bisexual Women
P.O. Box 6011
Boston, MA 02114
617-236-SAFE

Parents Anonymous
800-421-0353
www.parentsanonymous-natl.org

Perpetrators
Brother to Brother
1660 Broad St.
Providence, RI 02905
401-467-3710

Men Stopping Violence
1020 DeKalb Ave. NE
Atlanta, GA 30307
404-688-1376
www.menstoppingviolence.org

KEY CONCEPTS

Introduction

- Although the image of the ideal American family is one of happiness and harmony, in reality there is a great deal of domestic abuse and violence.

- Abuse refers to a pattern of behavior that dominates, controls, lowers self-esteem, or takes away freedom of choice.

- Nurses are required by law to report suspected incidents of child abuse in all states and most states also have mandatory reporting for elder abuse.

- The most common and unrecognized form of domestic violence occurs between siblings.

- Each year, 2.8 million American children experience at least one act of physical violence. Shaken baby syndrome causes permanent brain damage or death to many children.

- In the United States, homicide is one of the five leading causes of death before the age of 18. Sixty percent of children who are killed by their parents are under the age of four.

- In most cases of adolescents killing their parents, the teens have been severely abused.

- In Munchausen syndrome by proxy the parent persistently fabricates or induces illness in a child with the intent of keeping in contact with health care providers and hospitals.

- Violence is the single, largest cause of injury to women in the United States.

- The first acts of partner violence usually occur in dating relationships.

- Domestic violence occurs in some gay and lesbian relationships, for the same reasons as in heterosexual relationships.

- Elder abuse includes neglecting basic needs, psychological abuse, violation of rights, financial abuse, sexual, and physical abuse.

- Pregnancy is a time of increased risk for abuse, and a past history of abuse is one of the strongest predictors of the likelihood that pregnant women will be abused.

- Stalking is the act of following, viewing, communicating with, or moving threateningly toward another person.

Knowledge Base

- Domestic violence is the deliberate and systematic pattern of abuse used to gain control over the victim. The behavior is always intentional.

- Domestic violence can happen without warning and without a buildup of tension. A pattern or cycle develops consisting of begging for forgiveness, hope on the part of the victim, and a return to violence.

- Abused children often try to please the parent in order to stop the violence.

- The abuser has total control over the victim, who lives in a constant state of fear.

- Some 50 percent of the women who are murdered, are killed by a past or present husband or lover. The risk of death increases as the victims resist or try to take control over their lives by leaving the abuser.

- Violent people are extremely jealous and possessive and view others in terms of property and ownership.

- Victims may be immobilized by anxiety, helplessness, depression, self-blame, and guilt.

KEY CONCEPTS (continued)

- The abuser is often most dangerous when threatened with or faced with separation.

- Anger may turn to violence when children are unable to fulfill the unrealistic expectations of parents.

- Severe and ongoing domestic violence has been documented in almost every country.

- Risk factors for violence related to ethnicity in the United States include financial strain, unemployment/underemployment, and undereducation.

- There appears to be a genetic–environmental link to violence involving low levels of serotonin (5-HT).

- Domestic violence is frequently transgenerational; as many as 80 percent of male abusers have grown up in violent homes.

- If the use of violence is rewarded by a gain in power, the behavior is reinforced.

- The cultural values and economic system help entrap women, who are often forced to choose between poverty and abuse.

The Nursing Process

Assessment

- Clients in all clinical settings should be routinely assessed for evidence of violence.

- Assessment questions should be adapted to the client's age, gender, and family situation.

Diagnosis

- The most important outcome of nursing assessment is identifying the existence of domestic violence. Priority must be given to critical and serious physical injuries.

- The severity and potential fatality of the situation must be considered, as well as the needs of dependent children and legal issues surrounding the case.

Outcome Identification and Goals

- The most important outcome for victims of domestic violence is remaining safe and free from harm.

Nursing Interventions

- The treatment of families experiencing domestic violence requires a multidisciplinary approach.

- The priority for care is assuring the victim's physical safety.

- Victims need to develop an escape plan to use when their safety is threatened.

- Families must learn to use effective communication.

- Family members must identify methods to manage anger appropriately.

- Parents need help in developing and improving their parenting skills.

- Feminist-sensitive therapy is a survivor-centered approach. Adult victims are supported and empowered to take charge of their own lives.

- Most abusers do not seek treatment unless it is court ordered or there are custody issues involved. Group therapy is more helpful than individual therapy for abusers.

Evaluation

- Short-term evaluation focuses on the identification of domestic violence, the family's ability to recognize that a problem exists, the willingness of the family to follow through with referrals, and the removal of the victim from a volatile situation.

- Long-term evaluation focuses on the victim's recognition of blamelessness, ending denial of the problem, awareness of competence, sense of power over his or her own life, recognition of personal rights, and decreased isolation and secrecy.

- Evaluation of nursing practice focuses on actions taken to combat violence both within families and in society, preventive teaching strategies, and advocating for increased bilingual/bicultural professionals to intervene with families.

EXPLORE MediaLink

- Interactive resources, including animations, for this chapter can be found on the Companion Web site at *http://www.prenhall.com/fontaine*. Click on Chapter 21 and select the activities for this chapter.

- For NCLEX review questions and an audio glossary, access the accompanying CD-ROM in this book.

REFERENCES

Adelman, R. D., Lachs, M. S., & Breckman, R. (1999). Elder abuse and neglect. In R. T. Ammerman, & M. Hersen (Eds.), *Assessment of family violence: A clinical and legal sourcebook* (pp. 271–286). New York: John Wiley & Sons.

Bauman, L., & Friedman, S. (1998). Corporal punishment. *Pediatric Clinics of North America, 45,* 403–414.

Bloom, S. L., & Reichert, M. (1998). *Bearing witness: Violence and collective responsibility.* New York: Haworth Press.

Busby, D. M., & Smith, G. L. (2000). Family therapy with children who are victims of physical violence. In C. E. Bailey (Ed.), *Children in therapy* (pp. 164–191). New York: Norton.

Centers for Disease Control and Prevention. (2000). National Center for Injury Prevention and Control. Dating Violence. *www.cdc.gov/ncipc/factsheets/datviol.htm.*

Desjarlais, R., Eisenberg, L., Good, B., & Kleinman, A. (1995). *World mental health.* New York: Oxford University Press.

Dowdell, E. B., & Foster, K. L. (1999). Munchausen syndrome by proxy: Recognizing a form of child abuse. *Nursing Spectrum, 12*(20), 20–22.

Ewing, C. P. (1997). *Fatal families.* Thousand Oaks, CA: Sage.

Gamache, D. (1998). Domination and control: The social context of dating violence. In B. Levy (Ed.), *Dating violence* (pp. 69–83). Seattle, WA: Seal Press.

Gershater-Molko, R. M., & Lutzker, J. R. (1999). Child neglect. In R. T. Ammerman & M. Hersen (Eds.), *Assessment of family violence: A clinical and legal sourcebook* (2nd ed.) (pp. 157–183). New York: John Wiley & Sons.

Hall, J. M. (2000). Women survivors of childhood abuse: The impact of traumatic stress on education and work. *Issues in Mental Health Nursing, 21*(5), 443–471.

Hansen, D. J., Sedlar, G., & Warner-Rogers, J. E. (1999). Child physical abuse. In R. T. Ammerman & M. Hersen (Eds.), *Assessment of family violence: A clinical and legal sourcebook* (2nd ed.) (pp. 127–156). New York: John Wiley & Sons.

Heim, C., Newport, D. J., Bonsall, R., & Miller, A. H. (2001). Altered pituitary–adrenal axis responses to provocative challenge tests in adult survivors of childhood abuse. *American Journal of Psychiatry, 158*(4), 575–581.

Horan, D. L., Hill, L. D., & Schulkin, J. (2000). Childhood sexual abuse and preterm labor in adulthood: An endocrinological hypothesis. *Women's Health Issues, 10*(1), 27–33.

Johnson, M., Maas, M., & Moorhead, S. (2000). *Nursing outcomes classification (NOC)* (2nd ed.). St. Louis, MO: Mosby.

Kamphuis, J. H., & Emmelkamp, P. M. G. (2001). Traumatic distress among support-seeking female victims of stalking. *American Journal of Psychiatry, 158*(5), 795–798.

Levy, B., & Lobel, K. (1998). Lesbian teens in abusive relationships. In B. Levy (Ed.), *Dating violence* (pp. 203–208). Seattle, WA: Seal Press.

McCloskey, J. C., & Bulechek, G. M. (1996). *Nursing interventions classification (NIC)* (2nd ed.). St. Louis, MO: Mosby.

McCloskey, L. A., & Eisler, R. (1999). Family structure and family violence and nonviolence. In L. Kurtz (Ed.), *Encyclopedia of violence, peace, and conflict,* Vol. 2 (pp. 1–11). San Diego: Academic Press.

Mullen, P. E., Pathe, M., Purcell, R., & Stuart, G. W. (1999). Study of stalkers. *American Journal of Psychiatry, 156*(8), 1244–1249.

O'Keefe, M. (1998). Factors mediating the link between witnessing interparental violence and dating violence. *Journal of Family Violence, 13*(1), 39–57.

O'Leary, K. D., & Murphy, C. (1999). Clinical issues in the assessment of partner violence. In R. T. Ammerman & M. Hersen (Eds.), *Assessment of family violence: A clinical and legal sourcebook* (2nd ed.) (pp. 24–47). New York: John Wiley & Sons.

Raphel, S. M., & Berry, A. W. (1998). Culturally competent assessment for family violence. Washington, DC: American Nurses Association.

Ratey, J. J. (2001). *A user's guide to the brain.* New York: Pantheon Books.

Reno, J. (1999). Cyberstalking: A new challenge for law enforcement and industry. *www.usdoj.gov/criminal/cybercrime/cyberstalking.htm.*

Spector, R. E. (2000). *Cultural diversity in health & illness* (5th ed.). Upper Saddle River, NJ: Prentice Hall.

Straus, M. A. (1994). *Beating the devil out of them: Corporal punishment in American families.* Lexington, MA: Lexington Books.

Sudermann, M., & Jaffe, P. G. (1999). Child witnesses of domestic violence. In R. T. Ammerman & M. Hersen (Eds.), *Assessment of family violence: A clinical and legal sourcebook* (2nd ed.) (pp. 343–366). New York: John Wiley & Sons.

Taylor, J. Y. (2000). Sisters of the yam: African American women's healing and self-recovery from intimate male partner violence. *Issues in Mental Health Nursing, 21*(5), 515–531.

Torres, S., & Han, H. R. (2000). Psychological distress in non-Hispanic white and Hispanic abused women. *Archives of Psychiatric Nursing, 14*(1), 19–29.

U.S. Department of Health & Human Services. (2000). *Healthy people 2010. www.health.gov/healthypeople/lhi/lhiwhat.htm.*

West, C. M. (1998a). Leaving a second closet: Outing partner violence in same-sex couples. In J. L. Jasinski & L. M. Williams (Eds.), *Partner violence* (pp. 163–183). Newbury Park, CA: Sage.

West, C. M. (1998b). Lifting the "political gag order": Breaking the silence around partner violence in ethnic minority families. In J. L. Jasinski & L. M. Williams (Eds.), *Partner violence* (pp. 184–209). Newbury Park, CA: Sage.

Widom, C. S. (1999). Posttraumatic stress disorder in abused and neglected children grown up. *American Journal of Psychiatry, 156*(8), 1223–1229.

Woods, S. J. (2000). Prevalence and patterns of posttraumatic stress disorder in abused and postabused women. *Issues in Mental Health Nursing, 21*(3), 309–324.

CHAPTER 22

Sexual Violence

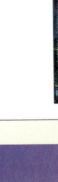

OBJECTIVES

After reading this chapter, you will be able to:

- EXPLAIN the factors contributing to sexual violence.
- ASSESS a survivor's behavioral, affective, and cognitive responses to assault.
- PARTICIPATE in a multidisciplinary intervention for child or adult victims of assault.
- REFER clients to appropriate community resources.
- REPORT suspected incidents of child sexual abuse.

MediaLink

CD-ROM
- *Audio Glossary*
- *NCLEX Review*

Companion Web site
www.prenhall.com/fontaine
- *Critical Thinking*
- *More NCLEX Review*
- *Case Study*
- *Care Map Activity*
- *Links to Resources*

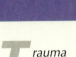

*T*rauma

split off
to endure

left with parts
to pull together

an internal family
to work with

separate feelings
with a united force

to win

to heal

—Heather, Age 30

Sexual violence includes criminal behaviors such as sexual harassment, rape, and child sexual abuse. It is defined as the use of threat, intimidation, force, and exploitation of authority with the goal of imposing one's will on a nonconsenting person for the purpose of personal gratification that may or may not be predominantly sexual in nature. Sexual violence is, first and foremost, an act of violence, hatred, and aggression. Like other acts of violence (assault and battery or murder), there is a violation of and injury to the victims. The injuries may be physical and/or psychological. Victims are overwhelmed and overpowered and are violated as human beings. During the harassment, attack, or abuse, victims are not only out of control of their situation, but they are also assaulted in the most vulnerable dimension of the self. Sexual violence is not an occasional, isolated incident experienced by people in extraordinary situations. Sexual violence is a widespread problem, taking place in a broad social context, which allows and even encourages it to occur. When we encourage gender role differences that accentuate masculine aggression and feminine passivity and when we confuse sexual activity with sexual violence, we create a climate of tolerance of sexual violence in our society.

SEXUAL HARASSMENT

Sexual harassment of women in the workplace and in schools has always existed as a hidden crime. Only recently has it been recognized for what it is—discrimination against and violation of women. Prevalence rates, reported by women, range between 30 and 55 percent. However, women frequently do not report harassment because they do not expect to be believed and fear that they will be accused of contributing to the problem. Nurses are not immune to sexual harassment as they practice their profession. Studies have found that 60 to 80 percent of staff nurses report multiple incidents of sexual harassment most frequently by male clients, followed by co-workers and physicians (Madison & Minichiello, 2000).

Sexual harassment is unwanted and unwelcome sexual behavior that interferes with everyday life. It is one end of the continuum of sexual violence against women with the other end of the continuum being rape (Berman, McKenna, Arnold, Taylor, & MacQuarrie, 2000). Sexual harassment behaviors include:

- Sexual teasing, jokes, remarks, or demeaning comments
- Making sexually stereotypical comments
- Showing offensive pictures
- Asking invasive questions regarding personal life
- Persistent pressure for dates
- Letters, telephone calls, or e-mail of a sexual nature
- Sexual gestures
- Deliberate touching, cornering, or pinching
- Invasive watching

■ Pressure for sexual favors

■ Actual or attempted rape

Studies of girls and boys age 9 to 19 years indicate that 87 percent of girls and 71 percent of boys have experienced sexual harassment in school. The belief that this is normal adolescent behavior ignores the effects on the victims as well as the criminal aspects of the behavior (Fineran & Bennett, 1999). Peer sexual harassment includes the above behaviors as well as:

■ Calling someone gay or lesbian in a malicious manner

■ Spreading sexual rumors

■ Flashing or mooning someone

■ "Spiking"—pulling down someone's pants

■ "Snuggies"—pulling underwear up at the waist so it goes in between the buttocks

The United States Equal Employment Opportunity Commission (EEOC) is the government agency that interprets and enforces employment laws. In 1980, the EEOC issued a position statement clearly stating that sexual harassment is considered a form of sexual discrimination and, therefore, an unlawful employment act. Although most cases of sexual harassment have traditionally involved a male harasser and a female victim, the EEOC also determined that the sexual harasser, as well as the victim, can be either a man or a woman. Research indicates, however, that the vast majority of harassers are male and that the behavior is more about dominance than about sex.

There are two distinctive categories of sexual harassment: quid pro quo and hostile environment. *Quid pro quo* (translated as "this for that") means that an employer or other person of authority suggests that he will give her this job, promotion, or salary, in return for that sexual favor. This form of sexual harassment is the most well known. *Hostile environment* sexual harassment is unwelcome sexual conduct that has the purpose or effect of creating an intimidating, hostile, or offensive working environment. This type of sexual harassment can involve supervisors, co-workers, and even customers or vendors. The intent of the law is to give people the opportunity to work in an environment that is free from sex-based discrimination, taunts, jeers, and insults.

Sexual harassment can lead to severe stress in the victims. Many victims experience depression, isolation,

---

BOX 22.1

Steps Toward Harassment Prevention and Response

■ Give verbal notice to the offender. Respond directly and simply, for example, "I don't like . . . and I want you not to do it again."
■ Give stronger warnings and notice that you will report the behavior, for example, "If this happens again, I'm going to discuss this with human resources."
■ Issue a written warning.
■ Keep a detailed record of the behavior you find objectionable, when it occurred, and what you did in response.
■ Make an informal harassment inquiry—discuss the situation with your supervisor or human resources person. The goal is not punishment but problem solving, education, and consciousness raising.
■ File a formal complaint within the organization. At this point, the harasser faces serious personal and professional damage. The situation cannot be kept completely confidential and the company or school is obliged to investigate.
■ File with the EEOC in the United States: 800-669-4000.
■ In Canada, file with the Canadian Human Rights Commission: 613-995-1151. It is highly advisable to have an attorney at this point.
■ Go to court. This tends to be a long, painful battle. It may be settled before trial.

---

feelings of powerlessness, helplessness, fear, restlessness, inability to concentrate, somatic complaints, sexual problems, and loss of self-esteem. At its most severe, harassment resembles the other sexual traumas of rape and child sexual abuse and may result in post-traumatic stress disorder. Filing a complaint of sexual harassment is never easy. Regardless of the outcome, the investigation can be extremely stressful for all people involved (Lips, 2001). See Box 22.1 for the steps toward harassment response.

RAPE

Rape is a crime of violence. It is second only to homicide in its violation of a person. The issue is not one of sex but rather one of force, domination, and humiliation. If you think rape is about sex, you have confused the weapon with the motivation. **Rape** refers to any forced sexual activity; the key factor is the absence of consent. Forcible rape by juveniles in both the United States and the United Kingdom has been on the increase, and teens now account for 18 to 20 percent of rapes (Murphy & Page, 1999).

There is no typical rape victim. Of reported rapes, however, 93 percent of the victims are female and 90 percent of the perpetrators are male. One can be a victim of rape at any age, from childhood through old age. Police records indicate that a woman is raped every six minutes in the United States. Experts believe that 84 percent of rapes are unreported. It is believed that one out of every three or four American women will be raped or sexually assaulted at least once in her lifetime; 60 to 80 percent of victims are raped by a spouse, partner, relative, or friend (Draucker & Madsen, 1999; McLeer & Rose, 1999; Smith & Kelly, 2001).

Of all women raped on college campuses, 50 percent are *date rapes.* In surveys of college men, 10 to 15 percent admitted that they had committed date rape on at least one occasion, and another 22 percent admitted they had used verbal coercion and deception to pressure a date into having sex. Women very rarely report rapes when they know their attackers, especially if they are or were in a dating relationship with the attacker. The victim is often blamed by herself and others for being naive or provocative. A cultural value, slow to die, is: If a woman accepts a date and allows the man to pay all the expenses, she somehow "owes" him sexual access and has no right to refuse (Shaw, 1999). For ways to minimize the risk of date rape see Box 22.2.

Traditionally, husbands have not been charged when they raped their wives. It was not until 1974 in the United States and 1991 in Great Britain that the first cases of marital rape were prosecuted. In 1993, **marital rape** became a crime in all 50 states. Some states, however, still have exemptions from prosecuting husbands for rape. Marital rape is the most prevalent and underreported form of rape, with estimates of 2 million instances per year in the United States. Between one third and one half of battered women are raped by their partners. The attacks range from assaults that are relatively quick to those that involve sadistic,

---

BOX 22.2

Minimizing the Risk of Date Rape

- Be cautious in relationships based on dominant-male, submissive-female stereotypes. Date rapists usually have macho attitudes and believe women to be inferior.
- Be cautious when a date tries to control your behavior—who you can meet, where you can go, what you can do. This indicates a need to dominate and control and increases your vulnerability by isolating you.
- Do not drink any drink at a party that you have set down.
- Do not stay in a situation in which you feel uncomfortable.
- Be very clear in your communication. If a simple no is not respected, leave or insist he leave. Speak forcefully.
- Avoid giving mixed messages. For example, do not say no and then continue petting.
- Do not go to a place that is so private that help is not available.

---

torturous episodes that last for hours. In some instances, wives are forced to have sex with other people while their husbands watch. Women who are raped by their husbands or partners are less likely to report the assault or to seek professional help (Draucker & Stern, 2001).

Some men who rape their wives see the rape as punishment for perceived wrongs. Others believe they have a right to sex on demand and that when sex is refused they have a right to take it. For other perpetrators, rape is a way to assert power and control. Some may even try to impregnate their wives to ensure that they will not leave the relationship. Others become angered over pregnancy and increase the level of violence in an attempt to abort the fetus.

The myth of male rape has been that it occurs only where heterosexual contact is not possible, such as in prisons or in isolated living conditions. As more **male rape** victims report the crime, however, this myth is being exploded. It is estimated that 5 to 10 percent of all sexual assault victims are men. Male victims as a group are more likely to have been beaten and are more reluctant to reveal the sexual component of their assaults. Homosexual victims fear police prejudice, and heterosexual victims feel shame and confusion regarding their own sexuality. Male rape is not a homosexual attack. Just as in female rape, the issue is one of *violence* and *domination* rather than one of sex. Some perpetrators are gay males who coerce partners or dates into sexual activity by use of threats or intimidation, as in date rape. Other perpetrators are heterosexual males who rape other males as a way of punishing and degrading them. Often, the assaults involve more than one offender. This type of assault can occur among prison inmates or as part of gay bashing. Inmates who are sexually assaulted are often viewed by the public as deserving of their fate because of the crimes they have committed against society. Similarly, many people believe that gay men deserve to be raped as punishment for their "perverse" lifestyle (Hodge & Canter, 1998; Lips, 2001).

CHILDHOOD SEXUAL ABUSE

Childhood sexual abuse is defined as inappropriate sexual behavior, instigated by a perpetrator, for purposes of the perpetrator's sexual pleasure or for economic gain through child prostitution or pornography. Behavior ranges from exhibitionism, peeping, explicit sexual talk, touching, caressing, masturbation, oral sex, vaginal sex, and anal sex, to forcing children to engage in sex with one another or with animals.

Childhood sexual abuse must be distinguished from *natural* and healthy *sexual exploration* during childhood. It is natural that children of similar age and developmental status explore one another's bodies by looking and touching, often referred to as "playing doctor." This is not considered to be problematic behavior.

Childhood sexual abuse does not discriminate. It occurs in all ethnic, religious, economic, and cultural subgroups. Affinity systems—immediate family, relatives, friends, neighbors, clergy members, scout leaders, coaches—account for 75 to 80 percent of the abusers. Male perpetrators account for 90 percent of the reported cases. Children with mental retardation or physical disability are four to ten times more vulnerable to sexual victimization than nondisabled children since they may have difficulty asserting their rights or informing an adult protector. Although father–daughter incest is most reported, it is believed that **sibling**

incest is the most widespread. Some siblings turn to each other for emotional nurturance and acceptance. In other instances, a sibling uses coercion or violence to perpetrate (National Center for Victims of Crime, 2001; Sholevar & Schwoeri, 1999).

Sexually abused children and adult survivors of childhood sexual abuse (hereafter referred to as adult survivors) are crying out for help. A few cry out loudly in protest, but the majority cry inwardly in silence. It is thought that as many as one in three girls and one in seven boys are abused sexually before the age of 18. Many of these are single incidents. Boys are more frequently molested outside the family system than are girls. The period of abuse tends to begin and end at a younger age in boys (Morrell, Mendel, & Fischer, 2001; Shaw, 1999).

Childhood sexual abuse is a major health problem in the United States. The majority of cases are probably unreported. Health care professionals, as well as families, have used denial to cope with ambiguous evidence of the cultural taboos of incest and sex with children. In order to respond appropriately to cues that signal sexual abuse, you must understand the characteristics and dynamics of the perpetrators, victims, and families involved. A note of caution must be added, however. With increased publicity, there is a real danger of a witch hunt's developing; any hint or accusation of sexual abuse may be interpreted as absolute proof of guilt. Individuals and families have been destroyed by rumors and false accusations. You must assess carefully and maintain a balance between the extremes of denial and automatic belief of guilt.

TYPES OF OFFENDERS

Some offenders prefer girls, others prefer boys, and some abuse both, as long as the victim is a child. Some are interested in adolescents or preteens, some in toddlers, and some in infants. Some offenders do not abuse until they are adults, but more than half start in their teens.

Juvenile Offenders

Many, if not most, of these cases are unreported. Family members often want to protect and shield the young offender. At other times, the behavior is rationalized as adolescent male experimentation. Fifty to sixty percent of juvenile offenders were sexually abused as children; they gradually develop offending behaviors as they reach adolescence. The other forty to fifty percent show fairly high rates of other delinquent behaviors and most are diagnosed with conduct disorder. Generally, these individuals have problems in all areas of their lives (Johnson, 2000). (See Chapter 17 for information on conduct disorder.)

Those offenders who were child victims tend to have an earlier age at onset of abusing, to have more victims, and to have male victims when compared with nonabused teen sex offenders. Juvenile offenders may seek victims within or outside the family system. The type of sexual offense often parallels their own experiences of abuse. Sexuality and aggression are closely linked in the thoughts and actions of these young people. The most frequent offense is sexual touching, which may escalate to rape and other sex crimes (Murphy & Page, 1999; Ryan, 2000).

Just as most juveniles who commit delinquent acts do not go on to adult criminal behavior, the majority of juveniles who commit sexual offenses and receive treatment do not continue their molesting behavior. For those in treatment the sexual relapse rate is only 10 to 15 percent. This information is not meant to minimize the seriousness of their offenses, the impact on victims, and the nature of their psychological disturbances but to recognize the differences between adolescent and adult offenders (Brown, 2000).

Male Offenders

One research project that studied fathers who abused their daughters established five types of incestuous fathers. *Sexually preoccupied* abusers (26 percent of the fathers) have a conscious and often obsessive sexual interest in their daughters. Many of them regard their daughters as sex objects, in some cases as early as birth. *Adolescent regressors* (33 percent of the fathers) become sexually interested in their daughters when they begin puberty. These men sound and act like adolescents around their daughters. *Self-gratifiers* (20 percent of the fathers) are not sexually attracted to their daughters per se, and during the abuse, they fantasize about someone else. In effect, they are simply using their daughters' bodies. *Emotional dependents* (10 percent of the fathers) see themselves as failures and feel very lonely and depressed. They see their daughters as romantic figures in their lives. *Angry retaliators* (10 percent of the fathers) abuse out of anger, either at the daughter or at the mother. This type of offender is most likely to have a criminal history of assault and rape (Schetky, 1999).

Female Offenders

Female perpetrators have been largely overlooked but commit between 3 and 13 percent of sexual abuse cases. The most common types of sexual abuse by women are fondling, oral sex, and group sex.

Female sex offenders fall into four major types. *Teacher–lovers* are older women who teach children about lovemaking. *Experimenter–exploiters* are often girls who have had no sex education growing up. Babysitting is often an opportunity to explore younger children. Many of the girls in this group do not even realize what they are doing or that it is inappropriate. *Predisposers* usually come from a family with a long history of physical and sexual abuse. These families have been dysfunctional over many generations. *Women coerced by males* are those who abuse children because men have forced them to abuse. Usually, they have been victims as children and are easily manipulated and intimidated (Green, 1999).

KNOWLEDGE BASE: RAPE

Rape is a violent act against an innocent person. It changes lives forever because once people become victims they never again feel completely safe. The victim's response to this act of violence is referred to as **rape-trauma syndrome**. Some rape survivors do not develop major symptoms in response to the trauma, while as many as 25 percent continue to have signs of impairment a year after the assault. A variety of factors contribute to the response, including age or developmental state, a history of prior victimization, the relationship to the offender, precrisis coping abilities, and the ability to use support resources. Response factors related to the rape itself include the severity of the rape, the duration, the frequency, the number of offenders, and the degree of violence. Environmental factors contributing to a rape victim's response are the quality and continuity of social supports, and community attitudes and values (American Psychiatric Association, 2000).

BEHAVIORAL CHARACTERISTICS

Many victims of rape *do not report* the crime. Sometimes this is due to guilt or embarrassment about what has occurred. Other victims are fearful of how their families or the police will react. Some perpetrators threaten victims by saying they will return to rape them again if the police are notified. Because many of the crimes are committed by acquaintances, friends, dates, or husbands, victims fear they will not be believed.

Some victims respond immediately with *agitated and nonpurposeful behavior*. They are brought to the emergency department emotionally distraught and unable to respond to questions about what has occurred. Their level of anxiety may be so high that they may not be able to follow simple directions. Some rape victims may shower or bathe before notifying the police or going to the hospital. This cleaning-up behavior is often an attempt to regain control of oneself and counteract the feelings of helplessness induced by the rape.

The majority of victims appear in good control of their feelings and behavior immediately after the rape. This *appearance of outward calmness* usually indicates a state of numbness, disbelief, and emotional shock. They may say such things as "This whole thing doesn't seem real," "I must be dreaming. This couldn't have happened," and "I just can't believe this has happened to me." You must recognize that underneath the calmness is acute distress. If you assume that the calmness implies no distress, you will overlook the person's need for emotional support and intervention.

There may be *long-term behavioral characteristics* of the rape-trauma syndrome. Some survivors are prone to crying spells that they may or may not be able to explain. Some may have difficulty establishing or maintaining personal relationships, especially with people who remind them of the perpetrator. Many develop problems at work or school. Some report nightmares and have difficulty sleeping. Others develop secondary phobic reactions to people, objects, or situations that remind them of the rape. Sexual dysfunctions are not unusual. A woman who is a survivor of partner rape suffers additional problems. Often, she must continue to interact with her rapist because she is dependent on him. She may be forced to pretend, to herself and to family members and friends, that the rape never occurred. Until it becomes more socially acceptable and legally feasible to report rape by an intimate partner, many of these survivors will suffer in silence.

AFFECTIVE CHARACTERISTICS

Victims of rape suffer immediate and long-lasting emotional trauma. After a period of shock and disbelief, many experience episodes of *fear*. Fear can result from a stimulus directly associated with the attack, such as a penis, the act of oral sex, or a person who looks like the offender. There are also fears of rape consequences such as pregnancy; sexually transmitted infections, especially HIV; talking to the police; and testifying in court. In addition, there are fears related to potential future attacks, which underlie fears of getting close to men, of being alone, and of being in a strange place. Typically, the level of fear peaks around the third week, but it may take a long time for the level to decrease.

Depression frequently develops within a few weeks of the assault. This posttrauma depression usually lasts about three months, and it is not unusual for the survivor to experience suicidal ideation. For some, the depression will develop into a major depressive disorder requiring medical intervention (Symes, 2000).

Rape victims feel physically and emotionally violated, as well as unclean and contaminated. The loss of control over their bodies and their autonomy leads to feelings of *helplessness and vulnerability*. They may feel alienated from friends and family, particularly if there is not a strong supportive network. Anger is a healthy response to the violation that has occurred, but the energy of anger must be appropriately discharged so the person does not later become obsessed with fantasies of revenge.

COGNITIVE CHARACTERISTICS

During the actual rape, some victims use the defense mechanism of *depersonalization* or *dissociation* to cope with the attack. By perceiving the attack as "not really happening to me," a victim protects her sense of integrity. Other victims rely on *denial* to block out the traumatic experience. The use of these defense mechanisms may continue through initial treatment and should be supported until the person is able to face the reality of the attack.

Jaime, a graduate student at the local university, was brought to the hospital by the police who found her running down the street half-clothed. In the hospital she was able to tell the staff that
(continued)

she had been raped by her date, Jovan, another graduate student. She exhibited outward calmness but kept repeating: "This cannot have happened to me. My friends introduced us and he seemed so nice." She was unable to decide who to call to take her back to the dorm or what to tell her friends about what had happened.

If victims are in a state of emotional shock, they will have great *difficulty making decisions*. Uncertain of how their significant others will react to the situation, they may hesitate to tell family or friends. They need a great deal of support in using the problem-solving process to make decisions.

There may be a period during which victims *blame themselves* for the rape. This self-blame may be heard in such statements as "If only I had taken a different way home," "I should have been able to escape because he didn't have a gun," and "If I were a better wife, he wouldn't have raped me." Remember that the victim is never to blame for this violent crime.

Some survivors develop *obsessional thoughts* about the rape, which may be severe enough to interfere with daily functioning. Some experience flashbacks, some have violent dreams, and others may be preoccupied with thoughts of future danger. Rape profoundly affects a person's beliefs about the environment. If the assault occurred in the home, the normal feeling of safety within the home will most likely be destroyed. Belief in an inability to protect themselves in the future may lead to *social withdrawal* or phobic avoidance. Young female survivors, especially, may generalize their fear to the point that it applies to all men or all strange men. Women who have been raped by their husbands often state that their ability to trust the husband or any other man has been destroyed. Box 22.3 describes the phases of response to rape.

SOCIAL CHARACTERISTICS

Families of rape survivors experience many of the same thoughts and emotions as the victims themselves. They may talk about guilt, doubts, fear, anger, hatred of the perpetrator, and feelings of helplessness. They need to be educated about the nature and trauma of rape and the immediate and potential long-term reactions of the survivors. They require direction in how to best support the survivor so that they neither overprotect nor minimize the impact of the rape.

BOX 22.3

Phases of Response to Rape

Anticipatory Phase
- Begins when the victim realizes the situation is potentially dangerous
- The victim may think about how to get away, may reason or argue with the offender, and recall advice people have given about rape
- Use of dissociation, suppression, or rationalization to preserve the illusion of invulnerability
- Possible physical action

Impact Phase
- The period of actual assault and immediate aftermath
- Intense fear of death or serious injury
- Expressive styles
  - Open expression of feelings—crying, sobbing, pacing
  - Controlled style—numbness, shock, disbelief
  - Compound reaction—reactivated symptoms of previous conditions, for example, psychotic behavior, depression, suicidal behavior, substance abuse
- Somatic reactions—tension headache, fatigue, increased startle reaction, nausea, gagging

Reconstitution Phase
- Outward appearance of adjustment with an attempt to restore equilibrium
- Life activities are renewed, but superficially and mechanically
- Periods of anxiety, fear, nightmares, depression, guilt, shame, vulnerability, helplessness, isolation, sexual dysfunctions

Resolution Phase
- Anger at the assailant, at society, and at the judicial system
- The need to talk to resolve feelings
- The survivor seeks family and professional support

Many cultural *myths* have surrounded the crime of rape for a long time. Some of these myths are the following:

- "Good girls" don't get raped.
- Women ask to be raped by the clothes they wear

such as going braless or wearing short skirts and tight tops.

- Women ask to be raped by going to their date's apartment on the first date.
- The average healthy woman can escape a potential rapist if she really wants to.
- A woman who is stuck-up and thinks she is too good deserves to be taught a lesson.
- If a woman engages in petting and lets things get out of hand, it is her own fault if she gets raped.
- Women cry rape after they have consented to sex with a friend.
- Among males, only homosexuals get raped.
- Any man could resist rape if he really tried.

Changing the misconceptions of the general public has been a slow process. Many people continue to believe the myths that blame the victim rather than the perpetrator. Steps have been taken to abolish these myths from the legal system and to treat rape as the crime of violence it is. However, there is still much work to be done.

CULTURE-SPECIFIC CHARACTERISTICS

Rape occurs cross-culturally and is one of the most underreported crimes worldwide. Thus, it is very difficult to calculate the prevalence rate. Rape is a significant concern for women in all cultures. Many societies believe that women, not men, are responsible for rape. Female rape victims are sometimes more scorned than their male perpetrators on the premise that the men could not control themselves but the women should have been able to avoid the rape. People cling to stereotyped and prejudicial views of victims of sexual violence, which compounds the agony of the victims (Lefley, 1999).

The consequences of rape in societies where young women's worth is equated with their virginity are especially disastrous. Their ruined reputation cannot be revised. In some countries women are forced to marry their rapist to erase the stigma of "spoiled goods." Others turn to prostitution to survive, and some commit suicide. Women victims are blamed rather than perpetrators punished. In some instances women may even be killed by male family members to cleanse the family (Lefley, 1999).

Throughout history, rape has been a part of war

and civil strife. The right to rape women and children has been seen as the booty of war for the victors. Wars in Bangladesh, Bosnia, Kuwait, Somalia, South Africa, and El Salvador give evidence of many cases of systematic and repeated rape of civilian and refugee women. Torture of political prisoners is also gender based, with women being raped repeatedly by different men. Involuntary prostitution or female sexual slavery has a long history, and recent attention has been drawn to this problem in the Philippines, Thailand, Nepal, Burma, and India.

Rape is also used as a weapon of ethnic cleansing as enemies humiliate the women and attempt to exterminate a particular group. Unwanted impregnation results in botched abortions, psychological torture, unwanted children, stigmatized children, and abandoned children. Unfortunately, many of these women also suffer subsequent persecution from their own families and societies. They may be thought to have dishonored their family, questions are raised concerning their consent to sex, and they are no longer marriageable (Lefley, 1999; Turpin, 1999).

PHYSIOLOGICAL CHARACTERISTICS

Rape usually results in a number of physical injuries. The victim may be beaten, stabbed, or shot. Profuse bleeding and trauma to vital organs may be critical problems. Nongenital physical injuries occur in about 40 percent of rape cases. Most likely, the vagina or rectum will be sore or swollen. There may be tearing of the vaginal or rectal wall from forceful insertion of the penis or a foreign object. The throat may be traumatized from forced oral sex (Centers for Disease Control and Prevention [CDC], 2001).

Female victims of childbearing age may become pregnant as a result of the rape. The adult pregnancy rate associated with rape is estimated to be almost 5 percent. Victims of all ages and both sexes may contract a sexually transmitted infection from the perpetrator, via any mucous membrane area such as the vagina, rectum, mouth, or throat. This transmission rate ranges from 4 to 30 percent (CDC, 2001).

Sexual problems are one of the longest-lasting effects of rape. Nearly all adult rape survivors feel the need to withdraw from sexual activity for a period of time. For some, a period of celibacy is necessary to reestablish control and autonomy. Others may choose abstinence because they feel unclean or contaminated.

Both the survivor and the sex partner must understand that the need for closeness and nondemanding physical contact continues. Expressing caring and affection through nonsexual touching minimizes the partner's feelings of rejection and reduces the survivor's feelings of self-blame and uncleanliness.

CONCOMITANT DISORDERS

As a direct result of the rape, survivors may experience posttraumatic stress disorder (PTSD) or may turn to alcohol or drugs to numb the emotional pain. Survivors are more likely to experience major depression, anxiety disorders, or eating disorders. They are more likely to attempt suicide than are individuals who have not been raped (Draucker & Stern, 2001; Symes, 2000).

CAUSATIVE THEORIES

Theorists in many disciplines have studied the crime of rape in an effort to understand the causes and develop preventive measures. Most agree that rape is a crime of violence generated by issues of power and anger rather than by sex drive.

Intrapersonal Theory

The intrapersonal perspective views rapists as emotionally immature individuals who feel powerless and unsure of themselves. They are incapable of managing the normal stresses of everyday life. The causes of rape are many, but the dynamics of the act are that perpetrators abuse their own and others' sexuality as a method of discharging anger and frustration. From this perspective, there are five types of rape: anger rape, power rape, sadistic rape, gang rape, and date/acquaintance rape (Holmes, 1991).

An **anger rape** is distinguished by physical violence and cruelty to the victim. Believing that he is the victim of an unjust society, the rapist takes revenge on others by raping. He uses extreme force and viciousness to debase the victim. The ability to injure, traumatize, and shame the victim provides an outlet for his rage and temporary relief from his turmoil. Rapes occur episodically as the rage builds up and he strikes out at others to relieve his pain.

In a **power rape**, the intent of the rapist is not to injure someone but to command and master another person sexually. The rapist has an insecure self-image, with feelings of incompetency and inadequacy. The

rape becomes the vehicle for expressing power and strength. Seeing his victim as a conquest, the rapist temporarily feels omnipotent.

A **sadistic rape** involves brutality, bondage, and torture as stimulants for the rapist's own sexual excitement. For the rapist, the assault is an erotic experience. He plans very carefully, and the process of rape may be ritualized. The victims are often murdered after being raped.

A **gang rape** involves a number of perpetrators and may be part of a group ritual that confirms masculinity, power, and authority. The perpetrators may range in age from 10 to 30, but they are most typically adolescents. Victims are usually the same age as the gang members.

A **date rape**, or **acquaintance rape**, is forced sexual activity by a perpetrator who is known to the victim. Typically, there is less physical violence and more coercion and deception involved. Even during the high school years, it is estimated that 30 percent of female students are sexually or physically abused in their dating relationships.

Not all rapists are alike. Their motives and expectations vary. The majority of convicted sex offenders do not suffer from major mental disorders. Many do meet the criteria for antisocial, schizoid, paranoid, and narcissistic personality disorders. Rapists are typically young; 80 percent are under the age of 30, and 75 percent are under age 25. The majority report having been sexually and physically abused as children or adolescents (Burton & Rasmussen, 1998; Koss & Boeschen, 2000).

Interpersonal Theory

Most rapists do not have normal interpersonal involvements. Preoccupied with their own fantasies, they want to control and dominate others rather than engage in mutually satisfying relationships. With this model in mind, a rapist sees no need for consent to sexual activity, particularly from his wife or partner. The husband may view the rape as merely a disagreement over sexual behavior. If the wife has said she does not want to engage in sex and the husband uses force, her control and autonomy have been violated. When sex occurs without consent, it is, in fact, rape.

Social Learning Theory

The acceptance of interpersonal violence in a culture contributes to a higher incidence of rape. Society's approval of the use of intimidation, coercion, and force to achieve a goal promotes an excessive level of violence. Violent behavior is an expression of power and strength, and individual rights are disregarded.

Aggression is learned through three primary sources: family and peers, culture/subculture, and the mass media. The modeling effect occurs when potential offenders see rape scenes and other acts of violence against women in real life or in the media, in slasher and horror films, and in violent pornography. The media contribute to the process of desensitization; with repeated exposure, viewers become numb to the pain, fear, and humiliation of sexual aggression (Shaw, 1999).

Feminist Theory

From the feminist perspective, rape is the result of long and deeply rooted socioeconomic traditions. Men dominate most political and economic activities, and women are viewed as subservient and relatively powerless. At the furthest extreme, women are viewed as property. Sexual gratification is not the prime motive in rape; rather, sex is used to establish or maintain *control* of one person by another. When women are considered inferior to men, tacit approval is given for coercion and force. These stereotypes support the false beliefs that at times women deserve to be raped, that they may want or need to be raped, and that rape does not cause them much physical or emotional damage.

Sexist values affect people of all ages, both female and male. When school children are asked questions regarding rape, many believe it is acceptable for a man to force a woman to have sex if they are in a dating relationship. Some college students believe forced sex is acceptable if a woman agrees and then changes her mind, if the couple is engaged in heavy petting, or if both people willingly have their clothes off (Koss & Boeschen, 2000).

NURSING PROCESS

Assessment

Rape victims must be assessed physiologically from head to toe for any serious or critical injuries that may have resulted from the assault. Critical injuries have the highest priority of care.

Before any further medical intervention occurs, clients must be informed of their right to have a *rape crisis advocate* with them during the assessment process. The victim must also be informed of their *rights* to have:

- Family or friends present during the questioning and examination
- Their personal physician notified
- Privacy during the assessment and treatment process
- Confidentiality maintained by all members of the staff
- Gentle and sensitive treatment
- Detailed explanations of, and giving consent for, all tests and procedures, including photographs
- Referrals for follow-up treatment and counseling

Victims who respond to rape in a controlled manner may be able to answer assessment questions, but those in a state of emotional shock and disbelief may find it difficult to engage actively in the assessment process. The method by which you complete the assessment depends on the person's response to the trauma.

As a nurse, you must *respect the victim's autonomy* in order to prevent revictimization. Give the client as much control as possible through every step of the assessment and treatment process. With the victim's permission, a vaginal or rectal examination is performed to determine necessary treatment and to provide evidence for legal action. With permission, photographs of the injuries may be taken for legal documentation. The physiological assessment process must be carefully documented in writing to assist with possible prosecution of the perpetrator. See the Focused Nursing Assessment feature for guidance in the assessment process of people who have been raped.

In the 1990s, *Sexual Assault Nurse Examiner (SANE)* programs were established to improve the community response to sexual assault victims. The retraumatization of victims in the medical setting in

Behavior Assessment	Affective Assessment	Cognitive Assessment
Nursing observations: Is the client able to respond verbally to questions? Is the client able to follow simple directions? Have you bathed, douched, changed clothes, or done any self-treatment before coming to the hospital?	Could you explain ways in which you are experiencing any of the following emotions? ■ Disbelief ■ Shame ■ Embarrassment ■ Humiliation ■ Helplessness ■ Vulnerability ■ Anxiety ■ Fear ■ Guilt ■ Anger ■ Depression	Nursing observations: Is there any evidence of the use of defense mechanisms? Describe the client's attention span. Can you tell me where you are? What is today's date? Can you describe what occurred? Have you been informed of your rights? Who have you informed about the rape? Family? Friends? Police? Do you need help in telling others about the rape? In what way, if any, do you feel responsible for the attack?

the past included long waits in busy public areas, not being allowed to eat, drink, or urinate to avoid destroying evidence, and health care professionals untrained in forensic evidence collection procedures.

A SANE is a registered nurse who has advanced education and clinical preparation in forensic examination of sexual assault victims. SANEs provide respectful and prompt emergency medical–legal treatment. They offer victims compassionate care of both physical and psychological traumas. SANEs know what forensic evidence to collect and how to document injuries and other legal evidence. SANE programs provide improved medical and legal response to sexual assault victims (U.S. Department of Justice, 2001). Such data can be viewed on the U.S. Department of Justice Web site, which can be accessed through a resource link on the Companion Web site for this book.

Diagnosis

The assessment process provides the data from which you develop your nursing diagnoses. Physical and mental status priorities must be quickly established by the health care team. Attention must then be given to the long-range physical, emotional, social, and legal concerns of the survivor.

The nursing diagnosis for clients who have been raped is *Rape-trauma syndrome*. If clients suffer from reactivated symptoms of a previous physical illness or mental disorder, or if they rely on alcohol or drugs to manage their trauma, they are given the more specific nursing diagnosis of *Rape-trauma syndrome: Compound reaction*. The nursing diagnosis of *Rape-trauma syndrome: Silent reaction* is applied when the client experiences high levels of anxiety, an inability to discuss the trauma, abrupt changes in relationships with men and/or changes in sexual behavior, and the onset of phobic reactions.

Outcome Identification and Goals

Based on the assessment data, you select outcomes appropriate to the nursing diagnoses. See the Nursing Diagnoses with NOC and NIC feature for outcomes associated with the rape-trauma diagnosis.

Once you have established outcomes, you and the client mutually identify goals for change. Goals are

Social Assessment

Who do you think are your most available support systems? Family? Friends? Clergy? Rape advocate?

Are you in need of temporary shelter?

May I provide you with information about available counseling?

Physiological Assessment

Have physical injuries such as scratches, bruises, and cuts been recorded and photographed?

Have fingernail scrapings been taken and preserved?

Has blood typing been done?

Have smears been taken of the mouth, throat, vagina, and rectum for detection of sexually transmitted infections?

Have combings been made of the pubic hair and preserved?

Has genital trauma been recorded and photographed?

Has rectal trauma been recorded and photographed?

Have semen specimens been preserved?

If applicable, when was the client's last menstrual period?

Has the clothing been inspected and preserved?

All questions in the Physiological Assessment section are nursing observations; they are not asked of the client.

specific behavioral measures by which you, clients, and significant others have identified as realistic and attainable. The following are examples of some of the goals appropriate to victims of rape:

- Identifies immediate concerns
- Verbalizes anticipated problems
- Utilizes the problem-solving process to make own decisions
- Has control over remembering
- Utilizes community resources
- Verbalizes an improved ability to trust others
- Describes some tolerable meaning to the trauma
- Verbalizes feelings of empowerment

Nursing Interventions

Safety: Crisis Management

Rape-Trauma Treatment

It is important to *support defense mechanisms* until clients are able to cope with the reality of the assault.

Give them ample time to respond to simple questions; anxiety will decrease their ability to perceive input, thereby slowing down their response time. If clients are unable to express feelings, acknowledge the difficulty by saying, "I understand that it's difficult for you to describe your feelings right now. That's okay. You may be able to talk about them later." Communicate your knowledge and understanding of the usual emotional responses to rape. Statements such as "People usually experience a number of feelings, like anxiety, fear, embarrassment, guilt, and anger" will reassure clients that their feelings are a normal reaction to rape.

Encourage the client to *talk about the rape* to help them through the stage of disbelief. Many clients will have a compulsive need to recount the assault. The emotional arousal of the trauma contributes to this intense pressure to talk. Listen patiently and supportively, understanding that compulsive retelling is a natural way by which the victim is gradually desensitized to the trauma.

Identify specific *coping behaviors* clients used during the rape such as screaming, fighting, talking, blacking

NURSING DIAGNOSES with NOC & NIC

Victims of Rape

DIAGNOSIS	OUTCOMES	INTERVENTIONS
Rape-Trauma Syndrome	*Abuse Recovery:* Emotional: Healing of psychologic injuries due to abuse	Rape-Trauma Treatment
	Abuse Recovery: Sexual: Healing following sexual abuse or exploitation	
	Coping: Action to manage stressors that tax an individual's resources	Support Group
	Fear Control: Personal actions to eliminate or reduce disabling feelings of alarm aroused by an identifiable source	Anticipatory Guidance

SOURCES: Johnson, M., Maas, M., & Moorhead, S. (2000). *Nursing outcomes classification (NOC)* (2nd ed.). St. Louis, MO: Mosby; McCloskey, J. C., & Bulechek, G. M. (1996). *Nursing interventions classification (NIC)* (2nd ed.). St. Louis, MO: Mosby; and North American Nursing Diagnoses Association (1999). *Nursing diagnoses definitions and classification 1999–2000*. Philadelphia: Author.

out, and/or remaining passive. Initially, clients may experience distortions related to self-blame or guilt. Recognizing that their behavior was an adaptive mechanism for survival will raise their self-esteem and

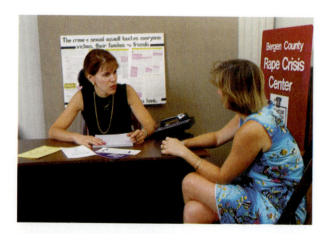

PHOTO 22.1 ■ Rape crisis centers offer women support in dealing with sexual assault.

SOURCE: R. Sidney/The Image Works.

decrease their feelings of guilt. Repeatedly tell clients it was not their fault. It is critical to stress that *survival is the most important outcome*. Reassure them that their responses were all that was possible under the degree of fear that rape induces. A helpful statement might be, "I know you handled the situation right because you are alive."

The next step is to help the clients *identify immediate concerns* and prioritize them. Focusing on immediate problems lessens the client's confusion and feelings of being overwhelmed. Next, help the client use the *problem-solving process*. Clients need to be empowered to make their own decisions and act on their own behalf. Restoring personal choice is a primary antidote to rape trauma. Informed choices help clients regain control and autonomy, both of which were violated during the rape.

Rape is both a personal and a family crisis. Clients may need help in *identifying who to tell* about the rape. Victims often fear how family and friends will respond to the situation. Anticipatory guidance on your part will help them take advantage of available support systems. When significant others are involved, prepare them before they join the victim because they may not know how to best support their loved one.

Discuss beliefs about postcoital contraception and abortion if appropriate. Pregnancy may result from the rape, and clients must have information about available options. The most common medical intervention is a course of hormonal treatment. Elevated doses of oral contraceptive or DES (diethylstilbestrol) may be administered if the woman chooses to prevent conception. Mifepristone (RU-486) is a chemical that greatly diminishes the chance that a fertilized ovum will be implanted or that a placenta will develop. Clients should be informed about the need for follow-up medical evaluation and treatment for sexually transmitted infections, including a test for HIV/AIDS.

A *written list of referrals* of community resources should be provided before clients are discharged from the emergency department. Sexual assault advocacy programs address a wide range of victim needs including crisis counseling and emotional support to victims and their families. Crisis intervention counseling can help minimize the long-term emotional and spiritual impact of sexual assault. See the Community Resources feature at the end of this chapter for a list of national resources that can provide local referrals.

Behavioral: Coping Assistance

Support Groups

Support groups provide an opportunity for victims to meet with other survivors of rape in a safe, supportive, and egalitarian setting. In this therapeutic environment, clients have their feelings validated as normal reactions to the assault and receive confirmation of their survival behaviors. Support groups may help moderate depression by providing an opportunity to speak openly and network with other survivors and supportive people. Individuals may be able to redirect the energy that is often spent on anger and pain into compassionate acts of supporting others. The long-term goal of support groups is to help survivors understand their distress and take charge of their own recovery. Recovery is accomplished by counteracting self-blame, sharing grief, and affirming self and life.

Anticipatory Guidance

Girls and women must be empowered to deal with sexual harassment. Teaching them how to resist unwanted comments and behaviors may minimize the effect of

harassment. Teach them to speak out their thoughts and feelings regarding the cultural sanctions of sexual harassment in a patriarchal society. Help them identify that even subtle harassment is damaging to one's self-esteem. What is often called "teasing" is, in fact, harassment (Berman et al., 2000). Refer back to Box 22.1 for steps to take when dealing with harassment at school or on the job.

As a nurse, you must challenge cultural values and beliefs that promote and condone sexual violence. Myths that support rape in any way must be confronted, and a new understanding of rape and rape victims must be developed. Changing the stereotypes of gender roles and the inequality of power inherent in heterosexual relationships can decrease the prevalence of sexual violence. It is only through this process that long-term changes will occur.

Evaluation

The long-term goal of intervention is to help rape victims return to their precrisis level or achieve a higher level of functioning. The road to recovery is profoundly personal and uniquely individual. Finally, *it is the victim/survivor who determines if recovery is complete.* To complete the nursing process you evaluate clients' responses to nursing interventions based on the outcomes you selected. You should determine the appropriate intervals for measurement and documentation of the outcomes according to each individual's status. The following are examples of indicators (Johnson, Maas, & Moorhead, 2000).

Abuse Recovery: Emotional

Those who have recovered from emotional abuse report a substantial or extensive sense of confidence, self-esteem, self-empowerment feelings, and positive interpersonal relationships. Symptom mastery is an indication that the crisis has been resolved in an adaptive fashion. This is evidenced by a decrease in anxiety and depression. Behaviors that are extinguished include suicide attempts, self-injurious actions, trauma-induced behaviors, and impulsive actions. Another indicator of recovery is the client's ability to trust and attach to others.

Abuse Recovery: Sexual

Those who have recovered from sexual abuse report a substantial or extensive ability to verbalize feelings, identify inappropriate guilt, and express hope and empowerment. They will be free from sleep disturbances, depression, suicidal ideation, sexual problems, and inappropriate expression of anger.

Coping

Recovery from sexual violence includes clients' ability to demonstrate, often or consistently, effective coping strategies, modification of lifestyle as necessary, a decrease in negative feelings, and a decrease in physical symptoms. They will demonstrate a control over remembering in that they can elect to recall or not recall the rape and experience fewer flashbacks. Clients utilize available social supports and verbalize any needs for assistance. Spiritual coping is evidenced by their discovery of some tolerable meaning to the trauma and to themselves as trauma survivors.

Fear Control

Sexual assault survivors learn to avoid, when possible, stimuli that remind them of their trauma. They also anticipate fearful situations and develop coping strategies. Their feelings can be felt, named, and endured without overwhelming arousal or numbing. Fearful episodes become less frequent, have a shorter duration, and are less intense. Clients also maintain a sense of purpose despite their fear. They are able to maintain interpersonal relationships and perform their social roles.

KNOWLEDGE BASE: CHILDHOOD SEXUAL ABUSE

Childhood sexual abuse is a process, not just an event. Not all children become symptomatic following sexual abuse—some may never have symptoms and some may not experience difficulties until adulthood. A single traumatic experience does not usually lead to mental disorders. To the extent that other life experiences are positive, children are likely to have no or few long-term effects. To the extent that other life experiences are also negative, the effects of the sexual abuse are amplified.

There is no identified "sexual abuse syndrome," and reactions vary greatly from one person to another. The effects of sexual abuse are most severe when the incidents are frequent and occur over a long period of time, the activities are wide ranging and extensive, there is more than one perpetrator, the relationship to

the perpetrator is close, and when sexual abuse is combined with physical and emotional abuse. There are behavioral, cognitive, and physical problems, as well as difficulties with emotional stability and interpersonal relationships during childhood, adolescence, and adulthood (Paris, 1999).

Abuse disrupts the smooth progression of development in several ways. For some there is an intensification and fixation of the current developmental stage. Others regress to an earlier stage. And some prematurely accelerate and develop a pseudo-maturity. The earlier the abuse occurs, the more profound the damage (Sholevar & Schwoeri, 1999).

BEHAVIORAL CHARACTERISTICS

Typically, *adult perpetrators* initiate sexual behavior in a *manipulative or coercive manner*. Often, the adult misrepresents the abuse as a game or "fun" activity. The behavior usually follows a progression of sexual activity, from exposure and fondling to oral, vaginal, and/or anal sex. *Secrecy* is imposed on the child by persuasion or threat. The abuser may say such things as "If you tell, you'll be sent away," "If you tell, I won't love you anymore," "If you tell, I will kill you," and "If you tell, I'll do the same thing to your baby brother." Children know adults have absolute power over them, so they obey. When they have been threatened with abandonment or harm, they frequently choose to protect others. When asked, "Why didn't you tell sooner?" the answers are, "I didn't know who to tell," "I was scared," or "I did tell and no one believed me."

Donell describes his sexual abuse by his Boy Scout leader in this way: "Whenever we would go on camping trips, he would pick out which boy would share his tent for that trip. Until it was "our turn," we had no idea what was going on. When it happened to me, I couldn't believe it! He made me promise not to tell. I just can't figure out why no one noticed. From that time on I acted out at school all the time."

Sometimes, adult perpetrators use "grooming behaviors" to prepare or persuade victims to comply with the abuse. **Grooming behaviors** are used to gain the trust of children or family members before the abuse begins. Behaviors include hanging out with and participating in

BOX 22.4

Sexual Behavior Clues of Abused Children

Sexual Behavior

- With children of different ages or different developmental levels; the wider the age range, the greater the concern
- That is significantly different from other children of the same age
- That continues in spite of the child's having been given consistent and clear messages to stop
- That occurs in public or other places where the child has been told is not acceptable
- That is adult-type activities with other children; other children may complain about it
- Initiated by the child toward an adult that is in the manner of adult–adult sexual contact
- That increases in frequency, intensity, or intrusiveness.

SOURCES: Burton, J. E., & Rasmussen, L. A. (1998). *Treating children with sexually abusive behavior problems.* New York: Haworth Press; Damon, L. L., & Card, J. A. (1999). Incest in young children. In R. T. Ammerman & M. Hersen (Eds.), *Assessment of family violence: A clinical and legal sourcebook* (2nd ed.). New York: John Wiley & Sons; and Johnson, T. C. (1999). Development of sexual behavior problems in childhood. In J. A. Shaw (Ed.), *Sexual aggression* (pp. 41–74). Washington, DC: American Psychiatric Press.

activities with the children, baby-sitting for the parents, or buying gifts for the children or other family members.

Some *children* who have been sexually abused form a clinging attachment to one or both parents. Some become extremely affectionate both inside and outside the family system, while others have problems with impulse control and aggression toward others. Some children isolate themselves at school or in the neighborhood and limit most of their interactions to family members. They may *act out sexually*, by initiating oral or genital sex with other children or adults, for example. Some children, in an effort to master their trauma and regain a sense of personal control, victimize others as they were victimized. In addition, sexually abused children often engage in *self-destructive behaviors* such as head banging, self-mutilation, and suicide (Johnson, 1999). See Box 22.4 for behavioral characteristics of children who have been abused.

Adolescent victims may *run away* from home to escape an intolerable situation. Because they have learned, at home, that sexual behavior is rewarded by affection, love, and attention, some turn to prostitution. Others are forced into *prostitution* as a way to support themselves while living on the streets. Adolescents may unconsciously seek to repeat the trauma as a way of mastering it. This repetition may take the form of revictimization or perpetrating against others.

Some *adult survivors* engage in *self-mutilation*, as in cutting, slashing, or burning themselves. It is important to understand the meaning of such behavior. For some, the pain of self-mutilation proves their existence and reassures them that they are alive and real. Self-mutilation may be a plea for nurturance, as they come to the emergency department seeking care. Others nurture them by cleaning up the wounds after self-mutilating. For those who dissociate, self-mutilation may be a way to stop the dissociation with physical pain. Other adult survivors self-mutilate as a form of self-punishment and as a way to decrease feelings of guilt. And finally, some self-mutilate as a way to reduce emotional pain through the feeling of physical pain. It is important to understand the function of the behavior in order to replace it with healthier behaviors that satisfy the same need. (See Chapter 9 for further information on self-mutilation.)

There are a number of possible *sexual effects* for adult survivors. Sexual behaviors are a trigger for some abuse survivors who only develop symptoms once they become sexually active. Some have a very strong aversion to sex and are filled with terror in sexual situations. Some are sexually inhibited and experience discomfort with sexual thoughts, feelings, and behaviors. Some engage in compulsive sexual behavior, perhaps as an unconscious way to validate their shame and guilt or a way to feel powerful. Other sexual symptoms include anger or disgust associated with touch, feeling emotionally distant during sex, experiencing intrusive sexual thoughts or images, and experiencing orgasmic, erectile, or ejaculatory difficulties. Many adult survivors go through a period of celibacy as they try to manage fear, anger, and distrust.

AFFECTIVE CHARACTERISTICS

Behind a facade of dominance, *perpetrators* often feel weak, afraid, and inadequate. They inappropriately view the child as a safe and less threatening source of caring than an adult. They are unable to distinguish between nonsexual and sexual affection for children. *Lack of empathy* for the victim is typical of perpetrators. Many perpetrators experience intense pleasure based on their sense of *power* and *domination*.

Child victims experience many *fears*. They fear if they tell another adult, they will not be believed, and they fear that they themselves will be blamed. If the abuse is occurring within the family, they may have fantasies of being rejected by family members. They may fear that the family will be separated, especially if this threat was made by the abuser.

Children often *feel responsible* for the adult's behavior and ashamed that they have not been able to stop the abuse. Secrecy and guilt keep these children isolated, causing them to feel alienated from their peers. The feeling of *powerlessness* is extremely prevalent because what the victim says and does makes no difference. The associated rage typically does not emerge until *adolescence*. When the suppressed *rage* comes to the surface, it may be directed against the self in self-defeating and self-destructive ways.

Many *adult survivors* continue to believe that they were to blame for the abuse and should have been able to resist the adult. This *self-blame* often contributes to depression and anxiety and to panic attacks. Distrusting and fearing men, many survivors have *multiple fears* relating to sexual interactions. For some, *anger* is the only emotion experienced and expressed, all other feelings being severely repressed. Many adult survivors continue to hate their perpetrators, as well as nonabusing significant adults for not protecting them (Sholevar & Schwoeri, 1999).

COGNITIVE CHARACTERISTICS

Cognitive distortions are self-statements *perpetrators* use to deny, minimize, justify, and rationalize their behavior. In addition, they have an impaired capacity for empathy or bonding with children. They view their victims as objects and they focus primarily on their own pleasure and satisfaction.

Secrecy and silence are used by perpetrators to escape accountability. When secrecy fails and the child victims or adult survivors begin to talk to others about the abuse, perpetrators usually *attack the credibility* of the victims and try to make sure no one will listen.

Perpetrators make such statements as "It never happened, She's lying," "He's exaggerating some innocent touching," and "Even if it did happen, it's time to forget the past and move on." Other perpetrators acknowledge the abuse but *minimize the impact* with statements such as "We didn't have intercourse, so it really wasn't sex" and "She didn't really mind; in fact, we have a very close relationship," and "It was just a game, I would never have forced myself on her." Others use the defense mechanism of *projection* and *blame* the child for the abuse, as evidenced by such statements as "She's a very provocative child, and she seduced me" and "If he hadn't enjoyed it so much, I wouldn't have continued."

Some *child victims* use *denial* to cope with the trauma. Acknowledging the abuse would mean acknowledging that the world is dangerous and that those who are supposed to protect and nurture failed and caused harm. Other victims *minimize the impact* and say it was not important, saying things like "It's not so bad; it only happens once a month" and "It's all right because it stopped when I was 11 years old."

Family members may use denial to protect the *family system*. Denial functions to keep the incest a secret while appearing to be a cohesive, "normal" family. When the secret comes out, the *process of denial* usually follows four stages. In stage one, the family denies the facts of the incest, believing that it never happened. Stage two is denial of awareness. The mother may say she was never told by the child. Denial of responsibility and blaming factors external to the family is the third stage. The final or fourth stage of family denial is denial of the impact on the victim. In this stage, the family minimizes the traumatic effects. As the family works through the stages of denial, they come to realization and acknowledgment of the facts and the seriousness of the abuse (Sholevar & Schwoeri, 1999).

Frequently, *dissociation* is the victim's major defense. The mind is "separated" from the body, so the victim is not emotionally present during the sexual attack. It prevents the feelings attached to the trauma from reaching conscious awareness in order to survive the trauma. Dissociation is evidenced by such statements as "I put myself in the wall, where he couldn't reach all of me" and "When he would come into my room, I would close my eyes and go to my favorite place. Only my body stayed on the bed; the rest of me wasn't there." When sexual abuse is severe and sadistic, the victim may develop dissociative identity disorder (DID). (See Chapter 11 for a discussion of DID.)

Research shows that many memories of past events are not reports but *reconstructions*. It is the difference between remembering facts and remembering events. What is remembered is the overall impression rather than the specific details. The details we add when we reconstruct our experience depend on our personality traits and cognitive styles. We may also create pseudo-memories of events that never actually occurred, especially after being told of such "events" by trusted individuals. That is the reason why reports of remembered child abuse in adults should ideally be corroborated by other people (Chu, Frey, Ganzel, & Matthews, 1999; Paris, 1999).

There is widespread belief that the mother always knows when her husband is sexually involved with one or more of the children. In reality, mothers are *often unaware of the sexual abuse*. Some deny any evidence of the abuse because they feel inadequate to cope with the family problems. Others use denial because they fear their husbands' retaliation against them if the accusation of incest is brought into the open. Denial may be a defense mechanism used by women who fear financial, social, and emotional problems if their husbands are removed from the family. When cues to sexual abuse are discovered, some women question their own thinking processes. Believing their husbands are incapable of this type of behavior, they, therefore, believe something must be wrong with themselves.

Cherenia has recently become somewhat suspicious that her husband Joe may be sexually abusing their daughter. In response to her fears, she says the following things to herself: "You must really have a dirty mind, Cherenia. How could you possibly think those things about Joe? He's a very good husband. He works hard and loves all of us. He goes to church every week, and everyone knows what a good family man he is. How could you even consider that he might be doing something so awful? You must be really sick, Cherenia."

It is not unusual for *adult survivors* to have *total amnesia* for the childhood sexual abuse. In such a case, amnesia is considered a defense mechanism in response to the trauma and is more likely to occur when the abuse began at a very young age. Recall of the abuse may be triggered by a significant life event such as marriage or pregnancy, or during the process of psychotherapy.

Self-blame contributes to *low self-esteem* in adult survivors. They feel worthless and different from other people. Survivors often feel alienated from or even hate their bodies. They may believe they are only sex objects to be used and abused by others. They may suffer from *flashbacks* and nightmares. Many adult survivors have very little sense of self since their boundaries were so profoundly violated as children. This makes them more vulnerable to revictimization as adults.

Confusion about sexuality is very common among *male survivors*. Victimization of a male carries a hidden implication of being less than a man. Heterosexual survivors fear that the abuse has made, or will make, them homosexual. Intense homophobia and/or hypermasculine behavior may be an effort to disprove their fears. Gay survivors worry that their sexual preference may have caused the abuse. It must be remembered that childhood sexual abuse is not related to adult sexual orientation.

SOCIAL CHARACTERISTICS

Male survivors are affected by different social values than women. Men are expected to be powerful, active, and competent. They often equate being abused with being weak, female, or gay. Society believes that men are always sexually willing and eager and therefore sex cannot be abusive. The general thought is that he must have sought it or at least welcomed the sexual activity (Hodge & Canter, 1998).

Many *adult survivors* have difficulties with relationships. Superficial relationships are usually much easier than intimate relationships. As children, these adults learned that those who love you are the ones who hurt you, and that living in a family is not safe. There is a sense of *betrayal* by those they are dependent upon, a sense of *powerlessness* since they could do nothing to stop the abuse, and finally, a sense of *stigmatization* when they incorporate the shame and guilt that has been communicated to them. As a result, in adulthood they may be incapable of trusting others and feel trapped by intimate relationships. Adult survivors also struggle with *control issues*. Anyone who has been raised in an environment that was out of control or dangerous grows up with a strong need to control the environment as much as possible. Such a need for control can contribute to conflict in relationships.

Sasha, age 19, describes her relationship with her father when she was 12 years old in this way: "I don't remember how it started, but my father conned me into soaping up his stomach, testicles, and erect penis when he was in the bathtub. This took place at his apartment when my brothers and I went there for the weekend. I didn't particularly enjoy it, but my father encouraged it. I got completely turned off by it when he offered to do it to me. One time, while I was sleeping on the bed, I woke up from a violent shaking of the bed. I was dressed in a shirt and shorts. I realized my father was rubbing his penis between my thighs and feeling on my vagina. I didn't let him know I was awake, and I turned slightly, hoping he would stop. I never wore that tee shirt or shorts again. I've never told anyone. Even my father doesn't know that I know. I think my experiences have had a deep effect on my relationships. Every time I get close to a man, I become afraid. I think what I'm most afraid of is being used. My childhood experiences seem to bother me the most when my friends talk about their childhood with their fathers and how they were 'Daddy's little girl.' Feelings of rage, anger, and total disgust burn deep inside me."

There is a significant connection between being sexually abused as a child and being *revictimized* as an adult. This in no way implies, however, that an adult survivor is responsible for being abused, as there is never a legitimate excuse for emotional or physical violence. Adults who were sexually abused as children become victims again in adulthood for many reasons. One thing a person learns from sexual abuse is how to be abused. In order to survive, children teach themselves to endure assaults. They learn they cannot protect themselves. They learn to keep the abuse a secret and to "forgive and forget" each violent incident. All of these survival techniques make them vulnerable to abuse in adulthood.

CULTURE-SPECIFIC CHARACTERISTICS

Any consideration of sexual abuse must take into account cultural views of appropriate and inappropriate sexual behavior. The aspects of culture relating to child sexual abuse include family structures, moral and reli-

gious principles, and child-rearing practices. Other aspects include the relative value of interdependence, treatment of sexuality, gender roles, and interpersonal boundaries. The ways in which communities view violence and sexual assault, and the action that is taken when these occur, reflect cultural values. It is only when we understand cultural diversity that we are able to develop effective prevention programs (Raphel & Berry, 1998).

There is no such thing as a generic African American, Asian American, Hispanic American, or member of any other minority group. There are differences not only between groups but also among members of the same group. These differences are based on gender, socioeconomic status, and level of acculturation to Euro-American norms. The cultural solidifying factor is the experience of racism perpetrated by the majority culture. Members of minority cultures are less likely to report the abuse as the result of both fear of blame and rejection by their community and fear of retaliation in the form of more severe legal penalties. Box 22.5 gives some culture-specific information on child sexual abuse.

PHYSIOLOGICAL CHARACTERISTICS

The obvious physical signs of sexual abuse in a child are the presence of a sexually transmitted infection, irritated or swollen genitals or rectal tissue, or both. Chronic vaginal or urinary tract infections with no known medical cause may be indicators that the child is being sexually abused. Among female victims, 12 to 24 percent become pregnant as a result of the abuse. The pregnant adolescent victim often has only vague stories regarding the father of her baby (Sholevar & Schwoeri, 1999).

Some children will, consciously or unconsciously, attempt to abuse their bodies to either prevent or stop the sexual abuse. The child may gain a great deal of weight, hoping to become so unattractive that the abuser will leave the child alone. If an older child is being abused, a younger sister may become anorexic in an attempt not to mature and experience the same abuse. This lack of care for the body may continue into adult life in an unconscious attempt to maintain distance and avoid intimate relationships.

Corticotropin-releasing hormone (CRH) is associated with the "fight or flight" response to a threat. Animal studies demonstrate that traumatic experiences early in life change how the CRH gene is expressed in the brain. Increased CRH in the amygdala contributes to a chronic sense of fear that accompanies depression, anxiety, and PTSD in victims and survivors. Because there is an oversecretion of CRH, certain stressful life events may trigger symptoms in adult survivors. There is an accompanying increase in glucocorticoids that may also be neurotoxic to the hippocampus. Stress also increases the turnover of norepinephrine, which may affect areas of the brain involved in the regulation of emotion and memory (Horan, Hill, & Schulkin, 2000; Schetky, 1999).

Adult female survivors may have concerns about having a "normal" child and fears regarding pregnancy. For some, it is a difficult to decision to bring a child into the world. Labor and delivery can be very difficult because, once again, their body is out of control and in pain. If health professionals are aware of the history of

---

BOX 22.5

Culture-Specific Characteristics of Sexual Abuse

Euro-Americans

- The keeping of family secrets is a traditional value.
- Sex is a taboo subject.
- Many believe that satisfying one's own needs at the expense of others is a moral right.
- Sexual domination may be a manifestation of power.

African Americans

- Prevalence appears to be the same as for Euro-Americans.
- More likely to be physically abused and less likely to be sexually abused than Euro-American or Latino children
- Many have had negative encounters with the criminal justice system and/or social service agencies, which impedes reporting of child sexual abuse.
- May be reluctant to identify an African American perpetrator and turn him over to a system that administers harsher legal consequences to African Americans for criminal behavior

Puerto Ricans

- The reaction to sexual abuse is often geared toward maintaining the family's homeostasis; family loyalty is very important.
- If the daughter is a victim, the mother is perceived as being responsible.
- The popular beliefs are that sexually abused males become homosexuals and sexually abused females are considered promiscuous.

Mexican Americans

- There is a tendency for perpetrators to be more closely related to the victim.
- Both boys and girls are more likely than African American children to report rectal penetration.
- Boys are less likely to report abuse than girls.

Asian, Pacific Island, and Filipino Americans

- Sexuality is seldom discussed openly.
- Family structure is authoritarian and children are expected to be obedient to all authority figures.
- Physical abuse is more common than sexual abuse.
- When child discloses, the family often directs its anger at the child and intervening adults; family will deny the abuse to save the family's reputation.
- Children may recant stories of sexual abuse, thus sacrificing their individual needs for family integrity.

American Jews

- Often have traditional gender roles
- Believe that family togetherness provides a safe haven from inevitable persecution
- Sexual abuse is seen as "the way of the gentiles," which burdens victims who anguish about revealing the family secret.

SOURCES: Abney, V. D., & Priest, R. (1995). African Americans and sexual child abuse. In L. A. Fontes (Ed.), *Sexual abuse in nine North American cultures* (pp. 11–30). Newbury Park, CA: Sage; Comas-Diaz, L. (1995). Puerto Ricans and sexual child abuse. In L. A. Fontes (Ed.), *Sexual abuse in nine North American cultures* (pp. 31–66). Newbury Park, CA: Sage; Featherman, J. M. (1995). Jews and sexual child abuse. In L. A. Fontes (Ed.), *Sexual abuse in nine North American cultures* (pp. 128–155). Newbury Park, CA: Sage; Huston, R. L., et al., (1995). Characteristics of childhood sexual abuse in a predominantly Mexican American population. *Child Abuse & Neglect, 19*(2), 165–176; Lefley, H. P. (1999). Transcultural aspects of sexual victimization. In J. A. Shaw (Ed.), *Sexual aggression* (pp. 129–166). Washington, DC: American Psychiatric Press; and Okamura, A., Heras, P., & Wong-Kerberg, L. (1995). Asian, Pacific Island, and Filipino Americans and sexual child abuse. In L. A. Fontes (Ed.), *Sexual abuse in nine North American cultures* (pp. 67–96). Newbury Park, CA: Sage.

childhood sexual abuse, they can be more supportive during labor and delivery.

CONCOMITANT DISORDERS

Having suffered sexual abuse in childhood is often a hidden feature of adult mental disorders (see Table 22.1 ■). As many as 60 to 70 percent of psychiatric clients have a history of abuse. Repeated trauma in childhood distorts the personality. Since child victims cannot protect themselves, they must adapt to the trauma as well as they can. Behaviors that were originally adaptive become symptoms in adulthood. These people have a bewildering combination of symptoms, including anger, depression, anxiety, insomnia, suspicion, eating disorders, substance abuse, and self-mutilation. Adult survivors often collect many different diagnoses before the underlying problem of PTSD is correctly identified (Ray, 2001; Sholevar & Schwoeri, 1999).

Adolescent sex offenders are at risk for the above dis-orders if they are also victims. Of all adolescent offenders, 48 percent are diagnosed with conduct disorder and 19 percent with substance abuse (Shaw, 1999).

CAUSATIVE THEORIES

There is no single cause of childhood sexual abuse. Rather, the abuse results from a combination of personality, family, and cultural factors.

Intrapersonal Theory

There are many types of perpetrators of childhood sexual abuse. Some traits are contradictory, and there is no agreement on a composite personality. Certain characteristics apply to many people, not just abusers. The descriptions are guidelines for assessment, not proof that the person actually committed sexual abuse.

Perpetrators usually have low self-esteem and feel more secure in interactions with children than with adults. Some were emotionally deprived as children

TABLE 22.1

Cues to Sexual Abuse

Perpetrator	Child/Adolescent	Adult Survivor
Behavioral cues		
Dominating, coercive, inappropriate affection, poor impulse control	Extremely affectionate, sexual acting out, isolative, self-destructive, running away, prostitution, suicide	Sexual dysfunction, compulsive sexual behavior, self-mutilation, substance abuse
Affective cues		
Feelings of weakness, inadequacy; inability to distinguish between nonsexual and sexual affection; lack of empathy	Multiple fears, guilt, powerlessness, rage	Anxiety, panic attacks, rage, distrust, fear of men
Cognitive cues		
Denial, minimization of blame, impact, projection	Denial, minimization of impact, dissociation	Amnesia for events, self-worthlessness, flashbacks/nightmares, confusion about sexual orientation
Mental disorders		
Impulse control disorders	Dissociative disorders, including DID; anxiety disorders; mood disorders	Dissociative disorders, including DID; anxiety disorders; mood disorders; substance abuse; personality disorders; PTSD

and thus have a great need for constant, unconditional love, which is more easily obtained from children than from adults. Some perpetrators are described as lacking impulse control and the ability to experience feelings of guilt. Others are described as rigid and overcontrolled, while others are dominant and aggressive.

If perpetrators were themselves sexually abused as children, they may have learned to associate all feelings of love with sexual behavior. Most people who were sexually abused as children do *not* go on to sexually abuse others. However, some victimized children develop offending behavior in late childhood, adolescence, or adulthood. Most likely, there are a number of factors involved in why some abuse and others do not. The world of abuse is comprised only of victims (powerless) and perpetrators (powerful). Victims become perpetrators in an unconscious attempt to master the trauma of their own experiences and take over the power. The move from victim to offender may also result when anger and hostility are externalized and projected onto new victims (Sholevar & Schwoeri, 1999).

Family Systems Theory

Family systems theory considers structure, cohesion, adaptability, and communication patterns of families in which children are being sexually abused. Refer to Chapter 3 for more detailed information on families.

Family structure is usually hierarchical according to age, roles, and distribution of power. Typically, the adults, who are older, assume the parental roles and are the most influential. The structure of incestuous families, however, is often quite different as the result of dysfunctional boundary patterns. An adult may move "down" in the structure or a child may move "up" in terms of roles and influence (boundaries). If the father moves downward, he assumes a childlike role and is cared for and nurtured like a child in the family. In this position, the father assumes little parental responsibility. He may then turn to the daughter, as a "peer," for sexual

and emotional gratification. As another example, the daughter may move upward and replace the mother in the hierarchy. The mother does not usually move downward but rather moves out of the structure by distancing herself emotionally or physically from the family. As the daughter assumes the parental role and responsibilities, the father may turn to her for fulfilling his emotional and sexual needs (Burton & Rasmussen, 1998).

Family cohesion refers to the degree of emotional bonding that occurs within a family. At one end of the cohesion continuum is the family system that is disengaged; that is, the family members are isolated and alienated from one another. At the other end of the continuum is the enmeshed family system, in which the members are immersed in and absorbed by one another. The healthiest family systems function between these two extremes. Sexual abuse in families usually occurs in an enmeshed family. The need to be overinvolved in each other's lives is accompanied by intense fears of abandonment.

Family adaptability is also described along a continuum. At one extreme is the rigid family system and at the other end, the chaotic family system. Families involved in sexual abuse tend to function at either end of the continuum. Rigid family systems have strict rules and stereotyped gender-role expectations, with minimal emotional interaction. Children have no power and authority, even over their own bodies. They are not allowed to question or protest inappropriate sexual behavior. In contrast, chaotic family systems have either no rules or constantly changing rules. Within the chaotic system, there may be no assigned roles or no rules regarding appropriate sexual behavior, which may contribute to the incidence of sexual abuse.

Communication patterns within the family system may contribute to the occurrence of sexual abuse. Incest depends on keeping the secret within the family. In family systems that avoid conflict, accusations of sexual abuse are not tolerated. Peace must be kept at all costs.

NURSING PROCESS

Assessment

It is vitally important that you acknowledge the reality of childhood sexual abuse. Nurses who deny the existence of the problem will miss the cues and fail to complete a detailed assessment. If you are knowledgeable about the incidence and the characteristics of the

Behavior Assessment	Affective Assessment	Cognitive Assessment
Child Victim		
Are there signs of regressive behavior in the child?	Do you get enough love from other family members?	How would you describe the family's problems?
Is the child exhibiting clinging behavior?	Tell me about the fears you may have if any family secrets are told: Not being believed? Being blamed for the problems? Your parents will not love you? Your parents will be taken away? You will be moved to a foster home? Physical punishment?	Who do you believe is responsible for these problems?
Does the child have friendships with other children?		What happens or might happen when you tell the family secrets?
Has there been any sexual acting out on the part of the child?		Are you able to separate your mind from your body while you are being hurt?
Has the child ever run away or threatened to run away?		
Has the child ever attempted suicide?		
Adult Survivor		
When growing up, who had which type of responsibilities in the home?	Describe the relationships in your family of origin.	Have you always remembered the abuse or was there a period of amnesia?
How were family secrets kept within the family?	In what ways do you continue to blame yourself for the childhood abuse?	What are the things you value most about yourself?
When you were young, who was (were) the closest family member(s) with whom you had any sexual activity?	Describe those people in your life who you are able to trust.	Do you have concerns about your sexual orientation?
Describe any self-mutilating behavior.	In what situations do you feel angry and out of control?	
Describe your present state of sexual functioning.		

problem, you will be alert for cues that demand nursing assessment. See the Focused Nursing Assessment feature for the types of questions to ask of both child victims and adult survivors.

When assessing *children*, remember that some will exhibit most of the characteristics presented in this chapter, others will exhibit only some, and still others will exhibit none of the characteristics. Also remember that these same behavioral, affective, and cognitive characteristics may be symptoms of other emotional problems in children. Once it has been discovered that one child in a family is a victim of sexual abuse, suspect the abuse of siblings, both boys and girls, as well. Sometimes entire families are sexually abused before someone "tells."

You must appreciate the power of secrecy and how difficult it is for *adult survivors* to disclose such information, especially for men, who, in our society, are expected to be anything other than victimized. Routine questions on nursing histories may provide an opportunity for survivors to share their pain and obtain treatment as adults. As a nurse, you are responsible for initiating the topic, as shame and confusion may keep the adult survivor from doing so. If you

Social Assessment	Physiological Assessment
Child Victim	
Who are your friends? Do they come over to play at your home?	Smears of mouth, throat, vagina, and rectum for sexually transmitted infections
Who are the people in your life who hurt you?	HIV testing
	Throat irritation
	Genital irritation or trauma
	Rectal irritation or trauma
	Chronic vaginal and/or urinary tract infections
	Pregnancy
Adult Survivor	
Describe the most important relationships in your life.	Weight and nutritional status
Has it been easier for you to maintain superficial relationships as opposed to intimate relationships?	Sleeping problems
	Evidence of substance abuse
In what ways do you need to be in control in relationships?	Evidence of self-mutilation
In what ways have you been abused as an adult? Emotionally? Physically? Sexually?	

All questions in the Physiological Assessment section are nursing observations; they are not asked of the client.

avoid the topic, you will be contributing to pathology by supporting the client's denial of reality. Failure to initiate a discussion of sexual abuse sends a message to clients that such abuse does not occur or does not matter. Now that childhood sexual abuse has been identified as a major health problem, nurses in every clinical setting must be alert for cues from both individuals and families. When working with adult survivors, you must continuously assess the client's comfort level with the physical setting. Closed doors will increase anxiety in some clients, while others will request that doors never remain open. Some will be uncomfortable in a room with a couch or a bed rather than chairs. How close you sit can be an issue for some clients. Even normally appropriate physical contact, such as a handshake, may increase anxiety. Always ask permission before touching a client.

Diagnosis

There are many potential nursing diagnoses for victims, survivors, and families suffering from childhood sexual abuse. In synthesizing the assessment data, consider how well clients are functioning in daily life. See

NURSING DIAGNOSES with NOC & NIC

Victims, Survivors, and Families of Child Sexual Abuse

DIAGNOSIS	OUTCOMES	INTERVENTIONS
Child Victim Diagnoses Ineffective individual coping related to being a victim of sexual abuse	*Coping:* Action to manage stressors that tax an individual's resources	Coping Enhancement
Powerlessness related to being a victim of sexual abuse	*Abuse Recovery:* Emotional: Healing of psychologic injuries due to abuse	Self-Esteem Enhancement
Post-trauma syndrome related to being a victim of sexual abuse	*Abuse Recovery:* Sexual: Healing following sexual abuse or exploitation	Abuse Protection: Child Play Therapy; Art Therapy; Music Therapy
Social isolation related to keeping the family secret of sexual abuse	*Social Support:* Perceived availability and actual provision of reliable assistance from other persons	Support Group Spiritual Support
Family Diagnoses Altered family process related to disruption of the family unit when abuse is discovered	*Family Coping:* Family actions to manage stressors that tax family resources	Family Integrity Promotion

the Nursing Diagnoses with NOC and NIC feature for common nursing diagnoses.

Outcome Identification and Goals

Based on the assessment data, you select outcomes appropriate to the nursing diagnoses. See the Nursing Diagnoses with NOC and NIC feature for outcomes.

Once you have established outcomes, you, the client, and the family mutually identify goals for change. Goals are specific behavioral measures by which you, clients, and significant others determine progress toward healing. The following are examples of

some of the goals appropriate to people who have experienced childhood sexual abuse:

- Remains safe and free from harm
- Utilizes a variety of therapies to express feelings about the sexual abuse
- Verbalizes improved self-esteem
- Manages negative emotions in an appropriate manner
- Verbalizes a feeling of connectedness to significant others
- Verbalizes improvement in sexual functioning

DIAGNOSIS	OUTCOMES	INTERVENTIONS
Adult Survivor Diagnoses Post-trauma syndrome related to being an adult survivor	***Abuse Recovery:*** Emotional: Healing of psychological injuries due to abuse	Art therapy Guilt Work Facilitation Coping Enhancement Simple Relaxation Therapy
Spiritual distress related to asking questions about fairness and justice in life or not being protected by a supreme being	***Spiritual Well-Being:*** Personal expressions of connectedness with self, others, higher power, all life, nature, and the universe that transcend and empower the self	Spiritual Support
Chronic low self-esteem related to self-blame for the abuse	***Self-Esteem:*** Personal judgment of self-worth	Self-Esteem Enhancement
Social isolation related to difficulty in forming intimate relationships, mistrust of others	***Social Support:*** Perceived availability and actual provision of reliable assistance from other persons	Support Group
Sexual dysfunction related to the trauma of abuse	***Abuse Recovery:*** Sexual: Healing following sexual abuse or exploitation	Sexual Counseling

SOURCES: Johnson, M., Maas, M., & Moorhead, S. (2000). *Nursing outcomes classification (NOC)* (2nd ed.). St. Louis, MO: Mosby; McCloskey, J. C., & Bulechek, G. M. (1996). *Nursing interventions classification (NIC)* (2nd ed.). St. Louis, MO: Mosby; and North American Nursing Diagnoses Association (1999). *Nursing diagnoses definitions and classification 1999–2000*. Philadelphia: Author.

■ Utilizes community resources

Nursing Interventions

Although as a culture we say that we protect our children, we do not in reality live out this value. We do not invest many of our energies—time, caring, and money—in the prevention of childhood sexual abuse. Our present approaches to treatment and to the social control of sexual abuse are not yet effective enough that we can be assured of the long-term safety of children. As nurses, we must all become active in the battle to stop child sexual abuse.

Safety: Risk Management
Abuse Protection: Child

The first priority of care with child victims is to *ensure the safety of the child*. Nurses are *mandated by law to report any suspected child sexual abuse.* Complaints of abuse by a family member are generally investigated by civil authorities such as child protective services. Sexual abuse complaints are also referred to the police. If the investigation finds sufficient evidence, criminal prosecution of the alleged perpetrator may follow.

Protective services will implement one of four plans

if they find that a child has been sexually abused by a family member:

1. The most frequent option is one in which the abuser is removed from the family. The nonabusing parent must be able to protect the child from any contact with the abuser.

2. When the nonabusing parent is unable to protect the child, both the child and the abuser are removed from the home. This option maximizes the safety of the child and decreases the child's feelings of responsibility.

3. In a few cases in which families have not used physical violence, where there is no substance abuse, and there is someone who can ensure the child's safety, the family may be allowed to remain intact while participating in intensive therapy.

4. In a few instances, the child may be removed from the family when that appears to be the safest option. Unfortunately, this decision may place additional guilt on the child.

Family: Life Span Care
Family Integrity Promotion

Throughout the process of family intervention, you collaborate with family members in problem solving and attaining and maintaining positive relationships. When families are enmeshed and either rigid or chaotic, you help family members move to a *moderate position between the extremes*. With a rigid family, you will problem-solve ways in which the members can increase their flexibility of roles and rules. With a chaotic family, you will problem-solve ways to organize appropriate roles and formulate consistent rules. You may refer families to family therapy for more intense intervention.

Behavioral: Behavior Therapy
Play Therapy; Art Therapy; Music Therapy

An important goal of nursing intervention is to facilitate the child's ability to talk and to think about the abuse with decreasing anxiety. It is up to you to create a safe and predictable environment in which the child feels supported. Make it clear to the child that you understand that talking about the abuse is difficult. Plan interventions that will *encourage affective release in a supportive environment*. Child victims must be able to experience a range of emotions. *Play therapy* helps

these children play out traumatic themes, fears, and distorted beliefs. It is a nonthreatening way to process thoughts and feelings associated with the abuse, both symbolically and directly. *Therapeutic stories* present the traumatic issues of abuse, link victims' feelings and behavior, and describe new coping methods. *Journal writing* can help children over age 10 cope with intrusive thoughts and feelings. They often choose to bring their journal into the one-to-one sessions with their therapist.

Art therapy provides an opportunity to *express feelings* for which there are no words. Art therapy helps adults in the healing process. Making group murals to express both individual progress and a sense of unity among clients can be very effective. Sitting and looking at soothing art works may be effective in reducing anxiety. *Music therapy*, combined with movement or dance, may be a way for clients to experience very early memories. *Anxiety may be lessened* by singing or humming a song, or playing a musical instrument. Journal writing is used more than any other expressive therapy and can be expanded to include poetry, songs, and plays.

Behavioral: Coping Assistance
Guilt Work Facilitation

Feminist-sensitive therapy can and should be practiced by all professionals dealing with sexual abuse. Because the process of sexual abuse is disempowering, it is important to empower survivors. The focus on *traumatic stress therapy* treats the trauma while acknowledging the process and result of victimization. *Developmental therapy* focuses on the "gaps" in the personality that occurred during the abuse process, such as trust issues, identity issues, and relationship issues. *Loss therapy* focuses on helping survivors identify and grieve over things lost during childhood sexual abuse, such as innocence, trust, nurturing, and memories.

Self-Esteem Enhancement

In working with adult survivors, remember that they have been robbed of a sense of power and feel detached from others. Recovery includes *restoring power and control*. Be sure to avoid becoming a "rescuer," as that might send the message that clients are not capable of acting for themselves. Also be careful not to set yourself up as a powerful authority because that might recreate the type of relationship in which the abuse occurred. The most helpful approach is being ally, collaborator, and supporter as clients struggle through the healing process. Point out ways they have taken control of their lives, and help them identify situations in which they are able to make self-respecting choices. As Glaister and Abel (2001, p. 193) describe the appropriate nurse therapist, "It was essential they find someone who could be present, who could understand, who could listen, and who could provide information on what to expect and on ways to grow. They needed supporters to step aside and allow them to be in control of their healing."

Interventions are designed to *increase self-esteem*. Adult survivors have a continuous internal monologue of negative statements like "You're weak, stupid, incompetent, unlovable, and unattractive." Negative statements become self-administered abuse and keep the survivor weak and powerless. You can help clients become aware of the frequency and intensity of these negative thoughts. Teach them to consciously replace negative thoughts with positive ones. Often difficult at first, it becomes easier with practice. Self-esteem is enhanced through the use of assertive skills. Survivors need to learn how to state their own opinions, interests, and needs directly and clearly. They need to calmly and rationally set limits of others' demands on them. As these new skills increase, so does self-esteem.

Coping Enhancement

Adult survivors also need to learn *skills for managing negative emotions, thoughts, and memories*. You can instruct them to do simple breathing exercises while focusing their attention on something in the room. Teach them to say to themselves: "Take the next few minutes to let go of the past and let go of your worries about the future. Come into this time and place." Sensory counting is another skill you can teach clients. Ask them to name one thing they can see in the room, then one thing they can hear, then one thing they can sense in their bodies. Continue on with two things they can see, hear, and sense. They can decide if they want to repeat observations or try to find new things. Repeat this process again and again, increasing the number each time. Usually, by the time they reach four or five, they are back in the here and now. This is a very powerful self-help technique for managing memory flooding and dissociation.

You can also ask clients to imagine a safety "container" in their minds. This container then becomes a receptacle in which they can "put and lock away" unpleasant thoughts. You can teach them to do the same process with a safe place—somewhere they can go to "get away and rest."

Sexual healing is important for many adult survivors. It is an empowering process that enables the survivors to reclaim their sexuality as positive and pleasurable. This process may take several months to several years. It is usually not undertaken until the more general issues such as depression, anger, self-blame, and self-destructive behaviors are resolved. The program of recovery is best guided by a sex therapist with expertise in working with adult survivors. For survivors caught up in compulsive and addictive sexual behaviors, participation in 12-step recovery programs is often essential.

Spiritual Support

Betrayal by abusing adults is a spiritual issue. As nurses, we sometimes ignore a client's need for spiritual healing. Especially with adult survivors, you must support **spiritual recovery**. The sense of purpose in life is disrupted for victims and survivors. They also experience a loss in faith in a divine being as well as in other people. They are consumed with spiritual questions like "Why did it happen to me?," "What's wrong with me?," and "Am I some evil person?" When people are sexually abused, they must struggle with questions of a God or some higher power who either overlooked their pain and did not respond or did not even see their pain at all. It is not unusual for survivors to be angry with the Divine and hold God responsible for the abuse. This anger may in turn trigger fear and guilt for hating someone so powerful.

To recover from sexual abuse, survivors must place responsibility for the abuse where it belongs—100 percent with the offender. If they fail to do this, they will continue to be paralyzed by self-blame and guilt. The adult self needs to reach out and care for the hurt inner child by breaking down the walls that have isolated that child. Fully experiencing the rage and grief enables the survivor to move on to self-forgiveness and more complete healing. Spirituality includes a *sense of connectedness to others*. Survivors must begin the long journey of developing trusting relationships. They need to experience human contact and the warmth of the nurse–client relationship. Approach each client individually and remember that the paths of human spirituality are as varied as the people taking them. Life events often shape belief systems in dramatic ways. The crisis and trauma of sexual abuse challenges victims and survivors to reflect on their values, beliefs, and their search for meaning. Approach each person with a sense of compassion and *encourage this spiritual reflection*. When requested, refer clients to religious/spiritual counselors who understand the emotional issues surrounding sexual abuse and who are sensitive to the need of survivors to work slowly through their spiritual struggles.

Support Groups

Support groups allow survivors to share their feelings and experiences with others who believe their stories. The group setting fosters mutual understanding and decreases the sense of isolation. Many adult survivors find self-help groups to be very supportive in the process of healing. They are given a better idea of how their behavior affects others while helping others makes them feel more competent. They are reassured by seeing others recover. The Community Resources feature at the end of this chapter lists national groups designed for survivors as well as perpetrators of child sexual abuse.

Behavioral: Psychological: Comfort Promotion

Simple Relaxation Therapy

Because adult survivors are often anxious, interventions to reduce anxiety are also necessary. Clients who learn progressive relaxation and controlled breathing are often able to avoid full-blown panic attacks. Teach the process, and talk clients through the stages of relaxation until they are able to reduce anxiety by themselves. When they are relaxed, instruct them to imagine a scene in which they feel safe and comfortable. Any time they need to, they can return to this safe scene where they are in total control. Daily practice facilitates the usefulness of these techniques.

Evaluation

Nurses in the acute care setting may not have the opportunity for long-term evaluation. Short-term evaluation focuses mainly on identifying child victims and adult survivors and referrals to appropriate community resources. Nurses in long-term or community settings have the opportunity to evaluate the effectiveness of the multidisciplinary treatment plan over an extended period.

To complete the nursing process, you evaluate clients' responses to nursing interventions based on the outcomes you selected. You determine the appropriate intervals for measurement and document the condition of clients according to each individual's status. Johnson, Maas, and Moorhead (2000) is the resource for identifying measurement scales and specific indicators for each outcome.

Abuse Recovery: Emotional

Victims identify intrapersonal and interpersonal strengths. They determine what aspects of life are under their control. They utilize assertive skills in interactions with others. Victims report a sense of empowerment. Survivors acknowledge that the responsibility for the abuse belongs with the perpetrator.

Coping

Clients differentiate effective from ineffective coping patterns. They use the process of guided self-dialog to think through situations before responding to them. Clients use techniques such as deep breathing, sensory counting, and "thought containers" to manage intrusive thoughts and flashbacks.

Family Coping

Dependent children who have been sexually abused remain free from harm and exhibit normal growth and development. All family members participate in family therapy. They communicate openly and directly with one another, avoiding secret keeping within the family system. Families demonstrate flexibility in roles and rules within the family.

Self-Esteem

Children and adult survivors identify their own strengths and abilities. They replace negative thoughts with positive ones. Clients state their own opinions, interests, and needs directly and clearly. They set limits on others' demands on them.

Social Support

Clients and families utilize group therapy and self-help support groups in managing their responses to sexual abuse. They verbalize increased trust in others, behave more assertively, and communicate directly.

Spiritual Well-Being

Individuals with adequate spiritual well-being express a sense of hope and of meaning and purpose in life.

CRITICAL THINKING

Ann is working in an emergency department in her community hospital. One of her jobs is to care for rape victims who may come into the emergency department and to provide community education on sexual violence. The job is a new one for Ann, though she has six years of emergency nursing experience. She is a little nervous about the new position, as she has never been required to assess a community problem, plan, and implement services for a community. Her supervisor has offered her support and guidance.

One of the first things that Ann does is to gather data on the number of rape victims who have been admitted to the emergency service in the past year and the circumstances around their rapes. She learns very quickly that the number has increased since the previous year. Ann is also aware that many rape victims do not report the crime, so the number she has is probably not an accurate number for the community.

Ann decides that she wants to provide a multiprong program that focuses on prevention as well as treatment. She will develop some educational programs for the emergency department staff so that they are better able to care for rape victims. Recognizing the importance of prevention, she will develop a program that could be offered to various groups in the community, such as school staff and faculty, students, and other community groups. After she gets this pulled together, she plans on beginning a crisis management group for rape victims. The latter intervention will be the most difficult for Ann, but she has had some psychiatric experience and led groups before. You have been assigned to work with Ann during your clinical rotation. As you listen to her plans, you are excited about participating.

1. Ann's program for students will focus on date rape and anticipatory guidance. How would you incorporate these topics into an educational program?

2. A major focus of the emergency department staff is assessment of the rape victim. This is a very difficult time for the rape victim. Ann asks you to think about what content is critical for her to include in an educational program on assessment for the emergency department staff. What would be the most therapeutic way for the staff to assess the client and meet the client's complex needs in the emergency department?

3. What impact does a rape have on the victim psychologically?

4. Ann has just helped with the assessment of a rape victim and is telling you about the client. She tells you that the client is in the impact phase. What are some of the possible characteristics of this phase?

5. During one of the group meetings that you are sitting in on, the members and Ann discuss recovery. After the meeting, you tell Ann that you are surprised by the self-confidence and empowerment that some of the women in the group exhibit compared to the recent rape victims. How can you explain these attitudes?

For an aditional Case Study, please refer to the Companion Web site for this book.

They participate in spiritual experiences such as meditation, prayer, worship, song, and/or spiritual reading. Clients express feelings of serenity and a connectedness with others.[*]

Abuse Recovery: Sexual

Child victims and adult survivors disclose the facts of and their feelings about the abusive situation. They process their expectations of protection in the therapeutic setting. Concomitant problems such as mood disorders, sleep disturbances, self-destructive anger, eating disorders, self-mutilation, and suicidal ideation, resolve. Clients verbalize a sense of empowerment and age-appropriate sexual behavior or improved sexual functioning.[*]

---

[*]These selected outcome indicators are from Johnson, M., Maas, M., & Moorhead, S. (2000). *Nursing outcomes classification (NOC)* (2nd ed.). St. Louis, MO: Mosby.

CHAPTER REVIEW

COMMUNITY RESOURCES

Links to these Web sites can be accessed on the Companion Web site for this book.

Children and Adult Survivors

Center for Constitutional Rights
606 Broadway, 7th Floor
New York, NY 10012
212-614-6464
www.crr-ny.org

Survivors of Incest Anonymous World Service Office
P.O. Box 190
Benson, MD 21018
410-893-3322
www.siawso.org

Incest Survivors
Resource Network International
P.O. Box 7375
Las Cruces, NM 88006-7375
505-521-4260
www.zianet.com/ISRNI

Mending the Sacred Hoop
Violence Against Indian Women
202 East Suoerior St.
Duluth, MN 55802
888-305-1650
www.msh-ta.org

National Center for Victims of Crime
2000 M St. NW, Suite 48
Washington, DC 20036

800-FYI-CALL
800-211-7996 (hearing impaired)
www.ncvc.org

Rape, Abuse, and Incest National Network (RAINN)
635-B Pennsylvania Ave., SF
Washington, DC 20003
800-656-4673
www.rainn.org

Rape Treatment Center
www.911rape.org

VOCAL (Victims of Clergy Abuse Linkup)
5315 N Clark St. #214
Chicago, IL 60640-2113
847-475-4622
www.Thelinkup.com

VOICES (Victims of Incest Can Emerge Survivors)
P.O. Box 148309
Chicago, IL 60614
800-786-4238
www.voices-action.org

Perpetrators

Safer Society Foundation
P.O. Box 340
Brandon, VT 05733-0310
802-247-5141
www.safersociety.org

BOOKS FOR CLIENTS AND FAMILIES

Ainscough, C., & Toon, K. (2000). *Surviving childhood sexual abuse workbook.* Tucson, AZ: Fisher Books.

Davis, L. (1990). *The courage to heal workbook: For women and men survivors of child sexual abuse.* New York: HarperPerennial.

Haines, S. (1999). *The survivors guide to sex: How to have an empowered sex life after child sexual abuse.* San Francisco, CA: Cleis Press.

Ledray, L. E. (1994). *Recovering from rape* (2nd ed.). New York: Henry Holt.

Raine, N. V. (1998). *After silence: Rape and my journey back.* New York: Crown.

U.S. Department of Education. (1999). *Protecting students from harassment and hate crimes.* www.ed.gov/pubs/Harassment.

Wasserman, B. (1998). *Feeling good again: A workbook for children who have been sexually abused.* Brandon, VT: The Safer Society Press.

KEY CONCEPTS

Introduction

■ Sexual violence is an act of violence, hatred and aggression with physical and/or psychological injury to the victims.

Sexual Harassment

■ Sexual harassment is unwanted and unwelcome sexual behavior that interferes with everyday life. It can be either quid pro quo or a hostile environment.

■ Sexual harassment can lead to severe stress in the victims.

Rape

■ Rape is a crime of violence perpetrated against innocent victims of all ages.

■ Ninety-three percent of rape victims are female and 90 percent of the perpetrators are male.

■ Date rape and marital rape are often unreported because victims may feel responsible or fear the disbelief of others.

■ Male victims, as a group, are more likely to have been beaten and are more reluctant to reveal the sexual component of their assaults.

Childhood Sexual Abuse

■ Sexual abuse is defined as inappropriate sexual behavior, instigated by a perpetrator, for purposes of the perpetrator's sexual pleasure or for economic gain through child prostitution or pornography.

■ Sexual abuse occurs in all ethnic, religious, economic, and cultural subgroups in the United States. The vast majority of victims know their abusers.

■ Fifty to sixty percent of juvenile offenders were sexually abused as children; the other 40 to 50 percent usually have conduct disorder.

■ There are five types of incestuous fathers: sexually preoccupied abusers, adolescent regressors, self-gratifiers, emotional dependents, and angry retaliators.

■ There are four major types of female offenders: teacher-lovers, experimenter-exploiters, predisposers, and women coerced by males.

Knowledge Base: Rape

■ Rape-trauma syndrome is characterized by symptoms of, or specific responses to, the experience of being raped.

■ Behavioral characteristics of rape victims include agitation, outward calmness, crying, nightmares, sleep problems, phobias, and relationship difficulties.

■ Affective characteristics of rape victims include shock, anxiety, fear, depression, and a sense of helplessness and vulnerability.

■ Cognitive characteristics of rape victims include depersonalization, dissociation, denial, difficulty making decisions, self-blame, obsessions, and concerns for future safety.

■ Families of rape victims experience many of the same thoughts and emotions as the victims themselves. They must be educated about rape and the immediate and potential long-term reactions of the victims.

■ Rape occurs cross-culturally and is one of the most underreported crimes worldwide.

■ In some countries, women are forced to marry their rapist or go into prostitution so they may survive, or they may even be put to death by their families to cleanse the family name.

■ Physiological characteristics include trauma and injuries, pregnancy, sexually transmitted infections (STIs), and difficulties with sexual functioning.

■ As a direct result of the rape, survivors may experience PTSD, substance abuse, depression, anxiety disorders, eating disorders, and suicidal behavior.

■ Most theorists agree that rape is a crime of violence generated by issues of power and anger. Theories relating to rape include revenge, dominance, eroticized assault, gang rituals, inadequate relationships, acceptance of violence within a culture, and sexist cultural values.

The Nursing Process

Assessment

■ Clients must be immediately assessed for any serious or critical injuries. Prior to any further assessment, clients must be informed of their rights including the right to have a rape crisis advocate, family, or friends with them during the assessment process.

■ The client must be given as much control as possible through every step of the assessment and treatment process.

■ A SANE is a registered nurse who has advanced education and clinical preparation in forensic examination of sexual assault victims.

Diagnosis

■ The nursing diagnosis is Rape-trauma syndrome, which may be further classified as compound or silent reaction.

Outcome Identification and Goals

■ The most common outcomes include abuse recovery: emotional; abuse recovery: sexual; coping; and fear control.

Nursing Interventions

■ It is important to support defense mechanisms until clients are able to cope with the reality of the abuse.

■ Many clients have a compulsive need to recount the abuse as a way to gradually desensitize the trauma.

■ Stress that survival is the most important outcome and the act of violence was not their fault.

■ Help clients identify immediate concerns and prioritize them.

■ Help them identify who to tell about the rape through the process of anticipatory guidance.

■ Discuss beliefs about postcoital contraception and abortion if appropriate.

■ Provide a written list of community resources.

■ Support groups provide an opportunity for victims to have their feelings validated as normal reactions to the assault, to speak openly, to network with other survivors, and to take charge of their own recovery.

■ Girls and women must be empowered to deal with sexual harassment.

Evaluation

■ To complete the nursing process, you evaluate clients' responses to nursing interventions based on the outcomes you selected.

■ Nursing interventions are evaluated as effective when clients return to their precrisis level, or achieve a higher level, of functioning.

Knowledge Base: Childhood Sexual Abuse

■ The effects of sex abuse are most severe when the incidents are frequent and occur over a long period of time, the activities are extensive, there is more than one perpetrator, the relationship to the perpetrator is close, and when sex abuse is combined with physical and emotional abuse.

■ Adult perpetrators initiate sexual behavior in a manipulative or coercive manner. They often feel weak, afraid, and inadequate. They use secrecy and silence to escape accountability. If confronted by others, they will often deny the abuse.

■ Child victims are at the mercy of adult perpetrators. Some become extremely affectionate, while others have problems with impulse control and aggression toward others. They may act out sexually with other children or adults.

■ Child victims are filled with fears of not being believed, being blamed, and/or being rejected by the family. Secrecy and guilt often keep them isolated from their peers.

■ In order to survive the trauma, child victims may use denial, minimization, or dissociation.

■ Adolescent victims may run away from home and may turn to prostitution for a variety of reasons.

■ Some adult survivors engage in self-mutilation for a number of reasons: to prove their existence, as a plea for nurturance, as a way to self-nurture, to stop dissociation, to punish the self, and/or to reduce emotional pain through physical pain.

■ Many adult survivors have sexual problems such as aversion, inhibition, and compulsive sexual behavior. Others suffer from confusion about their sexual orientation.

■ Many adult survivors continue to believe that they were to blame for the abuse. They suffer from low self-esteem, depression, anxiety, and rage.

■ Some adult survivors have total amnesia about the abuse, which is a response to the trauma.

■ Intimate relationships are often difficult for adult survivors. Survivors of childhood sexual abuse remain vulnerable and may be revictimized as adults.

■ Physiological characteristics of sexual abuse include STIs, trauma to the genitals, chronic vaginal or urinary tract infections, and pregnancy.

■ Having suffered sexual abuse in childhood is often a hidden feature of adult mental disorders. Adult psychiatric clients with a history of abuse have a bewildering combination of symptoms, including anger, depression, anxiety, insomnia, suspicion, eating disorders, substance abuse, and self-mutilation.

■ There is no single cause of childhood sexual abuse. Perpetrators may lack impulse control, or they may be rigid and overcontrolled. Many of them were sexually abused as children.

■ In incestuous families, hierarchical lines are crossed; for example, the father moves down to the child's level, or the child moves up to replace the mother. These families are often enmeshed, and the family system is either chaotic or rigid.

The Nursing Process

Assessment

- It is very difficult for both child victims and adult survivors to break the silence and respond to nursing assessment questions.

- When it is discovered that one child in a family is a victim of sexual abuse, all other children in the family must also be assessed for abuse.

- You must continually be aware of the client's comfort level with the physical environment during the assessment process.

Diagnosis

- Nursing diagnoses are formulated for the child victim, the family members, and the adult survivor. The most common are: Ineffective individual coping, powerlessness, post-trauma syndrome, social isolation, ineffective family coping, disabling, altered parenting, altered family process, spiritual distress, chronic low self-esteem, social isolation, and sexual dysfunction.

Outcome Identification and Goals

- The most common outcomes include abuse recovery, sexual, coping, family integrity, self-esteem, social support, and spiritual well-being.

Nursing Interventions

- The priority of care with child victims is to ensure the safety of the child.

- Nurses help families move toward a moderate position between the extremes of rigid and chaotic; they learn to increase their flexibility of roles or implement consistent rules.

- Child victims learn to manage their feelings through verbalization, play therapy, art therapy, and journal writing.

- Types of therapy useful with adult survivors include feminist-sensitive therapy, traumatic stress therapy, developmental therapy, and loss therapy.

- The most helpful approach with adult survivors is being ally, collaborator, and supporter as they struggle through the healing process.

- It is important to restore power and control to adult survivors.

- Spiritual recovery is part of the healing process.

- Both child victims and adult survivors must place responsibility for the abuse where it belongs—100 percent with the offender.

- Interventions are designed to help the adult survivor increase self-esteem and reduce anxiety.

- Adult survivors heal through the use of art therapy, music therapy, journal writing, group therapy, and self-help groups.

Evaluation

- To complete the nursing process, you evaluate clients' responses to nursing interventions based on the outcomes you selected.

EXPLORE *MediaLink*

- Interactive resources, including animations, for this chapter can be found on the Companion Web site at *http://www.prenhall.com/fontaine.* Click on Chapter 22 and select the activities for this chapter.

- For NCLEX review questions and an audio glossary, access the accompanying CD-ROM in this book.

REFERENCES

American Psychiatric Association. (2000). *Diagnostic and statistical manual of mental disorders* (4th ed., Text Revision). Washington, DC: Author.

Berman, H., McKenna, K., Arnold, C. T., Taylor, G., & MacQuarrie, B. (2000). Sexual harassment: Everyday violence in the lives of girls and women. *Advances in Nursing Science, 22*(4), 32–46.

Brown, S. M. (2000). Healthy sexuality and the treatment of sexually abusive youth. *SIECUS Report, 29*(1), 40–46.

Burton, J. E., & Rasmussen, L. A. (1998). *Treating children with sexually abusive behavior problems.* New York: Haworth Press.

Centers for Disease Control and Prevention. (2001). *www.cdc.gov/ncipc/factsheets/rape.htm.*

Chu, J. A., Frey, L. M., Ganzel, B. L., & Matthews, J. A. (1999). Memories of

REFERENCES *(continued)*

childhood abuse: Dissociation, amnesia, and corroboration. *American Journal of Psychiatry, 156*(5), 749–755.

Draucker, C. B., & Madsen, C. (1999). Women dwelling with violence. *IMAGE, 31*(4), 327–332.

Draucker, C. B., & Stern, P. N. (2001). Women's responses to sexual violence by male intimates. *Western Journal of Nursing, 22*(4), 385–397.

Fineran, S., & Bennett, L. (1999). Gender and power issues of peer sexual harassment among teenagers. *Journal of Interpersonal Violence, 14*(6), 626–641.

Glaister, J. A., & Able, E. (2001). Experiences of women healing from childhood sexual abuse. *Archives of Psychiatric Nursing, 15*(4), 188–194.

Green, A. H. (1999). Female sex offenders. In J. A. Shaw (Ed.), *Sexual aggression* (pp. 195–210). Washington, DC: American Psychiatric Press.

Hodge, S., & Canter, D. (1998). Victims and perpetrators of male sexual assault. *Journal of Interpersonal Violence, 13*(2), 222–239.

Holmes, R. M. (1991). *Sex crimes.* Newbury Park, CA: Sage.

Horan, D. L, Hill, L. D., & Schulkin, J. (2000). Childhood sexual abuse and preterm labor in adulthood: An endocrinological hypothesis. *Women's Health Issues, 10*(1), 27–33.

Johnson, M., Maas, M., & Moorhead, S. (2000). *Nursing outcomes classification (NOC)* (2nd ed.). St. Louis, MO: Mosby.

Johnson, T. C. (1999). Development of sexual behavior problems in childhood. In J. A. Shaw (Ed.), *Sexual aggression* (pp. 41–74). Washington, DC: American Psychiatric Press.

Johnson, T. C. (2000). Sexualized children and children who molest. *SIECUS Report, 29*(1), 35–37.

Koss, M. P., & Boeschen, L. (2000). Rape. In A. E. Kazdin (Ed.), *Encyclopedia of psychology,* Vol. 7 (pp. 1–6). Oxford, UK: Oxford University Press.

Lefley, H. P. (1999). Transcultural aspects of sexual victimization. In J. A. Shaw (Ed.), *Sexual aggression* (pp. 129–166). Washington, DC: American Psychiatric Press.

Lips, H. M. (2001). *Sex and gender* (4th ed.). Mountain View, CA: Mayfield.

Madison, J., & Minichiello, V. (2000). Recognizing and labeling sex-based and sexual harassment in the health care workplace. *Journal of Nursing Scholarship, 32*(4), 405–410.

McLeer, S. V., & Rose, M. (1999). Extrafamilial child sexual abuse. In J. A. Shaw (Ed.), *Sexual aggression* (pp. 210–242). Washington, DC: American Psychiatric Press.

Morrell, B., Mendel, M. P., & Fischer, L. (2001). Object relations disturbances in sexually abused males. *Journal of Interpersonal Violence, 16*(9), 851–864.

Murphy, W. D., & Page, I. J. (1999). Adolescent perpetrators of sexual abuse. In J. A. Shaw (Ed.), *Sexual aggression* (pp. 367–389). Washington, DC: American Psychiatric Press.

National Center for Victims of Crime. (2001). *www.ncvc.org.*

Paris, J. (1999). *Nature and nurture in psychiatry.* Washington, DC: American Psychiatric Press.

Raphel, S. M., & Berry, A. W. (1998). *Culturally competent assessment for family violence.* Washington, DC: American Nurses Association.

Ray, S. L. (2001). Male survivors' perspectives on incest/sexual abuse. *Perspectives in Psychiatric Care, 37*(2), 49–59.

Ryan, G. (2000). Perpetration prevention. *SIECUS Report, 29*(1), 28–34.

Schetky, K. H. (1999). Sexual victimization of children. In J. A. Shaw (Ed.), *Sexual aggression* (pp. 107–128). Washington, DC: American Psychiatric Press.

Shaw, J. A. (1999). Sexually aggressive behavior. In J. A. Shaw (Ed.), *Sexual aggression* (pp. 3–40). Washington, DC: American Psychiatric Press.

Sholevar, G. P., & Schwoeri, L. D. (1999). Sexual aggression within the family. In J. A. Shaw (Ed.), *Sexual aggression* (pp. 75–105). Washington, DC: American Psychiatric Press.

Smith, M. E., & Kelly, L. M. (2001). The journey of recovery after a rape experience. *Issues in Mental Health Nursing, 22,* 337–352.

Symes, L. (2000). Arriving at readiness to recover emotionally after sexual assault. *Archives of Psychiatric Nursing, 14*(1), 30–38.

Turpin, J. (1999). Women and war. In L. Kurtz (Ed.), *Encyclopedia of violence, peace & conflict,* Vol. 3 (pp. 801–811). San Diego: Academic Press.

U.S. Department of Justice. (2001). Sexual assault nurse examiner (SANE) programs: Improving the community response to sexual assault victims. *www.ojp.usdoj.gov/ovc/pub lications/bulletins/sane_4_2001/welcome. html.*

CHAPTER 23

Community Violence

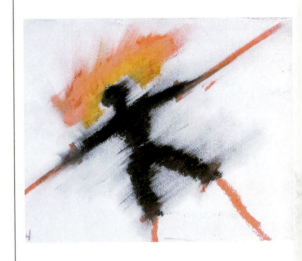

OBJECTIVES

After reading this chapter, you will be able to:

- DISCUSS the prevalence of violence in the United States.

- DESCRIBE types of predatory violence.

- DIFFERENTIATE between the four types of personal-cause homicides.

- DESCRIBE violence in the workplace, schools, and on the street.

- DISCUSS the interaction of neurobiological, personality, and societal factors that correlate with community violence.

- APPLY the nursing process to potential perpetrators of community violence.

MediaLink

CD-ROM
- *Audio Glossary*
- *NCLEX Review*

Companion Web site www.prenhall.com/fontaine
- *Critical Thinking*
- *More NCLEX Review*
- *Case Study*
- *Care Map Activity*
- *Links to Resources*

N ights come
Dreams advance
Terror strikes
Then loneliness

Emptiness consumes me
Hopelessness surrounds me
Despair drowns me

I'm lost in a hollow wheel
With no light showing me the way

—Kate, Age 19 (drawing)
—Anna, Age 19 (poetry)

The extreme acts of violence on September 11, 2001, in New York, Virginia, and Pennsylvania, and the acts of **bioterrorism** that followed, increased the awareness of international terrorism for people throughout the world. Bioterrorism can be described as "the use, or threatened use, of biological agents to promote or spread fear or intimidation upon an individual, a specific group, or the population as a whole for religious, political, ideological, financial or personal purposes" (Arizona Department of Health Services, 2001). These incidents have dramatically changed the way Americans view the security of their world as the illusion of invulnerability was lost. In addition to mourning the loss of thousands of innocent victims,

people must manage their shock, fear, and despair. The images will haunt all of us to some degree or another. They also give us a new perspective as we come together and bond over the disaster. **Terrorism** has been defined as the "deliberate creation and exploitation of fear through violence of the threat of violence in the pursuit of political change" (Hoffman, 1998, p. 43). Terrorism is very different from the types of community violence presented in this chapter. The purpose, the dynamics, and the aftereffects of terrorism are beyond the scope of this chapter.

We, in the United States, live in a violent culture. It is a culture that promotes, supports, and even encourages and romanticizes violence. Violence is a common theme in computer games, movies, television dramas, and the lyrics and visual images of rock music videos. The mass media is filled with reports of Americans killing one another. Recent events, such as youths who have committed violent murders at their schools, have drawn unprecedented attention to the problem of violent preteens and adolescents. Handgun ownership is at an all-time high while confidence in protection from law enforcement is at an all-time low. Acts of violence remind us that no community can be complacent in its efforts to make neighborhoods, workplaces, and schools safer than they are at the current time.

According to the FBI, one violent crime occurs every 18 seconds in the United States. Every day, 15 Americans between the ages of 15 and 24 commit suicide and 23 are murdered. Five out of six people living in the United States will be victims of a violent crime at least one time in their lives. A child dies every two hours from a gunshot wound and many more are seriously wounded. Armed assailants are becoming significantly younger with almost half between the ages of 11 and 20. Every day, 316 children are arrested for violent crimes. A survey of 500 elementary school children reported that 40 percent had witnessed a shooting and 34 percent had observed a stabbing. Another survey reported that one third of a sample of school age children in Chicago reported witnessing a homicide and two thirds a serious assault. In New Orleans, 91 percent of 9- to 12-year-olds reported witnessing at least one violent incident. In Washington, D.C., 61 percent of a sample of first- and second-grade children and 72 percent of fifth- and sixth-grade children reported witnessing violence in their community. It is only in the last few years that researchers have looked at the effects of community violence on children (Hoffman & Summers, 2001; Levi, 1999; Shahinfar, Fox, & Leavitt, 2000; Veenema, 2001).

Serious violent delinquency is at its peak during adolescence and early adulthood. Almost half of the victims of violent crime are between 12 and 25 years of age, and one third are 12 to 19 years old. Homicide is the second leading cause of death for all teens and young adults. In the United States, more people are in state and federal prisons than in any other country in the world. For every 100,000 persons, 344 are jailed, giving the United States the highest ratio of prisoners in the Western world (Arseneault et al., 2000; Bloom & Reichert, 1998).

Young males are the chief perpetrators and are also the chief victims of violent acts. Males are twice as likely as females to be victimized by other males. Males also hurt themselves at a much higher rate, with a suicide rate four times that of teen girls. This disproportionate number continues through adulthood so that by age 85, men have a 1,350 percent greater suicide rate than their female peers (Bloom & Reichert, 1998; Gustavsson & MacEachron, 1998; Hoffman & Summers, 2001). See Chapter 20 for information about suicide.

Violent adults were often violent children, and violent children often learn about violence at home. The U.S. Advisory Board on Child Abuse and Neglect (1992, p. 10) stated: "Adult violence against children leads to childhood terror, childhood terror leads to teenage anger, and teenage anger too often leads to adult rage, both destructive toward others and self-destructive. Terror, anger, and rage—these are not the ingredients of safe streets, strong families, and caring communities."

This chapter focuses primarily on perpetrators of violence who are children and adolescents since these are the majority in terms of numbers. Youth also reflect the social, economic, moral, and ethical problems in the larger society. The hope is that prevention strategies directed toward youth will decrease the level of violence throughout the United States.

TYPES OF VIOLENCE

AFFECTIVE VIOLENCE

Affective violence is the verbal expression of intense anger and emotions. It is bullying, ugly taunts, disre-spect, alienation, scapegoating, and physical threats that many people experience every day. Injury of the target is the primary goal. Typically, the behavior is impulsive and in response to interpersonal stress and frequently under the influence of alcohol and drugs (Shea, 1998).

PREDATORY VIOLENCE

Predatory violence includes hate crimes that are motivated by bias and hatred of minority groups. People, who typically do nothing to provoke the attack, are harassed, tortured, and even killed just because they are different. Hate crimes occur in rural, suburban, and urban communities alike, targeting racial or ethnic minorities, religious minorities, and gay, lesbian, bisexual, or transgendered (GLBT) people. Following the terrorists attacks of September 11, 2001, there were scattered incidents of violence against people presumed to be from Muslim countries. Apart from this situation, African Americans are the most frequent targets, GLBT individuals the next most frequent, followed by Euro-Americans and Jews. Euro-Americans commit 63 percent and African Americans commit 19 percent of the reported hate crimes. A large number—60 percent—of hate crime perpetrators are youthful thrill-seekers who commit the crime for the thrill associated with the victimization. A part of this reflects the desire to live up to friends' expectations and to prove toughness and heterosexuality to friends. Some perpetrators are driven by racial or religious ideology or ethnic bigotry. They reflect the negative cultural attitudes and justify their actions as righteous responses (Franklin, 2000; Smith, 1999).

Perpetrators of hate crimes often plan the acts out beforehand, frequently get pleasure from the violent act itself, and feel little, if any, remorse. Hate crimes may end in murder, with two recent notable examples: The torture and crucifixion-style killing of Matthew Shepard, a gay college student in Wyoming; and the dragging death of James Byrd Jr., an African American adult male, in Texas.

Many teens live in a violent world. Some are victims of this "typical" violence and are also at an increased risk for violence unique to their minority status. Ideally, the school setting could offer a temporary haven where all students feel safe. The reality, however, is that hate crimes often occur during school hours. For example, 90 percent of gay youth report verbal abuse and as many as half are physically harassed. Gay adults do not fare much better, with 41 percent reporting being the target of verbal harassment, threats, vandalism of property, and physical assaults as the result of their sexual or gender orientation. Sexual orientation harassment is not legally equivalent to sexual harassment based on gender (see Chapter 22). Because sexual orientation and gender identity are not protected by federal and most state regulations, it is legal to discriminate against these individuals (Gustavsson & MacEachron, 1998; Kuehnle & Sullivan, 2001; Sloan, King, & Sheppard, 1998).

Another form of predatory violence involves the phenomenon of **stalking**, which can be viewed on a continuum from nondelusional to delusional. In nondelusional stalking, there is a relationship between the victim and the perpetrator, which tends to be or have been one of close interpersonal involvement. (See Chapter 21 for information on stalking and domestic violence.) At the delusional end of the continuum, the relationship exists only in the mind of perpetrators who may have a delusion that a famous person is in love with them (erotomanic delusion). Stalkers may also be motivated by religious delusions or hallucinations directing them to target a particular person. There is often a preoccupation with the victim that becomes consuming and ultimately could lead to the victim's death.

In between these two extremes of stalking is a mixture of relationships. The victim and perpetrator may have dated only one or two times; the victim may have only smiled or said hello in passing; or they may be in some way socially or vocationally acquainted. In some instances, the stalker may make obscene or harassing phone calls or send letters professing love or knowledge of the victim's movements. The behavior may eventually move to threats and menacing comments. At some point, stalkers may make their identity known through appearing at the victim's work or residence.

Cyberstalking refers to the use of the Internet, e-mail, or other electronic communications to stalk another person. It is a serious problem that is likely to become more widespread. Similar to other forms of stalking, cyberstalkers wish to establish control over the victim. In many cases, there was a prior relationship between perpetrator and victim, but there are also a number of situations of cyberstalking by strangers. Electronic harassment of adults is not a federal crime and is not a crime in most states. Thus, there are no reliable statistics on how many people have been victimized online (Reno, 1999).

There are a small number of psychiatric inpatients who stalk, threaten, or harass hospital staff after discharge. Those who engage in this type of predatory violence typically limit their behavior to oral or written threats or unwanted telephone calls. The problem behavior is usually limited to the period shortly after discharge with a low risk of physical harm (Sandberg, McNiel, & Binder, 1998).

TYPES OF HOMICIDE

Burgess and Dowdell (1999) have identified four types of *personal-cause homicide*: nonspecific homicide, revenge homicide, patricide/matricide homicide, and authority killing. Personal-cause homicides are not driven by material gain or sexual intention, unlike other types of homicide motivated by a need for money, political concerns, organized crime or gangs, or violence for pleasure.

In **nonspecific homicide**, only the perpetrator, who seems to want as many victims as possible, knows the motive. The crime often becomes a massacre with little regard for the value of life. The crime, although planned, is often unorganized, with no arrangements for escaping the police.

On December 1, 1997, in West Paducah, Kentucky, Michael Carneal, age 14, entered his high school and opened fire on a group of students at a prayer meeting, killing three and wounding five. When another teen grabbed him to stop him, he said, "Kill me please. I can't believe I did that."

On February 29, 2000, in Mount Morris Township, Michigan, a 6-year-old boy went to school, told first-grader Kayla Rolland that he didn't like her, and then shot her with a handgun he had brought from home. The boy was reportedly made to stay after school nearly every day for violent behavior.

Perpetrators of **revenge homicide** retaliate for real or imagined offenses brought on by the victim.

Depending on the event that triggered the act of revenge, there may be multiple victims. Perpetrators of revenge homicide are often the victims of bullying, teasing, humiliation, and physical assault. Killing those who torment them is an act of revenge. The murder is prearranged and organized, including plans for escaping the scene of the crime. A recent stressful event or the accumulation of chronic stress often motivates these individuals.

On March 24, 1998, in Jonesboro, Arkansas, Andrew Golden, age 11, and Mitchell Johnson, age 13, sat on a hill 100 yards away from the school. As the children and teachers left the building in response to a false fire alarm, they fired 22 rounds of ammunition, killing five and wounding 15 people.

On March 5, 2001, in Santee, California, Charles Andrew Williams, 15, opened fire from a bathroom at the high school, killing two and wounding 13. Other students said he was picked on all the time because he was "scrawny." Peers called him freak, dork, and nerd.

Patricide/matricide homicide may be in response to many years of physical and sexual abuse, or from a defiance of rules, a dare from a peer group, or other causes not related to parental behavior. Typically, children and adolescents who kill parents flee the scene only to be captured fairly quickly. Of all youth who commit murder each year in the United States, only 8 percent murder one or both parents. Juveniles who have killed a parent are typically Euro-American, middle-class boys who have had little contact with law enforcement. Some are loners who are anxious for acceptance by peers and adults. Others kill as the result of a family-related argument. Less often, parents are killed for money, possessions, or freedom. Children who kill their parents often do so in a sudden, uncontrollable rage and do so in a mindless brutal fashion (Kelleher, 1998).

In February 1996, Joshua Jenkins, age 15, killed his mother, father, both grandparents, and his 10-year-old sister. Although he had no prior history of violence, he had a long history of bizarre and unpredictable behavior.

In October 1997, Luke Woodham, age 16, stabbed his mother to death and then went to his high school with a rifle hidden beneath his trench coat. He opened fire, killing his former girlfriend and another student and injured seven. He tried to escape in his mother's car but crashed it near the scene of his crimes. His explanation to the arresting police was, "I am not insane. I am angry."

On May 21, 1998, in Springfield, Oregon, Kipland Kinkel, age 15, shot his parents to death at home. He then went to the local high school and opened fire, killing two students and wounding 20 others. He asked the police officer who led him away to shoot him.

Those who commit an **authority killing** frequently do so in response to real or imagined offenses. The targets may be individuals or a building or structure that symbolizes the authority. The killer may desire to commit suicide or die at the hands of police to attain martyrdom for the murders.

On May 26, 2000, Nathaniel Brazill, 13, was sent home for throwing water balloons. He returned with a handgun, went into an English class, and shot and killed his teacher, Barry Grunow.

SETTINGS OF COMMUNITY VIOLENCE

Violence occurs in all the usual places we turn to for security—home, workplace, school, and neighborhood. (Family violence is discussed in Chapter 21.)

WORKPLACE VIOLENCE

Workplace violence has become a major social and economic problem, with thousands of people a year being victims of violent crime on the job. About 40 percent of the victims of nonfatal violence in the workplace report that they know the offender. Workplace homicide is one of the fastest-growing types of homicide with 20 workplace deaths each week in the United States. Overall, homicide is the second leading cause of fatal occupational injuries (Crime Characteristics, 2001).

Seventy-five percent of these homicides are committed by strangers or intruders and are related to robbery and 80 percent of the victims die from gunshot wounds. Those at highest risk are males who are self-employed or those working in law enforcement, grocery stores, restaurants, gas stations, taxis, and government service (Denenberg & Braverman, 1999).

Workplace homicides not related to robbery are either acts of domestic violence or stalking, acts by former or current disgruntled employees, or acts by customers or clients. In those situations in which the perpetrator was someone the victim knew, 97 percent died from gunshot injuries (Bloom & Reichert, 1998).

In November 1999, Byron Uyesugi opened fire at a Xerox office in Honolulu. A repairman for the company, Uyesugi killed seven co-workers.

In December 2000, Michael McCermott, who was upset about an IRS request to garnish his wages to pay back taxes, came to work as usual and then opened fire, killing seven co-workers.

Violence in hospitals has grown along with violence in society, In one study of 103 hospitals in California, 58 percent of the staff had suffered injuries from visitors or patients, usually with a gun or a knife. Half of these events occurred in the emergency department, and the major trigger was a prolonged wait. Generally, the perpetrator was under the influence of alcohol or drugs or was mentally ill. A survey conducted by the Emergency Nurses Association found that 97 percent of staff is exposed to verbal abuse twice a month, 87 percent exposed to assault without weapons one to five times a year, and 24 percent said they were exposed to physical violence with weapons one to five times a year. According to the 1993 American Psychiatric Association's Task Force on Clinician Safety, approximately 40 percent of psychiatrists, and an even higher percentage of psychiatric–mental health nurses, have been assaulted by patients. The most common setting for these situations is inpatient units and emergency

rooms, where the most acutely ill persons are generally treated (Bloom & Reichert, 1998; Sandberg, McNiel, & Binder, 1998).

SCHOOL VIOLENCE

Though the nation's schools actually are safer than ever, the legacy of the killings at schools across the country— from Oregon to Colorado to Virginia, from Arkansas to Pennsylvania, from Mississippi to Kentucky—looms large in the minds of Americans. In spite of the fact that 100,000 guns are brought to school every year, fewer than 1 percent of all violent deaths of children occur in or around school property. Every year, 160,000 students skip classes because they fear physical harm, and 40 children are hurt or killed. Teachers are also victims of **school violence**, with 6,250 threatened with bodily harm and 260 physically assaulted yearly (Bloom & Reichert, 1998).

A nonscientific, volunteer survey of 129,593 students in grades 6 through 12 found that 25 percent of the students reported that they do not feel safe from violence in school, 30 percent said they have been threatened physically at school, 25 percent said they have been hit, and 20 percent said they have been robbed at school. Almost half of the respondents said there is a gun in their home, and of those, more than half said they have access to it (Rhule, 2000). Another study of suburban high school students found that 20 percent believed it was okay to shoot someone who has stolen something from you and 8 percent believed it was okay to shoot a person who has done something to offend or insult you. Those attitudes reflect the continuing potential for violence in our schools. The *Gun Free Schools Act of 1994* requires schools to expel for at least one year any student who brings a firearm to school as well as referring the student to the criminal justice or juvenile justice system (Bloom & Reichert, 1998).

STREET VIOLENCE

Teens are much more likely than adults to be victims of **street violence**. No longer can they expect to be safe at school or in their neighborhoods. Sixty-three percent of thefts and 50 percent of all violent crimes are against 12- to 19-year-olds. Thirty-six percent of Euro-American teens and 54 percent of African American teens worry about being a victim of a crime much or some of the time (Moore & Cook, 1999).

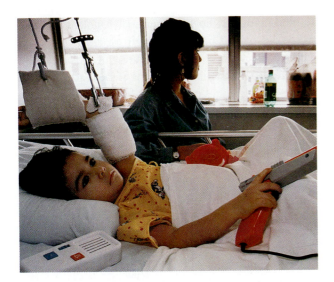

PHOTO 23.1 ■ Societal influences on children's behavior are pervasive. This 3-year-old boy suffered a gunshot wound during a drive-by shooting. Still, the boy plays with a toy pistol while recuperating in his hospital bed.

SOURCE: Rick Hunter/Corbis/Sygma.

Violent **gangs** now operate in 94 percent of all medium- and large-sized cities and small towns are not exempt from this situation. It is estimated that there are 28,700 gangs with 780,000 members active in the United States. Most or all gang members are involved in drug sales and in a variety of serious and violent crimes. Many acts of violence are the result of bad drug deals, infringement on drug territory, or in response to an event perceived as disrespect by a rival gang member—referred to in gang slang as "dis." In the past, fists may have established the determination of the gang leader. Now it is settled by flying lead (Moore & Cook, 1999). Innocent bystanders are often harmed or killed by violent gang members by being victims of drive-by shootings, cross-fire gang shooting, and murder as part of gang initiation.

KNOWLEDGE BASE

As a nurse, you must be involved in the prevention, detection, and treatment of community violence. Development of the knowledge base and the ability to identify factors that contribute to community violence will help you arrive at early detection and an accurate diagnosis of the problem.

BEHAVIORAL CHARACTERISTICS

Corporal punishment, the hitting or spanking of children, gives the message that violence is acceptable. Children are spanked when parents are usually very angry and thus children learn that extreme anger justifies abuse. Other underlying messages are: If you are small and weak, you deserve to be hit; people who love you hit you; and violence is appropriate if the end result is good. Being hit as a child increases the probability that aggression will be used to handle conflicts in the child's life. The inherent message is that authority figures should be feared, not trusted and respected. The message of violence is continued in some school systems. In those states where teachers are allowed to hit children, there is a significantly higher rate of student violence (Bloom & Reichert, 1998; Koch, 2000).

Several studies have shown that children who witness violence display more internalizing (withdrawn, anxious, depressed) behavior while those who are victims display more externalizing (aggressive, disruptive) behavior. Those children who witness community violence watch from the sidelines, recognizing their own inability to change the situation. This sense of helplessness contributes to internalizing behavior. On the other hand, children who are victimized by community violence are more likely to learn aggressive, externalizing behavior as a means of self-protection or a way of relating to others (Shahinfar, Fox, & Leavitt, 2000).

At one end of the continuum of violent behavior are the numerous citizen militias and other assorted individuals who believe that violence targeted against representative members of groups is a legitimate protest. The most dramatic example of this type of community violence in the United States is the Oklahoma City bombing of the federal building in 1995.

AFFECTIVE CHARACTERISTICS

Violent people have often been denied normal emotional experiences as they were growing up. Hearing messages such as "Big boys don't cry" and "The past is the past, just let it be" denies children the opportunity to experience emotional support from their caregivers. Some children, especially boys, are expected not to show any emotion, talk about feelings, and least of all cry. What usually stops most of us from striking out is empathy, imagining the hurt that the victim would feel. The process of denying one's own feelings makes it impossible for some individuals to learn how to relate to others with empathy. The pressure to bottle up emotions leads some people to violence against the self—substance abuse and suicide—and to violence against others—assault and homicide (Smith & Thomas, 2000).

When people have little bonding with others and live an isolated life, they must rely on their own internal psychological and social world. In the case of violent people, that internal world is filled with bitterness, resentment, and rage. There is no supportive network to correct or modify the misperceptions of people in their environment. This situation can precipitate violent acting out (Burgess & Dowdell, 1999).

COGNITIVE CHARACTERISTICS

Thinking drives behavior, and violent individuals think of violent solutions to perceived offenses against them. They may live in an inner fantasy world with frequent thoughts of anger, revenge, and justifiable rage. They may rationalize their behavior or project their anger by saying, in essence, "You were disrespectful to me; that is why I had to blow your head off." Some perpetrators believe that if they commit violent acts they will become famous. The Columbine killers—in videos found after their deaths—basked in the attention they knew would come their way, even discussing which movie director should be entrusted to tell their story, Steven Spielberg or Quentin Tarantino (Burgess & Dowdell, 1999).

SOCIAL CHARACTERISTICS

Violence in the United States is gender related. Males inflict violence on other males both overtly and covertly. Males are more likely to be involved in wars, physical battery, and economic and cultural subjugation of minority, gay, and lower-class men. "Might makes right" in playgrounds, athletic fields, homes, and boardrooms. Boys are expected and permitted to push, pull, threaten, bully, and hurt each other. Many researchers who study violence believe that only hurt people hurt others. In other words, there is some systematic "hurting" of boys that underlies and contributes to the prevalence of violent acting out by males.

The myth that boys are "naturally" violent is a very dangerous one to believe. Though we know that boys are most likely to be the perpetrators of violent crime, they are also the frightened victims of those acts. It is not biology that makes boys violent. Rather, it is the environment in which we raise them. Boys are bombarded daily with professional wrestling, movie heroes who solve their problems with guns, and an ever-growing stream of hard-core violent video games. And then we call this "healthy" adult masculinity. Boys say they are forced to lead a double life: strong and brave on the outside, yet full of worries and agitation on the inside (Pollack, 2000).

More people kill each other with guns than by all other methods combined. An important social issue is the alarming increase in the number of guns purchased in the United States. The dramatic increase in homicides and suicides is almost solely due to this easy access to guns. The presence of guns in violent interactions increases the likelihood that one or more participants will be killed. As firearms with greater firing powers are increasingly available, the lethality has also increased.

CULTURE-SPECIFIC CHARACTERISTICS

The rate of firearm deaths among children 14 years and younger is nearly 12 times higher in the United States than in 25 other industrialized countries combined. Teens in the United States are at least four times as likely to be murdered then their counterparts in these same countries. The United States has strong laws against violence, but they are inconsistently applied and compete with pervasive pro-violence messages (Bloom & Reichert, 1998).

The leading cause of death for persons in the United States varies according to age and ethnic group. At highest risk are African American males and at lowest risk are Euro-American females and males (see Table 23.1 ■). These data support the earlier discussion regarding the impact of racism and poverty on violent behavior.

Cross-culturally, males are more physically aggressive than are females. They assault more frequently and severely and commit more homicides. In the United States, Spain, and Russia, teen crime associated with gangs is a significant problem. Unemployment of youth is a contributing factor of violence in Jamaica, St. Lucia, and South Africa. An increase in juvenile

TABLE 23.1

Homicide as Leading Cause of Death

Group	Age				
	10–14	*15–24*	*25–34*	*35–44*	*45–54*
Black males	2	1	1	5	8
Black females	2	2	4	6	11
Hispanic males	2	2	2	5	8
Hispanic females	4	2	4	5	10
White males	4	3	3	7	11
White females	6	4	5	7	11
American Indian males	3	3	3	6	9
American Indian females	2	3	5	6	8
Asian males	3	2	4	5	7
Asian females	4	4	4	6	7

SOURCE: Centers for Disease Control and Prevention. (2000). Leading Causes of Death Reports. *www.cdc.gov.*

crime is associated with rapid political change and modernization in South Africa, Russia, Slovenia, and Jamaica (Hoffman & Summers, 2001).

Violence against the self is not common in Latin American countries compared with other countries. Latin Americans do not kill themselves, but they do kill each other. The rate of homicide, however, is much higher than in North America or Europe. Among men in Guatemala, homicide is the most frequent cause of death. Homicide is the second leading cause of death in Ecuador, Mexico, Brazil, El Salvador, Venezuela, Paraguay, Panama, and other countries. The epidemic of violence is traced to guerrilla warfare, drug lords, poverty, inequalities, and social unrest. Violence is now the number one health priority in Latin America (Arboleda-Florez & Weisstub, 2000).

CONCOMITANT DISORDERS

It is very common for youth with conduct problems to also display symptoms of attention deficit/hyperactivity disorder (ADHD), the most commonly diagnosed behavioral disorder of children. (See Chapter 17 for more information on ADHD and conduct disorder.)

This co-occurrence is often associated with an early onset of aggression and impairment in personal, interpersonal, and family functioning.

Exposure to community violence, through witnessing violence or being victimized, is significantly related to posttraumatic stress disorder (PTSD). (See Chapter 11 for more information on PTSD.) Many studies indicate that one third of children and teens who are exposed to community violence develop PTSD. Traumatic experiences, such as violence in the community, challenge people's basic belief that the world is safe, predictable, and controllable. When these basic assumptions are called into question, feelings of helplessness and hopelessness are likely to emerge (Duckworth, Hale, Clair, & Adams, 2000; Overstreet & Braun, 2000).

CAUSATIVE THEORIES

Community violence is easy to describe but difficult to explain. There is no single cause of this type of violence. It results from an interaction of neurobiological, personality, and societal factors that have an impact on individuals and groups of people.

Some people believe that violence within the community is related to a *lack of something* such as discipline, religion, mothers at home, involved fathers, poverty, fair play, or rights of all sorts. Others believe that violence is related to an *excess of something* such as welfare, permissiveness, attention, material goods, or rights of all sorts. Only where there is the presence of a number of risk factors does violent behavior occur.

Neurobiological Theory

Neurobiological theorists propose that genes and neurotransmitters may contribute to causing violent behavior. Although a genetic predisposition may make certain behaviors more likely, it does not make them inevitable. Serotonin (5-HT) exerts inhibitory control over aggression and is inversely correlated with the level of aggression. Low levels of 5-HT are implicated in a lack of control, loss of temper, and explosive rage. The relationship of dopamine (DA) and norepinephrine (NE) to aggression is less clear. DA appears to be inversely correlated with aggression. NE may be correlated with affective aggression through its sensitizing effects, which prepare a person to respond to threatening environmental stimuli (Berkowitz, 1999; LeMarquand, Benkelfut, & Pihl, 1999).

The association between hormones and violence is more subtle and complex than formerly thought. Hormones are *consequences* as well as *causes* of behavior. In other words, hormones do not switch behaviors on or off. At times, hormones may change the probability that certain behaviors that can be labeled "aggression" will occur in particular situations by people with history of psychosocial risk factors. Low cortisol has been associated with greater antisocial behavior. The male brain is organized by testosterone in such a way that males are more apt to react aggressively to annoyances and offenses. Much of the testosterone effects on aggression may involve 5-HT. It is also believed that mood itself may alter levels of testosterone. In sporting events, testosterone levels rise in the victors and fall in the losers. This may result from the individual's experience of dominance (Berkowitz, 1999; LeMarquand et al., 1999).

Studies have shown that a higher number of minor physical anomalies of the mouth, ears, eyes, head, hands, and feet are found in groups of individuals with chronic violent antisocial behavior. Minor physical anomalies are considered indicators of disruption in fetal development. It is thought that the central nervous system may also be affected since it develops at the same time as the affected organs. Further research will be needed to determine if a person is at higher risk for the development of violent delinquency as a result of atypical brain development (Arseneault, Tremblay, Boulerice, Sequin, & Saucier, 2000).

Social Learning Theory

Social learning theory proposes that violence is a learned behavior and people are conditioned to respond aggressively and violently. Children learn about violence from observation, from being victims, and from behaving violently themselves. If the use of violence is rewarded by a gain in power, the behavior is reinforced. If there is immediate negative reinforcement from individuals and institutions within the community, a decrease in violent behavior will result.

Aggression, as a way of interacting with others and solving problems, is learned very early in life and usually is learned very well. The payoff in the experience of power and control often is high, so that despite occasional or even more frequent punishment, it is difficult to unlearn; and so the behavior persists. This is probably why most interventions and rehabilitation programs that target adolescents and young adults have been unsuccessful.

Contextual Sensitivity Hypothesis

The **contextual sensitivity hypothesis** is based on the belief that human behavior is highly sensitive to social contexts. Certain social contexts are considered to be toxic as they contribute to violent perpetration and victimization. This toxicity can be understood from the perspective of socioeconomic factors, parent/family factors, and peer influences.

Socioeconomic Factors Community violence is associated with *economic inequality*. Extremes of poverty and racism contribute to the trauma of children and become breeding grounds for violence as evidenced by a higher incidence of violence in poor communities. In the United States, 1 in 10 adults and 1 in 5 children live in poverty. Poverty is not an equal-opportunity condition: African American and Latino children as well as children from mother-only families are disproportionately poor. Families who are struggling to just put food on the table may have minimal time to supervise the children, who are then more likely to act out.

Poverty also affects the child's chance for school success. Poor academic performance, expulsion, and dropout rates are common indicators of unsuccessful youth functioning. The more children and adolescents are turned off by and turned away from the school system, the more they tend to associate with and seek approval from antisocial peers. Those who are subject to racism experience humiliation, powerlessness, and rage and may act out in retaliatory violence. Racism and poverty create chaotic environments, making children vulnerable to violence as victims, witnesses, and perpetrators (Duckworth et al., 2000; Shelton, 2000).

Parent and Family Factors Research has demonstrated that youths who engage in high levels of **antisocial behavior** are much more likely than other youths to have a biological parent who also engages in antisocial behavior. This association is thought to reflect both the genetic transmission of predisposing temperament, modeling of aggression, and lack of control over expression of negative emotions. It is also believed that ineffective and inconsistent discipline and poor supervision contributes to antisocial behavior in children (Kelleher, 1998).

Research examining the mental health outcomes of child abuse and neglect has demonstrated that childhood victimization places children at increased risk for violent criminal behavior. Child abuse and neglect often occur in chronically dysfunctional families, and it may be difficult to disentangle the effect of abuse and neglect from the impact of other stressors. Children living in abusive and neglectful families may also experience parental separations, poor physical and emotional health of their caretakers, and the need to cope with financial and social problems (Bloom & Reichert, 1998; Kelleher, 1998).

Peer Influences All children tend to make friends with peers who are similar to themselves. This becomes socially significant when *antisocial children form groups* and reinforce one another's antisocial behavior. By adolescence, violence can be the membership card for entry into some adolescent peer groups. Most studies that compare the relative effects of parental supervision and peer deviance find that peer deviance is a stronger predic-tor of delinquency than the family (Hoffman & Summers, 2001)

NURSING PROCESS

The focus in this section is on potential perpetrators of community violence. This section suggests steps you can take to prevent violence and other troubling behaviors and to intervene and get help for troubled individuals. In the words of Carol Easley Allen, PhD, RN (2000, p. 2), we must all "advocate for a peaceful society, remove sources that teach violence to children, impose strict controls on firearms, provide resources to support family economic stability, . . . and ensure access to care for victims of violence."

Assessment

Given the incidence of community violence, it is logical to assume that you will encounter potential perpetrators in a variety of clinical settings. Violence can by inflicted by very different types of people in many different types of settings. There are clues, however, that you need to recognize that would indicate the possibility of a violent outburst. See Box 23.1 for risk factors

for violent behavior. Box 23.2 describes work-related behavior that is cause for concern regarding workplace violence.

BOX 23.1

Risk Factors for Violent Behavior

- Past history of aggressive and violent behavior
- Serious threats of violence
- Psychosis
- Romantic obsessions or erotomanic delusions
- Chemical dependency
- Depression and suicidality
- Pathological blaming, feelings of persecution
- Impaired neurological functioning
- Personality disorder
- Interest in firearms, bombs
- Affiliation with gangs

Cues for Workplace Violence

- Attendance problems
- Increased demands for supervisor's time
- Decreased productivity
- Inconsistent work patterns
- Poor on-the-job relationships
- Blames others for life problems
- Unusual or changed behavior
- Preoccupation with weapons
- Substance abuse on the job
- Continual excuses or blaming others

The Focused Nursing Assessment feature is designed for assessing children and adolescents. Early warning signs are just that—indicators that a child may need help. We must assess the situation and get help for the child before problems escalate. It is important, however, to avoid inappropriately labeling or stigmatizing because individuals appear to fit a specific profile. Early warning signs should not be used as a rationale to exclude, isolate, or punish a child. It is important to be aware of false cues—including race, socioeconomic status, cognitive or academic ability, or physical appearance. Children who are at risk for violence typically exhibit multiple warning signs, repeatedly, and with increasing intensity over time. Thus, it is important not to overreact to single signs, words, or actions (Dwyer, Osher & Warger, 1998).

Imminent warning signs indicate that a person is very close to behaving in a way that is potentially dangerous to self and/or others. These signs require an immediate response. No single sign can predict that a dangerous act will occur. Usually, they are presented as a sequence of serious, hostile threats or behaviors directed at peers, family, staff, or other individuals. Imminent warning signs may include (Dwyer et al., 1998):

- Serious physical fighting with family or peers
- Severe destruction of property
- Severe rage for seemingly minor reasons
- Detailed threats of lethal violence
- Possession and/or use of firearms or other weapons
- Other self-injurious behaviors or threats of suicide

Diagnosis

Based on assessment data, nursing diagnoses are formulated for the potential perpetrators of community violence. See the Nursing Diagnoses with NOC and NIC feature for possible nursing diagnoses for selected nursing diagnoses for potential perpetrators.

Outcome Identification and Goals

Based on the assessment data, you select outcomes appropriate to the client's current state and the identified nursing diagnoses. Possible outcomes for potential perpetrators are found in the Nursing Diagnoses with NOC and NIC feature.

Client goals are specific behavioral prescriptions that you, the client, and significant others identify as realistic and attainable. The following are examples of goals appropriate to potential perpetrators of community violence:

- Verbalizes an internal locus of control
- Relates appropriately to several peers
- Verbalizes an improved self-esteem
- Accepts responsibility for own behavior
- Attends school or work
- Improves academic performance
- Interacts with others with less prejudicial behavior
- Exhibits no threats of violence and no violent behavior

Nursing Interventions

Everyone has a personal responsibility for reducing the risk of violence. We must take steps to maintain order, demonstrate mutual respect and caring for one another, and ensure that children who are troubled get the help they need.

The Nursing Diagnoses with NOC and NIC feature lists the nursing interventions classification for potential perpetrators of community violence.

Behavioral: Behavioral Therapy

Behavior Modification: Social Skills

Some violence prone individuals alienate their peers by interrupting others, intruding in particular situations, invading personal space, and treating others' property as if it were their own. When youth experience conflict with peers or adults, they often refuse to back down, even on little points. It is important that you *avoid power struggles*, which can be damaging to children's self-esteem. It is better to role model how to negotiate differences and how to admit to errors.

Nursing interventions are also directed at helping these children establish and maintain social relationships. *Role modeling* is an effective way to demonstrate social skills such as giving and receiving compliments, sharing, conflict resolution, and personal boundary issues. Because these children often use anger to control people, they may become abusive, aggressive, or threatening. *Feedback* and *consequences* must be immediate to avoid reinforcing this inappropriate behavior.

As the nurse, you structure the child's environment to allow for success and *clearly state the rules and expectations*. It is important that you provide frequent, immediate, and consistent feedback regarding both appropriate and inappropriate social behavior. You may select particular peers to interact with the child. It is best to begin with one-on-one interactions. You might suggest the client–child work with one child at the computer, another child while problem solving, and a different child in free play. As the child's social skills improve, two or more children can be included in each of the groups.

Behavior Modification: Limit Setting

When working with children and adolescents who have limited self-control, it is critical that you *set appropriate limits*. Limit setting reinforces the predictability of the environment. As these individuals learn about and accept external limits, they are assisted in developing internal controls. The staff should adopt a *solution focus* rather than a problem focus such as "What can we do to solve this problem?" rather than "What is the cause of this problem?" When unwanted behavior occurs, staff should help children identify clearly what the desirable, positive alternative is, in behavioral terms. You may find it helpful to develop *behavioral contracts* with some children. The contract, which is mutually created, has clear behavioral expectations, states how these are to be achieved, and relates achievement to particular rewards. Consequences for inappropriate behavior must be immediate, logical, and appropriate to the child's age. *Time-out procedures* are used as a cooling-off period as well as providing the necessary time for reflection. As a general rule, time-outs should be no longer than one minute per year of development. During this time, the child receives no

attention and no environmental stimulation. A time-out is always accompanied by a clear statement of the reasons why it is necessary and a statement of what the desirable alternative behavior would be. After it is over, you review the incident with the child, who then returns to the normal milieu.

Behavior Modification: Self-Responsibility Facilitation

The goal of the interventions is to help children overcome their defensiveness and tendency to project blame on others. Children who are at risk for becoming violent often are unable or unwilling to accept responsibility for their choices and behaviors. When things go wrong, they blame others. You may hear, "She started it," or "I couldn't help it, he made me do it." Even young children can be taught the concept of good choices versus bad choices. As the nurse, you need to *establish reasonable and meaningful consequences* for both good and bad decisions. Excuses are not accepted for bad choices and the focus returns to that child's personal decisions regarding behavior.

Behavioral: Cognitive Therapy

Anger Control Assistance

Since violence prone children often experience explosive outbursts, they need to learn *coping skills* to help them avoid aggression in the future. Giving the acting-out child choices is often effective. "There are two quieter places you may go to: your room or the deck. Which one would you like?" Each time a choice is given, the child must pause and consider the options. Each pause decreases the amount of energy behind the anger. Giving choices also helps children to feel they have some control in the situation. It is best to intervene before the behavior escalates to out-of-control aggression. Assist in identifying the source of the anger, and establish the expectation that the child can control the behavior. Direct the child to seek assistance before lashing out with aggressive behavior. If appropriate, provide physical outlets for the expression of anger or tension. Help the child identify the benefits of expressing anger in an adaptive, nonviolent way as well as identifying the consequences of inappropriate expression of anger. Teach the child calming measures such as deep breathing and self-controlled time-outs when beginning to feel aggressive.

When a child is out of control, reasoning with that

Behavior Assessment	Affective Assessment	Cognitive Assessment
How does this child/teen manage stress? Is there evidence of positive coping skills?	Is there an inappropriate expression of feelings?	Does this child/teen believe that she or he is picked on and persecuted?
Are there patterns of impulsive or intimidating behavior?	Does this child experience uncontrolled anger?	Is there a lack of responsibility for own behavior and a pathological blaming of others?
Is there a history of discipline problems?	Are there excessive feelings of isolation and rejection from peers?	Is there low interest in school and poor academic performance?
Is there a past history of violent and aggressive behavior?	Are there signs of depression?	Does the child show a strong interest in firearms and other weapons?
Is there an expression of violence in writings and drawings?	Is the child suicidal?	
Is there access to, possession of, and use of firearms?		
Does this child use alcohol and/or drugs?		
Have there been serious threats of violence?		
Is there evidence that the child is affiliated with a gang?		

child is useless and you may need to institute a therapeutic hold. To prevent injury, this hold should never be attempted without additional training in the use of the technique. With both of you sitting on the floor, get behind the child with your back against the wall. Put your legs over the child's legs. With your arms enclosing the child's arms, cross them at the waist and hold them against the child's sides. In a calm voice say, "I am going to hold you until your outburst is over. I will not let you hurt yourself or me or destroy anything. I will hold you until this is over and you are safe."

Behavioral: Communication Enhancement

Socialization Enhancement

The inability to develop empathy for others decreases children's social sensitivity and leads to peer disapproval and conflict. Since they are unable to put themselves in another's place, they demonstrate little or no empathy unless it is to manipulate someone. They often have no concept of how they have hurt another's feelings.

Since some of these children have learned violence from being treated disrespectfully, it is helpful if you role model positive interactions. Treat the child with warmth, friendliness, humor, empathy, and unconditional positive regard. Minimize the amount of attention given for negative behavior and maximize the amount of attention given for desirable and positive behavior. A kindergarten through twelfth grade program called *Resolving Conflict Creatively Program (RCCP)* may be instituted in the clinical setting. The goal of RCCP is to help children learn to care about others, resolve conflicts nonviolently, solve problems cooperatively, value diversity, make responsible decisions, confront prejudice, and to take positive, meaningful action. See the Community Resources feature at the end of the chapter for address information.

Children need to learn the process of practicing

Social Assessment

Are there environmental risk factors such as poverty, parental stress, or a dangerous neighborhood?

Has the child been a victim of being teased, bullied, ridiculed, or humiliated?

Has the child been a victim of violence?

Is there an intolerance for diversity among peers and prejudicial attitudes?

Physiological Assessment

Is the growth and development normal for the child's age?

Are there any minor physical anomalies of the mouth, ears, eyes, head, hands, or feet?

Is there any impaired neurological functioning?

Is the child experiencing a psychosis?

---

democracy in the home, in the neighborhood, and in school. As they learn how to *solve problems without violence*, they will be better prepared for healthy adult interactions and relationships. Youth need to be encouraged to express their views, listen attentively, and seek mutually acceptable solutions to conflict.

Behavioral: Coping Assistance

Crisis Interventions

Responding to the aftermath of a violent tragedy is a component of a violence prevention and response plan. The first step, debriefing, provides the structure for people to talk about the experience in a way that helps them feel safe. As a nurse, you can encourage the people involved in the incident to describe what they experienced. The more they talk about what happened, the more they will be able to process the event. Follow-up sessions allow individuals to reflect on the incident and its meaning in their lives, which is part of the

recovery process. See Chapter 10 for more information on crisis intervention. Anytime a trauma occurs, the potential to develop posttraumatic stress disorder, which is discussed in Chapter 11.

Safety: Risk Management

Environmental Management: Community

Cooperative community action is needed to halt the violence in schools, in the workplace, and on the street. Because of their expertise in working with residents and leaders, community health nurses are often called on to collaborate in the development of community action programs. Nurses can help community leaders study violence prevention programs that have already been established (see the Community Resources feature). Nurses can encourage neighborhoods to become active participants in community safety. Nurses may also conduct educational programs targeted at people who are at risk for becoming perpetrators of violence (Riner & Flynn, 1999).

NURSING DIAGNOSES with NOC & NIC

Violent or Potentially Violent Youth

DIAGNOSIS	OUTCOMES	INTERVENTIONS
Risk for loneliness related to excessive feelings of isolation and rejection from peers	*Social Interaction Skills:* An individual's use of effective interaction behaviors	Behavior Modification: Social Skills
Self-esteem disturbance related to beliefs of being persecuted	*Self-Esteem:* Personal judgment of self-worth	Self-Esteem Enhancement
Ineffective individual coping related to a lack of responsibility for own behavior and a pathological blaming of others	*Self-Esteem:* Personal judgment of self-worth	Behavior Modification: Self-Responsibility Facilitation
Altered role performance related to a low interest in school and poor academic performance	*Role Performance:* Congruence of an individual's role behavior with role expectations	
Fear related to being a victim of being teased, bullied, ridiculed, or humiliated	*Fear Control:* Personal actions to eliminate or reduce disabling feelings of alarm aroused by an identifiable source	
Impaired social interaction related to an intolerance for diversity among peers and prejudicial attitudes	*Social Involvement:* Frequency of an individual's social interactions with persons, groups, or organizations	Socialization Enhancement
Risk for violence, directed at others related to threats of violence, past violent behavior, uncontrolled anger, and possession of firearms or other weapons	*Abusive Behavior Self-Control:* Self-restraint of own behaviors to avoid abuse and neglect of dependents or significant others *Aggression Control:* Self-restraint of assaultive, combative, or destructive behavior toward others	Behavior Modification: Limit Setting Anger Control Assistance

SOURCE: Johnson, M., Maas, M., & Moorhead, S. (2000). *Nursing outcomes classification (NOC)* (2nd ed.). St. Louis, MO: Mosby; McCloskey, J. C., & Bulechek, G. M. (1996). *Nursing interventions classification (NIC).* St. Louis, MO: Mosby; and North American Nursing Diagnoses Association (1999). *Nursing diagnoses definitions and classification 1999–2000.* Philadelphia: Author.

BOX 23.3

Family Education

Tips for Parents

- Involve your child in setting rules for appropriate behavior at home.
- Spend time with your child.
- Talk with your child about the violence she or he sees—on television, in video games, and possibly in the neighborhood. Help your child understand the consequences of violence.
- Teach your child how to solve problems. Praise your child when she or he follows through.
- Help your child find ways to show anger that do not involve verbally or physically hurting others. When you get angry, use it as an opportunity to model these appropriate responses for your child—and talk about it.
- Note any disturbing behaviors in your child. Get help for your child.
- Listen to your child if she or he shares concerns about friends who may be exhibiting troubling behaviors. Share this information with a trusted professional such as the school nurse, principal, or teacher.

The Centers for Disease Control and Prevention (CDC) has published a 216-page guide called *Best Practices in Youth Violence Prevention*. This publication can serve as a sourcebook as you become involved in family, neighborhood, and school violence prevention programs. For a free copy, call 888-252-7751. See Box 23.3 on tips for parents in the prevention of violence. See Box 23.4 for tips for peer education for prevention of school violence.

Evaluation

To complete the nursing process, you evaluate clients' responses to nursing interventions based on the outcomes you selected. You determine the appropriate intervals for measurement and document the condition of clients according to each individual's status. Johnson, Maas, and Moorhead (2000) is the resource for identifying measurement scales and specific indicators for each outcome.

Abusive Behavior Self-Control

Clients identify thoughts of anger, revenge, and rage that are unreasonable for the situation. They do not have access to firearms or other weapons. Clients exhibit no threats of violence and no violent behavior. They accept external limits as they learn to develop internal controls.

Aggression Control

Perpetrators refrain from emotionally, financially, or physically violating other individuals. Clients identify feelings of anger, frustration, hostility, and aggression. Clients identify alternatives to aggression and maintain self-control without supervision. They communicate their needs appropriately and verbalize control of impulses.*

BOX 23.4

Tips for Peer Education

- Listen to your friends if they share troubling feelings or thoughts. Encourage them to get help from a trusted adult. Share your concerns with your parents.
- Participate in violence prevention programs such as peer mediation and conflict resolution. Employ your new skills in other settings, such as home, neighborhood, and community.
- Break the deadly code of silence. Work with your teachers and administrators to create a safe process for reporting threats, intimidation, weapon possession, drug selling, gang activity, graffiti, and vandalism. Use the process.
- Help to develop and participate in activities that promote student understanding of differences and that respect the rights of all.
- Be a role model—take personal responsibility by reacting to anger without physically or verbally harming others.

SOURCE: Adapted from Dwyer, K., Osher, D., & Warger, C. (1998). *Early warning, timely response: A guide to safe schools*. Washington, DC: U.S. Department of Education.

---

*These selected outcome indicators are from Johnson, M., Maas, M., & Moorhead, S. (2000). *Nursing outcomes classification (NOC)* (2nd ed.). St. Louis, MO: Mosby.

CRITICAL THINKING

The school nurses for a suburban community are meeting for their monthly discussion of current issues and to plan future continuing education for the group. Sue, who is the school nurse at one of the large middle schools, comes in late to the meeting and is clearly stressed. Since one of the purposes of the group is to offer support and a place for the nurses to discuss their problems, the group asks Sue if she needs some time to discuss any issues. She tells the group that early in the schoolday a 7th grader was found with a gun. The gun was found when the boy took the gun out of his locker and told the students around him that this gun would save him. The students reported him to their homeroom teacher. The principal called the police, and the student was expelled as is required by the Gun Free Schools Act.

Sue is asked about the student. She tells the group that the student is quiet, isolated, and has been prone to angry outbursts when criticized. His grades are below average, and his parents have not shown much interest in his school activities. None of his teachers have had any contact with his parents. The student is new to the school system as he moved into the area one year ago from out of state. His record indicates that he has been in four different schools in different locations. The teachers are very upset and frightened. This is the first time there has been an incident related to a gun at the school. The students were talking about it all day. Sue comments that she has been seeing an increase in violence in the school (e.g., several fights, verbal arguments, and threats).

1. What factors may impact the risk of violence in a school?

2. The student with the gun comes from a family in which neither of the parents is employed and lives in a housing unit. What is the relationship between poverty and violence?

3. If Sue had known that this student might be heading for problems, an assessment would be an important step to take. Considering what is known about the student, what further data would be needed?

4. Due to the fact that Sue has noted that aggression is increasing in the school, one of the school nurses suggests that Sue consider conducting an anger control assistance program. How can she help the students reduce their anger?

5. As the school nurses are all concerned about the increasing trend of violence, they decide to develop an educational program for teachers and school staff. Formulate a plan for what content they might include in this program.

For an additional Case Study, please refer to the Companion Web site for this book.

Role Performance

Academic performance is at grade level. They attend school on a daily basis.

Self-Esteem

Adolescent males show emotions and discuss feelings with peers and supportive adults. They verbalize an internal locus of control and an improved self-esteem.

Social Interaction Skills

Adolescents verbalize feelings of connectedness to others. They avoid deviant peer groups and associate with teens who are socially appropriate. Clients avoid power struggles with other adolescent males. They utilize the problem solving process to negotiate differences with others.

Social Involvement

Adolescents identify the benefits of interpersonal relationships. They participate in extra-curricular activities and community groups and verbalize a sense of belonging.

CHAPTER REVIEW

COMMUNITY RESOURCES

Links to these Web sites can be accessed on the Companion Web site for this book.

Bilingual Hot Line for Victims of Trauma
P.O. Box 161810
Austin, TX 78716
800-799-SAFE
www.ndvh.org

Anti-Defamation League
823 United Nations Plaza
New York, NY 10017
212-885-7700
www.adl.org

Center to Prevent Handgun Violence
Sarah Brady, Chair
12251 St. NW, Suite 1100
Washington, DC 20005
202-289-7319
www.handguncontrol.org

Human Rights Campaign
919 18th St. NW
Washington, DC 20006
202-628-4160
www.hrc.org

National School Safety Center
www.nssc1.org

National Youth Gang Center
Institute for Intergovernmental Research
P.O. Box 12729
Tallahassee, FL 32327
850-385-0600
www.iir.com/nygc

RCCP National Center
40 Exchange Place, Suite 1111
New York, NY 10005
212-509-0022
www.esrnational.org

Prevention Programs

Best Practices for Youth Violence
Centers for Disease Control and Prevention
888-252-7751
www.cdc.gov/ncipc/dup/bestpractices.htm

Communities That Care
130 Nickerson St., Suite 107
Seattle, WA 98109
800-736-2630

Rising Above Gangs and Drugs: How to Start a Community
    Reclamation Project
Juvenile Justice Clearinghouse
P.O. Box 6000
Rockville, MD 20849-6000
800-638-8736
www.ncjrs.org

Steps to Prevent (STOP) Firearm Injury Center to Prevent
    Handgun Violence
P.O. Box 425
Bladensburg, MD 20710-9974

Violence Prevention Curriculum for Adolescents
EDC Publishing Center
55 Chapel St., Suite 24
Newton, MA 02160
800-225-4276
www.hamfish.org/program/id/362

BOOKS FOR CLIENTS AND FAMILIES

Herman, J. (1997). *Trauma and recovery.* New York: Basic Books.

Rosenbloom, D., & Williams, M. B. (1999). *Life after trauma: A workbook for healing.* New York: Guilford Press.

KEY CONCEPTS

Introduction

- The U.S. culture is one that promotes, supports, and even encourages and romanticizes violence.

- Males are the chief perpetrators and also the chief victims of violent acts.

- Affective violence is the verbal expression of intense anger and emotions. It is the bullying, ugly taunts, disrespect, and physical threats that many people experience every day.

- Hate crimes are motivated by bias and hatred of minority groups and may even end in murder.

- Stalking ranges from delusional to nondelusional, and there may or may not be a relationship with the victim.

- In nonspecific homicides, the motive is known only to the perpetrator, and there may be a massacre with little regard for life.

- Revenge killings retaliate for real or imagined offenses by the victim.

- Patricide and/or matricide may be in response to many years of physical and sexual abuse.

- Authority killing may be targeted at individuals or at building or institutions that symbolize the authority.

- Nearly 1 million people a year are victims of workplace violence.

- The most common settings for violence in hospitals are the emergency room and psychiatric inpatient units.

- Fewer than 1 percent of all violent deaths of children occur in or around school property.

- Teens are much more likely than adults to be victims of violence.

Knowledge Base

- Hitting or spanking children gives the message that violence is acceptable.

- Children who witness violence display more internalizing behavior, while those who are victims display more externalizing behavior.

- When individuals live in isolation and have no supportive network, their internal world may be filled with bitterness, resentment, and rage, which can precipitate violent acting out.

- Violent people may rationalize their behavior or project their anger onto the victim.

- The rate of firearm deaths among children 14 years and younger is nearly 12 times higher in the United States than in 25 other industrialized countries combined.

- Co-morbid disorders for violent people include ADHD and PTSD.

- There is no single cause of violence. It results from an interaction of neurobiological, personality, and societal factors.

- Violent people may have low levels of 5-HT, which is implicated in a lack of control, loss of temper, and explosive rage.

- Low cortisol has been associated with greater antisocial behavior.

- Social learning theory states that children learn about violence from observation, from being victims, and from behaving violently themselves.

- Extremes of poverty and racism contribute to the trauma of children and become breeding grounds for violence.

- Violent youths are more likely than other youths to have a biological parent who also engages in antisocial behavior, which is thought to reflect both the genetic transmission of temperament and modeling of aggression.

- Antisocial and violent children tend to make friends with peers similar to themselves through which antisocial behavior is reinforced.

The Nursing Process

Assessment

- Early warning signs are indicators for doing an in-depth assessment of children who may become violent.

- Imminent warning signs indicate that a person is very close to behaving in a dangerous way and include serious physical fighting, severe destruction of property, detailed threats of lethal violence, possession of weapons, and threats of suicide.

Diagnosis

- Nursing diagnoses include: risk for loneliness, self-esteem disturbance, ineffective individual coping, altered role performance, fear, posttrauma response, impaired social interaction, and risk for violence directed at others.

Outcome Identification and Goals

- Outcomes include abusive behavior self-control, aggression control, role performance, self-esteem, social interaction skills, and social involvement.

Nursing Interventions

- Nursing interventions are directed at helping violence-prone children establish and maintain social relationships.

- It is critical that you set appropriate limits.

- Feedback and consequences for behavior must be immediate to avoid reinforcing inappropriate behavior.

- Time-outs are used as a cooling-off period as well as providing the necessary time for reflection.

- Excuses are not accepted for bad choices, and children are held responsible for personal decisions regarding behavior.

- When nursing interventions are successful, the outcomes reflect that they demonstrate impulse control; identify factors that contribute to their violent behavior; meet role expectations in the family, at school, in the community, and with peers; demonstrate a positive regard for others and themselves; and use social interaction skills appropriately.

Evaluation

- Provide the child with limited choices to both deescalate the situation and provide the child with some sense of control.

- If the child is out of control, you may need to institute a therapeutic hold.

- Model positive interactions by treating the child with warmth, friendliness, humor, and empathy.

- Cooperative community action is needed to halt the violence in schools, in the workplace, and on the street. Nurses can be leaders in this area.

EXPLORE *MediaLink*

- Interactive resources, including animations, for this chapter can be found on the Companion Web site at *http://www.prenhall.com/fontaine*. Click on Chapter 23 and select the activities for this chapter.

- For NCLEX review questions and an audio glossary, access the accompanying CD-ROM in this book.

REFERENCES

Allen, A. C. (2000, April). Veterans, victims and violence. *The Nation's Health*, p. 2.

Arboleda-Florez, J., & Weisstub, D. N. (2000). Conflicts and crises in Latin America. In A. Okasha, J. Arboleda-Florez, & N. Sartorius (Eds.), *Ethics, culture, and psychiatry* (pp. 29–46). Washington, DC: American Psychiatric Press.

Arizona Department of Health Services. (2001). Epidemiology and surveillance. Retrieved November 25, 2001, from the World Wide Web, *http://www.hs.state.us/phs/edc/edrp/es/bthistor1.htm*.

Arseneault L., Tremblay, R. E., Boulerice, B., Sequin, J. R., Saucier, J. F. (2000). Minor physical anomalies and family adversity as risk factors for violent delinquency in adolescents. *American Journal of Psychiatry, 157*(6), 917–923.

Berkowitz, L. (1999). Psychology of aggression. In L. Kurtz (Ed.), *Encyclopedia of violence, peace, and conflict*. Vol. 1 (pp. 35–45). San Diego: Academic Press.

Bloom, S. L., & Reichert, M. (1998). *Bearing witness: Violence and collective responsibility*. New York: Haworth Press.

Burgess, A. W., & Dowdell, E. B. (1999, January 25). Forensic nursing and violent schoolboys. *Nursing Spectrum, 12*(2), 12–14.

Crime Characteristics. (2001). Bureau of Justice Statistics. *www.ojp.gov/bjs/evict_c.htm*.

Denenberg, R. V., & Braverman, M. (1999). *Violence-prone workplace*. Ithaca, NY: Cornell University Press.

Duckworth, M. P., Hale, D. D., Clair, S. D., & Adams, H. E. (2000). Influence of interpersonal violence and community chaos on stress reactions in children. *Journal of Interpersonal Violence, 15*(8), 806–826.

Dwyer, K., Osher, D., & Warger, C. (1998). *Early warning, timely response: A guide to safe schools*. Washington, DC: U.S. Department of Education.

Franklin, K. (2000). Antigay behaviors among young adults. *Journal of Interpersonal Violence, 15*(4), 339–362.

Gustavsson, N. S., & MacEachron, A. E. (1998). Violence and lesbian and gay youth. In L. M. Sloan & N. S. Gustavsson (Eds.), *Violence and social injustice against lesbian, gay and bisexual people* (pp. 41–50). New York: Haworth Press.

Hoffman, B. (1998). *Inside terrorism*. New York: Columbia University Press.

Hoffman, A. M., & Summers, R. W. (2001). *Teen violence: A global view*. Westport, CT: Greenwood Press.

Johnson, M., Maas, M., Moorhead, S. (2000). *Nursing outcomes classification (NOC)* (2nd ed.). St. Louis, MO: Mosby.

Kelleher, M. D. (1998). *When good kids kill*. Westport, CT: Praeger.

Koch, K. (2000). School violence. In D. M. Bonilla (Ed.), *School violence* (pp. 5–33). New York: Wilson.

Kuehnle, K., & Sullivan, A. (2001). Patterns of anti-gay violence. *Journal of Interpersonal Violence, 16*(9), 928–943.

LeMarquand, D., Benkelfut, C., & Pihl, R. O. (1999). Biochemical factors. In L. Kurtz (Ed.), *Encyclopedia of violence, peace, and conflict*. Vol. 1 (pp. 197–211). San Diego: Academic Press.

Levi, P. (1999). Sustainability of healthcare environments. *Image, 31*(4), 395–398.

Moore, J. P., & Cook I. L. (1999). *Highlights of the 1998 national youth gang survey*. Washington DC: Office of Juvenile Justice and Delinquency Prevention.

Overstreet, S., & Braun, S. (2000). Exposure to community violence and posttraumatic stress syndrome. *American Journal of Orthopsychiatry, 70*(2), 263–271.

Pollack, W. (2000). *Real boys' voices*. New York: Random House.

REFERENCES *(continued)*

Reno, J. (1999). Cyberstalking: A new challenge for law enforcement and industry. *www.usdoj.gov/criminal/cybercrime/cyber stalking.htm.*

Rhule, P. (2000, April 14–16). Our kids are afraid: 13th Annual Teen Survey. *USA WEEKEND,* pp. 8–10.

Riner, M. E., & Flynn, B. C. (1999). Creating violence-free healthy cities for our youth. *Holistic Nursing Practice, 14*(1), 1–11.

Sandberg, D. A., McNiel, D. E., & Binder, R. L. (1998). Characteristics of psychiatric inpatients who stalk, threaten, or harass hospital staff after discharge. *American Journal of Psychiatry, 155*(8), 1102–1105.

Shahinfar, A., Fox, N. A., & Leavitt, L. A. (2000). Preschool children's exposure to violence. *American Journal of Orthopsychiatry, 70*(1), 115–125.

Shea, S. C. (1998). *Psychiatric interviewing: The art of understanding* (2nd ed.). Philadelphia: Saunders.

Shelton, D. (2000). Health status of young offenders and their families. *Journal of Nursing Scholarship, 32*(2), 173–178.

Sloan, L. M., King, L., & Sheppard, S. (1998). Hate crimes motivated by sexual orientation. In L. M. Sloan & N. S. Gustavsson (Eds.), *Violence and social injustice against lesbian, gay and bisexual people* (pp. 25–39). New York: Haworth Press.

Smith, H. (1999). *Seeking solutions.* Public Broadcasting Service, *www.pbs.org/seeking solutions.*

Smith, H., & Thomas, S. P. (2000). Violent and nonviolent girls. *Issues in Mental Health Nursing, 21*(5), 547–575.

U.S. Advisory Board on Child Abuse and Neglect. (1992). *The continuing child protection emergency: A challenge to the nation.* Washington, DC: U.S. Government Printing Office.

Veenema, T. G. (2001). Children's exposure to community violence. *Journal of Nursing Scholarship, 33*(2), 167–173.

NOS = Not Otherwise Specified

An *x* appearing in a diagnostic code indicates that a specific code number is required.

An ellipsis (. . .) is used in the names of certain disorders to indicate that the name of a specific mental disorder or general medical condition should be inserted when recording the name (e.g., 293.0 Delirium Due to Hypothyroidism).

If criteria are currently met, one of the following severity specifiers may be noted after the diagnosis:

Mild
Moderate
Severe

If criteria are no longer met, one of the following specifiers may be noted:

In Partial Remission
In Full Remission
Prior History

Disorders Usually First Diagnosed in Infancy, Childhood, or Adolescence

MENTAL RETARDATION
Note: These are coded on Axis II.
317   Mild Mental Retardation
318.0   Moderate Mental Retardation
318.1   Severe Mental Retardation
318.2   Profound Mental Retardation
319   Mental Retardation, Severity Unspecified

LEARNING DISORDERS
315.00 Reading Disorder
315.1   Mathematics Disorder
315.2   Disorder of Written Expression
315.9   Learning Disorder NOS

MOTOR SKILLS DISORDER
315.4   Developmental Coordination Disorder

COMMUNICATION DISORDERS
315.31 Expressive Language Disorder
315.32 Mixed Receptive-Expressive Language Disorder
315.39 Phonological Disorder
307.0   Stuttering
307.9   Communication Disorder NOS

PERVASIVE DEVELOPMENTAL DISORDERS
299.00 Autistic Disorder
299.80 Rett's Disorder
299.10 Childhood Disintegrative Disorder
299.80 Asperger's Disorder
299.80 Pervasive Developmental Disorder NOS

ATTENTION-DEFICIT AND DISRUPTIVE BEHAVIOR DISORDERS
314.xx Attention-Deficit/Hyperactivity Disorder
   .01   Combined Type
   .00   Predominantly Inattentive Type
   .01   Predominantly Hyperactive-Impulsive Type
314.9   Attention-Deficit/Hyperactivity Disorder NOS

312.xx Conduct Disorder
   .81   Childhood-Onset Type
   .82   Adolescent-Onset Type
   .89   Unspecified Onset
313.81 Oppositional Defiant Disorder
312.9   Disruptive Behavior Disorder NOS

FEEDING AND EATING DISORDERS OF INFANCY OR EARLY CHILDHOOD
307.52 Pica
307.53 Rumination Disorder
307.59 Feeding Disorder of Infancy or Early Childhood

TIC DISORDERS
307.23 Tourette's Disorder
307.22 Chronic Motor or Vocal Tic Disorder
307.21 Transient Tic Disorder
        Specify if: Single Episode/Recurrent
307.20 Tic Disorder NOS

ELIMINATION DISORDERS
___.__ Encopresis
787.6   With Constipation and Overflow Incontinence
307.7   Without Constipation and Overflow Incontinence
307.6   Enuresis (Not Due to a General Medical Condition)
        Specify type: Nocturnal Only/Diurnal Only/Nocturnal and Diurnal

OTHER DISORDERS OF INFANCY, CHILDHOOD, OR ADOLESCENCE
309.21 Separation Anxiety Disorder
        Specify if: Early Onset
313.23 Selective Mutism
313.89 Reactive Attachment Disorder of Infancy or Early Childhood
        Specify type: Inhibited Type/Disinhibited Type
307.3   Stereotypic Movement Disorder
        Specify if: With Self-Injurious Behavior

313.9   Disorder of Infancy, Childhood, or Adolescence
          NOS

Delirium, Dementia, and Amnestic and Other Cognitive Disorders

DELIRIUM

293.0   Delirium Due to . . . *[Indicate the General Medical Condition]*

____.__   Substance Intoxication Delirium *(refer to Substance-Related Disorders for substance-specific codes)*

____.__   Substance Withdrawal Delirium *(refer to Substance-Related Disorders for substance-specific codes)*

____.__   Delirium Due to Multiple Etiologies *(code each of the specific etiologies)*

780.09   Delirium NOS

DEMENTIA

294.xx*   Dementia of the Alzheimer's Type, With Early Onset *(also code 331.0 Alzheimer's disease on Axis III)*
   .10   Without Behavioral Disturbance
   .11   With Behavioral Disturbance

294.xx*   Dementia of the Alzheimer's Type, With Late Onset *(also code 331.0 Alzheimer's disease on Axis III)*
   .10   Without Behavioral Disturbance
   .11   With Behavioral Disturbance

290.xx   Vascular Dementia
   .40   Uncomplicated
   .41   With Delirium
   .42   With Delusions
   .43   With Depressed Mood
          Specify if: With Behavioral Disturbance

Code presence or absence of a behavioral disturbance in the fifth digit for Dementia Due to a General Medical Condition:

   0 = Without Behavioral Disturbance
   1 = With Behavioral Disturbance

294.1x*   Dementia Due to HIV Disease *(also code 042 HIV on Axis III)*

294.1x*   Dementia Due to Head Trauma *(also code 042 HIV on Axis III)*

294.1x*   Dementia Due to Head Trauma *(also code 854.00 head injury on Axis III)*

294.1x*   Dementia Due to Parkinson's Disease *(also code 332.0 Parkinson's disease on Axis III)*

294.1x*   Dementia Due to Huntington's Disease *(also code 333.4 Huntington's disease on Axis III)*

294.1x*   Dementia Due to Pick's Disease *(also code 331.1 Pick's disease on Axis III)*

294.1x*   Dementia Due to Creutzfeldt-Jakob Disease *(also code 046.1 Creutzfeldt-Jakob disease on Axis III)*

---

* ICD-9-CM code valid after October 1, 2000.

294.1x*   Dementia Due to . . . *[Indicate the General Medical Condition not listed above] (also code the general medical condition on Axis III)*

____.__   Substance-Induced Persisting Dementia *(refer to Substance-Related Disorders for substance-specific codes)*

____.__   Dementia Due to Multiple Etiologies *(code each of the specific etiologies)*

294.8   Dementia NOS

AMNESTIC DISORDERS

294.0   Amnestic Disorder Due to . . . *[Indicate the General Medical Condition]*
          Specify if: Transient/Chronic

____.__   Substance-Induced Persisting Amnestic Disorder *(refer to Substance-Related Disorders for substance-specific codes)*

294.8   Amnestic Disorder NOS

OTHER COGNITIVE DISORDERS

294.9   Cognitive Disorder NOS

Mental Disorders Due to a General Medical Condition Not Elsewhere Classified

293.89   Catatonic Disorder Due to . . . *[Indicate the General Medical Condition]*

310.1   Personality Change Due to . . . *[Indicate the General Medical Condition]*
          Specify type: Labile Type/Disinhibited Type/Aggressive Type/Apathetic Type/Paranoid Type/Other Type/Combined Type/Unspecified Type

293.9   Mental Disorder NOS Due to . . . *[Indicate the General Medical Condition]*

Substance-Related Disorders

The following specifiers apply to Substance Dependence as noted:

   [a]With Physiological Dependence/Without Physiological Dependence
   [b]Early Full Remission/Early Partial Remission/Sustained Full Remission/Sustained Partial Remission
   [c]In a Controlled Environment
   [d]On Agonist Therapy

The following specifiers apply to Substance-Induced Disorders as noted:

   [I]With Onset During Intoxication/[W]With Onset During Withdrawal

ALCOHOL-RELATED DISORDERS

Alcohol Use Disorders

303.90   Alcohol Dependence[a,b,c]
305.00   Alcohol Abuse

Alcohol-Induced Disorders

303.00   Alcohol Intoxication
291.81   Alcohol Withdrawal
          Specify if: With Perceptual Disturbances
291.0   Alcohol Intoxication Delirium

291.0   Alcohol Withdrawal Delirium
291.2   Alcohol-Induced Persisting Dementia
291.1   Alcohol-Induced Persisting Amnestic
        Disorder
291.x   Alcohol-Induced Psychotic Disorder
  .5   With Delusions[I,W]
  .3   With Hallucinations[I,W]
291.89 Alcohol-Induced Mood Disorder[I,W]
291.89 Alcohol-Induced Anxiety Disorder[I,W]
291.89 Alcohol-Induced Sexual Dysfunction[I]
291.89 Alcohol-Induced Sleep Disorder[I,W]
291.9   Alcohol-Related Disorder NOS

AMPHETAMINE (OR AMPHETAMINE-LIKE)–RELATED DISORDERS

Amphetamine Use Disorders
304.40 Amphetamine Dependence[a,b,c]
305.70 Amphetamine Abuse

Amphetamine-Induced Disorders
292.89 Amphetamine Intoxication
        Specify if: With Perceptual Disturbances
292.0   Amphetamine Withdrawal
292.81 Amphetamine Intoxication Delirium
292.xx Amphetamine-Induced Psychotic Disorder
  .11   With Delusions[I]
  .12   With Hallucinations[I]
292.84 Amphetamine-Induced Mood Disorder[I,W]
292.89 Amphetamine-Induced Anxiety Disorder[I]
292.89 Amphetamine-Induced Sexual Dysfunction[I]
292.89 Amphetamine-Induced Sleep Disorder[I,W]
292.9   Amphetamine-Related Disorder NOS

CAFFEINE-RELATED DISORDERS

Caffeine-Induced Disorders
305.90 Caffeine Intoxication
292.89 Caffeine-Induced Anxiety Disorder[I]
292.89 Caffeine-Induced Sleep Disorder[I]
292.9   Caffeine-Related Disorder NOS

CANNABIS-RELATED DISORDERS

Cannabis Use Disorders
304.30 Cannabis Dependence[a,b,c]
305.20 Cannabis Abuse

Cannabis-Induced Disorders
292.89 Cannabis Intoxication
        Specify if: With Perceptual Disturbance
292.81 Cannabis Intoxication Delirium
292.xx Cannabis-Induced Psychotic Disorder
  .11   With Delusions[I]
  .12   With Hallucinations[I]
292.89 Cannabis-Induced Anxiety Disorder[I]
292.9   Cannabis-Related Disorder NOS

COCAINE-RELATED DISORDERS

Cocaine Use Disorders
304.20 Cocaine Dependence[a,b,c]
305.60 Cocaine Abuse

Cocaine-Induced Disorders
292.89 Cocaine Intoxication
        Specify if: With Perceptual Disturbances
292.0   Cocaine Withdrawal
292.81 Cocaine Intoxication Delirium
292.xx Cocaine-Induced Psychotic Disorder
  .11   With Delusions[I]
  .12   With Hallucinations[I]
292.84 Cocaine-Induced Mood Disorder[I,W]
292.89 Cocaine-Induced Anxiety Disorder[I,W]
292.89 Cocaine-Induced Sexual Dysfunction[I]
292.89 Cocaine-Induced Sleep Disorder[I,W]
292.9   Cocaine-Related Disorder NOS

HALLUCINOGEN-RELATED DISORDERS

Hallucinogen Use Disorders
304.50 Hallucinogen Dependence[b,c]
305.30 Hallucinogen Abuse

Hallucinogen-Induced Disorders
292.89 Hallucinogen Intoxication
292.89 Hallucinogen Persisting Perception Disorder
        (Flashbacks)
292.81 Hallucinogen Intoxication Delirium
292.xx Hallucinogen-Induced Psychotic Disorder
  .11   With Delusions[I]
  .12   With Hallucinations[I]
292.84 Hallucinogen-Induced Mood Disorder[I]
292.89 Hallucinogen-Induced Anxiety Disorder[I]
292.9   Hallucinogen-Related Disorder NOS

INHALANT-RELATED DISORDERS

Inhalant Use Disorders
304.60 Inhalant Dependence[b,c]
305.90 Inhalant Abuse

Inhalant-Induced Disorders
292.89 Inhalant Intoxication
292.81 Inhalant Intoxication Delirium
292.82 Inhalant-Induced Persisting Dementia
292.xx Inhalant-Induced Psychotic Disorder
  .11   With Delusions[I]
  .12   With Hallucinations[I]
292.84 Inhalant-Induced Mood Disorder[I]
292.89 Inhalant-Induced Anxiety Disorder[I]
292.9   Inhalant-Related Disorder NOS

NICOTINE-RELATED DISORDERS

Nicotine Use Disorder
305.1   Nicotine Dependence[a,b]

Nicotine-Induced Disorder
292.0   Nicotine Withdrawal
292.9   Nicotine-Related Disorder NOS

OPIOID-RELATED DISORDERS

Opioid Use Disorders
304.00 Opioid Dependence[a,b,c,d]
305.50 Opioid Abuse

Opioid-Induced Disorders

292.89　Opioid Intoxication
　　　　Specify if: With Perceptual Disturbances
292.0　　Opioid Withdrawal
292.81　Opioid Intoxication Delirium
292.xx　Opioid-Induced Psychotic Disorder
　.11　　　With Delusions[I]
　.12　　　With Hallucinations[I]
292.84　Opioid-Induced Mood Disorder[I]
292.89　Opioid-Induced Sexual Dysfunction[I]
292.89　Opioid-Induced Sleep Disorder[I,W]
292.9　　Opioid-Related Disorder NOS

PHENCYCLIDINE (OR PHENCYCLIDINE-LIKE)–RELATED DISORDERS

Phencyclidine Use Disorders

304.60　Phencyclidine Dependence[b,c]
305.90　Phencyclidine Abuse

Phencyclidine-Induced Disorders

292.89　Phencyclidine Intoxication
　　　　Specify if: With Perceptual Disturbances
292.81　Phencyclidine Intoxication Delirium
292.xx　Phencyclidine-Induced Psychotic Disorder
　.11　　　With Delusions[I]
　.12　　　With Hallucinations[I]
292.84　Phencyclidine-Induced Mood Disorder[I]
292.89　Phencyclidine-Induced Anxiety Disorder[I]
292.9　　Phencyclidine-Related Disorder NOS

SEDATIVE-, HYPNOTIC-, OR ANXIOLYTIC-RELATED DISORDERS

Sedative, Hypnotic, or Anxiolytic Use Disorders

304.10　Sedative, Hypnotic, or Anxiolytic Dependence[a,b,c]
305.40　Sedative, Hypnotic, or Anxiolytic Abuse

Sedative-, Hypnotic-, or Anxiolytic-Induced Disorders

292.89　Sedative, Hypnotic, or Anxiolytic Intoxication
292.0　　Sedative, Hypnotic, or Anxiolytic Withdrawal
　　　　Specify if: With Perceptual Disturbances
292.81　Sedative, Hypnotic, or Anxiolytic Intoxication Delirium
292.81　Sedative, Hypnotic, or Anxiolytic Withdrawal Delirium
292.82　Sedative, Hypnotic, or Anxiolytic-Induced Persisting Dementia
292.83　Sedative-, Hypnotic-, or Anxiolytic-Induced Persisting Amnestic Disorder
292.xx　Sedative-, Hypnotic-, or Anxiolytic-Induced Psychotic Disorder
　.11　　　With Delusions[I,W]
　.12　　　With Hallucinations[I,W]
292.84　Sedative-, Hypnotic-, or Anxiolytic-Induced Mood Disorder[I,W]

292.89　Sedative-, Hypnotic-, or Anxiolytic-Induced Anxiety Disorder[W]
292.89　Sedative-, Hypnotic-, or Anxiolytic-Induced Sexual Dysfunction[I]
292.89　Sedative-, Hypnotic, or Anxiolytic-Induced Sleep Disorder[I,W]
292.9　　Sedative-, Hypnotic, or Anxiolytic-Related Disorder NOS

POLYSUBSTANCE-RELATED DISORDER

304.80　Polysubstance Dependence[a,b,c,d]

OTHER (OR UNKNOWN) SUBSTANCE-RELATED DISORDERS

Other (or Unknown) Substance Use Disorders

304.90　Other (or Unknown) Substance Dependence[a,b,c,d]
305.90　Other (or Unknown) Substance Abuse

Other (or Unknown) Substance-Induced Disorders

292.89　Other (or Unknown) Substance Intoxication
　　　　Specify if: With Perceptual Disturbances
292.0　　Other (or Unknown) Substance Withdrawal
　　　　Specify if: With Perceptual Disturbances
292.81　Other (or Unknown) Substance-Induced Delirium
292.82　Other (or Unknown) Substance-Induced Persisting Dementia
292.83　Other (or Unknown) Substance-Induced Persisting Amnestic Disorder
292.xx　Other (or Unknown) Substance-Induced Psychotic Disorder
　.11　　　With Delusions[I,W]
　.12　　　With Hallucinations[I,W]
292.84　Other (or Unknown) Substance-Induced Mood Disorder[I,W]
292.89　Other (or Unknown) Substance-Induced Anxiety Disorder[I,W]
292.89　Other (or Unknown) Substance-Induced Sexual Dysfunction[I]
292.89　Other (or Unknown) Substance-Induced Sleep Disorder[I,W]
292.9　　Other (or Unknown) Substance-Related Disorder NOS

POLYSUBSTANCE-RELATED DISORDER

304.80　Polysubstance Dependence[a,b,c,d]

OTHER (OR UNKNOWN) SUBSTANCE-RELATED DISORDERS

Other (or Unknown) Substance Use Disorders

304.90　Other (or Unknown) Substance Dependence[a,b,c,d]
305.90　Other (or Unknown) Substance Abuse

Other (or Unknown) Substance-Induced Disorders

292.89　Other (or Unknown) Substance Intoxication
　　　　Specify if: With Perceptual Disturbances
292.0　　Other (or Unknown) Substance Withdrawal
　　　　Specify if: With Perceptual Disturbances

292.81 Other (or Unknown) Substance-Induced Delirium

292.82 Other (or Unknown) Substance-Induced Persisting Dementia

292.83 Other (or Unknown) Substance-Induced Persisting Amnestic Disorder

292.xx Other (or Unknown) Substance-Induced Psychotic Disorder
.11 With Delusions[I,W]
.12 With Hallucinations[I,W]

292.84 Other (or Unknown) Substance-Induced Mood Disorder[I,W]

292.89 Other (or Unknown) Substance-Induced Anxiety Disorder[I,W]

292.89 Other (or Unknown) Substance-Induced Sexual Dysfunction[I]

292.89 Other (or Unknown) Substance-Induced Sleep Disorder[I,W]

292.9 Other (or Unknown) Substance-Related Disorder NOS

Schizophrenia and Other Psychotic Disorders

295.xx Schizophrenia

The following Classification of Longitudinal Course applies to all subtypes of Schizophrenia:

Episodic With Interepisode Residual Symptoms (*Specify if:* With Prominent Negative Symptoms)/Episodic With No Interepisode Residual Symptoms

Continuous (*Specify if:* With Prominent Negative Symptoms)

Single Episode in Partial Remission (*Specify if:* With Prominent Negative Symptoms)/Single Episode in Full Remission

Other or Unspecified Pattern

.30 Paranoid Type
.10 Disorganized Type
.20 Catatonic Type
.90 Undifferentiated Type
.60 Residual Type

295.40 Schizophreniform Disorder
Specify if: Without Good Prognostic Features/With Good Prognostic Features

295.70 Schizoaffective Disorder
Specify type: Bipolar Type/Depressive Type

297.1 Delusional Disorder
Specify type: Erotomanic Type/Grandiose Type/Jealous Type/Persecutory Type/Somatic Type/Mixed Type/Unspecified Type

298.8 Brief Psychotic Disorder
Specify if: With Marked Stressor(s)/Without Marked Stressor(s)/With Postpartum Onset

297.3 Shared Psychotic Disorder

293.xx Psychotic Disorder Due to . . . *[Indicate the General Medical Condition]*
.81 With Delusions
.82 With Hallucinations

___.__ Substance-Induced Psychotic Disorder *(refer to Substance-Related Disorders for substance-specific codes)*
Specify if: With Onset During Intoxication/With Onset During Withdrawal

298.9 Psychotic Disorder NOS

Mood Disorders

Code current state of Major Depressive Disorder or Bipolar I Disorder in fifth digit:

1 = Mild
2 = Moderate
3 = Severe Without Psychotic Features
4 = Severe With Psychotic Features
    Specify: Mood-Congruent Psychotic Features/Mood-Incongruent Psychotic Features
5 = In Partial Remission
6 = In Full Remission
0 = Unspecified

The following specifiers apply (for current or most recent episode) to Mood Disorders as noted:

[a]Severity/Psychotic/Remission Specifiers/[b]Chronic/[c]With Catatonic Features/[d]With Melancholic Features/[e]WIth Atypical Features/[f]With Postpartum Onset

The following specifiers apply to Mood Disorders as noted:

[g]With or Without Full Interepisode Recovery/[h]With Seasonal Pattern/[i]With Rapid Cycling

DEPRESSIVE DISORDERS

296.xx Major Depressive Disorder
.2x Single Episode[a,b,c,d,e,f]
.3x Recurrent[a,b,c,d,e,f,g,h]

300.4 Dysthymic Disorder
Specify if: Early Onset/Late Onset
Specify if: With Atypical Features

311 Depressive Disorder NOS

BIPOLAR DISORDERS

296.xx Bipolar I Disorder
.0x Single Manic Episode[a,c,f]
Specify if: Mixed
.40 Most Recent Episode Hypomanic[g,h,i]
.4x Most Recent Episode Manic[a,c,f,g,h,i]
.6x Most Recent Episode Mixed[a,c,f,g,h,i]
.5x Most Recent Episode Depressed[a,b,c,d,e,f,g,h,i]
.7 Most Recent Episode Unspecified[g,h,i]

296.89 Bipolar II Disorder[a,b,c,d,e,f,g,h,i]
Specify (current or most recent episode):
Hypomanic/Depressed

301.13 Cyclothymic Disorder

296.80 Bipolar Disorder NOS

293.83 Mood Disorder Due to . . . *[Indicate the General Medical Condition]*
Specify type: With Depressive Features/With Major Depressive-Like Episode/With Manic Features/With Mixed Features

___.__ Substance-Induced Mood Disorder *(refer to Substance-Related Disorders for substance-specific codes)*
Specify type: With Depressive Features/With Manic Features/With Mixed Features
Specify if: With Onset During Intoxication/With Onset During Withdrawal

296.90 Mood Disorder NOS

Anxiety Disorders

300.01 Panic Disorder Without Agoraphobia
300.21 Panic Disorder With Agoraphobia
300.22 Agoraphobia Without History of Panic Disorder
300.29 Specific Phobia
Specify type: Animal Type/Natural Environment Type/Blood-Injection-Injury Type/Situational Type/Other Type
300.23 Social Phobia
Specify if: Generalized
300.3 Obsessive-Compulsive Disorder
Specify if: With Poor Insight
309.81 Posttraumatic Stress Disorder
Specify if: Acute/Chronic
Specify if: With Delayed Onset
308.3 Acute Stress Disorder
300.02 Generalized Anxiety Disorder
293.84 Anxiety Disorder Due to . . . *[Indicate the General Medical Condition]*
Specify if: With Generalized Anxiety/With Panic Attacks/With Obsessive-Compulsive Symptoms
___.__ Substance-Induced Anxiety Disorder *(refer to Substance-Related Disorders for substance-specific codes)*
Specify if: With Generalized Anxiety/With Panic Attacks/With Obsessive-Compulsive Symptoms/With Phobic Symptoms
Specify if: With Onset During Intoxication/With Onset During Withdrawal
300.00 Anxiety Disorder NOS

SOMATOFORM DISORDERS

300.81 Somatization Disorder
300.82 Undifferentiated Somatoform Disorder
300.11 Conversion Disorder
Specify type: With Motor Symptom or Deficit/With Sensory Symptom or Deficit/With Seizures or Convulsions/With Mixed Presentation
307.xx Pain Disorder
.80 Associated With Psychological Factors
.89 Associated With Both Psychological Factors and a General Medical Condition
Specify if: Acute/Chronic
300.7 Hypochondriasis
Specify if: With Poor Insight
300.7 Body Dysmorphic Disorder
300.82 Somatoform Disorder NOS

Factitious Disorders

300.xx Factitious Disorder
.16 With Predominantly Psychological Signs and Symptoms
.19 With Predominantly Physical Signs and Symptoms
.19 With Combined Psychological and Physical Signs and Symptoms
300.19 Factitious Disorder NOS

Dissociative Disorders

300.12 Dissociative Amnesia
300.13 Dissociative Fugue
300.14 Dissociative Identity Disorder
300.6 Depersonalization Disorder
300.15 Dissociative Disorder NOS

Sexual and Gender Identity Disorders

SEXUAL DYSFUNCTIONS

The following specifiers apply to all primary Sexual Dysfunctions:

Lifelong Type/Acquired Type
Generalized Type/Situational Type
Due to Psychological Factors/Due to Combined Factors

SEXUAL DESIRE DISORDERS

302.71 Hypoactive Sexual Desire Disorder
302.79 Sexual Aversion Disorder

SEXUAL AROUSAL DISORDERS

302.72 Female Sexual Arousal Disorder
302.72 Male Erectile Disorder

ORGASMIC DISORDERS

302.73 Female Orgasmic Disorder
302.74 Male Orgasmic Disorder
302.75 Premature Ejaculation

SEXUAL PAIN DISORDERS

302.76 Dyspareunia (Not Due to a General Medical Condition)
306.51 Vaginismus (Not Due to a General Medical Condition)

SEXUAL DYSFUNCTION DUE TO A GENERAL MEDICAL CONDITION

625.8 Female Hypoactive Sexual Desire Disorder Due to . . . *[Indicate the General Medical Condition]*
608.89 Male Hypoactive Sexual Desire Disorder Due to . . . *[Indicate the General Medical Condition]*
607.84 Male Erectile Disorder Due to . . . *[Indicate the General Medical Condition]*
625.0 Female Dyspareunia Due to . . . *[Indicate the General Medical Condition]*
608.89 Male Dyspareunia Due to . . . *[Indicate the General Medical Condition]*
625.8 Other Female Sexual Dysfunction Due to . . . *[Indicate the General Medical Condition]*
608.89 Other Male Sexual Dysfunction Due to . . . *[Indicate the General Medical Condition]*

____.__ Substance-Induced Sexual Dysfunction *(refer to Substance-Related Disorders for substance-specific codes)*
    Specify if: With Impaired Desire/With Impaired Arousal/With Impaired Orgasm/With Sexual Pain
    Specify if: With Onset During Intoxication
302.70 Sexual Dysfunction NOS

PARAPHILIAS
302.4   Exhibitionism
302.81 Fetishism
302.89 Frotteurism
302.2   Pedophilia
    Specify if: Sexually Attracted to Males/Sexually Attracted to Females/Sexually Attracted to Both
    Specify if: Limited to Incest
    Specify type: Exclusive Type/Nonexclusive Type
302.83 Sexual Masochism
302.84 Sexual Sadism
302.3   Transvestic Fetishism
    Specify if: With Gender Dysphoria
302.82 Voyeurism
302.9   Paraphilia NOS

GENDER IDENTITY DISORDERS
302.xx Gender Identity Disorder
  .6   in Children
  .85   in Adolescents or Adults
    Specify if: Sexually Attracted to Males/Sexually Attracted to Females/Sexually Attracted to Both/Sexually Attracted to Neither
302.6   Gender Identity Disorder NOS
302.9   Sexual Disorder NOS

Eating Disorders
307.1   Anorexia Nervosa
    Specify type: Restricting Type; Binge-Eating/Purging Type
307.51 Bulimia Nervosa
    Specify type: Purging Type/Nonpurging Type
307.50 Eating Disorder NOS

Sleep Disorders
PRIMARY SLEEP DISORDERS
Dyssomnias
307.42 Primary Insomnia
307.44 Primary Hypersomnia
    Specify if: Recurrent
347   Narcolepsy
780.59 Breathing-Related Sleep Disorder
307.45 Circadian Rhythm Sleep Disorder
    Specify type: Delayed Sleep Phase Type/Jet Lag Type/Shift Work Type/Unspecified Type
307.47 Dyssomnia NOS

Parasomnias
307.47 Nightmare Disorder
307.46 Sleep Terror Disorder
307.46 Sleepwalking Disorder

307.47 Parasomnia NOS

SLEEP DISORDERS RELATED TO ANOTHER MENTAL DISORDER
307.42 Insomnia Related to . . . *[Indicate the Axis I or Axis II Disorder]*
307.44 Hypersomnia Related to . . . *[Indicate the Axis I or Axis II Disorder]*

OTHER SLEEP DISORDERS
780.xx Sleep Disorder Due to . . . *[Indicate the General Medical Condition]*
  .52   Insomnia Type
  .54   Hypersomnia Type
  .59   Parasomnia Type
  .59   Mixed Type
____.__ Substance-Induced Sleep Disorder *(refer to Substance-Related Disorders for substance-specific codes)*
    Specify type: Insomnia Type/Hypersomnia Type/Parasomnia Type/Mixed Type
    Specify if: With Onset During Intoxication/With Onset During Withdrawal

Impulse-Control Disorders Not Elsewhere Classified
312.34 Intermittent Explosive Disorder
312.32 Kleptomania
312.33 Pyromania
312.31 Pathological Gambling
312.39 Trichotillomania
312.30 Impulse-Control Disorder NOS

Adjustment Disorders
309.xx Adjustment Disorder
  .0   With Depressed Mood
  .24   With Anxiety
  .28   With Mixed Anxiety and Depressed Mood
  .3   With Disturbance of Conduct
  .4   With Mixed Disturbance of Emotions and Condut
  .9   Unspecified
    Specify if: Acute/Chronic

Personality Disorders
Note: These are coded on Axis II.
301.0   Paranoid Personality Disorder
301.20 Schizoid Personality Disorder
301.22 Schizotypal Personality Disorder
301.7   Antisocial Personality Disorder
301.83 Borderline Personality Disorder
301.50 Histrionic Personality Disorder
301.81 Narcissistic Personality Disorder
301.82 Avoidant Personality Disorder
301.6   Dependent Personality Disorder
301.4   Obsessive-Compulsive Personality Disorder
301.9   Personality Disorder NOS

Other Conditions That May Be a Focus of Clinical Attention

PSYCHOLOGICAL FACTORS AFFECTING MEDICAL CONDITION

316 . . . *[Specified Psychological Factor] Affecting . . . [Indicate the General Medical Condition]*
Choose name based on nature of factors:
Mental Disorder Affecting Medical Condition
Psychological Symptoms Affecting Medical Condition
Personality Traits or Coping Style Affecting Medical Condition
Maladaptive Health Behaviors Affecting Medical Condition
Stress-Related Physiological Response Affecting Medical Condition
Other or Unspecified Psychological Factors Affecting Medical Condition

MEDICATION-INDUCED MOVEMENT DISORDERS

332.1 Neuroleptic-Induced Parkinsonism
333.92 Neuroleptic Malignant Syndrome
333.7 Neuroleptic-Induced Acute Dystonia
333.99 Neuroleptic-Induced Acute Akathisia
333.82 Neuroleptic-Induced Tardive Dyskinesia
333.1 Medication-Induced Postural Tremor
333.90 Medication-Induced Movement Disorder NOS

OTHER MEDICATION-INDUCED DISORDER

995.2 Adverse Effects of Medication NOS

RELATIONAL PROBLEMS

V61.9 Relational Problem Related to a Mental Disorder or General Medical Condition
V61.20 Parent-Child Relational Problem
V61.10 Partner Relational Problem
V61.8 Sibling Relational Problem
V62.81 Relational Problem NOS

PROBLEMS RELATED TO ABUSE OR NEGLECT

V61.21 Physical Abuse of Child
(code 995.54 if focus of attention is on victim)
V61.21 Sexual Abuse of Child
(code 995.53 if focus of attention is on victim)

V61.21 Neglect of Child
(code 995.52 if focus of attention is on victim)
___.__ Physical Abuse of Adult
V61.12 (if by partner)
V62.83 (if by person other than partner) *(code 995.81 if focus of attention is on victim)*
___.__ Sexual Abuse of Adult
V61.12 (if by partner)
V62.83 (if by person other than partner) *(code 995.83 if focus of attention is on victim)*

ADDITIONAL CONDITIONS THAT MAY BE A FOCUS OF CLINICAL ATTENTION

V15.81 Noncompliance With Treatment
V65.2 Malingering
V71.01 Adult Antisocial Behavior
V71.02 Child or Adolescent Antisocial Behavior
V62.89 Borderline Intellectual Functioning
Note: This is coded on Axis II.
780.9 Age-Related Cognitive Decline
V62.82 Bereavement
V62.3 Academic Problem
V62.2 Occupational Problem
313.82 Identity Problem
V62.89 Religious or Spiritual Problem
V62.4 Acculturation Problem
V62.89 Phase of Life Problem

Additional Codes

300.9 Unspecified Mental Disorder (nonpsychotic)
V71.09 No Diagnosis or Condition on Axis I
799.9 Diagnosis or Condition Deferred on Axis I
V71.09 No Diagnosis on Axis II
799.9 Diagnosis Deferred on Axis II

Multiaxial System

Axis I   Clinical Disorders
          Other Conditions That May Be a Focus of Clinical Attention
Axis II   Personality Disorders
          Mental Retardation
Axis III General Medical Conditions
Axis IV   Psychosocial and Environmental Problems
Axis V   Global Assessment of Functioning

A multiaxial system involves an assessment on several axes, each of which refers to a different domain of information that may help the clinician plan treatment and predict outcome. There are five axes included in the DSM-IV multiaxial classification:

Axis I   Clinical Disorders
          Other Conditions That May Be a Focus of Clinical Attention
Axis II   Personality Disorders
          Mental Retardation
Axis III General Medical Conditions
Axis IV   Psychosocial and Environmental Problems
Axis V   Global Assessment of Functioning

The use of the multiaxial system facilitates comprehensive and systematic evaluation with attention to the various mental disorders and general medical conditions, psychosocial and environmental problems, and level of functioning that might be overlooked if the focus were on assessing a single presenting problem. A multiaxial system provides a convenient format for organizing and communicating clinical information, for capturing the complexity of clinical situations, and for describing the heterogeneity of individuals presenting with the same diagnosis. In addition, the multiaxial system promotes the application of the biopsychosocial model in clinical, educational, and research settings.

The rest of this section provides a description of each of the DSM-IV axes. In some settings or situations, clinicians may prefer not to use the multiaxial system. For this reason, guidelines for reporting the results of a DSM-IV assessment without applying the formal multiaxial system are provided at the end of this section.

AXIS I

Clinical Disorders

Other Conditions That May Be a Focus of Clinical Attention

Disorders Usually First Diagnosed in Infancy, Childhood, or Adolescence (*excluding Mental Retardation, which is diagnosed on Axis II*)

Delirium, Dementia, and Amnestic and Other Cognitive Disorders

Mental Disorders Due to a General Medical Condition

Substance-Related Disorders

Schizophrenia and Other Psychotic Disorders

Mood Disorders

Anxiety Disorders

Somatoform Disorders

Factitious Disorders

Dissociative Disorders

Sexual and Gender Identity Disorders

Eating Disorders

Sleep Disorders

Impulse-Control Disorders Not Elsewhere Classified

Adjustment Disorders

Other Conditions That May Be a Focus of Clinical Attention

AXIS I: Clinical Disorders— Other Conditions That May Be a Focus of Clinical Attention

Axis I is for reporting all the various disorders or conditions in the Classification except for the Personality Disorders and Mental Retardation (which are reported on Axis II). The major groups of disorders to be reported on Axis I are listed in the box below. Also reported on Axis I are Other Conditions That May Be a Focus of Clinical Attention.

When an individual has more than one Axis I disorder, all of these should be reported. If more than one Axis I disorder is present, the principal diagnosis or the reason for visit should be indicated by listing it first. When an individual has both an Axis I and an Axis II disorder, the principal diagnosis or the reason for visit will be assumed to be on Axis I unless the Axis II diagnosis is followed by the qualifying phrase "(Principal Diagnosis)" or "(Reason for Visit)." If no Axis I disorder is present, this should be coded as V71.09. If an Axis I diagnosis is deferred, pending the gathering of additional information, this should be coded as 799.9.

AXIS II: Personality Disorders and Mental Retardation

Axis II is for reporting Personality Disorders and Mental Retardation. It may also be used for noting prominent maladaptive personality features and defense mechanisms. The listing of Personality Disorders and Mental Retardation on a separate axis ensures that consideration will be given to the possible presence of Personality Disorders and Mental Retardation that might otherwise be overlooked when attention is directed to the usually more florid Axis I disorders. The coding of Personality Disorders on Axis II should not be taken to imply that their pathogenesis or range of appropriate treatment is fundamentally different from that for the disorders coded on Axis I. The disorders to be reported on Axis II are listed in the box below.

In the common situation in which an individual has more than one Axis II diagnosis, all should be reported. When an individual has both an Axis I and an Axis II diagnosis and the Axis II diagnosis is the principal diagnosis or the reason for visit, this should be indicated by adding the qualifying phrase "(Principal Diagnosis)" or "(Reason for Visit)" after the Axis II diagnosis. If no Axis II disorder is present, this should be coded as V71.09. If an Axis II diagnosis is deferred, pending the gathering of additional information, this should be coded as 799.9.

Axis II may also be used to indicate prominent maladaptive personality features that do not meet the threshold for a Personality Disorder (in such instances, no code number should be used). The habitual use of maladaptive defense mechanisms may also be indicated on Axis II.

AXIS II

Personality Disorders

Mental Retardation

Paranoid Personality Disorder	Narcissistic Personality Disorder
Schizoid Personality Disorder	Avoidant Personality Disorder
Schizotypal Personality Disorder	Dependent Personality Disorder
Antisocial Personality Disorder	Obsessive-Compulsive Personality disorder
Borderline Personality Disorder	Personality Disorder Not Otherwise Specified
Histrionic Personality Disorder	Mental Retardation

AXIS III: General Medical Conditions

Axis III is for reporting current general medical conditions that are potentially relevant to the understanding or management of the individual's mental disorder. These conditions are classified outside the "Mental Disorders" chapter of ICD-9-CM (and outside Chapter V of ICD-10). A listing of the broad categories of general medical conditions is given in the box below.

As discussed in the "Introduction," the multiaxial distinction among Axis I, Axis II, and Axis III disorders does not imply that there are fundamental differences in their conceptualization, that mental disorders are unrelated to physical or biological factors or processes, or that general medical conditions are unrelated to behavioral or psychosocial factors or processes. The purpose of distinguishing general medical conditions is to encourage thoroughness in evaluation and to enhance communication among health care providers.

General medical conditions can be related to mental disorders in a variety of ways. In some cases it is clear that the general medical condition is directly etiological to the development or worsening of mental symptoms and that the mechanism for this effect is physiological. When a mental disorder is judged to be a direct physiological consequence of the general medical condition, a Mental Disorder Due to a General Medical Condition should be diagnosed on Axis I and the general medical condition should be recorded on both Axis I and Axis III. For example, when hypothyroidism is a direct cause of depressive symptoms, the designation on Axis I is 293.83 Mood Disorder Due to Hypothyroidism, With Depressive Features, and the hypothyroidism is listed again and coded on Axis III as 244.9.

In those instances in which the etiological relationship between the general medical condition and the mental symptoms is insufficiently clear to warrant an Axis I diagnosis of Mental Disorder Due to a General Medical Condition, the appropriate mental disorder (e.g., Major Depressive Disorder) should be listed and coded on Axis I; the general medical condition should only be coded on Axis III.

There are other situations in which general medical conditions are recorded on Axis III because of their importance to the overall understanding or treatment of the individual with the mental disorder. An Axis I disorder may be a psychological reaction to an Axis III general medical condition (e.g., the development of 309.0 Adjustment Disorder With Depressed Mood as a reaction to the diagnosis of carcinoma of the breast). Some general medical conditions may not be directly related to the mental disorder but nonetheless have important prognostic or treatment implications (e.g., when the diagnosis on Axis I is 296.30 Major Depressive Disorder, Recurrent, and on Axis III is 427.9 arrhythmia, the choice of pharmacotherapy is influenced by the general medical condition; or when a person with diabetes mellitus is admitted to the hospital for an exacerbation of Schizophrenia and insulin management must be monitored).

When an individual has more than one clinically relevant Axis III diagnosis, all should be reported. If no Axis III disorder is present, this should be indicated by the notation "Axis III: None." If an Axis III diagnosis is deferred, pending the gathering of additional information, this should be indicated by the notation "Axis III: Deferred."

AXIS III

General Medical Conditions (with ICD-9-CM codes)

Infectious and Parasitic Diseases (001–139)

Neoplasms (140–239)

Endocrine, Nutritional, and Metabolic Diseases and immunity Disorders (240–279)

Diseases of the Blood and Blood-Forming Organs (280–289)

Diseases of the Nervous System and Sense Organs (320–389)

Diseases of the Circulatory System (390–459)

Diseases of the Respiratory System (460–519)

Diseases of the Digestive System (520–579)

Diseases of the Genitourinary System (580–629)

Complications of Pregnancy, Childbirth, and the Puerperium (630–676)

Diseases of the Skin and Subcutaneous Tissue (680–709)

Diseases of the Musculoskeletal System and Connective Tissue (710–739)

Congenital Anomalies (740–759)

Certain Conditions Originating in the Perinatal Period (760–779)

Symptoms, Signs, and Ill-Defined Conditions (780–799)

Injury and Poisoning (800–999)

AXIS IV: Psychosocial and Environmental Problems

Axis IV is for reporting psychosocial and environmental problems that may affect the diagnosis, treatment, and prognosis of mental disorders (Axes I and II). A psychosocial or environmental problem may be a negative life event, an environmental difficulty or deficiency, a familial or other interpersonal stress, an inadequacy of social support or personal resources, or other problem relating to the context in which a person's difficulties have developed. So-called positive stressors, such as job promotion, should be listed only if they constitute or lead to a problem, as when a person has difficulty adapting to the new situation. In addition to playing a role in the initiation or exacerbation of a mental disorder, psychosocial problems may also develop as a consequence of a person's psychopathology or may constitute problems that should be considered in the overall management plan.

When an individual has multiple psychosocial or environmental problems, the clinician may note as many as are judged to be relevant. In general, the clinician should note only those psychosocial and environmental problems that have been present during the year preceding the current evaluation. However, the clinician may choose to note psychosocial and environmental problems occurring prior to the previous year if these clearly contribute to the mental disorder or have become a focus of treatment—for example, previous combat experiences leading to Posttraumatic Stress Disorder.

In practice, most psychosocial and environmental problems will be indicated on Axis IV. However, when a psychosocial or environmental problem is the primary focus of clinical attention, it should also be recorded on Axis I, with a code derived from the section "Other Conditions That May Be a Focus of Clinical Attention."

For convenience, the problems are grouped together in the following categories:

■ **Problems with primary support group**—e.g., death of a family member; health problems in family; disruption of family by separation, divorce, or estrangement; removal from the home; remarriage of parent; sexual or physical abuse; parental overprotection; neglect of child; inadequate discipline; discord with siblings; birth of a sibling
■ **Problems related to the social environment**—e.g., death or loss of friend; inadequate social support; living alone; difficulty with acculturation; discrimination; adjustment of life-cycle transition (such as retirement)

- **Educational problems**—e.g., illiteracy; academic problems; discord with teachers or classmates; inadequate school environment
- **Occupational problems**—e.g., unemployment; threat of job loss; stressful work schedule; difficult work conditions; job dissatisfaction; job change; discord with boss or co-workers
- **Housing problems**—e.g., homelessness; inadequate housing; unsafe neighborhood; discord with neighbors or landlord
- **Economic problems**—e.g., extreme poverty; inadequate finances; insufficient welfare support
- **Problems with access to health care services**—e.g., inadequate health care services; transportation to health care facilities unavailable; inadequate health insurance
- **Problems related to interaction with the legal system/crime**—e.g., arrest; incarceration; litigation; victim of crime
- **Other psychosocial and environmental problems**—e.g., exposure to disasters, war, other hostilities; discord with nonfamily caregivers such as counselor, social worker, or physician; unavailability of social service agencies

When using the Multiaxial Evaluation Report Form, the clinician should identify the relevant categories of psychosocial and environmental problems and indicate the specific factors involved. If a recording form with a checklist of problem categories is not used, the clinician may simply list the specific problems on Axis IV.

AXIS IV

Psychosocial and Environmental Problems

Problems with primary support group
Problems related to the social environment
Educational problems
Occupational problems
Housing problems
Economic problems
Problems with access to health care services
Problems related to interaction with the legal system/crime
Other psychosocial and environmental problems

AXIS V: Global Assessment of Functioning

Axis V is for reporting the clinician's judgment of the individual's overall level of functioning. This information is useful in planning treatment and measuring its impact, and in predicting outcome.

The reporting of overall functioning on Axis V can be done using the Global Assessment of Functioning (GAF) Scale. The GAF Scale may be particularly useful in tracking the clinical progress of individuals in global terms, using a single measure. The GAP Scale is to be rated with respect only to psychological, social, and occupational functioning. The instructions specify, "Do not include impairment in functioning due to physical (or environmental) limitations."

The GAF scale is divided into 10 ranges of functioning. Making a GAF rating involves picking a single value that best reflects the individual's overall level of functioning. The description of each 10-point range in the GAF scale has two components: the first part covers symptom severity, and the second part covers functioning. The GAF rating is within a particular decile if **either** the symptom severity **or** the level of functioning falls within the range. For example, the first part of the range 41–50 describes "serious symptoms (e.g., suicidal ideation, severe obsessional rituals, frequent shoplifting)" and the second part includes "any serious impairment in social, occupational, or school functioning (e.g., no friends, unable to keep a job)." It should be noted that in situations where the individual's symptom severity and level of functioning are discordant, the final GAF rating always reflects the worse of the two. For example, the GAF rating for an individual who is a significant danger to self but is otherwise functioning well would be below 20. Similarly, the GAF rating for an individual with minimal psychological symptomatology but significant impairment in functioning (e.g., an individual whose excessive preoccupation with substance use has resulting in loss of job and friends but no other psychopathology) would be 40 or lower.

In most instances, ratings on the GAF Scale should be for the current period (i.e., the level of functioning at the time of the evaluation) because ratings of current functioning will generally reflect the need for treatment or care. In order to account for day-to-day variability in functioning, the GAF rating for the "current period" is sometimes operationalized as the lowest level of functioning for the past week. In some settings, it may be useful to note the GAF Scale rating both at time of admission and

at time of discharge. The GAF Scale may also be rated for other time periods (e.g., the highest level of functioning for at least a few months during the past year). The GAF Scale is reported on Axis V as follows: "GAF =," followed by the GAF rating from 0 to 100, followed by the time period reflected by the rating in parentheses—for example, "(current)," "(highest level in past year)," "(at discharge)."

In order to ensure that no elements of the GAF scale are overlooked when a GAF rating is being made, the following method for determining a GAF rating may be applied:

STEP 1: Starting at the top level, evaluate each range by asking "is **either** the individual's symptom severity OR level of functioning worse than what is indicated in the range description?"

STEP 2: Keep moving down the scale until the range that best matches the individual's symptom severity OR the level of functioning is reached, **whichever is worse**.

STEP 3: Look at the next lower range as a double-check against having stopped prematurely. This range should be too severe on **both** symptom severity **and** level of functioning. If it is, the appropriate range has been reached (continue with step 4). If not, go back to step 2 and continue moving down the scale.

STEP 4: To determine the specific GAF rating within the selected 10-point range, consider whether the individual is functioning at the higher or lower end of the 10-point range. For example, consider an individual who hears voices that do not influence his behavior (e.g., someone with long-standing Schizophrenia who accepts his hallucinations as part of his illness). If the voices occur relatively infrequently (once a week or less), a rating of 39 or 40 might be most appropriate. In contrast, if the individual hears voices almost continuously, a rating of 31 or 32 would be more appropriate.

In some settings, it may be useful to assess social and occupational disability and to track progress in rehabilitation independent of the severity of the psychological symptoms.

GLOBAL ASSESSMENT OF FUNCTIONING (GAF) SCALE

Consider psychological, social, and occupational functioning on a hypothetical continuum of mental health-illness. Do not include impairment in functioning due to physical (or environmental) limitations.

TABLE A.1

Code	(Note: Use intermediate codes when appropriate, e.g., 45, 68, 72.)
100/91	Superior functioning in a wide range of activities, life's problems never seem to get out of hand, is sought out by others because of his or her many positive qualities. No symptoms.
90/81	Absent or minimal symptoms (e.g., mild anxiety before an exam), good functioning in all areas, interested and involved in a wide range of activities, socially effective, generally satisfied with life, no more than everyday problems or concerns (e.g., an occasional argument with family members).
80/71	If symptoms are present, they are transient and expectable reactions to psychosocial stressors (e.g., difficulty concentrating after family argument), no more than slight impairment in social, occupational, or school functioning (e.g., temporarily falling behind in schoolwork).
70/61	Some mild symptoms (e.g., depressed mood and mild insomnia) OR some difficulty in social, occupational, or school functioning (e.g., occasional truancy, or theft within the household), but generally functioning pretty well, has some meaningful interpersonal relationships.
60/51	Moderate symptoms (e.g., flat affect and circumstantial speech, occasional panic attacks) OR moderate difficulty in social, occupational, or school functioning (e.g., few friends, conflicts with peers or co-workers).
50/41	Serious symptoms (e.g., suicidal ideation, severe obsessional rituals, frequent shoplifting) OR any serious impairment in social, occupational, or school functioning (e.g., no friends, unable to keep a job).
40/31	Some impairment in reality testing or communication (e.g., speech is at times illogical, obscure, or irrelevant) OR major impairment in several areas, such as work or school, family relations, judgment, thinking, or mood (e.g., depressed man avoids friends, neglects family, and is unable to work; child frequently beats up younger children, is defiant at home, and is failing at school).
30/21	Behavior is considerably influenced by delusions or hallucinations OR serious impairment in communication or judgment (e.g., sometimes incoherent, acts grossly inappropriately, suicidal preoccupation) OR inability to function in almost all areas (e.g., stays in bed all day; no job, home, or friends).
20/11	Some danger of hurting self or others (e.g., suicide attempts without clear expectation of death; frequently violent; manic excitement) OR occasionally fails to maintain minimal personal hygiene (e.g., smears feces) OR gross impairment in communication (e.g., largely incoherent or mute).
10/1	Persistent danger of severely hurting self or others (e.g., recurrent violence) OR persistent inability to maintain minimal personal hygiene OR serious suicidal act with clear expectation of death.
0	Inadequate information.

The rating of overall psychological functioning on a scale of 0–100 was operationalized by Luborsky in the Health-Sickness Rating Scale (Luborsky L: "Clinicians' Judgments of Mental Health." *Archives of General Psychiatry* 7:407–417, 1962). Spitzer and colleagues developed a revision of the Health-Sickness Rating Scale called the Global Assessment Scale (GAS) (Endicott J, Spitzer RL, Fleiss JL, Cohen J: "The Global Assessment Scale: A Procedure for Measuring Overall Severity of Psychiatric Disturbance." *Archives of General Psychiatry* 33:766–771, 1976). A modified version of the GAS was included in DSM-ILL-R as the Global Assessment of Functioning (GAF) Scale.

INDEX

Page numbers followed by f indicate figure or box. Page numbers followed by t indicate table.

SINGLE PC LICENSE AGREEMENT AND LIMITED WARRANTY

READ THIS LICENSE CAREFULLY BEFORE OPENING THIS PACKAGE. BY OPENING THIS PACKAGE, YOU ARE AGREEING TO THE TERMS AND CONDITIONS OF THIS LICENSE. IF YOU DO NOT AGREE, DO NOT OPEN THE PACKAGE. PROMPTLY RETURN THE UNOPENED PACKAGE AND ALL ACCOMPANYING ITEMS TO THE PLACE YOU OBTAINED THEM. *THESE TERMS APPLY TO ALL LICENSED SOFTWARE ON THE DISK EXCEPT THAT THE TERMS FOR USE OF ANY SHAREWARE OR FREEWARE ON THE DISKETTES ARE AS SET FORTH IN THE ELECTRONIC LICENSE LOCATED ON THE DISK:*

1. GRANT OF LICENSE and OWNERSHIP: The enclosed computer programs and data ("Software") are licensed, not sold, to you by Pearson Education, Inc. ("We" or the "Company") and in consideration of your purchase or adoption of the accompanying Company textbooks and/or other materials, and your agreement to these terms. We reserve any rights not granted to you. You own only the disk(s) but we and/or our licensors own the Software itself. This license allows you to use and display your copy of the Software on a single computer (i.e., with a single CPU) at a single location for <u>academic</u> use only, so long as you comply with the terms of this Agreement. You may make one copy for back up, or transfer your copy to another CPU, provided that the Software is usable on only one computer.

2. RESTRICTIONS: You may <u>not</u> transfer or distribute the Software or documentation to anyone else. Except for backup, you may <u>not</u> copy the documentation or the Software. You may <u>not</u> network the Software or otherwise use it on more than one computer or computer terminal at the same time. You may <u>not</u> reverse engineer, disassemble, decompile, modify, adapt, translate, or create derivative works based on the Software or the Documentation. You may be held legally responsible for any copying or copyright infringement which is caused by your failure to abide by the terms of these restrictions.

3. TERMINATION: This license is effective until terminated. This license will terminate automatically without notice from the Company if you fail to comply with any provisions or limitations of this license. Upon termination, you shall destroy the Documentation and all copies of the Software. All provisions of this Agreement as to limitation and disclaimer of warranties, limitation of liability, remedies or damages, and our ownership rights shall survive termination.

4. LIMITED WARRANTY AND DISCLAIMER OF WARRANTY: Company warrants that for a period of 60 days from the date you purchase this SOFTWARE (or purchase or adopt the accompanying textbook), the Software, when properly installed and used in accordance with the Documentation, will operate in substantial conformity with the description of the Software set forth in the Documentation, and that for a period of 30 days the disk(s) on which the Software is delivered shall be free from defects in materials and workmanship under normal use. The Company does not warrant that the Software will meet your requirements or that the operation of the Software will be uninterrupted or error-free. Your only remedy and the Company's only obligation under these limited warranties is, at the Company's option, return of the disk for a refund of any amounts paid for it by you or replacement of the disk. THIS LIMITED WARRANTY IS THE ONLY WARRANTY PROVIDED BY THE COMPANY AND ITS LICENSORS, AND THE COMPANY AND ITS LICENSORS DISCLAIM ALL OTHER WARRANTIES, EXPRESS OR IMPLIED, INCLUDING WITHOUT LIMITATION, THE IMPLIED WARRANTIES OF MERCHANTABILITY AND FITNESS FOR A PARTICULAR PURPOSE. THE COMPANY DOES NOT WARRANT, GUARANTEE OR MAKE ANY REPRESENTATION REGARDING THE ACCURACY, RELIABILITY, CURRENTNESS, USE, OR RESULTS OF USE, OF THE SOFTWARE.

5. LIMITATION OF REMEDIES AND DAMAGES: IN NO EVENT, SHALL THE COMPANY OR ITS EMPLOYEES, AGENTS, LICENSORS, OR CONTRACTORS BE LIABLE FOR ANY INCIDENTAL, INDIRECT, SPECIAL, OR CONSEQUENTIAL DAMAGES ARISING OUT OF OR IN CONNECTION WITH THIS LICENSE OR THE SOFTWARE, INCLUDING FOR LOSS OF USE, LOSS OF DATA, LOSS OF INCOME OR PROFIT, OR OTHER LOSSES, SUSTAINED AS A RESULT OF INJURY TO ANY PERSON, OR LOSS OF OR DAMAGE TO PROPERTY, OR CLAIMS OF THIRD PARTIES, EVEN IF THE COMPANY OR AN AUTHORIZED REPRESENTATIVE OF THE COMPANY HAS BEEN ADVISED OF THE POSSIBILITY OF SUCH DAMAGES. IN NO EVENT SHALL THE LIABILITY OF THE COMPANY FOR DAMAGES WITH RESPECT TO THE SOFTWARE EXCEED THE AMOUNTS ACTUALLY PAID BY YOU, IF ANY, FOR THE SOFTWARE OR THE ACCOMPANYING TEXTBOOK. BECAUSE SOME JURISDICTIONS DO NOT ALLOW THE LIMITATION OF LIABILITY IN CERTAIN CIRCUMSTANCES, THE ABOVE LIMITATIONS MAY NOT ALWAYS APPLY TO YOU.

6. GENERAL: THIS AGREEMENT SHALL BE CONSTRUED IN ACCORDANCE WITH THE LAWS OF THE UNITED STATES OF AMERICA AND THE STATE OF NEW YORK, APPLICABLE TO CONTRACTS MADE IN NEW YORK, AND SHALL BENEFIT THE COMPANY, ITS AFFILIATES AND ASSIGNEES. THIS AGREEMENT IS THE COMPLETE AND EXCLUSIVE STATEMENT OF THE AGREEMENT BETWEEN YOU AND THE COMPANY AND SUPERSEDES ALL PROPOSALS OR PRIOR AGREEMENTS, ORAL, OR WRITTEN, AND ANY OTHER COMMUNICATIONS BETWEEN YOU AND THE COMPANY OR ANY REPRESENTATIVE OF THE COMPANY RELATING TO THE SUBJECT MATTER OF THIS AGREEMENT. If you are a U.S. Government user, this Software is licensed with "restricted rights" as set forth in subparagraphs (a)–(d) of the Commercial Computer-Restricted Rights clause at FAR 52.227-19 or in subparagraphs (c)(1)(ii) of the Rights in Technical Data and Computer Software clause at DFARS 252.227-7013, and similar clauses, as applicable.

Should you have any questions concerning this agreement or if you wish to contact the Company for any reason, please contact in writing: Prentice-Hall, New Media Department, One Lake Street, Upper Saddle River, NJ 07458.

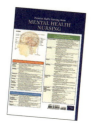

Quick Guide to Special Features